D0603122

CONTEMPORARY INTELLECTUAL ASSESSMENT

CONTEMPORARY INTELLECTUAL ASSESSMENT

THIRD EDITION

Theories, Tests, and Issues

Edited by
Dawn P. Flanagan
Patti L. Harrison

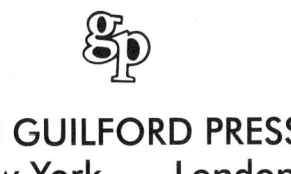

THE GUILFORD PRESS
New York   London

© 2012 The Guilford Press
A Division of Guilford Publications, Inc.
72 Spring Street, New York, NY 10012
www.guilford.com

Printed in the United States of America

This book is printed on acid-free paper.

Last digit is print number: 9   8   7   6   5   4   3   2   1

The authors have checked with sources believed to be reliable in their efforts to
provide information that is complete and generally in accord with the standards
of practice that are accepted at the time of publication. However, in view of the
possibility of human error or changes in behavioral, mental health, or medical
sciences, neither the authors, nor the editors and publisher, nor any other party who
has been involved in the preparation or publication of this work warrants that the
information contained herein is in every respect accurate or complete, and they are
not responsible for any errors or omissions or the results obtained from the use of
such information. Readers are encouraged to confirm the information contained in
this book with other sources.

Library of Congress Cataloging-in-Publication Data

Contemporary intellectual assessment : theories, tests, and issues / edited by Dawn
P. Flanagan, Patti L. Harrison.–3rd ed.
    p. cm.
    Includes bibliographical references and index.
    ISBN 978-1-60918-995-2 (hardcover)
    1. Intelligence tests.   2. Intelligence tests—History.   I. Flanagan, Dawn P.
II. Harrison, Patti L.
    BF431.C66 2012
    153.9′3—dc23
                                                                2011019751

About the Editors

Dawn P. Flanagan, PhD, is Professor of Psychology and Director of the School Psychology Training Programs at St. John's University in Queens, New York. She is also Assistant Clinical Professor at the Yale Child Study Center. Dr. Flanagan serves as an expert witness, learning disability consultant, and psychological test and measurement consultant and trainer, and has published widely on cognitive assessment, specific learning disabilities, and psychometric theories of the structure of cognitive abilities.

Patti L. Harrison, PhD, is Professor in the Department of Educational Studies in Psychology, Research Methodology, and Counseling at the University of Alabama. She has conducted research on intelligence, adaptive behavior, and preschool assessment. Dr. Harrison has published and presented on assessment topics in school psychology, clinical psychology, and special education venues. She is a past editor of *School Psychology Review.*

Contributors

Vincent C. Alfonso, PhD, Graduate School of Education, Fordham University, New York, New York

Kristina J. Andren, PsyD, School Psychology Program, University of Southern Maine, Gorham, Maine

Kathleen Armstrong, PhD, Department of Pediatrics, University of South Florida, Tampa, Florida

Erin Avirett, BA, Department of Psychology and Philosophy, Texas Women's University, Denton, Texas

Nayena Blankson, PhD, Department of Psychology, Spelman College, Atlanta, Georgia

Bruce A. Bracken, PhD, School of Education, College of William and Mary, Williamsburg, Virginia

Jeffery P. Braden, PhD, Department of Psychology, North Carolina State University, Raleigh, North Carolina

Kristina C. Breaux, PhD, The Psychological Corporation, San Antonio, Texas

Rachel Brown-Chidsey, PhD, School Psychology Program, University of Southern Maine, Gorham, Maine

John B. Carroll, PhD (deceased), Department of Psychology, University of North Carolina at Chapel Hill, Chapel Hill, North Carolina

Jie-Qi Chen, PhD, Erikson Institute, Chicago, Illinois

J. P. Das, PhD, Department of Educational Psychology, University of Alberta, Edmonton, Alberta, Canada

John L. Davis, MA, Department of Educational Psychology, Texas A&M University, College Station, Texas

Scott L. Decker, PhD, Department of Psychology, Barnwell College, University of South Carolina, Columbia, South Carolina

Melissa DeVries, PhD, Neurology, Learning, and Behavior Center, Salt Lake City, Utah

Felicia A. Dixon, PhD, Department of Educational Psychology, Ball State University, Muncie, Indiana

Shauna G. Dixon, MS, Graduate School of Education, Harvard University, Cambridge, Massachusetts

Lisa Whipple Drozdick, PhD, The Psychological Corporation, San Antonio, Texas

Agnieszka N. Dynda, PsyD, Department of
Psychology, St. John's University,
Jamaica, New York

Colin D. Elliott, PhD, Gervitz School
of Education, University of California,
Santa Barbara, California

Julia A. Englund, BA, Department of
Psychology, University of South Carolina,
Columbia, South Carolina

Catherine A. Fiorello, PhD, NCSP, School
Psychology Program, Department of Psychological
Studies in Education, College of Education,
Temple University, Philadelphia, Pennsylvania

Dawn P. Flanagan, PhD, Department of
Psychology, St. John's University,
Jamaica, New York

Randy G. Floyd, PhD, Department of
Psychology, University of Memphis,
Memphis, Tennessee

Laurie Ford, PhD, Department of Educational
and Counseling Psychology, University of British
Columbia, Vancouver, British Columbia, Canada

Howard Gardner, PhD, Graduate School of
Education, Harvard University,
Cambridge, Massachusetts

Sam Goldstein, PhD, Neurology, Learning, and
Behavior Center, Salt Lake City, Utah

James B. Hale, PhD, Department of Psychology,
University of Victoria, Victoria, British Columbia,
Canada

Jason Hangauer, EdS, Department of Pediatrics,
University of South Florida, Tampa, Florida

Julie N. Henzel, PsyD, The Nisonger Center,
Ohio State University, Columbus, Ohio

John L. Horn, PhD (deceased), Department of
Psychology, University of Southern California,
Los Angeles, California

Randy W. Kamphaus, PhD, College of
Education, Georgia State University,
Atlanta, Georgia

Alan S. Kaufman, PhD, Child Study Center,
Yale University, New Haven, Connecticut

James C. Kaufman, PhD, Department of
Psychology, California State University,
San Bernardino, California

Nadeen L. Kaufman, EdD, Child Study Center,
Yale University, New Haven, Connecticut

Timothy Z. Keith, PhD, Department of
Educational Psychology, University of Texas
at Austin, Austin, Texas

Sangwon Kim, PhD, Department of Child
Development, Ewha Womans University,
Seoul, South Korea

Laura Grofer Klinger, PhD, TEACCH Autism
Program, University of North Carolina at
Chapel Hill, Chapel Hill, North Carolina

Michelle L. Kozey, MA, Department of
Educational and Counseling Psychology,
University of British Columbia, Vancouver,
British Columbia, Canada

John H. Kranzler, PhD, Special Education
Program, College of Education, University of
Florida, Gainesville, Florida

Elizabeth O. Lichtenberger, PhD, private
practice, Carlsbad, California

Denise E. Maricle, PhD, Department of
Psychology and Philosophy, Texas Women's
University, Denton, Texas

Jennifer T. Mascolo, PsyD, Department
of Health and Behavior Studies,
Teachers College, Columbia University,
New York, New York

Nancy Mather, PhD, Department of Disability
and Psychoeducational Studies, College of
Education, University of Arizona,
Tucson, Arizona

Robb N. Matthews, MA, Department of
Educational Psychology, Texas A&M University,
College Station, Texas

R. Steve McCallum, PhD, Department of Educational Psychology and Counseling, University of Tennessee, Knoxville, Tennessee

George McCloskey, PhD, Department of Psychology, Philadelphia College of Osteopathic Medicine, Philadelphia, Pennsylvania

Kevin S. McGrew, PhD, Institute for Applied Psychometrics, St. Cloud, Minnesota

David E. McIntosh, PhD, Department of Special Education, Ball State University, Muncie, Indiana

Daniel C. Miller, PhD, Department of Psychology and Philosophy, Texas Women's University, Denton, Texas

Ryan Murphy, EdS, Department of Psychology, Philadelphia College of Osteopathic Medicine, Philadelphia, Pennsylvania

Joanna L. Mussey, MA, Department of Psychology, University of Alabama, Tuscaloosa, Alabama

Joshua Nadeau, MS, Department of Pediatrics, University of South Florida, Tampa, Florida

Jack A. Naglieri, PhD, ABAP, Curry School of Education, University of Virginia, Charlottesville, Virginia; Devereux Center for Resilient Children, Villanova, Pennsylvania

Juliana Negreiros, MA, Department of Educational and Counseling Psychology, University of British Columbia, Vancouver, British Columbia, Canada

Bradley C. Niebling, PhD, Midwest Instructional Leadership Council, Urbandale, Iowa

Salvador Hector Ochoa, PhD, Department of Educational Psychology, University of Texas–Pan American, Edinburg, Texas

Sarah E. O'Kelly, PhD, Civitan International Research Center, Sparks Clinics and Department of Psychology, University of Alabama at Birmingham, Birmingham, Alabama

Samuel O. Ortiz, PhD, Department of Psychology, St. John's University, Jamaica, New York

Tulio M. Otero, PhD, Clinical PsyD and School Psychology Programs, Chicago School of Professional Psychology, Chicago, Illinois

Eric E. Pierson, PhD, NCSP, Department of Educational Psychology, Ball State University, Muncie, Indiana

Mark Pomplun, PhD, Assessment and Accountability Department, St. Charles School District, St. Charles, Illinois

Tara C. Raines, PsyS, Gwinnett County Public Schools, Gwinnett County, Georgia

Cecil R. Reynolds, PhD, Department of Educational Psychology, Texas A&M University, College Station, Texas

Matthew R. Reynolds, PhD, Department of Psychology and Research in Education, University of Kansas, Lawrence, Kansas

Cynthia A. Riccio, PhD, Department of Educational Psychology, Texas A&M University, College Station, Texas

Alycia M. Roberts, BA, Department of Psychology, University of South Carolina, Columbia, South Carolina

Jane Rogers, MA, Department of Psychology, Philadelphia College of Osteopathic Medicine, Philadelphia, Pennsylvania

Gale H. Roid, PhD, Department of Institutional Research, Warner Pacific College, Portland, Oregon

Ellen W. Rowe, PhD, Center for Psychological Services, George Mason University, Fairfax, Virginia

Andrea N. Schneider, BA, Department of Psychology, University of Victoria, Victoria, British Columbia, Canada

W. Joel Schneider, PhD, Department
of Psychology, Illinois State University,
Normal, Illinois

Fredrick A. Schrank, PhD, ABPP, Woodcock–
Muñoz Foundation, Olympia, Washington

Jennie Kaufman Singer, PhD, Criminal
Justice Division, California State University,
Sacramento, California

Marlene Sotelo-Dynega, PsyD, Department
of Psychology, St. John's University,
Jamaica, New York

Robert J. Sternberg, PhD, Oklahoma State
University, Stillwater, Oklahoma

Dustin Wahlstrom, PhD, The Psychological
Corporation, San Antonio, Texas

John D. Wasserman, PhD, American Institute
of Psychology, Burke, Virginia

Lawrence G. Weiss, PhD, The Psychological
Corporation, San Antonio, Texas

Barbara J. Wendling, MA, Woodcock–Muñoz
Foundation, Dallas, Texas

James Whitaker, PsyD, Department of
Psychology, Philadelphia College of Osteopathic
Medicine, Philadelphia, Pennsylvania

Gabrielle Wilcox, PsyD, Providence Behavioral
Health, Lancaster, Pennsylvania

Anne Pierce Winsor, PhD, private practice,
Atlanta, Georgia

Kirby L. Wycoff, PsyD, NCSP, Milton Hershey
School, Hershey, Pennsylvania

Megan Yim, BA, Department of Psychology,
University of Victoria,
Victoria, British Columbia, Canada

Jianjun Zhu, PhD, The Psychological
Corporation, San Antonio, Texas

Preface

The history of intelligence testing has been well documented from the early period of mental measurement to present-day conceptions of the structure of intelligence and valid assessment methods. The foundations of psychometric theory and practice were established in the late 1800s and set the stage for the ensuing measurement of human cognitive abilities. The technology of intelligence testing was apparent in the early 1900s, when Binet and Simon developed a test that adequately distinguished children with mental retardation from children with normal intellectual capabilities, and was well entrenched when the Wechsler–Bellevue was published in the late 1930s. In subsequent decades, significant refinements and advances in intelligence testing technology have been made, and the concept of individual differences has remained a constant focus of scientific inquiry.

Although several definitions and theories have been offered in recent decades, the nature of intelligence, cognition, and competence continues to be elusive. Perhaps the most popular definition was that offered by Wechsler in 1958. According to Wechsler, intelligence is "the aggregate or global capacity of the individual to act purposefully, to think rationally and to deal effectively with his environment" (p. 7). It is on this conception of intelligence that the original Wechsler tests were built. Because for decades the Wechsler batteries were the dominant intelligence tests in the field of psychology and were found to measure global intelligence validly, they assumed "number one" status and remain in that position today. As such, Wechsler's definition of intelligence continues to guide and influence the present-day practice of intelligence testing.

In light of theoretical and empirical advances, however, it is clear that earlier editions of the Wechsler tests were not based on the most dependable and current evidence of science, and that overreliance on these instruments served to widen the gap between intelligence testing and cognitive science. From the 1980s through the 2000s, new intelligence tests have been developed to be more consistent with contemporary research and theoretical models of the structure of cognitive abilities. In addition, changes in services, programs, legislation, and policy in psychology and education have had many implications for practical uses of cognitive assessments and the client populations for whom they are applied. Since the publication of the first edition of *Contemporary Intellectual Assessment: Theories, Tests, and Issues* in 1997, there has been tremendous growth in research about cognitive constructs. Contemporary purposes of cognitive assessment in psychology and education have been framed in light of, for example, recent research in neuropsychology and executive functioning; multi-tiered service delivery for children experiencing learning problems; and increasing uses of cognitive and neuropsychological assessment for people who have autism spectrum disorders, attention-deficit/hyperactivity disorder (ADHD), and other challenges.

The information presented in this text on modern intelligence theory and assessment technology suggests that clinicians should be familiar with the many approaches to assessing intelligence that are now available. In order for the field of intellectual assessment to continue to advance, clinicians should use instruments that operationalize empirically supported theories of intelligence and should employ assessment techniques that are designed to measure the broad array of cognitive abilities represented in current theory and research. It is only through a broader measurement of intelligence, grounded in well-validated theories of the nature of human cognitive abilities, that professionals can gain a better understanding of the relationship between intelligence and important outcome criteria (e.g., school achievement, occupational success) and can continue to narrow the gap between the professional practice of intelligence and cognitive ability testing and theoretical, empirical, and practical advances in psychology and education.

PURPOSE AND OBJECTIVES

The purpose of the third edition of this book is to provide a comprehensive conceptual and practical overview of current theories of intelligence, individual measures of cognitive ability, and uses of intellectual assessments. This text summarizes the latest research in the field of intellectual assessment and includes comprehensive treatment of critical issues that should be considered when the use of intelligence tests is warranted. The three primary objectives of this book are as follows: (1) to present in-depth descriptions of prominent theories of intelligence, tests of cognitive abilities, and neuropsychological instruments, and issues related to the use of these tests; (2) to provide important information about the validity of contemporary intelligence, cognitive, and neuropsychological tests; and (3) to demonstrate the utility of a well-validated theoretical and research foundation for developing cognitive tests and interpretive approaches, and for guiding research and practice. The ultimate goal of this book is to provide professionals with the knowledge necessary to use the latest cognitive instruments effectively.

Practitioners, university faculty, researchers, undergraduate and graduate students, and other professionals in psychology and education will find this book interesting and useful. It would be appropriate as a primary text in any graduate (or advanced undergraduate) course or seminar on cognitive psychology, clinical or psychoeducational assessment, or measurement and psychometric theory.

ORGANIZATION AND THEMES

This book consists of 36 chapters, organized into six parts, as well as an appendix.

Part I, "The Origins of Intellectual Assessment," traces the historical roots of test conceptualization, development, and interpretation up to the present day. The updated chapters provide readers with an understanding of how current practices evolved, as well as a basis for improving contemporary approaches to test interpretation. Chapters provide a necessary foundation from which to understand and elucidate the contemporary and emerging theories, tests, and issues in the field of intellectual assessment that are presented in subsequent sections of this volume.

Part II, "Contemporary Theoretical Perspectives," updates several models presented in the previous editions of this text. These theories are described in terms of (1) how they reflect recent advances in psychometrics, neuropsychology, and cognitive psychology; (2) what empirical evidence supports them; and (3) how they have been operationalized and applied. A comprehensive description of each theory is provided, focusing specifically on its historical origins, as well as the rationale and impetus for its development and modification. The theories represent viable foundations from which to develop and interpret cognitive measures—measures that may lead to greater insights into the nature, structure, and neurobiological substrates of cognitive functioning.

Part III, "Contemporary Intelligence, Cognitive, and Neuropsychological Batteries (and Associated Achievement Tests)," includes comprehensive chapters on the most widely used individual intelligence batteries and their utility in understanding the cognitive capabilities of individuals from toddlerhood through adulthood. The third edition of *Contemporary Intellectual Assessment: Theories, Tests, and Issues* updates information found in the second edition and provides current research about the most recent revisions of the Wechsler intellectual, memory, and achievement scales; the Stanford–Binet Intelligence Scales, Fifth Edition; the Kaufman Assessment Battery for Children—Second Edition and the Kaufman Test of Educational Achievement—Second Edition; the Woodcock–Johnson III Normative Update; the Differential Ability Scales—Second Edition; the Universal Nonverbal Intelligence Test; the Cognitive Assessment System; and the Reynolds Intellectual Assessment Scales. A new chapter on the NEPSY-II, added to the third edition, provides a focus on assessment of neuropsychological components of cognition. In general, the authors provide descriptions of their assessment instruments and discuss the instruments' theoretical and research underpinnings, organization and format, and psychometric characteristics. The authors also summarize the latest research and practical uses and provide recommendations for interpreting the abilities measured by their instruments.

Part IV, "Contemporary Interpretive Approaches and Their Relevance for Intervention," includes chapters about the latest research and models for interpretation of intelligence test results. The third edition updates second edition chapters on topics such as the cross-battery approach to interpretation based on the Cattell–Horn–Carroll theory, information-processing approaches, interpretation that addresses needs of culturally and linguistically diverse populations, and linking cognitive assessment with academic interventions for students with learning disabilities. A new chapter in Part IV focuses on cognitive hypothesis testing. A key feature of the chapters in Part IV is the implications of contemporary psychometric research for practical and valid interpretive approaches.

Part V, "Assessment of Intelligence and Cognitive Functioning in Different Populations," addresses a number of the populations with whom individual intelligence, cognitive ability, and neuropsychological tests are widely used. Chapters on early childhood, giftedness, and learning disabilities were updated from the second edition. The third edition includes new chapters about individuals for which cognitive assessment is increasingly a key component of diagnoses and/or programming, including individuals with autism spectrum disorders, ADHD, sensory and physical disabilities, traumatic brain injury, and intellectual disabilities.

Part VI, "Contemporary and Emerging Issues in Intellectual Assessment," includes updated chapters related to the validity of intelligence batteries. In the third edition, Part VI also adds a number of important new chapters on significant current issues and new directions for individual intellectual assessment, including neuropsychological approaches, assessment of executive functions, and implications for problem-solving and multi-tiered approaches to learning problems of children in schools. Suggestions and recommendations regarding the appropriate use of intelligence, cognitive ability, and neuropsychological tests, as well as future research directions, are provided throughout this section of the book.

Because of the many significant contributions made by John B. Carroll (1916–2003) to our understanding of the structure of cognitive abilities, the chapter that he wrote for the first edition of this book is included in the Appendix. Likewise, John L. Horn's (1928–2006) contributions to and extensions of Cattell's original Gf-Gc theory were monumental. His chapter from the second edition of our book is reprinted here in Chapter 3. Both Carroll and Horn's landmark contributions to the field of cognitive psychology over a period of several decades paved the way for the present-day Cattell–Horn–Carroll theory of cognitive abilities, which is described in Chapter 4.

ACKNOWLEDGMENTS

We wish to thank the individuals who have contributed to or assisted in the preparation of this book. We are appreciative of the editorial assistance of Alla Zhelinsky, whose close attention to detail improved the quality of this work. We are also extremely grateful for the extraordinary contributions of our chapter authors. It has been a rewarding experience to work with such a dedicated group of people who are nationally recognized authorities in their respective areas. The contributions of Natalie Graham, Mary Beth Wood, Laura Specht Patchkofsky, and the rest of the staff at The Guilford Press are also gratefully acknowledged. Their expertise, and their pleasant and cooperative working style, made this project an enjoyable and productive endeavor.

DAWN P. FLANAGAN, PhD
PATTI L. HARRISON, PhD

REFERENCE

Wechsler, D. (1958). *The measurement and appraisal of adult intelligence* (4th ed.). Baltimore: Williams & Wilkins.

Contents

IV. CONTEMPORARY INTERPRETIVE APPROACHES AND THEIR RELEVANCE FOR INTERVENTION

PART I

THE ORIGINS
OF INTELLECTUAL ASSESSMENT

CHAPTER 1

A History of Intelligence Assessment
The Unfinished Tapestry

John D. Wasserman

When our intelligence scales have become more accurate and the laws governing IQ changes have been more definitively established it will then be possible to say that there is nothing about an individual as important as his IQ, except possibly his morals; that the greatest educational problem is to determine the kind of education best suited to each IQ level; that the first concern of a nation should be the average IQ of its citizens, and the eugenic and dysgenic influences which are capable of raising or lowering that level; that the great test problem of democracy is how to adjust itself to the large IQ differences which can be demonstrated to exist among the members of any race or nationality group.
—LEWIS M. TERMAN (1922b)

This bold statement by the author of the first Stanford–Binet intelligence scale captures much of both the promise and the controversy that have historically surrounded, and that *still* surround, the assessment of intelligence. Intelligence tests and their applications have been associated with some of the very best and very worst human behaviors. On the one hand, intelligence assessment can provide a meaningful basis for understanding the strengths and weaknesses of misunderstood children, adolescents, or adults—thereby providing data that can be used to design and implement interventions to help people reach their potential more effectively. On the other hand, intelligence assessment can be used to segregate and label people—treating their future as a fixed outcome, an unchangeable fate. The history of forced sterilizations of individuals with intellectual disabilities in the United States and many other countries is a tragic example of how intelligence tests may be misused, exceeded only by the systematic extermination of intellectually disabled individuals in Nazi Germany (e.g., Friedlander, 1995). The topic

of intelligence and its assessment deservedly elicits many strong feelings.

Intelligence is arguably the most researched topic in the history of psychology, and the concept of *general intelligence* has been described as "one of the most central phenomena in all of behavioral science, with broad explanatory powers" (Jensen, 1998, p. xii). Still, social, legal, and political forces have in some instances excluded intelligence test results from important types of educational and personnel decision-making processes. Tangible advances in assessment practices have been slow and episodic. Following Alfred Binet's initial successes, the beginning of the 20th century saw an accelerated pace of small- and large-scale applied intelligence testing, but many anticipated educational and occupational benefits were never realized. Buros (1977) considered 1927 as the "banner year" in which "the testing movement reached maturity" (p. 9). The middle of the century saw only incremental gains in testing, such as electronic scoring, analysis, and reporting of test results, but with comparatively "little progress" (Buros, 1977,

p. 10) and more than a little "stagnation" (Carroll, 1978, p. 93). A landmark quantitative review of factor-analytic investigations near the end of the 20th century (i.e., Carroll, 1993) stimulated a new school of thinking about intelligence assessment, but the story remains unfinished. In the United States, federal educational reforms and civil rights legislation have had pronounced effects upon the use of intelligence tests in education. It is possible to see the history of intelligence assessment as an unfinished tapestry depicting the rich saga of a developing discipline, with recurrent characters interwoven through different narratives, as well as more than a few loose and unresolved thematic threads.

In this chapter, the origins of intelligence assessment are recounted, with an emphasis on milestone events and seminal individuals. Thematic strands present from the early days are traced, including some that were resolved and some that remain unresolved. An effort has been made whenever possible to provide samples of primary source material. Finally, although we all tend to view history through the lens of our own experiences, it is helpful to appreciate the sociocultural context, institutional traditions, and professional *Zeitgeist* associated with historical events, as well as the experiences and personal motivations that may have driven the ideas and behaviors of historical figures.

PSEUDOSCIENTIFIC ANTECEDENTS: PHRENOLOGY IN THE 19TH CENTURY

The first science purporting to be a "true science of mind" that could measure mental qualities and functions was *cranioscopy*, introduced at the beginning of the 19th century by Franz Joseph Gall, and later renamed *phrenology* by Gall's associate, Johann Gaspar Spurzheim. Gall (1758–1828) was a Viennese physician and neuroanatomist, and Spurzheim (1776–1832) was a physician and colleague who would ultimately be responsible for the widespread dissemination of phrenology. But it would be a Scotsman, George Combe (1788–1858)—who developed and published a two-volume system of phrenology in 1824, as well as launching a phrenology journal with his brother—who would prove most instrumental in the popularization of phrenology. Combe's system appears in Figure 1.1. He also wrote the immensely successful book *The Constitution of Man*, which advanced the idea that all the laws of nature were in harmony with one

another, and that people could best fulfill God's will and obtain the greatest happiness by discovering these laws and obeying them. The book went through eight editions and sold approximately 350,000 copies between 1828 and 1900.

The basic tenets of phrenology can be summarized easily. In a letter to a Viennese official, Gall (1798/1857) asserted that the brain was the organ of the mind, that the mind could be reduced to a number of faculties, that the faculties were innate, that the faculties were located in distinct and particular organs of the brain, that the surface of the skull was determined by the external form of the brain, and that phrenologists could judge the development of individual faculties merely by examining the form of the skull. A well-developed faculty was thought to have a large cerebral organ that corresponded to a cranial protuberance. Gall originally described and localized 27 distinct faculties; Spurzheim (1815) increased the list to 32 faculties; Combe (1853) further expanded the list to 35; and others expanded the list to 43 (e.g., Payne, 1920).

Gall and Spurzheim traveled through Europe promoting phrenology, which Gall advocated as a science and Spurzheim as a way to reform education, religion, and penology. It quickly became popular in the United Kingdom, and Spurzheim came to the United States in 1832 to promote phrenology to a scientific community that was already quite familiar with it. By the time Combe conducted his 1839 American phrenology lecture tour, audiences averaged over 500 across each of the 16 lectures (Walsh, 1976). A satirical depiction of a phrenological examination from about the same time appears in Figure 1.2.

Gall and Spurzheim are today credited with recognizing the significance of gray matter as the source of nerve fibers; most importantly, they are credited with introducing the neuroscientific concept of functional localization in the cerebral cortex (Simpson, 2005). Dallenbach (1915) provides evidence that they should be credited with the terms *mental functions* and *faculties*. British philosopher and critic G. H. Lewes (1867) went a step further, asserting that Gall laid the groundwork for psychology as a science rather than philosophy: "Gall rescued the problem of mental functions from Metaphysics and made it one of Biology" (p. 407). Even so, there is a long history of disparaging efforts to localize mental functions in specific regions in the brain by calling them a new "phrenology" (e.g., Franz, 1912; Fuster, 2008, p. 346).

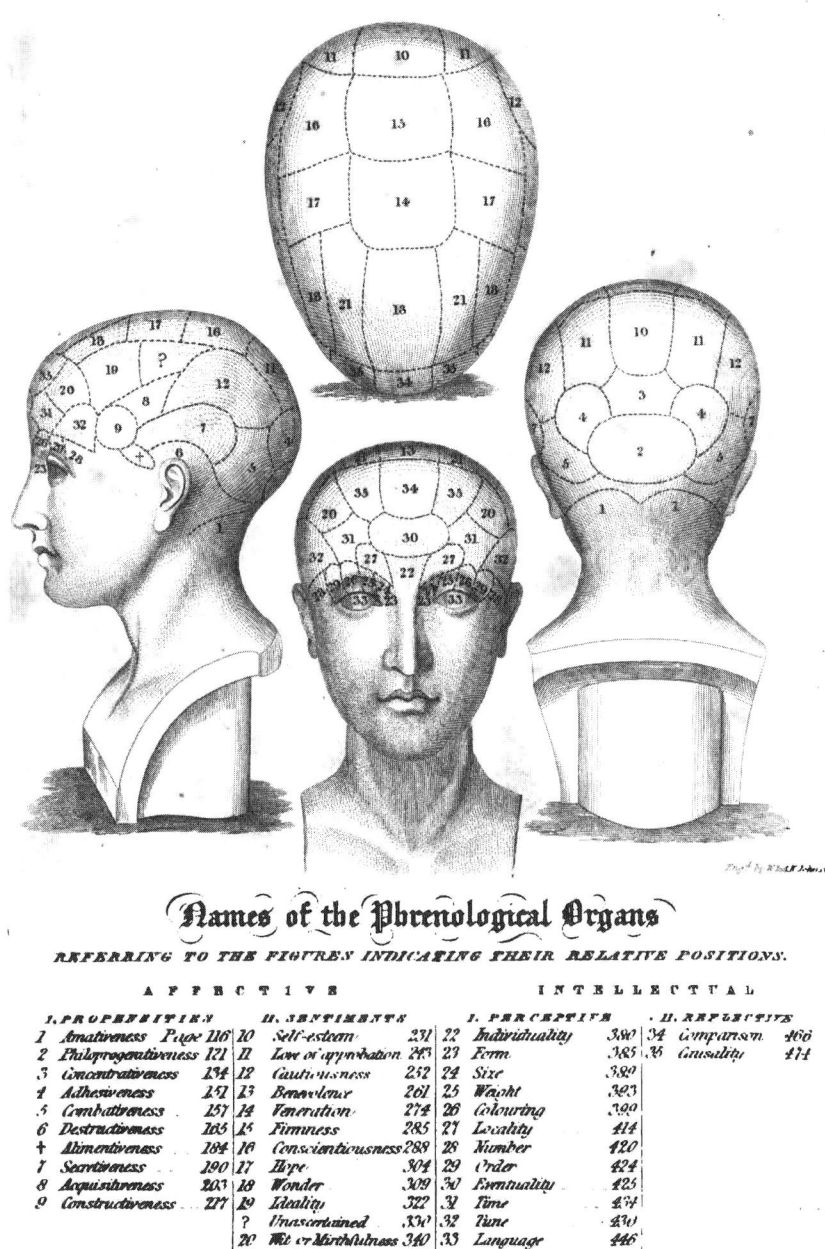

FIGURE 1.1. George Combe, the best-known phrenologist of the 19th century, divided the brain into intellectual faculties and feelings. The plate of the phrenological bust faces the title page in Combe (1830). In the public domain.

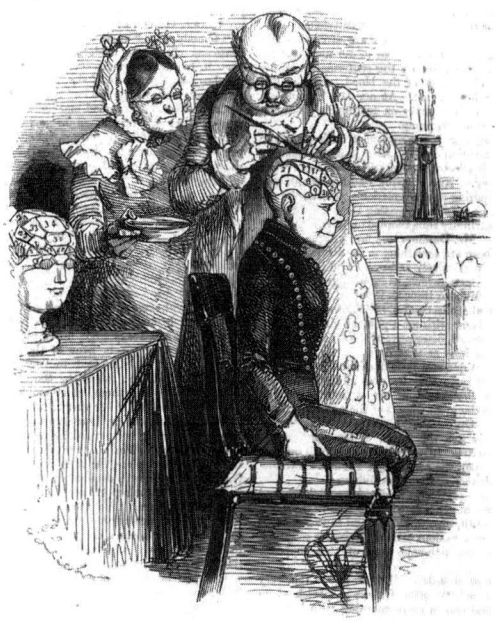

FIGURE 1.2. Illustration from a fictional story of a member of a phrenology society who decides to use phrenology to identify a possible thief in his household. The drawing shows a servant who was paid five shillings to shave his head so that the phrenological organs could be traced in ink, not a standard part of phrenology practice. From Prendergast (1844, p. 17). In the public domain.

PHILOSOPHICAL AND SCIENTIFIC ANTECEDENTS

The most prominent British philosopher of his era, Herbert Spencer (1820–1903) sought to synthesize universal natural laws (especially *evolution*) across the disciplines of biology, psychology, sociology, and ethics. Spencer coined the phrase "survival of the fittest" (p. 444) in *The Principles of Biology* (1864) after reading Charles Darwin (1859), although he was reluctant to accept Darwin's evolutionary mechanism of natural selection. In *The Principles of Psychology* (1855), Spencer described how the behavior of the individual organism adapts through interaction with the environment, and defined *intelligence* as a "continuous adjustment" of "inner to outer relations" (p. 486). Spencer's ideas persist in a number of ways to this day. Intelligence, as we shall see, is still widely considered to represent a capacity associated with adaptation to one's environment. In a critical review of Spencer's synthesis, John Dewey (1904) was struck

by the luck that Spencer and Darwin published almost simultaneously, thereby making their very different concepts of evolution indistinguishable to the public.

Beyond Spencer's philosophical influence, the foundation for psychology as a science, as well as for the scholarly study of intelligence, was laid by naturalist Charles Darwin (1809–1882), who is most remembered for his theory of evolution by natural selection. In his writings, Darwin frequently referred to adaptive behavior in animals and humans as "intelligent"; more importantly, he argued that the same forces that act on animal evolution also apply to human mental abilities: "There is no fundamental difference between man and the higher mammals in their mental faculties" (Darwin, 1871, p. 35). In *The Descent of Man*, Darwin (1871) went even further in applying his evolutionary theory to human mental characteristics—probably after reading the work of his half-cousin Francis Galton, the Victorian polymath, whose drive for scientific measurement of human capabilities would start the race to develop measures of intelligence in motion.

It is difficult to overstate the impact of Darwin's theory of evolution on psychology. By considering human behavior in an evolutionary context, Darwin treated the study of psychology as no less a science than biology and other natural sciences. His influence was substantial and may be seen, for example, in Joseph Jastrow's (1901) American Psychological Association (APA) presidential address to start the 20th century. Jastrow described psychology as both a laboratory science and an applied science, setting the study of intelligence in a somewhat Spencerian evolutionary context:

> Intelligence must first be realized as an advantage-gaining factor in the evolutionary struggle; that struggle is not merely, and indeed in all the stages that here come into consideration, not mainly a conflict of tooth and nail, a contest of strength of claw and fleetness of foot, but a war of wits, an encounter of skill and cunning, a measure of strategy and foresight. (p. 9)

Francis Galton and the Anthropometric Laboratory

If you lived in London in the mid-1880s or 1890s, you could pay three- or fourpence for you or your children to undergo a variety of physical measurements and tests, with the option to register results for future reference and follow-up. The measurements were available from Francis Galton's An-thropometric Laboratory, first located at the International Health Exhibition (see Figure 1.3), then at the University of Cambridge, the South Kensington Museum, and finally at the Clarendon Museum at Oxford. *Anthropometry* referred to the "measurement of man," and Galton's laboratory was, according to Diamond (1977), "a device to tease the public into providing the data he needed for his research" (p. 52). As a lifelong advocate for objective scientific measurement, Galton (1822–1911; see Figure 1.4) was a pioneer in the use of test batteries and questionnaires for data collection, the concept of control groups in research, and statistical methods (as developer of the techniques of regression and correlation).

Galton introduced his system of anthropometric measurements in *Inquiries into Human Faculty and Its Development* (1883), where he wrote, "It is needless for me to speak here about the differences in intellectual power between different men and different races, or about the convertibility of genius as shown by different members of the same gifted family achieving eminence in varied ways" (pp. 82–83). He conceptualized his measurements as constituting indicators of physical efficiency to complement performance on formal academic written literary examinations, which he thought were the best available measures of intelligence (e.g., Galton, 1884, 1891).

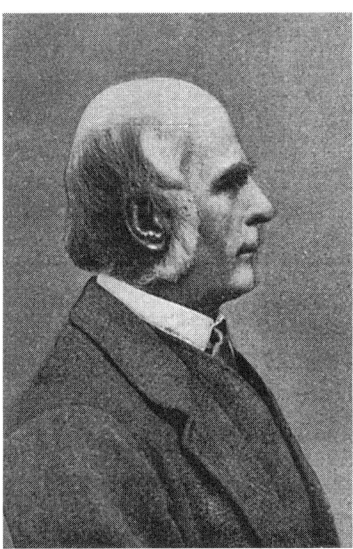

FIGURE 1.4. Francis Galton in 1888 at the age of 66, when the Anthropometric Laboratory remained active. From the copperplate prepared for *Biometrika*. In the public domain.

The examination took less than 1 hour. Although the makeup of the battery changed slightly over time, each session began with the examinee's completing a card recording age, birthplace, marital status (married, unmarried, or widowed), residence (urban, suburban, or country), and occupation. The examinee's name, birth date, and initials were collected in the laboratory's later years, with the full name indexed in a separate list. The examiner then recorded the color of the examinee's eyes and hair, followed by tests and measurements of sensory acuity, stature, strength, and lung capacity:

- Eyesight keenness, color sense, and judgment in estimating length and squareness
- Hearing keenness and highest audible note
- Height standing, without shoes
- Height sitting, from seat of chair
- Span of arms (between opposite fingertips, with arms fully extended)
- Weight, in usual indoor clothing
- Breathing capacity (volume of air exhaled after a deep breath)
- Strength of pull (as an archer draws a bow)
- Strength of grasp (squeeze with the strongest hand)
- Swiftness of blow with fist (against a flat bar with pad at one end)

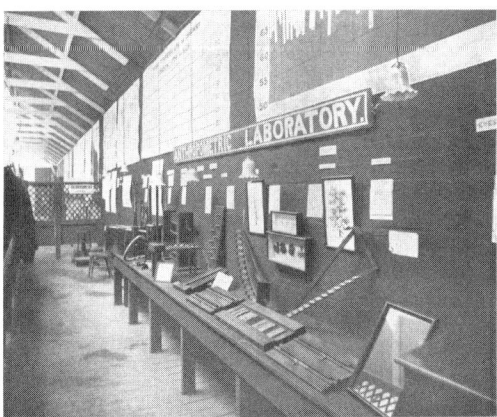

FIGURE 1.3. Francis Galton's first Anthropometric Laboratory was featured at the International Health Exhibition held in London in 1884–1885. Nearly 10,000 people paid threepence each to be examined and receive a copy of their measurements. From Pearson (1924, Plate L). Reprinted by permission of Cambridge University Press.

Specialized instruments (some invented by Galton) were employed, such as the spirometer, which required exhaling into a tube to measure the number of cubic inches of water displaced in a tank. Galton (1890b) interpreted breathing (lung) capacity as an indicator of energy level:

> The possession of a considerable amount of breathing capacity and of muscular strength is an important element of success in an active life, and the rank that a youth holds among his fellows in these respects is a valuable guide to the selection of the occupation for which he is naturally fitted, whether it should be an active or a sedentary one. (p. 238)

Galton constructed normative distributions for each measurement, including mean values and *percentile ranks* (i.e., the percentage of cases falling below the obtained score) in specified age ranges, differentiated by gender. Some measures, like breathing capacity and strength of grip, were assessed in relation to stature. It was possible to look at a normative chart and instantly know your approximate percentile rank. After collecting data on nearly 10,000 examinees at the International Health Exhibition, Galton's laboratory at South Kensington collected data on an additional 3,678 examinees (Galton, 1892), so adult norms were based on fairly large samples.

Galton never directly asserted that his tests measured *intelligence*. Instead, he observed that sensory measures are relevant in determining the breadth of experience upon which intelligence can operate:

> The only information that reaches us concerning outward events appears to pass through the avenue of our senses; and the more perceptive our senses are of difference, the larger is the field upon which our judgment and intelligence can act. (Galton, 1907, p. 19)

In 1890, he acknowledged that only research could reveal the most important areas of human functioning to measure, through careful examination of test results and correlations with external criteria:

> One of the most important objects of measurement is hardly if at all alluded to here and should be emphasized. It is to obtain a general knowledge of the capacities of a man by sinking shafts, as it were, at a few critical points. In order to ascertain the best points for the purpose, the sets of measures should be compared with an independent estimate of the man's powers. We thus may learn which of the measures are the most instructive. (Galton, 1890a, p. 380)

The uncertainty, of course, was where to sink the "shafts"—or, in other words, which abilities to measure.

With the methods proposed by Galton, a belief in scientifically based mental measurement of individual differences began to crystallize in the 1890s, and many independent research efforts were launched in the United States and Europe. Charles E. Spearman (1904, pp. 206–219) counted over 30 international investigators studying mental tests, and this was probably an underestimate. The quest for mental tests is generally agreed to have started in Great Britain with Galton's initiatives, but Spearman's (1904) discovery of a *general intellectual factor*, described in a later section, would almost immediately begin to guide theory development. The earliest U.S. efforts in mental testing came through large-scale studies from James McKeen Cattell (Cattell & Farrand, 1896) at Columbia University; Franz Boas, then at Clark University (see Bolton, 1892); J. Allen Gilbert (1894) at Yale University; and Joseph Jastrow (1893) at the University of Wisconsin, Madison. In France, Alfred Binet and his colleagues (principally Victor Henri and then Théodore Simon) were the pioneers. Germany's early contributors included Hermann Ebbinghaus and Emil Kraepelin, especially his student Axel Oehrn (1896).

It is debatable whether efforts to develop a working intelligence test ever became a scientific race, like the competitive quest to identify the molecular structure of deoxyribonucleic acid (DNA) or the pursuit of space travel technology to become the first nation to land a person on the moon. Certainly, there was constant comparison between test development efforts in different nations. For example, Sharp (1899) reviewed the competing perspectives of "M. Binet and the French psychologists," "Prof. Kraepelin and the German psychologists," and the American psychologists (p. 334), pitting the assertions of each research group against one another. In journals like *L'Année Psychologique*, Binet and his colleagues could be found reviewing work by all competing laboratories, even commenting on Sharp's paper. After Spearman (1904) described his statistical method of quantifying "general" intelligence, competition between research groups may have become even more pronounced because a more focused end goal had been specified (i.e., a test of "general" intelligence per se, rather than random tests of associated mental processes). As shown in Figure 1.5, the practice of intelligence assessment in the earliest years of the 20th century essentially consisted of an array of sensory

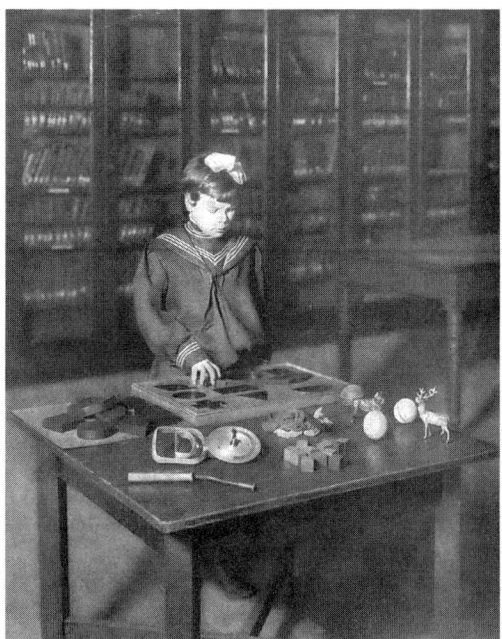

FIGURE 1.5. A photograph depicting the array of tasks used to measure intelligence at Lightner Witmer's Psychological Clinic at the University of Pennsylvania in about 1908. On the table are a Galton whistle for testing the upper limit of sound perception; a dynamometer for testing hand strength; colored yarns and blocks for testing counting skills and color perception; toys to test common knowledge, play, instinctive reactions, and coordination; and the formboard for identifying nonverbal problem solving and detecting feeble-mindedness. From Carter (1909, p. 166). In the public domain.

and motor measures, with a formboard to measure higher mental processes.

James McKeen Cattell and the End of Anthropometrics

If there were royalty in the field of psychology, James McKeen Cattell (1860–1944) might qualify. He was the son of a professor at (and later the president of) Lafayette College in Easton, Pennsylvania, where he graduated as valedictorian in 1880. After studying for 2 years in Germany, he won a fellowship at Johns Hopkins University, where he began researching the timing of various mental processes in G. Stanley Hall's "physiologico-psychological laboratory" (Sokal, 1981, p. 64). He left to study with Wilhelm Wundt, the father of experimental psychology, at the University of Leipzig, Germany,

where he worked from 1883 to 1886 before receiving his doctorate. His article "The Time It Takes to See and Name Objects" (Cattell, 1886) summarized two of his studies on basic reading processes, which are now considered to be the first research studies to support a whole-word, sight-reading approach to reading instruction (Venezky, 2002, p. 6). Rejecting Wundt's reliance on experimenter introspection, Cattell conducted reaction time experiments with some of his own instruments, growing interested in the measurement of individual differences. According to his biographer, Michael M. Sokal, Cattell "refocused psychological research away from experimenters' self-observation of their mental activity and toward subjects' behavior in a laboratory setting precisely defined by experimenters" (Sokal, 2006, p. 25). In just a few years, Cattell would become the leading American experimental psychologist of his time.

In 1887, Cattell took a position at the University of Cambridge, where he came to know and work closely with Francis Galton. Cattell's data card from his personal anthropometric measurements appears in Figure 1.6. Cattell helped Galton set up the Anthropometric Laboratory at South Kensington. Cattell would remain devoted to Galton for the rest of his life, acknowledging in his late 60s that Galton was "the greatest man whom I have known" (Cattell, 1930, p. 116). For 2 years, Cattell split his time between work in Galton's laboratory, lecturing and establishing a laboratory at Cambridge University, and lecturing also at Bryn Mawr College and the University of Pennsylvania in the United States. In 1888, Cattell became a professor of psychology at the University of Pennsylvania (the first such professorship established anywhere, he claimed). In 1891, Cattell relocated to Columbia University, where he became the administrative head—beginning Columbia's experimental psychology laboratory and mentoring doctoral students like Edward L. Thorndike, Robert S. Woodworth, and Harry L. Hollingworth, who would themselves become faculty and leading figures in psychology. Over 40 students would take their doctorates with Cattell, seven of them becoming presidents of the APA. Cattell himself served as president of the APA in 1895.

With respect to intelligence testing, Cattell is a seminal historical figure due to his tireless advocacy for psychology as a science, his own test development efforts, and his advocacy for psychometrics and testing, as well as his emphasis on statistical analyses of individual differences, all of

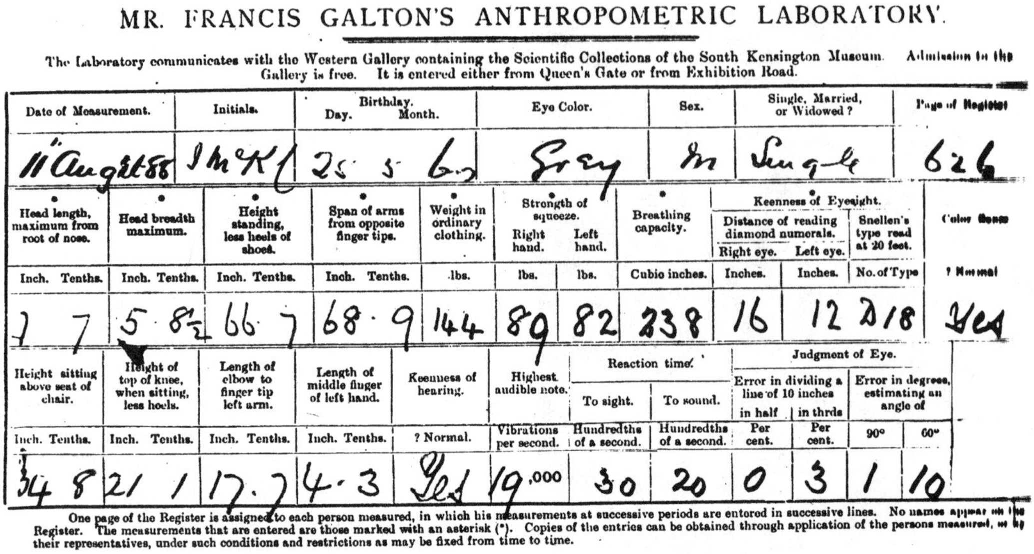

MR. FRANCIS GALTON'S ANTHROPOMETRIC LABORATORY.

The Laboratory communicates with the Western Gallery containing the Scientific Collections of the South Kensington Museum. Admission to the Gallery is free. It is entered either from Queen's Gate or from Exhibition Road.

Date of Measurement.	Initials.	Birthday. Day.	Birthday. Month.	Eye Color.	Sex.	Single, Married, or Widowed?	Page of Register
11 August 88	JMcK	25	5	Grey	M	Single	626

Head length, maximum from root of nose.	Head breadth maximum.	Height standing, less heels of shoes.	Span of arms from opposite finger tips.	Weight in ordinary clothing.	Strength of squeeze. Right hand.	Strength of squeeze. Left hand.	Breathing capacity.	Keenness of Eyesight. Distance of reading diamond numerals. Right eye.	Keenness of Eyesight. Distance of reading diamond numerals. Left eye.	Snellen's type read at 20 feet.	Color Sense
Inch. Tenths.	Inch. Tenths.	Inch. Tenths.	Inch. Tenths.	lbs.	lbs.	lbs.	Cubic inches.	Inches.	Inches.	No. of Type	? Normal
7 7	5 8½	66 7	68 · 9	144	89	82	238	16	12	D 18	Yes

Height sitting above seat of chair.	Height of top of knee, when sitting, less heels.	Length of elbow to finger tip left arm.	Length of middle finger of left hand.	Keenness of hearing.	Highest audible note.	Reaction time. To sight.	Reaction time. To sound.	Judgment of Eye. Error in dividing a line of 10 inches in half	Judgment of Eye. Error in dividing a line of 10 inches in thrds	Error in degrees, estimating an angle of 90°	Error in degrees, estimating an angle of 60°
Inch. Tenths.	Inch. Tenths.	Inch. Tenths.	Inch. Tenths.	? Normal.	Vibrations per second.	Hundredths of a second.	Hundredths of a second.	Per cent.	Per cent.		
34 8	21 1	17 . 7	4 · 3	Yes	19,000	30	20	0	3	1	10

One page of the Register is assigned to each person measured, in which his measurements at successive periods are entered in successive lines. No names appear on the Register. The measurements that are entered are those marked with an asterisk (*). Copies of the entries can be obtained through application of the persons measured, or by their representatives, under such conditions and restrictions as may be fixed from time to time.

FIGURE 1.6. Measurement data card recorded in 1888 at Galton's Anthropometric Laboratory for J. McKeen Cattell, who was deeply influenced by Francis Galton. Papers of James McKeen Cattell, 1835–1948, Library of Congress, Washington, D.C. In the public domain.

which established a fertile environment for test development at Columbia University and in American psychology in general. In the British journal *Mind*, Cattell (1890) used the term *mental tests* for the first time:

> Psychology cannot attain the certainty and exactness of the physical sciences, unless it rests on a foundation of experiment and measurement. A step in this direction could be made by applying a series of mental tests and measurements to a large number of individuals. The results would be of considerable scientific value in discovering the constancy of mental processes, their interdependence, and their variation under different circumstances. Individuals, besides, would find their tests interesting, and perhaps, useful in regard to training, mode of life or indication of disease. (p. 373)

Cattell made his principal research initiative at Columbia an investigation to determine whether a battery of Galtonian anthropometric tests and sensory, motor, and higher cognitive tasks could constitute a measure of intelligence. Beginning in 1894, the Cattell–Columbia Tests (as Cattell referred to them in 1924) were given to freshmen at Columbia's School of Arts and School of Mines. With student consent, the tests were to be repeated at the end of the sophomore and senior years. In the course of an hour, 26 measurements were made in the laboratory, and 44 observations were recorded. Later, each student sent in answers to 50 questions with regard to background, health, physical condition, habits (including coffee, smoking, alcohol use, and exercise), and interests. Cattell also had access to student academic records and athletic accomplishments.

Tests and measurements conducted in the laboratory included some of Galton's sensory measures; some of Cattell's reaction time measures; and some newer measures, including letter cancellation, rapid color naming, memory for digits, logical memory, self-reported retrieval of mental images, and a word association test. The battery was something of a hybrid between anthropometric, lower-order, and higher-order measures. Cattell had always relied on the experimental approach as producing descriptive results that would speak for themselves; he did not offer a priori hypotheses or even articulate his concept of intelligence. Cattell's commitment to quantitative measurement and statistical analysis of experimental results was unshakeable, and as late as 1924, Cattell, pictured in Figure 1.7, still expressed a belief that his test battery might correlate with long-term student accomplishments. He would not have the chance to find out, as two studies would put a conclusive end to Cattell's approach to intelligence testing and his experimental research efforts.

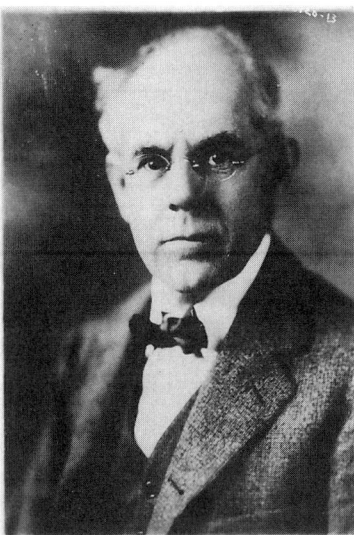

FIGURE 1.7. James McKeen Cattell at the age of 63 in December 1923. Long after the failure of his anthropometric testing program and after his 1917 dismissal from Columbia University, Cattell founded The Psychological Corporation and continued to edit several scientific journals. From the chapter author's collection.

First, a dissertation completed by Stella Sharp (1899) in Edward B. Titchener's laboratory at Cornell University sought to examine the variability of complex mental processes and the relations between complex mental processes, with the intention of demonstrating the practicality of testing complex processes rather than the simpler mental processes endorsed by Cattell and Galton. She assessed seven advanced philosophy students at the university with the test battery formulated by Binet and Henri (1895), including measures of memory, mental images, imagination, attention, observation/comprehension, suggestibility, and aesthetic tastes. Her results listed the scores of individual participants and described these results in terms of rank order and variability. Sharp concluded:

> We concur with Mm. Binet and Henri in believing that individual psychical differences should be sought for in the complex rather than in the elementary processes of mind, and that the test method is the most workable one that has yet been proposed for investigating these processes. (Sharp, 1899, p. 390)

She further concluded that the Binet–Henri measures required modification but were practical and yielded considerable variation in scores. She of-

fered only qualitative observations about relations between tests of different mental processes, however. Although she did not collect data on other assessment approaches, she was critical of the anthropometric tests as unproven and lacking an explanatory theory.

The second blow to Cattell's testing program, and its *coup de grâce*, came from a Columbia University psychology graduate student, Clark Wissler (1901). Wissler examined the correlations between the Cattell–Columbia Tests and student grades for 300 undergraduates at Columbia and Barnard Colleges. He reported that while isolated correlations were large (e.g., height and weight $r = .66$; Latin and Greek grades $r = .75$), the laboratory mental tests had negligible correlations with each other and with college class grades. The failure to correlate with academic grades was considered fatal to Cattell's testing program because academic performance had long been considered an independent criterion measure of intelligence. In the words of Cattell's biographer, Wissler's analysis would definitively "discredit anthropometric testing" (Sokal, 2006, p. 29).

It remains to note that over a century after Galton's and Cattell's testing programs were discredited, the relations of elementary cognitive processes (reaction time and sensory discrimination) to mental abilities and intelligence are now being revisited. Jensen (2006) has effectively summarized the literature relating reaction time to intelligence, while Deary and his colleagues (Deary, 1994; Deary, Bell, Bell, Campbell, & Fazal, 2004) have documented findings with sensory discrimination and intelligence. There is uniform agreement as to the serious methodological flaws in the Sharp and Wissler studies, including small sample size, restriction of range, and unreliability of measures (e.g., Buckhalt, 1991; Deary, 1994; Jensen, 2006).

THE ORIGINS OF CONTEMPORARY INTELLIGENCE TESTING

I have described the pseudoscience of phrenology and the visionary science of Galton, who inspired the search for effective ways to measure intelligence and who pioneered many statistical methods that would be critical for norm-referenced assessment. I have also recounted the tale of the psychologist that Galton so profoundly influenced, J. McKeen Cattell, who threw down a gauntlet of sorts when proposing that *mental tests* should constitute part of establishing psychology as a science that can measure individual differences. The unfortunate fate of Cattell's test battery has been told. Even after his assessment work was discredited, however, Cattell remained a highly connected institutional scientist and a pioneer in the development of scientific psychology in American universities.

Ironically, the problem of developing a working intelligence test would be solved by an outsider, a man with few friends, who worked without pay and who had no institutional connections of any benefit. He did have his own journal, however, where he reviewed the work of his contemporaries. His name was Alfred Binet.

Alfred Binet:
The Innovative Outsider

Alfred Binet (1857–1911) is generally acknowledged as the father of intelligence tests, having developed the first working measure of intelligence. Binet's remarkable history has been most definitively documented by biographer Theta Wolf (1973). He was educated as a lawyer but chose not to practice; some historical accounts also report that Binet studied medicine until his father, a physician, traumatized him by showing him a cadaver. As an only child of a wealthy family he could afford to pursue a career with little remuneration, and he developed a consuming interest in the study of psychology. He was a voracious reader across several languages who educated himself as a psychologist, spending considerable time studying in the Bibliothèque Nationale [French National Library]. He wrote his first article at age 23 and completed a doctorate in the natural sciences at age 37. According to long-time colleague Théodore Simon, for most of Binet's career "psychology was his sole occupation" (quoted by Wolf, 1973, p. 9).

Although he is remembered for his intelligence test (from which he does not appear to have profited financially), Alfred Binet was a remarkably productive and versatile researcher, authoring nearly 300 works during his career; he is now credited with pioneering experimental investigations in areas of abnormal, cognitive, developmental, educational, forensic, personality, and social psychology (e.g., Siegler, 1992; Wolf, 1973). Regrettably, most of his work has never been translated into English, although nearly all of it has been brought back into print in the last decade. Personally, he has been described as a loner, "a reserved man with few friends" (Tuddenham, 1974, p. 1071), and as a domineering individual who antagonized

many of his coworkers (cf. Henri Piéron, according to an interview with Wolf, 1961, p. 246). In 1901, Binet wrote a friend, "I educated myself all alone, without any teachers; I have arrived at my present scientific situation by the sole force of my fists; *no one*, you understand, no one, has ever helped me" (quoted by Wolf, 1973, p. 23). Lacking patronage, he was denied academic positions in France (Nicolas & Ferrand, 2002), and his efforts for educational reform and mental measurement in the military were resisted by a rigid French establishment (e.g., Carson, 2007; Zazzo, 1993). Several scholars have sought to explain why so much of his work was forgotten after his death (e.g., Fancher, 1998; Schneider, 1992; Siegler, 1992; Wolf, 1973), and the answer seems to lie in his disconnection from the professional and academic community in France: He did not present at conferences, he did not leave students to continue his work, and he preferred to work alone or with a collaborator. Only at the 2005 centennial of the first Binet–Simon scale did he begin to garner national recognition in his native France for his remarkable contributions.

A devastating early career setback left Binet careful to avoid preconceptions and reticent to form theories in his experimental work. In one of his first positions, Binet's work with collaborator Charles Féré at Jean Martin Charcot's clinic in the Salpêtrière Hospital in Paris was publicly discredited. In working with Charcot's hysterical patients in the 1880s (at a time when Sigmund Freud was also studying with Charcot), Binet and Féré thought they had proven that movements and perceptions could be shifted from one side of the body to the other, and that emotions could be reversed (e.g., from love to hate) through the application of magnets while participants were hypnotized. Their demonstrations could not be independently replicated, presumably because participants were prone to dissimulation or demand effects. Charcot's approach and the Binet–Féré studies were effectively challenged in a series of articles by a Belgian psychologist, Franz Joseph Delboeuf. Gradually Binet realized he had been "taken in" by Charcot's reputation; suitably chastened, he learned painful lessons about the need for careful experimentation, objective observation, and skepticism about a priori theoretical assumptions. Binet left the Salpêtrière in 1890, ending his connections with Charcot and Féré. For the rest of his life, he remained wary of theories that might bias his research findings.

From 1890 through his death, Binet published more than 200 articles, many in the journal *L'Année Psychologique*, which he cofounded and edited. In 1891, he became an unpaid staff member at the Laboratory of Physiological Psychology at the Sorbonne. Three years later, he became director of the laboratory, a position he held until his death. Between 1894 and 1898, Binet and Victor Henri sought new methods that would "substitute for vague notions of man in general, of the archetypal man, precise observations of individuals considered in all the complexity and variety of their aptitudes" (Binet & Henri, 1894, p. 167; translated and cited by Carson, 2007, p. 132). In 1899, Binet was approached by a young intern physician and *aliéniste* (psychiatrist), Théodore Simon, who had access to clinical populations (Wolf, 1961). Simon completed his doctoral thesis under Binet's supervision, and their subsequent collaborations included Binet's most important work in intelligence assessment.

The creative work that culminated in the intelligence scales began in 1890, when Binet published three papers describing experimental studies with his two young daughters, Madeleine and Alice (given the pseudonyms Marguerite and Armande), whom he had carefully observed and tested with a variety of cognitive and personality tasks. Binet's wife and daughters appear in Figure 1.8. In describing their attentional styles, he wrote that Madeleine was "silent, cool, concentrated, while Alice was a laugher, gay, thoughtless, giddy, and turbulent" (translated by Wolf, 1966, p. 234). Many of the tasks Binet gave his daughters will be familiar to contemporary psychologists—word generation, word association, sentence generation,

sentence completion, thematic composition for various pictures, description of objects or pictures, design reproduction, letter cancellation, digit repetition, reaction time after stimulation, recall of unrelated words, recall of prose passages, recall of pictured objects, recall of nonsense sentences (i.e., sentences presented in a foreign language unknown to the girls), and verbal responses to inkblots. Binet was careful to analyze the quality of response content. For example, he classified verbal responses as personal, unelaborated, abstract, or imagined; prose recall was scored according for verbatim recall and gist recall; thought processes were described according to linearity, conventionality, and originality. Binet continually made qualitative observations of performance styles that differentiated his daughters. Madeleine had greater "stability" and had better voluntary control of her attention; she could more effectively focus on assigned work and memorize neutral, uninteresting material; and she tended to respond with shorter and more constant reaction times. Alice presented more "variability"; she was more imaginative and emotional; and material to be learned had to be of interest to her, or she would have difficulty. She could not memorize long literary passages verbatim as her sister could, but she could accurately remember a series of ideas provided just once (see Wolf, 1973, p. 132). Binet continued to test his daughters through midadolescence with a battery of cognitive and personality tests, including measures of attention, language, reasoning, and memory (many repeated multiple times in alternative

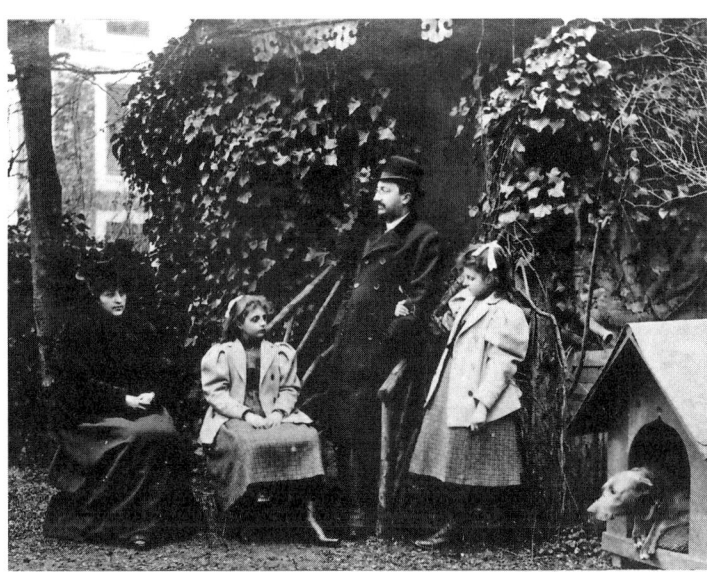

FIGURE 1.8. Alfred Binet; his wife, Laure Balbiani Binet; and his daughters, Madeleine and Alice, whom he tested extensively with cognitive and personality tasks through their midadolescence. In his writings, Binet described the girls under the pseudonyms Marguerite and Armande. Madeleine was said to be "silent, cool, concentrated, while Alice was a laugher, gay, thoughtless, giddy, and turbulent" (translated by Wolf, 1966, p. 234). Theta H. Wolf Papers, Archives of the History of American Psychology, Center for the History of Psychology, University of Akron. Reprinted by permission.

forms over several years), always accompanied by careful qualitative observation and interview inquiries. He reported the results in 1903 in *L'étude Expérimentale de l'Intelligence [The Experimental Study of Intelligence]*.

Comparison of his children's performances with each other and with those of adults led Binet to conclude that complex, multidimensional tasks were more sensitive to developmental changes than narrow, unidimensional tasks. He further concluded that a mental developmental progression from childhood through adulthood should be reflected in task performance:

> In case one should succeed in measuring intelligence—that is to say, reasoning, judgment, memory, the ability to make abstractions—which appears not absolutely impossible to me, the figure that would represent the average intellectual development of an adult would present an entirely different relation to that of the figure representing the intellectual development of a child. (Binet, 1890, p. 74, translated by Wolf, 1966, p. 235)

In 1895, Binet and Henri outlined the project for the development of an intelligence test, specifying 10 discrete mental faculties that would be measured: memory, imagery, imagination, attention, comprehension, suggestibility, aesthetic sentiment, moral sentiment, muscular strength/willpower, and motor ability/hand–eye coordination. Binet and Henri, along with other colleagues from Binet's laboratory, appear in Figure 1.9. Higher-order, complex processes were considered to show greater variability among individuals and to constitute better measures of intelligence than simpler sensory and motor processes:

> The higher and more complex a process is, the more it varies in individuals; sensations vary from one individual to another, but less so than memory; memory of sensations varies less than memories of ideas, etc. The result is, that if one wishes to study the differences existing between two individuals, it is necessary to begin with the most intellectual and complex processes, and it is only secondarily necessary to consider the simple and elementary processes. (Binet & Henri, 1895, p. 417; translated by Sharp, 1899, p. 335)

In a passage that made direct reference to the work of Galton and Cattell, Binet and Henri (1895) rebutted the claim that greater experimental precision was possible in the measurement of simpler mental processes:

> If one looks at the series of experiments made—the *mental tests* as the English say—one is astonished by the considerable place reserved to the sensations and the simple processes, and by the little attention lent to the superior processes. . . . The objection will be made that the elementary processes can be determined with much more precision than the superior processes. This is certain, but people differ in these elementary ones much more feebly than in the complex ones; there is no need, therefore, for as precise a method for determining the latter as for the former. . . . Anyway, it is only by applying one's self to this point that one can approach the study of individual differences. (Binet & Henri, 1895, pp. 426, 429; translated by Siegler, 1992, p. 181)

The formal mandate that led to the development of the intelligence test came in October 1904, when Joseph Chaumié, the Minister of Public Instruction, established a commission chaired

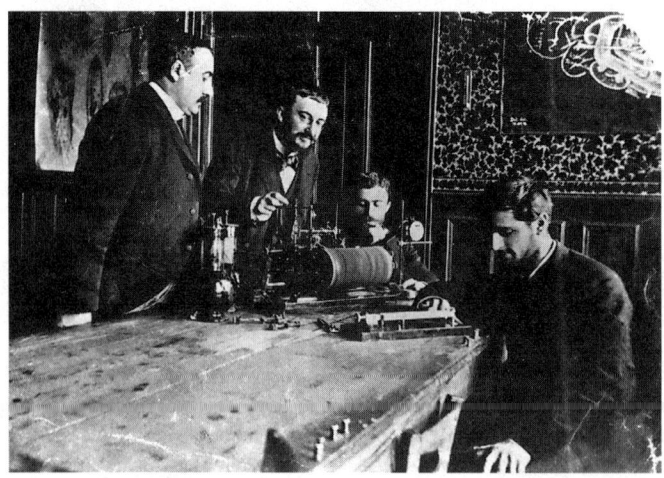

FIGURE 1.9. Alfred Binet and colleagues in the 1890s: J. Courtier, J. Philippe, and Victor Henri. This group collaborated in the work involved for Binet's (1894) book on experimental psychology. Photo from Binet's Laboratoire de Psychologie Physiologique de la Sorbonne (École des Hautes-Études). Theta H. Wolf Papers, Archives of the History of American Psychology, Center for the History of Psychology, University of Akron. Reprinted by permission.

by Léon Bourgeois and charged it with studying how France's 1882 mandatory public education laws could be applied to abnormal [*anormaux*] children, including students who were blind, deaf-mute, and backward [*arriérés*] (Carson, 2007; Wolf, 1969). The ministry was persuaded to take this initiative by public pressure, including a resolution from the 1903 Third National Congress of Public and Private Welfare held at Bordeaux, where critics noted France's failure to comply with its own special education laws. A resolution from an educational advocacy group, La Société Libre pour l'Étude Psychologique de l'Enfant [Free Society for the Psychological Study of the Child], was also a reason for creation of the Bourgeois Commission. Binet was a leader of La Société Libre and an author of the resolution, and he became a member of the commission, which began its work by circulating questionnaires to teachers and principals throughout France. The commission met on numerous occasions in 1904 and 1905, issuing its report in 1906.

Binet saw in the commission's mandate an opportunity to complete his efforts toward a norm-referenced standard for diagnosis and educational decision making. Building on the earlier work with Henri (who had departed), Binet and Simon developed and tested a series of cognitive tests. Their collaborations worked in tandem: One of them would talk with and question the examinee, while the other wrote the replies and noted salient behaviors. The assessments had "the air of a game" for children, with encouragement being constantly provided (Binet & Simon, 1905/1916a, p. 141). The work culminated in the 1905 publication of the Binet–Simon Intelligence Scale (Binet & Simon, 1905/1916c), consisting of 30 items that could be given in about 20 minutes; it was normed on some 50 children from ages 3 through 11 years; and one of its chief advances may have been to combine a wide range of cognitive tasks to obtain a global estimate of intelligence (e.g., DuBois, 1970). Binet and Simon (1905/1916c) sequenced tasks in a cognitive-developmental order from easy to hard and from simpler to more complex, while sampling a wide range of tasks tapping various abilities. In general, they sought tasks that tapped the higher-order ability of *judgment*—especially procedures that had demonstrated the capacity to differentiate groups on the basis of intelligence. For example, individuals considered *idiots* generally could not move beyond the 6th of the 30 tasks; individuals considered *imbeciles* rarely went beyond the 15th task (Binet & Simon, 1905/1916a).

The Bourgeois Commission issued its report early in 1906, based primarily on a subcommittee report drafted by Binet. Recommendations were that the *anormaux* be educated through *classes spéciales* annexed to ordinary primary schools and, in certain situations, through separate institutions. A five-part classification of exceptional students was proposed, identifying students who were blind, deaf, medically abnormal, intellectually backward, and emotionally unstable. The commission recommended that students who did not benefit from education, teaching, or discipline should receive a "medico-pedagogical examination" before being removed from primary schools, and that such children, if educable, should be placed in special classes. The examination was to be overseen by an examination committee consisting of an inspector of primary schools, a physician, and a director of the separate special school. The commission did not offer any specific content for the examination, recommending that the Minister of Public Instruction appoint a competent person to draw up a scientific guide for the school examination committee (Carson, 2007). Undoubtedly Binet hoped to draw up the scientific guide, and Binet and Simon's (1907/1914) book *Les Enfants Anormaux* was probably intended to serve as the guide; it even contained a preface by Léon Bourgeois, the head of the commission.

Unfortunately, Binet's efforts were almost completely rebuffed by the French establishment. When the French legislature enacted the law of April 15, 1909, on the education of the *anormaux*, it stated that the commission determining eligibility for special education should be composed of a physician, school inspector, and director or teacher at an *école perfectionnement*. It highlighted the medical examination and made no mention of any role for psychologists or use of special methods (i.e., intelligence tests) for assessing students (Carson, 2007). Binet's efforts had little visible impact on practice in his native France.

In the 1908 revision, the Binet–Simon Scale took its definitive revolutionary form, the "graded scale of intelligence" [*L'échelle métrique de l' intelligence*], which was easier to use and interpret (Binet & Simon, 1908/1916b). It featured 56 tests arranged by difficulty so that tests were placed at levels, or grades, corresponding to approximately a 75% pass rate for children of a given age, based on normative performances of about 200 children between the ages of 3 and 15. The 1908 scale permitted a student's mental level [*niveau mental*] to be estimated through what later became interpreted in the United States as a mental age level. The mental level was determined by the highest age at which a child passed four or five tests (the basal year), with an additional year credited for each of the five tests passed beyond the basal. By the completion of the 1911 edition (Binet, 1911/1916), the scale was extended from age 3 through adult-hood, with 11 levels and five items administered at each level. Table 1.1 lists content from the final 1911 scale. The Binet–Simon Scale never yielded an intelligence quotient (IQ), but Binet endorsed the convention of identifying intellectual disability [*arriérés*] for a mental level delay of "two years when the child is under [age] nine, and three

---

TABLE 1.1. Contents of the Binet–Simon (Binet, 1911/1916) Intelligence Scale [*L'Échelle Métrique de l' Intelligence*]

Three years

Show eyes, nose, mouth
Name objects in a picture
Repeat 2 figures
Repeat a sentence of 6 syllables
Give last name

Four years

Give sex
Name key, knife, penny
Repeat 3 figures
Compare 2 lines

Five years

Compare 2 boxes of different weights
Copy a square
Repeat a sentence of 10 syllables
Count 4 sous
Put together two pieces in a "game of patience"

Six years

Distinguish morning and evening
Define by use
Copy diamond
Count 13 pennies
Compare 2 pictures esthetically

Seven years

Right hand, left ear
Describe a picture
Execute 3 commissions
Count 3 single and 3 double sous
Name 4 colors

Eight years

Compare 2 objects from memory
Count from 20 to 0
Indicate omission in pictures
Give the date
Repeat 5 digits

Nine years

Give change out of 20 sous
Definitions superior to use
Recognize the value of 9 pieces of money
Name the months
Comprehend easy questions

Ten years

Place 5 weights in order
Copy a design from memory
Criticize absurd statements
Comprehend difficult questions
Place 3 words in 2 sentences

Twelve years

Resist the suggestion of lines
Place 3 words in 1 sentence
Give more than 60 words in 3 minutes
Define 3 abstract words
Comprehend a disarranged sentence

Fifteen years

Repeat 7 figures
Find 3 rhymes
Repeat a sentence of 26 syllables
Interpret a picture
Solve a problem composed of several facts

Adults

Comprehend a cut in a folded paper
Reversed triangle
Answer the question about the President
Distinguish abstract words
Give the sense of the quotation from Hervieu

Note. The final 1911 Binet–Simon Scale extended from 3 years into adulthood. In this edition, an individual's mental level [*niveau mental*] was estimated by identifying the highest age at which all the tests were passed (the basal year), to which is added one-fifth of a year for every test passed. The Binet–Simon Scale never yielded an intelligence quotient (IQ), but Binet endorsed the convention of identifying intellectual disability for a mental-level delay of 2 years when a child is under age 9, and 3 years past his or her 9th birthday. From Binet (1911/1916). In the public domain.

years when he is past his ninth birthday" (Binet & Simon, 1907/1914, p. 42). Long after Binet's death, Simon indicated that the use of a summary IQ score was a betrayal [*trahison*] of the scale's objective (cited by Wolf, 1973, p. 203).

In the spring of 1908, Henry H. Goddard, director of the psychological research laboratory at the New Jersey Training School for Feeble-Minded Girls and Boys (later known as the Vineland Training School), traveled to Europe. He visited doctors and teachers working in 19 different institutions and 93 special classes. Ironically, he did not even look up Binet in Paris, having been told by Pierre Janet that "Binet's Lab. is largely a myth . . . Not much being done—says Janet," according to his journal (cited by Zenderland, 1998, pp. 92–93). In Brussels, he met Ovide Decroly, a Belgian teacher, physician, and psychologist, engaged in a tryout of the 1905 Binet–Simon Scale. Decroly provided him with a copy of the test, and upon his return home, Goddard began to use the test on the children at the training school. In the words of Goddard's biographer Leila Zenderland (1998), Goddard immediately understood the significance of the Binet–Simon Scale:

> Two years of frustrating institutional experience had prepared him to see what Janet, Cattell, and even [G. Stanley] Hall, the most prescient of contemporary psychological entrepreneurs, had missed. Contained within Binet's articles, Goddard quickly realized, was an entirely new psychological approach toward diagnosing and classifying feeble minds. (p. 93)

In a short time, Goddard would become the United States' leading advocate for Binet's approach to assessment and diagnosing intellectually disabled individuals. He described his evaluation of the ease, simplicity, and the utility of the 1908 scale as "a surprise and a gratification" (Goddard, 1916, p. 5), and he promoted the test widely. The Binet–Simon Scale was both praised and criticized widely in professional journals; for example, several consecutive issues of the *Journal of Educational Psychology* in April, May, and June 1916 were dedicated to "Mentality Tests: A Symposium," a wide-ranging exchange of experiences with the Binet–Simon Scale (and other tests) by 16 leading psychologists. Goddard arranged for Elizabeth S. Kite, his laboratory's field worker and contributor to the famous Kallikak study, to complete the definitive translations into English of Binet and Simon's writings on their intelligence scale. By 1916, the Vineland laboratory had distributed 22,000 copies of a pamphlet describing administration of the Binet–Simon Scale and 88,000 record forms, as well as publishing a two-volume translation of the Binet–Simon articles (Goddard, 1916). By 1939, there were some 77 available adaptations and translations of the Binet–Simon Scale (Hildreth, 1939), including the most used psychological test of all, the Stanford–Binet. According to Théodore Simon, Binet gave Lewis M. Terman at Stanford University the rights to publish an American revision of the Binet–Simon Scale "for a token of one dollar" (cited by Wolf, 1973, p. 35). Terman's work would change the landscape for mental testing in the United States.

The Binet–Simon Intelligence Scale represented a major paradigm shift for the young field of psychology. It tapped intelligence through assessment of complex mental abilities, as opposed to the narrow sensory and motor measures dominating the Galton–Cattell batteries. It was standardized, with explicit procedures for administration and objective scoring guidelines. It was norm-referenced, permitting an individual's performance to be compared with that of his or her age peers. It was reliable, yielding consistent scores from one occasion to another. It was developmentally sensitive, recognizing that mental abilities in children develop in a meaningful progression and that the abilities of children differ substantially from that of adults. It was efficient and engaging, administered in an adaptive format in which content changed frequently. It offered clinical assessment, aimed at diagnosing intellectual disabilities, identifying cognitively advanced students, and describing the characteristics of both "normal" and "abnormal" individuals. Finally and most importantly, it seemed to work fairly well, providing an empirical foundation for the nascent study of intelligence and cognitive abilities.

Lewis M. Terman: Defender of the Discipline

I hate the impudence of a claim that in fifty minutes you can judge and classify a human being's predestined fitness in life. I hate the pretentiousness of that claim. I hate the abuse of scientific method which it involves. I hate the sense of superiority which it creates, and the sense of inferiority which it imposes.

—WALTER LIPPMANN (1923)

When journalist Walter Lippmann launched the first high-profile public attack on intelligence testing in a series of articles in *The New Republic* (Lippmann, 1922a, 1922b, 1922c, 1922d, 1922e,

1922f, 1923), it was Lewis M. Terman (1922a) who responded and defended the new discipline. He was the natural choice—developer of the Stanford University revision of the Binet–Simon Intelligence Scale (later called the Stanford–Binet Intelligence Scale); member of the National Research Council team that created the Army mental tests in 1917 and 1918; coauthor of the National Intelligence Tests and Terman Group Test of Mental Ability, released in 1920; principal investigator on the longitudinal Genetic Studies of Genius, initiated in 1921–1922; and coauthor of the Stanford Achievement Test, which would be released in 1923. For decades, Terman would be the living American most strongly associated with intelligence testing and its value for educational decision making.

The 12th of 14 children from a rural Indiana farming family, Lewis M. Terman (1877–1956) was a brilliant, hard-working, and determined student from an early age; he accelerated from first grade to third grade and memorized most of his textbooks. Graduating early from eighth grade (the conclusion of education in typical Midwest farming communities of that era), he began teacher's college at the age of 15, attending when he could and taking breaks to earn enough money to return. He pursued training in education, as teaching was the "only avenue of escape for the youth who aspired to anything beyond farm life" (Terman, 1932, p. 300); eventually he would teach for one year in a one-room schoolhouse. By the age of 21, he had earned three baccalaureate degrees from Central Normal College in Danville, Indiana, and he became a principal of a small high school. He then pursued a master's degree in psychology at Indiana University, followed by a doctorate at Clark University. In 1905, recurrent tubercular hemorrhages in his lungs (eventually the cause of his death) forced Terman to relocate his family to Southern California, where he worked again as a high school principal and then as a professor of pedagogy at Los Angeles State Normal School (later UCLA) before accepting a position in 1909 at Stanford University, where he remained for the duration of his career. Figure 1.10 shows Terman at about the time he started his career at Stanford University.

Terman is described by two biographers, Henry L. Minton (1988) and May V. Seagoe (1975), as having been a highly gifted man and voracious learner, who was tirelessly persistent, intense, and sensitive. As a rigorous and careful researcher, he became a pioneer in mental testing by creating the best of many adaptations of the Binet–Simon

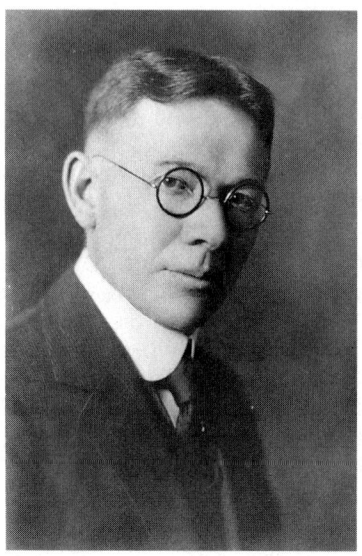

FIGURE 1.10. Lewis M. Terman in 1910, the year he arrived at Stanford University. Terman was the leading advocate for intelligence testing in the first half of the 20th century. Reprinted by courtesy of the Department of Special Collections and University Archives, Stanford University Libraries.

Scale. He also harbored a progressive vision of large-scale testing to identify the individual differences and needs of schoolchildren, as well as to identify intellectually gifted children (Chapman, 1988). Like Cattell, Terman had been seen by a phrenologist as a child; he was deeply impressed by the experience and remembered that the phrenologist "predicted great things of me" (Terman, 1932, p. 303). Having spent 6 months each year during his adolescence toiling at farmwork from 5:00 A.M. through about 7:00 or 8:00 P.M., Terman considered his intellectual abilities to have been inherited; he remembered his lengthy stints at farmwork as periods without mental stimulation, contributing to his conviction that environment was substantially less important than heredity in explaining intelligence.

Terman's master's thesis on leadership, his doctoral dissertation on genius, and his longitudinal study of gifted children beginning in 1921–1922 all contributed to his status as founder of the "gifted child" movement. Terman's thesis, published as a journal article in 1904, used experimental methodology (from Binet's suggestibility studies), teacher ratings, and questionnaires to examine leadership in male and female schoolchildren from grades 2 through 8. It is a qualitatively rich study that identifies different types of leaders and subtly links leadership with perceived intelligence. Terman's dissertation, completed in 1905 and published as a journal article in 1906, was entitled "Genius and Stupidity: A Study of Some of the Intellectual Processes of Seven 'Bright' and Seven 'Stupid' Boys." For his dissertation, Terman administered a variety of higher-order mental tests to seven boys identified by teachers as the "brightest" and seven boys identified as the "dullest," based upon a holistic review (i.e., not merely based on classwork) of willing boys. All of the boys were 10–13 years of age. Terman tested the boys for about 20–40 hours in each of eight areas: creative imagination, logical processes, mathematical ability, mastery of language, interpretation of fables, ease of learning to play chess, powers of memory, and motor abilities. Some tests were culled from the literature, including measures from Binet and Henri, Ebbinghaus, and others; other tests were tasks developed by Terman that would reappear in the Stanford–Binet. Terman found that the bright boys were superior to the dull boys in all but the motor tests, with creative imagination tests showing modest differences between bright and dull boys. Most tests administered tended to agree with one another—a finding that Terman interpreted as supporting the presence of Spearman's general factor. Bright children preferred to read, while dull children preferred to play games; there was little difference between the two groups in terms of persistence.

In 1910, Terman began his revision of the Binet–Simon Scale, a technical *tour de force* that would be published in 1916. Terman began initial studies by administering the 1908 Binet–Simon Scale to some 400 schoolchildren, as well as examining all available published studies of age-level placement for the Binet tests. It soon became evident that some tests were misplaced, with tests at the lower age levels too easy and those at the upper age levels too hard. He also wanted to add tests to reach six at each age level, eventually augmenting the Binet–Simon with 36 new tasks and clarifying administration and scoring criteria. Terman, his students, and his colleagues tested some 700 additional children in pilot studies. Some of Terman's new tasks were noteworthy, including a 100-word vocabulary test yielding full credit for correct definitions, half credit for partially correct definitions, and no credit for incorrect responses; and (arguably) the first executive function measure, the Ball and Field Test of Practical Judgment (see Littman, 2004, for an account of its origins). Terman and

Childs (1912a, 1912b, 1912c, 1912d) published a "tentative revision and extension" of the Binet–Simon Scale, but further revision was necessary, given the 1911 extension of the Binet–Simon Scale through adulthood. As Seagoe (1975) reports, Terman's "unfamiliarity with statistics" and dislike of the "drudgery of computation" (p. 47) caused him to rely heavily on Arthur S. Otis, and for later editions on Truman L. Kelley and Quinn McNemar, for statistical analyses and data management. Dahlstrom (1985) notes the contribution of Otis's statistical knowledge and skills for the 1916 Stanford–Binet: "The efforts of Arthur S. Otis . . . were particularly important in this entire venture. He carried out the work on the item analyses and try-outs of the various early combinations of these items in tentative scales" (p. 76). Otis would later make important contributions to the development of the Army mental tests.

Terman's final standardization sample for the 1916 Stanford–Binet included 905 participants between the ages of 5 and 14 years, all within 2 months of a birthday and drawn from public schools in California and Nevada. No foreign-born or minority children were included. Special population studies included 200 "defective" and "superior" children. The adult sample consisted of 150 adolescent delinquents, 150 unemployed men, 50 high school students, and 30 businessmen across California and Oregon. The overall sample was predominantly white, urban, and middle-class, with an average adult mental age of 15–17 years. The final 1916 Stanford–Binet consisted of 90 items—six at each age level from ages 3 to 10; eight items at age 12; six items at age 14; and six items at each of two adult levels (average adult, superior adult). Sixteen alternative tests were available for tests that were inappropriate or otherwise spoiled. Of the final 90 items, 60% were drawn from the Binet–Simon and 40% from Terman and other sources. Terman adapted William Stern's (1914) "mental quotient" to generate the IQ (mental age divided by chronological age, with the product multiplied by 100 to remove decimals). Although Terman was critical of Spearman's work, he explicitly stated that the Stanford–Binet measured general intelligence, in effect making the single IQ score a functional estimate of Spearman's *g* and treating intelligence as a unitary construct:

> The scale does not pretend to measure the entire mentality of the subject, but only *general intelligence*. There is no pretence of testing the emotions or the will beyond the extent to which these naturally dis-

play themselves in the tests of intelligence. (Terman, 1916, p. 48; emphasis in original)

Terman retained Binet's adaptive testing format, which permitted flexibility in determining at which level to start the test, and different item types were intermixed to make the testing experience a fast-moving experience with tasks changing frequently.

Terman's Stanford–Binet was a resounding success, becoming the most frequently used psychological test (and intelligence test) in the United States for decades (Louttit & Browne, 1947). The Stanford–Binet would be renormed and expanded to create two parallel forms (Form L for Lewis, and Form M for coauthor Maud A. Merrill) spanning the ages 2 years through Superior Adult III in a remarkable 1937 revision (Terman & Merrill, 1937). The best items from the two forms would be retained in a single form for two updates (Terman & Merrill, 1960, 1973). From sales of test record forms, R. L. Thorndike (1975) estimated that the Stanford–Binet was administered to an average of about 150,000 persons a year from 1916 to 1937, to about 500,000 persons a year from 1937 to 1960, and to about 800,000 a year from 1960 to 1972. The fourth edition would make radical changes,

including conversion to a point scale format and assessment of discrete factors of ability according to extended Gf-Gc theory (Thorndike, Hagen, & Sattler, 1986), but the fifth edition would endeavor to restore some of the features that distinguished the Stanford–Binet from its start (Roid, 2003).

Terman was also responsible, more than any other psychologist, for the rapid growth of intelligence and achievement tests in schools. The "Oakland experiment" of 1917–1918 was one of the first systematic attempts to use intelligence/ability tests as a basis for grouping students—a movement that is well documented in Chapman's *Schools as Sorters* (1988). Beginning in 1917, one of Terman's students, Virgil E. Dickson, became director of research for the Oakland Public Schools and organized the testing of 6,500 schoolchildren with the Stanford–Binet, the Otis Absolute Point Scale, and other tests in all of Oakland's 45 elementary schools. From his findings, Dickson concluded that many students fail because their ability levels make mastery of the ordinary curriculum impossible; furthermore, he asserted, the "mentally superior" are in need of accelerated curricula. Dickson called for segregation of students into special classes based on their ability levels. Figure 1.11 depicts the introduction of intelligence tests in

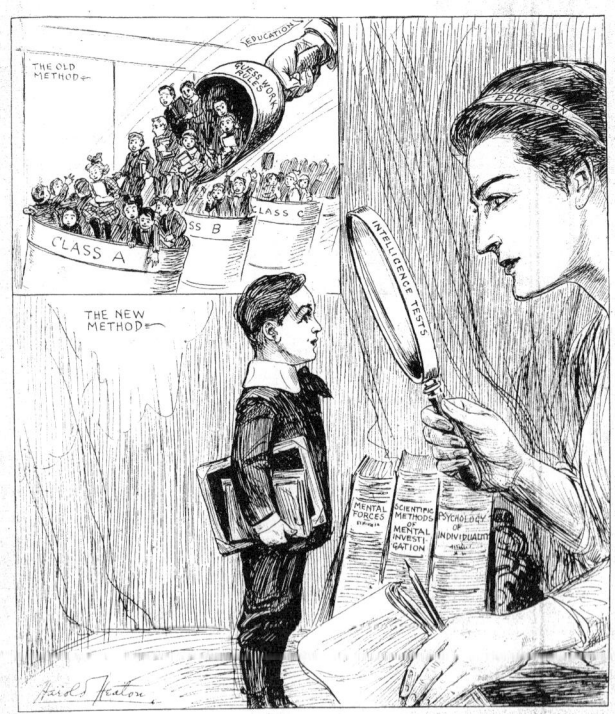

FIGURE 1.11. After the success of the "Oakland experiment" of 1917–1918, Terman and other psychologists advocated successfully for the use of intelligence tests to group students according to their ability levels. Educators recognized the value of measuring "individual differences" but were wary of the proliferating tests (e.g., Hines, 1922). From Heaton (1922). In the public domain.

the schools. Receiving enthusiastic endorsements from administrators and teachers, Dickson (1919) concluded:

> Standard tests, both psychological and pedagogical—group and individual—should be of great assistance in classification of pupils according to ability and capacity to do the work. They should inspire better teaching and better educational guidance through a more intimate knowledge of the individual child. (p. 225)

In 1923, Dickson published *Mental Tests and the Classroom Teacher*, the first in a series of "measurement and adjustment" books to be edited by Terman and published through the World Book Company. In 5 years, Terman would oversee nine additional titles, each focusing on problems of student testing and "adjustments to meet the problems of instruction and school administration arising out of individual differences" (see Chapman, 1988, p. 104, for a description of Terman's blueprint for the series).

Large-Scale Assessments and the Army Mental Tests

In retrospect, it was a remarkable accomplishment: In the span of only 18 months during World War I, a small team of psychologists developed, tried out, and then directed the administration of the first intelligence measures designed for large-scale adult testing. By the time the Armistice was signed in November 1918, an estimated 1,726,966 Army enlisted men and officers had been tested with the new group tests. More than 83,500 enlisted men were also given individual examinations. Although the military was not particularly appreciative of the testing program, psychologists used the perceived success of the Army mental tests to sell the general public on the value of mental testing; large-scale assessment thus found its way into American education system, where it remains prominent today. Accounts of World War I Army mental testing are available in official narratives from the psychologist directing the process (e.g., Yerkes, 1919, 1921; Yoakum & Yerkes, 1920), as well as a number of independent scholars (e.g., Camfield, 1969; Carson, 1993; Kevles, 1968; Napoli, 1981; Samelson, 1977; Sokal, 1987; Spring, 1972; von Mayrhauser, 1986, 1987, 1989). I draw on these sources and others for the following history.

The story of the Army mental tests begins with the United States' lack of preparation for the war. World War I, which started in 1914, was fought mainly in Europe between the Allied Powers (the Russian and British Empires, France, and later Italy and the United States) and the Central Powers (the Austro-Hungarian, German, and Ottoman Empires and Bulgaria). An isolationist United States, under the leadership of President Woodrow Wilson, sought neutrality in what was perceived as a European conflict, leaving the U.S. military unprepared to enter the war. As of April 1917, the strength of the U.S. Army was below 200,000 men, the smallest number since the Civil War (e.g., Yockelson, 1998).

Wilson finally asked Congress for a declaration of war against Germany on April 2, 1917 (Wilson, 1917). Congress declared war 4 days later. President Wilson signed the Selective Service Act into law on May 18, 1917; within a few months, 10 million men had registered for the draft, with almost 2.8 million men actually being drafted by the U.S. Army (Baker, 1918). Under General John J. Pershing, troops of the American Expeditionary Forces (AEF) began arriving in Europe in June 1917.

The draft, however, had no established procedures to identify and exclude men who were unfit for service. There was also no way to identify large numbers of potential officers, since the existing officers had been selected and trained through the U.S. Military Academy at West Point and fell far short of needs. Secretary of War Newton Baker (1918, p. 15) wrote that "one of the most serious problems confronting the War Department in April 1917, was the procurement of sufficient officers to fill the requirements of the divisions that were to be formed for overseas duty." Moreover, there was no systematic way to assign men to specialized military jobs similar to those they had held in civilian life (e.g., assigning a practicing accountant to military requisitions tracking or record keeping). The massive draft provided an opportunity for the young scientific discipline of psychology to demonstrate the value of its still-new technologies—the intelligence test and personnel selection procedures—to efficiently screen large numbers of enlisted men.

Yerkes and the Army Mental Tests

The involvement of psychologists in the war effort formally began on April 6, 1917, at the annual meeting of Edward B. Titchener's Society of Experimental Psychologists at Harvard University. When war was officially declared by the U.S. Congress on that day, Robert M. Yerkes, the president of the APA, asked the assembled psychologists how psychologists could assist the government in time of war. A committee was proposed under Yerkes's chairmanship, "to gather information concerning the possible relations of psychology to military problems" (Yerkes, 1921, p. 7). Almost 2 weeks later, on April 21, the executive council of the APA met in the Hotel Walton in Philadelphia. In preparation, Yerkes had been busy behind the scenes, touring Canadian hospitals, interviewing military doctors, and soliciting support from APA council members and members of the National Research Council. According to historian Richard T. von Mayrhauser (1987), Yerkes would use the military crisis to assert "near-dictatorial power within the profession" of psychology (p. 135).

The meeting at the Hotel Walton was misguided from the start because it involved a discussion among academic psychologists about what the military needed, rather than a request to the military as to how psychology might serve military needs. Moreover, a heavy-handed Yerkes sought to impose his narrow vision of mental testing on psychology, while suppressing input from another council member, Walter Dill Scott, who had more applied experience in personnel selection than anyone else at the meeting. With simultaneous authorization from the APA council and the National Research Council Psychology Committee, Yerkes appointed a dozen war-related psychology committees and chairs, dealing with areas such as aviation, recreation, propaganda, vision, acoustics, shellshock, emotional stability, and deception. Yerkes appointed himself chair of the "Committee on the Psychological Examining of Recruits," which was charged with preparation and standardization of testing methods and the demonstration of their effectiveness. Yerkes's initial testing plan—10-minute individual mental testing of at least 20% of "exceptional or unsatisfactory" recruits (von Mayrhauser, 1987, p. 141) by psychologists working under the supervision of military physicians—was in part a recapitulation of his own experiences working half-time directing research in the Psychopathic Department at Boston State Hospital under the supervision of Harvard psychiatrist Elmer Ernest Southard. At the same hospital, Yerkes had developed his own point scale adaptation of the Binet–Simon (Yerkes, Bridges, & Hardwick, 1915), which he probably hoped would be prominent in any testing program.

APA council member Walter V. Bingham later described his (and colleague Walter Dill Scott's) revulsion at events in Yerkes's meeting: "Meet-ing of the council in the smoke-filled room of a Philadelphia hotel. Midnight. Scott's utter disgust with the shortsighted self-interest revealed. His insurrection not previously told" (cited by von Mayrhauser, 1987, p. 139). Elsewhere in Bingham's papers appears the following disclosure:

> As the meeting proceeded it became clear to Scott and Bingham that Yerkes and the others were interested primarily in going into the army in order to acquire new psychological knowledge. They seemed to be more concerned with what the army could do for them than with what they could do for the army. Angrily, Scott and Bingham walked out in a huff. (cited by von Mayrhauser, 1987, p. 139)

With this divisive start, Yerkes alienated Scott, who had experience and skills he sorely needed. There was much at stake, as George Ellery Hale, famed astronomer and organizer of the National Research Council, warned Yerkes in May 1917:

> In the case of psychology, it is obvious that the first thing to do is to prove conclusively that the psychologists can perform service of unquestioned value to the government. . . . It is of fundamental importance that no tests be adopted which are not absolutely conclusive because if they were, the science of psychology would suffer an injury from which it would not recover for many years. (G. E. Hale to R. M. Yerkes, 1917; cited by Camfield, 1992, p. 107)

Yerkes's Committee and Arthur Otis

The Committee on the Psychological Examining of Recruits, made up of Robert M. Yerkes, Walter V. Bingham, Henry H. Goddard, Thomas H. Haines, Lewis M. Terman, F. Lyman Wells, and Guy M. Whipple, met at the Vineland Training School in New Jersey from May 28 to June 9 to develop the Army mental tests (see Figure 1.12). After reaching agreement that the tests had the goals of eliminating "unfit" recruits and identifying those with "exceptionally superior ability" (who might become officers), discussion turned to the merits of brief individually administered tests versus group-administered tests. Deciding that efforts should be made to test all recruits, the committee concluded that brief individual tests were problematic in terms of reliability and uniformity of method and interpretation, opting instead for group administration (Yerkes, 1921, p. 299). At this point, Lewis Terman presented the group-administered tests developed by his Stanford graduate student Arthur S. Otis. According to Yerkes (1921, p. 299), 4

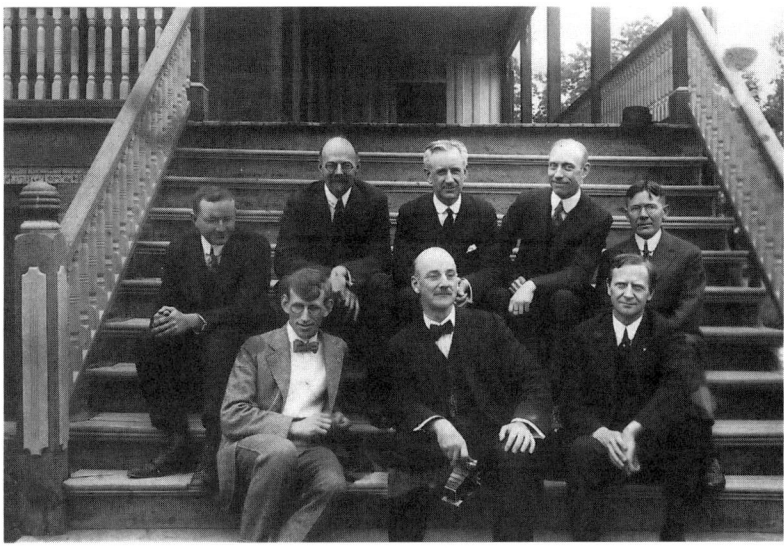

FIGURE 1.12. Robert M. Yerkes's Committee on the Psychological Examination of Recruits at a 1917 meeting, during development of the Army mental tests at the Vineland Training School in New Jersey. Back row, left to right: Frederic Lyman Wells, Guy M. Whipple, Yerkes (Chair), Walter V. Bingham, and Lewis M. Terman. Front row, left to right: Edgar A. Doll (not a committee member), Henry H. Goddard, and Thomas H. Haines. Henry H. Goddard Papers, Archives of the History of American Psychology, Center for the History of Psychology, University of Akron. Reprinted by permission.

of the 10 tests in the original Army scale for group testing were accepted with little change from the Otis scale, and certain other tests were shaped in part by the content and format of the Otis series.

Committee members identified a dozen criteria to use for selection of additional tests: suitability for group use; interest and appeal; economy of administration time; score range and variability; scoring objectivity; scoring ease and rapidity; minimal writing requirements; resistance to coaching; resistance to malingering; resistance to cheating; independence from educational influences; and convergent validity with independent measures of intelligence. Each test was to consist of 10–40 items, with a time limit not to exceed 3 minutes. Moreover, oral directions needed to be simple, and written instructions easy to read. All tests needed to be accompanied by two or three completed sample items to ensure that examinees understood task requirements.

Psychologists around the country were recruited to write additional items to create 10 parallel equivalent forms of the Army mental tests. The tests underwent a series of pilot studies with 400 examinees drawn from different settings across the country. After revisions were made, a larger trial with the 10 forms was conducted on 4,000 recruits in Army and Navy settings during July and August 1917. The final test occurred in the fall of 1917, when 80,000 men in four national Army cantonments were tested, along with 7,000 college, high school, and elementary school students to check the Army results. All processing of record forms and statistical analyses were conducted by a small group working out of Columbia University, directed by Edward L. Thorndike with assistance from Arthur Otis and Louis L. Thurstone. Thorndike and his statistical analysis group endorsed the psychometric properties of the group tests, although clearly not all forms were equivalent, and some had to be dropped in the end.

Examination Beta was developed after Alpha, when it became evident that a different approach was needed for valid assessment of recruits who were either illiterate or limited in their English proficiency. It included ideas from Otis, Terman, and others and was tested at several training camps and at the Vineland Training School. After some 15 tests were reduced to 8 tests, the Beta was completed in April 1918. It was designed to correlate well with Examination Alpha, to differentiate average from very low levels of ability, and to be easily understood and administered, yielding few zero scores.

In December 1917, the Surgeon General recommended to the Secretary of War the continuance and extension of psychological examining to the entire Army. In January 1918, the Secretary of War authorized creation of a division of psychology in the Sanitary Corps out of the Surgeon General's office and expansion of the psychological examining program. A school for military psychology was organized with the Medical Officers Training Camp in Fort Oglethorpe, Georgia. While the school was active in 1918, approximately 100 officers of the Sanitary Corps and 300 enlisted men were given special training in military psychology. By the end of the war, psychological examining occurred at 35 army training camps and several army hospitals (Yerkes, 1919, 1920). Figure 1.13 shows a group administration of the Army mental tests.

Examinations Alpha and Beta

The Army Alpha was intended for fluent and literate English-language speakers. Alpha was typically administered to men who could read newspapers and write letters home in English, with at least a fourth-grade education and five years of residency in the United States (Yerkes, 1921, p. 76). The Army Beta was a largely nonverbal scale intended for examinees with inadequate English-language proficiency or illiteracy (Yoakum & Yerkes, 1920). Beta was also given to low scorers on the Alpha. Men who had difficulty reading or writing in English were to be given both Alpha *and* Beta. E. G. Boring (1961) described the informal process of separating recruits into those suitable for Alpha or Beta: "You went down the line saying 'You read American newspaper? No read American newspaper?'—separating them in that crude manner into those who could read English and take the Alpha examination and those who must rely for instructions on the pantomime of the Beta examination" (p. 30).

Examination Alpha consisted of eight tests, required approximately 40–50 minutes to administer, and could be given to groups as large as 500. A sample test from Alpha appears in Figure 1.14. Examinees were provided with the test form and a pencil. Responses were scored with stencils based upon examinee responses (which usually involved writing numbers, underlining, crossing out, or checking a selected answer). After illiterate and non-English-speaking examinees were removed, and all recruits were seated with pencils and test forms, the examiner said:

> Attention! The purpose of this examination is to see how well you can remember, think, and carry out what you are told to do. We are not looking for crazy people. The aim is to help find out what you are best fitted to do in the Army. The grade you make in this examination will be put on your qualification card and will also go to your company commander. Some of the things you are told to do will be very easy. Some you may find hard. You are not expected to make a perfect grade, but do the very best you can. (Yoakum & Yerkes, 1920, p. 53; emphasis added)

Beta was typically administered with task performance modeled through pantomimed demonstrations and some brief verbal directions (e.g., "Fix it!" while pointing to the incomplete pictures on Pictorial Completion; Yoakum & Yerkes, 1920, p. 87). A sample test from Beta appears in Figure

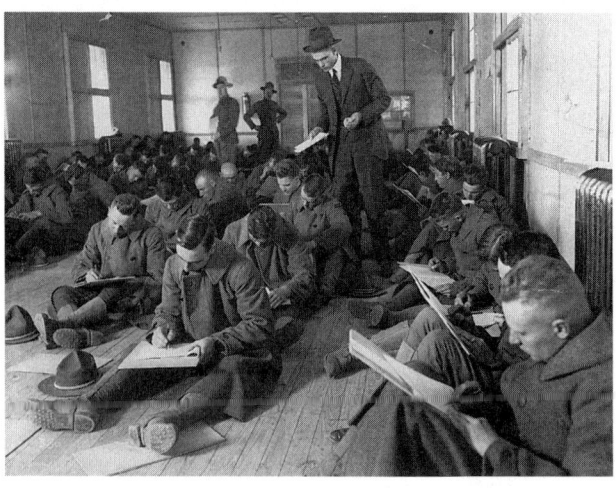

FIGURE 1.13. Group testing with the Army mental tests in a hospital ward, Camp Lee, Petersburg, Virginia, October 1917 Reproduced as Plate 5 (immediately after p. 90) in Yerkes (1921). Reprinted by permission of Time Life Pictures/Getty Images.

TEST 3

This is a test of common sense. Below are sixteen questions. Three answers are given to each question. You are to look at the answers carefully; then make a cross in the square before the best answer to each question, as in the sample:

SAMPLE
{
Why do we use stoves? Because
☐ they look well
☒ they keep us warm
☐ they are black
}

Here the second answer is the best one and is marked with a cross. Begin with No. 1 and keep on until time is called.

1 If plants are dying for lack of rain, you should
☐ water them
☐ ask a florist's advice
☐ put fertilizer around them

2 A house is better than a tent, because
☐ it costs more
☐ it is more comfortable
☐ it is made of wood

3 Why does it pay to get a good education? Because
☐ it makes a man more useful and happy
☐ it makes work for teachers
☐ it makes demand for buildings for schools and colleges

4 If the grocer should give you too much money in making change, what is the right thing to do?
☐ buy some candy of him with it
☐ give it to the first poor man you meet
☐ tell him of his mistake

5 Why should food be chewed before swallowing?
☐ it is better for the health
☐ it is bad manners to swallow without chewing
☐ chewing keeps the teeth in condition

6 If you saw a train approaching a broken track you should
☐ telephone for an ambulance
☐ signal the engineer to stop the train
☐ look for a piece of rail to fit in

7 If you are lost in a forest in the daytime, what is the thing to do?
☐ hurry to the nearest house you know of
☐ look for something to eat
☐ use the sun or a compass for a guide

8 It is better to fight than to run, because
☐ cowards are shot
☐ it is more honorable
☐ if you run you may get shot in the back

☞ Go to No. 9 above

9 Why are warships painted gray? Because gray paint
☐ is cheaper than other colors
☐ is more durable than other colors
☐ makes the ships harder to see

10 Why should all parents be made to send their children to school? Because
☐ it prepares them for adult life
☐ it keeps them out of mischief
☐ they are too young to work

11 The reason that many birds sing in the spring is
☐ to let us know spring is here
☐ to attract their mates
☐ to exercise their voices

12 Gold is more suitable than iron for making money because
☐ gold is pretty
☐ iron rusts easily
☐ gold is scarcer and more valuable

13 The cause of echoes is
☐ the reflection of sound waves
☐ the presence of electricity in the air
☐ the presence of moisture in the air

14 We see no stars at noon because
☐ they have moved around to the other side of the earth
☐ they are so much fainter than the sun
☐ they are hidden behind the sky

15 Some men lose their breath on high mountains because
☐ the wind blows their breath away
☐ the air is too rare
☐ it is always cold there

16 Why do some men who could afford to own a house live in a rented one? Because
☐ they don't have to pay taxes
☐ they don't have to buy a rented house
☐ they can make more by investing the money the house would cost

FIGURE 1.14. The Army Examination Alpha Practical Judgment Test. Soldiers were allowed 1½ minutes for this test. From Yerkes (1921). In the public domain.

1.15. Administered to groups as large as 60, it was typically completed in about 50–60 minutes and required a blackboard with chalk, eraser, curtain, and chart (on a roller to show 27 feet of pictorial instructions in panels). The examiner gave the brief instructions, while a demonstrator pantomimed how to complete tasks correctly on the blackboard panels corresponding to the test response form. There were seven final tests in Beta.

Reports of intelligence ratings derived from test scores were typically made within 24 hours and entered on service records and qualification cards that were delivered to commanding officers and personnel officers. Individual examinations with the Yerkes–Bridges Point Scale, the Stanford–Binet Intelligence Scale, or the Army Performance Scale were usually reserved as checks on questionable or problematic group examination results.

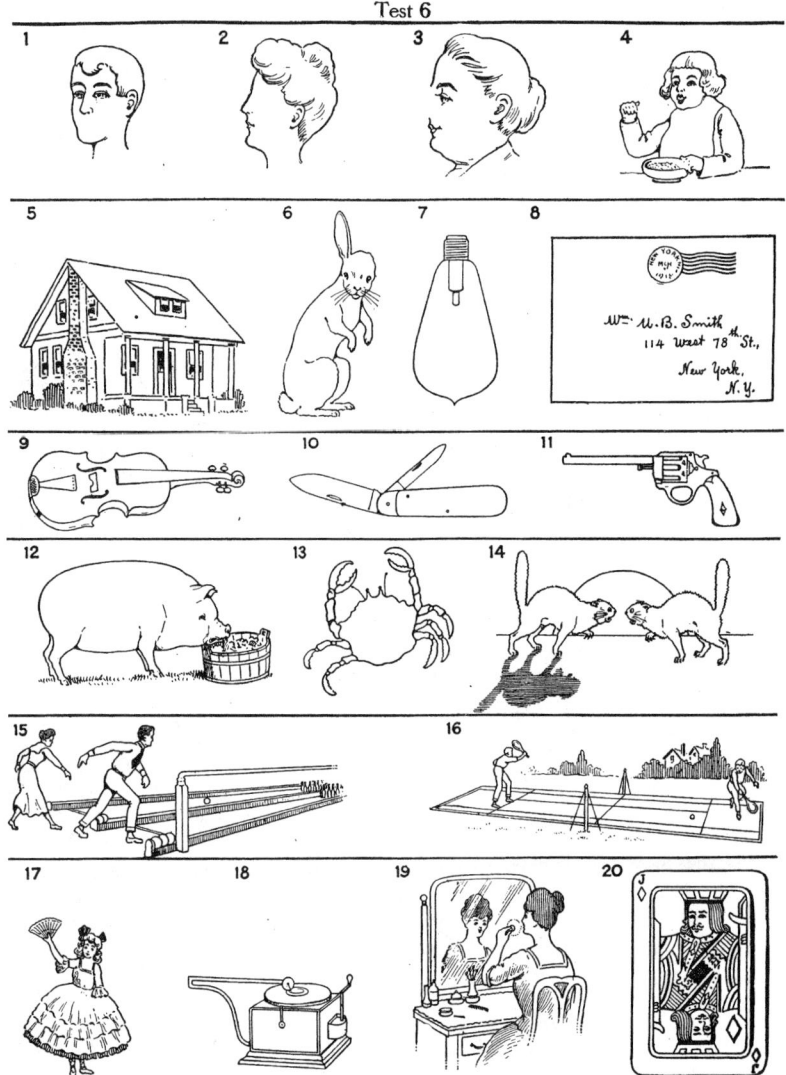

FIGURE 1.15. The Army Examination Beta Picture Completion Test. Instructions: "This is Test 6 here. Look. A lot of pictures . . . Now watch." Examiner points to separate sample at front of room and says to Demonstrator, "Fix it." After pausing, the Demonstrator draws in the missing part. Examiner says, "That's right." The demonstration is repeated with another sample item. Then Examiner points to remaining drawings and says, "Fix them all." Demonstrator completes the remaining problems. When the samples are finished, Examiner says to all examinees, "All right. Go ahead. Hurry up!" At the end of 3 minutes, Examiner says, "Stop!" From Yerkes (1921). In the public domain.

The test scores yielded grade ratings from A to E, with the following descriptions drawn from Yoakum and Yerkes (1920):

- A (Very Superior). An A grade was earned by only 4–5% of drafted men. These men were considered to have high officer characteristics

when they were also endowed with leadership and other necessary qualities. They were shown to have the ability to make a superior record in college or university.

- B (Superior). A B grade was obtained by 8–10% of examinees. This group typically contained many commissioned officers, as well as a large number of noncommissioned officers. A man with B-level intelligence was capable of making an average record in college.

- C+ *(High Average)*. The C+ group included 15–18% of all soldiers and contained a large number of recruits with noncommissioned officer potential and occasionally commissioned officer potential, when leadership and power to command were rated as being high.
- C *(Average)*. The C group included about 25% of soldiers who made excellent privates, with a certain amount of noncommissioned officer potential.
- C– *(Low Average)*. The C– group included about 20% of soldiers; these men usually made good privates and were satisfactory in routine work, although they were below average in intelligence.
- D *(Inferior)*. Men in the D group were likely to be fair soldiers, but they were usually slow in learning and rarely went above the rank of private. They were considered short on initiative and required more than the usual amount of supervision.
- D– and E *(Very Inferior)*. The last group was divided into two classes: D–, consisting of men who were very inferior in intelligence but who were considered fit for regular service, and E, consisting of men whose mental inferiority justified a recommendation for development battalion, special service organization, rejection, or discharge. The majority of men receiving these two grades had a mental age below 10 years. Those in the D– group were thought only rarely able to go beyond the third or fourth grade in primary school, however long they attended.

To his chagrin, Yerkes's division of psychology was appointed to the Sanitary Corps instead of the Medical Corps (where he had hoped psychologists would be classified), but he was still a member of the Surgeon General's staff. Yerkes encountered near-continual resistance to the testing program from the military establishment, and the Army mental examiners often had inadequate testing facilities or faced a deeply entrenched military establishment that did not see the value in intelligence tests. In response to queries about testing from Army officers, Yerkes gave the psychological examiners standard responses to provide as needed—specifying the potential value of the Alpha and Beta in military decision making, but also emphasizing that test scores alone should not constitute the sole basis for making military service decisions:

> The rating a man earns furnishes a fairly reliable index of his ability to learn, to think quickly and accurately, to analyze a situation, to maintain a state of mental alertness, and to comprehend and follow instructions. The score is little influenced by schooling. Some of the highest records have been made by men who had not completed the eighth grade. . . . The mental tests are not intended to replace other methods of judging a man's value to the service. It would be a mistake to assume that they tell us infallibly what kind of soldier a man will make. They merely help to do this by measuring one important element in a soldier's equipment, namely, intelligence. They do not measure loyalty, bravery, power to command, or the emotional traits that make a man "carry on." (Yoakum & Yerkes, 1920, pp. 22–24)

According to Yerkes (1918a, 1918b), the Army testing program was tasked with four military objectives: (1) aiding in the identification and elimination of "mentally defective" men who were unfit for service; (2) identifying men of exceptional intelligence for special responsibilities or possible officer training; (3) balancing military units in terms of intelligence; and (4) assisting personnel officers in the camps with the classification of men. The tests appear to have functioned well in identifying recruits of very high intelligence and very low intelligence, although research findings showed a disproportionate number of minority, foreign-born, and illiterate recruits as having very low intelligence, in spite of efforts to correct for the language and literacy demands of the Alpha with the Beta (Yerkes, 1921). There is little evidence that the Alpha and Beta were effectively used to balance the intellectual composition of military units. Although Army battalions ideally should be comparable and interchangeable in terms of effectiveness, individual battalion commanders no doubt wanted the best available recruits and held onto the recruit who received A and B grades. Yoakum and Yerkes (1920) described the challenge:

> In making assignments from the Depot Brigade to permanent organizations it is important to give each unit its proportion of superior, average, and inferior men. If this is left to chance there will inevitably be "weak links" in the army chain. Exception to this rule should be made in favor of certain arms of the service which require more than the ordinary number of mentally superior men; for example, Signal Corps, Machine Gun, Field Artillery and Engineers. These organizations ordinarily have about twice the

usual proportion of "A" and "B" men and very much less than the usual proportion of "D" and "D–" men. (p. 25)

With respect to the final objective, of assisting with personnel decisions, the Army mental tests provided a single piece of information—intelligence level—that was of considerable value. It would be Walter Dill Scott's Army Committee on Classification of Personnel that provided a context for the Army mental test scores in making military personnel decisions.

Scott's System of Personnel Selection

Walter Dill Scott (1869–1955) was a pioneering industrial psychologist, applying principles of experimental methodology to practical business problems (Ferguson, 1962, 1963a; Lynch, 1968; Strong, 1955). An interest in identifying and selecting successful salesmen led Scott (1916) to develop a multimethod quantitative personnel selection approach consisting of historical information from former employers (i.e., a model letter soliciting information and ratings, which was included in a *personal history record*); performance on tests of intellectual ability devised by Scott; performance on tests of technical ability (written calculation and clerical transcription) scored for accuracy, speed, and legibility; and multiple ratings based on a series of "interviews" with trained raters (in which the examinee was to introduce himself and try to sell merchandise to a series of interviewers posing as merchants). In 1916, Walter V. Bingham, the head of the division of applied psychology at Carnegie Institute of Technology, offered Scott the opportunity to direct the newly formed Bureau of Salesmanship Research and to become the first professor of applied psychology in the United States (Ferguson, 1964a). In a remarkable partnership between the Carnegie Bureau and 30 large national businesses, Scott had the opportunity to test his personnel selection methods with the hiring of 30,000 new salesmen each year, and comparison of personnel decisions against actual sales performances. It was a highly successful arrangement, possibly unprecedented in the history of psychology, and Scott's work was well regarded by the business community.

The history of Scott's personnel selection system in the military may be found in several resources, including official accounts from the Army (Committee on Classification of Personnel in the Army, 1919a, 1919b) and contemporary accounts from von Mayrhauser (1987, 1989); the most in-depth accounts are available from Ferguson (1963b, 1963c, 1964b, 1964c). When war was declared in 1917, Scott realized that his existing methods could readily be applied to personnel selection in the military. At the Hotel Walton meeting on April 21, Scott objected to Yerkes's positions on the war as an opportunity to advance the prominence of psychology. Scott and Bingham were the only psychologists at the meeting with experience in personnel selection, and they knew that Scott's system already had demonstrated effectiveness. In Scott's system, the mental test results had value, but Scott and Bingham were certain that interview ratings would be more important in the selection of officers. Moreover, Scott did not want to subordinate psychologists to psychiatrists, but instead thought they should report to a high official such as the Secretary of War. Offended by Yerkes's self-serving agenda, Scott and Bingham walked out.

Scott decided to launch his own initiative, independent of Yerkes. Scott revised his existing salesman rating scale, completing A Rating Scale for Selecting Captains by May 4, 1917. He shared with it several psychologists and asked Edward L. Thorndike to write a letter of support to Frederick P. Keppel, who had been a dean at Columbia and was now Third Assistant Secretary of War. Keppel invited Scott to Washington, D.C., where Scott presented his scale, did some testing with it, made some improvements, and overcame institutional resistance (including having his scale ripped "to tatters" by officers in Plattsburg who had been invited to suggest improvements [Committee on Classification of Personnel in the Army, 1919a, p. 50]). When he finally met directly with Secretary of War Newton D. Baker, Scott suggested that a group of psychologists and experienced employment managers be appointed to advise the Army on personnel selection, volunteering to assemble such a group. On August 5, 1917, Scott received approval of a plan to include scientific staff, a group of civilian experts for research and planning, and a board of military representatives to bring problems to the Committee on Classification of Personnel in the Army and help implement its recommendations. Within 6 weeks, the committee created and implemented a classification and assignment system for the Army where none had existed before. It was the largest program of personnel selection ever attempted to that time. Scott was the committee's director, Bingham was its executive secretary, and they answered directly to the Adjutant

General of the Army. They began with a single office that grew to 11 rooms in the War Building (then the central hub of military decision making, housing the offices of the Secretary of War, Chief of Staff, and Adjutant General).

Scott's personnel system for the army included a Soldier's (or Officer's) Qualification Card, grades on the Army mental tests and proficiency on specialized trade tests, and the Officers' Rating Scale in various forms for noncommissioned and commissioned officers. The Qualification Card relied on interviews to obtain occupational history, education, leadership experience, and military history. Test scores on the Army mental tests ranged from A through E and were provided by Yerkes's examiners. For recruits claiming experience in specific trades of value to the military, Scott's committee oversaw development of special trade tests that measured specific proficiencies, generating a range of scores from "Expert" through "Novice." Finally, the Officers' Rating Scale became the main tool used for the selection and promotion of officers, with all officers receiving quarterly ratings by the end of the war. This scale involved ratings in five areas: physical qualities, intelligence, leadership, personal qualities, and general value to the service.

If the Army mental tests were intended to measure general intelligence, the trade tests measured specific ability and knowledge related to the performance of several hundred specific occupations needed by the military. Vocational training was impractical, and men were frequently found to have misrepresented their civilian jobs and skills on the Soldier's Qualification Card. In order to identify personnel requirements for specific jobs, occupational titles were compiled and detailed personnel specifications were prepared by Scott's team. With the criteria of covering all trades rapidly and objectively by examiners who did not have to be knowledgeable about each individual trade, a series of oral, picture, and/or performance trade tests were administered and scored so that the number of questions correctly answered predicted status as a novice, apprentice, journeyman, or expert. There were 84 trade tests for jobs as varied as butchers, electricians, pipefitters, and most other specialties needed by the military. For example, the trade test officer issued driver's licenses for all drivers of touring cars, motorcycles, and trucks (Committee on Classification of Personnel in the Army, 1919a, p. 135). Examples of trade tests appear in the committee's personnel manual (1919b), and after the war compilations of

trade tests were published in Chapman (1921) and Toops (1921).

From the military's perspective, it is clear that Scott's personnel selection procedures were much more valued than Yerkes's testing program. At the end of the war, Yerkes's Division of Military Psychology was summarily and completely shut down. Scott's Committee on Classification of Personnel in the Army was transferred to the General Staff and merged with the newly created Central Personnel Branch, in effect institutionalizing Scott's personnel selection procedures within the Army (Yerkes, 1919). The War Department awarded Scott the Distinguished Service Medal when he left the service in 1919, and asked *him* to convey its appreciation to Major Yerkes. Scott became the highest-ranking psychologist in the Army, having been commissioned as a colonel in the Adjutant General's Department in November 1918.

Undoubtedly multiple factors explained the military's different responses to Scott and to Yerkes. Scott adapted his system to military needs, while Yerkes sought to impose academic know-how on an unreceptive army. Scott partnered with military personnel, while Yerkes's examiners were seen as unwelcome, externally imposed "pests" and "mental meddlers" by camp commanders (cited by Kevles, 1968, p. 574). No less than three independent investigations were launched by Army personnel, suspicious of Yerkes and his men (Zeidner & Drucker, 1988, p. 11). Scott worked initially in an advisory capacity, while Yerkes continually sought authority. Scott had considerable personal skills in persuasion and salesmanship (Strong, 1955), whereas Yerkes was a strong planner but a poor manager (Dewsbury, 1996). Scott's system had substantial and understandable face validity for military performance, while Yerke's Examinations Alpha and Beta did not have obvious relevance for soldiering. From the perspective of the history of intelligence testing, however, a broader argument should be considered: Yerkes's committee created the tests and his examiners generated scores, but Scott's committee provided a systematic context (including recruits' history and specific skills) within which the test scores made sense and could be used to make practical decisions by teams of military personnel not schooled in psychology.

World War II Assessment Procedures

In World War II, the plan developed by Scott was streamlined and implemented again, this time with Walter V. Bingham in charge of the personnel system and mental tests (Bingham, 1942, 1944). Bingham served as chair of the Committee on Classification of Military Personnel, the committee having been appointed in 1940 by the National Research Council at the request of the Adjutant General, months before passage of the Selective Service and Training Act (Bingham, 1944). In contrast to the unwelcome reception Yerkes had received in World War I, Bingham and the infrastructure he established were valued by the Army (Zeidner & Drucker, 1988). The Army Alpha was replaced by the Army General Classification Test, a shorter version of the Alpha; initial versions were administered in spiral omnibus form in about 40 minutes, and there were four parallel forms (Bittner, 1947; Staff, Personnel Research Section, 1945). Conceptualized as a test of "general learning ability," it consisted of vocabulary items (intended to tap verbal comprehension), arithmetic problems (thought to tap quantitative reasoning), and block-counting problems (intended to measure spatial thinking), all endeavoring to deemphasize speed somewhat. Grades of A to E were replaced with five levels of learning readiness, I to V. Terms like *mental age* and *IQ* were largely eliminated from group tests.

As in World War I, specialized Non-Language Tests were developed and standardized to test illiterate and non-English-speaking recruits (Sisson, 1948). In 1944, the Wechsler Mental Ability Scale, also known as the Army Wechsler, was replaced by the Army Individual Test, which included three verbal subtests (Story Memory, Similarities–Differences, and Digit Span) and three nonverbal subtests (Shoulder Patches, Trail Making, and Cube Assembly) (Staff, Personnel Research Section, 1944). Rapaport (1945) praised the Army Individual Test, noting that it was "admirably well-constructed" (p. 107) as a measure of general mental ability, but he also raised cautions about its diagnostic limitations. Numerous specialized trade tests and aptitude tests (e.g., mechanical aptitude, clerical aptitude) were developed as well. Most importantly, the Personnel Research Section of the Adjutant General's Office that Bingham established quickly earned the military's trust, leading to the creation of the Army Research Institute (which still exists). One of Bingham's charges was to put the "brakes on projects . . . of great scientific interest" if they did not help the Army "toward early victory" (Zeidner & Drucker, 1988, p. 24). It was a lesson in military priorities that Yerkes, whose agenda included advancing psychology as a science, may not have learned in World War I.

David Wechsler: The Practical Clinician

The practice of contemporary applied intelligence assessment in the second half of the 20th century may arguably be said to have been most strongly and directly influenced by the measurement instruments developed by David Wechsler (1896–1981). Beginning in the 1960s, the Wechsler intelligence scales supplanted the Stanford–Binet as the leading intelligence tests (Lubin, Wallis, & Paine, 1971). Surveys of psychological test usage decades after his death show that Wechsler's intelligence tests continue to dominate intelligence assessment among school psychologists, clinical psychologists, and neuropsychologists (Camara, Nathan, & Puente, 2000; Wilson & Reschly, 1996). The Wechsler scales for adults, children, and preschoolers are taught at much higher frequencies than any other intelligence tests in North American clinical and school psychology training programs (Cody & Prieto, 2000).

In many ways, David Wechsler was an unexpected success—coming to the United States as a child amid a flood of Eastern European immigrants, losing both parents by the age of 10, compiling a relatively ordinary academic record in high school and college (while graduating early), registering as a conscientious objector to the 1917 World War I draft (a risky decision at the time, when "slackers" were universally condemned), and not having become a naturalized citizen by the time of the war. Even so, these risk factors may have been somewhat ameliorated by the guidance of an accomplished older brother (pioneering neurologist Israel S. Wechsler), who became his caretaker and role model; by the opportunity to provide military service as an Army mental test examiner, thereby quickly learning about assessment and making key professional contacts; and by receiving his graduate education and professional psychology training at an opportune time and place in the development of what eventually would become "clinical" psychology.

Wechsler's Early Life and Education

David Wechsler was the youngest of three boys and four girls born in Romania to Moses Wechsler, a merchant, and Leah (Pascal) Wechsler, a shopkeeper (see, e.g., Matarazzo, 1972). At the time the Wechsler family emigrated in 1902, poor harvests in 1899 and 1900 had produced famine and an economic downturn in Romania, worsening the scapegoating of Jews and resulting in severe applications of existing anti-Jewish decrees (e.g., Kissman, 1948). The family's new life on the Lower East Side of New York City was marked by tragedy. Within 5 years of their arrival both Moses and Leah Wechsler passed away from malignancies ("Deaths reported Aug. 23," 1903; Wechsler, 1903; Wexler, 1906). The effects of these losses upon the family, particularly David as the youngest, are likely to have been profound. By 1910, David's older brother Israel S. Wechsler, then a physician in general practice, appears to have taken over as the head of the family.

Wechsler was educated in the public schools on the Lower East Side (see Wechsler, 1925, p. 181). After high school graduation, Wechsler attended the College of the City of New York (now known as City College) from 1913 to 1916, graduating with an AB degree but without honors at the age of 20 ("206 get degrees at City College," 1916). Following his graduation, Wechsler enrolled in graduate studies in psychology at Columbia University, where he would complete his master's degree in 1917 and his doctorate in 1925. His decision to continue his education beyond college had family precedent; his older brother, Israel, had graduated from New York University and Bellevue Medical College in 1907 at the age of 21. Israel would take a position in neurology at Mount Sinai Hospital in 1916 and begin teaching neurology at the outpatient clinic of the Columbia University College of Physicians and Surgeons in 1917 (Stein, 2004; see also "Israel Wechsler, Neurologist, Dies," 1962). Israel initially intended to become a psychiatrist and was self-taught in psychoanalysis, but personally identified as a neurologist because, as he later explained, "If the brain is the organ of thought and disturbance of its functions expresses itself in disorders which are called neuroses and psychoses, it seemed reasonable and necessary to know neurology" (Wechsler, 1957, pp. 1113–1114). Israel Wechsler was involved in the early-20th-century struggles between psychiatry and neurology, when each medical discipline was vying for control of the care of those with mental illness. David instead pursued psychology, but he would follow his brother's lead in becoming a practicing clinician, a hospital-based academic, and the author of professional textbooks.

Columbia was one of the few major universities that provided graduate experimental psychology training with a willingness to address applied problems, termed *experimental abnormal psychology* by Woodworth (1942, p. 11)—an educational orientation that would eventually evolve into clinical psychology (Routh, 2000). The Columbia graduate psychology department in this era was made up primarily of commuter students "who emerged from the subway for their classes and research and departed immediately into the subway afterwards" (Thorne, 1976, p. 164). Columbia University was the academic home of faculty J. McKeen Cattell (until his dismissal in October 1917), Robert S. Woodworth, and Edward L. Thorndike, three of the most influential psychologists of the early 20th century. "Cattell, Woodworth, and Thorndike were the trio at Columbia," said F. L. Wells, who had worked as an assistant to Cattell and Woodworth, adding, "Cattell might inspire awe, Thorndike admiration, and Woodworth affection. Affection toward Cattell and Thorndike was not possible" (quoted in Burnham, 2003, p. 34).

For his master's thesis, completed (and published as a journal article) in 1917, Wechsler (1917a) patched together a clinical memory battery from existing published and unpublished tests, closely following the memory framework suggested by Whipple (1915). Wechsler spent 2½ months conducting in-depth assessment of six patients with Korsakoff psychosis at the Manhattan State Hospital on Ward's Island. He saw each patient as many as 20 times, and he also had the opportunity to observe psychiatric assessment on the wards. Wechsler's master's thesis represented his first known attempt to build a test battery. He established a pattern he was later to follow with intelligence tests, memory tests, and a failed personality test: that of appropriating practical and clinically useful procedures from other authors, making slight improvements and modifications, and synthesizing them into a battery of his own.

World War I Service

After the U.S. Congress declared war on Germany in April 1917, Wechsler (1917b) completed his required registration for the draft, listing himself as a "Consciencious [sic] Objector" and as an alien who was a citizen of Romania, who was disabled by "Near Sightness [sic]" and "Physical Unfitness." To the item asking about his occupation, he wrote "Am student in school of philosophy." Wechsler's draft registration thus used multiple methods to avoid being drafted—claiming status as a conscientious objector, claiming exemption from military service by reason of alien (noncitizen) status, and claiming physical deficiencies that would disqualify him for military service. We do not know what motivated David Wechsler to try to avoid military service at age 21, but the public press treated conscientious objectors with contempt, and some were arrested and imprisoned. Even Army mental examiners considered conscientious objector status to be a form of psychopathology (May 1920). Wechsler's status as a noncitizen native of Romania, some 15 years after his arrival in the United States, also put him at risk. As an alien, he could not be drafted, but he could be deported. The U.S. Congress tried to close this draft loophole in response to the perceived "alien slacker" problem, but treaty obligations circumvented final passage ("Alien Slackers May Not Escape Service," 1917; "Pass Alien Slacker Bill," 1918). Within military training camps, however, some officers considered all aliens who had not become naturalized citizens as suspect.

Becoming an Army mental test examiner represented a way by which Wechsler could avoid seeing combat, and it was probably through back-channel communications from his professor Robert S. Woodworth to Robert M. Yerkes that Wechsler was identified as a prospective tester. In May 1918, Yerkes requested in writing that Wechsler and 13 others who had "qualifications for psychological service" be sent authorization for military induction and be assigned for course instruction in military psychology at Camp Greenleaf, Chickamauga Park, Georgia. Shown in Figure 1.16 at the time of his military service, Wechsler reported to the School for Military Psychology, where he was taught the Army Alpha, Army Beta, Stanford–Binet, Yerkes Point Scale, and other tests. Trainees also received instruction in military practices, including military law, field service, honors and courtesies, equipment, and gas attack defense instructions and drills. E. G. Boring, who reported to Camp Greenleaf as a captain in February 1918, described what may have also been Wechsler's experience:

> We lived in barracks, piled out for reveillé, stood inspection, drilled and were drilled, studied testing procedures, and were ordered to many irrelevant lectures. As soon as I discovered that everyone else resembled me in never accomplishing the impossible, my neuroses left me, and I had a grand time, with new health created by new exercise and many good friendships formed with colleagues under these intimate conditions of living. (Boring, 1961, p. 30)

In May 1918, Congress enacted legislation that allowed aliens serving in the U.S. armed forces to file a petition for naturalization without having made a declaration of intent or proving 5 years'

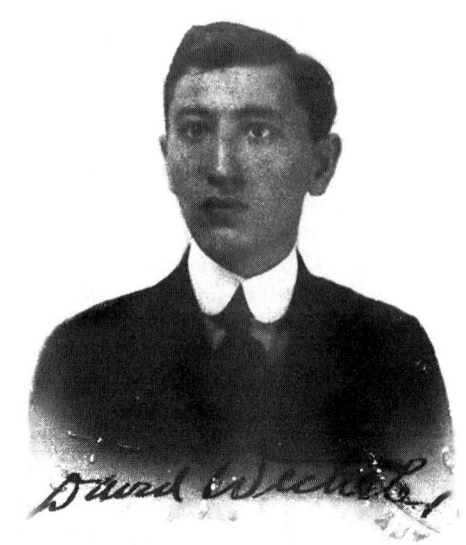

FIGURE 1.16. David Wechsler at the age of 23, from his 1918 passport application. Wechsler used a program designed to educate World War I veterans in Europe to pursue educational opportunities in France and London, including time with Charles E. Spearman and Karl Pearson. From Wechsler (1918b). National Archives and Records Administration, Washington, D.C. In the public domain.

residence (e.g., Scott, 1918). Under this new law, Wechsler became a naturalized citizen in June 1918, with Captain John E. Anderson and Lt. Carl A. Murchison, two psychologists who would have noteworthy careers, serving as his witnesses (Wechsler, 1918b). Wechsler completed his training at Camp Greenleaf in July, was promoted to the rank of corporal, and was assigned to Camp Logan in Houston, Texas, in early August 1918. There he would give individual psychological assessments to recruits who had failed the Alpha and/or the Beta, largely because of limited English proficiency or illiteracy. Conditions at Camp Logan were poor, with inadequate space and support, but the Army examiners administered over 300 individual assessments (Yerkes, 1921, p. 80).

It was during his time as an Army examiner that many of Wechsler's core ideas about assessment were born, especially his idea to construct an intelligence scale combining verbal and nonverbal tests, paralleling the Army Alpha and Army Beta/performance exams (Wechsler, 1981). Most of the assessment procedures appropriated by Wechsler for his intelligence scales appear in Yerkes (1921). Matarazzo (1981) relates that Wechsler realized the value of individual assessment when group tests yielded misleading results, as many of his examinees functioned adequately in civilian life in spite of their low group test scores. Wechsler also reportedly learned the value of nonverbal assessment and the limitations of the Stanford–Binet with adults. He even (Wechsler, 1932), described an approach to profile analysis of Army Alpha subtests—a clear antecedent to the intraindividual (ipsative) profile analyses still used in interpreting the Wechsler intelligence scales.

With the signing of the armistice, Wechsler participated in AEF University, a program created by order of General John J. Pershing and other military leaders to serve the 2 million idle (and bored) American servicemen who remained stationed in Europe, waiting to be shipped home (Cornebise, 1997; "Education for American Soldiers in France," 1919). Although Wechsler had never served overseas, he arranged to spend time in France (December 1918 to March 1919) and then in London (March 1919 through July 1919) as part of this program. Some 2,000 soldiers attended the Sorbonne, while about 2,000 soldier-students attended British universities, with 725 going to University College London ("U.S. Maintains Great Schools on Foreign Soil," 1919). At University College London, Wechsler had the opportunity to work for 3 months with Charles E. Spearman and to meet Karl Pearson, becoming familiar with Spearman's work on the general intelligence factor and Pearson's correlation statistic, as well as to note their professional rivalry (Wechsler, Doppelt, & Lennon, 1975). Wechsler was honorably discharged from the military in July 1919. Given his efforts to avoid military service in 1917, it might be considered ironic that the skills he acquired and contacts he made during his military service would shape his career in assessment and test development.

From 1919 to 1921, Wechsler studied and conducted research at the University of Montpelier and principally at the Sorbonne, under the supervision of Henri Pieron and Louis Lapicque (Rock, 1956, p. 675; Wechsler, 1925, p. 8). Wechsler used the research to complete his doctorate at Columbia, under the guidance of Robert Woodworth (Wechsler, 1925, p. 8). The opportunity to study at the Sorbonne came through Wechsler's application for an American Field Service fellowship from the Society for American Fellowships in French Universities (Wechsler, 1918b). In its first year (1919–1920), there were eight fellows, one of which was Wechsler.

Bellevue Psychiatric Hospital and Other Clinical Experiences

After completing his fellowship at the Sorbonne, Wechsler traveled through France, Switzerland, and Italy before reluctantly returning to the United States (Wechsler, 1921). Once he was settled in New York, he began practicing psychology, mostly conducting assessments, in a variety of clinical and industrial settings. His ambivalence about returning, as disclosed to Edwards (1974), was reflected in his 1922 paper on the psychopathology of indecision.

Wechsler spent the summer of 1922 working with F. L. Wells at the Psychopathic Hospital in Boston, followed by 2 years as a psychologist with the New York Bureau of Children's Guidance. The Bureau of Children's Guidance was a psychiatric clinic, operating under the aegis of the New York School of Social Work and reflecting the values of the popular child guidance movement. Directed by Bernard Glueck, the bureau served troubled children referred by school principals or selected teachers for problems in the areas of scholarship, attendance, behavior, or general welfare. It was staffed by social workers, psychiatrists, and psychologists. The bureau emphasized problems with delinquency, with the objective of "a keener understanding of the child as an individual, and assistance to the school in working out needed readjustments, whether they be physical, social or educational" ("Crime Clinics Growing," 1922).

From 1925 to 1927, Wechsler worked with J. McKeen Cattell as acting secretary and research associate of The Psychological Corporation (Wasserman & Maccubbin, 2002). Created by Cattell, The Psychological Corporation did not directly employ any psychologists at the time; instead, consulting psychologists worked in nonsalaried, commission-based arrangements, undertaking projects for businesses and dividing the payment between themselves and the corporation. A 29-year-old David Wechsler, having completed his dissertation, had difficulty finding a job and contacted his old professor, Cattell, who hired him; according to Wechsler, Cattell told him, "You can get the *pro tem* acting secretary here. You have to get your own business and whatever business you get, the company will get half of your remunerations" (Wechsler et al., 1975). Wechsler undertook two known projects at The Psychological Corporation: the development of an automobile driving simulator and psychometric tests for taxicab drivers (Wechsler, 1926), and a tabloid newspaper study with a *New York World* reporter to test the intelligence of Ziegfeld chorus girls with the Army Alpha.

In 1932, following the tragic death of two Bellevue Hospital staff psychologists in a boating accident ("*Sea Fox* Wreckage," 1931), Wechsler was hired as a psychologist by the Psychiatric Division of Bellevue Hospital, New York. Bellevue was the oldest public hospital in the United States, but its psychopathic wing was scheduled for replacement by the Bellevue Psychiatric Hospital, described at its groundbreaking as the "chief battle-ground in the war against diseases of the mind" ("Old Bellevue and New," 1930). When the new unit finally opened in 1933, its capacity was planned at 600 patients to "give wide scope and facility for modern methods of investigating and treating mental disorders" ("A Bellevue Unit Formally Opened," 1933). By 1941, Wechsler had become chief psychologist and a clinical faculty member at the New York University College of Medicine, supervising more than 15 clinical psychologists, five interns, and two research psychologists on grants (Weider, 2006). Wechsler would retire from Bellevue in 1967, after having pioneered the role of the psychologist in a psychiatric hospital (Wechsler, 1944), and his clinical experiences would help him remain oriented to the use of psychological testing as it relates to practical patient care.

Concept of Intelligence

In his earliest scholarly statement on intelligence in his brother's neurology book, Wechsler (1927) ventured a definition: "All definitions of intelligence refer essentially to ability to learn and adapt oneself to new conditions; that is, not knowledge and practical success, but ability to acquire knowledge and ability to cope with experience in a successful way" (p. 105). It is Wechsler's (1939) definition, which built on his previous efforts and borrowed elements from his predecessors, that remains best known among definitions of intelligence:

> Intelligence is the aggregate or global capacity of the individual to act purposefully, to think rationally and to deal effectively with his environment. It is global because it characterizes the individual's behavior as a whole; it is an aggregate because it is composed of elements or abilities which, though not entirely independent, are qualitatively differentiable. By measurement of these abilities, we ultimately evaluate intelligence. But intelligence is not identical with the mere sum of these abilities, however inclusive. (p. 3)

The long-standing popularity of this definition is probably due to the enduring popularity of the Wechsler intelligence scales with which it is associated. The definition reflects Wechsler's generally cautious writing style; it was exceptionally rare that he made any bold statement in writing that might alienate any colleagues. The phrase "aggregate or global capacity" appears to encompass Spearman's general factor, *g*—but Wechsler included an accommodation for the group factors, which, "though not entirely independent, are qualitatively differentiable." According to Wechsler (Wechsler et al., 1975), this definition also subsumes Binet's emphasis on adaptation. The phrase "to deal effectively with his environment" recapitulates Binet's (1911/1916) observation that "Intelligence marks itself by the best possible adaptation of the individual to his environment" (p. 301), as well as the use of adaptation in the definition of intelligence by others. In one of his final publications, Binet (1910) also took the position that intelligence is a dynamic synthesis, more than the different "pieces of the machine" that comprise it; this may have influenced Wechsler's statement that intelligence is more than the sum of its constituent abilities.

Creation and Development of the Wechsler Intelligence Scales

Of course, it is for his intelligence tests that David Wechsler is best remembered. Wechsler's gifts in the area of test development lay in his ability to synthesize the work of others—that is, to recognize clinically useful measurement procedures and to streamline and package them so as to be maximally useful for the practicing psychologist. His test work was unoriginal, and his intelligence tests consist entirely of tests (sometimes incrementally improved) that were originally devised by other psychologists. Several researchers have sought to trace the origins of the specific Wechsler intelligence subtests (e.g., Boake, 2002; Frank, 1983), a historically important endeavor, but it is notable that from the start Wechsler (1939) openly disclosed the sources he drew upon. As Boake (2002) suggested, it is most unfortunate that the names of the original innovators who created the Wechsler subtest procedures have been forgotten, omitted from mention in contemporary test manuals.

The Bellevue Intelligence Scale was originally subsidized by a Works Progress Administration grant during the Great Depression (Wechsler, 1981, Wechsler et al., 1975). Wechsler (1939, p. 137) reported that the test took 7 years to develop, and it first underwent trials in 1937 and 1938 at the Bellevue Psychiatric Hospital, the Court of General Sessions of New York City, and the Queens General Hospital. The need for a new adult test stemmed largely from the inadequacy of the Stanford–Binet, particularly its poor normative sample for adults, and the poor fit of the Army mental tests for clinical decision making. As the chief psychologist in a large public hospital, Wechsler had the opportunity to appreciate the needs and applications for an adult intelligence test. After careful review, Wechsler essentially cherry-picked his subtests from the most clinically useful and psychometrically adequate tests of his era; he thus provided practitioners with an easy transition to make from using many separate, independently normed tests with a variety of instructions and scoring rules to a single battery of co-normed tests, with streamlined administration and fairly uniform scoring rules. He acknowledged, "Our aim was not to produce a set of brand new tests but to select, from whatever source available, such a combination of them as would best meet the requirements of an effective adult scale" (Wechsler, 1939, p. 78). Most of the standardization sample of 1,586 participants was collected in the city and state of New York; the sample was stratified by age, sex, education, and occupation, but was limited to English-speaking white examinees.

The Bellevue consisted of 10 subtests, with the Vocabulary subtest serving as an alternate. With the exception of a single speeded subtest (Digit Symbol), items on each subtest were sequenced in approximate order of difficulty, from easiest to hardest. Performance on the first five subtests contributed to the Verbal IQ, and performance on the second five subtests contributed to the Performance IQ. Full Scale IQ scores ranged from 28 to 195. Subtest raw scores were converted to a mean of 10 and standard deviation of 3, while IQ scores approximated a mean of 100 and standard deviation of 15. Wechsler's subtests dichotomized the composition of his test battery into Verbal and Performance/nonverbal, just as the Army mental tests had distinguished between the Alpha and the Beta/performance tests. This dichotomy remained of value for the same reasons it was helpful with Army mental testing: It permitted valid assessment of individuals whose intelligence was likely to be underestimated by verbal intelligence tests alone (i.e., those who were poorly educated, from non-English-language origins, or otherwise disadvantaged by language-dependent tests). Moreover,

Wechsler considered distinctive Verbal and Performance intelligence tasks to sample behaviors in multiple areas of interest, generating important diagnostic information rather than representing different forms of intelligence (Wechsler, 1939). He considered the Verbal and Performance tests to be equally adequate measures of general intelligence, but he emphasized the importance of appraising people "in as many different modalities as possible" (Wechsler et al., 1975, p. 55).

The 1939 test battery (and all subsequent Wechsler intelligence scales) also offered a deviation IQ, the index of intelligence based on statistical distance from the normative mean in standardized units, as Arthur Otis (1917) had proposed. Wechsler deserves credit for popularizing the deviation IQ, although the Otis Self-Administering Tests and the Otis Group Intelligence Scale had already used similar deviation-based composite scores in the 1920s. Inexplicably, Terman and Merrill made the mistake of retaining a ratio IQ (i.e., mental age/chronological age) on the 1937 Stanford–Binet, even though the method had long been recognized as producing distorted IQ estimates for adolescents and adults (e.g., Otis, 1917). Terman and Merrill (1937, pp. 27–28) justified their decision on the dubious ground that it would have been too difficult to reeducate teachers and other test users familiar with the ratio IQ.

Wechsler first introduced the Bellevue Intelligence Scale at a meeting at the New York Academy of Medicine in 1937, and the first edition of *The Measurement of Adult Intelligence*—which would include the manual for the test soon known as the Wechsler–Bellevue Form I—was published in 1939. Early after its publication, Wechsler was approached by George K. Bennett, director of the Tests Division of The Psychological Corporation, who was impressed by the test and asked to produce the test materials (Edwards, 1974). Critics generally praised the "organization of well-known tests into a composite scale" with "considerable diagnostic as well as measurement value" (Lorge, 1943, p. 167), but Wechsler was faulted on technical errors (Anastasi, 1942; Cureton, 1941; McNemar, 1945) and theoretical shortcomings (e.g., Anastasi, 1942; Cronbach, 1949). Figure 1.17 shows Wechsler in the 1940s, after his test had become a success.

Among practicing psychologists and researchers working with adults, the Wechsler–Bellevue was a resounding success. In his review of research on the Wechsler–Bellevue in its first 5 years, Rabin (1945, p. 419) concluded:

The Wechsler–Bellevue Scales have stimulated considerable psychometric research and have supplanted some time-honored diagnostic tools. The reliability and validity of Wechsler's scales, as a whole and in part, have been proved in several studies. The consensus of opinion is that the test correlates highly with some of the best measures of intellect and that it tends to differentiate better than other measures between the dull and feebleminded. (p. 419)

In an update 6 years later, Rabin and Guertin (1951) noted the "vast popularity and wide usage of the test" (p. 239) and a "veritable flood" of research (p. 211), making the Wechsler–Bellevue "a commonly used measuring rod for comparison and validation, if not actual calibration of newer and more recent techniques" (p. 239).

From 1941 to 1945, Wechsler served as an expert civilian consultant to the Adjutant General's Office, preparing the Wechsler Mental Ability Scale, Form B (Wechsler, 1942, cited by Altus, 1945), also known as the Army Wechsler, and the Wechsler Self-Administering Test. These tests appear to have been of limited use for the military, in large part because they were too difficult for many Army recruits. The Wechsler Mental Abil-

ity Scale, Form B is of interest because it consisted of seven Verbal and nine Performance subtests, including Mazes and Series Completion (Altus, 1945), signaling possible additions to the battery. Wechsler also taught in the Army Psychological Training Program (Seidenfeld, 1942).

In the years and decades after the war, Wechsler developed the Wechsler–Bellevue Form II (Wechsler, 1946), the Wechsler Intelligence Scale for Children (WISC; Wechsler, 1949), the Wechsler Adult Intelligence Scale (WAIS; Wechsler, 1955), and the Wechsler Preschool and Primary Scale of Intelligence (WPPSI; Wechsler, 1967). Although David Wechsler died in 1981, most of these tests have gone through multiple editions, with staff test development specialists and external expert advisors substituting for a living author in recent years. In 1975, Wechsler expressed support for measuring intelligence in individuals older than age 65 "without exposing the older person to tests involving speed, perception, and so forth." He proposed to call this test the Wechsler Intelligence Scale for the Elderly, or the WISE (Wechsler et al., 1975; D. O. Herman, personal communication, November 9, 1993). Wechsler never proposed or wrote about achievement tests or nonverbal tests like those that currently carry his name.

In creating his intelligence scales, Wechsler combined popular and clinically useful existing tests into a streamlined, well-organized, and psychometrically innovative battery. Although his tests have become established as industry standards over many decades, Chattin and Bracken (1989) surveyed practicing school psychologists and reported that efficiency and practicality remain the central reasons why the Wechsler intelligence scales remain popular.

LOOSE THREADS: RESOLVED AND UNRESOLVED ISSUES IN INTELLIGENCE TESTING

Students of history are likely to find intelligence and its assessment a fascinating and frustrating subject—full of remarkable characters and events like those I have described—but also with many problems that surface over and over again. Because intelligence testing is a young science, it should be no surprise that so many strands in its story remain loose and unresolved, and there is sufficient diversity in thought among psychologists that even the most scientifically proven ideas will have dissenters. At the same time, it does not seem scientifically

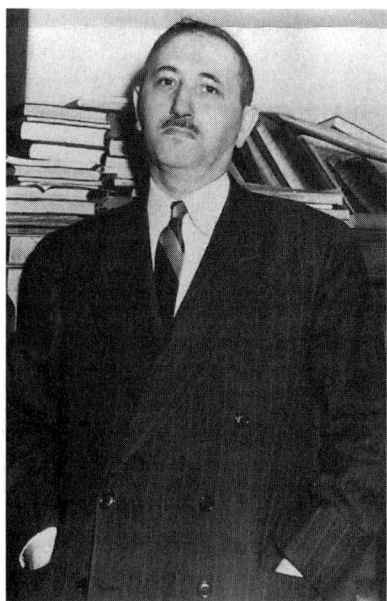

FIGURE 1.17. David Wechsler was chief psychologist at New York's Bellevue Psychiatric Hospital when he published his Bellevue Intelligence Scale (later known as the Wechsler–Bellevue), which quickly became the intelligence test of choice for adults. Reprinted by courtesy of Arthur Weider.

unreasonable to expect at some point a consensus-based definition of *intelligence*, agreement on the existence of a general factor of intelligence, and establishment of a uniform framework for understanding the structure of human cognitive abilities (all of which are discussed below). The historical association of intelligence testing with eugenics, however, is an ideological problem that may be harder to resolve; it may forever taint the tests with the appearance of social inequity and racism, in spite of many efforts to enhance the fairness of intelligence tests. In this section, I describe a few of many loose thematic threads that have contributed to breaks in the fabric of applied intelligence testing from its early days.

Before I begin describing long-standing unresolved issues in intelligence, it may be helpful first to note areas that appear to be resolved. In response to the public controversy associated with Herrnstein and Murray's (1994) book *The Bell Curve*, Linda S. Gottfredson of the University of Delaware contacted an editor at the *Wall Street Journal*, who agreed to publish a statement signed by experts about mainstream scientific thinking on intelligence. Gottfredson drafted the statement, had it reviewed by several authorities, and solicited signatures of agreement from experts across psychology and other disciplines. The resulting statement with 25 conclusions, "Mainstream Science on Intelligence," was published in late 1994 with 52 signatories (Gottfredson, 1994); it was later reprinted with supplemental information as an editorial in the journal *Intelligence* (Gottfredson, 1997). In another response to Herrnstein and Murray's book, the APA Board of Scientific Affairs created a task force to issue an authoritative scientific statement about intelligence and its assessment, entitled "Intelligence: Knowns and Unknowns" (Neisser et al., 1996). These two statements represent relatively rare scientific consensus statements about intelligence in the history of psychology. Ironically, there are many areas in which they appear to disagree.

The Definition of *Intelligence*

An initial step in any scholarly endeavor is to define one's terms, but the term *intelligence* still has no consensus-based definition. Efforts to arrive at a consensus date back about a century, as do criticisms that "psychologists have never agreed on a definition" (Lippmann, 1922c, p. 213). In a frequently quoted but much reviled definition, E. G. Boring (1923) wrote:

> Intelligence as a measurable capacity must at the start be defined as the capacity to do well in an intelligence test. Intelligence is what the tests test. This is a narrow definition, but it is the only point of departure for a rigorous discussion of the tests . . . no harm need result if we but remember that measurable intelligence is simply what the tests of intelligence test, until further scientific observation allows us to extend the definition. (p 35)

The failure to arrive at a consensus on defining *intelligence* after a century of research constitutes one of the most surprising loose threads in the history of psychology. Terman (1916) demurred, essentially arguing that we can work with the construct of intelligence without arriving at a definition:

> To demand, as critics of the Binet method have sometimes done, that one who would measure intelligence should first present a complete definition of it, is quite unreasonable. As Stern points out, electrical currents were measured long before their nature was well understood. Similar illustrations could be drawn from the processes involved in chemistry physiology, and other sciences. In the case of intelligence it may be truthfully said that no adequate definition can possibly be framed which is not based primarily on the symptoms empirically brought to light by the test method. (p. 36)

As demonstrated in the statements above, Boring and Terman expected that research would eventually lead to a definition of *intelligence*. How much longer must we wait?

As we have reported, the association of intelligence with evolutionary *adaptation* dates back to Spencer (1855), who described intelligence as "an adjustment of inner to outer relations" (p. 486). This definition may be understood as suggesting that intelligence confers a capacity to adapt to environmental change, but principles of neo-Darwinian evolution hold that natural selection favors adaptations that enhance survival and reproductive fitness. In order to validate a definition of intelligence featuring adaptation, then, the logical and empirical question is whether intelligence confers any advantages in terms of longer lifespans, fecundity, or other aspects of reproductive fitness. Studies relating intelligence to evolutionary fitness (e.g., family size, number of children) date back to the 1930s, and clearly a meta-analysis is needed to make sense of the many contradictory findings. Gottfredson (2007) recently reported evidence that higher intelligence may improve overall survival rate, and that lower intelligence may be associated with a disproportionately elevated risk of accidental death. Together with colleagues, she has also reported findings of a fitness factor that is related to intelligence (Arden, Gottfredson, Miller, & Pierce, 2009).

Several formal meetings or print symposia have sought a definition of *intelligence*, and the clear-cut conclusion from these efforts is that the experts do not agree on a definition. A list of proposed definitions for the term appears in Table 1.2. The earliest symposium I can identify, entitled "Instinct and Intelligence" (e.g., Myers, 1910), was held in London in July 1910, at a joint meeting of the Aristotelian and British Psychological Societies and the Mind Association, with resulting papers appearing in the *British Journal of Psychology*. The best-known print symposium is "Intelligence and Its Measurement: A Symposium," appearing in the *Journal of Educational Psychology* (Peterson, 1921; Pintner, 1921; Thorndike, 1921). The symposium asked 17 leading investigators explicitly what they conceived intelligence to be. Another symposium, "The Nature of General Intelligence and Ability," was conducted at the Seventh International Congress of Psychology, held at Oxford University in 1923 (e.g., Langfeld, 1924). In a follow-up to the 1921 *Journal of Educational Psychology* symposium, Sternberg and Detterman (1986) asked 25 authorities to write essays conveying what they believe intelligence to be. Sternberg and Berg (1986) tabulated facets of the definitions provided: In descending order, the most frequent attributes in definitions of intelligence were higher-level cognitive functions (50%), that which is valued by culture (29%), executive processes (25%), elementary processes (perception, sensation, and/ or attention; 21%), knowledge (21%), and overt behavioral manifestations of intelligence (such as effective or successful responses; 21%). By comparison, the most frequent attributes in definitions from the 1921 symposium were higher-level cognitive functions (57%), adaptation (29%), ability to learn (29%), physiological mechanisms (29%), elementary processes (21%), and overt behavioral manifestations of intelligence (21%). Even efforts to seek definitions of intelligence among laypeople have found that definitions vary; moreover, people can be self-serving and seem to offer definitions that also capture some quality readily found in themselves (e.g., Gay, 1948).

Never one to embrace diverse perspectives, Charles E. Spearman (1927) disparaged "repeated recourse to symposia" (p. 8) and surveys of expert opinion in efforts to define intelligence:

Chaos itself can go no further! The disagreement between different testers—indeed, even the doctrine and the practice of the selfsame tester—has reached its apogee. If they still tolerate each other's proceedings, this is only rendered possible by the ostrich-like policy of not looking facts in the face. In truth, "intelligence" has become a mere vocal sound, a word with so many meanings that it finally has none. (p. 14)

Jensen (1998) echoed Spearman's sentiment, recommending that psychologists "drop the ill-fated word from our scientific vocabulary, or use it only in quotes, to remind ourselves that it is not only scientifically unsatisfactory but wholly unnecessary" (p. 49).

The argument has also been made that a structural/statistical understanding of intelligence may serve as an adequate substitute for a verbal/ descriptive definition. Gottfredson and Saklofske (2009) suggest that definitional issues of intelligence are "now moot because the various empirical referents to which the term is commonly applied can be distinguished empirically and related within a common conceptual structure [i.e., the Cattell–Horn–Carroll model of human cognitive abilities]" (p. 188).

To *g* or Not to *g*?

Another long-standing unresolved thread in the history of intelligence testing has to do with the general factor of intelligence, psychometric *g*. General intelligence was affirmed in the 1994 "Mainstream Science on Intelligence" statement (Gottfredson, 1997), but the 1996 "Intelligence: Knowns and Unknowns" statement hedged on *g*, stating that "while the *g*-based factor hierarchy is the most widely accepted current view of the structure of abilities, some theorists regard it as misleading" (Neisser et al., 1996, p. 81). Here I describe some history for *g*.

In 1904, Charles E. Spearman (1863–1945) published a groundbreaking paper reporting the discovery of a factor of "general intelligence," derived from positive intercorrelations between individual scores on tests of sensory discrimination, musical talent, academic performance, and common sense. Although the correlation coefficient statistic was still relatively new, Spearman realized that previous studies (e.g., those by Gilbert and by Wissler) had failed to account for measurement error—that is, reduced score reliability, which invariably reduces the magnitude of correlations. He devised a method to correct the correlation coefficient for attenu-

TABLE 1.2. Selected Definitions of Intelligence (Arranged Chronologically)

Herbert Spencer (1855): "Instinct, Reason, Perception, Conception, Memory, Imagination, Feeling, Will, &c., &c., can be nothing more than either conventional groupings of the correspondences; or subordinate divisions among the various operations which are instrumental in effecting the correspondences. However widely contrasted they may seem, these various forms of intelligence cannot be anything else than either particular modes in which the adjustment of inner to outer relations is achieved; or particular parts of the process of adjustment" (p. 486).

Alexander Bain (1868): "The functions of Intellect, Intelligence, or Thought, are known by such names as Memory, Judgment, Abstraction, Reason, Imagination" (p. 82).

Hermann Ebbinghaus (1908): "Intelligence means organization of ideas, manifold interconnection of all those ideas which ought to enter into a unitary group because of the natural relations of the objective facts represented by them. The discovery of a physical law in a multitude of phenomena apparently unrelated, the interpretation of an historical event of which only a few details are directly known, are examples of intelligence thought which takes into consideration innumerable experiences neglected by the less intelligent mind. Neither memory alone nor attention alone is the foundation of intelligence, but a union of memory and attention" (pp. 150–151).

Charles S. Myers (1910): "As the organism becomes endowed with an increasingly larger number of mutually incompatible modes of reaction, the intelligent aspect apparently comes more and more to the fore while the instinctive aspect apparently recedes *pari passu* into the background" (p. 214).

C. Lloyd Morgan (1910): "I regard the presence of implicit expectation (in the lower forms) or explicit anticipation (in the higher forms) as distinguishing marks or criteria of intelligence. In other words for the intelligent organism the present experience at any given moment comprises more or less 'meaning' in terms of previously-gotten experience" (p. 220).

H. Wildon Carr (1910): "Intelligence is the power of using categories, it is knowledge of the relations of things. It is a knowledge that gives us the representation of a world of objects externally related to one another, a world of objects in space, or measurable actions and reactions. . . . Intelligence is an outward view of things, never reaching the actual reality it seeks to know" (pp. 232–233).

Alfred Binet and Théodore Simon (Binet, 1911/1916): "Intelligence serves in the discovery of truth. But the conception is still too narrow; and we return to our favorite theory; the intelligence marks itself by the best possible adaptation of the individual to his environment" (pp. 300–301).

William Stern (1914): "Intelligence is a general capacity of an individual consciously to adjust his thinking

to new requirements: it is general mental adaptability to new problems and conditions of life" (p. 3).

M. E. Haggerty (1921). "In my thinking the word intelligence does not denote a single mental process capable of exact analytic definition. It is a practical concept of connoting a group of complex mental processes traditionally defined in systematic psychologies as sensation, perception, association, memory, imagination, discrimination, judgment and reasoning "(p. 212).

V. A. C. Henmon (1921): "Intelligence . . . involves two factors—the capacity for knowledge and knowledge possessed" (p. 195).

Joseph Peterson (1921): "Intelligence seems to be a biological mechanism by which the effects of a complexity of stimuli are brought together and given a somewhat unified effect in behavior. It is a mechanism for adjustment and control, and is operated by internal as well as by external stimuli. The degree of a person's intelligence increases with his range of receptivity to stimuli and the consistency of his organization of responses to them" (p. 198).

Rudolf Pintner (1921): "I have always thought of intelligence as the ability of the individual to adapt himself adequately to relatively new situations in life. It seems to include the capacity for getting along well in all sorts of situations. This implies ease and rapidity in making adjustments and, hence, ease in breaking old habits and in forming new ones" (p. 139).

Lewis M. Terman (1921): "The essential difference, therefore, is in the capacity to form concepts to relate in diverse ways, and to grasp their significance: *An individual is intelligent in proportion as he is able to carry on abstract thinking*" (p. 128; emphasis in original).

Edward L. Thorndike (1921): "Realizing that definitions and distinctions are pragmatic, we may then define intellect in general as *the power of good responses from the point of view of truth or fact*, and may separate it according as the situation is taken in gross or abstractly and also according as it is experienced directly or thought of" (p. 124; emphasis in original).

L. L. Thurstone (1921): "Intelligence as judged in everyday life contains at least three psychologically differentiable components: a) the capacity to inhibit an instinctive adjustment, b) the capacity to redefine the inhibited instinctive adjustment in the light of imaginally experienced trial and error, c) the volitional capacity to realize the modified instinctive adjustment into overt behavior to the advantage of the individual as a social animal" (pp. 201–202).

Herbert Woodrow (1921): "Intelligence . . . is the capacity to acquire capacity" (p. 208).

(cont.)

TABLE 1.2. *(cont.)*

E. G. Boring (1923): "Intelligence as a measurable capacity must at the start be defined as the capacity to do well in an intelligence test. Intelligence is what the tests test" (p. 35).

Édouard Claparède (1924): "[Intelligence is] the ability to solve new problems" (quoted by Langfeld, 1924, p. 149).

Godfrey H. Thomson (1924): "[Intelligence is] the ability to meet new situations with old responses and to discard those responses which prove unsuccessful" (quoted by Langfeld, 1924, p. 149).

David Wechsler (1939): "Intelligence is the aggregate or global capacity of the individual to act purposefully, to think rationally and to deal effectively with his environment" (p. 3).

Anne Anastasi (1986): "Intelligence is not an entity within the organism but a quality of behavior. Intelligent behavior is essentially adaptive, insofar as it represents effective ways of meeting the demands of a changing environment" (pp. 19–20).

Jonathan Baron (1986): "I define intelligence as the set of whatever abilities make people successful at achieving their rationally chosen goals, whatever those goals might be, and whatever environment they are in. . . . To say that a person has a certain level of ability is to say that he or she can meet a certain standard of speed, accuracy, or appropriateness in a component process defined by the theory in question" (p. 29).

J. W. Berry (1986): "At the present time intelligence is a construct which refers to the end product of individual development in the cognitive-psychological domain (as distinct from the affective and conative domains); this includes sensory and perceptual functioning but excludes motor, motivational, emotional, and social functioning . . . it is also adaptive for the individual, permitting people to operate in their particular cultural and ecological contexts" (p. 35).

J. P. Das (1986): "Intelligence, as the sum total of all cognitive processes, entails planning, coding of information and attention arousal. Of these, the cognitive processes required for planning have a relatively higher status in intelligence. Planning is a broad term which includes among other things, the generation of plans and strategies, selection from among available plans, and the execution of those plans. . . . Coding refers to two modes of processing information, simultaneous and successive. . . . The remaining process (attention arousal) is a function basic to all other higher cognitive activities" (pp. 55–56).

Douglas K. Detterman (1986): "In my opinion, intelligence can best be defined as a finite set of independent abilities operating as a complex system" (p 57).

John Horn (1986): "'What do I conceive intelligence to be?' This is rather like asking me: 'What do I conceive invisible green spiders to be?' For current knowledge suggests to me that intelligence is not a unitary entity of any kind. Attempts to describe it are bound to be futile" (p. 91).

Earl Hunt (1986): "'Intelligence' is solely a shorthand term for the variation in competence on cognitive tasks that is statistically associated with personal variables. . . . Intelligence is used as a collective term for 'demonstrated individual differences in mental competence'" (p. 102).

James W. Pellegrino (1986): "The term intelligence denotes the general concept that individuals' responses to situations vary in quality and value as judged by their culture" (p. 113).

Sandra Scarr (1986): "To be an effective, intelligent human being requires a broader form of personal adaptation and life strategy, one that has been described in 'invulnerable' children and adults: They are copers, movers, and shapers of their own environments" (p. 120).

Richard E. Snow (1986): "[Intelligence can be defined in several ways:] . . . [1] the incorporation of concisely organized prior knowledge into purposive thinking—for short, call it *knowledge-based thinking*. . . . [2] *apprehension* captures the second aspect of my definition—it refers to Spearman's (1923, 1927) principle that persons (including psychologists) not only feel, strive, and know, but also *know* that they feel, strive, and know, and can anticipate further feeling, striving, and knowing; they monitor and reflect upon their own experience, knowledge, and mental functioning in the past, present, and future tenses. . . . [3] *adaptive purposeful striving*. It includes the notion that one can adopt or shift strategies in performance to use what strengths one has in order to compensate for one's weaknesses. . . . [4] agile, analytic reasoning of the sort that enables significant features and dimensions of problems, circumstances, and goals to be decontextualized, abstracted, and interrelated rationally . . . *fluid-analytic reasoning*. . . . [5] *mental playfulness* . . . able to find or create interesting problems to solve and interesting goals toward which to strive. This involves both tolerance of ambiguity and pursuit of novelty. . . . [6] *idiosyncratic learning* . . . Persons differ from one another in the way they assemble their learning and problem-solving performance, though they may achieve the same score. Persons differ *within* themselves in how they solve parts of a problem, or different problems in a series" (pp. 133–134; emphasis in original).

Robert J. Sternberg (1986): "Intelligence is mental self-government. . . . The essence of intelligence is that it provides a means to govern ourselves so that our thoughts and actions are organized, coherent, and responsive to both our internally driven needs and to the needs of the environment" (p. 141).

ation, reporting subsequently that his correlational analyses showed "all branches of intellectual activity have in common one fundamental function (or group of functions)" (p. 284), which he later described using concepts from physics such as "the amount of a general mental energy" (Spearman, 1927, p. 137). The *g* factor, or psychometric *g*, was a mathematically derived general factor, stemming from the shared variance that saturates batteries of cognitive/intelligence tests. Jensen (1998) has summarized the literature showing that correlates of *g* include scholastic performance, reaction time, success in training programs, job performance in a wide range of occupations, occupational status, earned income, and creativity, among others.

Critics of general intelligence appeared quickly. Edward L. Thorndike, who challenged Spearman's work for decades, reported no support for *g* on a set of measures similar to those originally used by Spearman, finding a weak correlation between sensory discrimination and general intelligence, and stating that "one is almost tempted to replace Spearman's statement by the equally extravagant one that there is *nothing whatever* common to all mental functions, or to any half of them" (Thorndike, Lay, & Dean, 1909, p. 368; emphasis in original).

Until Spearman's death, Thorndike; a Scotsman, Godfrey Thomson; and two Americans, Truman L. Kelley and Louis L. Thurstone, participated in an ongoing scholarly debate with him on the existence and nature of *g*, as well as other aspects of the structure of intelligence. Spearman devoted the rest of his career to elaboration and defense of his theory, authoring *The Nature of "Intelligence" and the Principles of Cognition* (Spearman, 1923), *The Abilities of Man: Their Nature and Measurement* (Spearman, 1927), and *Human Ability: A Continuation of "The Abilities of Man"* (Spearman & Wynn Jones, 1950). A good account of this debate may be found in R. M. Thorndike and Lohman (1990). Newly discovered exchanges among Thorndike, Thomson, and Spearman in the 1930s serve to highlight Spearman's dogmatism (Deary, Lawn, & Bartholomew, 2008).

The leading intelligence test developers generally accepted the existence of a psychometric *g* factor. After initial reticence, Alfred Binet eventually embraced a general factor; in *Les Idées Modernes sur les Enfants*, Binet (1909/1975) wrote that "the mind is unitary, despite the multiplicity of its faculties . . . it possesses one essential function to which all the others are subordinated" (p. 117). In the 1916 Stanford–Binet, Lewis M. Terman accepted the concept of general intelligence and conceded that the IQ score provided a good estimate of *g*:

> It is true that more than one mental function is brought into play by the test. The same may be said of every other test in the Binet scale and for that matter of any test that could be devised. It is impossible to isolate any function for separate testing. In fact, the functions called memory, attention, perception, judgment, etc., never operate in isolation. There are no separate and special "faculties" corresponding to such terms, which are merely convenient names for characterizing mental processes of various types. In any test it is "general ability" which is operative, perhaps now *chiefly* in remembering, at another time *chiefly* in sensory discrimination, again in reasoning, etc. (p. 194; emphasis in original)

David Wechsler, who had been deeply impressed with Spearman during his few months at University College London in 1919, wrote that Spearman's theory and its proofs constitute "one of the great discoveries of psychology" (Wechsler, 1939, p. 6). He further noted that "the only thing we can ask of an intelligence scale is that it measures sufficient portions of intelligence to enable us to use it as a fairly reliable index of the individual's global capacity" (p. 11).

What is the current status of *g*? When Reeve and Charles (2008) surveyed 36 experts in intelligence, they found a consensus that *g* is an important, nontrivial determinant (or at least predictor) of important real-world outcomes, and that there is no substitute for *g* even if performance is determined by more than *g* alone. With the leading authors of intelligence tests accepting psychometric *g*, and with authorities in intelligence research consensually accepting its importance, the thread of general intelligence would appear to be well secured in our metaphorical tapestry of the history intelligence.

Yet the concept of general intelligence continues to be challenged, most often on theoretical grounds but also on statistical grounds. Stephen J. Gould (1996) forcefully challenged *g*, associating it with many of the historically negative (and shameful) applications of intelligence testing. Several intelligence theorists, including Raymond B. Cattell, J. P. Das, Howard Gardner, and Robert J. Sternberg, have also rejected the concept of general intelligence. The most cogent challenges to *g* have come from John L. Horn (Horn & Noll, 1994, 1997), who pointed out fallacies of extracting *g* from the *positive manifold* (i.e., the finding that almost all tests that reliably measure a cognitive ability correlate positively with all other such tests).

The Structure of Intelligence

The struggle to construct a complex model of intelligence probably began with the phrenologists, who specified individual faculties (each corresponding to an "organ" of the brain) that together constituted intelligence. For example, Combe (1830) described faculties of perception (e.g., form, size, weight, eventuality, language) and faculties of reflection (e.g., comparison, causality) that altogether constituted intellectual faculties; he also described a separate set of affective faculties. With the discovery of *g* by Spearman (1904), the notion of a unitary intelligence gained traction, but by the end of the 1930s, psychologists and educators were again embracing the complexity of the mind (e.g., Ackerman, 1995). Current hierarchical models of intelligence feature broad ability factors, which have grown steadily in number: from the two factors enumerated by Cattell (1941) and Vernon (1950) to the eight specified by Carroll (1993) to about 10 factors specified by Carroll (2003) to about 15 or 16 broad factors in 2010 (e.g., McGrew, 2009; Newton & McGrew, 2010). The question that appears to be unresolved in this thread is this: Just how many group factors constitute the structure of intelligence?

For much of the 20th century and into the 21st, the complex structure of intelligence has been revealed through statistical methodologies that discover and define sources of test performance variance, usually through factor analyses. Factor analysis is a statistical technique capable of reducing many variables into a few underlying dimensions. The foundation for use of factor analysis in understanding the structure of cognition was laid with Spearman (1904). Spearman's theory encompassing general intelligence was originally called *two-factor theory* because it partitioned performance variance into a *general factor* shared across tasks, and *specific factors* that were unique to individual tasks. Following the contributions of Kelley, Thorndike, and Thurstone (among others), Spearman (1927) reluctantly came to acknowledge the existence of *group factors* formed by clusters of tests that yielded higher-than-expected intercorrelations by virtue of similarities in their content, format, or response requirements: "Any element whatever in the specific factor of an ability will be turned into a group factor, if this ability is included in the same set with some other ability which also contains this element" (p. 82). The extraction of a general factor and group factors (now called *broad ability factors*) contributed to the development of *hierarchical* structural analyses of intelligence. In hierarchical factor analyses, a general factor is first extracted; the residual variance is factored to extract any group factors; and the remaining variance is often said to be specific.

Although there have been well over 1,000 factor-analytic investigations in the literature of intelligence and cognitive abilities (see Carroll, 1993), many of which remain important in understanding the structure of cognitive abilities, space only permits coverage of a few prototypal models with distinctive characteristics.

Thurstone's Primary Mental Abilities

Louis L. Thurstone (1887–1955) developed the statistical technique of multiple factor analysis and is best remembered for his theory of primary mental abilities, a factor-analysis-derived model of multiple cognitive abilities that effectively challenged Spearman's single general factor of intelligence. Thurstone developed factor analysis techniques permitting the extraction of factors that are orthogonal to each other (i.e., separate, independent, and unrelated). From a battery of 56 paper-and-pencil tests administered in about 15 hours to each of 240 superior, college-level students, Thurstone (1938) extracted seven primary factors: spatial/visual, perception of visual detail, numerical, two verbal factors (logic and words), memory, and induction. From a study of over 700 students age 14, who were given 60 tests in 11 sessions lasting 1 hour each, Thurstone and Thurstone (1941) extracted six factors: verbal comprehension, word fluency, space, number, memorizing, and reasoning/induction. By 1945, Thurstone had settled on eight primary mental abilities, each denoted by a letter: Verbal Comprehension (V), Word Fluency (W), Number Facility (N), Memory (M), Visualizing or Space Thinking (S), Perceptual Speed (P), Induction (I), and Speed of Judgment (J). Although Thurstone (1947) eventually accepted the existence of a general factor, he considered the use of a single score such as the IQ to be inadequate, and urged the use of cognitive profiles describing strengths and weaknesses among the fundamental abilities (Thurstone, 1945)

Vernon's Hierarchical Model

In what has been called the first truly hierarchical model of intelligence, Philip E. Vernon (1905–1987) proposed that a higher-order g factor dominates two lower-order factors, v:ed (verbal:educational) and k:m (spatial:mechanical); in turn, v:ed and k:m subsume various minor group factors, which in turn dominate very narrow and specific factors. Based on his review of factor-analytic investigations through 1950, Vernon (1950, 1961) considered v:ed to dominate verbal, number, reasoning, attention, and fluency factors, while k:m dominates spatial ability, mechanical ability, psychomotor coordination, reaction time, drawing, handwork, and various technical abilities. He considered it a likely oversimplification to assume that there are just two factors at the level below g, although his simple dichotomy may be seen as having supported the verbal–performance dichotomy traditionally associated with the Wechsler intelligence scales.

Cattell, Horn, and Carroll's Model of Fluid and Crystallized Intelligence

Arguably the most important contemporary structural and hierarchical model of intelligence is based upon extensions of the theory of fluid (Gf) and crystallized (Gc) intelligence first proposed by Raymond B. Cattell (1905–1998) in a 1941 APA convention presentation. Cattell, who completed his doctorate in 1929 at University College London with Spearman, joined E. L. Thorndike's research staff at Columbia University in 1937, where he worked closely with proponents of multifactor models of intelligence. He authored over 500 articles and 43 books during his career. In his 1941 APA presentation, Cattell asserted the existence of two separate general factors: g_f (fluid ability or fluid intelligence) and g_c (crystallized ability or crystallized intelligence). The convention was later adopted that these factors would be represented by uppercase G, whereas a single general factor would be represented by lowercase g.

Fluid ability was described by Cattell (1963, 1971) and Horn (1976) as a facility in reasoning, particularly where adaptation to new situations is required and crystallized learning assemblies are of little use. Ability is considered to be fluid when it takes different forms or utilizes different cognitive skill sets according to the demands of the problem requiring solution. For Cattell, fluid ability is the most essential general-capacity factor, setting an upper limit on the possible acquisition of knowledge and crystallized skills. In contrast, *crystallized* intelligence refers to accessible stores of knowledge and the ability to acquire further knowledge via familiar learning strategies. It is typically measured by recitation of factual information, word knowledge, quantitative skills, and language comprehension tasks because these include the domains of knowledge that are culturally valued and educationally relevant in the Western world (Cattell, 1941, 1963, 1971, 1987; Horn & Cattell, 1966).

Cattell's model of fluid and crystallized intelligence was energized by the contribution of John L. Horn (1928–2006). Not only was Horn's (1965) dissertation the first empirical study of the theory since 1941; it also showed that fluid and crystallized abilities have different developmental trajectories over the lifespan (McArdle, 2007). Cattell and Horn expanded the number of ability factors from two to five (adding visualization, retrieval capacity, and cognitive speed; Horn & Cattell, 1966). In the next 25 years or so, Horn had arrived at nine ability factors (Horn & Noll, 1994, 1997), while Cattell's list had grown to six ability factors (adding distant memory and retrieval) plus three smaller provincial factors (visual, auditory, and kinesthetic; Cattell, 1998). The growth of the number of factors in this model continues, and a 2001 symposium at the University of Sydney enumerated even more potential ability factors (Kyllonen, Roberts, & Stankov, 2008). As noted earlier, McGrew (2009; see also Newton & McGrew, 2010) now lists 15 or 16 broad ability factors.

In 1993, John B. Carroll (1916–2003) built upon the work of Cattell and Horn by proposing a hierarchical, multiple-stratum model of human cognitive abilities with the general intelligence factor, g, at the apex (or highest stratum); eight broad factors of intelligence at the second stratum; and at least 69 narrow factors at the first (or lowest) stratum. Carroll was the author of nearly 500 books and journal articles over the span of 60 years; he had been mentored early in his career by L. L. Thurstone, and some years later after Thurstone's death he became director of the Thurstone Psychometric Laboratory at the University of North Carolina, Chapel Hill (Jensen, 2004). For a dozen years after his retirement, Carroll (1983, 1993, 1994) accumulated over a thousand archival datasets related to human cognitive test performance; 461 of the datasets were ultimately judged adequate for his analyses. He then conducted iterative principal-factor analyses requiring convergence to a strict criterion, followed by varimax rotation of the principal-factor matrix, with the requirement that each extracted factor contain salient loadings on at least two variables. If necessary, promax or other rotational procedures were used. Factorization was then carried up to the highest viable order. The data were subjected to the Schmid–Leiman orthogonalized hierarchical-factor procedure, and factor interpretations were based on the resulting hierarchical-factor matrix. Carroll's results showed general intelligence (g) as appearing in the highest stratum; the second stratum, listed in descending strength of association with g, consisted of fluid intelligence (Gf), crystallized intelligence (Gc), general memory and learning (Gsm), broad visual perception (Gv), broad auditory perception (Ga), broad retrieval ability (Gr), broad cognitive speediness (Gs), and processing speed (reaction time decision speed); finally, very narrow and specific factors were placed in the lowest stratum. Although Carroll's three-stratum model is historically young, its early reception suggests that it has quickly become a landmark study. The following samples from reviews are fairly representative:

- "Further research may alter details of the map, although it is unlikely that any research for some years to come will lead to a dramatic alteration in Carroll's taxonomy." (Brody, 1994, p. 65)
- "It is simply the finest work of research and scholarship I have read and is destined to be the classic study and reference work of human abilities for decades to come." (Burns, 1994, p. 35)
- "[It is] a truly monumental work." (Jensen, 2004, p. 3)
- "Carroll's work represents what may well be the most extensive, indeed, exhaustive analysis of a data case that has ever been attempted in the field of intelligence. The theory deserves to be taken seriously." (Sternberg, 1994, p. 65)

A note of caution for applied practitioners, however, comes from Carroll himself (1993): He indicated that his survey of cognitive abilities "paid very little attention to the importance, validity, or ultimate usefulness of the ability factors that have been identified" (p. 693). Carroll's three stratum theory has been integrated with extended Gf-Gc theory to form the Cattell–Horn–Carroll (CHC) framework, a name to which Horn and Carroll both agreed a few years after Cattell's death (Newton & McGrew, 2010). The CHC frame-

work already appears to have exerted a strong influence upon the development of contemporary intelligence tests (e.g., Keith & Reynolds, 2010). Shortly before his death, Carroll (2003) expanded his model to include 10 second-stratum factors, indicating that even this definitive model may be expanded.

Intelligence and Eugenics

We have seen more than once that the public welfare may call upon the best citizens for their lives. It would be strange if it could not call upon those who already sap the strength of the State for these lesser sacrifices, often not felt to be such by those concerned, in order to prevent our being swamped with incompetence. It is better for all the world, if instead of waiting to execute degenerate offspring for crime, or to let them starve for their imbecility, society can prevent those who are manifestly unfit from continuing their kind. The principle that sustains compulsory vaccination is broad enough to cover cutting the Fallopian tubes. Three generations of imbeciles are enough.
—OLIVER WENDELL HOLMES (*Buck v. Bell*, 1927)

So wrote Justice Oliver Wendell Holmes, Jr., for the majority opinion of the U.S. Supreme Court in 1927, in the case of Carrie Buck versus James Hendren Bell, Superintendent of the Virginia State Colony for Epileptics and Feeble Minded. Carrie Buck was an 18-year-old woman with the mental age equivalent of 9 when the superintendent of the Virginia State Colony petitioned to have her sterilized. She was reported to be the daughter of a feeble-minded mother in the same institution and the mother of a feeble-minded child—hence Holmes's statement that "Three generations of imbeciles are enough." By an 8-to-1 margin, the court upheld the 1924 Virginia statute, the Eugenical Sterilization Act of 1924, authorizing the compulsory sterilization of "mental defectives," including individuals who were "feeble-minded" (i.e., intellectually disabled). On October 19, 1927, Carrie Buck was sterilized. Although the Supreme Court ruling has never been challenged or reversed, the Commonwealth of Virginia repealed the 1924 sterilization law in 1974. Historian Paul A. Lombardo (2008) recently reexamined this case, finding that there was insufficient evidence ever to assert cognitive impairment in Buck or her daughter, based on their school records.

For our purposes, it may be enough to cite compulsory sterilization laws for those with intellectual disabilities as a historical illustration of how intelligence test results may be (mis)used. In the broader context are questions about the wisdom of making legal, political, and public policy decisions on the basis of intelligence test research. Scholars in intelligence are at risk when they stray too far from psychological science into the realm of social engineering.

Francis Galton coined the term *eugenics* in 1883, describing it as "the science of improving stock" and defining it as "all influences that tend in however remote a degree to give to the more suitable races or strains of blood a better chance of prevailing speedily over the less suitable than they otherwise would have had" (p. 25). In *Hereditary Genius* (1869), he had already presented evidence that superior abilities are found more often among eminent families (i.e., those of judges, statesmen, premiers, commanders, scientists, scholars, etc.), and he proposed to increase the proportion of individuals with superior genetic endowments and thereby benefit the national intelligence through selective early marriages. "A man's natural abilities are derived by inheritance," Galton (1869) wrote, "under exactly the same limitations as are the form and physical features of the whole organic world" (p. 1). He related his vision of a eugenics-practicing society in an unpublished fictional tale entitled "Kantsaywhere" (Galton, 1930). In this utopia, an individual's hereditary worth was measured by anthropometric tests, genetic failures were placed in labor colonies, enforced celibacy was the rule, and childbirth for the "unfit" was a crime. Karl Pearson noted in a footnote to this tale (p. 416 in Galton, 1930) that Galton's fictional laboratory in Kantsaywhere bears an uncanny resemblance to his anthropometric laboratory at South Kensington, one of the places where intelligence testing began. A photograph of Galton toward the end of his life, with his friend, colleague, and biographer, Karl Pearson, appears in Figure 1.18. Pearson, the renowned statistician, was also a dedicated eugenicist.

Almost all of the early authorities in the field of intelligence either wrote favorably about eugenics or belonged to organizations advocating eugenics. Some of the authorities on record as favoring eugenics in one form or another include J. McKeen Cattell, Raymond B. Cattell, Henry H. Goddard, Lewis M. Terman, Edward L. Thorndike, and Robert M. Yerkes. Until the horrors of Nazi genocide were exposed, including euthanasia of individuals with intellectual disabilities or mental disorders, eugenics was commonly seen as a contribution of

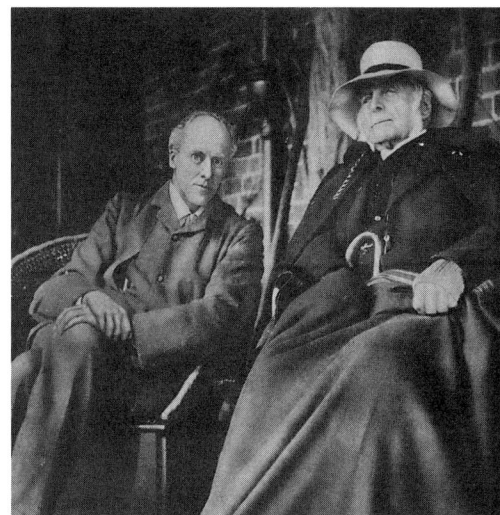

FIGURE 1.18. Francis Galton at age 87 with his biographer, Karl Pearson. Both were dedicated eugenicists. Photo from Pearson (1930, Plate 36). Reprinted by permission of The Pearson Papers, UCL Library Services, Special Collections.

science to human (and national) improvement. Lewis M. Terman, author of the Stanford–Binet, took a particularly active role in advocating for eugenics. For example, in a report to the California state legislature, Terman (1917) saw those with intellectual disabilities as having only negative impacts on society:

> Feeble-mindedness has always existed; but only recently have we begun to recognize how serious a menace it is to the social, economic, and moral welfare of the state. Extensive and careful investigations, in large numbers and in diverse parts of the United States, have furnished indisputable evidence that it is responsible for at least one-fourth of the commitments to state penitentiaries and reform schools, for the majority of cases of chronic and semi-chronic pauperism, and for much of our alcoholism, prostitution, and venereal diseases. (p. 45)

Terman's solutions were to segregate "feeble-minded" students in special classes so as not to "interfere with instruction" or "be a source of moral contagion" for other students (p. 51). He did not overtly recommend sterilization, but he implied that some action was necessary to prevent reproduction: "Three-fourths of the cases of feeble-mindedness are due to a single cause, heredity; and the one hopeful method of curtailing the increasing spawn of degeneracy is to provide additional care for our higher-grade defectives during the reproductive period" (p. 52).

Two of the most important 20th-century figures in applied intelligence testing, however, Alfred Binet and David Wechsler, are on record as having rejected perspectives associated with eugenics. Binet argued that intelligence can be changed, and he even developed a program of "mental orthopedics" to make educational interventions:

> I have often observed, to my regret, that a widespread prejudice exists with regard to the educability of intelligence. . . . A few modern philosophers seem to lend their moral support to these deplorable verdicts when they assert that an individual's intelligence is a fixed quantity, a quantity which cannot be increased. We must protest and react against this brutal pessimism. We shall attempt to prove that it is without foundation. (Binet, 1909/1975, pp. 105–106)

David Wechsler found a more oblique way to criticize the eugenicists—by associating them with totalitarianism. In a 1961 paper, shortly after defining the terms *eugenes* and *apartheid*, he wrote, "The belief in class distinctions, whether considered innate or acquired, is . . . an essential tenet of all groups who are afraid of being ousted or displaced, and in particular of totalitarian governments" (Wechsler, 1961, p. 421). As Wechsler was a member of an oppressed immigrant group (Eastern European Jews) threatened with genocide in Romania and Germany, his condemnation of eugenics should not be surprising.

How does eugenics constitute a loose thread in the history of intelligence? Although no mainstream authorities today advocate for eugenics of the type that led to tragedies in the past, scholarship in the biology and heredity of intelligence remains extremely controversial, with recent accounts including threats to the academic freedom and even loss of lifetime recognition of achievements in psychology for those who conduct research in associated areas, including heritability (e.g., APA, 1997; Gottfredson, 2010; Horn, 2001; Tucker, 2009). Moreover, it might be argued that the history of intelligence and eugenics has contributed to a public perception that intelligence is about elitism, racism, and exclusion. In spite of over a century of research, the study of intelligence remains controversial for its social applications and implications.

REFERENCES

Ackerman, M. (1995). Mental testing and the expansion of educational opportunity. *History of Education Quarterly, 35,* 279–300.

Alien slackers may not escape service. (1917, April 22). *New York Times,* p. E3.

Altus, W. D. (1945). The differential validity and difficulty of subtests of the Wechsler Mental Ability Scale. *Psychological Bulletin, 42,* 238–249.

American Psychological Association (APA). (1997). Gold Medal Award for Life Achievement in Psychological Science: Raymond B. Cattell. *American Psychologist, 52,* 797–799.

Anastasi, A. (1942). Review: *The Measurement of Adult Intelligence* by David Wechsler. *American Journal of Psychology, 55,* 608–609.

Anastasi, A. (1986). Intelligence as a quality of behavior. In R. J. Sternberg & D. K. Detterman (Eds.), *What is intelligence?: Contemporary viewpoints on its nature and definition* (pp. 19–21). Norwood, NJ: Ablex.

Arden, R., Gottfredson, L. S., Miller, G., & Pierce, A. (2009). Intelligence and semen quality are positively correlated. *Intelligence, 37,* 277–282.

Bain, A. (1868). *Mental science: A compendium of psychology, and the history of philosophy.* New York: Appleton.

Baker, N. D. (1918). *Annual report of the Secretary of War, 1918* (Vol. 1, pp. 5–65). Washington, DC: U.S. Government Printing Office.

Baron, J. (1986). Capacities, dispositions, and rational thinking. In R. J. Sternberg & D. K. Detterman (Eds.), *What is intelligence?: Contemporary viewpoints on its nature and definition* (pp. 29–33). Norwood, NJ: Ablex.

A Bellevue Unit formally opened. (1933, November 3). *New York Times,* p. 20.

Berry, J. W. (1986). A cross-cultural view of intelligence. In R. J. Sternberg & D. K. Detterman (Eds.), *What is intelligence?: Contemporary viewpoints on its nature and definition* (pp. 35–38). Norwood, NJ: Ablex.

Binet, A. (1890). The perception of lengths and numbers in some small children. *Revue Philosophique, 30,* 68–81.

Binet, A. (1894). *Introduction à la psychologie expérimentale.* Paris: Baillière et Cie.

Binet, A. (1903). *L'étude expérimentale de l'intelligence.* Paris: Schleicher Frères.

Binet, A. (1910). Avant-propos: Le bilan de la psychologie en 1910. *L'Année Psychologique, 17,* v–xi.

Binet, A. (1916). New investigations upon the measure of the intellectual level among school children. In H. H. Goddard (Ed.), *The development of intelligence in children (the Binet–Simon Scale)* (E. S. Kite, Trans.)

pp. 274–329). Baltimore: Williams & Wilkins. (Original work published 1911)

Binet, A. (1975). *Modern ideas about children* (S. Heisler, Trans.). Menlo Park, CA: Suzanne Heisler. (Original work published 1909)

Binet, A., & Henri, V. (1894). Le développement de la mémoire visuelle chez les enfants. *Revue Générale des Sciences Pures et Appliquées, 5,* 162–169.

Binet, A., & Henri, V. (1895). La psychologie individuelle. *L'Année Psychologique, 2,* 411–465.

Binet, A., & Simon, T. (1914). *Mentally defective children* (W. B. Drummond, Trans). New York: Longmans, Green. (Original work published 1907)

Binet, A., & Simon, T. (1916a). Application of the new methods to the diagnosis of the intellectual level among normal and subnormal children in institutions and in the primary schools. In H. H. Goddard (Ed.), *The development of intelligence in children (the Binet–Simon Scale)* (E. S. Kite, Trans; pp. 91–181). Baltimore: Williams & Wilkins. (Original work published 1905)

Binet, A., & Simon, T. (1916b). The development of intelligence in the child. In H. H. Goddard (Ed.), *The development of intelligence in children (the Binet–Simon Scale)* (E. S. Kite, Trans.; pp. 182–273). Baltimore: Williams & Wilkins. (Original work published 1908)

Binet, A., & Simon, T. (1916c). New methods for the diagnosis of the intellectual level of subnormals. In H. H. Goddard (Ed.), *The development of intelligence in children (the Binet–Simon Scale)* (E. S. Kite, Trans.; pp. 37–90). Baltimore: Williams & Wilkins. (Original work published 1905)

Bingham, W. V. (1942). The Army Personnel Classification System. *Annals of the American Academy of Political and Social Science, 220,* 18–28.

Bingham, W. V. (1944). Personnel classification testing in the Army. *Science (New Series), 100,* 275–280.

Bittner, R. H. (1947). The Army General Classification Test. In G. A. Kelly (Ed.), *New methods in applied psychology* (pp. 45–55). College Park: University of Maryland.

Boake, C. (2002). From the Binet–Simon to the Wechsler–Bellevue: Tracing the history of intelligence testing. *Journal of Clinical and Experimental Neuropsychology, 24,* 383–405.

Bolton, T. L. (1892). The growth of memory in school children. *American Journal of Psychology, 4,* 362–380.

Boring, E. G. (1923, June 6). Intelligence as the tests test it. *The New Republic, 35,* 35–37.

Boring, E. G. (1961). *Psychologist at large: An autobiography and selected essays.* New York: Basic Books.

Brody, N. (1994). Cognitive abilities. Reviewed work(s): *Human Cognitive Abilities: A Survey of Factor-Analytic Studies* by J. B. Carroll. *Psychological Science, 5,* 63, 65–68.

Buck v. Bell, 274 U.S. 200 (1927).

Buckhalt, J. A. (1991). Reaction time and intelligence: Contemporary research supports Cattell's abandoned hypothesis. *School Psychology International, 12,* 355–360.

Burnham, J. C. (2003). Interviewing as a tool of the trade: A not-very-satisfactory bottom line. In D. B. Baker (Ed.), *Thick description and fine texture: Studies in the history of psychology* (pp. 19–37). Akron, OH: University of Akron Press.

Burns, R. B. (1994). Surveying the cognitive terrain. Reviewed work(s): *Human Cognitive Abilities: A Survey of Factor-Analytic Studies* by John B. Carroll. *Educational Researcher, 23,* 35–37.

Buros, O. K. (1977). Fifty years in testing: Some reminiscences, criticisms, and suggestions. *Educational Research, 6*(7), 9–15.

Camara, W. J., Nathan, J. S., & Puente, A. E. (2000). Psychological test usage: Implications in professional psychology. *Professional Psychology: Research and Practice, 31,* 141–154.

Camfield, T. M. (1969). *Psychologists at war: The history of American psychology and the First World War.* Unpublished doctoral dissertation, University of Texas at Austin. (AAT No. 7010766)

Camfield, T. M. (1992). The American Psychological Association and World War I: 1914 to 1919. In R. B. Evans, V. S. Sexton, & T. C. Cadwallader (Eds.), *The American Psychological Association: A historical perspective* (pp. 91–118). Washington, DC: American Psychological Association.

Carr, H. W. (1910). Instinct and intelligence. *British Journal of Psychology, 3,* 230–236.

Carroll, J. B. (1978). On the theory-practice interface in the measurement of intellectual abilities. In P. Suppes (Ed.), *Impact of research on education: Some case studies* (pp. 1–105). Washington, DC: National Academy of Education.

Carroll, J. B. (1983). Studying individual differences in cognitive abilities: Through and beyond factor analysis. In R. F. Dillon & R. R. Schmeck (Eds.), *Individual differences in cognition* (pp. 1–33). New York: Academic Press.

Carroll, J. B. (1993). *Human cognitive abilities: A survey of factor analytic studies.* New York: Cambridge University Press.

Carroll, J. B. (1994). Cognitive abilities: Constructing a theory from data. In D. K. Detterman (Ed.), *Current topics in human intelligence: Vol. 4. Theories of intelligence* (pp. 43–63). Norwood, NJ: Ablex.

Carroll, J. B. (2003). The higher-stratum structure of cognitive abilities: Current evidence supports *g* and about ten broad factors. In H. Nyborg (Ed.), *The scientific study of general intelligence: Tribute to Arthur R. Jensen* (pp. 5–21). Boston: Pergamon Press.

Carson, J. (1993). Army Alpha, Army brass, and the search for Army intelligence. *Isis, 84,* 278–309.

Carson, J. (2007). *The measure of merit: Talents, intelligence, and inequality in the French and American republics, 1750–1940.* Princeton, NJ: Princeton University Press.

Carter, M. H. (1909). The conservation of the defective child. *McClure's Magazine, 33*(2), 160–171.

Cattell, J. M. (1886). The time it takes to see and name objects. *Mind, 11,* 63–65.

Cattell, J. M. (1890). Mental tests and measurements. *Mind, 15,* 373–381.

Cattell, J. M. (1924). The interpretation of intelligence tests. *Scientific Monthly, 18,* 508–516.

Cattell, J. M. (1930). Psychology in America. *Scientific Monthly, 30,* 114–126.

Cattell, J. M., & Farrand, L. (1896). Physical and mental measurements of the students of Columbia University. *Psychological Review, 3,* 618–648.

Cattell, R. B. (1941). Some theoretical issues in adult intelligence testing [Abstract]. *Psychological Bulletin, 38,* 592.

Cattell, R. B. (1963). Theory of fluid and crystallized intelligence: A critical experiment. *Journal of Educational Psychology, 54,* 1–22.

Cattell, R. B. (1971). *Abilities: Their structure, growth, and action.* Boston: Houghton Mifflin.

Cattell, R. B. (Ed.). (1987). *Intelligence: Its structure, growth and action.* New York: Elsevier Science.

Cattell, R. B. (1998). Where is intelligence?: Some answers from the triadic theory. In J. J. McArdle & R. W. Woodcock (Eds.), *Human cognitive abilities in theory and practice* (pp. 29–38). Mahwah, NJ: Erlbaum.

Chapman, J. C. (1921). *Trade tests: The scientific measurement of trade proficiency.* New York: Holt.

Chapman, P. D. (1988). *Schools as sorters: Lewis M. Terman, applied psychology, and the intelligence testing movement, 1890–1930.* New York: New York University Press.

Chattin, S. H., & Bracken, B. A. (1989). School psychologists' evaluation of the K-ABC, McCarthy scales, Stanford–Binet IV, and WISC-R. *Journal of Psychoeducational Assessment, 7,* 112–130.

Cody, M. S., & Prieto, L. R. (2000). Teaching intelligence testing in APA-accredited programs: A national survey. *Teaching of Psychology, 27,* 190–194.

Combe, G. (1830). *A system of phrenology* (3rd ed.). Edinburgh: Anderson.

Combe, G. (1853). *A system of phrenology* (5th ed.). Edinburgh: Maclachlan & Stewart.

Committee on Classification of Personnel in the Army. (1919a). *The personnel system of the United States Army: Vol. 1. History of the personnel system.* Washington, DC: U.S. Government Printing Office.

Committee on Classification of Personnel in the Army. (1919b). *The personnel system of the United States Army: Vol. 2. The personnel manual.* Washington, DC: U.S. Government Printing Office.

Cornebise, A. E. (1997). *Soldier-scholars: Higher education in the AEF, 1917–1919.* Philadelphia: American Philosophical Society.

Crime clinics growing. (1922, June 18). *New York Times,* p. 75.

Cronbach, L. J. (1949). *Essentials of psychological testing.* New York: Harper & Brothers.

Cureton, E. (1941). Reviewed work(s): *The Measurement of Adult Intelligence* by David Wechsler. *American Journal of Psychology, 54,* 154.

Dahlstrom, W. G. (1985). The development of psychological testing. In G. A. Kimble & K. Schlesinger (Eds.), *Topics in the history of psychology* (Vol. 2, pp. 63–113). Hillsdale, NJ: Erlbaum.

Dallenbach, K. M. (1915). The history and derivation of the word "function" as a systematic term in psychology. *American Journal of Psychology, 26,* 473–484.

Darwin, C. R. (1859). *On the origin of species by means of natural selection, or the preservation of favoured races in the struggle for life.* London: Murray.

Darwin, C. R. (1871). *The descent of man, and selection in relation to sex* (Vol. 1). London: Murray.

Das, J. P. (1986). On definition of intelligence. In R. J. Sternberg & D. K. Detterman (Eds.), *What is intelligence?: Contemporary viewpoints on its nature and definition* (pp. 55–56). Norwood, NJ: Ablex.

Deary, I. J. (1994). Sensory discrimination and intelligence: Postmortem or resurrection? *American Journal of Psychology, 107,* 95–115.

Deary, I. J., Bell, P. J., Bell, A. J., Campbell, M. L., & Fazal, N. D. (2004). Sensory discrimination and intelligence: Testing Spearman's other hypothesis. *American Journal of Psychology, 117,* 1–18.

Deary, I. J., Lawn, M., & Bartholomew, D. J. (2008). A conversation between Charles Spearman, Godfrey Thomson, and Edward L. Thorndike: The International Examinations Inquiry Meetings 1931–1938. *History of Psychology, 11,* 122–142.

Deaths reported Aug. 23. (1903, August 24). *New York Times,* p. 7.

Detterman, D. K. (1986). Human intelligence is a complex system of separate processes. In R. J. Sternberg & D. K. Detterman (Eds.), *What is intelligence?:*

Contemporary viewpoints on its nature and definition (pp. 57–61). Norwood, NJ: Ablex.

Dewey, J. (1904). The philosophical work of Herbert Spencer. *Philosophical Review, 13,* 159–175.

Dewsbury, D. A. (1996). Robert M. Yerkes: A psychobiologist with a plan. In G. A. Kimble, C. A. Boneau, & M. Wertheimer (Eds.), *Portraits of pioneers in psychology* (Vol. 2, pp. 87–105). Washington, DC: American Psychological Association.

Diamond, S. (1977). Francis Galton and American psychology. *Annals of the New York Academy of Sciences, 291,* 47–55.

Dickson, V. E. (1919). Report of the Department of Research. In *Superintendent's annual report, Oakland Public Schools, 1917–1918* (pp. 174–247). Oakland, CA: Tribune.

Dickson, V. E. (1923). *Mental tests and the classroom teacher.* Yonkers-on-Hudson, NY: World Book.

DuBois, P. H. (1970). Varieties of psychological test homogeneity. *American Psychologist, 25,* 532–536.

Ebbinghaus, H. (1908). *Psychology: An elementary textbook* (M. Meyer, Trans.). Boston: Heath.

Education for American soldiers in France. (1919). *Scientific Monthly, 8,* 475–477.

Edwards, A. E. (Ed.). (1974). *Selected papers of David Wechsler.* New York: Academic Press.

Fancher, R. E. (1998). Alfred Binet, general psychologist. In G. A. Kimble & M. Wertheimer (Eds.), *Portraits of pioneers in psychology* (Vol. 3, pp. 67–83). Washington, DC: American Psychological Association.

Ferguson, L. W. (1962). Walter Dill Scott: First industrial psychologist. *Heritage of Industrial Psychology, 1,* 1–10.

Ferguson, L. W. (1963a). Bureau of Salesmanship Research: Walter Dill Scott, Director. *Heritage of Industrial Psychology, 5,* 53–66.

Ferguson, L. W. (1963b). Psychology and the Army: Classification of personnel (1). *Heritage of Industrial Psychology, 10,* 141–167.

Ferguson, L. W. (1963c). Psychology and the Army: Introduction of the rating scale. *Heritage of Industrial Psychology, 9,* 125–139.

Ferguson, L. W. (1964a). Division of applied psychology: Carnegie Institute of Technology. *Heritage of Industrial Psychology, 3,* 25–34.

Ferguson, L. W. (1964b). Psychology and the Army: Classification of personnel (2). *Heritage of Industrial Psychology, 11,* 169–205.

Ferguson, L. W. (1964c). Psychology and the Army: Classification of personnel (3). *Heritage of Industrial Psychology, 12,* 209–246.

Frank, G. (1983). *The Wechsler enterprise: An assessment*

of the development, structure, and use of the Wechsler tests of intelligence. New York: Pergamon Press.

Franz, S. I. (1912). New phrenology. *Science (New Series), 35,* 321–328.

Friedlander, H. (1995). *The origins of Nazi genocide: From euthanasia to the final solution.* Chapel Hill: University of North Carolina Press.

Fuster, J. M. (2008). *The prefrontal cortex* (4th ed.). Amsterdam: Elsevier.

Gall, F. J. (1857). Letter to Joseph Fr[eiherr] von Retzer, upon the functions of the brain, in man and animals. In D. G. Goyder (Ed. & Trans.), *My battle for life: The autobiography of a phrenologist* (pp. 143–152). London: Simpkin, Marshall. (Original work published October 1, 1798)

Galton, F. (1869). *Hereditary genius: An inquiry into its laws and consequences.* London: Macmillan.

Galton, F. (1883). *Inquiries into human faculty and its development.* London: Macmillan.

Galton, F. (1884, June 5). Notes. "Rede" Lecture: The measurement of human faculty. *Nature, 30,* 129–131.

Galton, F. (1890a). Remarks [after J. M. Cattell's "Mental tests and measurements"]. *Mind, 15,* 380–381.

Galton, F. (1890b). Why do we measure mankind? *Lippincott's Monthly Magazine, 45,* 236–241.

Galton, F. (1891). Useful anthropometry. In *Proceedings of the American Association for the Advancement of Physical Education at its Sixth Annual Meeting, April 3 and 4, 1891* (pp. 51–58). Ithaca, NY: Andrus & Church.

Galton, F. (1892). Retrospect of work done at my anthropometric laboratory at South Kensington. *Journal of the Anthropological Institute, 21,* 32–35.

Galton, F. (1907). *Inquiries into human faculty and its development* (2nd ed.). London: Dent.

Galton, F. (1930). Kantsaywhere. In K. Pearson (Ed.), *The life, letters and labours of Francis Galton* (Vol. 3A, pp. 414–424). London: Cambridge University Press.

Gay, C. J. (1948). The blind look at an elephant: 10 experts, 25 "people" define "intelligence." *The Clearing House, 22,* 263–266.

Gilbert, J. A. (1894). Researches on the mental and physical development of school children. In E. W. Scripture (Ed.), *Studies from the Yale Psychological Laboratory* (Vol. 2, pp. 40–100). New Haven, CT: Yale University.

Goddard, H. H. (1916). Editor's introduction. In H. H. Goddard (Ed.), *The development of intelligence in children (the Binet–Simon Scale)* (pp. 5–8). Baltimore: Williams & Wilkins.

Gottfredson, L. S. (1994, December 13). Mainstream science on intelligence. *Wall Street Journal,* p. A18.

Gottfredson, L. S. (1997). Mainstream science on intelligence: An editorial with 52 signatories, history, and bibliography. *Intelligence, 24,* 13–23.

Gottfredson, L. S. (2007). Innovation, fatal accidents, and the evolution of general intelligence. In M. J. Roberts (Ed.), *Integrating the mind: Domain general versus domain specific processes in higher cognition* (pp. 387–425). Hove, UK: Psychology Press.

Gottfredson, L. S. (2010). Lessons in academic freedom as lived experience. *Personality and Individual Differences, 49,* 272–280.

Gottfredson, L. S., & Saklofske, D. H. (2009). Intelligence: Foundation and issues in assessment. *Canadian Psychology, 50,* 183–195.

Gould, S. J. (1996). *The mismeasure of man* (rev. ed.). New York: Norton.

Haggerty, M. E. (1921). Intelligence and its measurement: A symposium. *Journal of Educational Psychology, 12,* 212–216.

Heaton, H. [Artist] (1922). The pupil becomes an individual [Illustration]. *American School Board Journal, 64*(4), cover page.

Henmon, V. A. C. (1921). Intelligence and its measurement: A symposium. *Journal of Educational Psychology, 12,* 195–198.

Herrnstein, R. J., & Murray, C. (1994). *The bell curve: Intelligence and class structure in American life.* New York: Free Press.

Hildreth, G. H. (1939). *A bibliography of mental tests and rating scales* (2nd ed.). New York: Psychological Corporation.

Hines, H. C. (1922). Measuring the intelligence of school pupils. *American School Board Journal, 64*(4), 35–37, 135.

Horn, J. L. (1965). *Fluid and crystallized intelligence: A factor analytic study of the structure among primary mental abilities.* Unpublished doctoral dissertation, University of Illinois at Urbana–Champaign. (AAT 6507113)

Horn, J. L. (1976). Human abilities: A review of research and theory in the early 1970s. *Annual Review of Psychology, 27,* 437–485.

Horn, J. L. (1986). Some thoughts about intelligence. In R. J. Sternberg & D. K. Detterman (Eds.), *What is intelligence?: Contemporary viewpoints on its nature and definition* (pp. 91–96). Norwood, NJ: Ablex.

Horn, J. L. (2001). Raymond Bernard Cattell (1905–1998). *American Psychologist, 56,* 71–72.

Horn, J. L., & Cattell, R. B. (1966). Refinement and test of the theory of fluid and crystallized intelligence. *Journal of Educational Psychology, 57,* 253–270.

Horn, J. L., & Noll, J. (1994). A system for understanding cognitive capabilities: A theory and the evidence on which it is based. In D. K. Detterman (Ed.), *Current topics in human intelligence: Vol. 4. Theories of intelligence* (pp. 151–203). Norwood, NJ: Ablex.

Horn, J. L., & Noll, J. (1997). Human cognitive capabilities: Gf-Gc theory. In D. P. Flanagan, J. L. Genshaft, & P. L. Harrison (Eds.), *Contemporary intellectual assessment: Theories, tests, and issues* (pp. 53–91). New York: Guilford Press.

Hunt, E. (1986). The Heffalump of intelligence. In R. J. Sternberg & D. K. Detterman (Eds.), *What is intelligence?: Contemporary viewpoints on its nature and definition* (pp. 101–107). Norwood, NJ: Ablex.

Israel Wechsler, neurologist, dies. (1962, December 7). *New York Times,* p. 39.

Jastrow, J. (1893). The section of psychology. In M. P. Hardy (Ed.), *Official catalogue—World's Columbian Exposition* (Part 7, pp. 50–60). Chicago: Conkey.

Jastrow, J. (1901). Some currents and undercurrents in psychology. *Psychological Review, 8,* 1–26.

Jensen, A. R. (1998). *The g factor: The science of mental ability.* Westport, CT: Praeger.

Jensen, A. R. (2004). Obituary: John Bissell Carroll. *Intelligence, 32,* 1–5.

Jensen, A. R. (2006). *Clocking the mind: Mental chronometry and individual differences.* Amsterdam: Elsevier.

Keith, T. Z., & Reynolds, M. R. (2010). Cattell–Horn–Carroll abilities and cognitive tests: What we've learned from 20 years of research. *Psychology in the Schools, 47,* 635–650.

Kevles, D. J. (1968). Testing the Army's intelligence: Psychologists and the military in World War I. *Journal of American History, 55,* 565–581.

Kissman, J. (1948). The immigration of Romanian Jews up to 1914. In N. Shlomo (Ed.), *YIVO annual of Jewish social science* (Vols. 2–3, pp. 160–179). New York: Yiddish Scientific Institute.

Kyllonen, P. C., Roberts, R. D., & Stankov, L. (Eds.). (2008). *Extending intelligence: Enhancement and new constructs.* New York: Erlbaum.

Langfeld, H. S. (1924). The Seventh International Congress of Psychology. *American Journal of Psychology, 35,* 148–153.

Lewes, G. H. (1867). *The history of philosophy: From Thales to Comte* (Vol. 2, 3rd ed.). London: Longmans, Green.

Lippmann, W. (1922a). The abuse of the tests. *The New Republic, 32,* 297–298.

Lippmann, W. (1922b). A future for the tests. *The New Republic, 33,* 9–10.

Lippmann, W. (1922c). The mental age of Americans. *The New Republic, 32,* 213–215.

Lippmann, W. (1922d). The mystery of the "A" men. *The New Republic, 32,* 246–248.

Lippmann, W. (1922e). The reliability of intelligence tests. *The New Republic, 32,* 275–277.

Lippmann, W. (1922f). Tests of hereditary intelligence. *The New Republic, 32,* 328–330.

Lippmann, W. (1923). The great confusion: A reply to Mr. Terman. *The New Republic, 33,* 145–146.

Littman, R. A. (2004). Mental tests and fossils. *Journal of the History of the Behavioral Sciences, 40,* 423–431.

Lombardo, P. A. (2008). *Three generations, no imbeciles: Eugenics, the Supreme Court, and Buck v. Bell.* Baltimore: Johns Hopkins University Press.

Lorge, I. (1943). Review of *The measurement of adult intelligence. Journal of Consulting Psychology, 7,* 167–168.

Louttit, C. M., & Browne, C. G. (1947). The use of psychometric instruments in psychological clinics. *Journal of Consulting Psychology, 11,* 49–54.

Lubin, B., Wallis, R. R., & Paine, C. (1971). Patterns of psychological test usage in the United States: 1935–1969. *Professional Psychology, 2,* 70–74.

Lynch, E. C. (1968). Walter Dill Scott: Pioneer industrial psychologist. *Business History Review, 42,* 149–170.

Matarazzo, J. D. (1972). *Wechsler's measurement and appraisal of adult intelligence* (5th ed.). New York: Oxford University Press.

Matarazzo, J. D. (1981). Obituary: David Wechsler (1896–1981). *American Psychologist, 36,* 1542–1543.

May, M. A. (1920). The psychological examination of conscientious objectors. *American Journal of Psychology, 31,* 152–165.

McArdle, J. J. (2007). Obituary: John Leonard Horn 1928–2006. *Intelligence, 35,* 517–518.

McGrew, K. S. (2009). CHC theory and the human cognitive abilities project: Standing on the shoulders of the giants of psychometric intelligence research. *Intelligence, 37,* 1–10.

McNemar, Q. (1945). Reviewed work(s): *The Measurement of Adult Intelligence* by David Wechsler. *American Journal of Psychology, 58,* 420–422.

Minton, H. L. (1988). *Lewis M. Terman: Pioneer in psychological testing.* New York: New York University Press.

Morgan, C. L. (1910). Instinct and intelligence. *British Journal of Psychology, 3,* 219–229.

Myers, C. S. (1910). Instinct and intelligence. *British Journal of Psychology, 3,* 209–218.

Napoli, D. S. (1981). *Architects of adjustment; The history of the psychological profession in the United States.* Port Washington, NY: Kennikat Press.

Neisser, U., Boodoo, G., Bouchard, T. J., Boykin, A. W., Brody, N., Ceci, S. J., et al. (1996). Intelligence: Knowns and unknowns. *American Psychologist, 51,* 77–101.

Newton, J. H., & McGrew, K. S. (2010). Introduction to the special issue: Current research in Cattell–Horn–Carroll-based assessment. *Psychology in the Schools, 47,* 621–634.

Nicolas, S., & Ferrand, L. (2002). Alfred Binet and higher education. *History of Psychology, 5,* 264–283.

Oehrn, A. (1896). Experimentelle Studien zur Individualpsychologie. *Psychologische Arbeiten, 1,* 92–151.

Old Bellevue and new. (1930, June 20). *New York Times,* p. 19.

Otis, A. S. (1917). A criticism of the Yerkes–Bridges Point Scale, with alternative suggestions. *Journal of Educational Psychology, 8,* 129–150.

Pass alien slacker bill. (1918, February 28). *New York Times,* p. 5.

Payne, A. F. (1920). The scientific selection of men. *Scientific Monthly, 11,* 544–547.

Pearson, K. (Ed.). (1924). *The life, letters and labours of Francis Galton: Vol. 2. Researchers of middle life.* London: Cambridge University Press.

Pearson, K. (Ed.). (1930). *The life, letters and labours of Francis Galton: Vol. 3A. Correlation, personal identification and eugenics.* London: Cambridge University Press.

Pellegrino, J. W. (1986). Intelligence: The interaction of culture and cognitive processes. In R. J. Sternberg & D. K. Detterman (Eds.), *What is intelligence?: Contemporary viewpoints on its nature and definition* (pp. 113–116). Norwood, NJ: Ablex.

Peterson, J. (1921). Intelligence and its measurement: A symposium. *Journal of Educational Psychology, 12,* 198–201.

Pintner, R. (1921). Intelligence and its measurement: A symposium. *Journal of Educational Psychology, 12,* 139–143.

Prendergast, P. (1844). A "page" of phrenology. *The Illuminated Magazine, 11,* 17–20.

Rabin, A. I. (1945). The use of the Wechsler–Bellevue scales with normal and abnormal persons. *Psychological Bulletin, 42,* 410–422.

Rabin, A. I., & Guertin, W. H. (1951). Research with the Wechsler–Bellevue test: 1945–1950. *Psychological Bulletin, 48,* 211–248.

Rapaport, D. (1945). The new Army Individual Test of general mental ability. *Bulletin of the Menninger Clinic, 9,* 107–110.

Reeve, C. L., & Charles, J. E. (2008). Survey of opinions on the primacy of g and social consequences of ability testing: A comparison of expert and non-expert views. *Intelligence, 36,* 681–688.

Rock, G. (1956). *The history of the American Field Service, 1920–1955.* New York: American Field Service.

Roid, G. H. (2003). *Stanford–Binet Intelligence Scales, Fifth Edition.* Itasca, IL: Riverside.

Routh, D. K. (2000). Clinical psychology training: A history of ideas and practices prior to 1946. *American Psychologist, 55,* 236–241.

Samelson, F. (1977). World War I intelligence testing

and the development of psychology. *Journal of the History of the Behavioral Sciences, 13,* 274–282.

Scarr, S. (1986). Intelligence: Revisited. In R. J. Sternberg & D. K. Detterman (Eds.), *What is intelligence?: Contemporary viewpoints on its nature and definition* (pp. 117–120). Norwood, NJ: Ablex.

Schneider, W. H. (1992). After Binet: French intelligence testing, 1900–1950. *Journal of the History of the Behavioral Sciences, 28,* 111–132.

Scott, J. B. (1918). The amendment of the Naturalization and Citizenship Acts with respect to military service. *American Journal of International Law, 12,* 613–619.

Scott, W. D. (1916). Selection of employees by means of quantitative determinations. *Annals of the American Academy of Political and Social Science, 65,* 182–193.

Sea Fox wreckage. (1931, May 28). *New York Times,* p. 1.

Seagoe, M. V. (1975). *Terman and the gifted.* Los Altos, CA: Kaufmann.

Seidenfeld, M. A. (1942). The Adjutant General's School and the training of psychological personnel for the Army. *Psychological Bulletin, 39,* 381–384.

Sharp, S. E. (1899). Individual psychology: A study in psychological method. *American Journal of Psychology, 10,* 329–391.

Siegler, R. S. (1992). The other Alfred Binet. *Developmental Psychology, 28,* 179–190.

Simpson, D. (2005). Phrenology and the neurosciences: Contributions of F. J. Gall and J. G. Spurzheim. *Australian and New Zealand Journal of Surgery, 75,* 475–482.

Sisson, E. D. (1948). The Personnel Research Program of the Adjutant General's Office of the United States Army. *Review of Educational Research, 18,* 575–614.

Smith, M. L. (2000). By way of Canada: U.S. records of Immigration across the U.S.–Canadian border, 1895–1954 (St. Albans Lists). *Prologue, 32,* 192–199.

Snow, R. E. (1986). On intelligence. In R. J. Sternberg & D. K. Detterman (Eds.), *What is intelligence?: Contemporary viewpoints on its nature and definition* (pp. 133–139). Norwood, NJ: Ablex.

Sokal, M. M. (Ed.). (1981). *An education in psychology: James McKeen Cattell's journal and letters from Germany and England, 1880–1888.* Cambridge, MA: MIT Press.

Sokal, M. M. (Ed.). (1987). *Psychological testing and American society, 1890–1930.* New Brunswick, NJ: Rutgers University Press.

Sokal, M. M. (2006). James McKeen Cattell: Achievement and alienation. In D. A. Dewsbury, L. T. Benjamin, & M. Wertheimer (Eds.), *Portraits of pioneers in psychology* (Vol. 6, pp. 18–35). Mahwah, NJ: Erlbaum.

Spanier, M., & Spanier, D. (1902, September 17). Canadian passenger manifest for the S. S. *Lake Megantic* (sailed from Liverpool 9 September, arrived 17). *Québec Ports, Immigrant Passenger Lists, 1865–1935 (RG 76): Québec 1865–1921 (includes Montreal). Microfilm Reel T-481 (1902 25 Aug to 1903 July 28).* Ottawa: Library and Archives Canada.

Spearman, C. (1904). "General intelligence," objectively determined and measured. *American Journal of Psychology, 15,* 201–293.

Spearman, C. (1923). *The nature of "intelligence" and principles of cognition.* London: Macmillan.

Spearman, C. (1927). *The abilities of man: Their nature and measurement.* New York: Macmillan.

Spearman, C., & Wynn Jones, L. (1950). *Human ability: A continuation of "The Abilities of Man."* London: Macmillan.

Spencer, H. (1855). *The principles of psychology.* London: Longman, Brown, Green, & Longmans.

Spencer, H. (1864). *The principles of biology* (Vol. 1). London: Williams & Norgate.

Spring, J. H. (1972). Psychologists and the war: The meaning of intelligence in the Alpha and Beta tests. *History of Education Quarterly, 12,* 3–15.

Spurzheim, J. G. (1815). *The physiognomical system of Drs. Gall and Spurzheim; founded on an anatomical and physiological examination of the nervous system in general, and of the brain in particular; and indicating the dispositions and manifestations of the mind* (2nd ed.). London: Baldwin, Cradock, & Joy.

Staff, Personnel Research Section. (1942, March). *Analysis of Wechsler Self-Administering Test data* (PRS Report No. 286). Washington, DC: U.S. War Department, Adjutant General's Office.

Staff, Personnel Research Section. (1944). The new Army Individual Test of general mental ability. *Psychological Bulletin, 41,* 532–538.

Staff, Personnel Research Section. (1945). The Army General Classification Test. *Psychological Bulletin, 42,* 760–768.

Stein, M. (2004). The establishment of the Department of Psychiatry in the Mount Sinai Hospital: A conflict between neurology and psychiatry. *Journal of the History of the Behavioral Sciences, 40,* 285–309.

Stern, W. (1914). *The psychological methods of testing intelligence* (Educational Psychology Monographs No. 13; G. M. Whipple, Trans.). Baltimore: Warwick & York. (Original work published 1912)

Sternberg, R. J. (1986). Intelligence is mental self-government. In R. J. Sternberg & D. K. Detterman (Eds.), *What is intelligence?: Contemporary viewpoints on its nature and definition* (pp. 141–148). Norwood, NJ: Ablex.

Sternberg, R. J. (1994). 468 factor-analyzed data sets:

What they tell us and don't tell us about human intelligence. Reviewed work(s): *Human Cognitive Abilities: A Survey of Factor-Analytic Studies* by J. B. Carroll. *Psychological Science, 5*, 63–65.

Sternberg, R. J., & Berg, C. A. (1986). Quantitative integration: Definitions of Intelligence: A comparison of the 1921 and 1986 symposia. In R. J. Sternberg & D. K. Detterman (Eds.), *What is intelligence?: Contemporary viewpoints on its nature and definition* (pp. 155–162). Norwood, NJ: Ablex.

Sternberg, R. J., & Detterman, D. K. (Eds.). (1986). *What is intelligence?: Contemporary viewpoints on its nature and definition.* Norwood, NJ: Ablex.

Strong, E. K. (1955). Walter Dill Scott: 1869–1955. *American Journal of Psychology, 68*, 682–683.

Terman, L. M. (1904). A preliminary study in the psychology and pedagogy of leadership. *Pedagogical Seminary, 11*, 413–451.

Terman, L. M. (1906). Genius and stupidity: A study of some of the intellectual processes of seven "bright" and seven "stupid" boys. *Pedagogical Seminary, 13*, 307–373.

Terman, L. M. (1916). *The measurement of intelligence: An explanation of and a complete guide for the use of the Stanford revision and extension of the Binet–Simon Intelligence Scale.* Boston: Houghton Mifflin.

Terman, L. M. (1917). Feeble minded children in the schools. In F. C. Nelles (Chair), *Report of 1915 legislature committee on mental deficiency and the proposed institution for the care of feeble-minded and epileptic persons* (pp. 45–52). Whittier, CA: Whittier State School, Department of Printing Instruction.

Terman, L. M. (1921). Intelligence and its measurement: A symposium. *Journal of Educational Psychology, 12*, 127–133.

Terman, L. M. (1922a). The great conspiracy, or the impulse imperious of intelligence testers, psychoanalyzed and exposed by Mr. Lippmann. *The New Republic, 33*, 116–120.

Terman, L. M. (1922b). Were we born that way? *The World's Work, 44*, 655–660.

Terman, L. M. (1932). Trails to psychology. In C. Murchison (Ed.), *A history of psychology in autobiography* (Vol. 2, pp. 297–331). Worcester, MA: Clark University Press.

Terman, L. M., & Childs, H. G. (1912a). A tentative revision and extension of the Binet–Simon measuring scale of intelligence. *Journal of Educational Psychology, 3*, 61–74.

Terman, L. M., & Childs, H. G. (1912b). A tentative revision and extension of the Binet–Simon measuring scale of intelligence: Part II. Supplementary tests. 1. Generalization test: interpretation of fables. *Journal of Educational Psychology, 3*, 133–143.

Terman, L. M., & Childs, H. G. (1912c). A tentative revision and extension of the Binet–Simon measuring scale of intelligence: Part II. Supplementary tests—continued. *Journal of Educational Psychology, 3*, 198–208.

Terman, L. M., & Childs, H. G. (1912d). A tentative revision and extension of the Binet–Simon measuring scale of intelligence: Part III. Summary and criticisms. *Journal of Educational Psychology, 3*, 277–289.

Terman, L. M., & Merrill, M. A. (1937). *Measuring intelligence: A guide to the administration of the new Revised Stanford–Binet tests of intelligence.* Boston: Houghton Mifflin.

Terman, L. M., & Merrill, M. A. (1960). *Stanford–Binet Intelligence Scale: Manual for the third revision, Form L-M.* Boston: Houghton Mifflin.

Terman, L. M., & Merrill, M. A. (1973). *Stanford–Binet Intelligence Scale: Manual for the third revision, Form L-M (1972 table of norms by R. L. Thorndike).* Boston: Houghton Mifflin.

Thorndike, E. L. (1921). Intelligence and its measurement: A symposium. *Journal of Educational Psychology, 12*, 124–127.

Thorndike, E. L., Lay, W., & Dean, P. R. (1909). The relation of accuracy in sensory discrimination to general intelligence. *American Journal of Psychology, 20*, 364–369.

Thorndike, R. L. (1975). Mr. Binet's test 70 years later. *Educational Researcher, 4*, 3–7.

Thorndike, R. L., Hagen, E. P., & Sattler, J. M. (1986). *Stanford–Binet Intelligence Scale: Fourth Edition.* Chicago: Riverside.

Thorndike, R. M., & Lohman, D. F. (1990). *A century of ability testing.* Chicago: Riverside.

Thorne, F. C. (1976). Reflections on the golden age of Columbia psychology. *Journal of the History of the Behavioral Sciences, 12*, 159–165.

Thurstone, L. L. (1921). Intelligence and its measurement: A symposium. *Journal of Educational Psychology, 12*, 201–207.

Thurstone, L. L. (1938). *Primary mental abilities.* Chicago: University of Chicago Press.

Thurstone, L. L. (1945). Testing intelligence and aptitudes. *Hygeia, 23*, 32–36, 50, 52, 54.

Thurstone, L. L. (1947). *Multiple factor analysis: A development and expansion of the vectors of mind.* Chicago: University of Chicago Press.

Thurstone, L. L., & Thurstone, T. G. (1941). Factorial studies of intelligence. *Psychometric Monographs, 2*.

Toops, H. A. (1921). *Trade tests in education.* New York: Teachers College, Columbia University.

Tucker, W. H. (2009). *The Cattell controversy: Race, science, and ideology.* Urbana: University of Illinois Press.

Tuddenham, R. D. (1974). Review: Fame and oblivion. *Science (New Series)*, 183, 1071–1072.

206 get degrees at City College. (1916, June 23). *New York Times*, p. 7.

U.S. maintains great schools on foreign soil: Government trains soldiers for civilian life—thousands are enrolled. (1919, June 12). *Lima Daily News* [Lima, OH], p. 5.

Venezky, R. L. (2002). The history of reading research. In P. D. Pearson (Ed.), *Handbook of reading research* (Vol. 1, pp. 3–38). Mahwah, NJ: Erlbaum.

Vernon, P. E. (1950). *The structure of human abilities*. London: Methuen.

Vernon, P. E. (1961). *The structure of human abilities* (2nd ed.). London: Methuen.

von Mayrhauser, R. T. (1986). *The triumph of utility: The forgotten clash of American psychologies in World War I*. Unpublished doctoral dissertation, University of Chicago. (AAT T-29951)

von Mayrhauser, R. T. (1987). The manager, the medic, and the mediator: The clash of professional psychological styles and the wartime origins of group mental testing. In M. M. Sokal (Ed.), *Psychological testing and American society, 1890–1930* (pp. 128–157). New Brunswick, NJ: Rutgers University Press.

von Mayrhauser, R. T. (1989). Making intelligence functional: Walter Dill Scott and applied psychological testing in World War I. *Journal of the History of the Behavioral Sciences*, 25, 60–72.

Walsh, A. A. (1976). The "new science of the mind" and the Philadelphia physicians in the early 1800s. *Transactions and Studies of the College of Physicians of Philadelphia*, 43, 397–413.

Wasserman, J. D., & Maccubbin, E. M. (2002, August). *David Wechsler at The Psychological Corporation, 1925–1927: Chorus girls and taxi drivers*. Paper presented at the annual meeting of the American Psychological Association, Chicago.

Wechsler, D. (1917a). A study of retention in Korsakoff psychosis. *Psychiatric Bulletin*, 2, 403–451.

Wechsler, D. (1917b, June 5). *World War I Selective Service System Draft Registration Cards, 1917–1918* (Administration. M1509, Roll: 1765679, Draft Board: 96). Washington, DC: National Archives and Records.

Wechsler, D. (1918a, October 4). Passport Application No. 124984. In *Passport Applications, 1906–March 31, 1925*. Washington, DC: National Archives and Records Administration.

Wechsler, D. (1918b, June 7). *Petition for naturalization, David Wechsler*. United States District Court of the Northern District of Georgia, Rome Division. Morrow, GA: NARA Southeast Region.

Wechsler, D. (1921). Report of amendment of passport, August 18, 1921. In *Passport Applications, 1906–*

March 31, 1925. Washington, DC: National Archives and Records Administration.

Wechsler, D. (1922). Quelques remarques sur la psychopathologie de l'indecision [Some remarks on the psychopathology of indecision]. *Journal de Psychologie*, 19, 47–54.

Wechsler, D. (1925). The measurement of emotional reactions. *Archives of Psychology*, 76, 1–181.

Wechsler, D. (1926). Tests for taxicab drivers. *Journal of Personnel Research*, 5, 24–30.

Wechsler, D. (1927). Psychometric tests. In I. S. Wechsler, *Textbook of clinical neurology* (pp. 104–116). Philadelphia: Saunders.

Wechsler, D. (1932). Analytic use of the Army Alpha examination. *Journal of Applied Psychology*, 16, 254–256.

Wechsler, D. (1939). *The measurement of adult intelligence*. Baltimore: Williams & Wilkins.

Wechsler, D. (1944). The psychologist in the psychiatric hospital. *Journal of Consulting Psychology*, 8, 281–285.

Wechsler, D. (1946). *Wechsler–Bellevue Intelligence Scale, Form II. Manual for administering and scoring the test*. New York: The Psychological Corporation.

Wechsler, D. (1949). *Wechsler Intelligence Scale for Children (WISC)*. New York: Psychological Corporation.

Wechsler, D. (1955). *Wechsler Adult Intelligence Scale—Restandardized (WAIS)*. New York: Psychological Corporation.

Wechsler, D. (1961). Conformity and the idea of being well born. In I. A. Berg & B. M. Bass (Eds.), *Conformity and deviation* (pp. 412–423). New York: Harper & Row.

Wechsler, D. (1967). *Wechsler Preschool and Primary Scale of Intelligence (WPPSI)*. New York: The Psychological Corporation.

Wechsler, D. (1981). The psychometric tradition: Developing the Wechsler Adult Intelligence Scale. *Contemporary Educational Psychology*, 6, 82–85.

Wechsler, D., Doppelt, J. E., & Lennon, R. T. (1975). *A conversation with David Wechsler* (Unpublished transcript of interview). San Antonio, TX: The Psychological Corporation.

Wechsler, I. (1957). A neurologist's point of view. *Medical Clinics of North America*, 41, 1111–1121.

Wechsler, M. (1903, August 23). *Certificate and record of death, Certificate No. 24787. City of New York, Department of Health, State of New York*. New York: New York City Department of Records and Information Services Municipal Archives.

Weider, A. (2006). *A Weider Weltanschauung: A wider perspective of psychology*. Bloomington, IN: Xlibris.

Wexler, L. (1906, October 31). *Certificate and record of*

death, *Certificate No. 33534. City of New York, Department of Health, State of New York.* New York: New York City Department of Records and Information Services Municipal Archives.

Whipple, G. M. (1915). *Manual of mental and physical tests: Part 2. Complex processes* (2nd ed.). Baltimore: Warwick & York.

Wilson, M. S., & Reschly, D. J. (1996). Assessment in school psychology training and practice. *School Psychology Review, 25,* 9–23.

Wilson, W. (1917). Address of the President of the United States delivered at a joint session of the two houses of Congress, April 2, 1917. In *65th Congress, 1st Session, Senate* (Document No. 5, Serial No. 7264, pp. 3–8). Washington, DC: U.S. Government Printing Office.

Wissler, C. (1901). The correlation of mental and physical tests. *Psychological Monographs, 3*(6), 1–62.

Wolf, T. (1961). An individual who made a difference. *American Psychologist, 16,* 245–248.

Wolf, T. (1966). Intuition and experiment: Alfred Binet's first efforts in child psychology. *Journal of the History of the Behavioral Sciences, 2,* 233–239.

Wolf, T. (1969). The emergence of Binet's conceptions and measurement of intelligence: II. A case history of the creative process. *Journal of the History of the Behavioral Sciences, 5,* 207–237.

Wolf, T. (1973). *Alfred Binet.* Chicago: University of Chicago Press.

Woodrow, H. (1921). Intelligence and its measurement: A symposium. *Journal of Educational Psychology, 12,* 207–210.

Woodworth, R. S. (1942). *The Columbia University psychological laboratory.* New York: Columbia University.

Yerkes, R. M. (1918a). Measuring the mental strength of an army. *Proceedings of the National Academy of Sciences USA, 4,* 295–297.

Yerkes, R. M. (1918b, May 3). Memorandum for Mr. Garrett. *Records of the Office of the Surgeon General (Army) (RG 112).* College Park, MD: National Archives and Records Administration.

Yerkes, R. M. (1919). Report of the Psychology Committee of the National Research Council. *Psychological Review, 26,* 83–149.

Yerkes, R. M. (1920). What psychology contributed to the war. In R. M. Yerkes (Ed.), *The new world of science: Its development during the war* (pp. 364–389). New York: Century.

Yerkes, R. M. (Ed.). (1921). *Memoirs of the National Academy of Sciences: Vol. 15. Psychological examining in the United States Army.* Washington, DC: U.S. Government Printing Office.

Yerkes, R. M., Bridges, J. W., & Hardwick, R. S. (1915). *A point scale for measuring mental ability.* Baltimore: Warwick & York.

Yoakum, C. S., & Yerkes, R. M. (1920). *Army mental tests.* New York: Holt.

Yockelson, M. (1998). They answered the call: Military service in the United States Army during World War I, 1917–1919. *Prologue: Quarterly of the National Archives and Records Administration, 30,* 228–234.

Zazzo, R. (1993). Alfred Binet (1857–1911). *Prospects: The Quarterly Review of Comparative Education, 23,* 101–112.

Zeidner, J., & Drucker, A. J. (1988). *Behavioral science in the army: A corporate history of the Army Research Institute.* Arlington, VA: United States Army Research Institute for the Behavioral and Social Sciences.

Zenderland, L. (1998). *Measuring minds: Henry Herbert Goddard and the origins of American intelligence testing.* New York: Cambridge University Press.

CHAPTER 2

A History of Intelligence Test Interpretation

Randy W. Kamphaus
Anne Pierce Winsor
Ellen W. Rowe
Sangwon Kim

In this chapter, we focus exclusively on a histori-cal account of dominant methods of intelligence test interpretation, without critically evaluating each one. Although our research coverage is cur-sory, our topic is important. There is much to be learned from such an overview. As E. G. Boring (1929) wisely observed long ago, "Without such [historical] knowledge he sees the present in dis-torted perspective, he mistakes old facts and old views for new, and he remains unable to evaluate the significance of new movements and methods" (p. vii). Boring's wisdom remains valuable today, even when we consider the date and context in which his work was written, as reflected by his exclusively masculine phraseology. In recent de-cades, we have seen considerable new methods of intelligence test interpretation that are in fact merely reverberations of strategies that were either failed or questionable in a bygone era. Take, for example, the relatively widespread adoption of Howard Gardner's multiple-intelligences theory by schools around the United States and the world (see Chen & Gardner, Chapter 5, this volume). This potential "breakthrough" may yet be proven to be one, but Gardner's theory is definitely a clas-sic example of multiple-intelligence theory from the 1930s (Kamphaus, 2009), with the same atten-dant challenges to demonstrating valid inferences of test scores.

As would be expected, formal methods of in-telligence test interpretation emerged soon after Binet and Simon's creation of the first successful intelligence scale (Kamphaus, 2001). These early interpretive methods, sometimes referred to collo-quially as the "dipstick approach," attempted pri-marily to quantify a general level to intelligence—or, as Binet referred to it, *developmental level*. He preferred this qualitative description to yielding a test score (Kamphaus, 2001). With the addition of subtest scores to clinical tests and the emergence of group tests measuring different abilities, *clinical profile analysis* replaced the "dipstick approach" as the dominant heuristic for intelligence test in-terpretation. All scores were deemed appropriate for interpretation, in the hope of providing more "insight" into an individual's cognitive strengths and weaknesses. *Psychometric profile analysis* soon followed. However, as measurement approaches to intelligence test interpretation developed, validity problems with the interpretation of the panoply of subtest scores and patterns surfaced. Today, the gap between intelligence theory and test development has narrowed, and more validity evidence associ-ated with score inferences is available; thus test in-terpretation is becoming easier and more accurate. We trace all of these developments and look to the future in the remainder of this chapter.

QUANTIFICATION OF A GENERAL LEVEL: THE FIRST WAVE

The process of analyzing human abilities has intrigued scientists for centuries. Indeed, some method for analyzing people's abilities has existed for over 2,000 years, since the Chinese instituted civil service exams and formulated a system to classify individuals according to their abilities (French & Hale, 1990). Early work in interpretation of intelligence tests focused extensively on classification of individuals into groups. Early classification provided a way to organize individuals into specified groups based on scores obtained on intelligence tests—an organization that was dependent on the acceptance of intelligence tests by laypersons as well as by professionals. Today, professionals in the fields of psychology and education benefit from the use of well-researched and objective instruments derived through periods of investigation and development. The following discussion is a brief description of some of the early work leading to the development of instrumentation.

The Work of Early Investigators

At the beginning of the 20th century, practitioners in the fields of psychology and education were beginning to feel the compelling influence of Alfred Binet and his colleagues in France, most notably Théodore Simon. Binet's studies of the mental qualities of children for school placement led to the first genuinely successful method for classifying persons with respect to their cognitive abilities (Goodenough, 1949). Binet and Simon's development of the first empirical and practical intelligence test for applied use in the classification of students represented a technological breakthrough in the field of intelligence assessment. The first version of the Binet–Simon Intelligence Scale (Binet & Simon, 1905) would lead to future scales and, according to Anastasi (1988), an overall increase in the use of intelligence tests for a variety of purposes.

Binet's efforts reflected his great interest in certain forms of cognitive activity. These included the abilities related to thinking and reasoning, the development and application of strategies for complex problem solving, and the use and adaptation of abilities for success in novel experiences (Pintner, 1923). His work appeared to stem from an interest in the complex cognitive processes of children and would eventually lead to a series of popular instruments, most recently represented in the Stanford–Binet Intelligence Scales, Fifth Edition (SB5; Roid, 2003).

At the same time, scientists such as James McKeen Cattell in the United States were conducting equally important work of a different kind. Cattell's investigations frequently focused on measures of perception and motor skills. Although different in scope and purpose from that of Binet and Simon, Cattell's work would ultimately have a profound effect on the popularization and use of intelligence tests (Pintner, 1923). Cattell's experimentation resulted in the appointment of a special committee whose members, with the assistance of the American Psychological Association, were charged with developing a series of mental ability tests for use in the classification and guidance of college students (Goodenough, 1949). The development of these tests placed great emphasis on the need for standardized procedures.

Procedures for standardized test administration were introduced with the idea that the measurements associated with an individual would be even more informative when compared to the measurements of another person in the same age group who was administered the same test under the same standard conditions (Pintner, 1923). Indeed, the conditions of test administration must be controlled for everyone if the goal is scientific interpretation of the test data (Anastasi, 1988). Some of the earliest attempts at scientific test interpretation, used before and during World War II, included the classification of individuals into groups based on their test scores and accompanied by descriptive terminology.

Classification Schemes

The first well-documented efforts at intelligence test interpretation emphasized the assignment to a descriptive classification based on an overall intelligence test composite score. This practice seemed a reasonable first step, given that (1) the dominant scale of the day, the Stanford–Binet (Stanford Revisions and Extension of the Binet–Simon Scale [Terman, 1916] or the Revised Stanford–Binet [Terman & Merrill, 1937]), yielded only a global score; and (2) Spearman's (1927) general intelligence theory emphasized the preeminence of an underlying *mental energy*.

According to Goodenough (1949), the identification of mental ability was regarded as a purely physical/medical issue until the beginning of the 20th century. Wechsler (1944) made a similar statement, noting that the vocabulary of choice included medical–legal terms such as *idiot*, *imbecile*, and *moron*. Levine and Marks (1928, p. 131) provided an example of a classification system incorporating these terms (see Table 2.1).

TABLE 2.1. The Levine and Marks Intelligence Test Score Classification System

Level	Range in IQ
Idiots	0–24
Imbeciles	25–49
Morons	50–74
Borderline	75–84
Dull	85–94
Average	95–104
Bright	105–114
Very bright	115–124
Superior	125–149
Very superior	150–174
Precocious	175 or above

TABLE 2.2. Wechsler's Intelligence Classification According to IQ

Classification	IQ limits	% included
Defective	65 and below	2.2
Borderline	66–79	6.7
Dull normal	80–90	16.1
Average	91–110	50.0
Bright normal	111–119	16.1
Superior	120–127	6.7
Very superior	128 and over	2.2

This classification system used descriptive terms that were evaluative and pejorative (especially when employed in the vernacular), leading to stigmatization of examinees. In addition, the many category levels contained bands of scores with different score ranges. The top and bottom three levels comprised bands of 24 score points each, while those in the middle, from *borderline* to *very bright*, comprised bands of 9 points each. Although the band comprising the *average* range was not far from our present conceptions of *average* (except for this example's upper limit), the use of numerous uneven levels was potentially confusing to the layperson.

Wechsler (1944) introduced another classification scheme that attempted to formulate categories according to a specific structural rationale. Specifically, the system proposed by Wechsler was based on a definition of intelligence levels related to statistical frequencies (i.e., percentages under the normal curve), in which each classification level was based on a range of intelligence scores lying specified distances from the mean (Wechsler, 1944). In an effort to move away from somewhat arbitrary qualities, his classification scheme incorporated estimates of the prevalence of certain intelligence levels in the United States at that time (see Table 2.2).

Wechsler's system is notable for bands of IQ limits that are somewhat closer to those we use at the present time. Both the Levine and Marks (1928) and Wechsler (1944) schemes provide a glimpse at procedures used in early attempts at test interpretation. The potential for stigmatization has been lessened in the period since World War II; both scientists and practitioners have moved to a less evaluative vocabulary that incorporates parallel terminology around the mean, such as *above average* and *below average* (Kamphaus, 2001).

Considerations for Interpretation Using Classification Systems

We have made progress regarding the use of classification schemes in the evaluation of human cognitive abilities. The structure of classification systems appears to be more stable today than in the past. Previously, practitioners often applied Terman's classification system, originally developed for interpretation of the Stanford–Binet, in their interpretation of many different tests that measured a variety of different abilities (Wechsler, 1944). Fortunately, many test batteries today provide their own classification schemes within the test manuals, providing an opportunity to choose among appropriate tests and interpret the results accordingly. In addition, these classification systems are often based on deviation from a mean of 100, providing consistency across most intelligence tests and allowing comparison of an individual's performance on them.

Calculation of intelligence test scores, or IQs, became a common way of describing an individual's cognitive ability. However, test score calculation is only the first step in the interpretive process, which has been the case since the early days of testing (Goodenough, 1949). Although scores may fall neatly into classification categories, additional data should be considered when clinicians are discussing an individual's abilities. For example, individuals in the population who are assessed to have below average intellectual abilities do not necessarily manifest the same degree of disability and, in fact, may demonstrate considerable variability in capabilities (Goodenough, 1949). In a similar statement, Wechsler (1958) noted that an advantage to the use of scores in the classification process is to keep clinicians from forgetting that intelligence tests are completely relative and, moreover, do not assess absolute quantities.

These concerns of Goodenough and Wechsler have influenced intelligence test interpretation for decades. Clinicians continue to use classification schemes based on global IQ scores for diagnosis and interpretation, and the concerns of Goodenough and Wechsler are alive today. With the understanding that global IQ scores represent the most robust estimate of ability, they are frequently used in the diagnosis of intellectual disabilities, giftedness, learning disabilities, and other conditions. Still, we caution that global cutoff scores may not always be appropriate or adequate for the decisions typically made on the basis of intelligence test scores (Kaufman, 1990), since these scores constitute only one component of understanding an individual's range of talents, proclivities, and developed cognitive abilities.

CLINICAL PROFILE ANALYSIS: THE SECOND WAVE

Rapaport, Gil, and Schafer's (1945–1946) seminal work has exerted a profound influence on intelligence test interpretation to the present day. These authors, recognizing an opportunity provided by the publication of the Wechsler–Bellevue Scale (Wechsler, 1939), advocated interpretation of the newly introduced subtest scores to achieve a more thorough understanding of an individual's cognitive skills; in addition, they extended intelligence test interpretation to include interpretation of individual test items and assignment of psychiatric diagnoses.

Profiles of Subtest Scores

Rapaport and colleagues (1945–1946) espoused an entirely new perspective in the interpretation of intelligence tests, focusing on the shape of subtest score profiles in addition to an overall general level of intellectual functioning. Whereas the pre–World War II psychologist was primarily dependent on the Binet scales and the determination of a general level of cognitive attainment, the post-Rapaport and colleagues psychologist became equally concerned with the shape of a per-

son's profile of subtest scores. Specifically, patterns of high and low subtest scores could presumably reveal diagnostic and psychotherapeutic considerations:

> In our opinion, one can most fully exploit intelligence tests neither by stating merely that the patient was poor on some and good on other subtests, nor by trying to connect directly the impairments of certain subtest scores with certain clinical-nosological categories; but rather only by attempting to understand and describe the psychological functions whose impairment or change brings about the impairment of scores. . . . Every subtest score—especially the relationship of every subtest score to the other subtest scores—has a multitude of determinants. If we are able to establish the main psychological function underlying the achievement, then we can hope to construct a complex psychodynamic and structural picture out of the interrelationships of these achievements and impairments of functions . . . (Rapaport et al., 1945–1946, p. 106)

The Rapaport and colleagues' (1945–1946) system had five major emphases, the first of which involved interpretation of item responses. The second emphasis involved comparing a subject's item responses within subtests. Differential responding to the same item type (e.g., information subtest items assessing U.S. vs. international knowledge) was thought to be of some diagnostic significance. The third emphasis suggested that meaningful interpretations could be based on within-subject comparisons of subtest scores. Rapaport and colleagues introduced the practice of deriving diagnostic information from comparisons between Verbal and Performance scales, the fourth interpretive emphasis. They suggested, for example, that a specific Verbal–Performance profile could be diagnostic of depression (p. 68). The fifth and final emphasis involved the comparison of intelligence test findings to other test findings. In this regard, they noted, "Thus, a badly impaired intelligence test achievement has a different diagnostic implication if the Rorschach test indicates a rich endowment or a poor endowment" (p. 68).

The work of Rapaport and colleagues (1945–1946) was a considerable developmental landmark due to its scope. It provided diagnostic suggestions at each interpretive level for a variety of adult psychiatric populations. Furthermore, their work introduced an interpretive focus on intraindividual differences—a focus that at times took precedence over interindividual comparisons in clinical work with clients.

In addition to the breadth of their approach, the structure of the Rapaport and colleagues (1945–1946) approach gave clinicians a logical, step-by-step method for assessing impairment of function and for making specific diagnostic hypotheses. These authors directed clinicians to calculate a mean subtest score that could be used for identifying intraindividual strengths and weaknesses, and they gave desired difference score values for determining significant subtest fluctuations from the mean subtest score. The case of so-called "simple schizophrenia" (see Table 2.3) provides an example of the specificity of the diagnostic considerations that could be gleaned from a subtest profile.

Because of its thorough and clinically oriented approach, Rapaport and colleagues' (1945–1946) work provided a popular structure for training post-World War II clinical psychologists in the interpretation of intelligence test scores (i.e., the Wechsler–Bellevue Scale). This structure lingers today (Kamphaus, 2001).

Verbal–Performance Differences and Subtest Profiles

Wechsler (1944) reinforced the practice of profile analysis by advocating a method of interpretation that also placed a premium on shape over a general level, with particular emphasis on subtest profiles and Verbal–Performance differences (scatter). His interpretive method is highlighted in a case example presented as a set of results for what he called "adolescent psychopaths" (see Table 2.4). It is noteworthy that Wechsler did not provide a Full Scale IQ (FSIQ) for this case example, focusing instead on shape rather than level. Wechsler offered the following interpretation of this "psychopathic" profile of scores:

White, male, age 15, 8th grade. Continuous history of stealing, incorrigibility and running away. Several admissions to Bellevue Hospital, the last one after suicide attempt. While on wards persistently created disturbances, broke rules, fought with other boys and

TABLE 2.3. Diagnostic Considerations for the Case of "Simple Schizophrenia"

Subtest	Considerations
Vocabulary	Many misses on relatively easy items, especially if harder items are passed
	Relatively low weighted scores
	Parallel lowering of both the mean of the Verbal subtest scores (excluding Digit Span and Arithmetic) and the Vocabulary score
Information	Two or more misses on the easy items
	Relatively well-retained score 2 or more points above Vocabulary
Comprehension	Complete failure on any (especially more than one) of the seven easy items
	Weighted score 3 or more points below the Vocabulary score (or below the mean of the other Verbal subtests: Information, Similarities, and Vocabulary)
	Great positive Comprehension scatter (2 or more points superior to Vocabulary) is not to be expected
Similarities	Failure on easy items
	Weighted score 3 points below Vocabulary
Picture Arrangement	Tends to show a special impairment of Picture Arrangement in comparison to the other Performance subtests
Picture Completion	Weighted score of 7 or less
Object Assembly	Performance relatively strong
Block Design	No significant impairment from Vocabulary level
	Tends to be above the Performance mean
Digit Symbol	May show some impairment, but some "bland schizophrenics" may perform well

TABLE 2.4. Wechsler's Case Example for "Adolescent Psychopaths"

Subtest	Standard score
Comprehension	11
Arithmetic	6
Information	10
Digits	6
Similarities	5
Picture Arrangement	12
Picture Completion	10
Block Design	15
Object Assembly	16
Digit Symbol	12
Verbal IQ (VIQ)	90
Performance IQ (PIQ)	123

continuously tried to evade ordinary duties. Psychopathic patterning: Performance higher than Verbal, low Similarities, low Arithmetic, sum of Picture Arrangement plus Object Assembly greater than sum of scores on Blocks and Picture Completion. (p. 164)

This case exemplifies the second wave of intelligence test interpretation. This second wave was more sophisticated than the first, suggesting that intelligence test interpretation should involve more than mere designation of a general level of intelligence. However, methodological problems existed, eliciting one central question about these approaches: How do we know these various subtest profiles accurately differentiate between clinical samples, and thus demonstrate diagnostic utility? The next wave sought to answer this salient question by applying measurement science to the process of intelligence test interpretation.

PSYCHOMETRIC PROFILE ANALYSIS: THE THIRD WAVE

The availability of computers and statistical software packages provided researchers of the 1960s and 1970s greater opportunity to assess the validity of various interpretive methods and the psychometric properties of popular scales. Two research traditions—*factor analysis* and *psychometric profile analysis*—have had a profound effect on intelligence test interpretation.

Factor Analysis

Cohen's (1959) seminal investigation addressed the second wave of intelligence test interpretation by questioning the empirical basis of the intuitively based "clinical" methods of profile analysis. He conducted one of the first comprehensive factor analyses of the standardization sample for the Wechsler Intelligence Scale for Children (WISC; Wechsler, 1949), analyzing the results for 200 children from three age groups of the sample. Initially, five factors emerged: Factor A, labeled Verbal Comprehension I; Factor B, Perceptual Organization; Factor C, Freedom from Distractibility; Factor D, Verbal Comprehension II; and Factor E, quasi-specific. Cohen chose not to interpret the fourth and fifth factors, subsuming their loadings and subtests under the first three factors. Hence the common three-factor structure of the WISC was established as the de facto standard for conceptualizing the factor structure of the Wechsler scales. Eventually, Kaufman (1979) provided a systematic method for utilizing the three factor scores of the WISC-R (Wechsler, 1974) to interpret the scales as an alternative to interpreting the Verbal IQ (VIQ) and Performance IQ (PIQ), calling into question the common clinical practice of interpreting the Verbal and Performance scores as if they were measures of valid constructs. Cohen's labels for the first three factors were retained as names for the Index scores through the third revision of the Wechsler Intelligence Scale for Children (WISC-III; Wechsler, 1991). In addition, Cohen's study popularized the Freedom from Distractibility label for the controversial third factor (Kamphaus, 2001).

Cohen (1959) also introduced the consideration of subtest specificity prior to making subtest score interpretations. Investigation of the measurement properties of the subtests was crucial, as Cohen noted:

A body of doctrine has come down in the clinical use of the Wechsler scales, which involves a rationale in which the specific intellective and psychodynamic trait-measurement functions are assigned to each of the subtests (e.g., Rapaport et al., 1945–1946). Implicit in this rationale lies the assumption that a substantial part of a test's variance is associated with these specific measurement functions. (p. 289)

According to Cohen (1959), *subtest specificity* refers to the computation of the amount of subtest variance that is reliable (not error) and specific to the subtest. Put another way, a subtest's reliability coefficient represents both reliable specific and shared variance. When shared variance is removed, a clinician may be surprised to discover that little reliable specific variance remains to support interpretation. Typically, the clinician may draw a diagnostic or other conclusion based on a subtest with a reliability estimate of .80, feeling confident of the interpretation. However, Cohen cautioned this coefficient may be illusory because the clinician's interpretation assumes that the subtest is measuring an ability that is only measured by this subtest of the battery. The subtest specificity value for this same subtest may be rather poor if it shares considerable variance with other subtests. In fact, its subtest specificity value may be lower than its error variance (.20).

Cohen (1959) concluded that few of the WISC subtests could attribute one-third or more of their variance to subtest-specific variance—a finding that has been replicated for subsequent revisions of the WISC (Kamphaus, 2001; Kaufman, 1979). Cohen pointedly concluded that adherents to the "clinical" rationales would find no support in the factor-analytic studies of the Wechsler scales (p. 290). Moreover, he singled out many of the subtests for criticism; in the case of the Coding subtest, he concluded that Coding scores, when considered in isolation, were of limited utility (p. 295).

This important study set the stage for a major shift in intelligence test interpretation—that is, movement toward an emphasis on test interpretation supported by measurement science. Hallmarks of this approach are exemplified in Cohen's work, including the following:

1. Renewed emphasis on interpretation of the FSIQ (harkening back to the first wave), as a large second-order factor accounts for much of the variance of the Wechsler scales.
2. Reconfiguration of the Wechsler scales, proposing the three factor scores as alternatives or supplements to interpretation of the Verbal and Performance scales.
3. Deemphasis on individual subtest interpretation, due to limited subtest reliable specific variance (specificity).

Kaufman's Psychometric Approach

Further evidence of the influence of measurement science on intelligence test interpretation and the problems associated with profile analysis can be found in an influential book by Kaufman (1979), *Intelligent Testing with the WISC-R*. He provided a logically appealing and systematic method for WISC-R interpretation that was rooted in sound measurement theory. He created a hierarchy for WISC-R interpretation, which emphasized interpretive conclusions drawn from the most reliable and valid scores yielded by the WISC-R (see Table 2.5).

Although such interpretive methods remained "clinical," in the sense that interpretation of a child's assessment results was still dependent on the child's unique profile of results (Anastasi, 1988), the reliance on measurement science for the interpretive process created new standards for assessment practice. Application of such methods required knowledge of the basic psychometric properties of an instrument, and consequently required greater psychometric expertise on the part of the clinician.

These measurement-based interpretive options contrasted sharply with the "clinical" method espoused by Rapaport and colleagues (1945–1946)—an approach that elevated subtest scores and item responses (presumably the most unreliable and invalid scores and indicators) to prominence in the interpretive process. The measurement science approach, however, was unable to conquer some lingering validity problems.

TABLE 2.5. Kaufman's Hierarchy for WISC-R Interpretation

Source of conclusion	Definition	Reliability	Validity
Composite scores	Wechsler IQs	Good	Good
Shared subtest scores	Two or more subtests combined to draw a conclusion	Good	Fair to poor
Single subtest scores	A single subtest score	Fair	Poor

Diagnostic and Validity Problems

Publication of the Wechsler scales and their associated subtest scores created the opportunity for clinicians to analyze score profiles, as opposed to merely gauging an overall intellectual level from one composite score. Rapaport and colleagues (1945–1946) popularized this method, which they labeled *scatter analysis*:

> Scatter is the pattern or configuration formed by the distribution of the weighted subtest scores on an intelligence test . . . the definition of scatter as a configuration or pattern of all the subtest scores implies that the final meaning of the relationship of any two scores, or of any single score to the central tendency of all the scores, is derived from the total pattern. (p. 75)

However, Rapaport and colleagues (1945–1946) began to identify problems with profile analysis of scatter early in their research efforts. In one instance, they expressed their frustration with the Wechsler scales as a tool for profile analysis, observing that "the standardization of the [Wechsler–Bellevue] left a great deal to be desired so that the average scattergrams of normal college students, Kansas highway patrolmen . . . and applicants to the Menninger School of Psychiatry . . . all deviated from a straight line in just about the same ways" (p. 161).

Bannatyne (1974) constructed one of the more widely used recategorizations of the WISC subtests into presumably more meaningful profiles (see Table 2.6). Matheson, Mueller, and Short (1984) studied the validity of Bannatyne's recategorization of the WISC-R, using a multiple-group factor analysis procedure with three age ranges of the WISC-R and data from the WISC-R standardization sample. They found that the four categories had high reliabilities, but problems with validity. For example, the Acquired Knowledge category had sufficiently high reliabilities, but it was not independent of the other three categories, particularly Conceptualization. As a result, Matheson and colleagues advised that the Acquired Knowledge category not be interpreted as a unique entity; instead, they concluded that the Acquired Knowledge and Conceptualization categories were best interpreted as one measure of verbal intelligence, which was more consistent with the factor-analytic research on the WISC-R and other intelligence test batteries.

Similarly, Kaufman (1979) expressed considerable misgivings, based on a review of research designed to show links between particular profiles of subtest scores and child diagnostic categories (although he too had provided detailed advice for conducting profile analysis). Kaufman noted that the profiles proved to be far less than diagnostic:

> The apparent trends in the profiles of individuals in a given exceptional category can sometimes provide one piece of evidence to be weighed in the diagnostic process. When there is ample support for a diagnosis from many diverse background, behavioral, and test-related (and in some cases medical) criteria, the emergence of a reasonably characteristic profile can be treated as one ingredient in the overall stack of evidence. However, the lack of a characteristic profile should not be considered as disconfirming evidence. In addition, no characteristic profile, in and of itself, should ever be used as the primary basis of a diagnostic decision. We do not even know how many normal children display similar WISC-R profiles. Furthermore . . . the extreme similarity in the relative strengths and weaknesses of the typical profiles for mentally retarded, reading-disabled, and learning-disabled children renders differential diagnosis based primarily on WISC-R subtest patterns a veritable impossibility. (pp. 204–205)

Profile analysis was intended to identify intraindividual strengths and weaknesses—a process known as *ipsative interpretation*. In an ipsative interpretation, the individual client was used as his or her own normative standard, as opposed to making comparisons to the national normative

TABLE 2.6. Bannatyne's Recategorization of WISC Subtests

Spatial	Conceptualization	Sequencing	Acquired knowledge
Block Design	Vocabulary	Digit Span	Information
Object Assembly	Similarities	Coding	Arithmetic
Picture Completion	Comprehension	Arithmetic	Vocabulary
		Picture Arrangement	

sample. However, such seemingly intuitive practices as comparing individual subtest scores to the unique mean subtest score and comparing pairs of subtest scores are fraught with measurement problems. The clinical interpretation literature often fails to mention the poor reliability of a *difference score* (i.e., the difference between two subtest scores). Anastasi (1985) has reminded clinicians that the standard error of the difference between two scores is larger than the standard error of measurement of the two scores being compared. Thus interpretation of a 3- or 5-point difference between two subtest scores becomes less dependable for hypothesis generation or making conclusions about an individual's cognitive abilities. Another often-cited problem with ipsative interpretation is that the correlations among subtests are positive and often high, suggesting that individual subtests provide little differential information about a child's cognitive skills (Anastasi, 1985). Furthermore, McDermott, Fantuzzo, Glutting, Watkins, and Baggaley (1992), studying the internal and external validity of subtest strengths and weaknesses, found these measures to be wholly inferior to basic norm-referenced information.

Thus the long-standing practice of using profile analysis to draw conclusions about intraindividual strengths and weaknesses did not fare well in numerous empirical tests of its application. The lack of validity support for profile analysis remains unresolved (Kamphaus, 2009). Measurement problems remained, many of which were endemic to the type of measure used (e.g., variations on the Wechsler tradition). These validity challenges indicated the need for the fourth wave, wherein theory and measurement science became intermingled with practice considerations to enhance the validity of test score interpretation.

APPLYING THEORY TO INTELLIGENCE TESTS: THE FOURTH WAVE

Merging Research, Theory, and Intelligence Testing

Kaufman (1979) made among the first cogent arguments for the case that intelligence tests' lack of theoretical clarity and support constituted a critical issue of validity. He proposed reorganizing subtests into clusters that conformed to widely accepted theories of intelligence, thus allowing the clinician to produce more meaningful conclusions. The fourth wave has addressed intelligence test validity through the development of contemporary instruments founded in theory, and through integration of test results with multiple sources of information—hypothesis validation, as well as testing of rival hypotheses (Kamphaus, 2001).

Test Design for Interpretation

The history of intelligence test interpretation has been characterized by a disjuncture between the design of the tests and inferences made from those tests. A test, after all, should be designed a priori with a strong theoretical foundation, and supported by considerable validity evidence in order to measure a particular construct or set of constructs (and *only* those constructs). Prior to the 1990s, the interpretive process was conducted by clinicians who sometimes applied relatively subjective clinical acumen in the absence of empirically supported theoretical bases to interpret scores for their consumers. For more valid and reliable interpretation of intelligence tests, instrument improvement would now need to focus on constructing tests designed to measure a delimited and well-defined set of intelligence-related constructs.

During the second half of the 20th century, several theories of the structure of intelligence were introduced, promoting a shift to seeking theoretical support for the content of intelligence tests. Among the most significant theories have been Carroll's three-stratum theory of cognitive abilities, the Horn–Cattell fluid–crystallized (Gf-Gc) theory, the Luria–Das model of information processing, Gardner's multiple intelligences, and Sternberg's triarchic theory of intelligence (see Chapters 3–7 and the Appendix of the present volume for reviews).

Two popular theoretical models of intelligence have had the primary distinction of fostering this shift. First, the factor-analytic work of Raymond Cattell and John Horn (Horn & Cattell, 1966) describes an expanded theory founded on Cattell's (1943) constructs of *fluid intelligence* (Gf) and *crystallized intelligence* (Gc). Cattell described fluid intelligence as representing reasoning and the ability to solve novel problems, whereas crystallized intelligence was thought to constitute abilities influenced by acculturation, schooling, and language development. This fluid–crystallized distinction was supported by Horn (1988), who delineated additional contributing abilities such as visual–spatial ability, short-term memory, processing speed, and long-term retrieval.

Subsequent to this research was John Carroll's (1993) integration of findings from more than 460 factor-analytic investigations that led to the development of his three-stratum theory of intelligence. The three strata are organized by generality. Stratum III, the apex of the framework, consists of one construct only—general intelligence or *g*, the general factor that has been identified in numerous investigations as accounting for the major portion of variance assessed by intelligence test batteries. Stratum II contains eight broad cognitive abilities contributing to the general factor *g*, and is very similar to Gf-Gc abilities as described by Horn. Carroll's model proposes numerous narrow (specific) factors subsumed in stratum I. The two models are sometimes used together and are referred to in concert as the *Cattell–Horn–Carroll* (CHC) model of intelligence (see Chapters 3–4 and the Appendix in this volume).

Theory and Test Design Combined

Most modern intelligence tests are based in part or whole on a few widely accepted theories of intelligence—theories built upon and consistent with decades of factor-analytic studies of intelligence test batteries (Kamphaus, 2001). The commonality of theoretical development is demonstrated in the following brief descriptions of several widely used tests, many of which have been newly published or revised over the past few years. All are examples of a greater emphasis on theory-based test design. The intelligence tests are described in great detail in individual chapters of this book.

Among contemporary intelligence tests, the Woodcock–Johnson III (WJ III; Woodcock, McGrew, & Mather, 2001) is the instrument most closely aligned with the Cattell–Horn (Cattell, 1943; Horn, 1988; Horn & Cattell, 1966) and Carroll (1993) theories of intelligence. According to the WJ III technical manual (McGrew & Woodcock, 2001), Cattell and Horn's Gf-Gc theory was the theoretical foundation for the Woodcock–Johnson Psycho-Educational Battery—Revised (WJ-R; Woodcock & Johnson, 1989). Four years after publication of the WJ-R, Carroll's text was published; professionals interested in theories of intelligence began to think in terms of a combination or extension of theories, the CHC theory of cognitive abilities (McGrew & Woodcock, 2001). CHC theory, in turn, served as the blueprint for the WJ III. The WJ III developers designed their instrument to broadly measure seven of the eight stratum II factors from CHC theory, providing the following cognitive cluster scores:

Comprehension–Knowledge (crystallized intelligence), Long-Term Retrieval, Visual–Spatial Thinking, Auditory Processing, Fluid Reasoning (fluid intelligence), Processing Speed, and Short-Term Memory. Moreover, individual subtests are intended to measure several narrow abilities from stratum I. Finally, the General Intellectual Ability score serves as a measure of overall *g*, representing stratum III.

Similarly, the SB5 (Roid, 2003) is based on the CHC model of intelligence. The SB5 can be considered a five-factor model, in that it includes five of the broad stratum II factors having the highest loadings on *g*: Fluid Reasoning (fluid intelligence), Knowledge (crystallized knowledge), Quantitative Reasoning (quantitative knowledge), Visual–Spatial Processing (visual processing), and Working Memory (short-term memory). Among these factors, Visual–Spatial Processing is new to this revision—an attempt to enrich the nonverbal measures of the SB5, aiding in the identification of children with spatial talents and deficits. Moreover, the SB5 is constructed to provide a strong nonverbal IQ by creating nonverbal measures for all five factors.

The Wechsler Intelligence Scale for Children—Fourth Edition (WISC-IV; Wechsler, 2003) also emphasizes a stratified approach by replacing the VIQ and PIQ dichotomy with the four factor-based index scores that were supplemental in previous editions. The Index scores have been retitled to more accurately reflect the new theoretical structure, as well as new subtests introduced in this version. For example, the Perceptual Organization Index from the WISC-III has evolved into the Perceptual Reasoning Index, with new subtests designed to assess fluid reasoning abilities while reducing the effects of timed performance and motor skills. The controversial Freedom from Distractibility Index has become the Working Memory Index, reflecting research demonstrating working memory's essential role in fluid reasoning, learning, and achievement (Fry & Hale, 1996). Ten subtests contribute to the four index scores, which in turn contribute to the FSIQ; however, the primary focus of interpretation is on the index scores.

The Reynolds Intellectual Assessment Scales (RIAS; Reynolds & Kamphaus, 2003) battery exemplifies this movement to design intelligence tests on the basis of current theory and research, as well as for ease of interpretation. The following paragraphs use the RIAS to demonstrate a theoretical approach that supports modern intelligence test construction and interpretation.

The factor-analytic work of Carroll (1993) informed the creation of the RIAS by demonstrating many of the latent traits assessed by intelligence test were test-battery-independent. The RIAS focuses on the assessment of stratum III and stratum II abilities from Carroll's three-stratum theory. The RIAS is designed to assess four important aspects of intelligence: general intelligence (stratum Ill), verbal intelligence (stratum II, crystallized abilities), nonverbal intelligence (stratum II, visualization/spatial abilities), and memory (stratum II, working memory, short-term memory, or learning). These four constructs are assessed by combinations of the six RIAS subtests.

Although most contemporary tests of intelligence seek to measure at least some of the components from the extended Gf-Gc (Horn & Cattell, 1966) and the three-stratum (Carroll, 1993) models of intelligence, some tests based on different theories of intelligence are available. An example of an intelligence theory not aligned with Carroll's model is the *planning, attention, simultaneous, and successive* (PASS; Das, Naglieri, & Kirby, 1994) theory of cognitive functioning. The PASS theory is founded on Luria's (1966) neuropsychological model of integrated intellectual functioning, and a description of the PASS theory is presented by Naglieri, Das, and Goldstein in Chapter 7 of this volume.

Naglieri and Das (1990) have argued that traditional models of intelligence and means of assessing intelligence are limited. From the PASS theory's focus on cognitive processes, Naglieri and Das (1997) have created the Cognitive Assessment System (CAS). The PASS theory and the CAS offer an expansion of the more traditional conceptualizations of intelligence. Moreover, the CAS is a prime example of an instrument guided by theory in both development and interpretation. The four CAS scales were designed to measure the four constructs central to the theory. Hence the composite scales are labeled Planning, Attention, Simultaneous, and Successive. For those who subscribe to a Gf-Gc theory or a more traditional approach to the assessment of intelligence, the interpretation of results from the CAS may seem awkward or difficult. For example, most intelligence tests include a verbal scale or a scale designed to measure crystallized intelligence. The CAS has no such scale. On the other hand, interpretation of the CAS flows directly from the theory on which it was based.

The effects of basing intelligence tests on the confluence of theory and research findings are at least threefold. First, test-specific training is of less value. Once a psychologist knows these theories, which are marked by numerous similarities, he or she can interpret most modern intelligence tests with confidence. In other words, it is now important for a clinician to understand the constructs of intelligence, as opposed to receiving specific "Wechsler" or "Binet" training. Second, pre- and postprofessional training priority shifts to sufficient knowledge of theories of intelligence that inform modern test construction and interpretation. Third, as intelligence tests seek to measure similar core constructs, they increasingly resemble commodities (Kamphaus, 2009). A psychologist's decision to use a particular test may be based not so much on differences in validity as on differences in preference; intelligence test selection can now be based on issues of administration time, availability of scoring software, packaging, price, and other convenience-oriented considerations.

Theory and Hypothesis Validation

To address the meager reliability and validity of score profiles, Kamphaus (2001) has suggested an integrative method of interpretation that has two central premises. First, intelligence test results can only be interpreted meaningfully in the context of other assessment results (e.g., clinical findings, background information, and other sources of quantitative and qualitative information). Second, all interpretations made should be supported by research evidence and theory. Presumably, these two premises should mitigate against uniform interpretations that do not possess validity for a particular case (i.e., standard interpretations that are applied to case data but are at odds with information unique to an individual), as well as against interpretations that are refuted by research findings (i.e., interpretations that are based on clinical evidence but contradicted by research findings).

Failure to integrate intelligence test results with other case data is the main culprit in flawed interpretations. Matarazzo (1990) offered the following example from a neuropsychological evaluation in which the clinician failed to integrate test results with background information:

> There is little that is more humbling to a practitioner who uses the highest one or two Wechsler subtest scores as the only index of a patient's "premorbid" level of intellectual functioning and who therefore interprets concurrently obtained lower subtest scores as indexes of clear "impairment" and who is then

shown by the opposing attorney elementary and high school transcripts that contain several global IQ scores, each of which were at the same low IQ levels as are suggested by currently obtained lowest Wechsler subtest scaled scores. (p. 1003)

To protect against such failures to integrate information, Kamphaus (2001) has advised the intelligence test user to establish a standard for integrating intelligence test results with other findings. He suggests a standard of at least two pieces of corroborating evidence for each test interpretation made. Such a standard "forces" the examiner to carefully consider other findings and information before offering conclusions. A clinician, for example, may calculate a WISC-IV FSIQ score of 84 (below average) for a young girl and conclude that she possesses below-average intelligence. Even this seemingly obvious conclusion should be corroborated by two external sources of information. If the majority of the child's achievement scores fall into this range, and her teacher reports that the child seems to be progressing more slowly than the majority of the children in her class, the conclusion of below-average intelligence has been corroborated by two sources of information external to the WISC-IV. On the other hand, if this child has previously been diagnosed with an anxiety disorder, and if both her academic achievement scores and her progress as reported by her teacher are average, the veracity of the WISC-IV scores may be in question. If she also appears highly anxious and agitated during the assessment session, the obtained scores may be even more questionable.

The requirement of research (i.e., validity) support for test-based interpretation is virtually mandatory in light of the publication of the *Standards for Educational and Psychological Testing* (American Educational Research Association, American Psychological Association, & National Council on Measurement in Education, 1999) and the increased expectations of consumers for assessment accuracy (Kamphaus, 2001). Clinical "impressions" of examiners, although salient, are no longer adequate for supporting interpretations of a child's intelligence scores (Matarazzo, 1990). Consider again the example above in which the young girl obtains a WISC-IV FSIQ score of 84. Let us assume that she has been independently found to have persistent problems with school achievement. Given the data showing the positive relationship between intelligence and achievement scores, the results seem consistent with the research literature

and lend support to the interpretation of below-average developed cognitive abilities. Should it become necessary to support the conclusion of below-average intelligence, the clinician could give testimony citing studies supporting the correlational relationship between intelligence and achievement test scores (Matarazzo, 1990).

TESTING RIVAL HYPOTHESES

Some research suggests that clinicians routinely tend to overestimate the accuracy of their conclusions. There is virtually no evidence to suggest that clinicians underestimate the amount of confidence that they have in their conclusions (Dawes, 1995). Therefore, intelligence test users should check the accuracy of their inferences by challenging them with alternative inferences.

A clinician may conclude, for example, that a client has a personal strength in verbal intelligence relative to nonverbal. An alternative hypothesis is that this inference is merely due to chance. The clinician may then use test manual discrepancy score tables to determine whether the difference between the two standard scores is likely to be reliable (i.e., statistically significant) and therefore not attributable to chance. Even if a difference is reliable, however, it may not be a "clinically meaningful" difference if it is a common occurrence in the population. Most intelligence test manuals also allow the user to test the additional hypothesis that the verbal–nonverbal score inference is reliable, but too small to be of clinical value for diagnosis or intervention, by determining the frequency of the score difference in the population. If a difference is also rare in the population, the original hypothesis (that the verbal–nonverbal difference reflects a real difference in the individual's cognitive abilities) provides a better explanation than the alternative rival hypothesis (that the verbal–nonverbal difference is not of importance) for understanding the examinee's cognitive performances.

Knowledge of theory is important above and beyond research findings, as theory allows the clinician to do a better job of conceptualizing an individual's scores. Clearer conceptualization of a child's cognitive status, for example, allows the clinician to better explain the child's test results to parents, teachers, colleagues, and other consumers of the test findings. Parents will often want to know the etiology of the child's scores. They will question, "Is it my fault for not reading to her?" or

"Did he inherit this problem? My father had the same problems in school." Without adequate theoretical knowledge, clinicians will find themselves unprepared to give reasonable answers to such questions.

CONCLUSIONS

In this chapter, we have presented several overarching historical approaches to the interpretation of intelligence tests. For heuristic purposes, these approaches are portrayed as though they were entirely separate in their inception, development, and limitations. In the reality of clinical practice, however, much overlap exists. Moreover, aspects of each of these approaches continue to date. For example, since Spearman's (1927) publication of findings in support of a central ability underlying performance on multiple tasks, clinicians typically have interpreted a single general intelligence score. Most intelligence tests yield a general ability score, and research continues to provide evidence for the role of a general ability or g factor (McDermott & Glutting, 1997). In Carroll's (1993) hierarchical theory, g remains at the apex of the model. Therefore, the ongoing practice of interpreting this factor seems warranted, and elements of what we describe as the first wave remain. At the same time, clinicians continue to consider an individual's profile of scores. For the most part, the days of making psychiatric diagnoses or predictions of psychiatric symptoms on the basis of intelligence test scores as Rapaport and his colleagues (1945–1946) suggested are past, but profiles are still discussed—that is, in terms of ability profiles related to achievement or educational outcomes.

Furthermore, as was the case in what we describe as the third wave, results from psychometric analyses still inform and guide our interpretations. Now, however, they are also integrated into broad descriptions and theories of intelligence. Carroll's theory is the result of factor-analytic research, and writers have labeled many of the dominant theories of intelligence as *psychometric* in their approach (Neisser et al., 1996). Thus we see the progress in the area of intellectual assessment and interpretation as an evolution, rather than a series of disjointed starts and stops. This evolution has culminated in the integration of empirical research, theory development, and test design, resulting in more accurate and meaningful test interpretation.

What Will Be the Fifth Wave of Intelligence Test Interpretation?

Of course, the substance and direction of the next wave in intelligence test interpretation remain unknown. What seems safe to predict is that ongoing educational reform and public policy mandates will continue to shape intellectual assessment and their associated interpretations. The influence of educational needs and public policy were present when the first formal intelligence tests were introduced over a century ago, and their influence has not abated.

We hypothesize that the next wave will focus on the publication of new tests with stronger evidence of content validity; if the ultimate purpose of intelligence testing is to sample behavior representing a construct and then to draw inferences about that construct, the process of interpretation is limited by the clarity of the construct(s) being measured. It may also be time to apply a broader concept of *content validity* to intelligence test interpretation (e.g., Flanagan & McGrew, 1997). Cronbach (1971) suggested such an expansion of the term more than four decades ago, observing:

> Whether the operations that finally constitute the test correspond to the specified universe is the question of content validity. It is so common in education to identify "content" with the subject matter of the curriculum that the broader application of the word here must be stressed. (p. 452)

The nature–nurture debate in intelligence testing will continue to fade, thanks to findings indicating that cognitive ability is essentially "developed" through experience (Hart & Risley, 1995). Although the use of the term *IQ* has lessened, it is still popular among the general public. It has been replaced by terms such as *cognitive ability* and others, which have indirectly muted debates about the "excessive meanings" that have accompanied the IQ score, particularly its "native ability" interpretation among some segments of the public. It may now be time, in light of recent evidence, to adopt Anastasi's (1988) preferred term of long ago: *developed cognitive ability*.

We will also be likely to interpret intelligence tests in a more evidence-based manner. The evidence for the overall intelligence test score yielded by measures of developed cognitive ability is among the most impressive in the social sciences. Lubinski (2004) summarizes some enduring findings:

Measures of *g* covary .70–.80 with academic achievement measures, .70 with military training assignments, .20–.60 with work performance (correlations are moderated by job complexity), .30–.40 with income, and −.20 with unlawfulness. General intelligence covaries .40 with SES of origin and .50–.70 with achieved SES. As well, assortative mating correlations approach .50. These correlations indicate that *g* is among the most important individual differences dimensions for structuring the determinants of Freud's two-component characterization of life, *lieben* and *arbeiten*, working and loving (or resource acquisition and mating). (p. 100)

As intelligence tests incorporate current research-based theories of intelligence into their design, psychological interpretations will become ever more valid. This trend will be modified as changes occur in intelligence-testing technology, fostered by breakthrough theories (e.g., neurological) or empirical findings. Although it is difficult to draw inferences about the vast and somewhat undefined "universe" of cognitive functioning, it is also *de rigueur*. Psychologists make such interpretations about the complex universe of human behavior and functioning on a daily basis. The emergence of tests that better measure well-defined constructs will allow psychologists to provide better services to their clients than were possible even a decade ago.

ACKNOWLEDGMENTS

We would like to express our gratitude to Martha D. Petoskey and Anna W. Morgan for their contributions to the first edition of this chapter.

REFERENCES

American Educational Research Association, American Psychological Association, and National Council on Measurement in Education. (1999). *Standards for educational and psychological testing*. Washington, DC: American Educational Research Association.

Anastasi, A. (1985). Interpreting results from multiscore batteries. *Journal of Counseling and Development, 64,* 84–86.

Anastasi, A. (1988). *Psychological testing* (6th ed.). New York: Macmillan.

Bannatyne, A. (1974). Diagnosis: A note on recategorization of the WISC scale scores. *Journal of Learning Disabilities, 7,* 272–274.

Binet, A., & Simon, T. (1905). Methodes nouvelles pour le diagnostic du niveau intellectuel des anormaux [A new method for the diagnosis of the intellectual level of abnormal persons]. *L'Année Psychologique, 11,* 191–244.

Boring, E. G. (1929). *A history of experimental psychology*. New York: Century.

Carroll, J. B. (1993). *Human cognitive abilities: A survey of factor-analytic studies*. New York: Cambridge University Press.

Cattell, R. B. (1943). The measurement of adult intelligence. *Psychological Bulletin, 40,* 153–193.

Cohen, J. (1959). The factorial structure of the WISC at ages 7-6, 10-6, and 13-6. *Journal of Consulting Psychology, 23,* 285–299.

Cronbach, L. J. (1971). Test validation. In R. L. Thorndike (Ed.), *Educational measurement* (2nd ed., pp. 443–506). Washington, DC: American Council on Education.

Das, J. P., Naglieri, J. A., & Kirby, J. R. (1994). *Assessment of cognitive processes: The PASS theory of intelligence*. Needham Heights, MA: Allyn & Bacon.

Dawes, R. M. (1995). Standards of practice. In S. C. Hayes, V. M. Vollette, R. M. Dawes, & K. E. Grady (Eds.), *Scientific standards of psychological practice: Issues and recommendations* (pp. 31–43). Reno, NV: Context Press.

Flanagan, D. P., & McGrew, K. S. (1997). A cross-battery approach to assessing and interpreting cognitive abilities: Narrowing the gap between practice and cognitive science. In D. P. Flanagan, J. L. Genshaft, & P. L. Harrison (Eds.), *Contemporary intellectual assessment: Theories, tests, and issues* (pp. 314–325). New York: Guilford Press.

French, J. L., & Hale, R. L. (1990). A history of the development of psychological and educational testing. In C. R. Reynolds & R. W. Kamphaus (Eds.), *Handbook of psychological and educational assessment of children* (pp. 3–28). New York: Guilford Press.

Fry, A. F., & Hale, S. (1996). Processing speed, working memory and fluid intelligence: Evidence for a developmental cascade. *Psychological Science, 7*(4), 237–241.

Goodenough, F. L. (1949). *Mental testing: Its history, principles, and applications*. New York: Rinehart.

Hart, B., & Risley, T. R. (1995). *Meaningful differences in the everyday experience of young American children*. Baltimore: Brookes.

Horn, J. L. (1988). Thinking about human abilities. In J. R. Nesselroade & R. B. Cattell (Eds.), *Handbook of multivariate psychology* (2nd ed., pp. 645–865). New York: Academic Press.

Horn, J. L., & Cattell, R. B. (1966). Refinement and

test of the theory of fluid and crystallized general intelligences. *Journal of Educational Psychology, 57,* 253–270.

Kamphaus, R. W. (2001). *Clinical assessment of children's intelligence.* Needham Heights, MA: Allyn & Bacon.

Kamphaus, R. W. (2009). Assessment of intelligence and achievement. In T. B. Gutkin & C. R. Reynolds (Eds.), *The handbook of school psychology* (4th ed., pp. 230-246). Hoboken, NJ: Wiley.

Kaufman, A. S. (1979). *Intelligent testing with the WISC-R.* New York: Wiley-Interscience.

Kaufman, A. S. (1990). *Assessing adolescent and adult intelligence.* Needham Heights, MA: Allyn & Bacon.

Levine, A. J., & Marks, L. (1928). *Testing intelligence and achievement.* New York: Macmillan.

Lubinski, D. (2004). Introduction to the special section on cognitive abilities: 100 years after Spearman's (1904) "'General Intelligence,' Objectively Determined and Measured." *Journal of Personality and Social Psychology, 86*(1), 96–199.

Luria, A. R. (1966). *Human brain and higher psychological processes.* New York: Harper & Row.

Matarazzo, J. D. (1990). Psychological assessment versus psychological testing?: Validation from Binet to the school, clinic, and courtroom. *American Psychologist, 45*(9), 999–1017.

Matheson, D. W., Mueller, H. H., & Short, R. H. (1984). The validity of Bannatyne's acquired knowledge category as a separate construct. *Journal of Psychoeducational Assessment, 2,* 279–291.

McDermott, P. A., Fantuzzo, J. W., Glutting, J. J., Watkins, M. W., & Baggaley, A. R. (1992). Illusions of meaning in the ipsative assessment of children's ability. *Journal of Special Education, 25,* 504–526.

McDermott, P. A., & Glutting, J. J. (1997). Informing stylistic learning behavior, disposition, and achievement through ability subtests—or, more illusion of meaning? *School Psychology Review, 26*(2), 163–176.

McGrew, K. S., & Woodcock, R. W. (2001). *Woodcock–Johnson III technical manual.* Itasca, IL: Riverside.

Naglieri, J. A., & Das, J. P. (1990). Planning, attention, simultaneous, and successive (PASS) cognitive processes as a model for intelligence. *Journal of Psychoeducational Assessment, 8,* 303–337.

Naglieri, J. A., & Das, J. P. (1997). *Das–Naglieri Cognitive Assessment System.* Itasca, IL: Riverside.

Neisser, U., Boodoo, G., Bouchard, T. J., Boykin, A. W., Brody, N., Ceci, S. J., et al. (1996). Intelligence: Knowns and unknowns. *American Psychologist, 51,* 77–101.

Pintner, R. (1923). *Intelligence testing.* New York: Holt, Rinehart & Winston.

Rapaport, D., Gil, M., & Schafer, R. (1945–1946). *Diagnostic psychological testing* (2 vols.). Chicago: Year Book Medical.

Reynolds, C. R., & Kamphaus, R. W. (2003). *Reynolds Intellectual Assessment Scales.* Lutz, FL: Psychological Assessment Resources.

Roid, G. H. (2003). *Stanford–Binet Intelligence Scales, Fifth Edition.* Itasca, IL: Riverside.

Spearman, C. (1927). *The abilities of man.* New York: Macmillan.

Terman, L. M. (1916). *The measurement of intelligence: An explanation and a complete guide for the use of the Stanford revision and extensions of the Binet–Simon Intelligence Scale.* Boston: Houghton Mifflin.

Terman, L. M., & Merrill, M. A. (1937). *Measuring intelligence: A guide to the administration of the new Revised Stanford–Binet Tests of Intelligence.* Boston: Houghton Mifflin.

Wechsler, D. (1939). *The measurement of adult intelligence.* Baltimore: Williams & Wilkins.

Wechsler, D. (1944). *The measurement of adult intelligence* (3rd ed.). Baltimore: Williams & Wilkins.

Wechsler, D. (1949). *Wechsler Intelligence Scale for Children.* San Antonio, TX: Psychological Corporation.

Wechsler, D. (1958). *The measurement and appraisal of adult intelligence* (4th ed.). Baltimore: Williams & Wilkins.

Wechsler, D. (1974). *Wechsler Intelligence Scale for Children—Revised.* New York: Psychological Corporation.

Wechsler, D. (1991). *Wechsler Intelligence Scale for Children—Third Edition.* San Antonio, TX: Psychological Corporation.

Wechsler, D. (2003). *Wechsler Intelligence Scale for Children—Fourth Edition.* San Antonio, TX: Psychological Corporation.

Woodcock, R. W., & Johnson, M. B. (1989). *Woodcock–Johnson Psycho-Educational Battery—Revised.* Allen, TX: DLM Teaching Resources.

Woodcock, R. W., McGrew, K. S., & Mather, N. (2001). *Woodcock–Johnson III.* Itasca, IL: Riverside.

PART II

CONTEMPORARY THEORETICAL PERSPECTIVES

CHAPTER 3

Foundations for Better Understanding of Cognitive Abilities

John L. Horn
A. Nayena Blankson

PURPOSES AND PROVISOS

The extended theory of fluid and crystallized (Gf and Gc) cognitive abilities is wrong, of course, even though it may be the best account we currently have of the organization and development of abilities thought to be indicative of human intelligence. All scientific theory is wrong. It is the job of science to improve theory. That requires identifying what is wrong with it and finding out how to change it to make it more nearly correct. That is what we try to do in this chapter. First, we lay out the current theory. Then we indicate major things that we think are wrong with it. We end by suggesting some lines of research that may lead to improvement of the theory.

In laying out the theory, we speak of what we think we know. We say that something is known if there is evidence to support the claim that it is known. Since such evidence is never fully adequate or complete, we do not imply that what we say "is known" is really (*really*) known to be true. We do not provide full critiques to indicate why what we say is not necessarily true, but we provide provisos and cautions, and put research in a context such that major limitations can be seen.

Since the publication of the second edition of this text, John L. Horn has passed away. The present chapter is therefore a reprint of the chapter in the second edition.

Among the provisos are some we can point to immediately in this introduction.

First, because we depend on developmental evidence to a considerable extent, we point out that research on the development of human abilities is seriously lacking in major features of design required for strong inference about cause and effect. None of the research employs a controlled, manipulative (experimental) design in which age, genes, gender, or any of a host of other quite relevant independent variables are randomly assigned. Such design is, of course, impossible in studies of human development. But the fact that it is impossible does not correct for its limitations. The design is weak. Many relevant independent variables, including age, are confounded. Effects cannot be isolated. For this reason, what we say "is known" can only be a judgment call.

A second major proviso stems from the fact that most of the research we refer to as indicating "what is known about development" is cross-sectional. This means that usually we are referring to findings of age differences, not findings of age changes. Age differences may suggest age changes, but they do not establish them. Yet we speak of such differences in ways that imply that they indicate age changes. Our statements of "what is known" are judgments based on such incomplete evidence.

A third proviso stems from the fact that almost all the results we review are derived from averages calculated across measures, not on changes within individuals. This is no less true of the findings from repeated-measures longitudinal research than of the findings from cross-sectional research. It means that the evidence is not directly indicative of change within persons.

This is a rather subtle point, often not well recognized. It is worthwhile to take a moment to consider it in more detail. To do this, look at a simple example that illustrates the problem.

Suppose $N1$ people increase in an ability by $k1$ units from age $A1$ to $A2$, while $N2$ people decrease $k2$ in this ability over the same age period; assume no error. If $N1 = N2$ and $k1 = k2$, the net effect of averaging the measures at $A1$ and $A2$ is zero, which fosters the clearly wrong conclusion that there is no change. Yet this is the kind of finding on which we base our statements about what is known. Averages at different ages or times of measurement are the findings. Findings such as that of this example are regarded as indicating "no aging change." The correct conclusion is that some people have increased in the ability, while other people have decreased.

In this simple, balanced example, it is easy to see that the conclusion is incorrect. But the incorrectness of this conclusion is no less true when it is not so easily seen—as when $N1$ and $N2$ and $k1$ and $k2$ are not perfectly balanced. If there are more $N1$ people than $N2$ people, for example, and $k1$ and $k2$ are equal, then the incorrect conclusion is that the ability has increased from $A1$ to $A2$. On the other hand, if $N1$ equals $N2$ but $k2$ is larger than $k1$, the incorrect conclusion is that the ability has decreased from $A1$ to $A2$. Every other possible combination of these N's and k's is also incorrect. Most important, none of the results directly indicate what is true (assuming no error)—namely, that some people have increased in the ability and others have decreased. In regard to what is lawfully happening, it is not a matter of averaging over those who improve by $k1$ amounts and those who decline by $k2$ amounts. It's a matter of whether there is nonchance improvement and/or decline—and if so, by how much, over how long, and (most important) in relation to what variables that might indicate why. Indeed, it takes only one individual's reliable improvement in some function to disprove a generalization based on averages that the function necessarily declines.

In general, then, as we report "what is known," readers should remain aware that what we say is known may not be true. But readers should also remain aware that what we say is known may be true. The evidence of averages for groupings of individuals *may* indicate processes of age changes within individuals. The fact that such findings do not necessarily indicate such changes does not prove the opposite. Indeed, the findings provide a basis for reasonable judgments. We judge (with provisos) that most likely the averages indicate what we say is known.

What is known about human cognitive capabilities derives primarily from two kinds of research: (1) *structural research* (studies of the covariation patterns among tests designed to indicate basic features of human intelligence) and (2) *developmental research* (studies designed to indicate the ways in which cognitive capabilities develop over age). Our own particular understanding of development has derived primarily from the study of adults, but we use some evidence from research on children as well. We also use bits of evidence derived from research on genetic, neural, academic, and occupational correlates of abilities and their development.

EVIDENCE OF STRUCTURAL ORGANIZATION

The accumulated results from over 100 years of research on covariations among tests, tasks, and paradigms designed to identify fundamental features of human intelligence indicate no fewer than 87 distinct, different elementary capacities. Almost entirely, the covariation model has been one of linear relationship—and to a major extent and in the final analyses, this work has been based on a common-factor, simple-structure factor-analytic model. Thus the implicit theory has been that relationships indicating order among abilities are linear, and that a relatively small number of separate, independently distributed (although often interrelated) basic capacities account for the myriad of individual differences in abilities that thus far have been observed and measured. The findings of this research and the resulting structural theory are working assumptions—first approximations to the description and organization of human cognitive capacities.

The 80-some abilities indicated in this work are regarded as first-order factors among tests. They are often referred to as *primary mental abilities*. There are likely to be many more such elementary capacities, but this is the number indicated thus far by structural evidence (Carroll, 1993; Horn, 1991).

The same kind of factor-analytic evidence on

which the theory of primary abilities is based has also indicated some eight (or nine) broader, second-order factors among the primary factors.[1] Rather full descriptions of these abilities are given in Carroll (1993), Flanagan, Genshaft, and Harrison (1997), McGrew (1994), McGrew and Flanagan (1998), McGrew, Werder, and Woodcock (1991), and elsewhere in the current volume. Here we indicate the nature of these abilities and the relationships between first-order and second-order abilities in Table 3.1, with descriptions of primary abilities under headings of the second-order ability with which each primary ability is most closely associated.

Most of what is known about the development of abilities, and most theories about the nature of human intelligence, pertain to the second-order abilities. These can be described briefly as follows:

Acculturation knowledge (Gc), measured in tests indicating breadth and depth of knowledge of the language, concepts, and information of the dominant culture.

Fluid reasoning (Gf), measured in tasks requiring reasoning. It indicates capacities for identifying relationships, comprehending implications, and drawing inferences within content that is either novel or equally familiar to all.

Short-term apprehension and retrieval (SAR), also referred to as *short-term memory (Gsm)* and *working memory*. It is measured in a variety of tasks that require one to maintain awareness of elements of an immediate situation (i.e., the span of a minute or so).

Fluency of retrieval from long-term storage (TSR), also labeled *long-term memory (Glm)*. It is measured in tasks indicating consolidation for storage and tasks that require retrieval through association of information stored minutes, hours, weeks, and years before.

Processing speed (Gs), although involved in almost all intellectual tasks, is measured most purely in rapid scanning and comparisons in intellectually simple tasks in which almost all people would get the right answer if the task were not highly speeded.

Visual processing (Gv), measured in tasks involving visual closure and constancy, as well as fluency in recognizing the way objects appear in space as they are rotated and flip-flopped in various ways.

Auditory processing (Ga), measured in tasks that involve perception of sound patterns under distraction or distortion, maintaining aware-

ness of order and rhythm among sounds, and comprehending elements of groups of sounds.

Quantitative knowledge (Gq), measured in tasks requiring understanding and application of the concepts and skills of mathematics.

The structural evidence indicating that the primary abilities are parts of these distinct higher-order common factors has been obtained in samples that differ in gender, level of education, ethnicity, nationality, language, and historical period. The higher-order abilities account for the reliable individual-differences variability measured in conglomerate IQ tests and neuropsychological batteries. What is known about IQ, and what is referred to as Spearman's *g*, are known analytically in terms of the second-order abilities of which IQ and *g* are composed.

The higher-order abilities are positively correlated, but independent. Independence is indicated in a first instance by structural evidence: A best-weighted linear combination of any set of seven of the second-order abilities does not account for the reliable covariance among the elements of the eighth such ability.[2] More fundamentally, independence is indicated by evidence of distinct construct validities—that is, the evidence that measures representing different factors have different relationships with a variety of other variables (principally age, but also variables of neurology, behavioral genetics, and school and occupational performance).

This indication of structural organization of human abilities is referred to as *extended Gf-Gc theory*. This theory was derived in the first instance from Spearman's (1927) theory of a general, common *g* factor pervading all cognitive capabilities. It was modified notably by Thurstone's (1938, 1947) theory of some six or seven primary mental abilities. It was then altered by Cattell's (1941, 1957, 1971) recognition that while the Thurstone primary abilities were positively correlated and this positive manifold might indicate Spearman's *g*, still the general factor did not describe the evidence; there had to be at least two independent and broad common factors—Gf and Gc—because some of the abilities thought to indicate the *g* factor were associated in quite different ways with neurological damage and aging in adulthood. The extended theory then grew out of Cattell's theory, as evidence accumulated to indicate that two broad abilities did not represent relationships for visual, auditory, and basic memory functions. Abilities in these domains, too, were associated in

TABLE 3.1. Primary Abilities Described under Headings Indicating Second-Order Abilities

Primary ability label		Description
Gv: Visualization and spatial orientation abilities		
Vz	Visualization	Mentally manipulate forms to "see" how they would look under altered conditions
S	Spatial orientation	Visually imagine parts out of place and put them in place (e.g., solve jigsaw puzzles)
Cs	Speed of closure	Identify Gestalt when parts of the whole are missing—Gestalt closure
Cf	Flexibility of closure	Find a particular figure embedded within distracting lines and figures
Ss	Spatial planning	Survey a spatial field to find a path through it (e.g., pencil mazes)
Xa	Figural flexibility	Try out possible arrangements of visual pattern to find one that satisfies conditions
Le	Length estimation	Estimate length of distances between points
DFI	Figural fluency	Produce different figures, using the lines of a stimulus figure
DFS	Seeing illusions	Report illusions in such tests as the Muller–Lyer, Sanders, and Poggendorf
Ga: Abilities of listening and hearing		
ACV	Auditory comprehend	Demonstrate understanding of oral communications
TT	Temporal tracking	Demonstrate understanding of sequencing in sounds (e.g., reorder sets of tones)
AR	Auditory relations	Demonstrate understanding of relations among tones (e.g., identify notes of a chord)
TP	Identify tone patterns	Show awareness of differences in arrangements of tones
RYY	Judging rhythms	Identify and continue a beat
AMS	Auditory span memory	Immediately recall a set of notes played once
DS	Hear distorted speech	Show understanding of speech that has been distorted in different ways
Gc: Acculturational knowledge abilities		
V	Verbal comprehension	Demonstrate understanding of words, sentences, paragraphs
Se	Seeing problems	Suggest ways to deal with problems (e.g., fix a toaster)
Rs	Syllogistic reasoning	Given stated premises, draw logical conclusions even when nonsensical
VSI	Verbal closure	Show comprehension of sentences when parts are missing—verbal Gestalt
CBI	Behavioral relations	Judge interaction between persons to estimate how one feels about a situation
Mk	Mechanical knowledge	Identify tools, equipment, principles for solving mechanical problems
Vi	General information	Indicate understanding of a wide range of information
Gf: Abilities of reasoning under novel conditions		
I	Inductive reasoning	Indicate a principle of relationships among elements
R	General reasoning	Find solutions to verbal problems
CFR	Figural relations	Solve problems of relationships among figures
CMR	Semantic relations	Demonstrate awareness of relationships among pieces of information
CSC	Semantic classification	Show how symbols do not belong in class of several symbols
CFC	Concept formation	Given several examples of a concept, identify new instances
SAR: Abilities of short-term apprehension and retrieval		
Ma	Associate memory	When presented with one element of associated pair, recall the other element
Ms	Span memory	Immediately recall sets of elements after one presentation
Mm	Meaningful memory	Immediately recall items of a meaningfully related set
MMC	Chunking memory	Immediately recall elements by categories in which they are classified
MSS	Memory for order	Immediately recall the position of an element within a set of elements
DRM	Disrupted memory	Recall last word in previous sentence after being presented with other sentences

(cont.)

TABLE 3.1. *(cont.)*

Primary ability label		Description
TSR: Abilities of long-term storage and retrieval		
DLR	Delayed retrieval	Recall material learned hours before
DMT	Originality	Produce clever expressions or interpretations (e.g., story plots)
DMC	Spontaneous flexibility	Produce diverse functions and classifications (e.g., uses of a pencil)
Fi	Ideational fluency	Produce ideas about a stated condition (e.g., lady holding a baby)
Fe	Expression fluency	Produce different ways of saying much the same thing
Fa	Association fluency	Produce words similar in meaning to a given word
Gs: Speed of thinking abilities		
P	Perceptual speed	Quickly distinguish similar but different visual patterns
CDS	Correct decision speed	Quickly find or state correct answers to easy problems
FWS	Flexible writing speed	Quickly copy printed mixed upper- and lowercase letters and words
Gq: Quantitative mathematical abilities		
CMI	Estimation	Indicate information required to solve mathematical problems
Ni	Number facility	Do basic operations of arithmetic quickly and accurately
CMS	Algebraic reasoning	Find solutions for problems that can be framed algebraically

notably different ways with genetic, environmental, biological, and developmental variables. The two-factor theory had to be extended to a theory of several dimensions, as suggested by the listings above and in Table 3.1.

The broad abilities appear to represent behavioral organizations founded in neural structures and functions. The abilities are realized through a myriad of learning and biological/genetic influences operating over the course of a lifetime. Although there are suggestions that some of the abilities are somewhat more related to genetic determinants than are others, the broad patterns do not define a clean distinction between genetic and environmental determinants. Each broad ability involves learning, and is manifested as a consequence of many factors that can affect learning over years of development. Similarly, each ability is affected by genetic factors, as these can be expressed at different times throughout development. More detailed and scholarly accounts of the structural evidence are provided in Carroll (1993), Cattell (1971), Detterman (1993), Flanagan and colleagues (1997), Horn (1998), Masunaga and Horn (2000), McArdle, Hamagami, Meredith, and Bradway (2001), McArdle and Woodcock (1998), McGrew (1994), McGrew and Flanagan (1998), McGrew and colleagues (1991), and Perfect and Maylor (2000).

DEVELOPMENTAL EVIDENCE

The structural evidence indicates what is associated with what. The developmental evidence indicates what is correlated with age.[3] The structural evidence—showing how abilities indicate distinct factors—has informed the design of developmental research aimed at identifying how abilities relate to age. Variables that correlate to indicate a factor should relate to age in a manner indicating that they represent the same function or process. Similarly, the evidence indicating how different abilities correlate with age has informed the design of structural studies. Variables that change together over age should correlate to indicate the same factor. To the extent that variables both correlate to indicate the same factor and change together to indicate the same function, the two lines of evidence converge to provide evidence of cognitive processes. For the most part, this is the kind of evidence that has produced extended Gf-Gc theory. To a lesser extent, the theory is based on evidence derived from studies of behavioral-genetic and neurological relationships.

The second-order abilities of structural research are positively correlated. This suggests that there must be some higher-order organization among them. It is widely believed that this higher-order organization must be Spearman's g, or something very like it (Jensen, 1998). It turns out, however, that this is not a good explanation of the evidence. The interrelationships among the second-order abilities and their relationships with indicators of development and neurological functioning do not indicate a single factor. Rather, they suggest something along the following lines:

1. *Vulnerable abilities.* Gf, SAR, and Gs constitute a cluster of abilities to which much of Spearman's theory does indeed apply—in particular, his descriptions of capacities for apprehension and the education of relations and correlates. The abilities of this cluster are interrelated and associated in much the same way with variables indicating neurological, genetic, and aging effects.

2. *Expertise abilities.* Gc, TSR, and Gq constitute a cluster of abilities that correspond to the outcomes specified in the investment hypothesis of Cattell's theory of fluid and crystallized intelligence. It turns out that what Cattell described in investment theory is largely the same as what is described as the development of expertise in cognitive capabilities (which can be distinguished from various other kinds of expertise and from expertise in general). An important new twist on this integration of theory is recognition of new abilities in this cluster that in some ways parallel the abilities of the vulnerable cluster, but are developmentally independent of the vulnerable abilities. These new abilities differ from the vulnerable abilities not only in terms of structural relationships, but also in terms of their relationships to learning and socialization determinants. It is hypothesized that they have different relationships, also, with neurological, genetic, and aging influences.

3. *Sensory-perceptual abilities.* Mainly, the evidence in this case indicates that the abilities defining Gv and Ga are distinct from the other two clusters. They have some of the qualities of the vulnerable abilities, but they also have qualities of the expertise abilities; their relationships do not put them clearly in either class. More than this, they are closely linked to sensory modalities and appear to represent particular characteristics, strengths, and weaknesses of these modalities.

Most of the developmental evidence of which we speak derives from studies of adulthood. To a very considerable extent, this research has been directed at describing declines, and the findings consistent with this view are for the abilities of Gf, Gs, and SAR. Almost incidentally, the research directed at identifying adulthood declines has adduced evidence of age-related improvements and maintenance of some abilities; the findings in this case are primarily in respect to the abilities of Gc, TSR, and Gq. The aging curves for the sensory-perceptual abilities generally fall between those for the vulnerable and expertise abilities—not declining as early, as regularly, or as much as the former, and not improving as consistently or as much as the latter. Also, the declines in sensory-perceptual abilities often can be linked directly to declines in a sensory modality or damage to a particular function of the neural system.

The research producing the developmental evidence has been both cross-sectional and longitudinal. Although these two kinds of research have different strengths and weaknesses, and control for and reveal different kinds of influences, in studies of abilities they have most often led to very similar conclusions (Schaie, 1996). The results differ somewhat in detail—the average age at which plateaus and declines in development are reached,[4] for example—but as concerns which abilities decline and which improve and the general phases of development through which such changes occur, the evidence of repeated-measures longitudinal and cross-sectional research is essentially the same. In the following section, we summarize this evidence within an explanatory framework.

Research of the future should probably be directed at understanding abilities that are maintained or that improve with age in adulthood, and our thought is that expertise abilities in particular should be most carefully studied. To provide perspective for this view, we first review evidence on abilities that do not decline, or decline little and late in adulthood, and then consider the more extensive evidence and theory pertaining to aging decline.

Capabilities for Which There Is Little or No Aging Decline

The results indicating improvement and maintenance of abilities has come largely from the same studies in which evidence of aging decline was sought and found. The two most prominent kinds of abilities for which there is replicated evidence of improvement in adulthood are those of Gc (indicating breadth of knowledge of the dominant culture) and those of TSR (indicating fluency in retrieval of information from this store of knowledge).

Gc: Knowledge

The abilities of Gc are often referred to in efforts to specify what is most important about human intelligence. They are indicative of the intelligence of a culture, inculcated into individuals through systematic influences of acculturation. The range of such abilities is large. No particular battery of tests is known to sample the entire range. The sum of the achievement tests of the Woodcock–Johnson Psycho-Educational Battery—Revised (WJ-R) has probably provided the most nearly representative measure. The Verbal IQ of the Wechsler Adult Intelligence Scales (WAIS) has been a commonly used estimate. Indicators of the factor are measures of vocabulary, esoteric analogies, listening comprehension, and knowledge in the sciences, social studies, and humanities. Such measures correlate substantially with socioeconomic status, amount and quality of education, and other indicators of acculturation.

On average, through most of adulthood, there is increase with age in Gc knowledge (e.g., Botwinick, 1978; Cattell, 1971; Harwood & Naylor, 1971; Horn, 1998; Horn & Cattell, 1967; Horn & Hofer, 1992; Kaufman, 1990; Rabbitt & Abson, 1991; Schaie, 1996; Stankov & Horn, 1980; Woodcock, 1995). Results from some studies suggest improvement into the 80s (e.g., Harwood & Naylor, 1971, for WAIS Information, Comprehension, and Vocabulary). Such declines as are indicated show up in the averages late in adulthood—age 70 and beyond—and are small (Schaie, 1996). If differences in years of formal education are statistically controlled for, the increment of Gc with advancing age is increased (Horn, 1989; Kaufman, 1990).

TSR: Tertiary Storage and Retrieval

Two different kinds of measures indicate TSR abilities. Both kinds of indicators involve encoding and consolidation of information in long-term storage, and both involve fluency of retrieval from that storage. The parameters of association that characterize encoding and consolidation also characterize retrieval (Bower, 1972, 1975; Estes, 1974).

The first kind of test to identify TSR involves retrieval through association over periods of time that range from a few minutes to a few hours or longer. The time lapse must be sufficient to ensure that consolidation occurs, for this is what distinguishes these measures from indicators of SAR. For example, if a paired-associates test were to be used to measure the factor, recall would need to be obtained at least 5 minutes after presentation of the stimuli; if recall were obtained immediately after presentation, the test would measure SAR.

The second kind of test indicates associations among pieces of information that would have been consolidated and stored in a system of categories (as described by Broadbent, 1966) in the distant past, not just a few hours earlier. In a word association test, for example, an individual provides words similar in meaning to a given word. The person accesses an association category of information and pulls information from that category into a response mode.

Tests to measure TSR may be given under time limits, but these limits must be generous, so that subjects have time to drain association categories. If given under highly speeded conditions, the tests will measure cognitive speed (Gs), not TSR.

The retrieval of TSR is from the knowledge store of Gc, but facility in retrieval is independent of measures of Gc—independent in the sense that the correlation between TSR and Gc is well below their respective internal consistencies, and in the sense that they have different patterns of correlations with other variables.

For TSR abilities, as for Gc, the research results usually indicate improvement or no age differences throughout most of adulthood (Horn, 1968; Horn & Cattell, 1967; Horn & Noll, 1994, 1997; Schaie, 1996; Stankov & Horn, 1980; Woodcock, 1995).

Abilities That Decline with Age

Research on human abilities initially focused on infancy and childhood development and was directed at identifying abilities that characterize the intelligence of the human species. Research on adults focused from the start on abilities that, it was feared, declined with age in adulthood, and the abilities considered were those that had been identified in research on children. This research did not seek to identify abilities that characterize the intelligence of adults. That focus shifted a bit with the discovery that some of the abilities identified in childhood research improved with age in adulthood. In recent years the emphasis has shifted somewhat yet again, with recognition that cognitive expertise emerges in adulthood. Even today, however, the predominant view of human intelligence is that it is something that develops primarily only in childhood and declines with age in adulthood. The predominant view is that human intelligence is best characterized by the vulnerable abilities—Gf, SAR, and Gs.

The term *vulnerable* to characterize the Gf, SAR, and Gs abilities was adopted largely because the averages for these abilities were found to decrease with age in adulthood and to decline irreversibly with deleterious neurological and physiological changes—such as those that occur when high fever persists, or blood pressure drops to low levels, or anoxia is induced (as by alcoholic inebriation), or parts of the brain are infected or damaged (as by stroke). When it was found that in the same persons in whom vulnerable abilities declined, there were other abilities that improved (as in the case of adulthood aging) or either did not decline or the decline was reversible (as in the case of brain damage), the term *maintained* was coined to characterize these abilities—largely those of Gc, TSR, and Gq. What the research findings indicate is that when there is damage to particular parts of the brain (as in stroke), these abilities either do not decline (depending on the ability and where the damage is), or if there is decline, it is relatively small and does not persist. Thus the terms *vulnerable* and *maintained* signal a finding that in groups of people in whom some abilities decline, other abilities do not, and still other abilities improve. Though we must keep in mind that the findings are for averages, the suggestion is that within each of us some abilities are declining, others are being maintained, and some are improving. We have some reasonable ideas about "what" the vulnerable and maintained abilities are; we have less clear ideas about "why."

The findings are consistent in indicating that Gf, SAR, and Gs abilities are interrelated in a manner that calls for them to be considered together: Over most of the period of adulthood and in respect to many malfunctions of the central nervous system, there is decline in all three classes of abilities. Some notable differences, however, distinguish the three vulnerable abilities from one another.

Gf: Fluid Reasoning

The age-related decline in the Gf abilities is seen with measures of syllogisms and concept formation (McGrew et al., 1991); in reasoning with metaphors and analogies (Salthouse, 1987; Salthouse, Kausler, & Saults, 1990); with measures of comprehending series, as in letter series, figural series, and number series (Noll & Horn, 1998; Salthouse et al., 1990); and with measures of mental rotation, figural relations, matrices, and topology (Cattell,

1979). In each case, the decline is indicated most clearly if the elements of the test problems are novel—such that no advantage is given to people with more knowledge of the culture, more information, or better vocabulary.

The Gf abilities represent a kind of opposite to the Gc abilities: Whereas measures of Gc indicate the extent to which the knowledge of the culture has been incorporated by the individual, measures of Gf indicate abilities that depend minimally on knowledge of the culture.

But the feature that most clearly distinguishes the Gf abilities from the other vulnerable abilities is reasoning. All of the measures that most clearly define the Gf factor require, in one sense or another, reasoning. This is not to say that other measures do not fall on the factor, but it is to say that those other measures fall on other factors and are not the sine qua non of Gf. This will be seen more clearly as we consider how other abilities can account for some but not all of the reliable developmental changes in Gf.

SAR: Short-Term Memory

Memory is one of the most thoroughly studied constructs in psychology. There are many varieties of memory. The SAR factor indicates covariability among most of the many rather distinct kinds of short-term memory. This is the form of memory that has been most intensively studied in psychology.

There are two principal features of short-term memory. One is that it is memory over retrieval and recognition periods of less than 2 minutes. Retrieval and recognition over longer periods of time bring in other factors (largely the TSR factor), which we discuss later. The second feature is that it is memory for largely unrelated material; that is, most people usually do not have a logical system for organizing of—or making sense out of—the elements to be remembered. We have more to say about this later, too, particularly when we discuss expertise.

Over and above these two distinguishing characteristics of SAR, there is considerable heterogeneity among the various different short-term memory indicators of the factor. The different indicators have somewhat different relations to age in adulthood, for example, and thus are indicative of different aspects of a short-term memory function. It's as if SAR were an organ—say, analogous to the heart—in which different parts are more and less susceptible to the ravages of age. It is rather as if the right auricle of the heart were more susceptible than the left auricle to damages produced by coarctation of the aorta (which, indeed, is true).

Clang Memory

One notable way in which these different indicators of short-term memory are distinguished is in respect to the period of time over which retrieval or recognition is required. Characterized in this way, short-term memory ranges from apprehension (retrieval after milliseconds) (Sperling, 1960) to very short-term memory (recency), to somewhat longer short-term memory (primacy), to short-term span memory (retrieval after as much as a minute), and to what we have referred to above as not being short-term, and not indicating the SAR factor at all, but rather intermediate-term memory (retrieval after 2–10 minutes) and long-term memory (Atkinson & Shiffrin, 1968; Waugh & Norman, 1965—retrieval after hours, days, weeks, months, years). The intermediate-term and long-term kinds of memory indicate TSR, not SAR. The TSR factor does not decline with age in adulthood. Its correlates with other variables are generally different from those of SAR.

Recency and primacy are serial-position memory functions. These have been studied in considerable detail (Glanzer & Cunitz, 1966). *Recency* is memory for the last elements in a string of elements presented over time. It dissipates quickly; if there is delay of as much as 20 seconds, it is usually absent in most people. *Primacy* is memory for the first elements in a string of elements (retention being somewhat longer—30 seconds). Primacy seems to be an early indication of the consolidation that can lead to long-term memory. There is some aging decline in both recency and primacy, but the decline is small.

The total forward memory span encompasses both primacy and recency, and also the memory for elements in between the first and the last elements in a string. This component of SAR is often referred to as indicating a "magical number seven plus or minus two" (Miller, 1956). Most of us are able to remember only about seven things that we do not organize (i.e., unrelated things). But there are individual differences in this: Some can remember up to about nine unrelated things; others can remember only as many as five such things. The aging decline of this memory is small, too, but somewhat larger than the decline for either primacy or recency (Craik, 1977; Craik & Trehub, 1982; Horn, Donaldson, & Engstrom, 1981).

Short-Term Working Memory

Backward memory span helps define SAR, but is also often a prominent indicator of Gf. A backward span memory test requires recall of a string of elements in the reverse of the order in which they were presented (e.g., recall of a telephone number in the reverse of the order in which it would be dialed). The average span for such memory is about five elements, plus or minus two. Age-related differences in backward span memory are substantial and in this respect notably different from age-related differences in forward span memory. Not only is the age-related decline for this memory much larger than the decline for forward span memory, but also it is more correlated with the aging decline of Gf.

Backward span memory is one of several operational definitions of *short-term working* memory (STWM) (Baddeley, 1993, 1994; Carpenter & Just, 1989; Stankov, 1988). STWM is an ability to hold information in the span of immediate apprehension while doing other cognitive things, such as converting the order of things into a different order (as in backward span), searching for particular symbols, or solving problems. Another operational definition of STWM that illustrates this characteristic is a test that requires one to remember the last word in each sentence as one reads a passage of several sentences under directions to be prepared to answer questions about the passage; the measure of STWM is the number of last words recalled.

Indicators of STWM are dual-factor measures, as much related to Gf as they are to SAR. As noted, they also have larger (absolute-value) negative relationships to age (Craik, 1977; Craik & Trehub, 1982; Salthouse, 1991; Schaie, 1996).

An Exception: Expertise Wide-Span Memory (EWSM)

This is a form of short-term memory that is not indicative of SAR and that appears to increase, not decline, over much of adulthood (Ericsson & Kintsch, 1995; Masunaga & Horn, 2000, 2001). In some respects EWSM appears to be operationally the same as STWM (or even forward span memory); it is memory for a set of what can appear to be quite unrelated elements. There is a crucial difference, however: In EWSM the elements that can appear to be quite unrelated (and are quite unrelated for some people) can be seen to be related by an expert. For example, chess pieces arranged on a chessboard can seem to be quite unrelated to one who is not expert in understanding chess, but to a chess expert there can be relationships in the configuration of such pieces. Such relationships enable the expert to remember many more than merely seven plus or minus two pieces and their locations.[5] Also, such memories can be retained by experts (to varying degrees for varying levels of expertise) for much longer than a minute or two. In blindfold chess, for example, the expert retains memory for many more than seven elements for much more than 2 minutes.

Thus, EWSM does not meet the two criteria for defining SAR abilities that decline with age—namely, the criterion of short time between presentation and retrieval, and the criterion of no basis for organizing or making sense of the to-be-remembered elements. This suggests that EWSM will not be among the vulnerable abilities that irreversibly decline with age and neural damage. Indeed, evidence from recent studies suggests that if efforts to maintain expertise continue to be made in adulthood, there is no aging decline in EWSM. We return to a consideration of this matter in a later section of this chapter, when we discuss expertise in some detail.

Summary of Evidence on SAR

Thus, what we know about aging in relation to short-term apprehension and retrieval memory (SAR) is that decline is small for measures that primarily require retention over very short periods of time (i.e., measures that are largely indicative of apprehension). There are virtually no age differences for memory measured with the Sperling (1960) paradigm. The retention in this case is for a few milliseconds, but the span is relatively large—9 to 16 elements. As the amount of time one must retain a memory and the span of memory are increased, the negative relation between age and the measure of SAR increases (Cavanaugh, 1997; Charness, 1991; Craik & Trehub, 1982; Ericsson & Delaney, 1998; Gathercole, 1994; Kaufman, 1990; Salthouse, 1991; Schaie, 1996). As long as the memory measure is not a measure of working memory, however, the correlation with age never becomes terribly large: It is less than .25 for measures of reasonable reliability over an age range from young (in the 20s) to old (in the 70s) adulthood. Also, such a memory measure is not much involved in the reasoning of Gf and does not account for much of the aging decline in Gf. As a measure of SAR takes on the character of

working memory, however, the relationship of the measure to age becomes substantial—$r = .35$ and up for backward span measures of approximately the same reliability as forward span measures and over the same spread of ages—and the measure relates more to Gf and to the aging decline in Gf.

What we also know is that it is not simply the short period of presentation of elements to be remembered that defines the SAR factor; it is that coupled with the condition that the retriever has no organization system with which to make sense of the elements. When there is a system for making sense out of the presented elements, and the retriever knows and can use that system, the resulting memory is not particularly short term, nor is the span limited to seven plus or minus two. Decline with age in adulthood and decline with neurological damage may not occur, or may not occur irreversibly, with such memory. There is need for further evidence on this point.

The elements of short-term memory tasks are presented one after another under speeded conditions. It may be that speed of apprehension is partially responsible for correlations of SAR measures with other variables. To bring this possibility more fully into focus, let us turn now to a consideration of the rather complex matter of cognitive speed as it relates to aging in adulthood.

Gs: Cognitive Speed—A Link to General Factor Theories?

Most tests of cognitive abilities involve speed in one form or another—speed of apprehending, speed of decision, speed of reacting, movement speed, speed of thinking, and generally speed of behaving. Usually these different kinds of speed are mixed (confounded) in a given measure. There are positive intercorrelations among measures that are in varying degrees confounded in this manner. Generally, measures that are regarded as indicating primarily only speed per se (what we refer to as *chronometric measures*, such as reaction time and perceptual speed [Gs]) correlate positively with measures of cognitive capabilities that are not regarded as defined primarily by speed of performance (what we refer to as *cognitive capacity measures*). But there is confounding: The cognitive capacity measures require one or more of the elementary forms of speed mentioned above.

Chronometric measures have often been found to be negatively correlated with age in adulthood. There has been a great amount of research documenting these relationships and aimed at understanding just how speed is involved in human cognitive capability and aging (Birren, 1974; Botwinick, 1978; Eysenck, 1987; Hertzog, 1989; Jensen, 1987; Nettelbeck, 1994; Salthouse, 1985, 1991; Schaie, 1990).

Salthouse (1985, 1991) has provided comprehensive reviews of the evidence showing positive interrelationships among measures of speediness and negative correlation with age. The chronometric tasks that indicate these relationships are varied—copying digits, crossing off letters, comparing numbers, picking up coins, zipping a garment, unwrapping Band-Aids, using a fork, dialing a telephone number, sorting cards, digit–symbol substitution, movement time, trail making, and various measures of simple and complex reaction time. In studies in which young and old subjects were provided opportunity to practice complex reaction time tasks, practice did not eliminate the age differences, and no noteworthy age × practice interactions were found (Madden & Nebes, 1980; Salthouse & Somberg, 1982).

These kinds of findings have spawned a theory that slowing, particularly cognitive slowing, is a general feature of aging in adulthood (Birren, 1974; Kausler, 1990; Salthouse, 1985, 1991, 1992, 1993). This evidence has also been cited in support of a theory that there is a general factor of cognitive capabilities (e.g., Eysenck, 1987; Jensen, 1982, 1987, 1993; Spearman, 1927). That is, Spearman had proposed that neural speed is the underlying function governing central processes of g (his concept of general intelligence), and investigators such as Eysenck and Jensen (among many others), citing the evidence relating chronometric measures to cognitive capacity measures, have regarded the evidence as supportive of Spearman's theory. Salthouse (1985, 1991), coming at the matter primarily from the perspective of age relationships, has proposed that speed of information processing, reflecting speed of transmission in the neural system, is the essence of general intelligence.

These investigators bring a great deal of information to the table in coming to these conclusions. Still, we think that in the end they come to wrong conclusions. The evidence, when all of it is considered, does not indicate one common factor of g, the essence of which is cognitive speed. Indeed, evidence of this kind does not support a theory of one general factor of intelligence, a theory of one general factor of cognitive speed, or a theory of one general factor of aging.

The basic argument for these theories of a general factor is that the intercorrelations among reliable variables measuring that which is said to be general are all positive. One problem with this argument is that not all such intercorrelations are positive. But that's not the principal problem.[6] The problem is that even if the correlations were all positive, that evidence is not sufficient to establish a general common factor. Many, many variables are positively correlated, but that fact does not indicate one cause, or only one influence operating, or only one common factor (Horn, 1989, 2002; Thomson, 1916; Thurstone, 1947).

Research Examining Evidence for a Theory of *g*

Let us consider, first, structural evidence pertaining to a theory of *g*. This evidence indicates that many variables related to human brain function are positively correlated, both as seen within any given person and as seen in measures of individual differences. Indeed, there are many variables associated more generally with human body function that are positively correlated, and correlated with variables related to brain function. More than this, many variables of personality are positively intercorrelated and correlated with measures of brain and body functions. Indeed, positive intercorrelations are ubiquitous among between-person measures of various aspects of human function. Most of the measures of individual differences—everything from morality to simple reaction time—can (with reflection) be fitted within a quadrant of positive intercorrelations.

Thus, if the only requirement for a *g* factor is positive intercorrelations among variables, then many variables that are not abilities and not indicative of intelligence must be accepted as indicating that factor: It would be defined by a huge variety of questionnaire measures of temperament, attitudes, beliefs, values, motives, and indicators of social and ethnic classifications, as well as ability variables. Such a broad definition of a factor does not indicate the nature of human intelligence.

Spearman, both from the start (Spearman, 1904) and as his theory fully developed (Spearman, 1927), required more than simply positive intercorrelations to support his theory of *g*. The model to test the theory required that not only should the variables of *g* correlate positively; they should correlate with that common factor *alone* (i.e., they should correlate with no other common factor). Also, the different variables of a battery designed to provide evidence of the *g* factor should comprehensively represent the capabilities regarded as indicative of human intelligence. The basic capabilities were described as capacity for apprehension, capacity for education of relationships, and capacity for education of correlates. These were expected to reflect speed of neural processing and to be manifested in capabilities measured with cognitive tests designed to indicate human intelligence.

Thus, to provide evidence of the *g* factor, an investigator would need to assemble a battery of variables that together comprehensively represented human intelligence, and each variable considered on its own would have to uniquely indicate an aspect of *g*, and could not at all indicate any other common factor. The model is demanding, but it's testable. That's a beauty of Spearman's theory.

Indeed, the theory has been tested quite a number of times. There have been direct tests, in which very careful attention was given to selecting one and only one test to represent the capacities specified in the theory (Alexander, 1935; Brown & Stephenson, 1933; Burt, 1909, 1949; El Kousey, 1935; Horn, 1965, 1989; Rimoldi, 1948; Spearman, 1927, 1939). And there have been indirect tests, in which comprehensive batteries of cognitive tests hypothesized to be indicative of intelligence were submitted to common-factor analysis, and evidence of one common factor was sought at one level or another (e.g., Carroll, 1993; Cohen, 1959; Guilford, 1956; Gustafsson, 1984; Jackson, 1960; McArdle & Woodcock, 1998; Saunders, 1959; Stephenson, 1931; Thurstone, 1938; Vernon, 1950). The results from these various analyses are clear in indicating that one common factor will not suffice to represent the intercorrelations among all variables that represent the abilities thought to be indicative of human intelligence. In the direct tests, it is found that one common factor will not reproduce the intercorrelations. In the indirect tests, it is found that while one factor at a second or third order is indicated, it either is not a one-and-only-one common factor or is identical to a factor that is separate from other factors at a lower level (e.g., in Gustafsson's [1984] results).

The common factor that was separate from other factors at the second order and identical with a factor identified at the third order in Gustafsson's (1984) study was interpreted as Gf. This factor corresponds most closely to the construct Spearman described. It has been shown that it is possible to assemble indicators of this factor (reasoning, concentration, working memory, careful apprehension, and comparison speed) that very nearly satisfy the conditions of the Spearman

model: one and only one common factor (uncorrelated uniquenesses) that accounts for the variable intercorrelations (Horn, 1991, 1998). This Gf factor does not, however, account for the intercorrelations for other variables that are indicative of human intelligence—in particular, variables indicative of Gc, TSR, Ga, and Gv.

The structural evidence thus does not support a theory of *g*. The developmental evidence is even less supportive. In general, construct validation evidence is counter to a theory that human intelligence is organized in accordance with one common principle or influence. The evidence from several sources points in the direction of several distinct kinds of factors.

Many of the tests that have indicated adulthood aging decline of Gf are administered under time-limited, speeded conditions. This accounts in part for the age-related relationship usually found between Gf and Gs. However, when the confounding of cognitive speed and cognitive capability measures is reduced to a minimum (it is probably never eliminated entirely), the correlations between the two kinds of measures are not reduced to near-chance levels. Nonzero relationships remain for measures of Gs with measures of Gf and SAR (Horn et al., 1981; Horn & Noll, 1994). The relationships for simple (one-choice) reaction time measures become near zero (chance-like), but for two-choice and several-choice reaction time measures the correlation is clearly above that expected by chance.

The more any speeded measure involves complexity—in particular, the more a chronometric measure involves complexity—the higher the correlation is with other cognitive measures and with age. Simple reaction time, in which one reacts as quickly as possible to a single stimulus, correlates at a low level ($r < .20$) with most measures regarded as indicating some aspect of cognitive ability. For complex reaction time, in which one reacts as quickly as possible to one or another of several stimuli, the correlations with cognitive ability measures increase systematically with increases in the number of different stimuli and patterns of stimuli one needs to take into account before reacting (Jensen, 1987).

The aging decline in Gf can be clearly identified with tests that minimize speed of performance—provided (and this is important) that the tests have a high ceiling of difficulty in the sample of people under investigation, and thus that score on the test is a measure of the level of difficulty of the problems solved, not a measure of the speed of obtaining solutions (Horn, 1994; Horn et al., 1981; Noll & Horn, 1998).

Research Examining Evidence for a General Factor of Cognitive Speed

The structural evidence does not support this theory. Carroll (1993) has done a comprehensive review of the research bearing on this point. He found replicated evidence for factors of movement time, reaction time, correct decision speed (CDS), incorrect decision speed, perceptual speed (Gs), short-time retrieval speed, and fluency/speed of retrieval from long-term memory (TSR). Several different lines of evidence suggest that these factors do not relate to each other or to other variables in a manner that indicates a measure of one process of cognitive speed or one process of aging.

First, one line of evidence indicates that the Gs factor correlates negatively with age and positively with Gf and SAR, both of which decline with age, while moderately speeded retrieval tests (i.e., TSR) correlate positively with Gs and other speeded measures, but not negatively, with age. TSR also relates positively to Gc, which correlates positively, not negatively, with age. The TSR measures of speed thus have notably different correlations with age and other variables than do other Gs measures.

Second, the evidence of Walsh's (1982) careful studies of speed of visual perception shows that speed measures indicating peripheral functions (at the level of each eye—optic neural processing) correlate at only a near-zero (chance-like) level with speed measures indicating central nervous system functioning, although each of these two unrelated kinds of measures correlates negatively and substantially with age in adulthood. The aging decline in one kind of factor is not indicative of the decline in the other. It appears that just as hair turning gray and going bald are related to aging but are quite separate processes, so declines in peripheral processing speed and central processing speed are related to aging but are separate processes.

Third, although chronometric measures have often been found to relate positively to cognitive capacity measures (when these are confounded with speed), such relationships are found to sink to zero in homogeneous samples—people of the same age and education level. In particular, highly speeded simple-decision tests correlate at the chance level, or even negatively, with low-speed tests that require solving of complex intellectual

problems (Guilford, 1964). Thus, cognitive speed and cognitive capability are not positively related; they are negatively related when cognitive capability is measured in terms of the difficulty of the problems solved. Speed in solving problems is not intrinsically indicative of the complexity of the problems one is able to solve.

Capacity for Sustaining Attention: The Link between Cognitive Speed and Vulnerable Abilities

The evidence now suggests that the kind of cognitive speed that relates to decline of vulnerable abilities is a capacity for focusing and maintaining attention, not speed per se. This leads to a conclusion that cognitive speed measures relate to cognitive capability and aging primarily because they require focused attention, not because they require speed. This is indicated by evidence that chronometric measures relate to unspeeded measures of capacity for focusing and maintaining attention. In part-correlation analyses, it is shown that the unspeeded measures of attention account for most of the aging decline in speeded measures and for most of the relationship between cognitive speed and cognitive capacities. The evidence adds up as follows. First, measures of behaving as quickly as possible correlate substantially with measures of behaving as slowly as possible (Botwinick & Storandt, 1997). Second, these two kinds of measures correlate substantially (negatively) with age in adulthood, and both correlate substantially with cognitive capacity measures that decline with age in adulthood. Next, when the slowness measures are partialed from the speediness measures, the resulting residualized speediness correlates only very modestly with age, and at a chance level with the cognitive capacity measures (of Gf) that decline with age in adulthood (Horn et al., 1981; Noll & Horn, 1998). The slowness measures also correlate substantially with other indicators of maintaining attention. Behaving slowly requires that one focus and maintain attention on a task. Conclusion: Focusing and maintaining attention appears to be an aspect of the capacity for apprehension that Spearman described as a major feature of *g* (see also Baddeley, 1993; Carroll, 1993; Cunningham & Tomer, 1990; Hertzog, 1989; Horn, 1968, 1998, 2002; Horn et al., 1981; Hundal & Horn, 1977; Madden, 1983; Noll & Horn, 1998; Salthouse, 1991; Walsh, 1982).

The evidence thus suggests that the relationships of chronometric measures to age and to cognitive capacity are not due primarily to speed per se, but to the fact that speeded measures require focused and sustained attention. It is not cognitive speed that is at the core of cognitive capability; it is a capacity for focusing and maintaining attention. This is required in speedy performance, and it is required in solving complex problems. It accounts for the correlation between these two kinds of measures. This capacity declines with age in adulthood.

Age-related declines have been found for other sustained-attention tasks. Measures of vigilance, for example (in which subjects must detect a stimulus change imbedded in an otherwise invariant sequence of the stimuli), decline with age (Kausler, 1990; McDowd & Birren, 1990). Age-related declines have been found for divided-attention and selective-attention tasks (Bors & Forrin, 1995; Horn et al., 1981; Horn & Noll, 1994; Madden, 1983; McDowd & Birren, 1990; McDowd & Craik, 1988; Plude & Hoyer, 1985; Rabbitt, 1965; Salthouse, 1991; Wickens, Braune, & Stokes, 1987). When separate measures of concentration (slow tracing) and divided attention are partialed separately and together from measures of working memory, it is found that each independently accounts for some, but not all, of the aging decline in working memory.

Older adults perform more poorly than their younger counterparts on the Stroop test, a measure of resisting interference (Cohn, Dustman, & Bradford, 1984), and on distracted visual search tasks (Madden, 1983; Plude & Hoyer, 1985; Rabbitt, 1965). Hasher and Zacks (1988) suggest that aging decline in cognitive capability is due to distractibility and susceptibility to perceptual interference. These investigators found that the manifest retrieval problems of older adults were attributable to inability to keep irrelevant information from obscuring relevant information. Horn and colleagues (1981) also found that measures of eschewing irrelevancies in concept formation were related to measures of short-term memory, working memory, and Gf, and accounted for some of the age differences in these measures. All of these measures require concentration to maintain focused attention on a task. Hasher and Zacks concluded that a basic process in working memory is one of maintaining attention. Baddeley (1993) argued that working memory can be described as *working attention.*

It is concluded from a number of these partialing studies that Gf (which so resembles Spearman's g) involves processes of (1) gaining awareness of information (attention) and (2) holding different aspects of information in the span of awareness (working memory), both of which are dependent on (3) a capacity for maintaining concentration. Capacity for concentration may be dependent on *neural recruitment* (i.e., synchronous firing of many neurons in patterns that correspond to the patterns of abilities involved in solving a complex problem). If neurons of a neural recruitment pattern are lost, the synchrony and hence the efficiency of the firing pattern are reduced. Grossly, this is seen in the decline of Gf, SAR, and Gs.

AN EMERGING THEORY OF HUMAN INTELLIGENCE: ABILITIES OF EXPERTISE

The results we have just reviewed provide some glimmerings of the nature of human intelligence. But these are only glimmerings; some important things are missing. The picture is one of aging decline, but decline doesn't characterize everyday observations of adult intelligence. These observations are of adults who do most of the work of maintaining and advancing the culture—people who are the intellectual leaders in science, politics, business, and academics, people who raise children and are regarded as smarter than their teenagers and young adults. This picture is one of maturing adults functioning at ever-higher intellectual levels. Granted that the research results for Gc and TSR are consistent with this view, they seem insufficient to describe the thinking of high-functioning adults. There is reason to question whether the description of human intelligence that is provided by the extant research is accurate.

Inadequacies of Current Theory

Indeed, there are problems with the tests that are assumed to indicate human intelligence. Consider the tests defining Gc, the factor that does indeed show intelligence improving in adulthood. This factor should be a measure of the breadth and depth of cultural knowledge, but the tests that define the factor (e.g., vocabulary, information, and analogies) measure only surface knowledge, not depth of knowledge, and the knowledge sampled by these tests is narrow relative to the broad and diverse range of the knowledge of a culture.

The fundamental problem is that the tests thus far identified as indicating Gc measure only introductory, dilettante knowledge of a culture. They don't measure the depth of knowledge, or the knowledge that is most difficult to acquire. Difficult reasoning is not measured in the factor. This can be seen in esoteric analogies, a test used to estimate a reasoning aspect of Gc. The items of such a test sample understanding of relationships in several areas of knowledge, but the reasoning involved in the relationships of each area is simple, as in an item of the form "*Annual* is to *perennial* as *deciduous* is to ___." If one has a cursory knowledge of botany or horticulture, completing the analogy is simple; it doesn't take much reasoning. The variance of the analogies test thus mainly indicates the extent to which one has such introductory knowledge in several areas of scholarship. It does not represent ability in dealing with difficult abstractions in reasoning in any area. But difficult reasoning is what is called for in the work of a scientist, legislator, engineer, or plumber. Difficult reasoning is called for in measures of intelligence.

Thus, in-depth knowledge and in-depth reasoning are not assessed in current measures of Gc. A dilettante, flitting over many areas of knowledge, will score higher on the measure than a person who has developed truly profound understanding in an area of knowledge. It is the latter individual, not the dilettante, who is most likely to make significant contributions to the culture and to be judged as highly intelligent. Such a person is otherwise referred to as an *expert*. An expert best exemplifies the capabilities that indicate the nature and limits of human intelligence.

Defining Intelligence in Terms of Expertise

After childhood, adolescence, and young adulthood, people continue to think and solve problems, but usually (to an ever-larger extent as development proceeds) this thinking is directed to solving novel problems in fields of work. Adults develop abilities that help them to become expert. They come to understand a great deal about some things, to the detriment of increasing understanding other things. They neglect the work of maintaining and improving previously developed abilities that are not presently relevant for developing expertise. Thus, the intelligence of maturing adults becomes manifested in abilities of expertise more and more as development proceeds.

We conclude that (1) the measures currently used to estimate intelligence probably do not assess all the important abilities of human intelligence; (2) abilities that come to fruition in adulthood

represent the quintessential expression of human intellectual capacity; (3) these abilities are abilities of expertise; and (4) the principal problems of research for describing these abilities are problems of identifying areas of expertise, designing measures of the abilities of expertise in these areas, and obtaining samples of people who can represent the variation needed to demonstrate the presence and range of expertise abilities.

Expertise Abilities of Intelligence

Intellectual expertise depends on effective application of a large amount of knowledge in reasoning to cope with novel problems. The abilities exemplified in different domains of expertise are indicative of human intelligence. The levels of complexities in reasoning resolved in expressions of expertise are comparable to the levels of complexities resolved in expressions of Gf abilities, and the problems solved often appear to be novel.

In contrast to the reasoning that characterizes Gf, which is largely inductive, the reasoning involved in exercise of expertise is largely knowledge-based and deductive. This is seen in descriptions of the thinking in several areas of expertise—in chess, financial planning, and medical diagnosis (Charness, 1981a, 1981b, 1991; de Groot, 1978; Ericsson, 1996; Walsh & Hershey, 1993). For example, de Groot (1978) found that those at the highest level of expertise in chess chose the next move by evaluating the current situation in terms of principles derived from vast prior experience, rather than by calculating and evaluating the many move possibilities. Other work (Charness, 1981a, 1981b, 1991; Ericsson, 1996, 1997; Masunaga & Horn, 2001; Morrow, Leirer, Altieri, & Fitzsimmons, 1994; Walsh & Hershey, 1993) has similarly demonstrated that the expert characteristically uses deductive reasoning under conditions where the novice uses inductive reasoning. The expert is able to construct a framework within which to organize and effectively evaluate presented information, while the novice, with no expertise basis for constructing a framework, searches for patterns and does reasoning by trial-and-error evaluations. The expert apprehends large amounts of organized information; comprehends many relationships among elements of this information; infers possible continuations and extrapolations; and, as a result, is able to select the best from among many possibilities in deciding on the most likely outcome, consequence, or extension of relationships. The expert goes from the general (comprehension of relations, knowledge of principles) to the most likely specifics.

Expertise in problem solving also appears to involve a form of wide-span memory that is different from the forms of memory described (in current descriptions of intelligence) under the headings of *short-term memory, short-term apprehension and retrieval* (SAR), *instantaneous memory* (Sperling, 1960), and *working memory* (e.g., Baddeley, 1994). de Groot (1946, 1978) may have been the first to recognize a distinction between this expert memory and other forms of memory. He described how, with increasing expertise, subjects became better able to rapidly access alternative chess moves of increasingly higher quality, and then base their play on these complex patterns rather than engage in extensive search. Ericsson and Kintsch (1995) described such memory as a capacity that emerges as expertise develops. It becomes a defining feature of advanced levels of expertise (Ericsson & Delaney, 1998; Ericsson & Kintsch, 1995). It is a form of working memory, but it is functionally independent of what heretofore has been described as working memory. As noted earlier in this chapter, to distinguish it in language from this latter—which has been referred to as *short-term working memory* (STWM)—it is referred to as *expertise wide-span memory* (EWSM). It is a capacity for holding relatively large amounts of information (large relative to STWM) in immediate awareness for periods of several minutes. It functions as an aid to solving problems and behaving expertly. EWSM is different from STWM in respect to two major features: apprehension–retention limits and access in a sequence.

The apprehension–retention limits of STWM are small and of short duration. For example, the apprehension limits for the recency effect in serial position memory, which is often taken as an indicator of short-term memory, are only about three (plus or minus one), and this retention fades to zero in less than a few (estimated to be 10) seconds (Glanzer & Cunitz, 1966). The apprehension limits for the primacy effect also are only about three (plus or minus one), with duration less than a few seconds. In a near-classic article, Miller (1956) characterized the apprehension limits for forward span memory as the "magical number seven plus or minus two," and the duration of this memory (without rehearsal) is no more than 30 seconds. These kinds of limits have been demonstrated under conditions of competition for a limited resource, as in studies in which subjects are required to retain information while performing another

task (Baddeley, 1993; Carpenter & Just, 1989; Stankov, 1988). The limits seen in the Sperling (1960) effect are larger than seven, but there is no consolidation of this memory and the span fades within milliseconds; it is regarded as indicator of apprehension alone, not a measure of short-term retention (memory).

For EWSM, the apprehension limits are substantially larger, and the retention limits are substantially longer, than any of the limits accepted as indicating STWM. Just how much larger and longer these limits are is not clear, but chess experts, for example, appear to be able to hold many more than seven elements of separate games within the span of immediate awareness for as long as several minutes (Ericsson & Kintsch, 1995; Gobet & Simon, 1996). In playing blindfold chess (Ericsson & Staszewski, 1989; Holding, 1985; Koltanowski, 1985), the expert is literally never able to see the board; all the outcomes of sequences of plays must be kept within a span of immediate apprehension. The number of elements the expert retains in such representations is much more than seven, and this retention lasts over several minutes.

It has been argued that successive chunking in STWM is sufficient to account for feats of memory displayed by experts, and thus to obviate any need for a concept of EWSM (Chase & Simon, 1973; Gobet & Simon, 1996). Chase and Simon (1973) reasoned that high-level chess memory was mediated by a large number (10,000, they estimated) of acquired patterns regarded as chunks, which could be hierarchically organized. The analyses of Richman, Gobet, Staszewski, and Simon (1996) suggested that the number of such chunks would have to be in excess of 100,000, rather than 10,000. In any case, the mechanism suggested by Chase and Simon was direct retrieval of relevant moves cued by perceived patterns of chess positions that are stored in a form of STWM. They rejected a suggestion (Chase & Ericsson, 1982) that storage of generated patterns in long-term memory is possible within periods as brief as the 5-second presentations that were observed. Cooke, Atlas, Lane, and Berger (1993) and Gobet and Simon (1996), however, showed that this assumption is plausible. They found that highly skilled chess players could recall information from up to nine chess positions that had been presented one after the other as rapidly as one every 5 seconds without pauses. In the retrievals of blindfold chess, the number of chunks would appear to be larger than seven—and if chunks are maintained in a hierarchy or other such template, the representation would be changed with successive moves, and the number of sequences of such changes is larger than seven. Yet experts were able to use information of moves that were more than seven sequences removed from the point of decision.

Similarly, in studies of experts playing multiple games of chess presented on a computer screen, Saariluoma (1991) found that a chess master could simultaneously play six different games, each involving more than seven relationships. The expert appeared to retain representations of many more than seven chess positions in a flexibly accessible form while moving from one game to another.

STWM is characterized by sequencing in retention, but such sequencing seems to be unimportant in EWSM. In STWM, maximum span is attained only if items are retained and retrieved in the temporal order of apprehension. If a task requires retrieval in a different order, the number of elements recalled is substantially reduced; memory span backward, for example, is only about three to four, compared with the seven of forward span. In descriptions of chess experts displaying EWSM, on the other hand, information is almost as readily accessed from the middle or end of a sequence as from the beginning (Charness & Bosman, 1990).

The Ericsson and Kintsch (1995) analyses thus make the case that while chunking helps to explain short-term memory that is somewhat larger than seven plus two, it is not fully adequate to account for the very large apprehension, long retention, and flexibility of access that experts display. In particular, if the different sequences experts access are regarded as chunks that must be maintained if the retrieval of experts is to be adequately described, the number of such chunks must be considerably larger than seven plus two, and they must be retained longer than a few seconds. Thus chunking cannot be the whole story (Ericsson & Kintsch, 1995; Gobet & Simon, 1996).

How might EWSM work? Our theory is that the development of expertise sensitizes the person to become more nearly aware of the large amount of information that is, for a very short period of time, available to all people (not just experts), but ordinarily is not accessed. Sperling's (1960) work indicates that for a split second, the human is aware of substantially more information than is indicated by estimates of the limits of STWM. Similarly, the studies of Biederman (e.g., 1995) demonstrate that we can recognize complex visual stimuli involving many more than seven elements and retain them for longer than 60 seconds. However, most of the information that comes into immediate awareness fades from awareness very quickly. It fades partly because new information enters awareness to take the place of previous information; it fades also because meaningful organizing systems are not immediately available to enable a perceiver to organize the incoming information. Biederman's findings demonstrate that information that is seen only briefly but is organized by the perceiver can be retained for long periods of time. Thus, if meaningful systems for organizing information are built up through expertise development (the systems of EWSM), and such systems are available in the immediate situation, then large amounts of briefly seen information might be organized in accordance with this system and retained for long periods of time for use in problem solving in an area of expertise. Such organized information (seen only briefly) would not be replaced by other incoming information. However, the briefly seen information would need to be that of a domain of expertise. The development of expertise would not, in general, improve memory; it would do so only in a limited domain.

Further Notes on the Development of Expertise

What we now know about expertise suggests that it is developed through intensive practice over extended periods of time and is maintained through continued efforts in regular, well-structured practice (Anderson, 1990; Ericsson, 1996; Ericsson & Charness, 1994; Ericsson, Krampe, & Tesch-Romer, 1993; Ericsson & Lehmann, 1996; Walsh & Hershey, 1993). What is described as *well-structured practice* is essential for effective development of expertise. Such practice is not simply repetition and is not measured simply by number of practice trials. The practice must be designed to identify and correct errors and to move one to ever-higher levels of performance. There should be goals and appropriate feedback. It was found that in developing expertise in chess, self-directed practice (using books and studying sequences of moves made by expert players) could be as effective as coach-directed practice (Charness, 1981a, 1981b, 1991; Ericsson, 1996).

Just how long it takes to reach the highest levels of expertise—one's own asymptote—is not known with precision for any domain. A "10-year rule" has been given as an approximation for domains characterized by complex problem solving, but this has been much debated (Anderson, 1990; Charness, Krampe, & Mayr, 1996; Ericsson & Charness,

1994; Ericsson, Krampe, & Tesch-Romer, 1993). The upshot of the debate is that the time it takes to become expert varies with domain, the amount and quality of practice and coaching, the developmental level at which dedication to becoming an expert begins, health, stamina, and a host of other variables. Ten years is a very rough estimation for some domains, such as chess and medical diagnosis (Ericsson, 1996).

Since it takes time (i.e., years) to reach high levels of expertise in complex problem solving, and expertise in such domains is developed (at least partially) through the period of adulthood, it follows that expertise abilities can improve in adulthood. Indeed, the research literature is consistent in showing that across different domains of expertise, people beginning at different ages in adulthood advance from low to asymptotic high levels of expertise (Ericsson, Krampe, & Heizmann, 1993). Advanced levels of expertise in certain games (e.g., chess and go) and in financial planning have been attained and maintained by older adults (Charness & Bosman, 1990; Charness et al., 1996; Ericsson & Charness, 1994; Kasai, 1986; Walsh & Hershey, 1993). Rabbitt (1993) found that among novices, crossword-solving ability was positively correlated with test scores indicating Gf ($r = .72$) and negatively correlated with age ($r = -.25$), just as Gf is so correlated; however, among experts, crossword-solving ability was positively associated with age ($r = +.24$) and correlated near zero with Gf. The results of Bahrick (1984), Bahrick and Hall (1991), Conway, Cohen, and Stanhope (1991), Walsh and Hershey (1993), and Krampe and Ericsson (1996) indicate that continued practice is required to maintain a high level of expert performance: If the abilities of expertise are not used, they decline. To the extent that practice is continued, expertise is maintained over periods of years and decades.

It also appears from the extant (albeit sparse) evidence that high levels of EWSM can be maintained into advanced age. Baltes (1997) found that in domains of specialization, older adults could access information more rapidly than young adults. Charness (1981a, 1981b, 1991) found no age decrement in the depth of search for the next move and the quality of the resulting moves in chess. Such findings suggest that there may be little or no decline with age for complex thinking abilities if these abilities are developed within a domain of expertise.

Also suggesting that expertise abilities indicative of intelligence can be developed and maintained in adulthood are results obtained by Krampe and Ericsson (1996) for speeded abilities. They obtained seven operationally independent measures of speed in a sample of classical pianists who ranged from amateurs to concert performers with international reputations, and who ranged in age from the mid-20s to the mid-60s. Regardless of age, experts performed better than amateurs on all music-related speeded tasks. Age-related decline was found at the highest level of expertise, but reliably for only one of the seven measures, and the decline was notably smaller than for persons at lower levels of expertise. The single best predictor of performance on all music-related tasks was the amount of practice participants had maintained during the previous 10 years.

In samples of practicing typists of different ages, Salthouse (1985) found that although abilities of finger-tapping speed, choice reaction time, and digit–symbol substitution that would seem to be closely related to typing ability declined systematically with age, typing ability as such did not: Older typists attained the same typing speed as younger typists. The older typists had longer eye spans, which enabled them to anticipate larger chunks of the material to be typed. Salthouse interpreted this as a compensatory mechanism. It can also be viewed as indicating a more advanced level of expertise, for, seemingly, it would relate to improving the skill of a typist of any age.

In a study of spatial visualization in architects of different ages and levels of expertise, Salthouse (1991) found that high-level experts consistently scored above low-level experts at every age. In the abilities of expertise, elderly high-level experts scored higher than youthful low-level experts. With practice to increase and maintain expertise, cognitive abilities (of expertise) increased with advancing age.

Expertise: Conclusions, Implications, and Extrapolations

Thus, it seems that some kinds of expertise require, and indicate, high levels of the abilities that indicate human intelligence. Attaining such expertise involves developing deductive reasoning ability to solve very difficult problems. Also developed is EWSM, which enables one to remain aware of, and work with, large amounts of information in the area of expertise. This facilitates expertise deductive reasoning. Cognitive speed ability also develops in the domain of expertise as high levels of expertise are attained. Very possibly there are other abilities that develop under the press to acquire expertise. Research should be directed at identifying such abilities. These expertise abilities are different from the somewhat comparable abilities of fluid reasoning (Gf), working memory (SAR), and cognitive speed (Gs) that also characterize human intelligence.

It takes many years to develop a high level of expertise. Ten years is a rough estimate. Even more time is needed to develop the highest levels. Much of this development must occur in adulthood. High levels of the abilities of expertise are displayed primarily in adults (not younger people). Expertise abilities of older high-level experts exceed the comparable abilities of younger persons at lower levels of expertise.

Expertise abilities of intelligence are expected to increase (on average) in adulthood; that is, such abilities will increase at least in some people and during some parts of adulthood (perhaps mainly the early parts—the first 20 years, say). Burnout is common in activities that require intense dedication and work. After working intensely for years to develop expertise, one can reach a limit, begin to lose interest and focus, and become lax in maintaining and continuing to develop the abilities of one's expertise. Those abilities would then decline. People often switch fields after burning out in a particular field, and such switching might be accompanied by launching a program to develop expertise in the new field. This could occur at fairly advanced ages in adulthood. In this way, too, abilities of expertise could be expected to increase through much of adulthood.

Thus, our theory specifies that the deductive reasoning, EWSM, and cognitive speediness abilities associated with the development of expertise increase concomitantly with the decreases that have been found for Gf, STWM, and speediness defined outside a domain of expertise. It is possible that increase in expertise abilities necessarily results in decline in nonexpertise abilities, for the devotion of time, energy, and other resources to the development of expertise may of necessity take time, energy, and other resources away from maintenance of Gf, SAR, and Gs.

Such hypothesizing flows from sparse findings. The hypotheses may be correct, but perhaps for only a small number of people. The extant results have often come from studies of small samples. The adults in these cases may be exceptional. There have been no longitudinal follow-up studies to determine the extent to which people become exceptional and maintain that status. If such de-velopment occurs only in a few cases, there are good questions to ask about how the development might be fostered in most people. There is need for further research.

GENERAL SUMMARY

The present state of science thus indicates that human intelligence is a melange of many abilities that are interrelated in many ways. The abilities and their interrelationships are determined by many endogenous (genetic, physiological, neurological) and exogenous (experiential, nutritional, hygienic) influences. These influences operate over many minutes, months, and years of life; they may be more and less potent in some developmental periods than in others. There is very little we know, and much more we don't know, about these interrelationships and determinants.

It is unlikely that there is one central determinant running through the entire melange of abilities. If there is one such influence, the extant evidence suggests it must be weak, barely detectable among a chorus of other determinants. If g exists, it will be difficult to ferret it out from all the other influences that operate to produce intellectual abilities. Small influences can be hugely important, of course, but we have no inkling that is true for g (if, indeed, there is a g). Assertions that g has been discovered do nothing to help locate a possible g, or to indicate the importance of such an agent if it were to be found.

It is known that almost any task that can be made up to measure a cognitive ability correlates positively with tests of almost every other cognitive ability. Very few exceptions to this generalization have been found, but there are a couple. The first is found in samples of very young children—under 2–3 years of age. In such samples, measures involving motor skill and speediness have been found to be correlated near zero or perhaps even negatively with measures of awareness of concepts (i.e., the beginnings of vocabulary). The second exception is found in very homogeneous samples of young adults—all very nearly of the same age, same educational level, same ethnicity, same socioeconomic status, and so forth. Again, measures in which there is much emphasis on speediness correlate near zero, perhaps negatively, with tests that require solving difficult problems. With these two exceptions, cognitive ability tests are positively intercorrelated. This is referred to as a condition of *positive manifold*.

It is the evidence of positive manifold that is referred to in assertions that *g* has been discovered. But a positive manifold is not sufficient evidence of a single process. There are many ways for positive manifold to occur that do not involve one common factor (as described particularly well by Thomson, 1916, many decades ago).

Many variables that are not ability variables are positively correlated with ability variables (as well as among themselves). This does not indicate *g*. Variables scored in the "good" direction generally correlate positively with other things scored in the "good" direction (high ability correlates positively with ego strength, ambition, morale, family income, healthful habits, etc.), and variables scored in the "not good" direction generally correlate positively with other things scored in the "not good" direction (low ability correlates positively with neuroticism, other psychopathologies, inattentiveness, hyperactivity, boredom, lack of energy, delinquency, poverty, birth stress, etc.). Just as it is argued (e.g., by Jensen, 1998) that one can obtain a good measure of *g* by adding up scores on different ability tests that are positively intercorrelated, so one might argue that by taking into account the presence of a long list of the above-mentioned negative things and the absence of a long list of positive things, one can obtain a good measure of a *c* factor—*c* standing for *crud*.[7] The evidence for such a *c* factor is of the same form as the evidence said to exist for a *g* factor. The problems with the science of the *c* factor are the same as the problems with the science of the *g* factor. In both cases, many, many things can operate to produce the positive manifold of variable intercorrelations. In both cases, it is not a scientific simplification to claim (or imply) that one thing produces this positive manifold. In both cases, something like a bond theory of many causes (Thomson, 1916) is a more plausible model of the data than a one-common-factor model.

The extant evidence indicates that within the manifold of positive intercorrelations among cognitive abilities, there are pockets of substantially higher intercorrelations among some abilities, coupled with lower correlations of these abilities with other abilities. Such patterns of intercorrelations give rise to theories that separate sets of influences produce distinct common factors. Results from many studies now point to 80-some such distinct common factors operating at a primary level, and some eight or nine common factors operating at a second-order level.

Several indicators of primary-level influences interrelate to indicate a second-order factor that rather well represents Spearman's hypotheses that human intelligence is characterized by keenness of apprehension, ability to discern extant relationships, and ability to extrapolate to generate new, implied relationships. It seems that a capacity for attaining and maintaining focused attention is an integral part of this clutch of abilities. This capacity for concentration appears to enable speed in apprehending and scanning fundaments and possible relationships among fundaments in working toward solutions to complex problems. This capacity, coupled with abilities for apprehending the elements of problems, holding them in a span of awareness, identifying relationships among the elements, and working out the implications of these relationships, define *fluid reasoning* (Gf).

Gf does not represent one and only one common-factor influence running through all abilities that indicate the nature of human intelligence. Certain other primary-level indicators interrelate to indicate a second-order factor of ready acquisition of information. It is manifested in acquisition of knowledge about the language, concepts, and information of the dominant culture. The abilities of the factor are the abilities the society seeks to pass from one generation to the next through various processes of acculturation, particularly those of formal education. This set of abilities is labeled *crystallized knowledge* and symbolized as Gc.[8]

Gc and Gf together do not represent two and only two common-factor influences running through all abilities that indicate the nature of human intelligence. There are also common-factor influences representing separate forms of memory. One of these, labeled *short-term working memory* (STWM) or *short-term apprehension and retrieval* (SAR), indicates span and capacity for holding information in awareness for very short periods of time (less than a minute) while, for example, working on a problem such as would be solved through the processes of Gf. A second form of memory indicates a facility for consolidating information in a manner that enables it to be stored and retrieved minutes, hours, and days later. This facility is labeled *tertiary storage and retrieval* (TSR). A third form of EWSM stems from extended intense practice in developing cognitive expertise.

Primary-level abilities also interrelate to indicate second-order factors representing cognitive functions associated with perceptual modalities. One such factor indicates functions that facilitate visualization; this is labeled *broad visualization* (Gv). Another set of relationships is for abilities of listening and hearing and comprehending intricacies of sounds; it is referred to as *auditory ability* (Ga). There are very possibly somewhat comparable cognitive functions spinning off from the other sensory modalities, but there has been virtually no study of such possibilities.

Speed of reacting, speed of deciding, speed of movement, speed of perceiving, various speeds in solving various different kinds of problems, speed in thinking, and other aspects of speed of responding and behaving are involved in very intricate ways in almost all the abilities that are regarded as indicating human intelligence. Five common factors involving different sets of indicators of speediness have been identified at what is approximately a second-order level among primary factors of speediness. These indicators of speediness do not indicate a general factor for speed of thinking, however. Nor do any of the speed factors represent a sine qua non of the other second-order systems. Indeed, as concerns Gf in particular, a capacity for behaving slowly (which seems to indicate focused concentration) largely accounts for any relationship between reasoning and speed of thinking; that is, an ability to concentrate seems to determine quick thinking in solving the difficult, abstract problems that characterize Gf. It may be true that capacity for focusing concentration largely accounts for the speediness of the speed factors and their relationships to other broad cognitive factors, but these hypotheses have not been examined. Good research is needed in this area.

The systems involved in retaining information in immediate awareness, concentration, and reasoning with novel problems decline, on average, in adulthood. Yet an important referent for the concept of intelligence is expertise: high-level ability to deal successfully with complex problems in which the solutions require advanced, deep understanding of a knowledge domain. Cognitive capability systems involved in retrieving information from the store of knowledge (TSR) and the store of knowledge itself (Gc) increase over much of the period of adulthood development. These increases point to the development of expertise, but the Gc and TSR measures tap only surface-like indictors of expertise abilities. They do not indicate the depth of knowledge, the ability to deal with many aspects of a problem, the reasoning, and the speed in considering possibilities that characterize high-level expertise performances. Gc and TSR do not measure the feats of reasoning and memory that characterize the most sublime expressions of adult intelligence. These capabilities have been described in studies of experts in games (e.g., chess and go), in medical diagnosis, and in financial planning. Factor-analytic studies have demonstrated that expert performances depend on abilities of deductive reasoning and EWSM, abilities that are quite independent of the Gf, SAR, and Gs abilities of intelligence. Within a circumscribed domain of knowledge, EWSM provides an expert with much more information in the immediate situation than is available through the system for STWM. EWSM appears to sublimate to a form of deductive reasoning that utilizes a complex store of information to effectively anticipate, predict, evaluate, check, analyze, and monitor in problem solving within the knowledge domain. These abilities appear to characterize mature expressions of intelligence. Years of intensive, well-structured learning and regular practice are needed to develop and maintain these abilities. To the extent that such practice occurs through the years of adulthood, these abilities will increase; to this extent, important abilities of intelligence will not decline with advancing age.

NOTES

1. It is realized that what is considered first-order or second-order in a factor analysis depends on what is to be put into the analysis. If items are put into analysis, for example, the first-order factors are likely to be equivalent to the tests that are normally put into a first-order analysis, and the second-order factors among items correspond to the first-order factors among tests. Also, if tests are carefully chosen to represent one and only one first-order factor, the first-order factors will indicate the second-order factors among the usual factorings of tests. The order of a factor thus depends on the sampling of the elements to indicate that factor. It is with awareness of these possibilities that researchers have considered the sampling of elements and arrived at the classifications here referred to as *primary abilities* and *second-order* abilities.

2. This is the case, too, when nine second-order factors are considered.

3. That is, age is the primary marker for development, although by no means the only such marker (Nesselroade & Baltes, 1979).

4. The longitudinal findings generally suggest that declines set in somewhat earlier than is indicated by cross-sectional findings.

5. If the elements of the memory are not arranged in

accordance with patterns that are part of expertise understanding—as when chess pieces are located in a quite arbitrary manner on a chessboard—the expert's memory is no better than the nonexpert's, and the memory span is approximately seven plus or minus two, as it is for other unrelated material.

6. Indeed, a large majority of the intercorrelations are positive.

7. Indeed, Herrnstein and Murray (1994) obtained such a composite, scored in the opposite direction, and called it "The Middle Class Values Index." The thought of calling it a *crud* factor is owed to Paul Meehl, who referred to it in this manner in a conversation with Horn many years ago.

8. The terms *crystallized* and *fluid* in the labels for Gc and Gf, respectively, were affixed by Cattell (1957) to represent his hypothesis that Gf is a necessary determinant of Gc—it "flows" into production of a Gc that then becomes fixed, rather in the way that polyps produce the calcareous skeletons that constitute a coral reef. The sparse evidence at hand suggests that something like this process may operate in the early years of development, but that as development proceeds, Gc may precede and do more to determine Gf than the reverse.

REFERENCES

Alexander, H. B. (1935). Intelligence, concrete and abstract. *British Journal of Psychology* (Monograph Suppl. No. 19).

Anderson, J. R. (1990). *Cognitive psychology and its implications* (3rd ed.). New York: Freeman.

Atkinson, R. C., & Shiffrin, R. M. (1968). Human memory: A proposed system and its control processes. In K. W. Spence & J. T. Spence (Eds.), *The psychology of learning and motivation* (Vol. 2, pp. 89–105). New York: Academic Press.

Baddeley, A. (1993). Working memory or working attention? In A. Baddeley & L. Weiskrantz (Eds.), *Attention: Selection, awareness, and control: A tribute to Donald Broadbent* (pp. 152–170). Oxford: Clarendon Press.

Baddeley, A. (1994). Memory. In A. M. Colman (Ed.), *Companion encyclopedia of psychology* (Vol. 1, pp. 281–301). London: Routledge.

Bahrick, H. P. (1984). Semantic memory content in permaslore: 50 years of memory for Spanish learned in school. *Journal of Experimental Psychology: General, 113*, 1–29.

Bahrick, H. P., & Hall, L. K. (1991). Lifetime maintenance of high school mathematics content. *Journal of Experimental Psychology: General, 120*, 20–33.

Baltes, P. B. (1997). On the incomplete architecture of human ontogeny: Selection, optimization, and compensation as foundation of developmental theory. *American Psychologist, 52*, 366–380.

Biederman, I. (1995). Visual object recognition. In S. F. Kosslyn & D. N. Osherson (Eds.), *An invitation to cognitive science: Vol. 2. Visual cognition* (2nd ed., pp. 121–165). Cambridge, MA: MIT Press.

Birren, J. E. (1974). Psychophysiology and speed of response. *American Psychologist, 29*, 808–815.

Bors, D. A., & Forrin, B. (1995). Age, speed of information processing, recall, and fluid intelligence. *Intelligence, 20*, 229–248.

Botwinick, J. (1978). *Aging and behavior: A comprehensive integration of research findings.* New York: Springer.

Botwinick, J., & Storandt, M. (1997). *Memory related functions and age.* Springfield, IL: Thomas.

Bower, G. H. (1972). Mental imagery and associative learning. In L. W. Gregg (Ed.), *Cognition in learning and memory* (pp. 213–228). New York: Wiley.

Bower, G. H. (1975). Cognitive psychology: An introduction. In W. K. Estes (Ed.), *Handbook of learning and cognitive processes* (Vol. 1, pp. 3–27). Hillsdale, NJ: Erlbaum.

Broadbent, D. E. (1966). The well-ordered mind. *American Educational Research Journal, 3*, 281–295.

Brown, W., & Stephenson, W. (1933). A test of the theory of two factors. *British Journal of Psychology, 23*, 352–370.

Burt, C. (1909). Experimental tests of general intelligence. *British Journal of Psychology, 3*, 94–177.

Burt, C. (1949). Subdivided factors. *British Journal of Statistical Psychology, 2*, 41–63.

Carpenter, P. A., & Just, M. A. (1989). The role of working memory in language comprehension. In D. Clahr & K. Kotovski (Eds.), *Complex information processing: The impact of Herbert A. Simon* (pp. 31–68). Hillsdale, NJ: Erlbaum.

Carroll, J. B. (1993). *Human cognitive abilities: A survey of factor analytic studies.* New York: Cambridge University Press.

Cattell, R. B. (1941). Some theoretical issues in adult intelligence testing. *Psychological Bulletin, 38*, 592.

Cattell, R. B. (1957). *Personality and motivation structure and measurement.* Yonkers, NY: World Book.

Cattell, R. B. (1971). *Abilities: Their structure, growth and action.* Boston: Houghton Mifflin.

Cattell, R. B. (1979). Are culture-fair intelligence tests possible and necessary? *Journal of Research and Development in Education, 12*, 1–13.

Cavanaugh, J. C. (1997). *Adult development and aging* (3rd ed.). New York: ITP.

Charness, N. (1981a). Search in chess: Age and skill differences. *Journal of Experimental Psychology: Human Perception and Performance, 7*(2), 467–476.

Charness, N. (1981b). Visual short-term memory and aging in chess players. *Journal of Gerontology, 36*(5), 615–619.

Charness, N. (1991). Expertise in chess: The balance between knowledge and search. In K. A. Ericsson & J. Smith (Eds.), *Toward a general theory of expertise: Prospects and limits* (pp. 30–62). Cambridge, UK: Cambridge University Press.

Charness, N., & Bosman, E. A. (1990). Expertise and aging: Life in the lab. In T. M. Hess (Ed.), *Aging and cognition: Knowledge organization and utilization* (pp. 343–386). New York: Elsevier.

Charness, N., Krampe, R., & Mayr, U. (1996). The role of practice and coaching in entrepreneurial skill domains: An international comparison of life-span chess skill acquisition. In K. A. Ericsson (Ed.), *The road to excellence* (pp. 51–80). Mahwah, NJ: Erlbaum.

Chase, W. G., & Ericsson, K. A. (1982). Skill and working memory. In G. H. Bower (Ed.), *The psychology of learning and motivation* (Vol. 16, pp. 1–58). New York: Academic Press.

Chase, W. G., & Simon, H. A. (1973). Perception in chess. *Cognitive Psychology, 4,* 55–81.

Cohen, J. (1959). The factorial structure of the WISC at ages 7.6, 10.6, and 13.6. *Journal of Consulting Psychology, 23,* 289–299.

Cohn, N. B., Dustman, R. E., & Bradford, D. C. (1984). Age-related decrements in Stroop color test performance. *Journal of Clinical Psychology, 40,* 1244–1250.

Conway, M. A., Cohen, G., & Stanhope, N. (1991). On the very long-term retention of knowledge acquired through formal education: Twelve years of cognitive psychology. *Journal of Experimental Psychology: General, 120,* 395–409.

Cooke, N. J., Atlas, R. S., Lane, D. M., & Berger, R. C. (1993). Role of high-level knowledge in memory for chess positions. *American Journal of Psychology, 106,* 321–351.

Craik, F. I. M. (1977). Age differences in human memory. In J. E. Birren & K. W. Schaie (Eds.), *Handbook of the psychology of aging* (pp. 55–110). New York: Van Nostrand Reinhold.

Craik, F. I. M., & Trehub, S. (Eds.). (1982). *Aging and cognitive processes.* New York: Plenum Press.

Cunningham, W. R., & Tomer, A. (1990). Intellectual abilities and age: Concepts, theories and analyses. In A. E. Lovelace (Ed.), *Aging and cognition: Mental processes, self awareness and interventions* (pp. 279–406). Amsterdam: Elsevier.

de Groot, A. D. (1946). *Het denken van den schaker* [*Thought and choice in chess*]. Amsterdam: North-Holland.

de Groot, A. D. (1978). *Thought and choice in chess.* The Hague, Netherlands: Mouton.

Detterman, D. K. (Ed.). (1993). *Current topics in human intelligence* (Vol. 1). Norwood, NJ: Ablex.

El Kousey, A. A. H. (1935). The visual perception of space. *British Journal of Psychology* (Monograph Suppl. No. 20).

Ericsson, K. A. (1996). The acquisition of expert performance. In K. A. Ericsson (Ed.), *The road to excellence* (pp. 1–50). Mahwah, NJ: Erlbaum.

Ericsson, K. A. (1997). Deliberate practice and the acquisition of expert performance: An overview. In H. Jorgensen & A. C. Lehmann (Eds.), *Does practice make perfect?: Current theory and research on instrumental music practice* (pp. 9–51). Oslo: Norges musikkhogskole, NMH-publikasjoner.

Ericsson, K. A., & Charness, N. (1994). Expert performance. *American Psychologist, 49,* 725–747.

Ericsson, K. A., & Delaney, P. F. (1998). Working memory and expert performance. In R. H. Logie & K. J. Gilhooly (Eds.), *Working memory and thinking: Current issues in thinking and reasoning* (pp. 93–114). Hove, UK: Psychology Press/Erlbaum.

Ericsson, K. A., & Kintsch, W. (1995). Long-term working memory. *Psychological Review, 105,* 211–245.

Ericsson, K. A., Krampe, R. T., & Heizmann, S. (1993). Can we create gifted people? In *CIBA Foundation Symposium: The origins and development of high ability* (pp. 22–249). Chichester, UK: Wiley.

Ericsson, K. A., Krampe, R. T., & Tesch-Romer, C. (1993). The role of deliberate practice in the acquisition of expert performance. *Psychological Review, 100,* 363–406.

Ericsson, K. A., & Lehmann, A. C. (1996). Expert and exceptional performance: Evidence of maximal adaptation to task constraints. *Annual Review of Psychology, 47,* 273–305.

Ericsson, K. A., & Staszewski, J. (1989). Skilled memory and expertise: Mechanisms of exceptional performance. In D. Klahr & K. Kotovsky (Eds.), *Complex information processing* (pp. 235–268). Hillsdale, NJ: Erlbaum.

Estes, W. K. (1974). Learning theory and intelligence. *American Psychologist, 29,* 740–749.

Eysenck, H. J. (1987). Speed of information processing, reaction time, and the theory of intelligence. In P. A. Vernon (Ed.), *Speed of information processing and intelligence* (pp. 21–68). Norwood, NJ: Ablex.

Flanagan, D. P., Genshaft, J. L., & Harrison, P. L. (Eds.). (1997). *Contemporary intellectual assessment: Theories, tests, and issues.* New York: Guilford Press.

Gathercole, S. E. (1994). The nature and uses of working memory. In P. Morris & M. Gruneberg (Eds.), *Theoretical aspects of memory* (pp. 50–78). London: Routledge.

Glanzer, M., & Cunitz, A. R. (1966). Two storage mechanisms in free recall. *Journal of Verbal Learning and Verbal Behavior, 5*, 351–360.

Gobet, F., & Simon, H. A. (1996). Templates in chess memory: A mechanism for recalling several boards. *Cognitive Psychology, 31*, 1–40.

Guilford, J. P. (1956). The structure of the intellect. *Psychological Bulletin, 53*, 276–293.

Guilford, J. P. (1964). Zero intercorrelations among tests of intellectual abilities. *Psychological Bulletin, 61*, 401–404.

Gustafsson, J. E. (1984). A unifying model for the structure of intellectual abilities. *Intelligence, 8*, 179–203.

Harwood, E., & Naylor, G. F. K. (1971). Changes in the constitution of the WAIS intelligence pattern with advancing age. *Australian Journal of Psychology, 23*, 297–303.

Hasher, L., & Zacks, R. T. (1988). Working memory, comprehension, and aging: A review and a new view. In G. H. Bower (Ed.), *The psychology of learning and motivation* (Vol. 22, pp. 193–225). San Diego, CA: Academic Press.

Herrnstein, R. J., & Murray, C. (1994). *The bell curve: Intelligence and class structure in American life.* New York: Free Press.

Hertzog, C. (1989). Influences of cognitive slowing on age differences. *Developmental Psychology, 25*, 636–651.

Holding, D. H. (1985). *The psychology of chess skill.* Hillsdale, NJ: Erlbaum.

Horn, J. L. (1965). *Fluid and crystallized intelligence: A factor analytic and developmental study of the structure among primary mental abilities.* Unpublished doctoral dissertation, University of Illinois.

Horn, J. L. (1968). Organization of abilities and the development of intelligence. *Psychological Review, 75*, 242–259.

Horn, J. L. (1989). Models for intelligence. In R. Linn (Ed.), *Intelligence: Measurement, theory and public policy* (pp. 29–73). Urbana: University of Illinois Press.

Horn, J. L. (1991). Measurement of intellectual capabilities: A review of theory. In K. S. McGrew, J. K. Werder, & R. W. Woodcock (Eds.), *Woodcock–Johnson technical manual* (pp. 197–246). Allen, TX: DLM.

Horn, J. L. (1994). The theory of fluid and crystallized intelligence. In R. J. Sternberg (Ed.), *The encyclopedia of intelligence* (pp. 443–451). New York: Macmillan.

Horn, J. L. (1998). A basis for research on age differences in cognitive capabilities. In J. J. McArdle & R.

Woodcock (Eds.), *Human cognitive abilities in theory and practice* (pp. 57–91). Chicago: Riverside.

Horn, J. L. (2002). Selections of evidence, misleading assumptions, and oversimplifications: The political message of *The bell curve.* In J. Fish (Ed.), *Race and intelligence: Separating science from myth* (pp. 297–325). Mahwah, NJ: Erlbaum.

Horn, J. L., & Cattell, R. B. (1967). Age differences in fluid and crystallized intelligence. *Acta Psychologica, 26*, 107–129.

Horn, J. L., Donaldson, G., & Engstrom, R. (1981). Apprehension, memory and fluid intelligence decline in adulthood. *Research on Aging, 3*, 33–84.

Horn, J. L., & Hofer, S. M. (1992). Major abilities and development in the adult period. In R. J. Sternberg & C. A. Berg (Eds.), *Intellectual development* (pp. 44–99). New York: Cambridge University Press.

Horn, J. L., & Noll, J. (1994). A system for understanding cognitive capabilities. In D. K. Detterman (Ed.), *Current topics in intelligence* (pp. 151–203). Norwood, NJ: Ablex.

Horn, J. L., & Noll, J. (1997). Human cognitive capabilities: Gf-Gc theory. In D. P. Flanagan, J. L. Genshaft, & P. I. Harrison (Eds.), *Contemporary intellectual assessment* (pp. 53–91). New York: Guilford Press.

Hundal, P. S., & Horn, J. L. (1977). On the relationships between short-term learning and fluid and crystallized intelligence. *Applied Psychological Measurement, 1*, 11–21.

Jackson, M. A. (1960). The factor analysis of the Wechsler Scale. *British Journal of Statistical Psychology, 33*, 79–82.

Jensen, A. R. (1982). Reaction time and psychometric g. In H. J. Eysenck (Ed.), *A model for intelligence* (pp. 93–132). New York: Springer-Verlag.

Jensen, A. R. (1987). Psychometric g as a focus of concerted research effort. *Intelligence, 11*, 193–198.

Jensen, A. R. (1993). Why is reaction time correlated with psychometric g? *Current Directions in Psychological Science, 2*(2), 53–56.

Jensen, A. R. (1998). *The g factor: The science of mental ability.* Westport, CT: Praeger.

Kasai, K. (1986). *Ido de atama ga yoku naru hon [Becoming smart with GO].* Tokyo: Shikai.

Kaufman, A. S. (1990). *Assessing adolescent and adult intelligence.* Boston: Allyn & Bacon.

Kausler, D. H. (1990). *Experimental psychology, cognition, and human aging.* New York: Springer.

Koltanowski, G. (1985). *In the dark.* Coraopolis, PA: Chess Enterprises.

Krampe, R. T., & Ericsson, K. A. (1996). Maintaining excellence: Deliberate practice and elite performance in young and older pianists. *Journal of Experimental Psychology: General, 125*, 331–359.

Madden, D. J. (1983). Aging and distraction by highly familiar stimuli during visual search. *Developmental Psychology, 19*, 499–507.

Madden, D. J., & Nebes, R. D. (1980). Aging and the development of automaticity in visual search. *Developmental Psychology, 16*, 277–296.

Masunaga, H., & Horn, J. L. (2000). Characterizing mature human intelligence: expertise development. *Learning and Individual Differences, 12*, 5–33.

Masunaga, H., & Horn, J. L. (2001). Expertise and age-related changes in components of intelligence. *Psychology and Aging, 16*, 293–311.

McArdle, J. J., Hamagami, F., Meredith, W., & Bradway, K. P. (2001). Modeling the dynamic hypotheses of Gf-Gc theory using life-span data. *Learning and Individual Differences, 12*, 53–79.

McArdle, J. J., & Woodcock, R. (Eds.). (1998). *Human cognitive abilities in theory and practice*. Itasca, IL: Riverside.

McDowd, J. M., & Birren, J. E. (1990). Aging and attentional processes. In J. E. Birren & K. W. Schaie (Eds.), *Handbook of the psychology of aging* (3rd ed., pp. 222–233). New York: Academic Press.

McDowd, J. M., & Craik, F. I. M. (1988). Effects of aging and task difficulty on divided attention performance. *Journal of Experimental Psychology: Human Perception and Performance, 14*(20), 267–280.

McGrew, K. S. (1994). *Clinical interpretation of the Woodcock–Johnson Tests of Cognitive Ability—Revised.* Boston: Allyn & Bacon.

McGrew, K. S., & Flanagan, D. P. (1998). *The intelligence test desk reference (ITDR)*. Boston: Allyn & Bacon.

McGrew, K. S., Werder, J. K., & Woodcock, R. W. (1991). *WJ-R technical manual*. Chicago: Riverside.

Miller, G. A. (1956) The magical number seven, plus or minus two: Some limits on our capacity for processing information. *Psychological Review, 63*, 81–97.

Morrow, D., Leirer, V., Altieri, P., & Fitzsimmons, C. (1994). When expertise reduces age differences in performance. *Psychology and Aging, 9*, 134–148.

Nesselroade, J. R., & Baltes, P. B. (Eds.). (1979). *Longitudinal research in the study of behavior and development*. New York: Academic Press.

Nettelbeck, T. (1994). Speediness. In R. J. Sternberg (Ed.), *Encyclopedia of human intelligence* (pp. 1014–1019). New York: Macmillan

Noll, J., & Horn, J. L. (1998). Age differences in processes of fluid and crystallized intelligence. In J. J. McArdle & R. W. Woodcock (Eds.), *Human cognitive abilities in theory and practice* (pp. 263–281). Chicago: Riverside.

Perfect, T. J., & Maylor, E. A. (Eds.). (2000). *Models of cognitive aging*. Oxford: Oxford University Press.

Plude, D. J., & Hoyer, W. J. (1985). Attention and performance: Identifying and localizing age deficits. In N. Charness (Ed.), *Aging and human performance* (pp. 47–99). New York: Wiley.

Rabbitt, P. (1965). An age-decrement in the ability to ignore irrelevant information. *Journal of Gerontology, 20*, 233–238.

Rabbitt, P. (1993). Crystal quest: A search for the basis of maintenance of practice skills into old age. In A. Baddeley & L. Weiskrantz (Eds.), *Attention: Selection, awareness, and control* (pp. 188–230). Oxford: Clarendon Press.

Rabbitt, P., & Abson, V. (1991). Do older people know how good they are? *British Journal of Psychology, 82*, 137–151.

Richman, H. B., Gobet, H., Staszewski, J. J., & Simon, H. A. (1996). Perceptual and memory processes in the acquisition of expert performance: The EPAM model. In K. A. Ericsson (Ed.), *The road to excellence* (pp. 167–188). Mahwah, NJ: Erlbaum.

Rimoldi, H. J. (1948). Study of some factors related to intelligence. *Psychometrika, 13*, 27–46.

Saariluoma, P. (1991). Aspects of skilled imagery in blindfold chess. *Acta Psychologica, 77*, 65–89.

Salthouse, T. A. (1985). Speed of behavior and its implications for cognition. In J. E. Birren & K. W. Schaie (Eds.), *Handbook of the psychology of aging* (2nd ed., pp. 400–426). New York: Van Nostrand Reinhold.

Salthouse, T. A. (1987). The role of representations in age differences in analogical reasoning. *Psychology and Aging, 2*, 357–362.

Salthouse, T. A. (Ed.). (1991). *Theoretical perspectives on cognitive aging*. Hillsdale, NJ: Erlbaum.

Salthouse, T. A. (1992). Influence of processing speed on adult age differences in working memory. *Acta Psychologica, 79*, 155–170.

Salthouse, T. A. (1993). Speed mediation of adult age differences in cognition. *Developmental Psychology, 29*, 727–738.

Salthouse, T. A., Kausler, D. H., & Saults, J. S. (1990). Age, self-assessed health status, and cognition. *Journal of Gerontology, 45*, 156–160.

Salthouse, T. A., & Somberg, B. L. (1982). Isolating the age deficit in speeded performance. *Journal of Gerontology, 37*, 59–63.

Saunders, D. R. (1959). On the dimensionality of the WAIS battery for two groups of normal males. *Psychological Reports, 5*, 529–541.

Schaie, K. W. (1990). Perceptual speed in adulthood: Cross sectional and longitudinal studies. *Psychology and Aging, 4*(4), 443–453.

Schaie, K. W. (1996). *Intellectual development in adulthood: The Seattle longitudinal study*. Cambridge, UK: Cambridge University Press.

Spearman, C. (1904). "General intelligence," objectively determined and measured. *American Journal of Psychology, 15,* 210–293.

Spearman, C. (1927). *The abilities of man: Their nature and measurement.* London: Macmillan.

Spearman, C. (1939). Thurstone's work re-worked. *Journal of Educational Psychology, 30*(1), 1–16.

Sperling, G. (1960). The information available in brief visual presentations. *Psychological Monographs, 74,* 498–450.

Stankov, L. (1988). Single tests, competing tasks, and their relationship to the broad factors of intelligence. *Personality and Individual Differences, 9,* 25–33.

Stankov, L., & Horn, J. L. (1980). Human abilities revealed through auditory tests. *Journal of Educational Psychology, 72,* 21–44.

Stephenson, W. (1931). Tetrad-differences for verbal sub-tests relative to non-verbal sub-tests. *Journal of Educational Psychology, 22,* 334–350.

Thomson, G. A. (1916). A hierarchy without a general factor. *British Journal of Psychology, 8,* 271–281.

Thurstone, L. L. (1938). *Primary mental abilities* (Psychometric Monographs No. 1). Chicago: University of Chicago Press.

Thurstone, L. L. (1947). *Multiple factor analysis.* Chicago: University of Chicago Press.

Vernon, P. E. (1950). *The structure of human abilities.* London: Methuen.

Walsh, D. A. (1982). The development of visual information processes in adulthood and old age. In F. I. M. Craik & S. Trehub (Eds.), *Aging and cognitive processes* (pp. 99–125). New York: Plenum Press.

Walsh, D. A., & Hershey, D. A. (1993). Mental models and the maintenance of complex problem solving skills in old age. In J. Cerella, J. Rybash, W. Hoyer, & M. Commons (Eds.), *Adult information processing: Limits on loss* (pp. 553–584). San Diego, CA: Academic Press.

Waugh, N. C., & Norman, D. A. (1965). Primary memory. *Psychological Review, 72,* 89–104.

Wickens, C. D., Braune, R., & Stokes, A. (1987). Age differences in the speed and capacity of information processing I: A dual-task approach. *Psychology and Aging, 2,* 70–78.

Woodcock, R. W. (1995). Theoretical foundations of the WJ-R measures of cognitive ability. *Journal of Psychoeducational Assessment, 8,* 231–258.

CHAPTER 4

The Cattell–Horn–Carroll Model of Intelligence

W. Joel Schneider
Kevin S. McGrew

The Cattell–Horn–Carroll (CHC) theory of cognitive abilities consists of two components. First, it is a *taxonomy*[1] of cognitive abilities. However, it is no mere list. The second component, embedded in the taxonomy, is a set of theoretical explanations of how and why people differ in their various cognitive abilities. This chapter is intended to make CHC theory useful and usable to practitioners. It also aims to provide a reflective account of CHC theory's historical roots and evolution; an introspective meditation on its current status, with a candid discussion of its virtues and shortcomings; and a tempered but hopeful projection of its future.

THE IMPORTANCE OF TAXONOMIES

SOCRATES: . . . but in these chance utterances were involved two principles, the essence of which it would be gratifying to learn, if art could teach it.

PHAEDRUS: What principles?

SOCRATES: That of perceiving and bringing together in one idea the scattered particulars, that one may make clear by definition the particular thing which he wishes to explain.

PHAEDRUS: And what is the other principle, Socrates?

SOCRATES: That of dividing things again by classes, where the natural joints are, and not trying to break any part, after the manner of a bad carver.

—PLATO, *Phaedrus* (§ 265d)

A useful classification system shapes how we view complex phenomena by illuminating consequential distinctions and obscuring trivial differences. A misspecified classification system orients us toward the irrelevant and distracts us from taking productive action. Imagine if we had to use astrological classification systems for personnel selection, college admissions, jury selection, or clinical diagnosis. The scale of inefficiency, inaccuracy, and injustice that would ensue boggles the mind. Classification is serious business.

Much hinges on classification systems being properly aligned with our purposes. Consider the role that the periodic table of elements has played in the physical sciences. First arranged by Mendeleev in 1869, it is not just a random collection of different elements. Embedded in the periodic table are a number of organizing principles (e.g., number of protons, valence electrons) that not only *reflected* the theoretical advances of the 19th century, but also *propelled* discoveries in physics and chemistry to the present day.

A well-validated taxonomy of cognitive abilities will not resemble the periodic table of elements, but it should have the same function of organizing past findings and revealing holes in our knowledge warranting exploration. It should give researchers a common frame of reference and nomenclature. It should suggest criteria by which disagreements can be settled. For now, there is no taxonomy of cognitive abilities that commands the same level of authority as the periodic table of elements. Should one emerge, it will happen via the only means any scientific theory should: The theoretical framework will withstand all attempts to knock it down. Because it is a systematic synthesis of hundreds of studies spanning more than a century of empirical investigations of cognitive abilities, CHC theory is put forward as a candidate for a common framework for cognitive ability researchers (McGrew, 2009). All are invited to help build it, and anyone is entitled to try to knock it down by subjecting it to critical tests of its assumptions.

THE EVOLUTION OF THE CHC THEORY OF COGNITIVE ABILITIES

The CHC theory of intelligence is the "tent" that houses the two most prominent psychometric theoretical models of human cognitive abilities (Daniel, 1997, 2000; Kaufman, 2009; McGrew, 2005, 2009; Snow, 1998; Sternberg & Kaufman, 1998). CHC theory represents the integration of the Horn–Cattell Gf-Gc theory (Horn & Noll, 1997; see Horn & Blankson, Chapter 3, this volume) and Carroll's three-stratum theory (Carroll, 1993; see Carroll, Appendix to this volume).

The study of cognitive abilities is intimately linked to historical developments in exploratory and confirmatory factor analysis, the primary methodological engine that has driven the psychometric study of intelligence for over 100 years (Cudek & MacCallum, 2007). However, it is also important to recognize that non-factor-analytic research, in the form of heritability, neurocognitive, developmental, and outcome prediction (occupational and educational) studies, provides additional sources of validity evidence for CHC theory (Horn, 1998; Horn & Noll, 1997). Space limitations necessitate a focus only on the factor-analytic portions of the contemporary psychometric approach to studying individual differences in human cognitive abilities.

The historical development of CHC theory is presented in the timeline depicted in Figure 4.1. The first portion of this chapter is organized according to the events in this timeline.

Early Psychometric Heritage

The developers of intelligence tests were not as narrow minded as they are often made out to be; and, as a necessary corollary, nor are we as clever as some would

have it. Those who have not themselves read widely from the books and articles of luminaries such as Binet, Spearman, Thorndike, and Stern are not so much condemned to repeat history (as Santayana claimed) as they are to say and write silly things.

—LOHMAN (1997, p. 360)

Historical accounts of the evolution of the psychometric approach to the study of human individual differences abound (e.g., see Brody, 2000; Carroll, 1993; Cudeck & MacCallum, 2007; Horn & Noll, 1997; see also Wasserman, Chapter 1, this volume).[2] We cannot possibly convey the full extent of the depth, breadth, and subtlety of thought characteristic of most of the great early theorists. We have tried to avoid Lohman's curse of saying silly things by consulting the original sources. A good rule of thumb is that whenever an important historical theory appears laughable when summarized, the stupidity is in the summary, not the source.

As illustrated in Figure 4.1, Francis Galton is generally considered the founder of the field of individual differences via his interests in measuring, describing, and quantifying human differences and the genetics of geniuses. The study of individual differences in reaction time is credited with originating in German psychologist Wilhelm Wundt's lab. Wundt is reported to have had little interest in the study of individual differences. However, an American student of Wundt's, James McKeen Cattell, was interested in the topic and is credited with coining the term *mental test* (Cattell, 1890).

Another student of Wundt's, Charles Spearman, had a similar interest in measuring individual differences in sensory discrimination (reflecting the influence of Galton). Spearman (1904) developed a "two-factor theory" (a general intelligence factor, *g*, plus specific factors) to account for correlations between measures of academic achievement, reasoning, and sensory discrimination (see Figure 4.2).

Carroll (1993) suggested that Spearman's theory might be better called a "one-general-factor theory." Spearman is generally credited with introducing the notion of factor analysis to the study of human abilities. Spearman and his students eventually began to study other possible factors beyond *g*. The Spearman–Holzinger model (Carroll, 1993), which was based on Holzinger's development of the bifactor method, suggested *g* plus five group factors (Spearman, 1939). In the final statement of Spearman's theories, Spearman and Wynn-Jones (1950) recognized many group factors: verbal

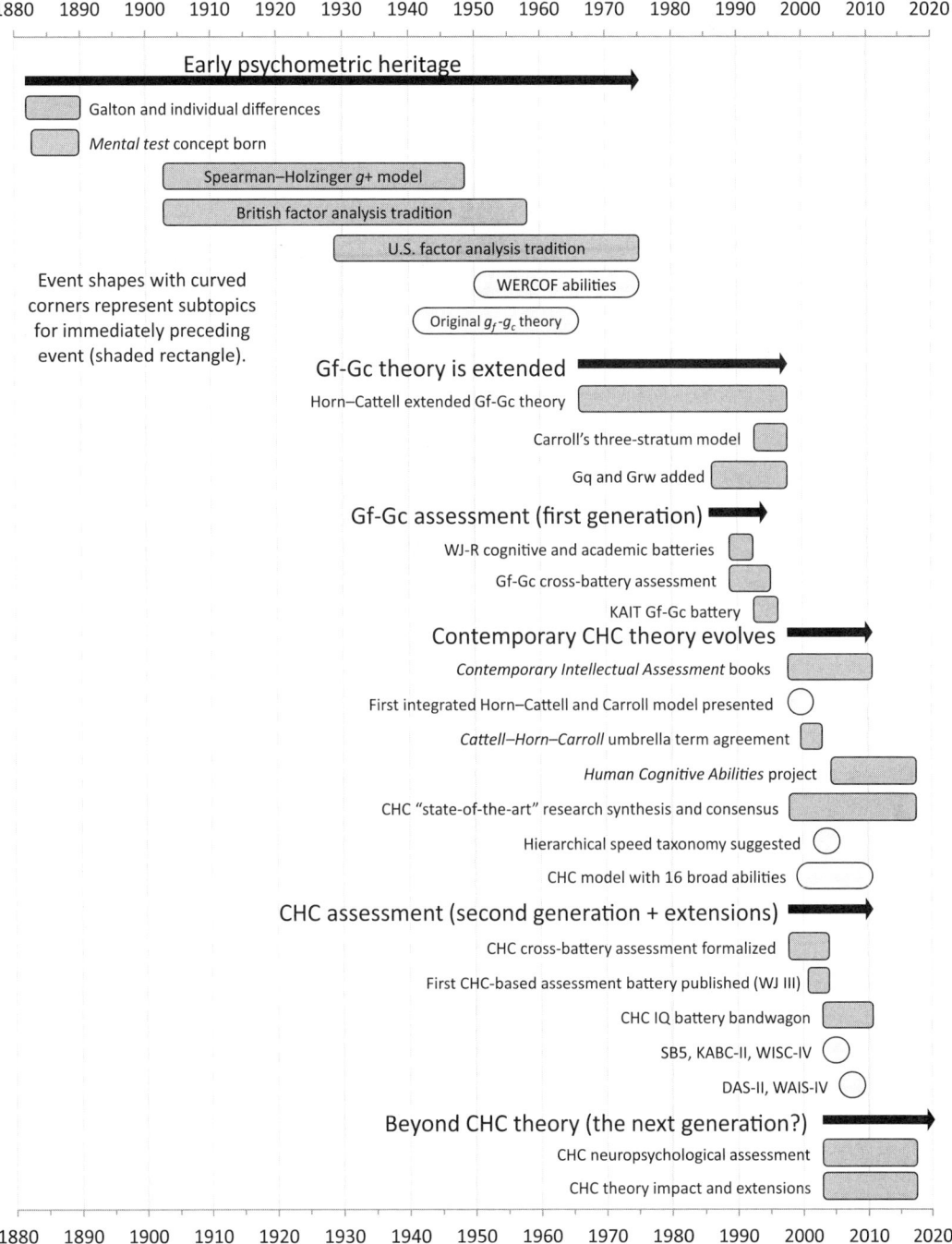

FIGURE 4.1. The evolution of CHC intelligence theory and assessment methods: A timeline.

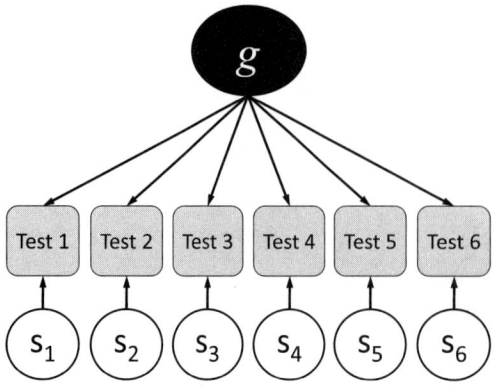

FIGURE 4.2. Spearman's two-factor theory.

(Gc), spatial (Gv), motor (Gp), memory (Glr and Gsm), mathematics (Gq), speed (Gs), and several others (abbreviations denote approximate correspondence with CHC theory). The definition and issues surrounding the construct of g are discussed in greater detail in Box 4.1.

Reflecting the seminal influence of Spearman, the British factor analysis tradition (see Figure 4.1) suggested that the lion's share of the variance of human intelligence was attributable to g and to very small group factors. The importance of the broader group factors was considered meager (Gustafsson, 1988).

Across the ocean, the factor analysis tradition in the United States focused on the use of early forms of multiple factor analysis that did not readily identify a g factor. Instead, the correlations among measures produced correlated (oblique) first-order factors that were typically factor analyzed again to produce second-order factors.

L. L. Thurstone is to factor analysis in the United States what Spearman is to the British tradition of factor analysis. Thurstone's theory posited seven to nine primary mental abilities (PMAs) that were independent of a higher-order g factor.[3] Thurstone's (1938) PMA theory included induction (I), deduction (D), verbal comprehension (V), associative memory (Ma), spatial relations (S), perceptual speed (P), numerical facility (N), and word fluency (Fw). Thurstone (1947) was willing to accept the possible existence of a g (general factor) above his PMAs. The primary Spearman–Holzinger/Thurstone disagreement was the perceived difference in relative importance of the first-order PMAs and the second-order g factor (Carroll, 1993).

From the 1940s to 1960s, numerous factor-analytic studies of human cognitive abilities were conducted using variants of Thurstone's multiple-factors method. The period from 1952 to approximately 1976 was particularly productive, as the Educational Testing Service (ETS) sponsored a series of activities and conferences with the goal to develop a standard kit of reference tests to serve as established factor "markers" in future factor analysis studies (Carroll, 1993). Summaries of the large body of PMA-based factor research suggested over 60 possible separate PMAs (Ekstrom, French, & Harman, 1979; French, 1951; French, Ekstrom, & Price, 1963; Guilford, 1967; Hakstian & Cattell, 1974; Horn, 1976). The ETS factor–reference group work established the well-replicated common factors (WERCOF) abilities (Horn, 1989). Carroll's (1993) model is strongly influenced by the 1976 edition of the ETS standard kit (Ekstrom et al., 1979). Of its 23 primary abilities, 16 have the same names in Carroll's list of stratum I (narrow) abilities. The remaining 7 ETS factors are all in Carroll's (1993) model but have different names.

Gf-Gc Theory Is Conceived

Raymond Cattell was a student of Spearman's who applied Thurstone-style factor-analytic methods to the WERCOF/PMA datasets.

Cattell (1941, 1943) concluded that Spearman's g was best explained by splitting g into general *fluid* (g_f) and general *crystallized* (g_c) intelligence. The positing of a hierarchical model of two equally important broad abilities (Gf and Gc) above the numerous lower-order WERCOF abilities represented the formal beginning of the Horn–Cattell Gf-Gc theory.[4]

The genius of Gf-Gc theory is not the idea that there was more than one factor, or that there were specifically two factors (both ideas had been previously articulated). The astounding achievement of the original Gf-Gc theory is that Cattell (1941, 1943) was able to describe the nature of both factors, model how Spearman's g arose from Gf and Gc, and explain many diverse and previously puzzling empirical observations. Most importantly, the findings have largely withstood the test of time. Cattell's (1943) first printed description of both factors is worth quoting here:

> Fluid ability has the character of a purely general ability to discriminate and perceive relations between any fundaments, new or old. It increases until adolescence and then slowly declines. It is associated with the action of the whole cortex. It is responsible for

BOX 4.1. Does *g* Exist?

The question of whether *g* exists causes more rancor amongst cognitive ability researchers than perhaps any other. For some, the mere mention of *g* brings to mind a rapid succession of frightful images that start with bureaucratic abuses of IQ tests and proceed straight to Hitler. For others, the fight for *g* is about preserving the last sanctuary of reason and liberty from the perverse and pervasive influence of showboating do-gooder muddleheads with a secret lust for worldwide domination via progressive education. Who can stay silent when the cords of one's identity are strained and the fate of nations hangs in the balance? Honor, dignity, pride, and justice demand otherwise. Of course, from time to time there are impassioned pleas for dispassionate discourse, but the sirens of serenity are seldom seductive.

Positive Manifold

In the beginning, Spearman (1904) discovered what has come to be known as the *positive manifold*—the tendency for all tests of mental ability to be positively correlated. Thousands of replicating studies later, Spearman's observation remains uncontroversial. What was then, what is now, and what will be controversial for a long time is Spearman's explanation for the positive manifold.

In many ways, Spearman's explanation was the simplest explanation possible. The reason that all tests are positively correlated is that performance on all tests is influenced by a common cause, *g*. Each test is influenced both by *g* and by its own *s* (specific) factor (see Figure 4.2). Spearman's two-factor theory has a misleading name because there are not just two factors; there is one general factor and as many *s* factors as there are tests. Thus the two-factor theory is really a theory about two different kinds of factors, general and specific.

Is *g* an Ability?

The controversy about the theoretical status of *g* may have less fire and venom if some misunderstandings are clarified. First, Spearman did not believe that performance on tests was affected by *g* and only *g*. He always accepted that specific factors were often important, and came to appreciate group factors (Spearman & Wynn-Jones, 1950). Second, Spearman (1927, p. 92) always maintained, even in his first paper about *g* (Spearman, 1904, p. 284), that *g* might consist of more than one general factor. Third, Spearman did not consider *g* to be an ability, or even a thing (Spearman, 1934, pp. 312–313; Spearman

& Wynn-Jones, 1950, p. 25). Yes, you read that last sentence correctly.

Horn (see Horn & Blankson, Chapter 3, this volume), Carroll (1998), and Cattell (1943) may have had different ideas about the nature of psychometric *g*, but they were all in agreement with Spearman that factors derived from factor analysis should not be reified prematurely. However, they believed that it was still useful to observe regularities in data and to hypothesize causes of those regularities. Cattell explained it thus:

> Obviously "*g*" is no more resident in the individual than the horsepower of a car is resident in the engine. It is a concept derived from the relations between the individual and his environment. But what trait that we normally project into and assign to the individual is not? The important further condition is that the factor is not determinable by the individual and his environment but only in relation to a group and its environment. A test factor loading or an individual's factor endowment has meaning only in relation to a population and an environment. But it is difficult to see why there should be any objection to the concept of intelligence being given so abstract a habitation when economists, for example, are quite prepared to assign to such a simple, concrete notion as "price" an equally relational existence. (p. 19)

We, like Spearman and essentially all other researchers who study this matter, are not sure about what causes statistical *g*. However, we suspect that Jensen (Bock, Goode, & Webb, 2000, p. 29) is correct in his judgment that *g* is not an ability itself, but the sum total of all forces that cause abilities within the same person to be more similar to each other than they otherwise would have been. Forces that simultaneously affect the whole brain may include individual differences in many individual genes and gene complexes, differential exposure to environmental toxins (e.g., lead, mercury, mold), parasites, childhood diseases, blunt-force trauma, large strokes, malnutrition, substance abuse, and many other forces. Furthermore, societal forces can act to cause otherwise uncorrelated abilities to become correlated. High socioeconomic status gives some people greater access to all of the things that enhance brain functioning and greater protection from all of the things that harm the brain. Low socioeconomic status is associated with exposure to a whole host of risk factors that can damage the whole brain. Put together, these forces seem more than enough to create the observed positive manifold and the *g* factor that emerges from factor analysis. Clinically, we view measures of *g* to be a useful point of reference, much like magnetic north. However, when we explore unfamiliar places, we do not restrict our view to lines of longitude. We like to look about in all directions.

the intercorrelations, or general factor, found among children's tests and among the speeded or adaptation-requiring tests of adults.

Crystallized ability consists of discriminatory habits long established in a particular field, originally through the operation of fluid ability, but no longer requiring insightful perception for their successful operation. (p. 178)

Cattell's (1963) Gf-Gc investment theory addressed the question "Why do some people know much more than others?" Cattell believed that differences in people's breadth and depth of knowledge are the joint function of two kinds of influences. Low fluid intelligence limits the rate at which a person can acquire and retain new knowledge. People with high fluid intelligence have far fewer constraints on their ability to learn.

Whether Gf is high or low, most learning comes about by effort. There are many non-ability-related reasons why some people engage in the learning process more than others, including availability and quality of education, family resources and expectations, and individual interests and goals. All of these differences in time and effort spent on learning were called *investment* by Cattell (1987). Cattell's original (1941, 1943) Gf-Gc theory has an explanation for the positive manifold: Gf and Gc are both general ability factors, and these factors are strongly correlated because Gf, in part, causes Gc via investment. However, for people with low Gf, investments in learning pay smaller dividends than for people with high Gf. This causes Gf and Gc to be highly correlated, and psychometric *g* emerges in the resulting positive manifold (see Figure 4.3).

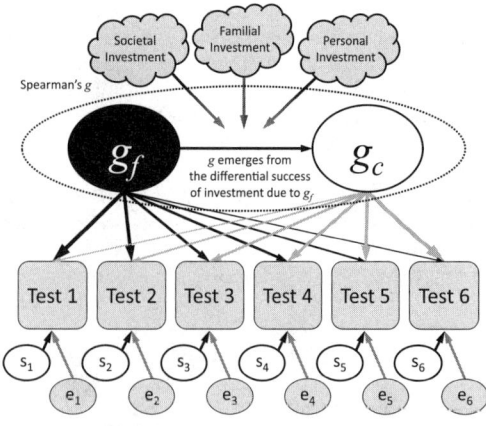

FIGURE 4.3. Cattell's investment theory.

Gf-Gc Theory Is Extended

However brilliant Cattell's original (1941, 1943) theory was, it remained a post hoc explanation of existing data until the first deliberate empirical test of the theory was conducted by John Horn (Cattell, 1963).[5] Horn's (1965) dissertation (supervised by Cattell) provided support for Cattell's theory, but also proposed that it be significantly expanded. It can be said that Horn reconceptualized and upgraded several of Thurstone's (1938, 1947) PMAs[6] to be coequal with Cattell's two general factors (e.g., space = Gv). Horn, Cattell, and others then worked to subdivide each of the general factors into narrower abilities that were even more primary than Thurstone's PMAs.

Horn's (1965) doctoral dissertation expanded Gf-Gc theory to several broad ability factors (Gf, Gc, Gv, Gs, SAR, TSR; Horn & Cattell, 1966). The change in notation from g_f and g_c to Gf and Gc was deliberate because in the extended Gf-Gc theory both Gf and Gc are narrower concepts than their counterparts in Cattell's original theory (see Horn & Blankson, Chapter 3, this volume).

From approximately 1965 to the late 1990s, Horn, Cattell, and others published systematic programs of factor-analytic research confirming the original Gf-Gc model and adding new factors. By 1991, Horn had extended the Gf-Gc theory to include 9–10 broad Gf-Gc abilities: fluid intelligence (Gf), crystallized intelligence (Gc), short-term acquisition and retrieval (SAR or Gsm), visual intelligence (Gv), auditory intelligence (Ga), long-term storage and retrieval (TSR or Glr), cognitive processing speed (Gs), correct decision speed (CDS), and quantitative knowledge (Gq). Woodcock's (1990, 1993) broad-ranging factor-analytic reviews of clinical measures of cognitive abilities strongly suggested the inclusion of a reading/writing (Grw) ability.

Carroll's (1993) Principia: *Human Cognitive Abilities*

Human Cognitive Abilities: A Survey of Factor-Analytic Studies (Carroll, 1993) represents in the field of applied psychometrics a work similar in stature to other so-called "principia" publications in other fields (e.g., Newton's three-volume *The Mathematical Principles of Natural Philosophy*, or *Principia* as it became known; Whitehead & Russell's *Principia Mathematica*). Briefly, Carroll summarized a reanalysis of more than 460 different datasets that included nearly all the more important and classic factor-analytic studies of human cognitive abilities since the time of Spearman. This important development is labeled *Carroll's three-stratum model* in the CHC timeline (see Figure 4.1).

We are not alone in elevating Carroll's work to such a high stature. Burns (1994) stated that Carroll's book "is simply the finest work of research and scholarship I have read and is destined to be *the classic study and reference work on human abilities for decades to come*" (p. 35; emphasis in original). Horn (1998) described Carroll's (1993) work as a "tour de force summary and integration" that is the "definitive foundation for current theory" (p. 58); he also compared Carroll's summary to "Mendeleev's first presentation of a periodic table of elements in chemistry" (p. 58). Jensen (2004) stated that "on my first reading this tome, in 1993, I was reminded of the conductor Hans von Bülow's exclamation on first reading the full orchestral score of Wagner's *Die Meistersinger*, 'It's impossible, but there it is!'" (p. 4). Finally, according to Jensen,

> Carroll's magnum opus thus distills and synthesizes the results of a century of factor analyses of mental tests. It is virtually the grand finale of the era of psychometric *description and taxonomy* of human cognitive abilities. It is unlikely that his monumental feat will ever be attempted again by anyone, or that it could be much improved on. It will long be the key reference point and a solid foundation for the *explanatory* era of differential psychology that we now see burgeoning in genetics and the brain sciences. (p. 5; emphasis in original)

The beauty of Carroll's (1993) book was that for the first time ever, an empirically based taxonomy of human cognitive abilities, based on the analysis (with a common method) of the extant literature since Spearman, was presented in a single, coherent, organized, systematic framework (McGrew, 2005, 2009). Briefly, Carroll proposed a three-tier model of human cognitive abilities that differentiates abilities as a function of breadth. At the broadest level (stratum III) is a general intelligence factor. Next in breadth are eight broad abilities that represent "basic constitutional and long-standing characteristics of individuals that can govern or influence a great variety of behaviors in a given domain" (Carroll, 1993, p. 634).

Stratum II includes the abilities of fluid intelligence (Gf), crystallized intelligence (Gc), general memory and learning (Gy), broad visual perception (Gv), broad auditory perception (Ga), broad retrieval ability (Gr), broad cognitive speediness (Gs), and reaction time/decision speed (Gt). Stratum I includes numerous narrow abilities subsumed by the stratum II abilities, which in turn are subsumed by the single stratum III g factor. Finally, Carroll recognized that his theoretical model built on the research of others, particularly Cattell and Horn. According to Carroll, the Horn–Cattell Gf-Gc model "appears to offer the most well-founded and reasonable approach to an acceptable theory of the structure of cognitive abilities" (p. 62).

In a sense, Carroll (1993) provided the field of intelligence with a much-needed "Rosetta stone" that would serve as a key for deciphering and organizing the enormous mass of literature on the structure of human cognitive abilities accumulated since the days of Spearman. Carroll's work was also influential in creating the awareness among intelligence scholars, applied psychometricians, and assessment professionals, that understanding human cognitive abilities required "three-stratum vision." As a practical benefit, Carroll's work provided a common nomenclature for professional communication—a nomenclature that would go "far in helping us all better understand what we are measuring, facilitate better communication between and among professionals and scholars, and increase our ability to compare individual tests across and within intelligence batteries" (McGrew, 1997, p. 171).

Gf-Gc Assessment: First Generation

The 1989 publication of the Woodcock–Johnson Psychoeducational Battery—Revised (WJ-R; Woodcock & Johnson, 1989), a revision of the original 1977 WJ battery (Woodcock, 1978; Woodcock & Johnson, 1977), represented the official "crossing over" of Gf-Gc theory to the work of applied practitioners, particularly those conducting assessments in educational settings. A personal account of the serendipitous events, starting in 1985, that resulted in the bridging of the intelligence theory–assessment gap can be found in the preceding edition of this chapter (McGrew, 2005), and additional historical context has been provided by Kaufman (2009).

Publication of the Horn–Cattell-Organized WJ-R Battery

The WJ-R test development blueprint was based on the Horn–Cattell extended Gf-Gc theory (McGrew, Werder, & Woodcock, 1991; Schrank,

Flanagan, Woodcock, & Mascolo, 2002). The WJ-R represented the first individually administered, nationally standardized, clinical cognitive and achievement battery to close the gap between contemporary psychometric theory (i.e., Horn–Cattell Extended Gf-Gc theory) and applied assessment practice. According to Daniel (1997), the WJ-R was "the most thorough implementation of the multifactor model" (p. 1039) of intelligence. As a direct result of the publication of the WJ-R, "Gf-Gc as a second language" emerged vigorously in educational and school psychology training programs, journal articles, books, and psychological reports, and became a frequent topic on certain professional and assessment-related electronic listservs.

First Proposal of Gf-Gc Cross-Battery Assessment

In 1990, Richard Woodcock planted the seed for the idea of Gf-Gc "battery-free" assessment, in which a common Gf-Gc taxonomy for assessment and interpretation was deployed across *all* intelligence batteries. In his seminal article summarizing his analysis of a series of joint confirmatory factor analysis (CFA) studies of the major intelligence batteries, Woodcock demonstrated how individual tests from each intelligence battery mapped onto the broad abilities of Horn–Cattell extended Gf-Gc taxonomy. More importantly, Woodcock suggested that in order to measure a greater breadth of Gf-Gc abilities, users of other instruments should use "cross-battery" methods to fill their respective Gf-Gc measurement voids. Practitioners were no longer constrained to the interpretive structure provided by a specific intelligence battery (see Flanagan, Alfonso, & Ortiz, Chapter 19, this volume, for a summary of their cross-battery approach).

Contemporary CHC Theory Evolves

The *Contemporary Intellectual Assessment* Books

The collective influence of the Horn–Cattell extended Gf-Gc theory, Carroll's (1993) treatise, and the publication of the WJ-R was reflected in nine chapters' being devoted to, or including significant treatment of, the Horn–Cattell extended Gf-Gc and Carroll three-stratum theories in Flanagan, Genshaft, and Harrison's (1997) first edition of *Contemporary Intellectual Assessment: Theories,* *Tests, and Issues* (often referred to informally as the "CIA book"). This publication, as well as its second edition (Flanagan & Harrison, 2005), was another key theory-to-practice bridging event (see Figure 4.1). The current volume (the third edition) continues the tradition.

The original CIA book contributed to the evolution of CHC theory for three primary reasons. First, it was the first intellectual assessment text intended for university trainers and assessment practitioners that included introductory chapters describing both the Horn–Cattell and Carroll models by the theorists themselves (Horn & Noll, 1997; Carroll's chapter is reprinted as the Appendix to the present volume).

Second, the *first* published integration of the Horn–Cattell and Carroll models was articulated in a chapter by McGrew (1997). Furthermore, Flanagan and McGrew (1998) articulated the need for tests in intelligence batteries to be classified at both the stratum I (narrow) and stratum II (broad) Gf-Gc ability levels. However, to do so, a single taxonomy was needed—yet the two major models contained some differences.[7] Instead of selecting one model over the other, McGrew (1997, p. 152) presented a "synthesized Carroll and Horn–Cattell Gf-Gc framework."

Finally, the original CIA text included the first formal description of the assumptions, foundations, and operational principles for implementing Gf-Gc cross-battery assessment (Flanagan & McGrew, 1997). The cross-battery seed planted by Woodcock (1990) had blossomed, and the intelligence theory-to-practice gap had narrowed fast. The CHC "tipping point" had begun.[8]

Formal "Branding" and Infusion of CHC Theory in Research and Practice

CHC theory represents *both* the Horn–Cattell and Carroll models, in their respective splendor. Much like the term *information-processing theories*, which provides an overarching theoretical umbrella for a spectrum of very similar (yet different) theoretical model variations (Lohman, 2001), the term *CHC theory* serves the same function for the "variations on a Gf-Gc theme" by Horn–Cattell and Carroll, respectively. The historical details of the origin of the umbrella *Cattell–Horn–Carroll (CHC)* term are described in McGrew (2005).

The recognition and influence of the CHC taxonomic umbrella increased steadily after 1999 (McGrew, 2009), particularly in professional fields engaged in applied intellectual assessment. The

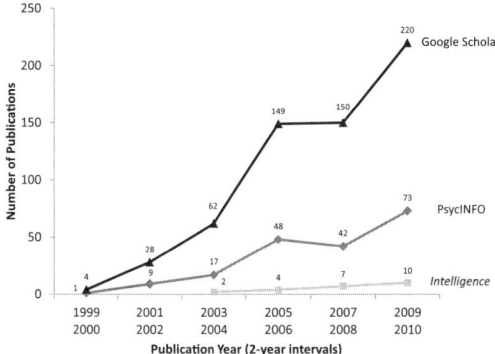

FIGURE 4.4. Number of publications including the terms *CHC* or *Cattell–Horn–Carroll* (by year) from two search sources.

adoption of the CHC umbrella model has been slower in publications in theoretical fields (e.g., *Intelligence*) outside the field of school psychology. As can be seen in Figure 4.4, the acceptance and use of the umbrella name *CHC theory* started in earnest in 2000–2001 and have steadily increased during the past decade.[9] It is clear that the professional discourse of intelligence theory and assessment literature is increasingly embracing CHC terminology.

CHC "State-of-the-Art" Research Syntheses

A major factor influencing the increasing recognition of the CHC framework has been a series of CHC "state-of-the-art" research syntheses (see Figure 4.1). In the second edition of the CIA text (Flanagan & Harrison, 2005), McGrew (2005) presented the most comprehensive historical treatment of the evolution of CHC theory. The second edition of the CIA included no fewer than 8 (of 29) chapters that specifically addressed the major components of CHC theory (McGrew, 2005, plus Horn & Blankson's and Carroll's chapters, reprinted here as Chapter 3 and the Appendix, respectively); CHC-grounded intelligence batteries (Elliott, 2005; Kaufman, Kaufman, Kaufman-Singer, & Kaufman, 2005; Roid & Pomplun, 2005; Schrank, 2005); and CHC theory's impact on test development and interpretation (Alfonso, Flanagan, & Radwan, 2005). CHC theory also received notable attention in chapters dealing with the history of intellectual assessment (Kamphaus, Winsor, Rowe, & Kim, 2005; Wasserman & Tulsky, 2005); information-processing approaches to intelligence

test interpretation (Floyd, 2005); interventions for students with learning disabilities (Mather & Wendling, 2005); assessment of preschoolers (Ford & Dahinten, 2005), gifted children (McIntosh & Dixon, 2005), and those with learning disabilities (Flanagan & Mascolo, 2005); and the use of CFA in the interpretation of intelligence tests (Keith, 2005). The current volume continues this tradition.

An acknowledged limitation of Carroll's (1993, p. 579) three-stratum model was the fact that Carroll's inferences regarding the relations between different factors at different levels (strata) emerged from data derived from a diverse array of largely independent studies and samples (McGrew, 2005). None of Carroll's datasets included the necessary breadth of variables to evaluate, in a single analysis, the general structure of his proposed three-stratum model. An important contribution of McGrew's (2005) review was the synthesis of a significant number of exploratory and confirmatory factor-analytic investigations completed since the publication of Carroll's seminal work. The reader is referred to McGrew (2005) and McGrew and Evans (2004) for detailed summaries. One contribution of these reviews was the recognition of the potential for internal elaborations and refinements of CHC theory and for external extensions of CHC theory through the addition of new constructs, such as the broad abilities of general knowledge (Gkn), tactile abilities (Gh), kinesthetic abilities (Gk), olfactory abilities (Go), and psychomotor speed (Gps).

Of particular interest, but largely ignored during the past several years, was the conclusion that the speed domains of Gs and Gt might best be represented within the context of a hierarchically organized speed taxonomy with a *g*-speed factor at the apex (McGrew, 2005; McGrew & Evans, 2004). This conclusion has been echoed by Danthiir, Roberts, Schulze, and Wilhelm (2005), who, after conducting much of the research that suggests a multidimensional speed hierarchy, suggested that "one distinct possibility is that mental speed tasks form as complex a hierarchy as level (i.e., accuracy) measures from psychometric tasks, with a general mental speed factor at the apex and broad factors of mental speed forming a second underlying tier" (p. 32). A slightly altered version of McGrew and Evans's (2004) hypothesized hierarchy of speed abilities is formally published here for the first time in Figure 4.5.

More recently, the journal *Psychology in the Schools* published a special issue (Newton &

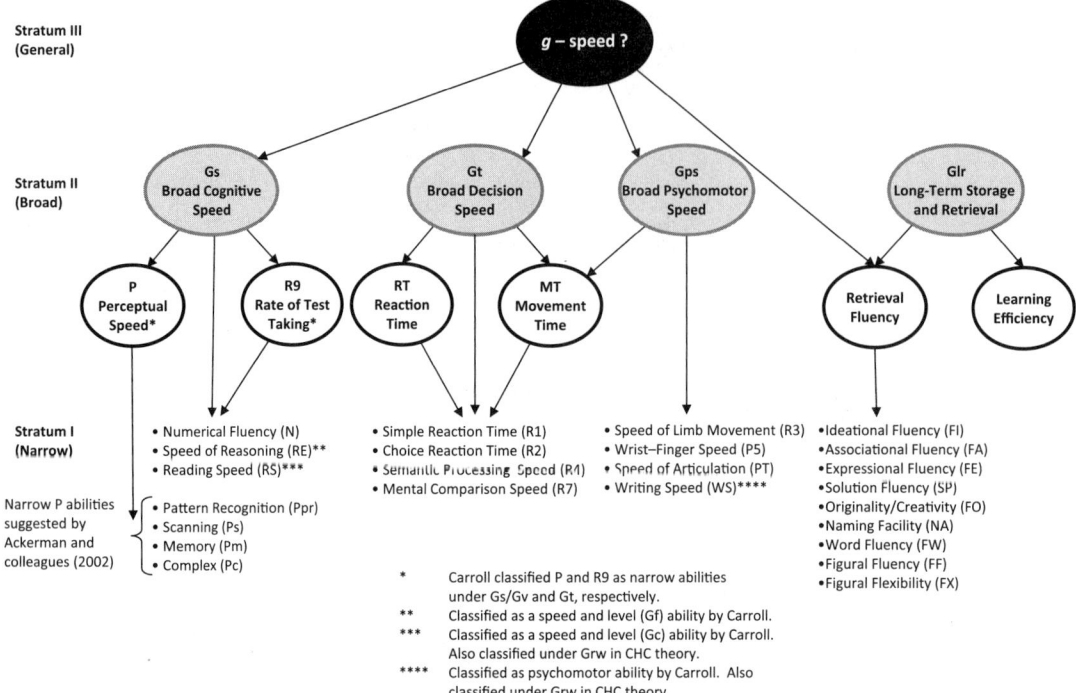

FIGURE 4.5. McGrew and Evans's (2004) hypothesized speed hierarchy, based on integration of Carroll's (1993) speed abilities with other research (Ackerman, Beier, & Boyle, 2002; O'Connor & Burns, 2003; McGrew & Woodcock, 2001; Roberts & Stankov, 1999; Stankov, 2000; Stankov & Roberts, 1997).

McGrew, 2010) that examined the contribution of the contemporary CHC theory in the applied fields of school psychology and special education. The core aim of the special issue was to "take stock" of the 20 years of CHC research jump-started by the 1989 publication of the WJ-R (see Figure 4.1). As articulated by the issue's editors (Newton & McGrew, 2010), the core question addressed was this: "Has the drawing of a reasonably circumscribed 'holy grail' taxonomy of cognitive abilities led to the promised land of intelligence testing in the schools—using the results of cognitive assessments to better the education of children with special needs?" (p. 631). Two broad overview articles were the central focus of the special issue.

Keith and Reynolds's (2010) article reviewed the factor-analytic research on seven different intelligence batteries from the perspective of the CHC model. Keith and Reynolds noted that most new and revised intelligence batteries were either grounded explicitly in CHC theory, or paid some form of implied "allegiance to the theory" (p. 635). Keith and Reynolds (2010) concluded that "although most new and revised tests of intelligence

are based, at least in part, on CHC theory, earlier versions generally were not. Our review suggests that whether or not they were based on CHC theory, the factors derived from both new and previous versions of most tests are well explained by the theory" (p. 635).

McGrew and Wendling's (2010) research synthesis in the special issue was designed to answer the question "What have we learned from 20 years of CHC COG–ACH [cognitive–achievement] relations research?" (p. 651). This review produced a number of important conclusions. First, cognitive abilities contribute to academic achievement in different proportions in different academic domains, and these proportions change over the course of development. For example, phonetic coding is relatively unimportant in the domain of mathematics, but is a major influence on the development of reading decoding. However, its influence changes over time. It is quite important in the first few years of schooling but its influence wanes in later childhood.

A second conclusion of McGrew and Wendling's review was that the most consistently salient CHC cognitive–achievement relations exist for narrow (stratum I) cognitive abilities. The authors recommended a refocusing of CHC school-based assessment on selective, referral-focused cognitive assessment of narrow cognitive and achievement abilities. Finally, McGrew and Wendling concluded that the developmentally nuanced relations between primarily narrow cognitive and achievement abilities argue "for more judicious, flexible, selective, 'intelligent' (Kaufman, 1979) intelligence testing where practitioners select sets of tests most relevant to each academic referral. Unless there is a need for a full-scale IQ *g* score for diagnosis (e.g., [intellectual disability], gifted[ness]), professionals need to break the habit of 'one complete battery fits all' testing" (p. 669).

In conclusion, a review of the extant intelligence theory and assessment literature published during the past 20+ years indicates that CHC theory has attained the status as the consensus psychometric model of the structure of human cognitive abilities. We are not alone in our conclusion. Ackerman and Lohman (2006) concluded that "the Cattell–Horn–Carroll (CHC) theory of cognitive abilities is the best validated model of human cognitive abilities" (p. 140).

Kaufman (2009) stated that CHC theory has formed the foundation for most contemporary IQ tests" (p. 91). Keith and Reynolds (2010) concluded that "we believe that CHC theory offers the best current description of the structure of human intelligence" (p. 642). Similarly, Detterman (2011) concluded that

> because the Carroll model is largely consistent with the model originally proposed by Cattell (1971), McGrew (2009) has proposed an integration of the two models which he calls the Cattell–Horn–Carroll (C-H-C) integration model. . . . Because of the inclusiveness of this model, it is becoming the standard typology for human ability. It is certainly the culmination of exploratory factor analysis. (p. 288)

Clearly, the CHC tipping point was reached during the past decade.

Beyond CHC Theory: The Next Generation?

A clear indication of the prominent stature achieved by the CHC theory of intelligence is the fact that it has increasingly been recognized and infused into related psychological assessment arenas and research on intelligence and psychometrics.

CHC-Based Neuropsychological Assessment

The most active CHC "spillover" has been in the area of neuropsychological assessment. A number of CHC-based neuropsychological assessment texts have been published, starting with Hale and Fiorello's *School Neuropsychology: A Practitioner's Handbook* (2004). Two texts by Miller, both with a school neuropsychology focus, are *Essentials of School Neuropsychology* (2007) and *Best Practices in School Neuropsychology: Guidelines for Effective Practice, Assessment, and Evidence-Based Intervention* (2010). It is our opinion that CHC-based neuropsychological assessment holds great potential. Much clinical lore within the field of neuropsychological assessment is tied to specific tests from specific batteries. CHC theory has the potential to help neuropsychologists generalize their interpretations beyond specific test batteries and give them greater theoretical unity.

However, many more CHC-organized factor-analytic studies of joint neuropsychological and CHC-validated batteries are needed before such a synthesis is possible (e.g., see Floyd, Bergeron, Hamilton, & Parra, 2010, and Hoelzle, 2008). Even more crucial are studies that describe the functioning of the brain (e.g., with functional magnetic resonance imaging) during performance on validated tests of CHC abilities.

Finally, it is not yet clear that the variations of ability observed in nondisabled populations are similar to the variations of ability observed in brain-injured populations. Much work needs to be done to verify that when brain injuries occur, CHC ability constructs provide a good framework to describe the kinds of symptoms and losses in function typically observed. If not, CHC theory must be revised or expanded before it can be the primary lens through which neuropsychologists interpret their findings. The potential of CHC-organized neuropsychological assessment is currently that—a yet-to-be-recognized potentiality.

CHC Theory Extensions and Impact

In McGrew's 2005 version of the current chapter, he stated that "older and lesser-used multivariate statistical procedures, such as multidimensional scaling (MDS), need to be pulled from psychometricians' closets to allow for the simultaneous examination of content (facets), processes, and processing complexity" (p. 172) of CHC measures. This recommendation recognized the value of the faceted hierarchical Berlin intelligence structure model (Beauducel, Brocke, & Liepmann, 2001; Süß, Oberauer, Wittmann, Wilhelm, & Schulze, 2002) as a promising lens through which to view CHC theory. Only a select few researchers have heeded this call, although Snow and colleagues (Marshalek, Lohman, & Snow, 1983; Snow, Kyllonen, & Marshalek, 1984) had clearly demonstrated the potential contribution of Guttman's (1954) MDS approach as early as the 1980s. Recent demonstrations of the "added value" that can occur when EFA/CFA intelligence test research is augmented by MDS analyses of the same data include the Cohen, Fiorello, and Farley (2006) three-dimensional (3-D) analysis and interpretation of the Wechsler Intelligence Scale for Children—Fourth Edition (WISC-IV); Tucker-Drob and Salthouse's (2009) MDS analysis of cognitive and neuropsychological test data aggregated across 38 separate studies ($N = 8,813$); and a series of unpublished 2-D and 3-D MDS analyses (and cluster analyses) of the Woodcock–Johnson III (WJ III) norm data, the Wechsler Adult Intelligence Scale—Fourth Edition (WAIS-IV) test correlations, and cross-battery datasets including the WJ III and WISC-R (Phelps, McGrew, Knopik, & Ford, 2005) and WJ III, WAIS-III, Wechsler Memory Scale—Third Edition (WMS-III), and Kaufman Adolescent and Adult Intelligence Test (KAIT) (McGrew, Woodcock, & Ford, 2002) by McGrew. When MDS methods are applied to data previously analyzed with structural EFA/CFA methods, new insights into the characteristics of tests and constructs previously obscured by the strong statistical machinery of factor analysis emerge (Süß & Beauducel, 2005; Tucker-Drob & Salthouse, 2009).

For example, McGrew (2010) has recently presented a multidimensional conceptual cognitive abilities framework based on the integration of (1) the extant CHC research literature, (2) mapping of CHC constructs to neuropsychological constructs and models, (3) results from his MDS-based analyses listed above, and (4) select theoretical constructs from cognitive neurosciences and cognitive information-processing theories.[10] The 16-domain CHC model presented by McGrew (2009) (defined in the second half of this chapter) is embedded in an *ability domain dimension* (along with, and mapped to, neuropsychological assessment domains) that includes (1) cognitive knowledge systems (Gc, Grw, Gq, Gkn); (2) cognitive operations (Gf, Glr, Gv, Ga); (3) cognitive efficiency

(Gsm, Gs) and cognitive control (executive functions, including controlled executive attention); (4) sensory functions (visual, auditory, tactile, kinesthetic, olfactory); and (5) motor functions (Gp, Gps). The contribution of cognitive neurosciences is incorporated in this ability domain dimension via the subcategorization of human abilities as type 1 (more automatic cognitive processing) and type II (more deliberate and controlled cognitive processing that is likely to place heavy demands on complex working memory) (see Evans, 2008). The MDS faceted insights into measures of intelligence, largely ignored by most proponents and users of CHC theory, are reflected in a *content/stimulus dimension* of the model, which includes (1) language or auditory–verbal, (2) quantitative or numerical, (3) visual–figural, (4) somatosensory, and (5) olfactory stimulus characteristics of tests of abilities. The *cognitive complexity dimension* incorporates the similar, yet complementary, characterization of cognitive abilities and tests in terms of degree of *cognitive complexity* as elucidated by tests' (or abilities') relative loading on psychometric g and nearness in proximity to the center of MDS radex models. The cognitive complexity dimension also indirectly represents the dimension of *breadth of ability domains* (general, broad, narrow).

The brief description of McGrew's multidimensional cognitive abilities framework is offered here in the spirit of positive skepticism articulated in Carroll's (1998) own critique of his 1993 seminal treatise and Jensen's (2004) sage advice that "an open-ended empirical theory to which future tests of as yet unmeasured or unknown abilities could possibly result in additional factors at one or more levels in Carroll's hierarchy" (p. 5). The importance of avoiding a premature "hardening" of the CHC categories has been demonstrated vis-à-vis the structural research on the domain of cognitive mental speed (see Figure 4.5), which suggests a domain characterized by a complex hierarchical structure with a possible g-speed factor at the same stratum level as psychometric g. The seductive powers of a neat and hierarchically organized CHC structural diagram of cognitive abilities must be resisted. Any theory that is derived primarily from a "rectilinear system of factors is . . . not of a form that well describes natural phenomena" (Horn & Noll, 1997, p. 84). By extension, assessment professionals must humbly recognize the inherent artificial nature of assessment tools built upon linear mathematical models.

Clearly, "intelligence is important, intelligence is complex" (Keith, 1994, p. 209). The current CHC taxonomy has benefited from over 100 years of research by a diverse set of scholars. Yet it is only a temporary "placeholder" taxonomy that is evolving through new research and theorizing, only a small part of which has been described above. Additional (r)evolutions in the constantly evolving taxonomy of human cognitive abilities are presented in the next section of this chapter.

CHC THEORY DESCRIBED AND REVISED

The "Human Cognitive Abilities" conference was held at the University of Virginia in 1994 to honor and discuss Carroll's (1993) masterwork. Cattell, Horn, Carroll, and many other luminaries in the field were in attendance. Published several years later, Carroll's address was called "Human Cognitive Abilities: A Critique" (Carroll, 1998). After reviewing some of the positive reviews of his book (and a few negative ones), he stated,

> Although all these reviews were in one sense gratifying, in another sense they were disappointing. They didn't tell me what I wanted to know: What was wrong with my book and its ideas, or at least what might be controversial about it? . . . Thus, ever since these reviews came out, I've been brooding about their authors might have said but didn't. (p. 6)

The critique of his own theory that followed this statement was a tour de force. Carroll possessed an extraordinarily rare combination of self-confidence, competence, and egoless commitment to truth!

We believe that Carroll's (1993) work is fundamentally sound, and that its major conclusions are as close to correct as current data allow. However, a number of minor inconsistencies in his model deserve some attention. We hope that he would have been gratified by our attempts to critique and improve upon his initial model.

In the sections that follow, we have multiple aims. First, we hope to define each of the constructs in CHC theory in terms that clinicians will find useful. Second, we hope to give some guidance as to which constructs are more central to the theory or have more validity data available. Third, we wish to alert readers to existing controversies and raise some questions of our own. Fourth, we propose a number of additions, deletions, and rearrangements in the list of CHC theory abilities.

We have organized the broad abilities in a way that draws on distinctions made by Cattell's (1971, 1987) triadic theory, Ackerman's (1996) process–personality–interests–knowledge (PPIK) theory, Woodcock's (1993) Gf-Gc information-processing theory, and Horn's (1985) remodeled Gf-Gc theory. There are numerous other valid ways in which this could have been accomplished.

General Intelligence (g)

At the apex of most models of CHC theory is the broadest of all cognitive ability constructs—general intelligence (g). Cattell, Horn, and Carroll each had different ideas about the origins and existence of psychometric g. Cattell (1963) explained the presence of the g factor via investment theory (see Figure 4.3 and related text). Carroll (1991) believed that the positive manifold is caused by general intelligence, a unitary construct. Horn (1985) believed there was sufficient evidence to reject the idea of g, but did not have strong opinions about any particular explanation of the positive manifold. CHC theory incorporates Carroll's (1993) notion of g, but users are encouraged to ignore it if they do not believe that theoretical g has merit, particularly in applied clinical assessment contexts.

Domain-Free General Capacities

Some CHC factors (Gf, Gsm, Glr, Gs, and Gt) are not associated with specific sensory systems. These diverse factors may reflect, respectively, different parameters of brain functioning that are relevant in most or all regions of the brain (Cattell, 1987). The fact that they are grouped together does not mean that clinicians should create composite scores with names like "Domain-Free General Capacity" because this is a conceptual grouping, not an implied functional unity.

Fluid Reasoning (Gf)

Definition of Gf

Fluid reasoning (Gf) can be defined as the deliberate but flexible control of attention to solve novel, "on-the-spot" problems that cannot be performed by relying exclusively on previously learned habits, schemas, and scripts. It is a multidimensional construct, but its parts are unified in their purpose: solving unfamiliar problems. Fluid reasoning is most evident in abstract reasoning that depends less on prior learning.[11] However, it is also present in day-to-day problem solving (Sternberg & Kalmar, 1998). Fluid reasoning is typically employed in concert with background knowledge and automatized responses (Goode & Beckman, 2010). That is, such reasoning is employed, even if for the briefest of moments, whenever current habits, scripts, and schemas are insufficient to meet the demands of a new situation. Fluid reasoning is also evident in inferential reasoning, concept formation, classification of unfamiliar stimuli, generalization of old solutions to new problems and contexts, hypothesis generation and confirmation, identification of relevant similarities, differences, and relationship among diverse objects and ideas, the perception of relevant consequences of newly acquired knowledge, and extrapolation of reasonable estimates in ambiguous situations.

Well-Supported Narrow Abilities within Gf

1. *Induction (I): The ability to observe a phenomenon and discover the underlying principles or rules that determine its behavior.* People good at inductive reasoning perceive regularities and patterns in situations that otherwise might seem unpredictable. In most inductive reasoning tests, stimuli are arranged according to a principle and the examinee demonstrates that the principle is understood (e.g., generating a new stimulus that also obeys the principle, identifying stimuli that do not conform to the pattern, or explaining the principle explicitly).

2. *General sequential reasoning (RG): The ability to reason logically, using known premises and principles.* This ability is also known as *deductive reasoning* or *rule application*. Whereas induction is the ability to use known facts to discover new principles, general sequential reasoning is the ability to use known or given principles in one or more logical steps to discover new facts or solve problems. A real-world example would be a judge or jury deciding, given presented facts and relevant laws, if the laws had been violated by certain actions in criminal cases.

3. *Quantitative reasoning (RQ): The ability to reason, either with induction or deduction, with numbers, mathematical relations, and operators.* Tests measuring quantitative reasoning do not require advanced knowledge of mathematics. The computation in such tests is typically quite simple. What makes them difficult is the complexity of reasoning required to solve the problems—for example, "Choose from among these symbols: $+ - \times \div =$ and insert them into the boxes to create a valid equation: $8\square4\square4\square8\square2$."

Assessment Recommendations for Gf[12]

Certain narrow abilities are more central to the broad factors than are others. Induction is probably the core aspect of Gf. No measurement of Gf is complete, or even adequate, without a measure of induction. If two Gf tests are given, the second should typically be a General Sequential (Deductive) Reasoning test. A Quantitative Reasoning test would be a lower priority unless there is a specific referral concern about mathematics difficulties or other clinical factors warranting such a focus.

Comments and Unresolved Issues Related to Gf

• *Are Piagetian reasoning (RP) and reasoning speed (RE) distinct aspects of Gf?* Carroll (1997) tendered the tentative hypotheses that reasoning speed and the kinds of tasks used to test Piagetian theories of cognitive development formed distinct narrow factors within Gf. There is little in the way of new evidence that these are distinct factors, and there is some evidence that they are not (Carroll, Kohlberg & DeVries, 1984; Danthiir, Wilhelm, & Schacht, 2005; Inman & Secrest, 1981). For these and other reasons too complicated to describe succinctly here, we have chosen to deemphasize these factors in the current description of CHC theory.

• *Are Gf and g identical?* Gf and *g* are sometimes reported to be perfectly correlated (e.g., Floyd, Evans, & McGrew, 2003; Gustafsson, 1984). Perhaps they are the same construct, although this hypothesis is the subject of considerable debate (see Ackerman, Beier, & Boyle, 2005; Kane, Hambrick, & Conway, 2005). Horn and Blankson (Chapter 3, this volume) note that Gf is theoretically congruent with Spearman's description of *g*. Carroll (2003) believed that there was sufficient evidence to reject the hypothesis that *g* and Gf are identical. Cattell's explanation for why *g* and Gf are so similar is that *g* is really the cumulative effects of a person's Gf from birth to the present ("this year's crystallized ability level is a function of last year's fluid ability level"; Cattell, 1987, p. 139). For this reason, his name for *g* was historical fluid intelligence, or $g_{f(h)}$.

Memory: General Considerations

From reading just the labels of memory abilities, it would appear that there is considerable disagreement among Cattell, Horn, and Carroll. Indeed, at first glance, it also appears that in the domain of memory, CHC theory does not even agree with its source theorists! Fortunately, almost all of the "disagreements" are resolved by the knowledge that the three source theorists sometimes used the same words differently (e.g., *short term*) or used different words to mean the same thing. A close reading of all the major works of CHC's source theorists will reveal that the differences are more apparent than real. The points of agreement are these:

1. It is important to distinguish between long-term memory and short-term memory, but it should not be forgotten that the two systems are interdependent. It is almost impossible to measure (with a single test) short-term memory without involving long-term memory, or to measure long-term memory without involving short-term memory.
2. It is important to distinguish between the ability to recall information stored in long-term memory and the fluency with which this information is recalled. That is, people who learn efficiently may not be very fluent in their recall of what they have learned. Likewise, people who are very fluent in producing ideas from their long-term memory may be slow learners. That is, learning efficiency and retrieval fluency are reasonably distinct abilities.

The scientific literature on memory is truly gigantic, and space does not permit us even to summarize all the topics in this body of research we think are relevant to CHC theory. We expect that this aspect of CHC theory will undergo continual refinement as researchers integrate basic research on memory processes with clinical applications of memory assessment. For now, we articulate a very basic model of how memory may work, so that different aspects of memory assessment can be understood more clearly. We use the terms *primary memory* and *secondary memory* here to avoid confusion that might arise by using analogous terms, such as *short-term memory* and *long-term memory*. Our discussion draws heavily from Unsworth and Engle (2007b).

Primary memory and secondary memory are not individual-difference variables. They are descriptive terms that refer to cognitive structures that everyone has. *Primary memory* refers to information that is in the current focus of attention (i.e., it is immediately accessible to consciousness). *Secondary memory* (also known as *long-term memory*) refers to memory that is not immediately accessible to consciousness. Information enters primary memory via sensory registers or is retrieved from secondary memory.

We will omit a discussion of how the properties of visual primary memory (also known as the *visuospatial sketchpad*) differ from those of auditory primary memory (also known as the *phonological loop*; Baddeley, 1986). What they have in common is a very limited capacity. For example, auditory primary memory holds about four chunks of information in the best of circumstances, and only one or two chunks in typical circumstances. If information is not maintained via rehearsal, it disappears from primary memory within seconds (although it can linger up to 30 seconds or more if no new information displaces it). If attention shifts, the information disappears from primary memory quite quickly. Although information in primary memory is fragile, it is very quickly manipulated and processed (much like RAM in a computer).

To be used (at least consciously), information stored in secondary memory must be retrieved back into primary memory. Some memories are more easily retrieved than others because they have been recently activated, they are more frequently activated, and they are associated with other memories to a greater degree. That is, memories that are unrelated to other memories are difficult to recall. Memories that are overly similar and indistinct (e.g., a string of random numbers) are very difficult to recall.

If primary memory holds only a few chunks of information, how is it that people can repeat back up to seven or more digits on a digits-forward memory span test? To answer this question, we must discuss one of the oldest findings in memory research: the serial position effect. The *serial position effect* consists of two effects, the primacy effect and the recency effect. The *primacy effect* refers to the fact that people are more likely to recall the first few parts of a list than the middle of the list. The typical explanation for this effect is that the first few items on a list are more likely to enter secondary memory. The *recency effect* refers to the tendency that the last two or three items on a list are more likely to be recalled than the middle part of the list.

On the easy items in a digits-forward memory span test, people are able to answer correctly by simply dumping the contents of primary memory. As they approach the limits of primary memory capacity, they begin mentally rehearsing the digits as they are being presented by the examiner. Rehearsal maintains information in primary memory, but also facilitates transfer of information into secondary memory. Most evidence suggests that as people approach their limits of performance on memory span tests, most of the information is pulled from recently activated items in secondary memory, not from primary memory (Unsworth & Engle, 2007a). Why? Because recalling the first part of this list actually displaces the contents of primary memory. If the string of digits is not mostly in secondary memory, the end of the string of digits will not be recalled correctly.

If examinees are allowed to recall any part of a list in any order, many people will adopt the strategy of saying the last few words of the list first and then saying the first part of the list. Thus they are using both primary and secondary memory optimally. This is the most likely reason that Carroll (1993) found evidence for a free-recall factor of memory. Performance on such tests reflects the combined use of primary and secondary memory to a greater degree than memory span tests. In addition, the single-exposure free-recall paradigm requires no memory of sequence, as does the forward memory span paradigm.

It should be noted that Carroll's (1993) free-recall factor was defined by tests in which there was only a single exposure to the list. This is also true of all of Horn's (1985) short-term memory abilities (e.g., associative memory and meaningful memory). These factors were defined mostly by *supraspan* tests (in which the lists to be recalled are longer than most people can recall after a single exposure), and people were given only one learning trial. Because most clinical tests of memory allow multiple learning trials, McGrew (1997) classified such tests as long-term memory tests. Thus neither theorist was wrong about the proper location of these factors. Different task demands alter the relative mix of short- and long-term memory abilities involved in a task. We clarify this confusing aspect of CHC theory for the first time here. In Figure 4.6, we present a conceptual map of the domain of memory in CHC theory.

Short-Term Memory (Gsm)

Definition of Gsm

Short-term memory (Gsm) can be defined as *the ability to encode, maintain, and manipulate information in one's immediate awareness.* Gsm[13] refers to

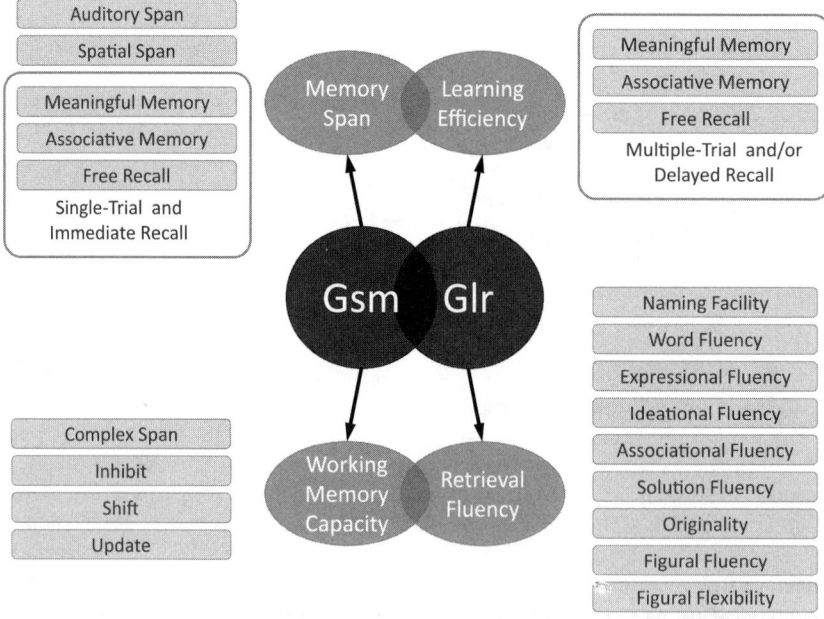

FIGURE 4.6. Conceptual map of memory-related abilities in CHC theory.

individual differences in both the capacity (size) of primary memory and to the efficiency of attentional control mechanisms that manipulate information within primary memory.

Well-Supported Narrow Abilities within Gsm

1. *Memory span (MS): The ability to encode information, maintain it in primary memory, and immediately reproduce the information in the same sequence in which it was represented.* Memory span tests are among the most commonly given tests in both research and clinical settings. In short items, performance is mostly determined by the capacity of primary memory. Participants simply dump the contents of primary memory. For most people, when the item length exceeds three or four, they deliberately engage their attention to maintain information in primary memory (e.g., they subvocally rehearse the list). As the maintenance-only strategy begins to fail, their attention is also directed to searching the contents of recently activated (i.e., just seconds ago) contents of secondary memory. For the most difficult items, there is little that distinguishes simple memory span tests from complex span tests that more directly measure the efficiency of attentional control mechanisms (Unsworth & Engle, 2007a). However, in clinical tests, the whole score represents a mix of several memory processes that are sometimes difficult to tease apart.

One way to get a purer measure of primary memory capacity is to give a test that minimizes the use of strategy (i.e., use of attentional control mechanisms to enhance performance). For example, the Comprehensive Test of Phonological Processing (CTOPP) Memory for Digits subtest presents two digits per second instead of the traditional rate of one digit per second. People who take both types of tests sometimes express surprise that the test with the faster rate was somehow easier than the memory span test with the slower rate. What they mean is that they just pulled information from primary memory (and a little bit from secondary memory) because they were simply unable to use attention-demanding strategies for maintaining information in primary memory or storing information in secondary memory.

It appears that auditory and visual (spatial) memory span tests draw on different abilities (Kane et al., 2004). We suspect that the two types of tests reflect the efficiency of Ga and Gv, respectively, in encoding the test stimuli. When the test stimuli become difficult to encode, visual memory tests load with Gv (such tests define Visual Memory, a narrow ability associated with Gv) and auditory memory tests load with Ga (e.g., the CTOPP Nonword Repetition subtest, in which examinees must repeat increasingly long nonsense words such as *haviormushkimelour*). However, when visual and auditory tests demand more attentional resources, the auditory–visual distinction becomes unimportant (Kane et al., 2004).

2. *Working memory capacity:*[14] *The ability to direct the focus of attention to perform relatively simple manipulations, combinations, and transformations of information within primary memory, while avoiding distracting stimuli and engaging in strategic/controlled searches for information in secondary memory.* These attentional control mechanisms are mostly under direct conscious control and are thus known by various terms containing the word *executive* (e.g., executive attention, executive control, central executive, executive functions, and many more). In this context, *executive* means that which *executes* (initiates, performs, controls) an action. Evidence that so-called "working memory capacity" tests and "executive function" tests belong in the same conceptual category is that a recent study rigorously designed to distinguish between the two constructs found that they were nearly perfectly correlated ($r = .97$) at the latent-variable level (McCabe, Roediger, McDaniel, Balota, & Hambrick, 2010).

Working memory capacity tests are typically measured by tasks in which information must be encoded (stored) and transformed (processed). The processing demands of these tasks is usually sufficient to bump information continuously out of primary memory. Thus successful performance on these tasks depends on efficient transfer of information to secondary memory and efficient retrieval of that information when it is needed (hence Horn's term *short-term apprehension and retrieval*). Most working memory capacity tests used in research are called "complex span" tests. Typically, participants must process information (e.g., verify whether a statement is true or false) and remember information (e.g., the last word in a sentence). The only clinical test that uses the complex span paradigm is the latter half of the Stanford–Binet Intelligence Scales, Fifth Edition (SB5) Verbal Working Memory subtest. However, many other clinical tests require encoding and attention-demanding processing of stimuli, such as the WISC-IV Letter–Number Sequencing subtest (among many others).

A number of attempts have been made to distinguish among various aspects of executive attentional control. One influential study distinguished between three functions: updating the contents of short-term memory, shifting of attention, and inhibition of responses/urges that are typically strongly cued by particular stimuli (Miyake et al., 2000). All three of these functions have to do with directing one's attention in the service of a goal, even when it is difficult to do so.

Assessment Recommendations for Gsm

We recommend using auditory Gsm tests for most purposes because most of the research showing relationships between Gsm and academic functioning have used auditory tests. We recommend using simple memory span tests and attention-demanding short-term memory tests to distinguish between short-term memory capacity problems and problems of executive attentional control.

Comments and Unresolved Issues Related to Gsm

• *Is Gsm g or Gf?* One important study suggested that Gf could be almost entirely explained by working memory capacity tests (Kyllonen & Christal, 1990). Replications using more refined methods have found that although the relationship between working memory capacity and Gf is substantial, the constructs are distinct (Unsworth & Engle, 2007b). It appears that adequate attentional resources are necessary for novel reasoning, but are not sufficient to explain entirely why some people are better than others at Gf tests.

• *Should Gsm be renamed?* Labels matter. A poorly named ability construct can cause misinterpretations, misdiagnoses, and therapeutic missteps—witness the confusion caused by naming one of the WISC-III's factor index scores "Freedom from Distractibility" (Kaufman, 1994, p. 212). Thankfully, this problem was resolved when the factor was renamed "Working Memory" on the WISC-IV. However, this new label highlights an ambiguity in the field of cognitive assessment. Many of us use the term *working memory capacity* to refer to the superordinate category of Gsm, whereas others use it to refer to a narrow ability within Gsm. For this reason, we considered eliminating this ambiguity from CHC theory by avoiding the term *working memory* altogether. The plan was to leave the name of Gsm unchanged,

and to change the name of the narrow CHC ability construct *working memory* to *attentional control*. There are many attractive features of this label, but like "freedom from distractibility," we believe that it would be likely to be misinterpreted, particularly in the context of diagnostic decisions related to ADHD. Although it is true that people with ADHD perform somewhat worse on measures of working memory capacity, the cognitive deficits associated with that disorder are more diverse than what is meant by attentional control (Barkley, 1997). Multidimensional constructs like attention are practically impossible to operationalize with a single type of test. Indeed, clinical measures of working memory capacity are merely a subset of a very diverse set of clinical measures of attention-related abilities. We worried that had we called the narrow ability "attentional control," that its meaning would be misinterpreted and it would be treated as if it represented "attention" in its totality. For all its faults, the term *working memory capacity* is so firmly established that it is likely to remain with us for quite some time. Even so, it is important to keep in mind that working memory capacity is not strictly a phenomenon of memory alone. By analogy, tests of working memory capacity are a bit like hurdling. Hurdling is the smooth alternation of running and jumping. However, there are many other kinds of running, and many other kinds of jumping than the kinds seen in hurdling events. Likewise, tests of working memory capacity involve the use of memory and attention in concert, but there are many other kinds of memory and many other kinds of attention than the kinds seen in these tests.

Long-Term Storage and Retrieval (Glr)

Definition of Glr

Long-term storage and retrieval (Glr) can be defined as *the ability to store, consolidate, and retrieve information over periods of time measured in minutes, hours, days, and years.* Short-term memory has to do with information that has been encoded seconds ago and must be retrieved immediately. What distinguishes Gsm tests from Glr tests is that in Gsm tests there is a continuous attempt to maintain awareness of that information. A Glr test involves information that has been put out of immediate awareness long enough for the contents of primary memory to be displaced completely. In Glr tests, continuous maintenance of information in primary memory is difficult, if not impossible.

Glr is distinguished from Gc and other acquired-knowledge factors in that Glr refers to the processes of memory (storage/learning efficiency and retrieval fluency), and Gc (and other acquired-knowledge factors) refers to the breadth of information stored in long-term memory. Presumably, people with high Gc acquired knowledge via Glr processes, but it is possible for highly motivated people to acquire quite a bit of knowledge even if their learning processes are inefficient.

There is a major division within Glr that was always implied in CHC theory, but we are making it more explicit here. Some Glr tests require efficient learning of new information, whereas others require fluent recall of information already in long-term memory.

Well-Supported Narrow Abilities within Glr

Glr LEARNING EFFICIENCY

Carroll (1993) noted that there was some evidence for learning abilities (his abbreviation for this ability was L1) but it was incomplete. We believe that factor analyses of the WJ III, WAIS-IV/WMS-IV, Kaufman Assessment Battery for Children—Second Edition (KABC-II), and other clinical batteries with learning tests now provide sufficient evidence that long-term learning is distinct from fluency on the one hand and from Gsm on the other. As noted previously, many memory test paradigms (paired associates, story recall, list learning) can be administered with only one exposure to the information to be learned. In such cases, they are measuring aspects of Gsm. If the tests require delayed recall or if they use multiple exposures to learn information, they are measures of Glr.

All tests of learning efficiency must present more information than can be retained in Gsm. This can be accomplished with the *repeated-supraspan* paradigm, in which evaluees are asked to remember more information than they can learn in one exposure and then the information is presented several more times. An example of this type of task is the Wide Range Assessment of Memory and Learning, Second Edition (WRAML2) Verbal Learning subtest, a free-recall list-learning test. This method is somewhat messy because part of the performance involves Gsm to a significant degree. A paradigm that minimizes the involvement of Gsm is the *structured learning task*. Such tasks have a teach–test–correct structure. First, a single bit of information is taught. That item is tested,

and corrective feedback is offered if required. Another item is taught, and both items are tested with corrective feedback if needed. Then another item is taught, and all three items are tested with corrective feedback if needed. Thus the test becomes longer and longer, but short-term memory is never overwhelmed with information. The WJ III Visual–Auditory Learning subtest is a good example of a structured learning task.

1. *Associative memory (MA): The ability to remember previously unrelated information as having been paired*. Pairs of items are presented together in the teaching phase of the test. In the testing phase, one item of the pair is presented, and the examinee recalls its mate. Item pairs must not have any previously established relationships (e.g., the word pairs *table–chair*, *woman–girl*), or the test is also a measure of meaningful memory.

2. *Meaningful memory (MM): The ability to remember narratives and other forms of semantically related information*. Carroll (1993) allowed for tests of meaningful memory to have a variety of formats (e.g., remembering definitions to unfamiliar words), but the core of this ability is the ability to remember the gist of a narrative. After hearing a story just once, most people can retell the gist of it fairly accurately. People who cannot do so are at a severe disadvantage in many domains of functioning. Stories are how we communicate values, transmit advice, and encapsulate especially difficult ideas. Much of the content of our interpersonal relationships consists of the stories we tell each other and the shared narratives we construct. Indeed, much of our sense of identity is the story we tell about ourselves (McAdams, Josselson, & Lieblich, 2006).

Many so-called "story recall" tests are barely concealed lists of disconnected information (e.g., "Mrs. Smith and Mr. Garcia met on the corner of Mulberry Street and Vine, where they talked about the weather, their favorite sports teams, and current events. Mr. Garcia left to buy gum, shoelaces, and paperclips. Mrs. Smith left to visit with her friends Karen, Michael, and Susan . . . "). A good story recall test has a story that has a true narrative arc. Because stories rely on conventions and require the listener to understand certain conventions of language and culture, many story memory tests have a strong secondary loading on Gc.

3. *Free-recall memory (M6): The ability to recall lists in any order*. Typically, this ability is measured by having evaluees repeatedly recall lists of

10–20 words. What distinguishes this ability from a method factor is that free-recall tests allow the evaluee to strategically maximize the primacy and recency effect by dumping the contents of primary memory first.

Glr RETRIEVAL FLUENCY

People differ in the rate at which they can access information stored in long-term memory. This aspect of ability has become increasingly recognized as important because of its role in reading comprehension. There is also a long-standing line of research showing that fluency of recall is an important precursor to certain forms of creativity. People who can produce many ideas from memory quickly are in a good position to combine them in creative ways. That said, high retrieval fluency is only a facilitator of creativity, not creativity itself.

The fluency factors in the following group are alike in that they involve the production of ideas.

4. *Ideational fluency (FI): The ability to rapidly produce a series of ideas, words, or phrases related to a specific condition or object.* Quantity, not quality or response originality, is emphasized. An example of such a test would be to think of as many uses of a pencil as possible in 1 minute.

5. *Associational fluency (FA): The ability to rapidly produce a series of original or useful ideas related to a particular concept.* In contrast to ideational fluency (FI), quality rather than quantity of production is emphasized. Thus the same question about generating ideas about uses of pencils could be used, but credit is given for creativity and high-quality answers.

6. *Expressional fluency (FE): The ability to rapidly think of different ways of expressing an idea.* For example, how many ways can you say that a person is drunk?

7. *Sensitivity to problems/alternative solution fluency (SP): The ability to rapidly think of a number of alternative solutions to a particular practical problem.* For example, how many ways can you think of to get a reluctant child to go to school?

8. *Originality/creativity (FO): The ability to rapidly produce original, clever, and insightful responses (expressions, interpretations) to a given topic, situation, or task.* This factor is quite difficult to measure for a variety of reasons. Because originality manifests itself in different ways for different people, such diversity of talent does not lend itself to standardized measurement. This factor is not strictly a

"retrieval" factor because it is by definition a creative enterprise. However, much of creativity is the combination of old elements in new ways. When we say that one idea sparks another, we mean that a person has retrieved a succession of related ideas from memory, and their combination has inspired a new idea.

The next two fluency abilities are related in that both are related to the fluent recall of words.

9. *Naming facility (NA): The ability to rapidly call objects by their names.* In contemporary reading research, this ability is called *rapid automatic naming* (RAN) or speed of lexical access. A fair measure of this ability must include objects that are known to all examinees; otherwise, it is a measure of lexical knowledge. This is the only fluency factor in which each response is controlled by testing stimulus materials. The other fluency factors are measured by tests in which examinees generate their own answers in any order they wish. In J. P. Guilford's terms, this is an ability involving *convergent production*, whereas the other fluency factors involve *divergent production* of ideas. In this regard, naming facility tests have much in common with Gs tests; they are self-paced tests in which an easy task (naming common objects) must be done quickly and fluently in the order determined by the test developer. Deficits in this ability are known to cause reading comprehension problems (in a sense, reading is the act of fluently "naming" printed words; Bowers, Sunseth, & Golden, 1999).

10. *Word fluency (FW): The ability to rapidly produce words that share a nonsemantic feature.* An example of a test that measures this ability is to name as many words as possible that begin with the letter *T*. This has been mentioned as possibly being related to the "tip-of-the-tongue" phenomenon (e.g., word-finding difficulties; Carroll, 1993). This is an ability that is well developed in Scrabble and crossword puzzle fans.

The next two fluency factors are related to figures.

11. *Figural fluency (FF): The ability to rapidly draw or sketch as many things (or elaborations) as possible when presented with a nonmeaningful visual stimulus (e.g., a set of unique visual elements).* Quantity is emphasized over quality. For example, in one part of the Delis–Kaplan Design Fluency test, examinees must connect dots with four straight lines in as many unique ways as they can within a time limit.

12. *Figural flexibility (FX): The ability to rapidly draw different solutions to figural problems.* An example of a test that measures this ability is to draw as many different ways as possible to fit several small shapes into a larger one.

Assessment Recommendations for Glr

We recommend measuring learning efficiency with structured learning tasks to minimize the contaminating effects of Gsm. However, repeated-supraspan tasks do allow a clinician to see how examinees use strategy to learn things. Structured learning tasks usually measure associative memory. We also recommend measuring meaningful memory because of its clear diagnostic value. Of the fluency measures, we recommend a measure of naming facility and a measure of ideational fluency, as the predictive validity of these factors is better understood than for the others.

Comments and Unresolved Issues Related to Glr

- *Is Glr retrieval fluency a distinct factor or a combination of Gs and attentional control?* In factor analyses, Glr retrieval fluency measures regularly load with Gs measures (e.g., in the Differential Ability Scales—Second Edition [DAS-II]) or with attentional control aspects of Gsm. Usually this happens where there are not enough fluency measures or Gs measures in the analysis for the two factors to emerge. When the two constructs are well represented in the correlation matrix, the factors appear as distinct abilities. Even so, it is likely that Gs and Glr share some variance, as both are speeded (see Figure 4.5). Theoretically, the attentional control aspects of Gsm are responsible for searching and retrieving from long-term memory. However, the two concepts appear to be reasonably distinct.

Cognitive Speed: General Considerations

Figure 4.5 displays an overview of how CHC speed abilities are believed to be related. This overview is mostly based on the model proposed by McGrew and Evans (2004), who integrated Carroll's (1993) model with more recent research (Ackerman, Beier, & Boyle, 2002; McGrew & Woodcock, 2001; O'Connor & Burns, 2003; Roberts & Stankov, 1999; Stankov, 2000; Stankov & Roberts, 1997). Both processing speed (Gs) and reaction and decision speed (Gt) are general abilities related to

speed. Both have to do with speed on very easy tests, although Gt tests are generally easier than Gs tests. What distinguishes Gs from Gt is fluency. Gt refers to the speed at which a single item can be performed, on average. That is, each item is presented singly, and the examiner controls the pace at which the next item is presented. Gs refers to the average speed at which a series of simple items is done *in succession* with *sustained concentration* over all items. That is, all items are presented at once, and the examinee determines when the next item will be attempted. In Gt tests the quickness of responding each time, with pauses between items, is critical. In Gs tests there are no pauses, and the examinee must sustain mental quickness and move swiftly from item to item until told to stop. This seemingly small difference makes a big difference. In Gs tests, the examinee is constantly shifting attention from item to item. Performance can be enhanced (or hindered) by looking ahead to the next several items. In Gt tests, this is not possible because the examiner determines when the next item is seen. Thus Gt is more purely about speed of perception or quickness of reactions, whereas Gs is more about the combination of sustained speed, fluency, and the adaptive allocation of attention. For this reason, Gs is more strongly correlated with *g* (and Gf) than is Gt.

Processing Speed (Gs)

Definition of Gs

Processing speed (Gs) can be defined as *the ability to perform simple, repetitive cognitive tasks quickly and fluently.* This ability is of secondary importance (compared to Gf and Gc) in predicting performance during the learning phase of skill acquisition. However, it becomes an important predictor of skilled performance once people know how to do a task. That is, once people know how to perform a task, they still differ in the speed and fluency with which they perform (Ackerman, 1987). For example, two people may be equally accurate in their addition skills, but one recalls math facts with ease, whereas the other has to think about the answer for an extra half-second and sometimes counts on his or her fingers.

Well-Supported Narrow Abilities within Gs

1. *Perceptual speed (P): The speed at which visual stimuli can be compared for similarity or difference.* Much as induction is at the core of Gf, perceptual

speed is at the core of Gs. One way to measure this factor is to present pairs of stimuli side by side, and the examinees judge them to be the same or different as quickly as possible. Another method of measuring this factor is to present a stimulus to examinees, and they must find matching stimuli in an array of heterogeneous figures. Research (Ackerman, Beier, & Boyle, 2002; Ackerman & Cianciolo, 2000; see McGrew, 2005) suggests that perceptual speed may be an intermediate-stratum ability (between narrow and broad) defined by four narrow subabilities: (a) pattern recognition (Ppr), the ability to quickly recognize simple visual patterns; (b) scanning (Ps), the ability to scan, compare, and look up visual stimuli; (c) memory (Pm), the ability to perform visual-perceptual speed tasks that place significant demands on immediate Gsm; and (d) complex (Pc), the ability to perform visual pattern recognition tasks that impose additional cognitive demands, such as spatial visualization, estimating and interpolating, and heightened memory span loads.

2. *Rate of test-taking (R9): The speed and fluency with which simple cognitive tests are completed.* Carroll's (1993) analyses of this factor included very heterogeneous variables (different contents, different task formats, different degrees of difficulty). Originally, there were no "rate-of-test-taking" tests. Instead, other tests measuring other abilities were given and the finishing times were recorded. It was found that there are individual differences in people's test-taking tempo, regardless of the type of test. Through the lens of CHC theory, the definition of this factor has narrowed to simple tests that do not require visual comparison (so as not to overlap with perceptual speed) or mental arithmetic (so as not to overlap with number facility). For example, the WISC-IV Coding subtest requires examinees to look up numbers in a key and produce an associated figure specified by the key.

The next three factors are related to the ability to perform basic academic skills rapidly.

3. *Number facility (N): The speed at which basic arithmetic operations are performed accurately.* Although this factor includes recall of math facts, number facility includes speeded performance of any simple calculation (e.g., subtracting 3 from a column of two-digit numbers). Number facility does not involve understanding or organizing mathematical problems and is not a major component of mathematical/quantitative reasoning or

higher mathematical skills. People with slow recall of math facts may be more likely to make computational errors because the recall of math facts is more effortful (i.e., consumes attentional resources) and is thus a source of distraction.

4. *Reading speed (fluency) (RS): The rate of reading text with full comprehension.* Also listed under Grw.

5. *Writing speed (fluency) (WS): The rate at which words or sentences can be generated or copied.* Also listed under Grw and Gps.

Assessment Recommendations for Gs

We recommend that the assessment of Gs primarily focus on perceptual speed and secondarily on rate of test taking. The three academic fluency factors should be assessed if they are relevant to the referral concern. These abilities sometimes act as predictors of more complex aspects of academic achievement (e.g., reading comprehension and math problem solving) and sometimes are considered academic outcomes themselves, depending on the referral concern. Many evaluees seek extended time on exams, and poor academic fluency is often considered sufficient justification for granting this accommodation.

Comments and Unresolved Issues Related to Gs

- *To what degree do the three academic fluency abilities depend on Glr fluency?* Each of the three academic fluency abilities requires fluent recall of information stored in long-term memory. Recalling math facts seems to be a close twin of naming facility (i.e., if the answer is remembered rather than computed). Once readers automatize reading of simple words (the words are recalled lexically rather than decoded phonetically), it would seem that this is also a special case of naming facility. Further research will clarify the degree to which these tasks call on the same cognitive processes.

Reaction and Decision Speed (Gt)

Definition of Gt

Reaction and decision speed (Gt) can be defined as the speed of making very simple decisions or judgments when items are presented one at a time. Tests of Gt differ from tests of Gs in that they are not self-paced. Each item is presented singly and there is a short period between items in which no response from the evaluee is required. The primary use of Gt measures has been in research settings. Researchers are interested in Gt, as it may provide some insight into the nature of *g* and some very basic properties of the brain (e.g., neural efficiency). One of the interesting aspects of Gt is that not only is faster reaction time in these very simple tasks associated with complex reasoning, but so is greater consistency of reaction time (less variability). People with more variable reaction times have lower overall cognitive performance (Jensen, 2006).

Well-Supported Narrow Abilities within Gt

1. *Simple reaction time (R1): Reaction time to the onset of a single stimulus (visual or auditory).* R1 is frequently divided into the phases of *decision time* (DT; the time to decide to make a response and the finger leaves a home button) and *movement time* (MT; the time to move the finger from the home button to another button where the response is physically made and recorded).

2. *Choice reaction time (R2): Reaction time when a very simple choice must be made.* For example, examinees see two buttons and must hit the one that lights up.

3. *Semantic processing speed (R4): Reaction time when a decision requires some very simple encoding and mental manipulation of the stimulus content.*

4. *Mental comparison speed (R7): Reaction time where stimuli must be compared for a particular characteristic or attribute.*

5. *Inspection time (IT): The speed at which differences in stimuli can be perceived.* For example, two lines are shown for a few milliseconds and then are covered up. The examinee must indicate which of the two lines is longer. If given sufficient time, all examinees are able to indicate which is the longer line. The difficulty of the task is determined by how much time the examinees have to perceive the lines. The inspection time paradigm is noteworthy because it does not require a rapid response and thus has no confounds with Gps. Measures of inspection time correlate with the *g* factor at approximately *r* = .4 (Jensen, 2006).

Assessment Recommendations for Gt

Tasks measuring Gt are not typically used in clinical settings (except perhaps in continuous-performance tasks). With the increasing use of low-cost mobile computing devices (smartphones; iPads and other slate notebook computers), we would not be surprised to see viable measures of Gt become available for clinical and applied use.

Psychomotor Speed (Gps)

Definition of Gps

Psychomotor speed (Gps) can be defined as *the speed and fluidity with which physical body movements can be made.* In Ackerman's (1987) model of skill acquisition, Gps is the ability that determines performance differences after a comparable population (e.g., manual laborers in the same factory) has practiced a simple skill for a very long time.

Well-Supported Narrow Abilities within Gps

1. *Speed of limb movement (R3). The speed of arm and leg movement.* This speed is measured after the movement is initiated. Accuracy is not important.

2. *Writing speed (fluency) (WS). The speed at which written words can be copied.* Also listed under Grw and Gps.

3. *Speed of articulation (PT). The ability to rapidly perform successive articulations with the speech musculature.*

4. *Movement time (MT).* Recent research (see summaries by Deary, 2003; Nettelbeck, 2003; see also McGrew, 2005) suggests that MT may be an intermediate-stratum ability (between narrow and broad strata) that represents the second phase of reaction time as measured by various elementary cognitive tasks (ECTs). The time taken to physically move a body part (e.g., a finger) to make the required response is MT. MT may also measure the speed of finger, limb, or multilimb movements or vocal articulation (*diadochokinesis*; Greek for "successive movements") (Carroll, 1993; Stankov, 2000) and is also listed under Gt.

Assessment Recommendations for Gps

Psychomotor speed is not generally used in clinical settings except for finger-tapping tests in neuropsychological settings. Although the speed of finger tapping is of some interest to neuropsychologists, they are more concerned with performance that is dramatically uneven on the right and left hands, as this may indicate in which hemisphere a brain injury may have occurred.

Acquired Knowledge

The next four abilities, Gc, Gkn, Grw, and Gq, are consistent with Cattell's (1943) original description of g_c. They all involve the acquisition of useful knowledge and understanding of important domains of human functioning. All of these factors represent information stored in long-term memory.

Comprehension–Knowledge (Gc)

Definition of Gc

Comprehension–knowledge (Gc) can be defined as *the depth and breadth of knowledge and skills that are valued by one's culture.* Every culture values certain skills and knowledge over others. For example, Gc-type verbal abilities have been found to be the first of three major factors considered to define intelligence when both experts in the field of intelligence and laypeople are surveyed (Sternberg, Conway, Ketron, & Bernstein, 1981). Gc reflects the degree to which a person has learned practically useful knowledge and mastered valued skills. Thus, by definition, it is impossible to measure Gc independent of culture. Gc is theoretically broader than what is measured by any existing cognitive battery (Keith & Reynolds, 2010).

Ideally, Gc is measured with tests that minimize the involvement of Gf. This means making the tests straightforward and less like puzzles. Gc tests typically do not require intense concentration. Items expected to be known only by experts in a field are avoided (e.g., "What is the difference between Pearson's r and Spearman's ρ?" "Who was William Henry Harrison's Secretary of the Treasury?" "What is the solvent most commonly used by dry cleaners?"). For typical Gc test items, almost anyone who graduates from high school has a reasonable chance of at least being exposed to the information. A good easy Gc item is not merely easy, but should reveal a serious knowledge deficit if not answered correctly. An adult who does not know why milk is stored in a refrigerator is probably not ready to live independently in unsupervised housing.

A good hard item on a Gc test is not merely obscure. It should reflect uncommon wisdom (e.g., "Explain what Voltaire might have meant when he said, 'To be absolutely certain about something, one must know everything or nothing about it'"), or it should be associated with deep knowledge of important aspects of one's local culture. For example, the question "Julius Caesar's nephew Octavian is also known as _____" may seem trivial

at first glance. However, the story of Rome's transition from a republic to an empire has long served as a cautionary tale of what might happen to the U.S. system of government if the citizenry does not vigilantly guard its liberties.

Compared to other cognitive abilities, Gc is relatively more easily influenced by factors such as experience, education, and cultural opportunities, but is also just as heritable as Gf (Horn & Noll, 1997). Gc is historically known as *crystallized intelligence.* Although it is featured prominently in CHC theory, Hunt (2000) has lamented the fact that researchers and intelligence scholars have largely ignored Gc recently in favor of studying more exciting or "sexy" CHC constructs (e.g., Gf). He has called it the "wallflower" ability.

Well-Supported Narrow Abilities within Gc

1. *General verbal information (K0): The breadth and depth of knowledge that one's culture deems essential, practical, or otherwise worthwhile for everyone to know.* This ability is distinguished from achievement tests and other domain-specific tests of specialized knowledge in that it refers to acquired knowledge across many domains. Although any particular item in a general verbal information test might look like an item from a more specialized test, the purpose of a general verbal information test is to measure the cumulative effects of exposure to and retention of diverse forms of culturally relevant information. Items testing general verbal information can require a very simple response (e.g., "Which country was formerly known as Rhodesia?"), or they can require a fairly in-depth explanation (e.g., "What does *comparative advantage* mean in economics?"). What distinguishes the first question from mere trivia is that a person who knows the answer probably also knows why the name of the country changed and has some idea as to why that country is currently so troubled.

2. *Language development (LD): General understanding of spoken language at the level of words, idioms, and sentences.* In the same way that induction is at the core of Gf, language development is at the core of Gc. Although LD is listed as a distinct narrow ability in Carroll's model, his description of his analyses make it clear that he meant language development as an intermediate category between Gc and more specific language-related abilities, such as lexical knowledge, grammatical sensitivity, and listening ability. Language development is separate from general information. It appears to be

a label for all language abilities working together in concert. Language development is an obvious precursor skill for reading comprehension. However, the influence between the two abilities is bidirectional: Children who understand language are able to enjoy reading, and are thereby exposed through print to complex aspects of language that only rarely occur in speech.

3. *Lexical knowledge (VL): Knowledge of the definitions of words and the concepts that underlie them.* Whereas language development is more about understanding words in context, lexical knowledge is more about understanding the definitions of words in isolation. This does not mean that it is a shallow skill, though. For people with deep lexical knowledge, each word in the dictionary is a cognitive aid or tool to help them understand and talk about the world around them. Lexical knowledge is also an obvious precursor skill for reading decoding and reading comprehension. As with language development, people who read more acquire vocabulary words that are more likely to appear in print than in speech.

4. *Listening ability (LS): The ability to understand speech.* This ability is typically contrasted with reading comprehension. Tests of listening ability typically have simple vocabulary, but increasingly complex syntax or increasingly long speech samples to listen to.

5. *Communication ability (CM): The ability to use speech to communicate one's thoughts clearly.* This ability is comparable to listening ability, except that it is productive (expressive) rather than receptive. Carroll's factor came from studies in which people had to communicate their thoughts in nontesting situations (e.g., giving a speech). Although there are many tests in which people are asked to compose essays, we are not aware of language tests in which people are asked to communicate orally in a comparable fashion.

6. *Grammatical sensitivity (MY): Awareness of the formal rules of grammar and morphology of words in speech.* This factor is distinguished from English usage in that it is manifested in oral language instead of written language, and that it measures more the *awareness* of grammar rules than correct usage.

Assessment Recommendations for Gc

Adequate measurement of Gc should include a measure of general information and a test of either language development or lexical knowledge (which is a facet of language development). If there is time to give three Gc tests, a test of listening ability is a good choice.

Comments and Unresolved Issues Related to Gc

- *Is oral production and fluency (OP) distinct from communication ability (CM)?* Carroll (1993) identified a very narrow oral speaking ability called *oral production and fluency.* What distinguished this factor from communication ability was that the former was measured in realistic settings (e.g., giving a speech in front of an audience). Given that the evidence for the OP factor is very weak, this distinction does not seem important enough to clutter up the model, at least until compelling evidence suggests otherwise.

- *Is foreign-language aptitude an ability?* Carroll listed foreign-language aptitude as an ability, but his definition did not match what he meant by stratum I abilities elsewhere. What he seemed to mean by it was the sum total of all the relevant cognitive predictors of success in learning foreign languages, which include grammatical sensitivity, phonetic coding, and lexical knowledge. Aptitudes are not abilities; they are combinations of abilities used to forecast achievement (Corno et al., 2002). For this reason, we have removed this factor from the list of CHC theory abilities. This does not mean that foreign-language aptitude "does not exist." It does exist. It is just a different kind of construct.

Domain-Specific Knowledge (Gkn)

Definition of Gkn

Domain-specific knowledge (Gkn) can be defined as *the depth, breadth, and mastery of specialized knowledge (knowledge not all members of a society are expected to have).* Specialized knowledge is typically acquired via one's career, hobby, or other passionate interests (e.g., religion, sports). Knowledge has been featured in a number of definitions of intelligence, particularly during adulthood. It has been described as a "central ingredient of adult intellect" (Ackerman, 1996, p. 241). Schank and Birnbaum (1994) stated that "The bottom line is that intelligence is a function of knowledge. One may have the potentiality of intelligence, but without knowledge, nothing will become of that intelligence" (p. 102).

The "G" in Gkn is somewhat paradoxical. There is no general ability called "Gkn" because all of the abilities within the Gkn domain are specific by definition. Yet when all possible specific Gkn domains are considered collectively, it is broader than Gc (Hambrick, Pink, Meinz, Pettibone, & Oswald, 2008). Ackerman and colleagues (Ackerman, 1996; Hambrick et al., 2008) have conducted the most systematic study of the domain of Gkn in adults. In addition to the importance of Gc and prior domain knowledge as predictors, these researchers have clearly demonstrated that learning new domain-specific knowledge (particularly declarative knowledge) is also influenced by a number of nonability (conative) variables. These conative variables include situational and individual interest and the Big Five personality characteristics of *openness to experience* and *typical intellectual engagement*. The *need for cognition* personality trait has also been implicated as a causal factor. The Ackerman intelligence-as-process, personality, interest, and intelligence-as-knowledge (PPIK) theory of intelligence is the best available empirically based comprehensive explanation of the development of Gkn abilities (Ackerman, 1996; Hambrick et al., 2008). The PPIK theory has its conceptual roots in Cattell's Investment hypothesis (see Figure 4.3).

Gkn is unusual in that the proper reference group is not a person's same-age peers in the general population. Rather, the basis of comparison for Gkn is a group of people expected to have the same kinds of specialized knowledge. For example, when measuring an oncologist's Gkn in oncology, it only makes sense to compare the oncologist's knowledge with the average score of other oncologists. Gkn is also unusual in that there are an infinite number of possible narrow factors of specialized knowledge (i.e., one for each potential specialization).

In Gc tests, there is a sense in which people are expected to know the answers to all of the test questions. In Gkn tests, there is no such expectation unless the person is a member of a certain profession or is considered an expert in a certain domain. The fact that a nurse does not know how to tune a guitar has no bearing on the evaluation of the nurse's abilities. However, if the nurse does not know how to administer a shot, the nurse would be considered incompetent, as would a guitarist who is unable to tune a guitar.

Another noteworthy distinction between Gc and Gkn is their differing relationships with working memory. When solving problems outside of their expertise, most experts are unable to perform extraordinary feats of working memory. However, in a phenomenon called *expertise wide-span memory* (see Horn & Blankson, Chapter 3, this volume), experts seem to be able to access large amounts of specialized knowledge very quickly in long-term memory, and are able to hold it in immediate awareness as if it were stored in working memory, so that it can be used to solve complex problems efficiently. Thus, instead of being able to hold a few chunks of information in working memory, experts seem to perform as if they are able to hold very large amounts of information in working memory, but only when working within their areas of specialization.

Well-Supported Narrow Abilities within Gkn

1. *Foreign-language proficiency (KL): Similar to language development, but in another language.* This ability is distinguished from foreign-language aptitude in that it represents achieved proficiency instead of potential proficiency. Presumably, most people with high foreign-language proficiency have high foreign-language aptitude, but not all people with high foreign-language aptitude have yet developed proficiency in any foreign languages. This ability was previously classified as an aspect of Gc. However, since Gkn was added to CHC theory, it is clear that specialized knowledge of a particular language should be reclassified. Although knowledge of English as a second language was previously listed as a separate ability in Gkn, it now seems clear that it is a special case of the more general ability of foreign-language proficiency. Note that this factor is unusual because it is not a single factor: There is a different foreign-language proficiency factor for every language.

2. *Knowledge of signing (KF): Knowledge of finger spelling and signing (e.g., American Sign Language).*

3. *Skill in lip reading (LP): Competence in the ability to understand communication from others by watching the movements of their mouths and expressions.*

4. *Geography achievement (A5): Range of geography knowledge (e.g., capitals of countries).* It is probably a quirk in the datasets available to Carroll that geography is singled out as a separate ability whereas other specific disciplines are lumped together in broad categories. It is quite likely that a factor analysis designed to distinguish among traditional academic disciplines (e.g., chemistry vs. biology) would succeed in doing so.

5. *General science information (K1): Range of scientific knowledge (e.g., biology, physics, engineering, mechanics, electronics).* This factor is quite broad, as it encompasses all of the sciences. It is likely that each discipline within science has a narrower subfactor.

6. *Knowledge of culture (K2): Range of knowledge about the humanities (e.g., philosophy, religion, history, literature, music, and art).* As with general science information, this factor is also quite broad. It is likely that this factor has many subfactors.

7. *Mechanical knowledge (MK): Knowledge about the function, terminology, and operation of ordinary tools, machines, and equipment.* There are many tests of mechanical knowledge and reasoning used for the purpose of personnel selection (e.g., the Armed Services Vocational Aptitude Battery, the Wiesen Test of Mechanical Aptitude).

8. *Knowledge of behavioral content (BC): Knowledge or sensitivity to nonverbal human communication/interaction systems (e.g., facial expressions and gestures).* The field of emotional intelligence research is very large, but it is not yet clear which constructs of emotional intelligence should be included in CHC theory. CHC theory is about abilities rather than personality, and thus the constructs within it are measured by tests in which there are correct answers (or speeded performance). Several ability-based measures of emotion recognition and social perception exist (e.g., Advanced Clinical Solutions for the WAIS-IV and WMS-IV, the Mayer–Salovey–Caruso Emotional Intelligence Test).

Assessment Recommendations for Gkn

In most situations, Gkn is measured informally by peer reputation, but there are many educational tests that can serve as reasonable markers of specific Gkn domains.

Reading and Writing (Grw)

Definition of Grw

Reading and writing (Grw) can be defined as *the depth and breadth of knowledge and skills related to written language.* People with high Grw read with little effort and write with little difficulty. When Grw is sufficiently high, reading and writing become perfect windows for viewing a person's language development. Whatever difficulties people

have understanding text or communicating clearly, it is most likely a function of Gc or Gkn. For people with low Grw, however, high language skills may not be evident in reading and writing performance. Although reading and writing are clearly distinct activities, the underlying sources of individual differences in reading and writing skills do not differentiate between the two activities cleanly. It appears that the ability that is common across all reading skills also unites all writing skills. It is important to note that when we administer tests of Grw, we are measuring much more than just Grw. Grw refers solely to the aspects of the tests that are related to reading and writing. A reading comprehension test draws on Grw, but also on Gc, Gsm, Glr, and perhaps Ga, Gs, Gf, and Gkn.

Well-Supported Narrow Abilities within Grw

1. *Reading decoding (RD): The ability to identify words from text.* Typically, this ability is assessed by oral reading tests with words arranged in ascending order of difficulty. Tests can consist of phonetically regular words (words that are spelled how they sound, such as *bathtub* or *hanger*), phonetically irregular words (words that do not sound how they are spelled, such as *sugar* or *colonel*), or phonetically regular pseudowords (fake words that conform to regular spelling rules, such as *gobbish* or *choggy*).

2. *Reading comprehension (RC): The ability to understand written discourse.* Reading comprehension is measured in a variety of ways. One common method is to have examinees read a short passage and then have them answer questions that can only be answered if the text was understood. A direct method of measuring Grw reading comprehension with reduced contamination of Gc (or Gf) is to ask questions about information that was stated directly in the text. However, we also wish to measure more complex aspects of reading comprehension, such as inference and sensitivity to the author's intent. Such skills draw deeply on Gc. A second method of measuring reading comprehension is the *cloze* technique, in which a key word has been omitted from a sentence or a paragraph. Examinees who understand what they are reading can supply the missing word.

3. *Reading speed (RS): The rate at which a person can read connected discourse with full comprehension.* There are various methods of measuring reading

speed, and there is no clear consensus about which method is best for which purposes. Should reading speed be measured by oral reading speed or silent reading speed? Should examinees be told to read as quickly as they can to measure maximal ability, or should they be told to read at their normal pace to measure their typical reading rate? How should the speed–accuracy (of comprehension) tradeoff be handled? Should the format be single words (to measure the efficiency of reading decoding) or full sentences or paragraphs (to measure the efficiency of reading comprehension)? We are certain that different kinds of reading speed tests measure different things that are important, but we are not sure exactly what is different about them. Clinicians are encouraged to think carefully about what exactly the test requires of examinees and to check to see if there is a logical connection between the apparent task demands and the referral concern. Reading speed is classified as a mixed measure of Gs (broad cognitive speed) and Grw in the hierarchical speed model (see Figure 4.5), although the amount of Gs and Grw measured most likely reflects the degree of difficulty of the reading involved in the task (e.g., reading lists of simple isolated words vs. reading short statements and indicating whether they are true or false).

4. *Spelling ability (SG): The ability to spell words.* This factor is typically measured with traditional written spelling tests. However, just as with reading decoding, it can also be measured via spelling tests consisting of phonetically regular nonsense words (e.g., *grodding*). It is worth noting that Carroll (1993) considered this factor to be weakly defined and in need of additional research.

5. *English usage (EU): Knowledge of the mechanics of writing (e.g., capitalization, punctuation, and word usage).*

6. *Writing ability (WA): The ability to use text to communicate ideas clearly.* There are various methods of assessing writing ability. Perhaps the most common method is to ask examinees to write an essay about an assigned topic. Another method is to have examinee write sentences that must include specific words or phrases (e.g., write a single sentence that includes *neither, although,* and *prefer*).

7. *Writing speed (WS): The ability to copy or generate text quickly.* Writing speed tasks are considered to measure both Grw and Gps (broad psychomotor speed) in the hierarchical speed hierarchy (see Figure 4.5). Similar to measures of reading speed,

the relative importance of Grw or Gps probably varies, depending on the format and level of writing skills involved.

Assessment Recommendations for Grw

Much more is known about reading assessment than writing assessment. For reading, it is recommended that assessments focus on the point of reading: comprehension. If a person comprehends text well, minor weaknesses in decoding and reading speed are of secondary concern (unless the assessment concern is about reading efficiency problems rather than reading comprehension problems). If there are comprehension deficits, the assessment should focus on the proximal causes of reading comprehension problems (decoding problems, slow reading speed) and then explaining the proximal causes with more distal causes (e.g., slow naming facility → slow reading speed → slow, labored, inefficient reading → comprehension problems). We recommend measuring reading decoding with both real words and pseudowords. Reading comprehension is probably best measured with a variety of methods, including the cloze method and answering both factual and inferential questions about longer passages.

Spelling ability is an important skill (especially in a phonetically irregular language like English) and is easily measured with a traditional spelling test. It is generally a good idea to select a test that allows the clinician to be able to understand the nature of spelling problems (e.g., phonetically regular misspellings?).

Writing tests are extremely varied and probably measure a wide variety of abilities other than just specific writing abilities. Observing a child's pattern of grammar, usage, and mechanics in responses to writing tests allow clinicians to distinguish between specific writing problems and more complex problems (e.g., general language difficulties). However, it is generally a good idea to examine a wide variety of samples of the evaluee's writing, both from formal tests (e.g., the Wechsler Individual Achievement Test—Third Edition [WIAT-III]) and from school writing assignments.

Comments and Unresolved Issues Related to Grw

• *Is cloze ability meaningfully distinct from reading comprehension?* No researcher, as far as we are aware, is interested in written cloze tests as measures of anything other than reading comprehension/language comprehension. McGrew's (1999) achievement battery cross-battery CFA of different forms of reading comprehension tests (which included the WJ III cloze Passage Comprehension test) across five different samples reinforces this recommendation, as the median reading comprehension factor test loadings ranged from .83 to .85. We speculate that when cloze tests form their own factor in a factor analysis, it is primarily due to method variance. Unless compelling evidence suggests otherwise, we suggest eliminating cloze ability from the list of stratum I abilities and consider the cloze format to be what it was always intended to be: a useful alternative method of assessing reading comprehension (RC).[15]

• *What is the nature of Carroll's verbal (printed) language comprehension factor?* This factor seems to emerge when there are not enough subtests in the battery for more differentiated models to emerge. Thus this factor appears to be a more general reading factor that combines decoding tests, reading comprehension tests (both long passages and cloze-type tests), reading speed measures, and printed vocabulary tests. There is no evidence that this is a distinct ability, and thus we recommend that it be dropped from CHC theory. In the cross-battery assessment worksheets (Flanagan, Ortiz, & Alfonso, 2007), the meaning of this factor has apparently narrowed to mean written vocabulary tests. Written vocabulary tests appear to be hybrids of reading decoding and lexical knowledge, and thus it appears that this factor is redundant.

• *Is Grw really just an aspect of Gc?* Many theorists, including Carroll and Horn, group Grw with Gc. There is no doubt that Gc and Grw are closely related and not connected solely via g. It is also clear that Grw tests are more closely related to each other than they are to traditional Gc tests. Developmental evidence (McGrew et al., 1991; McGrew & Woodcock, 2001) reveals a markedly different growth curve for Grw when compared to Gc—a form of construct evidence suggesting that they are not identical constructs.

Quantitative Knowledge (Gq)

Definition of Gq

Quantitative knowledge (Gq) can be defined as *the depth and breadth of knowledge related to mathematics*. Gq is distinct from quantitative reasoning (a facet of Gf) in the same way that Gc is distinct from the nonquantitative aspects of Gf. It consists of acquired knowledge about mathematics, such as knowledge of mathematical symbols (e.g., $\int$, π, Σ, ∞, $\neq$, $\leq$, $+$,$-$, $\times$, $\div$, $\sqrt{\ }$, and many others), operations (e.g., addition–subtraction, multiplication–division, exponentiation–nth rooting, factorials, negation, and many others), computational procedures (e.g., long division, reducing fractions, the quadratic formula, and many others), and other math-related skills (e.g., using a calculator, math software, and other math aids). Generally measures of Gq are selected as academic achievement tests and thus must be aligned with a student's curriculum in order for the score to be diagnostic of math difficulties. This is not the case when measures of Gq are used as aptitude tests (e.g., on the SAT, GRE, or ACT). Gq is unusual in that it consists of many subskills that are fairly well defined by curriculum guides and instructional taxonomies. Thus metrics of Gq tests can be specified in relative terms (e.g., index scores) and in terms of absolute standards (e.g., an examinee can multiply two-digit numbers, can use the quadratic equation). We believe that both forms of description are necessary to paint a vivid picture of a person's Gq abilities.

Well-Supported Narrow Abilities within Gq

1. *Mathematical knowledge (KM): Range of general knowledge about mathematics, not the performance of mathematical operations or the solving of math problems.* This factor involves "what" rather than "how" knowledge (e.g., "What does π mean?" "What is the Pythagorean theorem?")

2. *Mathematical achievement (A3): Measured (tested) mathematics achievement.* There are two ways that this factor is measured. The first method is to administer math calculation problems that are decontexualized (e.g., 67 + 45 = ___). This method gets at the heart of the factor: calculation with the demands of quantitative reasoning minimized. The second method is messier but focuses on the primary goal of mathematics: solving problems. Examinees are given a scenario and a problem, and they must use reasoning to translate the word problem into a mathematically tractable solution. Examinees then use their calculation skills to arrive at a solution. For example, how many square meters of flooring are needed to cover a 6-m by 8-m rectangular room? The examinee has to intuit (or use KM) that this problem is solved by setting up the equation $6 \times 8 = $ ___. Such tests clearly draw upon quantitative reasoning, a facet of Gf.

Assessment Recommendations for Gq

As with Grw, the selection of Gq tests for assessment will depend on the question being asked. Most assessments concentrate first on calculation skills and then on math problem solving. Calculation fluency is typically of secondary concern, but can yield important information about the proximal causes of calculation and problem-solving difficulties (e.g., a person who has to think about the answer to basic math facts can easily be distracted and make careless errors in the midst of an algebra problem). Math knowledge tests that have no calculation demands (e.g., WJ III Quantitative Concepts) can distinguish between people who do not know how to answer the question and people who do not know what the question is.

Comments and Unresolved Issues Related to Gq

- *Is Gq an aspect of Gc?* As originally defined by Cattell, Gq is clearly an aspect of Gc because it consists of acquired (mostly verbal) knowledge. However, since the extended Gf-Gc model was proposed, Gc has become a more narrowly focused construct, and Gq has needed to be defined separately. We propose that Gc (verbal comprehension–knowledge) is distinct from Gq, but that they are not connected solely by g. We believe that it is useful to think of a higher-order acquired-knowledge/expertise factor that unites Gc, Grw, Gq, and Gkn.

- *Are there more narrow Gq abilities?* Yes. Carroll (1993) only reported the narrow KM and A3 factors given their emergence in datasets that included mathematics measures in addition to the cognitive variables that were the primary target of Carroll's review. Carroll did not go out of his way to identify all possible data sets that included tests of mathematics. Thus, other Gq narrow abilities most likely exist, but have yet to be validated within the context of CHC theory. For example, there has been a recent explosion in research on "number sense" or "numerosity" (e.g., Berch, 2005; Butterworth, 2010; Fuchs et al., 2010; Hyde & Spelke, 2011; Jordon, Kaplan, Olah, & Locuniak, 2006). Lists of number sense skills vary tremendously, with Berch (2005) listing up to 30 different components. Geary (2007) suggests these primitive math competencies, which he organized into the classes of numerosity, ordinality, counting,

simple arithmetic, estimation, and geometry, are rooted in biology, selected by evolutionary processes, and serve as the foundation for the development of secondary mathematics skills (e.g., KM, A3). At this time it is not clear whether number sense represents the lower developmental end of the Gq narrow abilities of KM or A3 (or RQ in Gf), represents an ability below the narrow stratum in Gq or Gf (RQ), or should be considered a narrow ability outright. Given the importance of number sense in understanding math development and disabilities (Geary, 2007) and predicting both future reading and math performance (Jordan et al., 2006), we predict the publication of a number of standardized tests of number sense competencies. Thus, we would be remiss in not mentioning the need for research to determine the appropriate placement of number sense in the evolving CHC taxonomy.

Sensory- and Motor-Linked Abilities

Cattell, Horn, and Carroll all noted that there was something different about abilities that were directly associated with sensory modalities. Despite the G in their abbreviation, they are not as general as Gf, Gsm, Glr, Gs, and Gt; yet they are still very broad. What distinguishes these broad factors from other abilities in CHC theory is that they are linked to well-defined regions and functions of the cerebral cortex (i.e., primary regions of the cerebral cortex and their associated secondary regions).

One common theme in the discussion that follows is that these abilities are hard to define. We are not used to talking about sensory-related abilities without talking about the senses and sensory acuity. The distinction between sensation and perception is relevant here, but it is not fully adequate to describe these abilities. *Sensation* refers to the detection of a stimulus. *Perception* refers to complex processing of sensory information to extract relevant information from it (i.e., literally to make *sense* of it). These abilities do encompass perception, but also refer to higher-order and goal-directed processing of sensory information (e.g., imagining how a room might look different if it were painted a darker color).

The difficulty in defining and differentiating sensory abilities is captured in a statement regarding the Gv domain, which is likely to apply to each of these sensory-based domains. According to Eliot and Czarnolewski (2007),

One difficulty with defining spatial intelligence is that it is a dimension that is so fundamental and pervasive in people's everyday lives that they take it for granted. It is fundamental and pervasive in the sense that it may operate at any given moment at several levels of human consciousness and, in combination with other cognitive functions, may contribute to the solution process in different ways for many different types of problems. (p. 362)

Well stated!

Visual Processing (Gv)

Definition of Gv

Visual processing (Gv) can be defined as *the ability to make use of simulated mental imagery (often in conjunction with currently perceived images) to solve problems.* Once the eyes have transmitted visual information, the visual system of the brain automatically performs a large number of low-level computations (edge detection, light–dark perception, color differentiation, motion detection, etc.). The results of these low-level computations are used by various higher-order processors to infer more complex aspects of the visual image (object recognition, constructing models of spatial configuration, motion prediction, etc.). Tests measuring Gv are designed to measure individual differences in these higher-order processes as they work in tandem to perceive relevant information (e.g., a truck is approaching!) and solve problems of a visual–spatial nature (e.g., getting a large, ungainly piece of furniture through a narrow door).

Well-Supported Narrow Abilities within Gv

1. *Visualization (Vz): The ability to perceive complex patterns and mentally simulate how they might look when transformed (e.g., rotated, changed in size, partially obscured).* In the same way that induction is central to Gf and language development is central to Gc, this is the core ability of Gv. Almost all of the studies showing that Gv has predictive validity in forecasting important outcomes use measures of visualization as a proxy for Gv as a whole. A number of long-term longitudinal studies have shown that Gv (and visualization in particular) is an important yet often neglected precursor of high achievement in the so-called "STEM" domains (science, technology, engineering, mathematics; Lubinski, 2010; Wai, Lubinski, & Benbow, 2009).

2. *Speeded rotation (spatial relations; SR): The ability to solve problems quickly by using mental ro-*tation of simple images.* Whereas visualization is more about the difficulty of visualizing and rotating an image, speeded rotation is about the speed at which fairly simple images can be rotated. For example, a speeded rotation test might consist of an array of letters rotated from 1 to 360 degrees. After mentally rotating the letters to an upright position, the evaluee would discover that half of the letters are backward. The test measures the speed at which the correctly oriented letters can be distinguished from the backward letters.

3. *Closure speed (CS): The ability to quickly identify a familiar meaningful visual object from incomplete (e.g., vague, partially obscured, disconnected) visual stimuli, without knowing in advance what the object is.* This ability is sometimes called *Gestalt perception* because it requires people to "fill in" unseen or missing parts of an image to visualize a single percept.

4. *Flexibility of closure (CF): Ability to identify a visual figure or pattern embedded in a complex distracting or disguised visual pattern or array, when one knows in advance what the pattern is.* This factor is primarily defined by hidden-figures tests (examinees find simple figures embedded in complex backgrounds). Horn (1980) considered this type of test to be the best marker of Gv, probably because it correlates less with Gf than do many visualization tests.

5. *Visual memory (MV): The ability to remember complex images over short periods of time (less than 30 seconds).* The tasks that define this factor involve being shown complex images and then identifying them soon after the stimulus is removed. When the stimuli are simple, are numerous, and must be remembered in sequence, it becomes more of a Gsm test than a Gv test.

6. *Spatial scanning (SS): The ability to visualize a path out of a maze or a field with many obstacles.* This factor is defined by performance on paper-and-pencil maze tasks. It is not clear whether this ability is related to complex, large-scale, real-world navigation skills.

7. *Serial perceptual integration (PI): The ability to recognize an object after only parts of it are shown in rapid succession.* Imagine that a deer is walking behind some trees and that only a part of the deer can be seen at one time. Recognizing that this is a deer is an example of what this ability allows people to do.

8. *Length estimation (LE): The ability to visually estimate the length of objects.*

9. *Perceptual illusions (IL): The ability not to be fooled by visual illusions.*

10. *Perceptual alternations (PN): Consistency in the rate of alternating between different visual perceptions.* Some people are able to look at a figure such as a Necker Cube (a figure showing the edges of a cube such that it is unclear which face is forward) and very quickly switch back and forth between imagining it from one orientation to another. Other people have much more difficulty switching their perspective. Once seen in a particular way, the interpretation of the figure becomes fixed.

11. *Imagery (IM): The ability to mentally produce very vivid images.* Recent evidence confirmed the existence of this factor as separate from visualization and other narrow Gv constructs (Burton & Fogarty, 2003). Research has suggested that mental imagery is likely to be important for surgeons, the study of human anatomy, and piloting an airplane (Thompson, Slotnick, Burrage, & Kosslyn, 2009). One can further imagine that imagery may be important for artists and designers, packing a suitcase for a trip, interpreting graphs, solving geometry problems, and other activities, but we do not have compelling evidence that this is so. Small-scale brain imaging studies have suggested that visual spatial imagery may not be a single faculty; rather, "visualizing spatial location and mentally transforming locating rely on distinct neural networks" (Thompson et al., 2009, p. 1245). This research suggests a distinction between *transformational processing* and *memory for location.* An *objective* versus *spatial* imagery dichotomy has also been suggested (see Thompson et al., 2009), as well as the possibility of *quality* versus *speed* of imagery abilities (Burton & Fogarty, 2003). We believe that imagery is a promising CHC ability warranting more theoretical and psychometric research attention. We would not be surprised to see multiple imagery abilities validated. More importantly, if psychometrically well-developed practical imagery measures can be constructed, there is a good chance that they will be found to have diagnostic or predictive importance in select educational and occupational domains.

Assessment Recommendations for Gv

Adequate measurement of Gv should always include measures of visualization. If a visualization test utilizes manipulatives, it is important for it to minimize motor requirements (Gp, Gps). The physical manipulation of objects is not required to measure "in the mind's eye" visualization (see, e.g., the WJ III Spatial Relations and Block Rotation tests). If speeded tasks are used, they should be balanced by the inclusion of unspeeded tasks.

Comments and Unresolved Issues Related to Gv

• *Is visualization part of Gf?* In many factor-analytic studies, Gf is defined in part by tests considered to measure visualization (e.g., Woodcock, 1990). In Carroll's (1993) analyses, visualization tests often loaded on both Gf and Gv, and about a third of the time the loadings were higher on Gf. What might be happening? Studies of visualization tests suggest that people use a variety of strategies on spatial tests (Kyllonen, Lohman, & Woltz, 1984). Hegarty (2010) has classified these strategies broadly as either using mental imagery (on the Paper Folding Test: "I imagined folding the paper, punching the hole, and unfolding the paper in my mind") or analytic strategies (e.g., "I used the number of holes/folds to eliminate some of the answer choices"). We believe that the Gv loadings for visualization tests occur because many people use imagery to complete the tests some of the time, and that the Gf loadings occur because logical/analytic strategies are also employed by some people. Furthermore, Kyllonen and colleagues (1984) found that the best performers on visualization tests were flexible in their strategy use, adapting to the task demands of a particular item. This kind of judgment is invariably associated with Gf.

• *Why has the SR factor changed its name from spatial relations to speeded rotation?* Carroll defined the spatial relations factor by using Lohman's (1979) name and definition. Because Lohman, Pellegrino, Alderton, and Regian (1987) suggested that a better name might be "speeded rotation or reflection" (p. 267), Carroll (1993, p. 326) considered naming it that. Carroll acknowledged that all aspects of Gv deal with spatial relations, and thus the term *spatial relations* does not capture what is unique about the factor. Lohman (1996) subsequently renamed the factor *speeded rotation*, and we believe that it is time to make this switch as well. The term *spatial relations* has been used by many researchers to mean a variety of things, including what is meant by visualization. *Speeded rotation* is more descriptive of what the factor is and is thus more easily remembered. Fortuitously, it can keep the same abbreviation of SR. We believe that most of the SR (spatial relations) narrow-ability classifications of Gv tests during the first- and second-generation CHC development periods (see Figure 4.1) are wrong, and the second author offers his *mea culpas.*

• *Do spatial navigation abilities belong with Gv?* Many aspects of Gv are still unexplored. It seems highly likely that *spatial navigation ability,* defined here as the ability to find one's way and maintain a sense of direction and location while moving around in a complex real-world environment (Wolbers & Hegarty, 2010), should factor with Gv (Schoenfeld, Lehmann, & Leplow, 2010). Jansen's (2009) distinction between "small-scale" spatial abilities (visualization, mental rotation abilities as per the current CHC Gv domain) and "large-scale" spatial abilities (abilities involved in moving around a space that is not visible from the observer's standpoint)—latent factor abilities that correlated at a significant but low .30 in Wolbers and Hegarty's (2010) research—may prove useful in future research in this area. With the advent of 3-D computer graphics and virtual-reality software, we expect to see a variety of more realistic Gv tests.

Auditory Processing (Ga)

Definition of Ga

Auditory processing (Ga) can be defined as *the ability to detect and process meaningful nonverbal information in sound.* This definition is bound to cause confusion because we do not have a well developed vocabulary for talking about sound unless we are talking about speech sounds or music. Ga encompasses both of these domains, but also much more. There are two common misperceptions about Ga. First, although Ga depends on sensory input, it is not sensory input itself. Ga is what the brain does with sensory information from the ear, sometimes long after a sound has been heard (e.g., after he became deaf, Beethoven composed some of his best work by imagining how sounds would blend). The second extremely common misconception, even among professionals, is that Ga is oral language comprehension. It is true that one aspect of Ga (parsing speech sounds, or phonetic coding) is related to oral language comprehension—but this is simply a precursor to comprehension, not comprehension itself (in the

same way that adequate vision is a prerequisite for playing tennis, but vision is not normally thought of as a tennis skill).

If Gc is the wallflower (Hunt, 2000) at the CHC ball, then Ga is an adolescent social butterfly flitting from factor to factor, not readily defined or understood by others, and still in an awkward formative stage of adolescent theoretical and psychometric identity formation (with notable identity role confusion). Ga was the least studied factor in Carroll's (1993) treatise, largely because reliable and valid technology for measuring Ga abilities did not exist during most of the days of prolific psychometric factor-analytic research. This situation has been recently remedied by an explosion of wide-ranging (but not necessarily internally coherent or organized) research on a wide array of Ga characteristics (see Conway, Pisoni, & Kronenberger, 2009; Gathercole, 2006; Hubbard, 2010; Rammsayer & Brandler, 2007).

Well-Supported Narrow Abilities within Ga

1. *Phonetic coding (PC): The ability to hear phonemes distinctly.* This ability is also referred to as *phonological processing, phonological awareness, and phonemic awareness.* People with poor phonetic coding have difficulty hearing the internal structure of sound in words. This makes sounding out unfamiliar words while reading difficult. Poor phonetic coding is one of the major risk factors in reading disorders, specifically phonological dyslexia. Most people, even with very low Ga, can understand speech and speak perfectly well without awareness of the distinct phonemes they are hearing and saying. What they lack is the ability to separate phonemes mentally and hear them in isolation.

2. *Speech sound discrimination (US): The ability to detect and discriminate differences in speech sounds (other than phonemes) under conditions of little or no distraction or distortion.* The definition of this factor has been narrowed to nonphonemic aspects of speech sounds, in order to make it more distinct from phonetic coding. People who have poor speech sound discrimination are less able to distinguish variations in tone, timbre, and pitch in speech; this might reduce their ability to detect subtle emotional changes, or subtle changes in meaning due to differential emphasis.

3. *Resistance to auditory stimulus distortion (UR): The ability to hear words correctly even under con-*

ditions of distortion or loud background noise. It is not yet clear to what degree this ability depends on sensory acuity. As people age, they tend to complain that they have greater difficulty understanding speech in noisy public places or on a telephone with background noise. Speaking louder usually helps them understand better.

4. *Memory for sound patterns (UM): The ability to retain (on a short-term basis) auditory events such as tones, tonal patterns, and voices.* This ability is important for musicians, who need to be able to hold in mind a musical phrase they hear so that they can reproduce it later.

5. *Maintaining and judging rhythm (U8): The ability to recognize and maintain a musical beat.* This may be an aspect of memory for sound patterns, as short-term memory is clearly involved. However, it is likely that there is something distinct about rhythm that warrants a distinction. Future research is needed.

6. *Musical discrimination and judgment (U1 U9): The ability to discriminate and judge tonal patterns in music with respect to melodic, harmonic, and expressive aspects (phrasing, tempo, harmonic complexity, intensity variations).*

7. *Absolute pitch (UP): The ability to perfectly identify the pitch of tones.* As a historical tidbit, John Carroll had perfect pitch.

8. *Sound localization (UL): The ability to localize heard sounds in space.*

Assessment Recommendations for Ga

Ga may be unusual in CHC theory, in that psychologists are more interested in a narrow ability (phonetic coding) than in the broad ability (Ga). Some of the other Ga abilities are clearly related to musical achievement and are priorities if one is attempting to assess musical aptitude, or assess impairment for a brain-injured musician. We see promise for some yet to be clearly identified and understood Ga abilities (e.g., auditory imagery; auditory-based temporal processing measures; auditory gap detection; rhythm perception and production) for understanding general cognitive and language development.

Comments and Unresolved Issues Related to Ga

• *Does Carroll's (1993) temporal tracking (UK) belong in Ga?* Previously, this factor was listed as

part of Ga. *Temporal tracking* was defined as the ability to mentally track auditory temporal (sequential) events so as to be able to count, anticipate, or rearrange them (e.g., reorder a set of musical tones). This factor is measured by tests that require simultaneous storage and processing; thus it appears that such tests are methods of measuring working memory capacity (Stankov, 2000).[16]

• *Do Carroll's (1993) hearing and speech threshold (UA UT UU), sound frequency discrimination (U5), sound intensity/duration discrimination (U6), and general sound discrimination (U3) factors belong in CHC theory?* These are sensory acuity factors, and as such are outside the scope of CHC theory.

Olfactory Abilities (Go)

Definition of Go

Olfactory abilities (Go) can be defined as *the abilities to detect and process meaningful information in odors.* Go refers not to sensitivity of the olfactory system, but to the cognition one does with whatever information the nose is able to send. The Go domain is likely to contain many more narrow abilities than currently listed in the CHC model, as a cursory skim of Go-related articles reveals reference to such abilities as olfactory memory, episodic odor memory, olfactory sensitivity, odor specific abilities, odor identification and detection, odor naming, and olfactory imagery, to name but a few. Among the reasons why the Minnesota Multiphasic Personality Inventory has items about "peculiar odors" are that distorted and hallucinatory olfaction is a common early symptom of schizophrenia, and that poor olfaction is an associated characteristic of a wide variety of brain injuries, diseases and disorders (Doty, 2001; Dulay, Gesteland, Shear, Ritchey, & Frank, 2008). Clearly, olfactory processing is easily damaged and often acts as a "canary in the coal mine" for neurological insult or decline.

Hypothesized Narrow Abilities within Go

1. *Olfactory memory (OM): The ability to recognize previously encountered distinctive odors.* The oft-noted experience of smelling a distinctive smell and being flooded with vivid memories of the last time that odor was encountered does have some basis in research. Memory for distinctive odors has a much flatter forgetting curve than many other kinds of memory (Danthiir, Roberts, Pallier, & Stankov, 2001).

Assessment Recommendations for Go

Most practical and clinical applications of smell tests are actually sensory acuity tests. People who work where gas leaks are possible must be tested regularly to make sure that they can make potentially life-saving odor detections.

Comments and Unresolved Issues Related to Go

• *Does olfactory sensitivity (OS) belong in CHC theory?* This is the ability to detect and discriminate differences in odors. That is, it is a sensory acuity factor, and we believe it is thus outside the scope of CHC theory.

• *What about olfactory knowledge?* Surely there is an ability to name smells! There probably is, but it turns out that "blind" smelling identification tests are extremely difficult for most people. Fans of the television program *Top Chef* know that even high-end professional chefs are often laughably bad at identifying the smells of spices that the chefs work with daily. We await innovations in measurement and well-designed studies to include such a factor.

Tactile Abilities (Gh)

Definition of Gh

Tactile abilities (Gh) can be defined as the abilities to detect and process meaningful information in haptic (touch) sensations. Gh refers not to sensitivity of touch, but to the cognition one does with tactile sensations. Because this ability is not yet well defined and understood, it is hard to describe it authoritatively. We can speculate that it will include such things as tactile visualization (object identification via palpation), tactile localization (i.e., where has one been touched), tactile memory (i.e., remembering where one has been touched), texture knowledge (naming surfaces and fabrics by touch), and many others. Tests of Gh have long been used in neuropsychological batteries because of their ability to detect brain injury, especially to the somatosensory cortex.

Well-Supported Narrow Abilities within Gh

There are no well-supported cognitive ability factors within Gh yet. *Tactile sensitivity (TS)*, a sensory acuity ability, refers to the ability to make fine discriminations in haptic sensations. For example,

if two caliper points are placed on the skin simultaneously, we perceive them as a single point if they are close together. Some people are able to make finer discriminations than others.

Assessment Recommendations for Gh

Most practical and clinical applications of Gh tests actually use sensory acuity tests. There are no currently available tests of higher-order Gh processes that are clearly distinct from Gv. The Halstead–Reitan Neuropsychological Test Battery and the Dean–Woodcock Neuropsychological Battery include a number of Gh tests.

Comments and Unresolved Issues Related to Gh

• *How is Gh to be distinguished from Gv and Gf?* Two well-designed studies (Roberts, Stankov, Pallier, & Dolph, 1997; Stankov, Seizova-Cajic, & Roberts, 2001) found it difficult to distinguish between complex tests assumed to measure Gh and well-defined markers of Gv and Gf. Why might this be so? If the test involves identifying common objects (coins, keys, books, etc.) by handling them while blindfolded, the examinee is essentially using the hands instead of the eyes to *visualize* an object.

Kinesthetic Abilities (Gk)

Definition of Gk

Kinesthetic abilities (Gk) can be defined as *the abilities to detect and process meaningful information in proprioceptive sensations. Proprioception* refers to the ability to detect limb position and movement via *proprioreceptors* (sensory organs in muscles and ligaments that detect stretching). Gk refers not to the sensitivity of proprioception, but to the cognition one does with proprioceptive sensations. Because this ability is not yet well understood, we can only speculate that it will include such things as a dancer's ability to move into a certain position and visualize how it looks to another person (which would have Gv components), and knowledge of which body movements will be needed to accomplish a specific goal (e.g., passing through a narrow space). Such abilities are likely to be involved in Gardner's *bodily–kinesthetic intelligence* (see Chen & Gardner, Chapter 5, this volume).

One interesting possibility is that proprioceptive receptors and other mechanoreceptors in muscles are used in inferring characteristics of objects that are hefted and wielded (Turvey, 1996). That is, when an object is held and waved about (*dynamic touch*), one can get a sense of its length, weight, and mass distribution. Higher-order cognition occurs when this information informs potential uses (*affordances*) of the object (e.g., a hammer, a lever, a weapon).

Well-Supported Narrow Abilities within Gk

There are no well-supported cognitive ability factors within Gk yet. *Kinesthetic sensitivity (KS)*, a sensory acuity ability, refers to the ability to make fine discriminations in proprioceptive sensations (e.g., whether and how much a limb has been moved).

Assessment Recommendations for Gk

We are unaware of commercially available measures of Gk. Very little is known about the measurement of Gk. Readers are referred to Stankov and colleagues (2001) for ideas about Gk tests.

Comments and Unresolved Issues Related to Gk

• *How separate is Gk from Gp?* We suspect that Gk and Gp are so interconnected that they may form the same broad-ability construct. That is, although there is a clear physiological distinction between motor abilities and kinesthetic perception, motor performance is constantly informed by sensory feedback, and thus Gk and Gp can be considered an integrated functional unit.

Psychomotor Abilities (Gp)

Definition of Gp

Psychomotor abilities (Gp) can be defined as *the abilities to perform physical body motor movements (e.g., movement of fingers, hands, legs) with precision, coordination, or strength.*

Well-Supported Narrow Abilities within Gp

1. *Static strength (P3): The ability to exert muscular force to move (push, lift, pull) a relatively heavy or immobile object.*

2. *Multilimb coordination (P6): The ability to make quick specific or discrete motor movements of the arms or legs.*

3. *Finger dexterity (P2): The ability to make precisely coordinated movements of the fingers (with or without the manipulation of objects).*

4. *Manual dexterity (P1): The ability to make precisely coordinated movements of a hand or a hand and the attached arm.*

5. *Arm–hand steadiness (P7): The ability to precisely and skillfully coordinate arm–hand positioning in space.*

6. *Control precision (P8): The ability to exert precise control over muscle movements, typically in response to environmental feedback (e.g., changes in speed or position of object being manipulated).*

7. *Aiming (AI): The ability to precisely and fluently execute a sequence of eye–hand coordination movements for positioning purposes.*

8. *Gross body equilibrium (P4): The ability to maintain the body in an upright position in space or regain balance after balance has been disturbed.*

Assessment Recommendations for Gp

Psychologists are not usually interested in Gp for its own sake. Neuropsychologists use measures of Gp, such as various grip tests and pegboard tests, to measure uneven performance with the right and left hands as an indicator of lateralized brain injury. Industrial/organizational psychologists may use Gp measures for personnel selection in jobs that require manual dexterity. Occupational and physical therapists use measures of motor functioning with consistent regularity.

CHC THEORY VISUALIZED

In writing this chapter, we have become sensitized to the need for an overarching framework with which to understand CHC theory as a whole. When CHC theory consisted of 8–10 broad abilities, the sense of information overload it created upon initial encounter was already severe. Now that CHC theory consists of 16 broad abilities, the problem has increased exponentially. Some organizing principles are needed to manage the complexity of the taxonomy. In Figure 4.7, we show some higher-order groupings of the broad abilities in CHC theory. Some of these groupings (with solid boxes and overlapping ovals) are functional in nature. For example, Gsm and Glr have a common purpose. Some ability groupings (with dotted boxes) are merely conceptual groupings (e.g.,

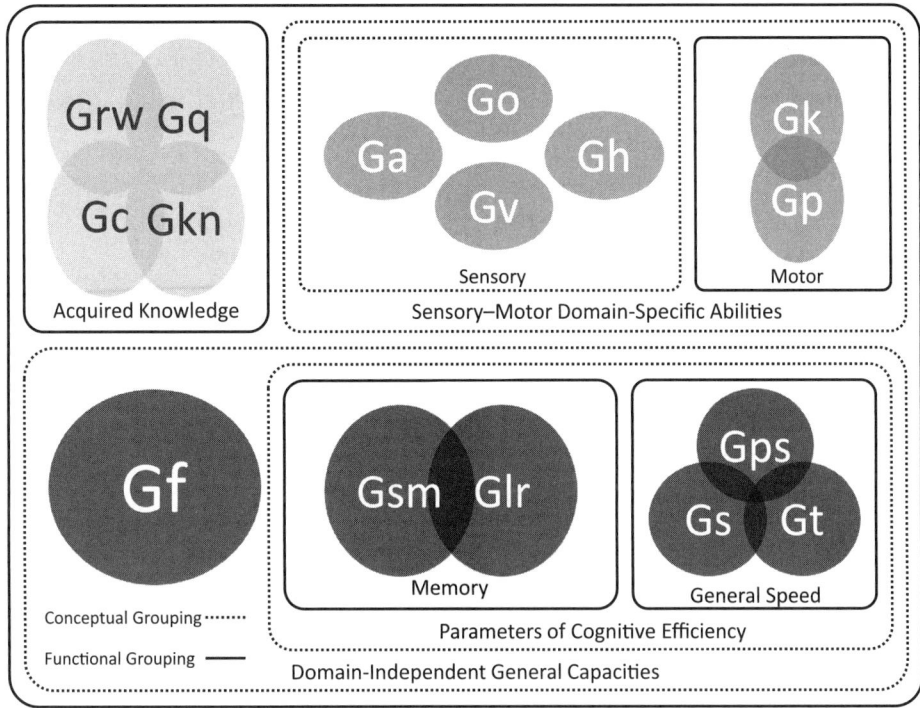

FIGURE 4.7. Conceptual and functional groupings of broad CHC abilities.

some abilities are related to sensory or motor functions).

In Figure 4.8, we present a highly speculative model of how CHC broad abilities might function as parameters of information processing. We have borrowed liberally from the information-processing models by Woodcock (1993) and Kyllonen (2002). We acknowledge that this information-processing model is not exactly cutting-edge, compared to current work in experimental cognitive psychology. However, we hope it stimulates research and theory that integrates knowledge from research on individual differences and experimental cognitive psychology.

The arrows represent the flow of information through different information-processing structures (represented as boxes). These structures are assumed to be invariant across normal humans, but their parameters (e.g., efficiency, speed, capacity, breadth, and power) differ from person to person. These parameters are hypothesized to map onto CHC constructs.

Information enters the mind via sensory receptors. Some people have more acute sensory receptors than others (and this varies from one sensory system to the other). The various sensory-linked

abilities (Gv, Ga, Go, Gh, Gk) determine the complexity of perceptual processing possible for any given person. Greater complexity of perceptual processing allows some people to perceive more nuance and complexity in everything. Gs and Gt represent general constraints on the speed of perception. Gsm places asymptotic limits on the capacity of working memory and the degree to which attention can be controlled within working memory. Gf and Gsm jointly determine the complexity of thought that is possible within working memory.

Glr learning efficiency determines how much effort is needed to store new information (of various kinds) in long-term memory. Gc, Gkn, Grw, and Gq are indices of the breadth of declarative knowledge stored in long-term memory. Nonverbal (procedural) knowledge is also presented, but little is known about its measurement. In part, the breadth of procedural knowledge may represent the degree to which the sensory–motor-linked abilities are influenced ("crystallized") by experience. For example, exposure to a particular language sensitizes us to perceive certain phonemes (part of Ga) and not others.

Glr retrieval fluency represents the speed at which information in long-term storage can be

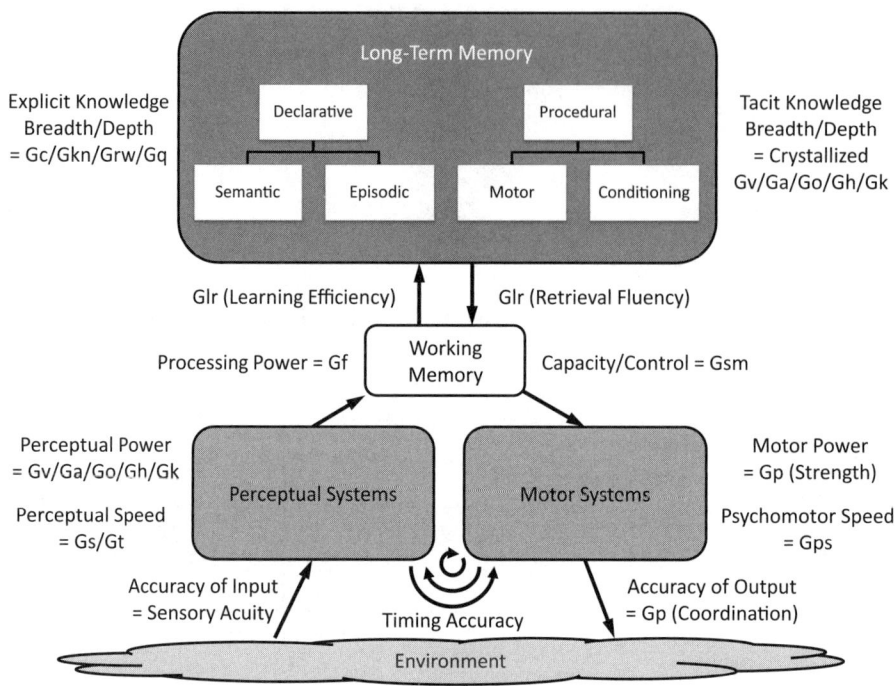

FIGURE 4.8. CHC abilities as parameters of information processing.

loaded into working memory structures for further cognitive processing and use. Gps represents the speed at which the central executive in working memory can execute motor commands. Gp represents parameters of motor performance, such as strength, coordination, and control. The accuracy of motor movement is thus analogous to sensory acuity. What would be analogous to Gv or Ga in the motor domain? It is not clear that there *must* be something, but it may have something to do with the complexity of movement possible for a person. Finally, because Kyllonen (2002) noted that perceptual and motor systems are constantly in dialogue, we represent differences in the accuracy and timing of this communication with the curved arrows. We speculate that individual differences in the accuracy and calibration of cerebellar and other brain-based timing mechanisms may turn out to be important determinants of cognitive and motor performance.[17]

Focusing on a subset of CHC abilities, in Figure 4.9 we present a conceptual map of how the four acquired-knowledge broad abilities may be related. This map is not a structural model (as seen in structural equation models), but rather a loose interpretation of ideas presented by Carroll (1993) and Ackerman (1996). At the top of the

conceptual map is all acquired knowledge, much of which is nonverbal (e.g., how to ride a bicycle). Acquired knowledge consists also of Gc and the two academic abilities, Grw and Gq. Gc is divided into two broad classes, language development and general information. Language development consists of many abilities, which can be roughly categorized by the degree to which the ability is oral or written and by the degree to which the language ability involves understanding language (receptive skills) or communicating with language (productive skills). The 2 × 2 matrix under language development is loosely based on a figure drawn by Carroll (1993, p. 147).

Under general information, we present Gkn (domain-specific knowledge). People who have broad Gc interests and knowledge are also likely to develop deep specialized knowledge in their particular field of interests. Gkn's symbol is empty because, by definition, Gkn is specialized, not unified. Because skills in Gkn develop according to specific interests and work experiences, we have drawn Gkn as a hexagon in honor of Holland's (1985) "RIASEC" (realistic, investigative, artistic, social, enterprising, and conventional) model of career interests. Holland's model is to the structure of interests what CHC theory is to cognitive

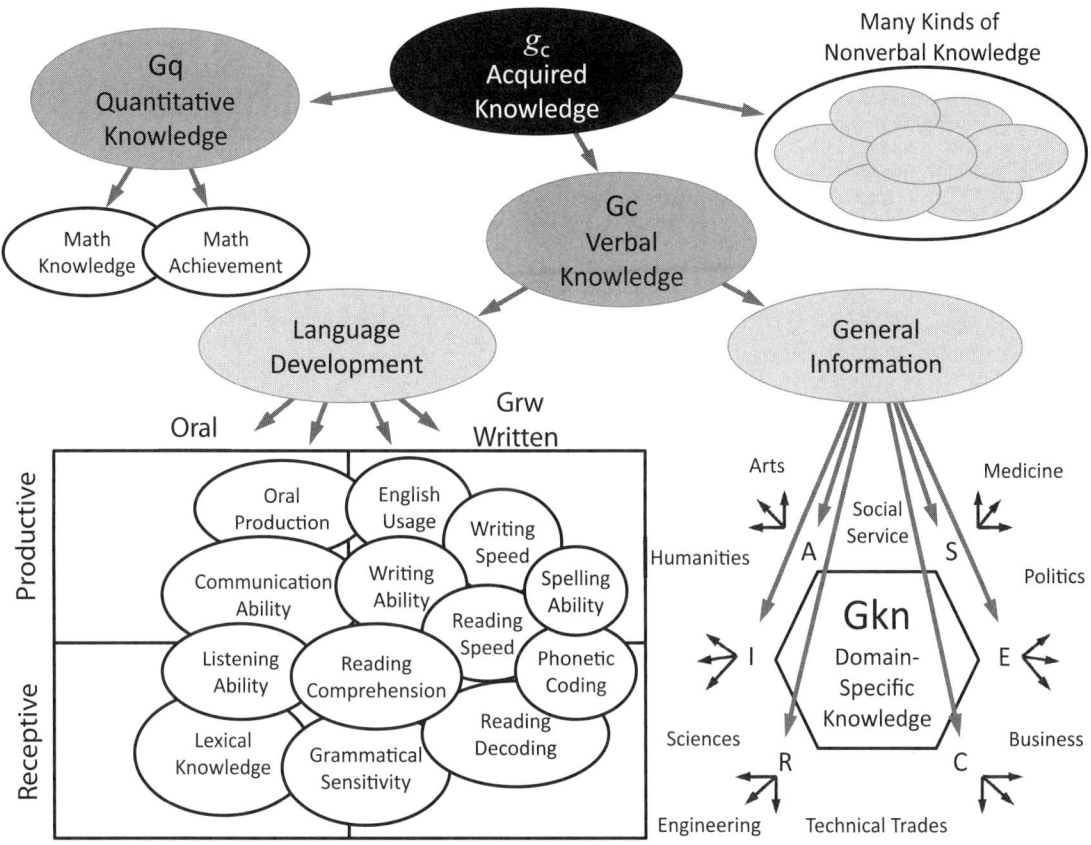

FIGURE 4.9. Conceptual map of acquired knowledge.

abilities. Holland's model suggests that interests that are adjacent to each other (e.g., social and enterprising interests) are likely to co-occur in the same person, and that interests that are further apart are less likely to co-occur in the same person (e.g., conventional and artistic interests). Once a person settles into a specific career path, his or her knowledge becomes extremely focused, symbolized by the scattering arrows jutting out from each of Holland's "big six" interests.

THE FUTURE EVOLUTION OF CHC THEORY

When the merger of the ideas of Cattell, Horn, and Carroll was first proposed by McGrew (1997), the hope was to facilitate the transfer of knowledge from these great thinkers to psychoeducational assessment practitioners. Gratifyingly, this hope has been realized in many ways. Had the purpose of CHC theory been simply to summarize the work of these grand masters of intelligence theory, the theory would quickly cease to be relevant, as new research causes older concepts to be refined or even superannuated. The ultimate goal, however, has always been for CHC theory to undergo continual upgrades, so that it would evolve toward an ever-more accurate summary of human cognitive diversity. With that end in mind, we have attempted to simplify the model where it needed simplification. We have also elaborated upon aspects of the model that needed elaboration. We hope that our research- and reasoning-based conclusions and hypotheses will make CHC theory more accurate, more understandable to practitioners, and ultimately more helpful to people who undergo psychoeducational assessment. We hope that many readers, especially long-time CHC users and researchers, are placed into a state of thoughtful disequilibrium regarding their understanding of the prevailing CHC model. Even if such users are unconvinced by our arguments, if the schemas of CHC users are broadened and refined by considering the ideas we have presented, our chapter will have been a success. The original source theorists of CHC theory would not idly stand by and let the current consensus-based theory calcify and suffer from hardening of the CHC categories. We believe that Cattell, Horn, and Carroll, and all the psychometric giants upon whose shoulders they stood, would smile on our efforts—and would then promptly engage us, and others, in spirited debates and empirical- and theory-based discourse.

NOTES

1. A *taxonomy* is a system of classification.
2. The "Factor Analysis at 100: Historical Developments and Future Directions" conference, held at the Thurstone Psychometric Laboratory, University of Carolina at Chapel Hill, May 13–15, 2004, produced a book and two interesting visual summaries of the factor analysis "genealogy" (academic backgrounds and relationships among individuals who have contributed to the field of factor analysis) and a timeline (significant publications in events in the 100-year history of factor analysis). Information is available online (*www.fa100.info*).
3. Different sources (Carroll, 1993; Horn & Noll, 1997; Jensen, 1998) list between seven and nine abilities, and also provide slightly different names for the Thurstone PMAs.
4. Cattell's original g_f-g_c notation utilized lowercase italic g's followed by subscripts. As described later in the chapter, these eventually changed to uppercase G (general) roman letters followed by lowercase letters that designated the specific cognitive ability domains. From this point forward in this chapter, the later convention is used.
5. Cattell (1963) was so excited by Horn's (1965) dissertation that he referenced many of its findings before it was even finished.
6. About Thurstone's PMA model, Horn and Noll (1997) noted that "to a considerable extent, modern hierarchical theories derive from this theory" (p. 62).
7. See McGrew (1997, 2005) for a discussion of the model differences.
8. A so-called "tipping point" is the "moment of critical mass, the threshold, the boiling point" (Gladwell, 2000, p. 12) where a movement that has been building over time, generally in small groups and networks, begins to influence a much wider audience.
9. The data in Figure 4.2 represent two different literature databases. The search terms CHC and *Cattell–Horn–Carroll* were submitted to the *PsycINFO* and the journal *Intelligence* reference archives. The searches identified any publications (journal articles, books, dissertations) where the two search terms occurred anywhere in the source (title, text, or references).
10. Background information and explanations of the evolution of McGrew's "beyond CHC theory" model work can be found online (*www.iqscorner.com/2010/10/pushing-edge-of-contemporary-cognitive.html*).
11. There is no such thing as reasoning that is completely independent of prior learning (Horn, 1985).
12. These recommendations are not based on hard evidence, but rather on our measured opinions. They do not obviate the need for sound clinical judgment. If there are specific referral concerns that require something other than what is recommended here, common sense should prevail.
13. Gsm is sometimes referred to as *working memory*, but we reserve this term to refer to Baddeley's (1986) theory of theoretical entities within short-term memory (central executive, phonological–articulatory loop, etc.). That is, there is a difference between a theory about species-invariant features of memory (i.e., working memory) and individual differences in the capacity and efficiency of those features (McGrew, 2005).
14. This factor was previously named *working memory*. However, as explained in McGrew (2005), this term does not refer to an individual-difference variable. *Working memory capacity* is an individual-difference variable, that is, a property of the working memory system as a whole.
15. Parallels for our hypothesis exist in all CHC domains. For example, the WJ III Concept Formation test is a miniature conceptual rule-learning task that includes corrective feedback. It has been established as a strong indicator of Gf I (induction). Most geometric or figural matrices tests similarly have been found to be strong indicators of Gf I (induction). Differences in performance between these two types of induction measures are likely due to the different methods used, unreliability inherent in each measure, and possible small amounts of reliable specific or unique variance.
16. McGrew attended the 1989 Minnesota Symposium on Learning and Individual Differences, and saw and heard Lazar Stankov stand up from his seat in the audience after listening to a presenter talk in detail about working memory, and make a strongly worded minispeech that the temporal tracking ability he and Horn had identified in 1980 (Stankov & Horn, 1980) should receive proper credit as being the first identification of what is now known as working memory.
17. A number of brain regions have been implicated in mental interval timing. These include, but are not limited to, the cerebellum, dorsolateral pre-

frontal cortex, parietal cortex, basal ganglia, and supplemental motor cortex. These brain areas are hypothesized to work together in a synchronized brain circuit or network to control precise mental timing and coordination of a wide array of cognitive and sensory–motor functions. The breadth of this mental timing literature is tremendous, with numerous "brain clock" models having been proposed and studied. Recent research by Rammsayer and colleagues has gone as far as suggesting that auditory-based temporal processing may be the essence of psychometric *g*, more so than traditional Jensenian-led research on reaction time *g*. This "IQ brain clock" literature is so large that McGrew devotes a special blog to reporting research on mental timing (the IQ Brain Clock blog; *ticktockbraintalk. blogspot.com*).

REFERENCES

Ackerman, P. L. (1987). Individual differences in skill learning: An integration of psychometric and information processing perspectives. *Psychological Bulletin, 102(1)*, 3–27.

Ackerman, P. L. (1996). A theory of adult intellectual development: Process, personality, interests, and knowledge. *Intelligence, 22*, 227–257.

Ackerman, P. L., Beier, M. E., & Boyle, M. O. (2002). Individual differences in working memory within a nomological network of cognitive and perceptual speed abilities. *Journal of Experimental Psychology: General, 131*, 567–589.

Ackerman, P. L., Beier, M. E., & Boyle, M. O. (2005). Working memory and intelligence: The same or different constructs? *Psychological Bulletin, 131*, 30–60.

Ackerman, P. L., & Cianciolo, A. T. (2000). Cognitive, perceptual speed, and psychomotor determinants of individual differences during skill acquisition. *Journal of Experimental Psychology: Applied, 6*, 259–290.

Ackerman, P. L., & Lohman, D. F. (2006). Individual differences in cognitive functions. In P. A. Alexander & P. Winne (Eds.), *Handbook of educational psychology* (2nd ed., pp. 139–161). Mahwah, NJ: Erlbaum.

Alfonso, V. C., Flanagan, D. P., & Radwan, S. (2005). The impact of the Cattell–Horn–Carroll theory on test development and interpretation of cognitive and academic abilities. In D. P. Flanagan & P. L. Harrison (Eds.), *Contemporary intellectual assessment* (2nd ed., pp. 185–202). New York: Guilford Press.

Baddeley, A. (1986). *Working memory*. New York: Clarendon Press/Oxford University Press.

Barkley, R. A. (1997). Behavioral inhibition, sustained attention, and executive functions. Constructing a unifying theory of ADHD. *Psychological Bulletin, 121*, 65–94.

Beauducel, A., Brocke, B., & Liepmann, D. (2001). Perspectives on fluid and crystallized intelligence: Facets for verbal, numerical, and figural intelligence. *Personality and Individual Differences, 30(6)*, 977–994.

Berch, D. B. (2005). Making sense of number sense: Implications for children with mathematical disabilities. *Journal of Learning Disabilities, 38(4)*, 333–339.

Bock, G., Goode, J. A., & Webb, K. (Eds.). (2000). *The nature of intelligence*. London: Novartis Foundation.

Bowers, P. G., Sunseth, K., & Golden, J. (1999). The route between rapid naming and reading progress. *Scientific Studies of Reading, 3(1)*, 31–53.

Brody, N. (2000). History of theories and measurements of intelligence. In R. J. Sternberg (Ed.), *Handbook of intelligence* (pp. 16–33). New York: Cambridge University Press.

Burns, R. B. (1994). Surveying the cognitive terrain. *Educational Researcher, 23(2)*, 35–37.

Burton, L., & Fogarty, G. (2003). The factor structure of visual imagery and spatial abilities. *Intelligence, 31*, 289–318.

Butterworth, B. (2010). Foundational numerical capacities and the origins of dyscalculia. *Trends in Cognitive Sciences, 14(12)*, 534–541.

Carroll, J. B. (1991). No demonstration that *g* is not unitary, but there is more to the story: Comment on Kranzler & Jensen. *Intelligence, 15*, 423–436.

Carroll, J. B. (1993). *Human cognitive abilities: A survey of factor-analytic studies*. New York: Cambridge University Press.

Carroll, J. B. (1997). Commentary on Keith and Witta's hierarchical and cross-age confirmatory factor analysis of the WISC-III. *School Psychology Quarterly, 12*, 108–109.

Carroll, J. B. (1998). Human cognitive abilities: A critique. In J. J. McArdle & R. W. Woodcock (Eds.), *Human cognitive abilities in theory and practice* (pp. 5–24). Mahwah, NJ: Erlbaum.

Carroll, J. B. (2003). The higher-stratum structure of cognitive abilities: Current evidence supports *g* and about ten broad factors. In H. Nyborg (Ed.), *The scientific study of general intelligence: Tribute to Arthur R. Jensen* (pp. 5–21). New York: Pergamon Press.

Carroll, J. B., Kohlberg, L., & DeVries, R. (1984). Psychometric and Piagetian intelligences: Toward resolution of controversy. *Intelligence, 8(1)*, 67–91.

Cattell, J. M. (1890). Mental tests and measurement. *Mind, 15*, 373–381.

Cattell, R. B. (1941). Some theoretical issues in adult intelligence testing. *Psychological Bulletin, 38*, 592.

Cattell, R. B. (1943). The measurement of adult intelligence. *Psychological Bulletin, 40*, 153–193.

Cattell, R. B. (1963). Theory for fluid and crystallized

intelligence: A critical experiment. *Journal of Educational Psychology, 54*, 1–22.

Cattell, R. B. (1971). *Abilities: Their structure, growth, and action.* Boston: Houghton Mifflin.

Cattell, R. B. (1987). *Intelligence: Its structure, growth, and action.* New York: Elsevier.

Cohen, A., Fiorello, C. A., & Farley, F. H. (2006). The cylindrical structure of the Wechsler Intelligence Scale for Children–IV: A retest of the Guttman model of intelligence. *Intelligence, 34*, 587–591.

Conway, C. M., Pisoni, D. B., & Kronenberger, W. G. (2009). The importance of sound for cognitive sequencing abilities. *Current Directions in Psychological Science, 18*(5), 275–279.

Corno, L., Cronbach, L. J., Kupermintz, H., Lohman, D. F., Mandinach, E. B., Porteus, A. W., et al. (2002). *Remaking the concept of aptitude: Extending the legacy of Richard E. Snow.* Mahwah, NJ: Erlbaum.

Cudeck, R., & MacCallum, R. C. (2007). *Factor analysis at 100: Historical developments and future directions.* Mahwah, NJ: Erlbaum.

Daniel, M. H. (1997). Intelligence testing: Status and trends. *American Psychologist, 52*(10), 1038–1045.

Daniel, M. H. (2000). Interpretation of intelligence test scores. In R. Sternberg (Ed.), *Handbook of intelligence* (pp. 477–491). New York: Cambridge University Press.

Danthiir, V., Roberts, R. D., Pallier, G., & Stankov, L. (2001). What the nose knows: Olfaction and cognitive abilities. *Intelligence, 29*, 337–361.

Danthiir, V., Roberts, R. D., Schulze, R., & Wilhelm, O. (2005). Mental speed: On frameworks, paradigms, and a platform for the future. In O. Wilhelm & R. W. Engle (Eds.), *Handbook of understanding and measuring intelligence* (pp. 27–46). Thousand Oaks, CA: Sage.

Danthiir, V., Wilhelm, O., & Schacht, A. (2005). Decision speed in intelligence tasks: Correctly an ability? *Psychology Science, 47*, 200–229.

Deary, I. (2003). Reaction time and psychometric intelligence: Jensen's contributions. In H. Nyborg (Ed.), *The scientific study of general intelligence: Tribute to Arthur R. Jensen* (pp. 53–76). Amsterdam: Pergamon Press.

Detterman, D. (2011). *The science of intelligence.* Manuscript in preparation.

Doty, R. L. (2001). Olfaction. *Annual Review of Psychology, 52*, 423–452.

Dulay, M. F., Gesteland, R. C., Shear, P. K., Ritchey, P. N., & Frank, R. A. (2008). Assessment of the influence of cognition and cognitive processing speed on three tests of olfaction. *Journal of Clinical and Experimental Neuropsychology, 30*, 327–337.

Ekstrom, R. B., French, J. W., & Harman, H. H. (1979). Cognitive factors: Their identification and replica-

tion. *Multivariate Behavioral Research Monographs, 79*(2), 3–84.

Eliot, J., & Czarnolewski, M. Y. (2007). Development of an Everyday Spatial Behavioral Questionnaire. *Journal of General Psychology, 134*(3), 361–381.

Elliott, C. D. (2005). The Differential Ability Scales. In D. P. Flanagan & P. L. Harrison (Eds.), *Contemporary intellectual assessment* (2nd ed., pp. 402–424). New York: Guilford Press.

Evans, J. (2008). Dual processing accounts of reasoning, judgment, and social cognition. *Annual Review of Psychology, 59*, 255–278.

Flanagan, D. P., Genshaft, J. L., & Harrison, P. L. (Eds.). (1997). *Contemporary intellectual assessment.* New York: Guilford Press.

Flanagan, D. P., & Harrison, P. L. (Eds.). (2005). *Contemporary intellectual assessment* (2nd ed.). New York: Guilford Press.

Flanagan, D. P., & Mascolo, J. T. (2005). Psychoeducational assessment and learning disability diagnosis. In D. P. Flanagan & P. L. Harrison (Eds.), *Contemporary intellectual assessment* (2nd ed., pp. 521–544). New York: Guilford Press.

Flanagan, D. P., & McGrew, K. S. (1997). A cross-battery approach to assessing and interpreting cognitive abilities: Narrowing the gap between practice and science. In D. P. Flanagan, J. L. Genshaft, & P. L. Harrison (Eds.), *Contemporary intellectual assessment* (pp. 314–325). New York: Guilford Press.

Flanagan, D. P., & McGrew, K. S. (1998). Interpreting intelligence tests from contemporary Gf-Gc theory: Joint confirmatory factor analysis of the WJ-R and the KAIT in a non-white sample. *Journal of School Psychology, 36*(2), 151–182.

Flanagan, D. P., Ortiz, S. O., & Alfonso, V. (2007). *Essentials of cross-battery assessment* (2nd ed.). Hoboken, NJ: Wiley.

Floyd, R. G. (2005). Information-processing approaches to interpretation of contemporary intellectual assessment instruments. In D. P. Flanagan & P. Harrison (Eds.), *Contemporary intellectual assessment* (2nd ed., pp. 203–233). New York: Guilford Press.

Floyd, R. G., Bergeron, R., Hamilton, G., & Parra, G. R. (2010). How do executive functions fit with the Cattell–Horn–Carroll model?: Some evidence from a joint factor analysis of the Delis–Kaplan Executive Function System and the Woodcock–Johnson III Tests of Cognitive Abilities. *Psychology in the Schools, 47*(7), 721–738.

Floyd, R. G., Evans, J. J., & McGrew, K. S. (2003). Relations between measures of Cattell–Horn–Carroll (CHC) cognitive abilities and mathematics achievement across the school-age years. *Psychology in the Schools, 40*, 155–171.

Ford, L., & Dahinten, V. S. (2005). Use of intelligence tests in the assessment of preschoolers. In D. P. Flanagan & P. L. Harrison (Eds.), *Contemporary intellectual assessment* (2nd ed., pp. 487–503). New York: Guilford Press.

French, J. W. (1951). *The description of aptitude and achievement tests in terms of rotated factors* (Psychometric Monographs No. 5). Chicago: University of Chicago Press.

French, J. W., Ekstrom, R. B., & Price, L. A. (1963). *Manual and kit of reference tests for cognitive factors.* Princeton, NJ: Educational Testing Service.

Fuchs, L. S., Geary, D. C., Compton, D. L., Fuchs, D., Hamlett, C. L., & Bryant, J. D. (2010). The contributions of numerosity and domain-general abilities to school readiness. *Child Development, 81*(5), 1520–1533.

Gathercole, S. E. (2006). Keynote article: Nonword repetition and word learning: The nature of the relationship. *Applied Psycholinguistics, 27,* 513–543.

Geary, D. C. (2007). An evolutionary perspective on learning disability in mathematics. *Developmental Neuropsychology, 32*(1), 471–519.

Gladwell, M. (2000). *The tipping point: How little things can make a big difference.* Boston: Little, Brown.

Goode, N., & Beckman, J. F. (2010). You need to know: There is a causal relationship between structural knowledge and control performance in complex problem solving tasks. *Intelligence, 38,* 345–352.

Guilford, J. P. (1967). *The nature of human intelligence.* New York: McGraw-Hill.

Gustafsson, J. E. (1984). A unifying model for the structure of intellectual abilities. *Intelligence, 8,* 179–203.

Gustafsson, J. E. (1988). Hierarchical models of individual differences in cognitive abilities. In R. J. Sternberg (Ed.), *Psychology of human intelligence* (Vol. 4, pp. 35–71). Hillsdale, NJ: Erlbaum.

Guttman, L. (1954). Some necessary conditions for common- factor analysis. *Psychometrika, 19,* 149–161.

Hakstian, A. R., & Cattell, R. B. (1974). The checking of primary ability structure on a basis of twenty primary abilities. *British Journal of Educational Psychology, 44,* 140–154.

Hale, J. B., & Fiorello, C. A. (2004). *School neuropsychology: A practitioner's handbook.* New York: Guilford Press.

Hambrick, D. Z., Pink, J. E., Meinz, E. J., Pettibone, J. C., & Oswald, F. L. (2008). The roles of ability, personality, and interests in acquiring current events knowledge: A longitudinal study. *Intelligence, 36,* 261–278.

Hegarty, M. (2010). Components of spatial intelligence. In B. H. Ross (Ed.), *The psychology of learning and motivation* (Vol. 52, pp. 265–297) San Diego, CA: Academic Press.

Hoelzle, J. B. (2008). Neuropsychological assessment and the Cattell–Horn–Carroll (CHC) cognitive abilities model. *Dissertation Abstracts International: Section B: The Sciences and Engineering, 69*(9B). (UMI No. AAI 3328214)

Holland, J. L. (1985). *Making vocational choices: A theory of vocational personalities and work environment.* Odessa, FL: Psychological Assessment Resources.

Horn, J. L. (1965). *Fluid and crystallized intelligence: A factor analytic study of the structure among primary mental abilities.* Unpublished doctoral dissertation, University of Illinois, Champaign.

Horn, J. L. (1976). Human abilities: A review of research and theory in the early 1970's. *Annual Review of Psychology, 27,* 437–485.

Horn, J. L. (1980). Concepts of intellect in relation to learning and adult development. *Intelligence, 4,* 285–317.

Horn, J. L. (1985). Remodeling old models of intelligence. In B. B. Wolman (Ed.), *Handbook of intelligence* (pp. 267–300). New York: Wiley.

Horn, J. L. (1991). Measurement of intellectual capabilities: A review of theory. In K. S. McGrew, J. K. Werder, & R. W. Woodcock (Eds.), *WJ-R technical manual* (pp. 197–232). Chicago: Riverside.

Horn, J. L. (1998). A basis for research on age differences in cognitive abilities. In J. J. McArdle & R. W. Woodcock (Eds.), *Human cognitive abilities in theory and practice* (pp. 57–92). Mahwah, NJ: Erlbaum.

Horn, J. L., & Cattell, R. B. (1966). Refinement and test of the theory of fluid and crystallized intelligence. *Journal of Educational Psychology, 57,* 253–270.

Horn, J. L., & Noll, J. (1997). Human cognitive capabilities: Gf-Gc theory. In D. P. Flanagan, J. L. Genshaft, & P. L. Harrison (Eds.), *Contemporary intellectual assessment: Theories, tests and issues* (pp. 53–91). New York: Guilford Press.

Hubbard, T. L. (2010). Auditory imagery: Empirical findings. *Psychological Bulletin, 136,* 302–329.

Hunt, E. (2000). Let's hear it for crystallized intelligence. *Learning and Individual Differences, 12,* 123–129.

Hyde, D. C., & Spelke, E. X. (2011). Neural signatures of number processing in human infants: Evidence for two core systems underlying numerical cognition. *Developmental Science, 14*(2), 360–371.

Inman, W. C., & Secrest, B. T. (1981). Piaget's data and Spearman's theory: An empirical reconciliation and its implications for academic achievement. *Intelligence, 5,* 329–344.

Jansen, P. (2009). The dissociation of small- and large-scale spatial abilities in school-age children. *Perceptual and Motor Skills, 109,* 357–361.

Jensen, A. R. (1998). *The g factor: The science of mental ability.* Westport, CT: Praeger.

Jensen, A. R. (2004). Obituary—John Bissell Carroll. *Intelligence, 32*(1), 1–5.

Jensen, A. R. (2006). *Clocking the mind: Mental chronometry and individual differences*. Amsterdam: Elsevier Science.

Jordan, N. C., Kaplan, D., Olah, L. N., & Locuniak, M. N. (2006). Number sense growth in kindergarten: A longitudinal investigation of children at risk for mathematical difficulties. *Child Development, 77*(1), 153–175.

Kamphaus, R. W., Winsor, A. P., Rowe, E. W., & Kim, S. (2005). A history of intelligence test interpretation. In D. P. Flanagan & P. L. Harrison (Eds.), *Contemporary intellectual assessment* (2nd ed., pp. 23–38). New York: Guilford Press.

Kane, M. J., Hambrick, D. Z., & Conway, A. R. A. (2005). Working memory capacity and fluid intelligence are strongly related constructs: Comment on Ackerman, Beier, and Boyle (2004). *Psychological Bulletin, 131*, 66–71.

Kane, M. J., Hambrick, D. Z., Tuholski, S. W., Wilhelm, O., Payne, T. W., & Engle, R. W. (2004). The generality of working-memory capacity: A latent-variable approach to verbal and visuo-spatial memory span and reasoning. *Journal of Experimental Psychology: General, 133*, 189–217.

Kaufman, A. S. (1979). *Intelligent testing with the WISC-R*. New York: Wiley.

Kaufman, A. S. (1994). *Intelligent testing with the WISC-III*. New York: Wiley.

Kaufman, A. S. (2009). *IQ testing 101*. New York: Springer.

Kaufman, J. C., Kaufman, A. S., Kaufman-Singer, J., & Kaufman, N. L. (2005). The Kaufman Assessment Battery for Children—Second Edition and the Kaufman Adolescent and Adult Intelligence Test. In D. P. Flanagan & P. L. Harrison (Eds.), *Contemporary intellectual assessment* (2nd ed., pp. 344–370). New York: Guilford Press.

Keith, T. Z. (1994). Intelligence is important, intelligence is complex. *School Psychology Quarterly, 9*(3), 209–221.

Keith, T. Z. (2005). Using confirmatory factor analysis to aid in understanding the constructs measured by intelligence tests. In D. P. Flanagan & P. L. Harrison (Eds.), *Contemporary intellectual assessment* (2nd ed., pp. 581–614). New York: Guilford Press.

Keith, T. Z., & Reynolds, M. R. (2010). Cattell–Horn–Carroll abilities and cognitive tests: What we've learned from 20 years of research. *Psychology in the Schools, 47*(7), 635–650.

Kyllonen, P. C. (2002). Knowledge, speed strategies, or working memory capacity?: A systems perspective. In R. J. Sternberg & E. L. Grigorenko (Eds.), *The general factor of intelligence: How general is it?* (pp. 415–465). Mahwah, NJ: Erlbaum.

Kyllonen, P. C., & Christal, R. E. (1990). Reasoning ability is (little more than) working memory capacity?! *Intelligence, 14*, 389–433.

Kyllonen, P. C., Lohman, D. F., & Woltz, D. J. (1984). Componential modeling of alternative strategies for performing spatial tasks. *Journal of Educational Psychology, 76*, 1325–1345.

Lezak, M. D., Howieson, D. B., & Loring, D. W. (2004). *Neuropsychological assessment* (4th ed.). New York: Oxford University Press.

Lohman, D. F. (1979). *Spatial ability: Review and re-analysis of the correlational literature* (Stanford University Technical Report No. 8). Stanford, CA: Stanford University.

Lohman, D. F. (1996). Spatial ability and *g*. In I. Dennis & P. Tapsfield (Eds.), *Human abilities: Their nature and assessment* (pp. 97–116). Hillsdale, NJ: Erlbaum.

Lohman, D. F. (1997). Lessons from the history of intelligence testing. *International Journal of Educational Research, 27*, 359–377.

Lohman, D. F. (2001). Issues in the definition and measurement of abilities. In J. M. Collis & S. Messick (Eds.), *Intelligence and personality: Bridging the gap in theory and measurement* (pp. 79–98). Mahwah, NJ: Erlbaum.

Lohman, D. F., Pellegrino, J. W., Alderton, D. L., & Regian, J. W. (1987). Dimensions and components of individual differences in spatial abilities. In S. H. Irvine & S. N. Newstead (Eds.), *Intelligence and cognition: Contemporary frames of reference* (pp. 253–312). Dordrecht: Martinus Nijhoff.

Lubinski, D. (2010). Spatial ability and STEM: A sleeping giant for talent identification and development. *Personality and Individual Differences, 49*, 344–351.

Marshalek, B., Lohman, D. F., & Snow, R. E. (1983). Complexity continuum in the radex and hierarchical models of intelligence. *Intelligence, 7*, 107–127.

Mather, N., & Wendling, B. (2005). Linking cognitive assessment results to academic interventions for students with learning disabilities. In D. P. Flanagan & P. L. Harrison (Eds.), *Contemporary intellectual assessment* (2nd ed., pp. 269–294). New York: Guilford Press.

McAdams, D. P., Josselson, R., & Lieblich, A. (2006). *Identity and story: Creating self in narrative*. Washington, DC: American Psychological Association.

McCabe, D. P., Roediger, H. L., McDaniel, M. A., Balota, D. A., & Hambrick, D. Z. (2010). The relationship between working memory capacity and executive functioning: Evidence for a common executive attention construct. *Neuropsychology, 24*, 222–243.

McGrew, K. S. (1997). Analysis of the major intelligence

batteries according to a proposed comprehensive Gf-Gc framework. In D. P. Flanagan, J. L. Genshaft, & P. L. Harrison (Eds.), *Contemporary intellectual assessment* (pp. 151–179). New York: Guilford Press.

McGrew, K. S. (1999). *The measurement of reading achievement by different individually administered standardized reading tests. Apples and apples, or apples and oranges?* (Research Report No. 1). St. Cloud, MN: Institute for Applied Psychometrics.

McGrew, K. S. (2005). The Cattell–Horn–Carroll theory of cognitive abilities. In D. P. Flanagan & P. L. Harrison (Eds.), *Contemporary intellectual assessment* (2nd ed., pp. 136–181). New York: Guilford Press.

McGrew, K. S. (2009). Editorial: CHC theory and the human cognitive abilities project: Standing on the shoulders of the giants of psychometric intelligence research. *Intelligence, 37*, 1–10.

McGrew, K. S. (2010). The Flynn effect and its critics: Rusty linchpins and "lookin' for g and Gf in some of the wrong places." *Journal of Psychoeducational Assessment, 28*, 448–468.

McGrew, K. S., & Evans, J. (2004). *Carroll Human Cognitive Abilities Project: Research Report No. 2. Internal and external factorial extensions to the Cattell–Horn–Carroll (CHC) theory of cognitive abilities: A review of factor analytic research since Carroll's seminal 1993 treatise.* St. Cloud, MN: Institute for Applied Psychometrics.

McGrew, K. S., & Wendling, B. J. (2010). Cattell–Horn–Carroll cognitive–achievement relations: What we have learned from the past 20 years of research. *Psychology in the Schools, 47*(7), 651–675.

McGrew, K. S., Werder, J. K., & Woodcock, R. W. (1991). *WJ-R technical manual.* Chicago: Riverside.

McGrew, K. S., & Woodcock, R. W. (2001). *Woodcock–Johnson III technical manual.* Itasca, IL: Riverside.

McGrew, K. S., Woodcock, R. W., & Ford, L. (2002). The Woodcock–Johnson Battery—Third Edition (WJ III). In A. S. Kaufman & E. O. Lichtenberger, *Assessing adolescent and adult intelligence* (2nd ed., pp. 561–628). Boston: Allyn & Bacon.

McIntosh, D. E., & Dixon, F. A. (2005). Use of intelligence tests in the identification of giftedness. In D. P. Flanagan & P. L. Harrison (Eds.), *Contemporary intellectual assessment* (2nd ed., pp. 504–510). New York: Guilford Press.

Mendeleev, D. (1869). On the relationship of the properties of the elements to their atomic weights. *Zhurnal Russkoe Fiziko- Khimicheskoe Obshchestvo, 1*, 60–77.

Miller, D. C. (2007). *Essentials of school neuropsychological assessment.* Hoboken, NJ: Wiley.

Miller, D. C. (2010). *Best practices in school neuropsychology: Guidelines for effective practice, assessment, and evidence-based intervention.* Hoboken, NJ: Wiley.

Miyake, A., Friedman, N. P., Emerson, M. J., Witzki, A. H., Howerter, A., & Wager, T. (2000). The unity and diversity of executive functions and their contributions to complex "frontal lobe" tasks: A latent variable analysis. *Cognitive Psychology, 41*, 49–100.

Nettelbeck, T. (2003). Inspection time and g. In H. Nyborg (Ed.), *The scientific study of general intelligence: Tribute to Arthur R. Jensen* (pp. 77–92). Amsterdam: Pergamon Press.

Newton, J. H., & McGrew, K. S. (2010). Introduction to the special issue: Current research in Cattell–Horn–Carroll-based assessment. *Psychology in the Schools, 47*(7), 621–634.

O'Connor, T. A., & Burns, N. R. (2003). Inspection time and general speed of processing. *Personality and Individual Differences, 35*, 713–724.

Phelps, L., McGrew, K. S., Knopik, S. N., & Ford, L. A. (2005). The general (g), broad, and narrow CHC stratum characteristics of the WJ III and WISC-III tests: A confirmatory cross-battery investigation. *School Psychology Quarterly, 20*, 66–88.

Rammsayer, T. H., & Brandler, S. (2007). Performance on temporal information processing as an index of general intelligence. *Intelligence, 35*(2), 123–139.

Roberts, R. D., & Stankov, L. (1999). Individual differences and human cognitive abilities: Toward a taxonomic model. *Learning and Individual Differences, 11*(1), 1–120.

Roberts, R. D., Stankov, L., Pallier, G., & Dolph, B. (1997). Charting the cognitive sphere: Tactile/kinesthetic performance within the structure of intelligence. *Intelligence, 25*, 111–148.

Roid, G. H., & Pomplun, M. (2005). Interpreting the Stanford–Binet Intelligence Scales, Fifth Edition. In D. P. Flanagan & P. L. Harrison (Eds.), *Contemporary intellectual assessment* (2nd ed., pp. 325–343). New York: Guilford Press.

Schank, R., & Birnbaum, L. (1994). Enhancing intelligence. In J. Khalfa (Ed.), *What is intelligence?* (pp. 72–106). Cambridge, UK: Cambridge University Press.

Schrank, F. A. (2005). Woodcock–Johnson III Tests of Cognitive Abilities. In D. P. Flanagan & P. L. Harrison (Eds.), *Contemporary intellectual assessment* (2nd ed., pp. 371–401). New York: Guilford Press.

Schrank, F. A., Flanagan, D. P., Woodcock, R. W., & Mascolo, J. T. (2002). *Essentials of WJ III cognitive abilities assessment.* New York: Wiley.

Schoenfeld, R., Lehmann, W., & Leplow, B. (2010). Effects of age and sex in mental rotation and spatial learning from virtual environments. *Journal of Individual Differences, 31*, 78–82.

Snow, R. E. (1998). Abilities and aptitudes and achievements in learning situations. In J. J. McArdle & R. W. Woodcock (Eds.), *Human cognitive abilities in theory and practice* (pp. 93–112). Mahwah, NJ: Erlbaum.

Snow, R. E., Kyllonen, P. C., & Marshalek, B. (1984). The topography of ability and learning correlation. In R. J. Sternberg (Ed.), *Advances in the psychology of human intelligence* (pp. 47–103). Hillsdale, NJ: Erlbaum.

Spearman, C. (1904). "General intelligence," objectively determined and measured. *American Journal of Psychology, 15*, 201–293.

Spearman, C. (1927). *The abilities of man: Their nature and measurement.* New York: Macmillan.

Spearman, C. (1934). The factor theory and its troubles. V. Adequacy of proof. *Journal of Educational Psychology, 25*, 310–319.

Spearman, C. (1939). Thurston's work reworked. *Journal of Educational Psychology, 30*, 1–16.

Spearman, C., & Wynn-Jones, L. (1950). *Human ability: A continuation of "The abilities of man."* London: Macmillan.

Stankov, L. (2000). Structural extensions of a hierarchical view on human cognitive abilities. *Learning and Individual Differences, 12*, 35–51.

Stankov, L., & Horn, J. L. (1980). Human abilities revealed through auditory tests. *Journal of Educational Psychology, 72*(1), 21–44.

Stankov, L., & Roberts, R. D. (1997). Mental speed is not the 'basic' process of intelligence. *Personality and Individual Differences, 22*(1), 69–84.

Stankov, L., Seizova-Cajic, T., & Roberts, R. (2001). Tactile and kinesthetic perceptual processes within the taxonomy of human abilities. *Intelligence, 29*, 1–29.

Sternberg, R. J., Conway, B. E., Ketron, J. L., & Bernstein, M. (1981). People's conceptions of intelligence. *Journal of Personality and Social Psychology, 41*, 37–55.

Sternberg, R. J., & Kalmar, D. A. (1998). When will the milk spoil?: Everyday induction in human intelligence. *Intelligence, 25*(3), 185–203.

Sternberg, R. J., & Kaufman, J. C. (1998). Human abilities. *Annual Review of Psychology, 49*, 1134–1139.

Süß, H.-M., Oberauer, K., Wittmann, W. W., Wilhelm, O., & Schulze, R. (2002). Working-memory capacity explains reasoning ability—and a little bit more. *Intelligence, 30*, 261–288.

Süß, H.-M., & Beauducel, A. (2005). Faceted models of intelligence. In O. Wilhelm & R. W. Engle (Eds.), *Handbook of understanding and measuring intelligence* (pp. 313–332). London: Sage.

Thompson, W. L., Slotnick, S. D., Burrage, M. S., & Kosslyn, S. M. (2009). Two forms of spatial imagery. *Psychological Science, 20*(10), 1245–1253.

Thurstone, L. L. (1938). *Primary mental abilities.* Chicago: University of Chicago Press.

Thurstone, L. L. (1947). *Multiple factor analysis.* Chicago: University of Chicago Press.

Tucker-Drob, E. M., & Salthouse, T. A. (2009). Confirmatory factor analysis and multidimensional scaling for construct validation of cognitive abilities. *International Journal of Behavioral Development, 33*(3), 277–285.

Turvey, M. T. (1996). Dynamic touch. *American Psychologist, 51*, 1134–1152.

Unsworth, N., & Engle, R. W. (2007a). The nature of individual differences in working memory capacity: Active maintenance in primary memory and controlled search from secondary memory. *Psychological Review, 114*, 104–132.

Unsworth, N., & Engle, R. W. (2007b). On the division or short-term and working memory: An examination of simple and complex span and their relation to higher order abilities. *Psychological Bulletin, 133*, 1038–1066.

Wai, J., Lubinski, D., & Benbow, C. P. (2009). Spatial ability for STEM domains: Aligning over fifty years of cumulative psychological knowledge solidifies its importance. *Journal of Educational Psychology, 101*, 817–835.

Wasserman, J. D., & Tulsky, D. S. (2005). A history of intelligence assessment. In D. P. Flanagan & P. L. Harrison (Eds.), *Contemporary intellectual assessment* (2nd ed., pp. 3–22). New York: Guilford Press.

Wolbers, T., & Hegarty, M. (2010). What determines our navigational abilities? *Trends in Cognitive Sciences, 14*, 138–146.

Woodcock, R. W. (1978). *Development and standardization of the Woodcock–Johnson Psycho-Educational Battery.* Hingham, MA: Teaching Resources.

Woodcock, R. W. (1990). Theoretical foundations of the WJ-R measures of cognitive ability. *Journal of Psychoeducational Assessment, 8*, 231–258.

Woodcock, R. W. (1993). An information processing view of the Gf-Gc theory. In *Journal of Psychoeducational Assessment Monograph Series: Woodcock–Johnson Psycho-Educational Assessment Battery—Revised* (pp. 80–102). Cordova, TN: Psychoeducational Corporation.

Woodcock, R. W., & Johnson, M. B. (1977). *Woodcock–Johnson Psycho-Educational Battery.* Hingham, MA: Teaching Resources.

Woodcock, R. W., & Johnson, M. B. (1989). *Woodcock–Johnson Psycho-Educational Battery—Revised.* Chicago: Riverside.

CHAPTER 5

Assessment of Intellectual Profile
A Perspective from Multiple-Intelligences Theory

Jie-Qi Chen
Howard Gardner

The theory of multiple intelligences (MI) was born in 1983 as the first edition of *Frames of Mind* by Howard Gardner of Harvard University appeared on our bookshelves. Nearly three decades have passed since its inception. The theory has touched numerous subfields of psychology and education, including counseling psychology, developmental therapy, gifted education, programs for at-risk children, museums, theme parks, and mass media, to name a few. As the book has been translated into more than 20 languages, the idea has traveled from one continent to another and one culture from another. MI-inspired educational practices have made noticeable impacts in many countries and regions around the world (Chen, Moran, & Gardner, 2009).

A central issue in MI-inspired educational practice is assessment. With MI's focus on individual differences, educators need tools to help detect these differences. It is unlikely that educators will be able to deliver effective personalized instruction without the knowledge of diverse ways of learning in individual students. Also, tradition dies hard. Our conception of intelligence as IQ is assessed by a variety of standardized tests. "If IQ can be measured, why can't MI be measured?" one might ask.

There is no lack of so-called "MI assessments" on the market. Most of them are designed to ascertain cognitive abilities and describe the intellectual profiles of individuals. The quality of the

instruments and the approaches to assessment vary enormously, ranging from self-reporting to observation checklists and performance-based instruments (Shearer, 2009). This chapter addresses the questions of what to assess and how to assess individual intellectual profiles from an MI-based perspective. We begin the chapter with an overview of MI theory. Moving from theory to practice, we identify several features of the MI approach to assessment of intellectual profiles. We then introduce several instruments that incorporate MI assessment features. Empirical studies based on these instruments are reported as well. Although the principles of MI assessment obtain across the age range, in this chapter we focus primarily on assessment during childhood. The chapter concludes with a discussion of the renewed significance of MI-based assessment in light of the accountability-driven movement in contemporary education.

AN OVERVIEW OF MI THEORY

A significant departure from the traditional view of intelligence as IQ, MI theory (Gardner, 1993a, 1999, 2006, 2011) presents at least three ideas that are revolutionary to our conceptualization of intelligence: definition of *intelligence*, methodology used to study intelligence, and identified intelligences. Growing from this revolutionary view of intelligences are the development and use of MI-based assessment for educational purposes.

Definition of Intelligence

Gardner (1999) defines *intelligence* as "a biopsychological potential to process information that can be activated in a cultural setting to solve problems or create products that are of value in a culture" (p. 33). By considering intelligence a potential, Gardner asserts its emergent and responsive nature, thereby differentiating his theory from traditional ones that view human intelligence as fixed and innate. Whether a potential can be activated depends on the values of the culture in which an individual grows up; the opportunities available in that culture; and personal choices made by individuals, their families, and others in their lives. These activating forces shape the development and expression of a range of intelligences from culture to culture and from individual to individual.

Gardner's definition of intelligence also differs from other formulations in that it considers the creation of products, such as musical scores, sculptures, or computer programs, to be as important an expression of intelligence as abstract problem solving. Traditional theories do not recognize created artifacts as manifestations of intelligence and therefore are limited in both conceptualization and measurement.

Methodology Used to Study Intelligence

In the process of developing MI theory, Gardner considered the range of adult end states that are valued in diverse cultures around the world. To identify the abilities that support these end states, he examined empirical data from disciplines that had not been considered previously for the purpose of defining human intelligence. His examination of these datasets yielded eight criteria for identifying an intelligence. The criteria took into consideration brain function, evolutionary history, special human populations, end-state adult performances, skill training, correlation of intelligence test results, development of symbol system, and core operations of intelligence (Gardner, 1993a). Of principal importance to Gardner in developing the criteria was capturing the range of purposes and processes entailed in human cognitive functioning.

The methodology Gardner used to develop MI theory represents a major departure from the psychological testing approach that has been used to study intelligence, and therefore has drawn great attention as well as strong criticism from the field of psychology (Gardner & Moran, 2006; Schaler, 2006; Waterhouse, 2006). Echoing Vygotsky (1978, p. 58), we argue that "any fundamentally new approach to a scientific problem inevitably leads to new methods of investigation and analysis. The invention of new methods that are adequate to the new ways in which problems are posed requires far more than a simple modification of previously accepted methods." As radically different as MI theory is, a departure from traditional means of studying intelligence is not an option but a necessity. The distinctive method Gardner used in studying intelligence is inseparable from his groundbreaking view of human intelligence.

Identified Intelligences

Gardner (1993a, 2006, 2011) has argued that standardized intelligence tests typically probe a limited number of intelligences, such as linguistic, logical–mathematical, and certain forms of spatial intelligences. MI theory has added five more candidates to the list: musical, bodily–kinesthetic, naturalistic, interpersonal, and intrapersonal intelligences. According to Gardner, all human beings possess all of the intelligences, but differ in relative strengths and weaknesses—an important source of individual differences.

The eight identified intelligences, according to Gardner, cannot be viewed merely as a group of raw computational capacities. They are subject to encoding in varied symbol systems created by various cultures. It is through symbol systems that intelligences are applied in specific domains or bodies of knowledge within a culture, such as mathematics, art, basketball, and medicine (Gardner, 1993a, 1999). As well, the world is wrapped in meanings. Intelligences can be implemented only to the extent that they partake of these meanings and enable individuals to develop into functioning, symbol-using members of their community. An individual's intelligences, to a great extent, are shaped by cultural influences and refined by educational processes. It is through the process of education that "raw" intellectual competencies are developed and individuals are prepared to assume mature cultural roles. Rich educational experiences are essential for the development of each individual's particular configuration of interests and abilities (Gardner, 1993b, 2006).

MI APPROACH TO ASSESSMENT OF INTELLECTUAL PROFILES

Assessment based on MI theory calls for a significant departure from traditional approaches to assessment. From the start, a distinctive hallmark of MI theory has been its spurning of one-shot, decontextualized, paper-and-pencil tests to rank individuals' "smartness" based on a single score (Gardner, 1993b, 2006). MI theory presents several basic principles for the assessment of intellectual profiles: (1) sampling intellectual capacities in a gamut of domains; (2) using media appropriate to each assessed domain; (3) choosing assessment materials that are meaningful to students; (4) attending to the ecological validity of assessment contexts; and (5) portraying complete intellectual profiles to support learning and teaching (Chen, 2004; Krechevsky, 1998) (see Table 5.1).

TABLE 5.1. MI Principles for the Assessment of Intellectual Profiles

- *Sample intellectual capacities in a range of domains* that include both traditionally defined academic areas such as reading, literacy, math, and science, as well as nonacademic areas such as visual arts, performing arts, movement, and understanding of others and self.

- *Use media appropriate to each domain of assessment* to engage in an intelligence-fair assessment process by looking at the problem-solving features and operational mechanisms of particular intelligences; such a process allows one to look directly at the functioning of each intellectual capacity.

- *Choose assessment materials that are meaningful to students* by supporting thinking, inviting questions, stimulating curiosity, facilitating discovery, and encouraging the use of imagination and multiple symbol systems in the students' problem-solving processes.

- *Attend to the ecological validity of assessment contexts* to ensure that the assessment environments are natural, familiar, and ongoing; use multiple samples of a child's performance; and incorporate clinical judgments from those who are knowledgeable about the child being assessed and directly responsible for using the results.

- *Portray complete intellectual profiles* that focus on students' strengths and include concrete, practical suggestions to help educators understand each child as completely as possible, and then mobilize the child's intelligences to achieve specific educational goals.

Sampling Intellectual Capacities in a Gamut of Domains

Because the fundamental principle of MI is that human intelligence is pluralistic, assessment based on MI theory incorporates a range of domains to tap different facets of each intellectual capacity. In addition to language, literacy, and mathematics—the primary foci of traditional intelligence tests and school achievement tests—MI-based assessment also looks at children's performance in areas often called nonacademic, such as music, arts, movement, and understanding of both self and others. The MI approach to assessment recognizes students who excel in linguistic and/or logical pursuits, as well as those who have cognitive and personal strengths in other intelligences. By virtue of the wider range they measure, MI types of assessment identify more students who are "smart," albeit in different ways (Gardner, 1993b, 2000).

It has been well documented that students who have trouble with some academic subjects, such as reading or math, are not necessarily inadequate in all areas (Chen, Krechevsky, & Viens, 1998; Diaz-Lefebvre, 2009; Levin, 2005). The challenge is to provide comparable opportunities for these students to demonstrate their strengths and interests. When students recognize that they are good at something, and their accomplishment is acknowledged by teachers, parents, and peers, they are far more likely to feel valued in the classroom and to experience further school success. In some instances, the sense of success in one area may make students more likely to engage in areas where they feel less comfortable. When that occurs, the systematic use of multiple measures goes beyond its initial purpose of identifying diverse cognitive abilities and becomes a means of bridging students' strengths from one area to other areas of learning (Chen et al., 1998; Dweck, 2007; Gardner, 1998).

Using Media Appropriate to Each Domain Being Assessed

On the basis of its contention that each intelligence exhibits particular problem-solving features and operational mechanisms, MI theory argues for *intelligence-fair* instruments to assess the unique capacities of each intelligence. Too often, language is the gatekeeper, forcing individuals to reveal their intelligence through the customary lens of linguistic ability; or logical analysis serves as a route to, or an obstacle thwarting, the measurement of non-scholastic abilities. In contrast, intelligence-fair instruments engage the key abilities of particular intelligences, allowing one to look directly at the functioning of each intellectual capacity.

When intelligence-fair instruments are used, bodily intelligence can be assessed by recording how a person learns a new dance or physical exercise. To consider a person's interpersonal intelligence, it is necessary to observe how he or she interacts with and influences others in different social situations. One situation might be the individual's interacting with a friend to offer extra support when the friend loses an art contest. Another relevant situation is observing an individual giving advice to a friend who is the target of a rumor. It is important to note that what is assessed is never an intelligence in pure form. Intelligences are always expressed in the context of specific tasks, domains, and disciplines. For example, there is no "pure" spatial intelligence; instead, there is spatial intelligence as expressed in a child's puzzle solution, route finding, block building, or basketball passing (Gardner, 1993b).

Choosing Assessment Materials Meaningful to Students

Materials are important in assessment because intelligence is manifested through a wide variety of artifacts. To be meaningful, the assessment materials first need to be familiar to children. Assessment based on MI theory is responsive to the fact that students' prior experience with assessment materials directly affects their performance on tasks. For example, children who have little experience with blocks are less likely to do well on a block design task. Likewise, it would be unfair to assess a child's musical ability by asking the child to play a music instrument that he or she has never experienced. In recognition of the role that experience plays, the MI approach to assessment emphasizes using materials that are familiar to children. If children are not familiar with materials, they are given ample opportunities to explore materials prior to any formal assessment.

The term *meaningful* also signifies the role of assessment materials in supporting a student's problem-solving process. To be fair, materials used in many current intelligence tests, such as pictures, geometric shapes, and blocks, are not unfamiliar to children in industrial societies. Yet such materials provide little intrinsic attraction because they have little meaning in children's daily lives. For assessment to be meaningful for students, the selection of materials must be a careful and deliberate process. Materials ought to be an integral part of students' problem solving processes, supporting thinking, inviting questions, and stimulating curiosity. Meaningful materials also facilitate students' discovery and encourage the use of imagination and multiple symbol systems (Rinaldi, 2001).

Attending to the Ecological Validity of Assessment Contexts

In the traditional intelligence assessment situation, a psychologist works with one child at a time, preferably in a relatively quiet room away from any distractions, including regular classroom activities. MI theory emphasizes the ecological validity of assessment contexts (Gardner, 1993b); that is, the assessment environments must be natural, familiar, and ongoing. When a child's ability is measured through a one-shot test using decontextualized tasks, the child's profile of abilities is often incomplete and may be distorted. In contrast, when assessment is naturally embedded in learning environments, it allows psychologists and educators to observe children's abilities in various situations over time. Such observations generate multiple samples of a child's ability that can be used to document variations of the child's performances within and across domains, and so to portray the child's intellectual profile more accurately.

Integrating authentic activities and observations over time, assessment based on MI theory does not typically function as a norm-referenced instrument does. Intelligence in the MI framework is defined as a potential, exhibiting various possible forms and subject to continuous changes in expression and strength. MI-based assessment involves performance standards or criterion references that educators can use to guide and evaluate their observations. In contrast to norm-referenced tests, which feature decontextualized and seemingly impartial judgments of students' performance, MI-based assessment is open to incorporating the clinical judgments of classroom teachers. In so doing, MI-based assessment places greater value on the experience and expertise of educators who are knowledgeable about the child being assessed and directly responsible for using the assessment results (Darling-Hammond & Ancess, 1996; Darling-Hammond & Snyder, 1992; Linn, 2000; Meisels, Bickel, Nicholson, Xue, & Atkins-Burnett, 2001; Moss, 1994).

Portraying Complete Intellectual Profiles to Support Learning and Teaching

Traditional tests—of achievement, readiness, intelligence, and the like—are often used to rank order and sort students on the basis of a single quantitative score. Seemingly objective scores on these standardized tests disguise the complex nature of human intelligence. In the process, the scores also limit a child's range of learning potentials and may narrow opportunities for success in school. Instead of ranking and labeling, the purpose of MI types of assessment is to support students on the basis of their complete intellectual profile. Such an intellectual profile portrays a child's strengths, interests, and weaknesses. It also includes concrete, practical suggestions to the student, such as how to build on the identified strengths, work on areas that need attention or intervention, and develop approaches to learning that are conducive to productive work (Kornhaber, Krechevsky, & Gardner, 1990; Krechevsky, 1998).

It is important to note that the identification of intellectual strengths and weaknesses of individuals is not the endpoint of MI types of assessment. The purpose of portraying a complete intellectual profile is to help educators understand each child as completely as possible and then mobilize his or her intelligences to achieve specific educational goals. MI-based assessments promote achievement of these goals by assisting educators in selecting appropriate instructional strategies and pedagogical approaches, based on a comprehensive and in-depth understanding of each child.

TOOLS USED FOR THE ASSESSMENT OF INTELLECTUAL PROFILES

Since MI theory was introduced, educators around the world have looked for an assessment that could be used to better understand students' intellectual profiles and inform instructional practice. The most widely used MI-based assessments include performance-based instruments, such as the Spectrum battery (Krechevsky, 1998), the Bridging assessment (Chen & McNamee, 2007), and Discovering Intellectual Strengths and Capabilities while Observing Varied Ethnic Responses (DISCOVER; Maker, 2005). In another MI-based approach to assessment, the New City School (1994) and the Key Learning Community (*www.616.ips.k12.in.us*)

use student portfolios and observational checklists to capture the full range and diversity of a child's intellectual profile. Lazear (1998, 1999) uses MI-based rubrics. With the Multiple Intelligences Developmental Assessment Scales (MIDAS; Shearer, 2007), survey data are collected and supplemented with interviews. Niccolini, Alessandri, and Bilancioni (2010) have developed the Web-Observation, an online assessment instrument based on an MI framework for educators. Below we briefly describe some of these instruments, focusing on those that have been studied empirically.

The Spectrum Battery

The Spectrum battery, designed by the staff of Project Spectrum at the Harvard Graduate School of Education, is the only MI-based assessment instrument developed with Gardner's direct involvement. Designed for preschool children, the Spectrum battery is composed of 15 activities in seven domains of knowledge: language, math, music, art, social understanding, sciences, and movement (for detailed descriptions of the instrument, see Chen, 2004; Krechevsky, 1998). The Spectrum name reflects its mission of recognizing diverse intellectual strengths in children.

During the assessment process, an assessor or a teacher works with children either individually or in small groups. Children engage in a range of activities, such as disassembling and assembling several house gadgets in the science domain; playing Montessori bells in the music domain; keeping track of passengers getting on and off a toy bus in the mathematics domain; and manipulating figures in a scaled-down, three-dimensional replica of the children's classroom to assess social understanding. Fun and challenging, these activities invite children to engage in problem-solving tasks. They are intelligence-fair, using materials appropriate to particular domains rather than relying only on language to assess multiple forms of competence and ability. They help to tap key abilities—abilities that are essential to the operation of particular intellectual domains in children's task performance. Each activity is accompanied by written instructions for task administration. These instructions include a score sheet that identifies and describes different levels of the key abilities assessed in the activity, making a child's performance on many activities quantifiable. Finally, upon completion of each assessment activity, the child's working style during the task is recorded. *Working style* refers to the way in which a child interacts with the materials of a domain, such as degree of engagement, confidence, or attention to detail (Chen, 2004; Krechevsky, 1998).

Spectrum assessment results are presented in the form of a Profile—a narrative report based on the information obtained from the assessment process (Chen & Gardner, 2005; Krechevsky, 1998). Using nontechnical language, the report focuses on the range of cognitive abilities examined by the Spectrum battery. It describes each child's relative strengths and weaknesses in terms of that child's own capacities, and only occasionally in relation to peers. Strengths and weaknesses are described in terms of the child's performance in different content areas. For example, a child's unusual sensitivity to different kinds of music may be described in terms of facial expressions, movement, and attentiveness during and after listening to various music pieces. It is important to note that the child's intellectual profile is described not only in terms of capacities, but also in terms of the child's preferences and inclinations. Furthermore, the Profile is not a static image, but a dynamic composition that reflects a child's interests, capabilities, and experiences at a particular point in time. Changes in it are inevitable as the child's life experience changes. The conclusion of the Profile typically includes specific recommendations to parents and teachers about ways to support identified strengths and improve weak areas (Krechevsky, 1998).

Empirical studies using the Project Spectrum materials have been revealing. In one study, Adams (1993) assessed 42 preschool children with a modified Spectrum battery and found that each individual's pattern of performance was highly likely to be distinct when a diverse set of abilities was measured. In another study, the staff of Project Spectrum worked with four first-grade classrooms in two local public schools (Chen & Gardner, 2005). The majority of students in these classrooms who had been identified as at risk for school failure (13 out of 15) demonstrated identifiable strengths on the Spectrum assessment. Also noteworthy, these students showed more strengths in nonacademic areas (such as mechanical, movement, and visual arts) than in academic areas (such as language and math). Had the assessment been limited to academic areas, these at-risk children's strengths would have gone undetected and could not have served as bridges for extending the children's interest and learning to other curricular areas. Most recently, Castejon, Perez, and Gilar

(2010) studied 393 children 4–7 years of age in two cities in Spain, using six Spectrum activities. They tested four models of the structure of intelligence, including a model with six uncorrelated factors and a model with one general cognitive factor or *g* factor. The results did not favor any one particular model or theory. On the one hand, results indicated that individual Spectrum tasks do tap into abilities other than *g*; on the other hand, they "are not so separate from general abilities as proposed by the original authors" (Castejon, Perez, & Gilar, 2010, p. 494).

Bridging

Bridging was developed by Chen and McNamee (2007) to help teachers portray intellectual profiles of children between the ages of 3 and 8. It shares certain features with the Spectrum assessment, including the identification of children's diverse cognitive strengths, the use of engaging activities, and a focus on guided observation and careful documentation. It differs from the Spectrum assessment by focusing on the operation of intellectual abilities in school curricular areas, such as language and literacy, number sense and geometry, physical, mechanical and natural sciences, performing arts, and visual arts. Bridging is organized in terms of school subject areas rather than intellectual domains, for several reasons: (1) Intelligences never function in abstract form, but rather are used in the context of specific disciplinary tasks; (2) school subject areas reflect intellectual abilities valued in our society; (3) children mobilize their intelligences in the pursuit of studying subject areas; and (4) aligning assessment areas with school subject areas facilitates teachers' incorporation of the assessment results into curriculum planning. The name of the instrument, Bridging, signifies its goal of building a bridge from assessment to teaching (Chen & McNamee, 2008).

Bridging includes a total of 15 regular classroom activities, such as reading a child's favorite book, constructing a model car with recycle materials, and experimenting with light and shadows (for a detailed description of Bridging, see Chen & McNamee, 2007). Children's performance in each of the 15 activities is scored according to a 10-level, criterion-referenced rubric developed specifically for 3- to 8-year-olds. As an example, the rubric used to measure performance on the "reading books" activity was based on the stages of pretend reading developed by Sulzby (1985) and work in guided reading by Fountas and Pinnell (1996). The rubric progresses from attending to pictures without forming stories at level 1 to reading for meaning independently at level 10 (Chen & McNamee, 2007).

In addition to children's performances, their approaches to learning in each activity are also measured. *Approaches to learning* are observable behaviors that describe ways children engage in classroom interactions and learning activities (Fantuzzo et al., 2007). Bridging includes five approaches to learning: initial engagement, focus, planfulness, goal orientation, and resourcefulness. Each approach is scored numerically on a scale from 1 to 5, with behavioral descriptors differentiating scores at levels 1, 3, and 5 (Chen & McNamee, 2011). Bridging assessment results for each child are depicted in a graphic chart. The chart illustrates the unique profile of the child's varied performance levels across a range of school subject areas and specifies the approaches to learning the child used during each activity. Teachers and parents can further look at the Bridging manual for a variety of curricular ideas based on their children's current levels of content skills and understanding.

Empirical data support the Bridging approach— both its conceptualization of children's abilities and the effective design of its assessment activities. In one study using Bridging, Chen, McNamee, and McCray (2011) examined the intellectual profiles of 92 preschool and kindergarten children. Results indicated that *within a child's profile*, levels of competence varied as a function of content area. A child's competence level was higher in some areas and lower in others. *Among children's profiles*, the patterns of their performance levels were distinctive. That is, the pattern in each child's profile differed from the pattern found in other children's profiles. Children's competence is thus domain-specific; so are their approaches to learning, as indicated in another study by Chen and McNamee (2011). Sixty-one children from preschool to second grade participated in the study. The results showed that children's approaches to learning varied as they participated in different activities in different content areas. Like intelligences, therefore, approaches to learning are not static traits located within an individual child, but a profile of tendencies describing the interaction of child, materials, and tasks.

In terms of Bridging's utility, over 400 preservice and inservice teachers from preschool through third grade have integrated it in their classrooms under the direct supervision of the instrument developers. An implementation study of 75 preservice teachers revealed that the construction of intellectual profiles for individual students using the Bridging assessment process was a key component in student teachers' understanding of diverse learners in their classrooms (Chen & McNamee, 2006). In another study, McNamee and Chen (2005) reported that teachers' understanding of individual students and content knowledge increased as the result of implementing Bridging in their classrooms. This increased understanding contributed to their ability to be more effective in curriculum planning and teaching.

The MIDAS and DISCOVER Assessments

Among the many MI-inspired assessments that others have designed independently, we describe two: the MIDAS and DISCOVER. Empirical data are reported for both instruments and both involve diverse populations. The MIDAS is designed to portray the profile of an individual's intellectual dispositions, based primarily on responses to a set of survey questions (Shearer, 2007; *www.MIResearch.org*). The MIDAS has four forms: Adult (19+), Teen (ages 15–18), All About Me (ages 9–14), and My Young Child (ages 4–8, parent report). The MIDAS profile consists of eight main scales and 26 subscales that describe the respondent's specific skills, capacities, and enthusiasms in each of the eight intellectual domains defined by Gardner (1993a). Responding to the criticism that the MIDAS results are questionable because they rely primarily on self-report, Shearer (2007) argues that one of the hallmarks of the MIDAS is attention to the intrapersonal intelligence reflected in the self-report process and profile interpretation. For the MIDAS, intrapersonal intelligence is the "royal road to learning, achievement, and personal growth" (Shearer, 2007).

The MIDAS has been translated into numerous foreign languages for use in countries such as Korea, Malaysia, Taiwan, Iran, Singapore, Ireland, and Chile. It has also been tested for its psychometric properties in the United States as well as internationally, including test–retest reliability, interrater reliability, concurrent validity, and level of independence among scales (Shearer, 2007). In an analysis of 23,000 individuals who completed the MIDAS profile, for example, Shearer (2005) found nine factors corresponding with the MIDAS main scale. He thus concluded that the MIDAS provides a reasonable estimate of the respondents' multiple intellectual dispositions.

The MIDAS has been used with diverse populations, including elementary, secondary, and university students, students with attention-deficit/hyperactivity disorder (ADHD) and learning disabilities; and adults seeking career help. In studies of 116 elementary children diagnosed with ADHD, for example, Shearer and colleagues found that, compared to typically developing peers, these students scored lower on the math, linguistic, and intrapersonal scales of the MIDAS, but higher on the naturalist, spatial and kinesthetic scales (Proulx-Schirduan, Shearer, & Case, 2009). The MIDAS profile provided a unique description of the students with ADHD, whose interests and strengths included artistic design, craft work, and recognizing different kinds of plants.

Another observation-based assessment in the spirit of MI theory is DISCOVER (Maker, 2005; *www.discover.arizona.edu*). Designed for the identification of gifted and talented students, the DISCOVER assessment focuses on a broad spectrum of problem-solving strategies in seven intellectual domains: spatial artistic, spatial analytical, logical mathematical, oral linguistic, written linguistic, interpersonal, and intrapersonal. During the DISCOVER assessment process, students participate in a series of active problem-solving exercises, using playful, age-appropriate materials. While students engage in a problem-solving process, trained and certified individuals observe, document, and rate the students' behavior, focusing on the problem-solving strategies they are using. The information is later compiled to produce "strength profiles" that summarize and interpret the assessment results. The DISCOVER assessment includes a total of seven different forms designed to accommodate age groups from preschoolers to adults.

The DISCOVER assessment has been used by a network of international partners from China, France, Hong Kong, Taiwan, Thailand, Saudi Arabia, and Egypt. Educators in these locations are eager to adapt the effective problem-solving strategies identified by DISCOVER to fit local contexts in their regions. Maker's work with Native American groups in the United States is particularly revealing. In a number of studies, Maker and her colleagues (Maker & Sarouphim, 2009; Sarouphim, 2004) found that children from these indigenous cultures are particularly apt at spatial

tasks, artistic abilities, and observational skills. Such strengths, however, are largely overlooked in the traditional assessment of gifted and talented students. With the DISCOVER assessment, more forms of giftedness can be identified, valued, and promoted.

RENEWED SIGNIFICANCE OF THE MI APPROACH TO ASSESSMENT

The testing of intelligence can be dated back to the beginning of the 20th century. Over a century later, many psychologists still adhere to the view of intelligence as a single, general faculty that can be accurately measured through norm-referenced, standardized intelligence tests. This view permeates our practice of education, including how we assess children and evaluate schools. As indicated before, the inappropriateness and danger of using one-shot, standardized tests to assess children's learning and achievement are considerable. Such tests sample only a small portion of children's intellectual abilities, typically their achievement in math and reading. Because a standard intelligence test ignores the wide range of abilities needed by society, it does little to help us recognize and nurture individuals' potentials. Furthermore, these tests categorize children on the basis of a single score. Children can be identified as "gifted" or deemed "at risk for school failure." Both labels can be assigned at a very early age, affecting the remainder of a child's school career and beyond. The possibility that an at-risk child has strengths in other areas is not considered relevant.

The belief in general intelligence drives not only the educational practice of standardized achievement testing, but also the more recent initiatives in school accountability. Students' mean scores on standardized tests are now used to rate schools. Some schools become exemplars; many more fall along a straight line between adequate performance and probationary status; some schools suffer penalties. Using standardized test scores to rate schools is problematic for the same reasons that using them is inappropriate for students. A mean score is a single number. It does not capture the full range of what a school achieves in a year. The successes that a school has can be hidden or obscured. As with individual students, mean test scores are practical for rank ordering, but they do little to help identify the strengths of a school. The success of an individual program in the school and the excellence of individual teachers are overshadowed by a low mean test score. As a final argument against this means of evaluating schools, there is little evidence that accountability systems focused on standardized test scores actually lead to higher student achievement in the long run (Baker et al., 2010).

The view of general intelligence as the basis for education has created a growing snowball of undesirable effects. Schools and children, particularly children from low-income and minority backgrounds, are losing traction. At every level in the school system, strengths are overlooked, and progress is too narrowly defined. With education constrained by limited vision and "teaching to the test," MI theory has a renewed significance. It calls our attention one more time to diversity, individuality, and multiple potentials for growth. It provides the foundation for moving beyond the view of general intelligence. It points the way to innovative forms of assessment that will integrate assessment, curriculum, and instruction.

According to MI theory, the primary purpose of conducting an assessment is to gather information for designing appropriate educational experiences and interventions. To serve this purpose, an assessment must sample more than a few narrow academic areas. All children are likely to have strengths in some areas and weaknesses in others when a range of areas is considered. Focusing on children's strengths is a pathway proven to be effective for fostering positive attitudes and engagement in learning (Chen et al., 1998). Looking at a range of intellectual domains makes it possible to construct profiles of individual capabilities, upending the tendency to describe differences among individuals in terms of a single score.

To assess a child's distinctive intellectual abilities is not to create another means of labeling the child. Rather, the ultimate goal of an MI approach to assessment is to help create environments that foster the development of individual as well as group potential and suggest alternative routes to the achievement of important educational goals (Gardner, 1993c). Clearly, this approach will require continued efforts to develop appropriate instruments and introduce them in school systems. We believe these efforts will help ensure that educators work not only to "leave no child behind," but also to inspire all children to move forward, developing their strengths and achieving their highest potential.

REFERENCES

Adams, M. (1993). *An empirical investigation of domain-specific theories of preschool children's cognitive abilities.* Unpublished doctoral dissertation, Tufts University.

Baker, E., Barton, P. E., Darling-Hammond, L., Haertel, E., Ladd, H. F., Linn, R. L., et al. (2010). *Problems with the use of student test scores to evaluate teachers.* Washington, DC: Economic Policy Institute. Retrieved from *epi.3cdn.net/724cd9a1eb91c40ff0_hwm6iij90.pdf*

Castejon, J. L., Perez, A. M., & Gilar, R. (2010). Confirmatory factor analysis of Project Spectrum activities: A second-order g factor or multiple intelligences? *Intelligence, 38,* 481–496.

Chen, J.-Q. (2004). The Project Spectrum approach to early education. In J. Johnson & J. Roopnarine (Eds.), *Approaches to early childhood education* (4th ed., pp. 251–179). Upper Saddle River, NJ: Pearson.

Chen, J.-Q., & Gardner, H. (2005). Assessment based on multiple-intelligences theory. In D. P. Flanagan & P. L. Harrison (Eds.), *Contemporary intellectual assessment* (2nd ed., pp. 77–102). New York: Guilford Press.

Chen, J.-Q., Krechevsky, M., & Viens, J. (1998). *Building on children's strengths: The experience of Project Spectrum.* New York: Teachers College Press.

Chen, J.-Q., & McNamee, G. (2006). Strengthening early childhood teacher preparation: Integrating assessment, curriculum development, and instructional practice in student teaching. *Journal of Early Childhood Teacher Education, 27,* 109–128.

Chen, J.-Q., & McNamee, G. (2007). *Bridging: Assessment for teaching and learning in early childhood classrooms.* Thousand Oaks, CA: Corwin Press.

Chen, J.-Q., & McNamee, G. (2008). From Spectrum to Bridging: Approaches to integrating assessment with curriculum and instruction in early childhood classrooms. In J. Johnson & J. Roopnarine (Eds.), *Approaches to early childhood education* (5th ed., pp. 251–279). Upper Saddle River, NJ: Pearson.

Chen, J.-Q., & McNamee, G. (2011). Positive approaches to learning in the context of preschool classroom activities. *Early Childhood Education Journal, 39*(1), 71–78.

Chen, J.-Q., McNamee, G., & McCray, J. (2011). The learning profile: A construct to understand learning and development of the whole child in content areas. *International Early Learning Journal, 1*(1), 1–24.

Chen, J.-Q., Moran, S., & Gardner, H. (Eds.). (2009). *Multiple intelligences around the world.* San Francisco: Jossey-Bass.

Darling-Hammond, L., & Ancess, L. (1996). Authentic

assessment and school development. In J. B. Baron & D. P. Wolf (Eds.), *Performance-based student assessment: Challenges and possibilities (95th yearbook of the National Society for the Study of Education)* (pp. 52–83). Chicago: University of Chicago Press.

Darling-Hammond, L., & Snyder, J. (1992). Reframing accountability: Creating learner-centered schools. In A. Lieberman (Ed.), *The changing contents of teaching (91st yearbook of the National Society for the Study of Education)* (pp. 11–36). Chicago: University of Chicago Press.

Diaz-Lefebvre, R. (2009). What if they learn differently? In J.-Q. Chen, S. Moran, & H. Gardner (Eds.), *Multiple intelligences around the world* (pp. 317–328). San Francisco: Jossey-Bass.

Dweck, C. (2007). *Mindset: The new psychology of success.* New York: Ballantine.

Fantuzzo, J. W., Bulotsky-Shearer, R., McDermott, P., McWayne, C., Frye, D., & Perlman, S. (2007). Investigation of dimensions of social-emotional classroom behavior and school readiness for low-income urban preschool children. *School Psychology Review, 36*(1), 44–62.

Fountas, I. C., & Pinnell, G. S. (1996). *Guided reading: Good first teaching for all children.* Portsmouth, NH: Heinemann.

Gardner, H. (1983). *Frames of mind: The theory of multiple intelligences.* New York: Basic Books.

Gardner, H. (1993a). *Frames of mind: The theory of multiple intelligences* (10th-anniversary ed.). New York: Basic Books.

Gardner, H. (1993b). *Multiple intelligences: The theory in practice.* New York: Basic Books.

Gardner, H. (1998). The bridges of Spectrum. In J.-Q. Chen, M. Krechevsky, & J. Viens (Eds.), *Building on children's strengths: The experience of Project Spectrum* (pp. 138–145). New York: Teachers College Press.

Gardner, H. (1999). *The disciplined mind.* New York: Simon & Schuster.

Gardner, H. (2000). *The disciplined mind: Beyond facts and standardized tests, the K–12 education that every child deserves.* New York: Penguin Books.

Gardner, H. (2006). *Multiple intelligences: New horizons.* New York: Basic Books.

Gardner, H. (2011). *Frames of mind: The theory of multiple intelligences* (30th-year ed.). New York: Basic Books.

Gardner, H., & Moran, S. (2006). The science of multiple intelligences theory: A response to Lynn Waterhouse. *Educational Psychologist, 41*(4), 227–232.

Kornhaber, M., Krechevsky, M., & Gardner, H. (1990). Engaging intelligence. *Educational Psychologist, 25*(3–4), 177–199.

Krechevsky, M. (1998). *Project Spectrum preschool assessment handbook.* New York: Teachers College Press.

Lazear, D. (1998). *The rubrics way: Using MI to assess understanding.* Tucson, AZ: Zephyr Press.

Lazear, D. (1999). *Multiple intelligence approaches to assessment: Solving the assessment conundrum.* Tucson, AZ: Zephyr Press.

Levin, H. M. (2005). *Accelerated schools: A decade of evolution.* New York: Springer.

Linn, R. (2000). Assessments and accountability. *Educational Researcher, 29*(2), 4–15.

Maker, C. J. (2005). *The DISCOVER Project: Improving assessment and curriculum for diverse gifted learners.* Storrs, CT: National Research Center on the Gifted and Talented.

Maker, C. J., & Sarouphim, K. M. (2009). Problem solving and the DISCOVER Project: Lessons from the Dine (Navajo) people. In J.-Q. Chen, S. Moran, & H. Gardner (Eds.), *Multiple intelligences around the world* (pp. 329–341). San Francisco: Jossey-Bass.

McNamee, G., & Chen, J.-Q. (2005). Dissolving the line between assessment and teaching. *Educational Leadership, 63*(3), 72–77.

Meisels, S. J., Bickel, D. D., Nicholson, J., Xue, Y. G., & Atkins-Burnett, S. (2001). Trusting teachers' judgments: A validity study of a curriculum-embedded performance assessment in kindergarten to grade 3. *American Educational Research Journal, 38*(1), 73–95.

Moss, P. (1994). Can there be validity without reliability? *Educational Researcher, 3*, 5–12.

New City School. (1994). *Multiple intelligences: Teaching for success.* St. Louis, MO: Author.

Niccolini, P., Alessandri, G., & Bilancioni, G. (2010). Web-Ob for multiple intelligences observation. *Procedia Social and Behavioral Sciences, 2*, 728–732.

Proulx-Schirduan, V., Shearer, C. B., & Case, K. I. (2009). *Mindful education for ADHD students: Differentiating curriculum and instruction using multiple intelligences.* New York: Teachers College Press.

Rinaldi, C. (2001). Introduction. In Project Zero & Reggio Children, *Making learning visible: Children as individual and group learners* (pp. 28–31). Reggio Emilia, Italy: Reggio Children.

Sarouphim, K. M. (2004). DISCOVER in middle school: Identifying gifted minority students. *Journal of Secondary Gifted Education, 10*, 61–69.

Schaler, J. (2006). *Howard Gardner under fire.* LaSalle, IL: Open Court.

Shearer, C. B. (2005). *Large scale factor analysis of the Multiple Intelligences Developmental Assessment Scales.* Paper presented at the annual meeting of the American Educational Research Association, Montreal, Canada.

Shearer, C. B. (2007). *The MIDAS: Professional manual* (rev. ed.). Kent, OH: MI Research and Consulting.

Shearer, C. B. (2009). The challenges of assessing the multiple intelligences around the world. In J.-Q. Chen, S. Moran, & H. Gardner (Eds.), *Multiple intelligences around the world* (pp. 353–362). San Francisco: Jossey-Bass.

Sulzby, E. (1985, Summer). Children's emergent reading of favorite storybooks: A developmental study. *Reading Research Quarterly, 20*(4), 458–481.

Vygotsky, L. S. (1978). *Mind in society: The development of higher psychological processes* (M. Cole, V. John-Steiner, S. Scribner, & E. Souberman, Trans.). Cambridge, MA: Harvard University Press.

Waterhouse, L. (2006). Multiple intelligences, the Mozart effect, and emotional intelligence: A critical review. *Educational Psychologist, 41*(4), 207–225.

CHAPTER 6

The Triarchic Theory of Successful Intelligence

Robert J. Sternberg

Some people seem to do what they do better than others, and so various cultures have created roughly comparable psychological constructs to try to explain, or at least to describe, this fact. The construct we have created we call *intelligence*. It is our way of saying that some people seem to adapt to the environments we both create and confront better than do others.

There have been numerous approaches to understanding the construct of intelligence, based on somewhat different metaphors for understanding the construct (Sternberg, 1990; see also essays in Sternberg, 2000). For example, some investigators seek to understand intelligence via what I have referred to as a geographic model, in which intelligence is conceived as a map of the mind. Such researchers have used psychometric tests to uncover the latent factors alleged to underlie intellectual functioning (see Schneider & McGrew, Chapter 4, this volume). Other investigators have used a computational metaphor, viewing intelligence in much the way they view the symbolic processing of a computer (see Naglieri, Das, & Goldstein, Chapter 7, this volume). Still others have followed an anthropological approach, viewing intelligence as a unique cultural creation. The approach I take in the triarchic theory proposed here can be viewed as a systems approach, in which many different aspects of intelligence are interrelated to each other in an attempt to understand how intelligence functions as a system.

The *triarchic theory of successful intelligence* (Sternberg, 1985a, 1988, 1997, 1999, 2004, 2005a, 2005b, 2008; Sternberg, Jarvin, & Grigorenko,

2011) explains in an integrative way the relationship between intelligence and (1) the internal world of the individual, or the mental mechanisms that underlie intelligent behavior; (2) experience, or the mediating role of the individual's passage through life between his or her internal and external worlds; and (3) the external world of the individual, or the use of these mental mechanisms in everyday life in order to attain an intelligent fit to the environment. The theory has three subtheories, one corresponding to each of the three relationships mentioned in the preceding sentence.

A crucial difference between this theory and many others is that the operationalizations (measurements) follow rather than precede the theory. Thus, rather than the theory's being derived from factor or other analyses of tests, the tests are chosen on the basis of the tenets of the theory. My colleagues and I have used many different kinds of tests (see Sternberg, 1985a, 1988, for reviews), such as analogies, syllogisms, verbal comprehension, prediction of future outcomes, and decoding of nonverbal cues. In every case, though, the choice of tasks has been dictated by the aspects of the theory that are being investigated, rather than the other way around.

DEFINITION OF SUCCESSFUL INTELLIGENCE

According to the proposed theory, *successful intelligence* is (1) the use of an integrated set of abilities needed to attain success in life, however an individual defines it, within his or her sociocultural context. People are successfully intelligent by virtue of (2) recognizing their strengths and making the most of them, at the same time that they recognize their weaknesses and find ways to correct or compensate for them. Successfully intelligent people (3) adapt to, shape, and select environments through (4) finding a balance in their use of analytical, creative, and practical abilities (Sternberg, 1997, 1999). Let us consider each element of the theory in turn.

The first element makes clear that there is no one definition of success that works for everyone. For some people, success is brilliance as lawyers; for others, it is originality as novelists; for others, it is caring for their children; for others, it is devoting their lives to God. For many people, it is some combination of things. Because people have different life goals, education needs to move away from single targeted measures of success, such as grade point average (GPA).

In considering the nature of intelligence, we need to consider the full range of definitions of success by which children can be intelligent. For example, in research we have done in rural Kenya (Sternberg et al., 2001), we have found that children who may score quite high on tests of an aspect of practical intelligence—knowledge of how to use natural herbal medicines to treat parasitic and other illnesses—may score quite poorly on tests of IQ and academic achievement. Indeed, we found an inverse relationship between the two skill sets, with correlations reaching the –.3 level. For these children, time spent in school takes away from time in which they learn the practical skills that they and their families view as needed for success in life. The same might be said, in the Western world, for many children who want to enter careers in athletics, theater, dance, art, music, carpentry, plumbing, entrepreneurship, and so forth. They may see time spent developing academic skills as time taken away from the time they need to develop practical skills relevant to meeting their goals in life.

The second element asserts that there are different paths to success, no matter what goal one chooses. Some people achieve success in large part through personal charm; others through brilliance of academic intellect; others through stunning originality; and yet others through working extremely hard. For most of us, there are at least a few things we do well, and our successful intelligence is dependent in large part upon making these things "work for us." At the same time, we need to acknowledge our weaknesses and find ways either to improve upon them or to compensate for them. For example, we may work hard to improve our skills in an area of weakness, or work as part of a team so that other people compensate for the kinds of things we do not do particularly well.

The third element asserts that success in life is achieved through some balance of adapting to existing environments, shaping those environments, and selecting new environments. Often when we go into an environment—as do students and teachers in school—we try to modify ourselves to fit that environment. In other words, we adapt. But sometimes it is not enough to adapt: We are not content merely to change ourselves to fit the environment, but rather, also want to change the environment to fit us. In this case, we shape the environment in order to make it a better one for us and possibly for others as well. But there may come times when our attempts to adapt and to shape the environment lead us nowhere—when we simply cannot find a way to make the environment work for us. In these cases, we leave the old environment and select a new environment. Sometimes the smart thing is to know when to get out.

Finally, we balance three kinds of abilities in order to achieve these ends: analytical abilities, creative abilities, and practical abilities. We need creative abilities to generate ideas, analytical abilities to determine whether they are good ideas, and practical abilities to implement the ideas and to convince others of the value of our ideas. Most people who are successfully intelligent are not equally endowed with these three abilities, but they find ways of making the three abilities work harmoniously together.

We have used five kinds of converging operations to test the theory of successful intelligence: cultural studies, factor-analytic studies, information-processing analyses, correlational analyses, and instructional studies (some of which are described below). This work is summarized elsewhere (e.g., Sternberg, 1985a, 1997, 2003a, 2003b). Examples of kinds of evidence in this work supporting the theory are the factorial separability of analytical, creative, and practical abilities; the substantial incremental validity of measures of practical intelligence over the validity of measures of academic (general) intelligence in predicting school and job performance; the usefulness of instruction based on the theory of successful intelligence, in comparison with other forms of instruction; and differences in the nature of what constitutes practical intelligence across cultures.

INTELLIGENCE AND THE INTERNAL WORLD OF THE INDIVIDUAL

Psychometricians, Piagetians, and information-processing psychologists have all recognized the importance of understanding the mental states or processes that underlie intelligent thought. In the triarchic theory, they seek this understanding by identifying and understanding three basic kinds of information-processing components, referred to as *metacomponents*, *performance components*, and *knowledge acquisition components*.

Metacomponents

Metacomponents are higher order, executive processes used to plan what one is going to do, to monitor it while one is doing it, and evaluate it after it is done. These metacomponents include (1) recognizing the existence of a problem, (2) deciding on the nature of the problem confronting one, (3) selecting a set of lower-order processes to solve the problem, (4) selecting a strategy into which to combine these components, (5) selecting a mental representation on which the components and strategy can act, (6) allocating one's mental resources, (7) monitoring one's problem solving as it is happening, and (8) evaluating one's problem solving after it is done. Let us consider some examples of these higher-order processes.

Deciding on the nature of a problem plays a prominent role in intelligence. For example, the difficulty for young children as well as older adults in problem solving often lies not in actually solving a given problem, but in figuring out just what the problem is that needs to be solved (see, e.g., Flavell, 1977; Sternberg & Rifkin, 1979). A major feature distinguishing people with intellectual disabilities from persons with typical functioning is the need of the former to be instructed explicitly and completely as to the nature of the particular task they are solving and how it should be performed (Butterfield, Wambold, & Belmont, 1973; Campione & Brown, 1979). The importance of figuring out the nature of the problem is not limited to persons with intellectual disabilities. Resnick and Glaser (1976) have argued that intelligence is the ability to learn from incomplete instruction.

Selection of a strategy for combining lower-order components is also a critical aspect of intelligence. In early information-processing research on intelligence, including my own (e.g., Sternberg, 1977), the primary emphasis was simply on figuring out what study participants do when confronted with a problem. What components do participants use, and into what strategies do they combine these components?

Soon information-processing researchers began to ask why study participants use the strategies they choose. For example, Cooper (1982) reported that in solving spatial problems, and especially mental rotation problems, some study participants seem to use a holistic strategy of comparison, whereas others use an analytic strategy. She sought to figure out what leads study participants to the choice of one strategy over another. Siegler (1986) proposed a model of strategy selection in arithmetic computation problems that links strategy choice to both the rules and the mental associations participants have stored in long-term memory. MacLeod, Hunt, and Mathews (1978) found that study participants with high spatial abilities tend to use a spatial strategy in solving sentence–picture comparison problems, whereas study participants with high verbal abilities are more likely to use a linguistic strategy. In my own work, I have found that study participants tend to prefer strategies for analogical reasoning that place fewer demands on working memory (Sternberg & Ketron, 1982). In such strategies, study participants encode as few features as possible of complex stimuli, trying to disconfirm incorrect multiple-choice options on the basis of these few features, and then choosing the remaining answer as the correct one. Similarly, study participants choose different strategies in linear–syllogistic reasoning (spatial, linguistic, mixed spatial–linguistic), but in this task, they do not always capitalize on their ability patterns to choose the strategy most suitable to their respective levels of spatial and verbal abilities (Sternberg & Weil, 1980). In sum, the selection of a strategy seems to be at least as important for understanding intelligent task performance as the efficacy with which the chosen strategy is implemented.

Intimately tied up with the selection of a strategy is the selection of a mental representation for information. In the early literature on mental representations, the emphasis seemed to be on understanding how information is represented. For example, can individuals use imagery as a form of mental representation (Kosslyn & Koenig, 1995)? Investigators have realized that people are quite flexible in their representations of information. The most appropriate question to ask seems to be not how such information is represented, but which representations are used in what circumstances. For example, I (Sternberg, 1977) found that analogy problems using animal names can draw on either spatial or clustering representations of the animal names. In the studies of strategy choice mentioned earlier, it was found that study participants can use either linguistic or spatial representations in solving sentence–picture comparisons (MacLeod et al., 1978) or linear syllogisms (Sternberg & Weil, 1980). We (Sternberg & Rifkin, 1979) found that the mental representation of certain kinds of analogies can be either more or less holistic, depending on the ages of the study participants. Younger children tend to be more holistic in their representations.

As important as any other metacomponent is the ability to allocate one's mental resources. Different investigators have studied resource allocation in different ways. Hunt and Lansman (1982), for example, have concentrated on the use of secondary tasks in assessing information processing and have proposed a model of attention allocation in the solution of problems that involve both a primary and a secondary task. In my work, I have found that better problem solvers tend to spend relatively more time in global strategy planning (Sternberg, 1981). Similarly, in solving analogies, better analogical reasoners seem to spend relatively more time encoding the terms of the problem than do poorer reasoners, but relatively less time in operating on these encodings (Sternberg, 1977; Sternberg & Rifkin, 1979). In reading as well, superior readers are better able than poorer readers to allocate their time across reading passages as a function of the difficulty of the passages to be read and the purpose for which the passages are being read (see Brown, Bransford, Ferrara, & Campione, 1983; Wagner & Sternberg, 1987).

Finally, monitoring one's solution process is a key aspect of intelligence (see also Brown, 1978). Consider, for example, the "missionaries and cannibals" problem, in which the study participants must "transport" a set of missionaries and cannibals across a river in a small boat without allowing the cannibals an opportunity to eat the missionaries—an event that can transpire only if the cannibals are allowed to outnumber the missionaries on either side of the river bank. The main kinds of errors that can be made are either to return to an earlier state in the problem space for solution (i.e., the problem solver goes back to where he or she was earlier in the solution process) or to make an impermissible move (i.e., the problem solver vio-

lates the rules, as in allowing the number of cannibals on one side to exceed the number of missionaries on that side) (Simon & Reed, 1976; see also Sternberg, 1982). Neither of these errors will result if a given subject closely monitors his or her solution processes. For young children, learning to count, a major source of errors in counting objects is to count a given object twice; again, such errors can result from failures in solution monitoring (Gelman & Gallistel, 1978). The effects of solution monitoring are not limited, of course, to any one kind of problem. One's ability to use the strategy of means–ends analysis (Newell & Simon, 1972)—that is, reduction of differences between where one is solving a problem and where one wishes to get in solving that problem—depends on one's ability to monitor just where one is in problem solution.

Performance Components

Performance components are lower-order processes that execute the instructions of the metacomponents. These lower-order components solve the problems according to the plans laid out by the metacomponents. Whereas the number of metacomponents used in the performance of various tasks is relatively limited, the number of performance components is probably quite large. Many of these performance components are relatively specific to narrow ranges of tasks (Sternberg, 1979, 1983, 1985a).

One of the most interesting classes of performance components is that found in inductive reasoning of the kind measured by tests such as matrices, analogies, series completions, and classifications. These components are important because of the importance of the tasks into which they enter: Induction problems of these kinds show the highest loading on the so-called *g*, or general intelligence factor (Carroll, Appendix, this volume; Horn & Blankson, Chapter 3, this volume; Jensen, 1980, 1998; Snow & Lohman, 1984; Sternberg & Gardner, 1982; see essays in Sternberg & Grigorenko, 2002). Thus identifying these performance components can give us some insight into the nature of the general factor. I am not arguing for any one factorial model of intelligence (i.e., one with a general factor) over others; to the contrary, I believe that most factor models are mutually compatible, differing only in the form of rotation that has been applied to a given factor space (Sternberg, 1977). The rotation one uses is a matter of theoretical or practical convenience, not of truth or falsity.

Two fundamental issues have arisen regarding the nature of performance components as a fundamental construct in human intelligence. The first, mentioned briefly here, is whether their number simply keeps expanding indefinitely. Neisser (1982), for example, has suggested that it does. As a result, he views the construct as of little use. But this expansion results only if one considers seriously those components that are specific to small classes of problems or to single problems. If one limits one's attention to the more important, general components of performance, the problem simply does not arise—as shown, for example, in our (Sternberg & Gardner, 1982) analysis of inductive reasoning or in Pellegrino and Kail's (1982) analysis of spatial ability. The second issue is one of the level at which performance components should be studied. In so-called "cognitive correlates" research (Pellegrino & Glaser, 1979), theorists emphasize components at relatively low levels of information processing (Hunt, 1978, 1980; Jensen, 1982). In so-called "cognitive components" research (Pellegrino & Glaser, 1979), theorists emphasize components at relatively high levels of information processing (e.g., Mulholland, Pellegrino, & Glaser, 1980; Snow, 1980; Sternberg, 1977). Because of the interactive nature of human information processing, it would appear that there is no right or wrong level of analysis. Rather, all levels of information processing contribute to both task and subject variance in intelligent performance. The most expeditious level of analysis depends on the task and subject population: Lower-level performance components may be more important, for example, in studying more basic information-processing tasks, such as choice reaction time, or in studying higher-level tasks in children who have not yet automatized the lower-order processes that contribute to performance of these tasks.

Knowledge Acquisition Components

Knowledge acquisition components are used to learn how to do what the metacomponents and performance components eventually do. Three knowledge acquisition components appear to be central in intellectual functioning: (1) selective encoding, (2) selective combination, and (3) selective comparison.

Selective encoding involves sifting out relevant from irrelevant information. When new information is presented in natural contexts, relevant information for one's given purpose is embedded in the midst of large amounts of purpose-irrelevant information. A critical task for the learner is that of sifting the "wheat from the chaff," recognizing just what among all the pieces of information is relevant for one's purposes (see Schank, 1980).

Selective combination involves combining selectively encoded information in such a way as to form an integrated, plausible whole. Simply sifting out relevant from irrelevant information is not enough to generate a new knowledge structure. One must know how to combine the pieces of information into an internally connected whole (see Mayer & Greeno, 1972).

Selective comparison involves discovering a nonobvious relationship between new information and already acquired information. For example, analogies, metaphors, and models often help individuals solve problems. The solver suddenly realizes that new information is similar to old information in certain ways, and then uses this information to form a mental representation based on the similarities. Teachers may discover how to relate new classroom material to information that students have already learned. Relating the new to the old can help students learn the material more quickly and understand it more deeply.

My emphasis on components of knowledge acquisition differs somewhat from the focus of some theorists in cognitive psychology, who emphasize what is already known and the structure of this knowledge (e.g., Chase & Simon, 1973; Chi, 1978; Keil, 1984). These various emphases are complementary. If one is interested in understanding, for example, differences in performance between experts and novices, clearly one would wish to look at the amount and structure of their respective knowledge bases. But if one wishes to understand how these differences come to be, merely looking at developed knowledge would not be enough. Rather, one would have to look as well at differences in the ways in which the knowledge bases were acquired. It is here that understanding of knowledge acquisition components will prove to be most relevant.

We have studied knowledge acquisition components in the domain of vocabulary acquisition (e.g., Sternberg, 1987; Sternberg & Powell, 1983). Difficulty in learning new words can be traced, at least in part, to the application of components of knowledge acquisition to context cues stored in long-term memory. Individuals with higher vocabularies tend to be those who are better able to apply the knowledge acquisition components to vocabulary-learning situations. Given the importance of vocabulary for overall intelligence, almost without respect to the theory or test one uses, utilization of knowledge acquisition components in vocabulary-learning situations would appear to be critically important for the development of intelligence.

Effective use of knowledge acquisition components is trainable. I have found, for example, that just 45 minutes of training in the use of these components in vocabulary learning can significantly and fairly substantially improve the ability of adults to learn vocabulary from natural language contexts (Sternberg, 1987). This training involves teaching individuals how to learn meanings of words presented in context. The training consists of three elements. The first is teaching individuals to search out certain kinds of contextual cues, such as synonyms, antonyms, functions, and category memberships. The second is teaching mediating variables. For example, cues to the meaning of a word are more likely to be found close to the word than at a distance from it. The third is teaching process skills—encoding relevant cues, combining them, and relating them to knowledge one already has.

To summarize, then, the components of intelligence are important parts of the intelligence of the individual. The various kinds of components work together. Metacomponents activate performance and knowledge acquisition components. These latter kinds of components in turn provide feedback to the metacomponents. Although one can isolate various kinds of information-processing components from task performance using experimental means, in practice the components function together in highly interactive, and not easily isolable, ways. Thus diagnoses as well as instructional interventions need to consider all three types of components in interaction, rather than any one kind of component in isolation. But understanding the nature of the components of intelligence is not in itself sufficient to understand the nature of intelligence because there is more to intelligence than a set of information-processing components. One could scarcely understand all of what it is that makes one person more intelligent than another by understanding the components of processing on, say, an intelligence test. The other aspects of the triarchic theory address some of the other aspects of intelligence that contribute to individual differences in observed performance, outside testing situations as well as within them.

INTELLIGENCE AND EXPERIENCE

Components of information processing are always applied to tasks and situations with which one has some level of prior experience (even if it is minimal experience). Hence these internal mechanisms are closely tied to one's experience. According to the experiential subtheory, the components are not equally good measures of intelligence at all levels of experience. Assessing intelligence requires one to consider not only components, but the level of experience at which they are applied.

Toward the end of the 20th century, a trend developed in cognitive science to study script-based behavior (e.g., Schank & Abelson, 1977), whether under the name of *script* or under some other name, such as *schema* or *frame*. There is no longer any question that much of human behavior is scripted in some sense. However, from the standpoint of the present subtheory, such behavior is nonoptimal for understanding intelligence. Typically, one's actions when going to a restaurant, doctor's office, or movie theater do not provide good measures of intelligence, even though they do provide good measures of scripted behavior. What, then, is the relation between intelligence and experience?

According to the experiential subtheory, intelligence is best measured at those regions of the experiential continuum involving tasks or situations that are either relatively novel on the one hand, or in the process of becoming automatized on the other. As Raaheim (1974) pointed out, totally novel tasks and situations provide poor measures of intelligence: One would not want to administer, say, trigonometry problems to a first grader roughly 6 years old. But one might wish to administer problems that are just at the limits of the child's understanding, in order to test how far this understanding extends. Related is Vygotsky's (1978) concept of the *zone of proximal development*, in which one examines a child's ability to profit from instruction to facilitate his or her solutions of novel problems. To measure automatization skill, one might wish to present a series of problems—mathematical or otherwise—to see how long it takes for their solution to become automatic, and to see how automatized performance becomes. Thus both the slope and the asymptote (if any) of automatization are of interest.

Ability to Deal with Novelty

Several sources of evidence converge on the notion that the ability to deal with relative novelty is a good way of measuring intelligence. Consider three such sources of evidence. First, we have conducted several studies on the nature of insight, both in children and in adults (Davidson & Sternberg, 1984; Sternberg & Davidson, 1982). In the studies with children (Davidson & Sternberg, 1984), we separated three kinds of insights: insights of selective encoding, insights of selective combination, and insights of selective comparison. Use of these knowledge acquisition components is referred to as *insightful* when they are applied in the absence of existing scripts, plans, or frames. In other words, one must decide what information is relevant, how to put the information together, or how new information relates to old in the absence of any obvious cues on the basis of which to make these judgments. A problem is insightfully solved at the individual level when a given individual lacks such cues. A problem is insightfully solved at the societal level when no one else has these cues, either. In our studies, we found that children who are intellectually gifted are so in part by virtue of their insight abilities, which represent an important part of the ability to deal with novelty.

The critical finding was that providing insights to the children significantly benefited the nongifted, but not the gifted, children. (None of the children performed anywhere near ceiling level, so that the interaction was not due to ceiling effects.) In other words, the gifted children spontaneously had the insights and hence did not benefit from being given these insights. The nongifted children did not have the insights spontaneously and hence did benefit. Thus the gifted children were better able to deal with novelty spontaneously.

Another source of evidence for the proposed hypothesis relating coping with novelty to intelligence derives from the large literature on fluid intelligence, which is in part a kind of intelligence that involves dealing with novelty (see Cattell, 1971). Snow and Lohman (1984; see also Snow, Kyllonen, & Marshalek, 1984) multidimensionally scaled a variety of such tests and found the dimensional loading to follow a radex structure. In particular, tests with higher loadings on *g*, or general intelligence, fall closer to the center of the spatial diagram. The critical thing to note is that those tests that best measure the ability to deal with novelty fall closer to the center, and tests tend to be more removed from the center as their assessment of the ability to deal with novelty becomes more remote. In sum, evidence from the laboratories of others as well as mine supports the idea that the various components of intelligence that are involved in dealing with novelty, as measured in particular tasks and situations, provide particularly apt measures of intellectual ability.

Ability to Automatize Information Processing

Several converging lines of evidence in the literature support the claim that automatization ability is a key aspect of intelligence. For example, I (Sternberg, 1977) found that the correlation between people–piece (schematic picture) analogy performance and measures of general intelligence increased with practice, as performance on these items became increasingly automatized. Skilled reading is heavily dependent on automatization of bottom-up functions (basic skills such as phonetic decoding), and the ability to read well is an essential part of crystallized ability—whether it is viewed from the standpoint of theories such as Cattell's (1971), Carroll's (1993), or Vernon's (1971), or from the standpoint of tests of crystallized ability, such as the verbal portion of the SAT. Poor comprehenders often are those who have not automatized the elementary, bottom-up processes of reading and hence do not have sufficient attentional resources to allocate to top-down comprehension processes. Ackerman (1987; Kanfer & Ackerman, 1989) has provided a three-stage model of automatization in which the first stage is related to intelligence, although the latter two appear not to be.

Theorists such as Jensen (1982) and Hunt (1978) have attributed the correlation between such tasks as choice reaction time and letter matching to the relation between speed of information processing and intelligence. Indeed, there is almost certainly some relation, although I believe it is much more complex than these theorists seem to allow for. But a plausible alternative hypothesis is that at least some of that correlation is due to the effects of automatization of processing: Because of the simplicity of these tasks, they probably become at least partially automatized fairly rapidly, and hence can measure both rate and asymptote of automatization of performance. In sum, then, although the evidence is far from complete, there is at least some support for the notion that rate and level of automatization are related to intellectual skill.

The ability to deal with novelty and the ability to automatize information processing are interrelated, as shown in the example of the automatization of reading described in this section. If one is well able to automatize, one has more resources left over for dealing with novelty. Similarly, if one is well able to deal with novelty, one has more resources left over for automatization. Thus performances at the various levels of the experiential continuum are related to one another.

These abilities should not be viewed in a vacuum with respect to the componential subtheory. The components of intelligence are applied to tasks and situations at various levels of experience. The ability to deal with novelty can be understood in part in terms of the metacomponents, performance components, and knowledge acquisition components involved in it. *Automatization* refers to the way these components are executed. Hence the two subtheories considered so far are closely intertwined. Now we need to consider the application of these subtheories to everyday tasks, in addition to laboratory ones.

INTELLIGENCE AND THE EXTERNAL WORLD OF THE INDIVIDUAL

According to the contextual subtheory, intelligent thought is directed toward one or more of three behavioral goals: *adaptation to an environment, shaping of an environment,* or *selection of an environment.* These three goals may be viewed as the functions toward which intelligence is directed. Intelligence is not aimless or random mental activity that happens to involve certain components of information processing at certain levels of experience. Rather, it is purposefully directed toward the pursuit of these three global goals, all of which have more specific and concrete instantiations in people's lives (Sternberg et al., 2000).

Adaptation

Most intelligent thought is directed toward the attempt to adapt to one's environment. The requirements for adaptation can differ radically from one environment to another—whether environments are defined in terms of families, jobs, subcultures, or cultures. Hence, although the components of intelligence required in these various contexts may be the same or quite similar, and although all of them may involve (at one time or another) dealing with novelty and automatization of information processing, the concrete instantiations that these processes and levels of experience take may differ substantially across contexts. This fact has an important implication for our understanding of the nature of intelligence. According to the triarchic theory in general, and the contextual subtheory in particular, the processes, experiential facets, and functions of intelligence remain essentially the same across contexts, but the particular instantiations of these processes, facets, and functions can differ radically. Thus the content of intelligent thought and its manifestations in behavior will bear no necessary resemblance across contexts. As a result, although the mental elements that an intelligence test should measure do not differ across contexts, the vehicle for measurement may have to differ. A test that measures a set of processes, experiential facets, or intelligent functions in one context may not provide equally adequate measurement in another context. To the contrary, what is intelligent in one culture may be viewed as unintelligent in another.

Different contextual milieus may result in the development of different mental abilities. For example, Puluwat navigators must develop their large-scale spatial abilities for dealing with cognitive maps to a degree that far exceeds the adaptive requirements of contemporary Western societies (Gladwin, 1970). Similarly, Kearins (1981) found that Australian Aboriginal children probably develop their visual–spatial memories to a greater degree than do Australian children of European descent. The latter are more likely to apply verbal strategies to spatial memory tasks than are the Aboriginal children, who employ spatial strategies. This greater development is presumed to be due to the greater need the Aboriginal children have for using spatial skills in their everyday lives. In contrast, members of Western societies probably develop their abilities for thinking abstractly to a greater degree than do members of societies in which concepts are rarely dealt with outside their concrete manifestations in the objects of the everyday environment.

One of the most interesting differences among cultures and subcultures in the development of patterns of adaptation is in the matter of time allocation, a metacomponential function. In Western cultures in general, careful allocation of time to various activities is a prized commodity. Our lives are largely governed by careful scheduling at home, school, work, and so on. There are fixed hours for certain activities and fixed lengths of time within which these activities are expected to be completed. Indeed, the intelligence tests we use show our prizing of time allocation to the fullest. Almost all of them are timed in such a way as to make completion of the tests a nontrivial challenge. A slow or cautious worker is at a distinct disadvantage.

Not all cultures and subcultures view time in the same way that we do. For example, among the Kipsigi, schedules are much more flexible; hence these individuals have difficulty understanding and dealing with Western notions of the time pressure under which people are expected to live (Super & Harkness, 1982). In Hispanic cultures, such as Venezuela, my own personal experience indicates that the press of time is taken with much less seriousness than it is in typical North American cultural settings. Even within the continental United States, though, there can be major differences in the importance of time allocation (Heath, 1983).

The point of these examples has been to illustrate how differences in environmental press and people's conception of what constitutes an intelligent response to it can influence just what counts as adaptive behavior. To understand intelligence, one must understand it not only in relation to its internal manifestations in terms of mental processes and its experiential manifestations in terms of facets of the experiential continuum, but also in terms of how thought is intelligently translated into action in a variety of different contextual settings. The differences in what is considered adaptive and intelligent can extend even to different occupations within a given cultural milieu. For example, I (Sternberg, 1985b) have found that individuals in different fields of endeavor (art, business, philosophy, physics) view intelligence in slightly different ways that reflect the demands of their respective fields.

Shaping

Shaping of the environment is often used as a backup strategy when adaptation fails. If one is unable to change oneself to fit the environment, one may attempt to change the environment to fit oneself. For example, repeated attempts to adjust to the demands of one's romantic partner may eventually lead to attempts to get the partner to adjust to oneself. But shaping is not always used in lieu of adaptation. In some cases, shaping may be used before adaptation is ever tried, as in the case of the individual who attempts to shape a romantic partner with little or no effort to shape him- or herself so as to suit the partner's wants or needs better.

In the laboratory, examples of shaping behavior can be seen in strategy selection situations where one essentially molds the task to fit one's preferred style of dealing with tasks. For example, in comparing sentence statements, individuals may select either a verbal or a spatial strategy, depending on their pattern of verbal and spatial ability (MacLeod et al., 1978). The task is "made over" in conformity to what they do best.

In some respects, shaping may be seen as the quintessence of intelligent thought and behavior. One essentially makes over the environment, rather than allowing the environment to make over oneself. Perhaps it is this skill that has enabled humankind to reach its current level of scientific, technological, and cultural advancement (for better or for worse). In science, the greatest scientists are those who set the paradigms (shaping), rather than those who merely follow them (adaptation). Similarly, the individuals who achieve greatest distinction in art and in literature are often those who create new modes and styles of expression, rather than merely following existing ones. It is not their use of shaping alone that distinguishes them intellectually, but rather a combination of their willingness to do it with their skill in doing it.

Selection

Selection involves renunciation of one environment in favor of another. In terms of the rough hierarchy established so far, selection is sometimes used when both adaptation and shaping fail. After attempting to both adapt to and shape a marriage, one may decide to deal with one's failure in these activities by "deselecting" the marriage and choosing the environment of the newly single. Failure to adjust to the demands of work environments, or to change the demands placed on one to make them a reasonable fit to one's interests, values, expectations, or abilities, may result in the decision to seek another job altogether. But selection is not always used as a last resort. Sometimes one attempts to shape an environment only after attempts to leave it have failed. Other times, one may decide almost instantly that an environment is simply wrong and feel that one need not or should not even try to fit into or to change it. For example, every now and then we get a new graduate student who realizes almost immediately that he or she came to graduate school for the wrong reasons, or who finds that graduate school is nothing at all like the continuation of undergraduate school he or she expected. In such cases, the intelligent thing to do may be to leave the environment as soon as possible, to pursue activities more in line with one's goals in life.

Environmental selection is not usually directly studied in the laboratory, although it may have relevance for certain experimental settings. Perhaps no research example of its relevance has been more salient than the experimental paradigm created by Milgram (1974), who, in a long series of studies, asked study participants to "shock" other study participants (who were actually confederates and who were not actually shocked). The finding of critical interest was how few study participants shaped the environment by refusing to continue with the experiment and walking out of it. Milgram has drawn an analogy to the situation in Nazi Germany, where obedience to authority created an environment whose horrors continue to amaze us to this day and always will. This example is a good one in showing how close matters of intelligence can come to matters of personality.

To conclude, adaptation, shaping, and selection are functions of intelligent thought as it operates in context. They may (although they need not) be employed hierarchically, with one path followed when another one fails. It is through adaptation, shaping, and selection that the components of intelligence, as employed at various levels of experience, become actualized in the real world. In this section, it has become clear that the modes of actualization can differ widely across individuals and groups, so that intelligence cannot be understood independently of the ways in which it is manifested.

INSTRUCTIONAL INTERVENTIONS BASED ON THE THEORY

The triarchic theory has been applied to instructional settings in various ways, with considerable success (Sternberg, 2010b; Sternberg & Grigorenko, 2004, 2007; Sternberg, Grigorenko, & Zhang, 2008; Sternberg, Jarvin, & Grigorenko, 2009). The componential subtheory has been applied in teaching the learning of vocabulary from context to adult study participants (Sternberg, 1987), as mentioned earlier. Experimental study participants were taught components of decontextualization. There were three groups, corresponding to three types of instruction that were given based on the theory (see Sternberg, 1987, 1988). Control study participants either received no relevant material at all, or else received practical items but without theory-based instruction. Improvement

occurred only when study participants were given the theory-based instruction, which involved teaching them how to use contextual cues, mediating variables such as matching parts of speech, and processes of decontextualization.

The experiential subtheory was the basis for the program (Davidson & Sternberg, 1984) that successfully taught insight skills (selective encoding, selective combination, and selective comparison) to children roughly 9–11 years of age. The program lasted 6 weeks and involved insight skills as applied to a variety of subject matter areas. An uninstructed control group received a pretest and a posttest, like the experimental group, but no instruction. We found that the experimental study participants improved significantly more than the controls, both when participants were previously identified as gifted and when they were not so identified. Moreover, we found durable results that lasted even 1 year after the training program, and we found transfer to types of insight problems not specifically used in the program.

The contextual subtheory served as the basis for a program called Practical Intelligence for Schools, developed in collaboration with a team of investigators from Harvard (Gardner, Krechevsky, Sternberg, & Okagaki, 1994; Sternberg, Okagaki, & Jackson, 1990) and based on Gardner's (2006) theory of multiple intelligences as well as on the triarchic theory. The goal of this program is to teach practical intellectual skills to children roughly 9–11 years of age in the areas of reading, writing, homework, and test taking. The program is completely infused into existing curricula. Over a period of years, we studied the program in a variety of school districts and obtained significant improvements for experimental versus uninstructed control study participants in a variety of criterion measures, including study skills measures and performance-based measures of performance in the areas taught by the program. The program has been shown to increase practical skills, such as those involved in doing homework, taking tests, or writing papers, as well as school achievement (Williams et al., 2002).

We have sought to test the theory of successful intelligence in the classroom. In a first set of studies, we explored the question of whether conventional education in school systematically discriminates against children with creative and practical strengths (Sternberg & Clinkenbeard, 1995; Sternberg, Ferrari, Clinkenbeard, & Grigorenko, 1996; Sternberg, Grigorenko, Ferrari, &

Clinkenbeard, 1999). Motivating this work was the belief that the systems in most schools strongly tend to favor children with strengths in memory and analytical abilities. However, schools can be unbalanced in other directions as well.

One school we visited in Russia in 2000 placed a heavy emphasis upon the development of creative abilities—much more so than on the development of analytical and practical abilities. While on this trip, we were told of yet another school (catering to the children of Russian businessmen) that strongly emphasized practical abilities, and in which children who were not practically oriented were told that eventually they would be working for their classmates who were practically oriented.

To validate the relevance of the theory of successful intelligence in classrooms, we have carried out a number of instructional studies. In one study, we used the Sternberg Triarchic Abilities Test (Sternberg, 1993). The test was administered to 326 children around the United States and in some other countries who were identified by their schools as gifted by any standard whatsoever (Sternberg et al., 1999). Children were selected for a summer program in (college-level) psychology if they fell into one of five ability groupings: *high-analytical, high-creative, high-practical, high-balanced* (high in all three abilities), or *low-balanced* (low in all three abilities). Students who came to Yale were then assigned at random to four instructional groups, with the constraint that roughly equal numbers with each ability pattern be assigned to each group. Students in all four instructional groups used the same introductory psychology textbook (a preliminary version of Sternberg, 1995) and listened to the same psychology lectures. What differed among them was the type of afternoon discussion section to which they were assigned. They were assigned to an instructional condition that emphasized either memory, analytical, creative, or practical instruction. For example, in the memory condition, they might be asked to describe the main tenets of a major theory of depression. In the analytical condition, they might be asked to compare and contrast two theories of depression. In the creative condition, they might be asked to formulate their own theory of depression. In the practical condition, they might be asked how they could use what they had learned about depression to help a friend who was depressed.

Students in all four instructional conditions were evaluated in terms of their performance on homework, a midterm exam, a final exam, and an independent project. Each type of work was evaluated for memory, analytical, creative, and practical quality. Thus all students were evaluated in exactly the same way. Our results suggested the utility of the theory of successful intelligence. This utility showed itself in several ways.

First, we observed when the students arrived at Yale that the students in the high-creative and high-practical groups were much more diverse in terms of racial, ethnic, socioeconomic, and educational backgrounds than were the students in the high-analytical group, suggesting that correlations of measured intelligence with status variables such as these may be reduced by using a broader conception of intelligence. Thus the kinds of students identified as strong differed in terms of the populations from which they were drawn, in comparison with students identified as strong solely by analytical measures. More importantly, just by expanding the range of abilities measured, we discovered intellectual strengths that might not have been apparent through a conventional test.

Second, we found that all three ability tests—analytical, creative, and practical—significantly predicted course performance. When multiple-regression analysis was used, at least two of these ability measures contributed significantly to the prediction of each of the measures of achievement. In particular, for homework assignments, significant beta weights were obtained for analytical (.25) and creative (.16) ability measures; for the independent project, significant weights were obtained for the analytical (.14), creative (.22), and practical (.14) measures; for the exams, significant weights were obtained for the analytical (.24) and creative (.19) measures (Sternberg et al., 1999). Perhaps as a reflection of the difficulty of deemphasizing the analytical way of teaching, one of the significant predictors was always the analytical score. (However, in a replication of our study with low-income African American students from New York, Deborah Coates of the City University of New York found a different pattern of results. Her data indicated that the practical tests were better predictors of course performance than were the analytical measures, suggesting that which ability test predicts which criterion depends on population as well as mode of teaching.)

Third and most important, there was an aptitude–treatment interaction, whereby students who were placed in instructional conditions that better matched their pattern of abilities outperformed students who were mismatched. In particular, repeated-measures analysis revealed statistically significant effects of match for analytical and creative tasks as a whole. Three of five practical tasks also showed an effect. In other words, when students are taught in a way that fits how they think, they do better in school (see Cronbach & Snow, 1977, for a discussion of the difficulties in eliciting aptitude–treatment interactions). Children who have high levels of creative and practical abilities, but who are almost never taught or assessed in a way that matches their pattern of abilities, may be at a disadvantage in course after course, year after year.

A follow-up study (Sternberg, Torff, & Grigorenko, 1998) examined learning of social studies and science by third graders and eighth graders. The 225 third graders were students in a very low-income neighborhood in Raleigh, North Carolina. The 142 eighth graders were largely middle- to upper-middle-class students studying in Baltimore, Maryland, and Fresno, California; these children were part of a summer program sponsored by the Johns Hopkins University for gifted students. In this study, students were assigned to one of three instructional conditions. Randomization was by classroom. In the first condition, they were taught the course that basically they would have learned had there been no intervention. The emphasis in the course was on memory. In a second condition, students were taught in a way that emphasized critical (analytical) thinking. In the third condition, they were taught in a way that emphasized analytical, creative, and practical thinking. All students' performance was assessed for memory learning (through multiple-choice assessments), as well as for analytical, creative, and practical learning (through performance assessments).

As expected, students in the successful-intelligence (analytical, creative, practical) condition outperformed the other students in terms of the performance assessments. For the third graders, respective means were highest for the triarchic (successful-intelligence) condition, second highest for the critical-thinking condition, and lowest for the memory condition for memory, analytical, and creative performance measures. For practical measures, the critical-thinking mean was insignificantly higher than the triarchic mean, but both were significantly higher than the memory mean. For the eighth graders, the results were similar. One could argue that this pattern of results merely reflected the way students were taught. Nevertheless, the result suggested that teaching for these kinds of thinking succeeded. More important, however, was the result that children in the successful-intelligence condition outperformed the other children even on the multiple-choice memory tests. In other words, to the extent that the goal is just to maximize children's memory for information, teaching for successful intelligence is still superior. It enables children to capitalize on their strengths and to correct or to compensate for their weaknesses, and it allows them to encode material in a variety of interesting ways.

We extended these results to reading curricula at the middle school and high school levels (Grigorenko, Jarvin, & Sternberg, 2002). In a study of 871 middle school students and 432 high school students, we taught reading either triarchically or through the regular curriculum. Classrooms were assigned randomly to treatments. At the middle school level, reading was taught explicitly. At the high school level, reading was infused into instruction in mathematics, physical sciences, social sciences, English, history, foreign languages, and the arts. In all settings, students who were taught triarchically substantially outperformed students who were taught in standard ways. Effects were statistically significant at the .001 level for memory, analytical, creative, and practical comparisons.

Thus the results of three sets of studies suggest that the theory of successful intelligence is valid as a whole. Moreover, the results suggest that the theory can make a difference not only in laboratory tests, but in school classrooms and even the everyday life of adults as well. At the same time, the studies have weaknesses that need to be remedied in future studies. The samples are relatively small and not fully representative of the entire U.S. population. Moreover, the studies have examined a limited number of alternative interventions. All interventions were of relatively short duration (up to a semester-long course). In addition, future studies should look at durability and transfer of training.

In sum, the triarchic theory serves as a useful basis for educational interventions and, in our own work, has shown itself to be a basis for interventions that improve students' performance relative to that of controls who do not receive the theory-based instruction.

ASSESSMENT STUDIES

One of the primary venues for assessing abilities is university admissions. When universities make decisions about selective admissions, the main quantitative data they have available to them are typically (1) GPA in high school or its equivalent, and

(2) scores on standardized tests (Lemann, 1999). Is it possible to create assessments that are psychometrically sound and that provide incremental validity over existing measures, without destroying the cultural and ethnic diversity that makes a university environment a place in which students can interact with and learn from others who are different from themselves?

The Rainbow Project

The Rainbow Project (for details, see Sternberg, 2009; Sternberg & the Rainbow Project Collaborators, 2005, 2006) was a first project designed to enhance university admissions procedures at the undergraduate level. The Rainbow measures were intended, in the United States, to supplement the SAT, but they can supplement any conventional standardized test of abilities or achievement. In the theory of successful intelligence, abilities and achievement are viewed as being on a continuum—abilities are largely achieved (Sternberg, 1998a, 1999)—so it is not clear that it matters greatly exactly what test is used, given that most of the tests used are highly g-loaded.

The SAT is a comprehensive examination currently measuring verbal comprehension and mathematical thinking skills, with a writing component recently added. A wide variety of studies have shown the utility of the SAT and similar tests as predictors of university and job success, with success in college typically measured by GPA (Schmidt & Hunter, 1998). Taken together, these data suggest reasonable predictive validity for the SAT in predicting undergraduate performance. Indeed, traditional intelligence or aptitude tests have been shown to predict performance across a wide variety of settings. But as is always the case for a single test or type of test, there is room for improvement. The theory of successful intelligence provides one basis for improving prediction and possibly for establishing greater equity and diversity, which is a goal of most higher-educational institutions (Bowen, Kurzweil, & Tobin, 2006). It suggests that broadening the range of skills tested to go beyond analytic skills, to include practical and creative skills as well, might significantly enhance the prediction of undergraduate performance beyond current levels. Thus the theory does not suggest *replacing*, but rather *augmenting*, the SAT and similar tests (such as the ACT or, in the United Kingdom, the A-levels) in the undergraduate admissions process. Our collaborative team of investigators sought to study how successful such an augmentation could be. Even if we did not use the SAT, ACT, or A-levels in particular, we still would need some kind of assessment of the memory and analytical abilities these tests measure.

Methodological Considerations

In the Rainbow Project, data were collected at 15 schools across the United States, including 8 four-year undergraduate institutions, 5 community colleges, and 2 high schools.

The participants were 1,013 students predominantly in their first year as undergraduates or their final year of high school. In this chapter, analyses only for undergraduate students are discussed because they were the only ones for whom my colleagues and I had data available regarding undergraduate academic performance. The final number of participants included in these analyses was 793.

Baseline measures of standardized test scores and high school GPAs were collected to evaluate the predictive validity of current tools used for undergraduate admission criteria, and to provide a contrast for the current measures. Students' scores on standardized university entrance exams were obtained from the College Board.

The measure of analytical skills was provided by the SAT, plus multiple-choice analytical items we added to measure inference of meanings of words from context, number series completions, and figural matrix completions.

Creative skills were measured by multiple-choice items and by performance-based items. The multiple-choice items were of three kinds. In one, students were presented with verbal analogies preceded by counterfactual premises (e.g., money falls off trees). They had to solve the analogies as though the counterfactual premises were true. In a second, students were presented with rules for novel number operations—for example, *flix*, which involves numerical manipulations differing as a function of whether the first of two operands is greater than, equal to, or less than the second. Participants had to use the novel number operations to solve presented math problems. In a third, participants were first presented with a figural series involving one or more transformations; they then had to apply the rule of the series to a new figure with a different appearance, and complete the new series. These measures are not typical of assessments of creativity and were included for relative quickness of participants' responses and relative ease of scoring.

Creative skills were also measured with open-ended measures. One measure required writing two short stories with a selection from among unusual titles, such as "The Octopus's Sneakers"; one required orally telling two stories based upon choices of picture collages; and the third required captioning cartoons from among various options. Open-ended performance-based answers were rated by trained raters for novelty, quality, and task-appropriateness. Multiple judges were used for each task, and satisfactory reliability was achieved (Sternberg & the Rainbow Project Collaborators, 2006).

Multiple-choice measures of practical skills were of three kinds. In one, students were presented with a set of everyday problems in the life of an adolescent and had to select the option that would best solve each problem. In another, students were presented with scenarios requiring the use of math in everyday life (e.g., buying tickets for a ballgame) and had to solve math problems based on the scenarios. In a third, students were presented with a map of an area (e.g., an entertainment park) and had to answer questions about navigating effectively through the area depicted by the map.

Practical skills were also assessed with three situational-judgment inventories: the Everyday Situational Judgment Inventory (Movies), the Common Sense Questionnaire, and the College Life Questionnaire, each of which taps different types of tacit knowledge. The general format of tacit-knowledge inventories has been described in Sternberg and colleagues (2000), so only the contents of the inventories used in this study are described here. The movies presented everyday situations that confront undergraduates, such as a student's asking for a letter of recommendation from a professor who shows, through nonverbal cues, that he does not recognize the student very well. Participants then had to rate various options for how well they would work in response to each situation. The Common Sense Questionnaire provided everyday business problems, such as being assigned to work with a coworker whom one cannot stand. The College Life Questionnaire provided everyday university situations for which a solution was required.

Unlike the creativity performance tasks, in the practical performance tasks the participants were not given a choice of situations to rate. For each task, participants were told that there was no "right" answer, and that the options described in each situation represented variations on how different people approach different situations.

Consider examples of the kinds of items participants might find on the Rainbow assessment. An example of a creative item might be to write a story using the title "3516" or "It's Moving Backward." Another example might show a collage of pictures in which people are engaged in different a wide variety of activities helping other people. A participant would then orally tell a story that took off from the collage. An example of a practical item might show a movie in which a student has just received a poor grade on a test. His roommate has had a health crisis the night before, and he has been up all night helping him. His professor hands him back the test paper, with a disappointed look on her face, and suggests to the student that he study harder next time. The movie then stops. Participants would then have to describe how the student might handle the situation. Or the participants might receive a written problem describing a conflict with another individual with whom a student is working on a group project. The project is getting mired down in the interpersonal conflict. The participants had to indicate how the student might resolve the situation to get the project done.

All materials were administered in either of two formats. A total of 325 of the university students took the test in paper-and-pencil format, whereas a total of 468 students took the test on the computer via the World Wide Web. No strict time limits were set for completing the tests, although the instructors were given rough guidelines of about 70 minutes per session. The time taken to complete the battery of tests ranged from 2 to 4 hours

As a result of the lengthy nature of the complete battery of assessments, participants were administered parts of the battery in an intentionally incomplete overlapping design. The participants were randomly assigned to the test sections they were to complete. Details about the use of this procedure are given in Sternberg and the Rainbow Project Collaborators (2006).

Creativity in the Rainbow Project (and the subsequent Project Kaleidoscope) was assessed on the basis of the novelty and quality of responses. Practicality was assessed on the basis of the feasibility of the products with respect to human and material resources.

Findings

The analysis described below is a conservative one that does not correct for differences in the selectivity of the institutions at which the study took place. In a study across so many undergraduate institutions differing in selectivity, validity coefficients will seem to be lower than is typical because an A at a less selective institution counts the same as an A at a more selective institution. When we corrected for institutional selectivity, the results described below became stronger. But correcting for selectivity has its own problems (e.g., on what basis does one evaluate selectivity?), and so uncorrected data are used in this chapter. We also did not control for university major: Different universities may have different majors, and the exact course offerings, grading, and populations of students entering different majors may vary from one university to another, rendering control difficult.

When we examined undergraduate students alone, the sample showed slightly higher mean SAT scores than those found in undergraduate institutions across the United States. The standard deviation was above the normal 100-point standard deviation, meaning that we did not suffer from restriction of range. Our means, although slightly higher than typical, were within the range of average undergraduate students.

Another potential concern was pooling data from different institutions. We pooled data because in some institutions we simply did not have large enough numbers of cases for the data to be meaningful.

Some scholars believe that there is only one set of skills that is highly relevant to school performance—what is sometimes called *general ability*, or *g* (e.g., Jensen, 1998). These scholars believe that tests may appear to measure different skills, but when statistically analyzed, show themselves just to be measuring the single general ability. Did the Rainbow tests actually measure distinct analytical, creative, and practical skill groupings? Factor analysis addressed this question. Three meaningful factors were extracted from the data: practical performance tests, creative performance tests, and multiple-choice tests (including analytical, creative, and practical). In other words, multiple-choice tests, regardless of what they were supposed to measure, clustered together. Thus method variance proved to be very important. The results show the importance of measuring skills using multiple formats, precisely because method is so important in determining factorial structure. The results show the limitations of exploratory factor analysis in analyzing such data, and also of dependence on multiple choice items outside the analytical domain. In the ideal situation, one wishes

to ensure that one controls for method of testing in designing aptitude and other test batteries.

Undergraduate admissions offices are not interested, exactly, in whether these tests predict undergraduate academic success. Rather, they are interested in the extent to which these tests predict school success *beyond* those measures currently in use, such as the SAT and high school GPA. In order to test the incremental validity provided by Rainbow measures above and beyond the SAT in predicting GPA, we conducted a series of hierarchical regressions that included the items analyzed above in the analytical, creative, and practical assessments.

If one looks at the simple correlations, the SAT (both verbal and math), high school GPA, and the Rainbow measures all predicted first-year undergraduate GPA. But how did the Rainbow measures fare on incremental validity? In one set of analyses, the SAT (both verbal and math) and high school GPA were included in the first step of the prediction equation because these are the standard measures used today to predict undergraduate performance. Only high school GPA contributed uniquely to prediction of undergraduate GPA. Inclusion of the Rainbow measures roughly doubled prediction (percentage of variance accounted for in the criterion) over that obtained with the SAT alone.

These results suggest that the Rainbow tests add considerably to the predictive power of the SAT alone. They also suggest the power of high school GPA in prediction, particularly because it is an atheoretical composite that includes within it many variables, including motivation and conscientiousness.

Studying group differences requires careful attention to methodology and sometimes has led to erroneous conclusions (Hunt & Carlson, 2007). Although one important goal of the Rainbow Project was to predict success in the undergraduate years, another important goal involved developing measures that would reduce ethnic group differences in mean levels. There has been a lively debate as to why there are socially defined racial group differences, and as to whether scores for members of underrepresented minority groups are over- or underpredicted by SATs and related tests (see, e.g., Bowen & Bok, 2000; Rushton & Jensen, 2005; Sternberg, Grigorenko, & Kidd, 2005; Turkheimer, Haley, Waldron, D'Onofrio, & Gottesman, 2003). There are a number of ways one can test for group differences in these measures, each of which involves a test of the size of the effect of ethnic group. Two different measures were chosen: ω^2 (omega squared) and Cohen's *d*.

There were two general findings. First, in terms of overall differences, the Rainbow tests appeared to reduce ethnic group differences, relative to traditional assessments of abilities like the SAT. Second, in terms of specific differences, it appears that the Hispanic American students benefited the most from the reduction of group differences. The African American students, too, seemed to show a reduction in difference from the European American mean for most of the Rainbow tests, although a substantial difference appeared to be maintained with the practical performance measures.

Although the group differences were not perfectly reduced, these findings suggest that measures can be designed that reduce ethnic and racial group differences on standardized tests, particularly for historically disadvantaged groups such as African American and Hispanic American students. These findings have important implications for reducing adverse impact in undergraduate admissions.

The SAT is based on a conventional psychometric notion of cognitive skills. Using this notion, it has had substantial success in predicting undergraduate academic performance. The Rainbow measures alone roughly doubled the predictive power of undergraduate GPA when compared to the SAT alone. In addition, the Rainbow measures predicted substantially beyond the contributions of the SAT and high school GPA. These findings, combined with encouraging results regarding the reduction of between-ethnicity differences, make a compelling case for furthering the study of the measurement of analytic, creative, and practical skills for predicting success at a university.

One important goal for this research was, and for future studies still is, the creation of standardized assessments that reduce the different outcomes between different groups as much as possible to maintain test validity. The measures described here suggest results toward this end. Although the group differences in the tests were not reduced to zero, the tests did substantially attenuate group differences relative to other measures such as the SAT. This finding could be an important step toward ultimately ensuring fair and equal treatment for members of diverse groups in the academic domain.

The principles behind the Rainbow Project apply at other levels of admissions as well. For example, we (Hedlund, Wilt, Nebel, Ashford, & Sternberg, 2006) have shown that the same principles can be applied in admissions to business schools, also with the result of increasing prediction and decreasing ethnic (as well as gender) group differences. Another study (Stemler, Grigorenko, Jarvin, & Sternberg, 2006) has found that including creative and practical items in augmented Advanced Placement psychology and statistics examinations can reduce ethnic group differences on the tests. Comparable results were found for the Advanced Placement physics examination (Stemler, Sternberg, Grigorenko, Jarvin, & Sharpes, 2009). And the same principles are being employed in a test for assessing the abilities of students in elementary school Chart, Grigorenko, & Sternberg, 2008).

It is one thing to have a successful research project, and another actually to implement the procedures in a high-stakes situation. We have had the opportunity to do so. The results of a second project, Project Kaleidoscope, are reviewed here.

Project Kaleidoscope

Tufts University in Medford, Massachusetts, has strongly emphasized the role of active citizenship in education. It has put into practice some of the ideas from the Rainbow Project. In collaboration with Dean of Admissions Lee Coffin, we instituted Project Kaleidoscope, which represents an implementation of the ideas of the Rainbow Project, but goes beyond that project to include in its assessment the construct of wisdom (for more details, see Sternberg, 2007, 2010a, 2010b, 2010c).

For all of the over 15,000 students applying to the School of Arts and Sciences and the School of Engineering at Tufts, we placed on the 2006–2007 application questions designed to assess wisdom, (analytical and practical), intelligence, and creativity synthesized (WICS), an extension of the theory of successful intelligence (Sternberg, 2003b). The program still continues, but the data reported here are for the first year, for which we have more nearly complete data (see Sternberg, 2010a).

The WICS theory extends the theory of successful intelligence on the basis of the notion that some people may be academically and even practically intelligent, but unwise—as in the case of corporate scandals such as those that have surrounded Enron, Worldcom, and Arthur Andersen, and in the case of numerous political scandals as well. In all these instances, the perpetrators were smart, well educated, and foolish. The conception of wisdom used here is the balance theory of wisdom (Sternberg, 2003b), according to which wisdom is the application of intelligence, creativity, and knowledge for the common good, by balancing intrapersonal, interpersonal, and extrapersonal interests over the long and short terms, through the infusion of positive ethical values.

The questions are optional. Whereas the Rainbow Project was done as a separate set of high-stakes tests administered with a proctor, Project Kaleidoscope was done as a section of the Tufts-specific supplement to the Common Application. It just was not practical to administer a separate high-stakes test battery such as the Rainbow measures for admission to one university. Moreover, the advantage of Project Kaleidoscope is that it got us away from the high-stakes testing situation in which students must answer complex questions in very short amounts of time under incredible pressure.

Students were encouraged to answer just a single question, so as not overly to burden them. Tufts University competes for applications with many other universities, and if the Tufts application had been substantially more burdensome than those of competitor schools, it would have put Tufts at a real-world disadvantage in attracting applicants. In the theory of successful intelligence, individuals with such intelligence capitalize on strengths and compensate for or correct weaknesses. Our format gave students a chance to capitalize on a strength.

As examples of items, a creative question asked students to write stories with titles such as "The End of MTV" or "Confessions of a Middle-School Bully." Another creative question asked students what the world would be like if some historical event had come out differently—for example, if Rosa Parks had given up her seat on the bus. Yet another creative question, a nonverbal one, gave students an opportunity to design a new product or an advertisement for a new product. A practical question queried how students had persuaded friends of an unpopular idea they held. A wisdom question asked students how a passion they had could be applied toward a common good.

Creativity and practicality were assessed in the same way as in the Rainbow Project. Analytical quality was assessed by the organization, logic, and balance of the essay. Wisdom was assessed by the extent to which the response represented the use of abilities and knowledge for a common good by balancing one's own, others', and institutional in-

terests over the long and short terms through the infusion of positive ethical values.

Note that the goal was (and still is) not to replace the SAT and other traditional admissions measurements (e.g., GPA and class rank) with some new test. Rather, it was to reconceptualize applicants in terms of academic/analytical, creative, practical, and wisdom-based abilities, using the essays as one but not the only source of information. For example, highly creative work submitted in a portfolio could also be entered into the creativity rating, as could evidence of creativity through winning of prizes or awards. The essays were major sources of information, but if other information was available, the trained admissions officers used it.

We now have some results from our first year of implementation, and they are very promising. Applicants were evaluated for creative, practical, and wisdom-based skills, if sufficient evidence was available, as well as for academic (analytical) and personal qualities in general.

Among the applicants who were evaluated as being academically qualified for admission, approximately half completed an optional essay in the first year and two-thirds in later years. Doing these essays had no meaningful effect on chances of admissions. However, *quality* of essays or other evidence of creative, practical, or wisdom-based abilities did have an effect. For those applicants given an A (top rating) by a trained admission officer in any of these three categories, average rates of acceptance were roughly double those for applicants not getting an A. Because of the large number of essays (over 8,000), only one rater rated applicants except for a sample to ensure that inter-rater reliability was sufficient, which it was.

Many measures do not look like conventional standardized tests, but have statistical properties that mimic them. We were therefore interested in convergent–discriminant validation of our measures. The correlation of our measures with a rated academic composite that included SAT scores and high school GPA were modest but significant for creative thinking, practical thinking, and wise thinking. The correlations with a rating of quality of extracurricular participation and leadership were moderate for creative, practical, and wise thinking. Thus the pattern of convergent discriminant validation was what we had hoped for.

The average academic quality of applicants in the School of Arts and Sciences rose slightly in 2006–2007, the first year of the project, in terms of both SAT and high school GPA. In addition, there were notably fewer students in what before had been the bottom third of the pool in terms of academic quality. Many of those students, seeing the new application, seem to have decided not to bother to apply. Many more strong applicants applied.

Thus adopting these new methods does not seem to result in less qualified applicants applying to the institution and being admitted. Rather, the applicants who are admitted are *more* qualified, but in a broader way. Perhaps most rewarding were the positive comments from large numbers of applicants that they felt our application gave them a chance to show themselves for who they were. Of course, many factors are involved in admissions decisions, and Project Kaleidoscope ratings were only one small part of the overall picture.

We did not get meaningful differences across ethnic groups—a result that surprised us, given that the earlier Rainbow Project reduced but did not eliminate differences. And after a number of years in which applications by underrepresented minorities were relatively flat in terms of numbers, during 2006–2007 they went up substantially. In the end, applications from African Americans and Hispanic Americans increased significantly, and admissions of African Americans were up 30% and of Hispanic Americans up 15%. So the Project Kaleidoscope results, like those of the Rainbow Project, showed that it is possible to increase academic quality and diversity simultaneously, and to do so for an entire undergraduate class at a major university, not just for small samples of students at some scattered schools. Most importantly, we sent a message to students, parents, high school guidance counselors, and others that we believe there is more to a person than the narrow spectrum of skills assessed by standardized tests, and that these broader skills can be assessed in a quantifiable way.

BEYOND TRADITIONAL THEORIES OF INTELLIGENCE

The triarchic theory consists of three interrelated subtheories that attempt to account for the bases and manifestations of intelligent thought; as such, it represents an expanded view of intelligence that departs from traditional, general, and dichotomous theoretical perspectives. The componential subtheory relates intelligence to the internal world of the individual. The experiential subtheory relates intelligence to the experience of the individual with tasks and situations. The contextual subtheory relates intelligence to the external world of the individual. The elements of the three subtheories are interrelated: The components of intelligence are manifested at different levels of experience with tasks, and in situations of varying degrees of contextual relevance to a person's life. The components of intelligence are posited to be universal to intelligence; thus the components that contribute to intelligent performance in one culture do so in all other cultures as well. Moreover, the importance of dealing with novelty and the automatization of information processing to intelligence are posited to be universal. But the manifestations of these components in experience are posited to be relative to cultural contexts. What constitutes adaptive thought or behavior in one culture is not necessarily adaptive in another culture. Moreover, thoughts and actions that would shape behavior in appropriate ways in one context might not shape them in appropriate ways in another context. Finally, the environment one selects will depend largely on the available environments and on the fit of one's cognitive abilities, motivation, values, and affects to the available alternatives.

REFERENCES

Ackerman, P. L. (1987). Individual differences in skill learning: An integration of psychometric and information processing perspectives. *Psychological Bulletin, 102,* 3–27.

Bowen, W. G., & Bok, D. (2000). *The shape of the river: Long-term consequences of considering race in college and university admissions.* Princeton, NJ: Princeton University Press.

Bowen, W. G., Kurzweil, M. A., & Tobin, E. M. (2006). *Equity and excellence in American higher education.* Charlottesville: University of Virginia Press.

Brown, A. L. (1978). Knowing when, where, and how to remember: A problem of metacognition. In R. Glaser (Ed.), *Advances in instructional psychology* (Vol. 1, pp. 77–165). Hillsdale, NJ: Erlbaum.

Brown, A. L., Bransford, J., Ferrara, R., & Campione, J. (1983). Learning, remembering, and understanding. In P. H. Mussen (Series Ed.) & J. Flavell & E. Markman (Vol. Eds.), *Handbook of child psychology: Vol. 3. Cognitive development* (4th ed., pp. 77–166). New York: Wiley.

Butterfield, E. C., Wambold, C., & Belmont, J. M. (1973). On the theory and practice of improving short-term memory. *American Journal of Mental Deficiency, 77,* 654–669.

Campione, J. C., & Brown, A. L. (1979). Toward a theory of intelligence: Contributions from research with retarded children. In R. J. Sternberg & D. K. Detterman (Eds.), *Human intelligence: Perspectives on its theory and measurement* (pp. 139–164). Norwood, NJ: Ablex.

Carroll, J. B. (1993). *Human cognitive abilities: A survey of factor-analytic studies.* New York: Cambridge University Press.

Cattell, R. B. (1971). *Abilities: Their structure, growth, and action.* Boston: Houghton Mifflin.

Chart, H., Grigorenko, E. L., & Sternberg, R. J. (2008). Identification: The Aurora Battery. In J. A. Plucker & C. M. Callahan (Eds.), *Critical issues and practices in gifted education* (pp. 281–301). Waco, TX: Prufrock.

Chase, W. G., & Simon, H. A. (1973). The mind's eye in chess. In W. G. Chase (Ed.), *Visual information processing* (pp. 215–281). New York: Academic Press.

Chi, M. T. H. (1978). Knowledge structure and memory development. In R. S. Siegler (Ed.), *Children's thinking: What develops?* (pp. 73–96). Hillsdale, NJ: Erlbaum.

Cooper, L. A. (1982). Strategies for visual comparison and representation: Individual differences. In R. J. Sternberg (Ed.), *Advances in the psychology of human intelligence* (Vol. 1, pp. 77–124). Hillsdale, NJ: Erlbaum.

Cronbach, L. J., & Snow, R. E. (1977). *Aptitudes and instructional methods.* New York: Irvington.

Davidson, J. E., & Sternberg, R. J. (1984). The role of insight in intellectual giftedness. *Gifted Child Quarterly, 28,* 58–64.

Flavell, J. H. (1977). *Cognitive development.* Englewood Cliffs, NJ: Prentice-Hall.

Gardner, H. (2006). *Multiple intelligences: New horizons.* New York: Basic Books.

Gardner, H., Krechevsky, M., Sternberg, R. J., & Okagaki, L. (1994). Intelligence in context: Enhancing students' practical intelligence for school. In K. McGilly (Ed.), *Classroom lessons: Integrating cognitive theory and classroom practice* (pp. 105–127). Cambridge, MA: Bradford Books.

Gelman, R., & Gallistel, C. R. (1978). *The child's understanding of number.* Cambridge, MA: Harvard University Press.

Gladwin, T. (1970). *East is a big bird.* Cambridge, MA: Harvard University Press.

Grigorenko, E. L., Jarvin, L., & Sternberg, R. J. (2002). School-based tests of the triarchic theory of intelligence: Three settings, three samples, three syllabi. *Contemporary Educational Psychology, 27,* 167–208.

Heath, S. B. (1983). *Ways with words: Language, life, and work in communities and classrooms.* New York: Cambridge University Press.

Hedlund, J., Wilt, J. M., Nebel, K. R., Ashford, S. J., & Sternberg, R. J. (2006). Assessing practical intelligence in business school admissions: A supplement to the Graduate Management Admissions Test. *Learning and Individual Differences, 16,* 101–127.

Hunt, E., & Carlson, J. (2007). Considerations relating to the study of group differences in intelligence. *Perspectives on Psychological Science, 2,* 194–213.

Hunt, E. B. (1978). Mechanics of verbal ability. *Psychological Review, 85,* 109–130.

Hunt, E. B. (1980). Intelligence as an information-processing concept. *British Journal of Psychology, 71,* 449–474.

Hunt, E. B., & Lansman, M. (1982). Individual differences in attention. In R. J. Sternberg (Ed.), *Advances in the psychology of human intelligence* (Vol. 1, pp. 207–254). Hillsdale, NJ: Erlbaum.

Jensen, A. R. (1980). *Bias in mental testing.* New York: Free Press.

Jensen, A. R. (1982). The chronometry of intelligence. In R. J. Sternberg (Ed.), *Advances in the psychology of human intelligence* (Vol. I, pp. 255–310). Hillsdale, NJ: Erlbaum.

Jensen, A. R. (1998). *The g factor.* Westport, CT: Praeger.

Kanfer, R., & Ackerman, P. L. (1989). Dynamics of skill acquisition: Building a bridge between intelligence and motivation. In R. J. Sternberg (Ed.), *Advances in the psychology of human intelligence* (Vol. 5, pp. 83–134). Hillsdale, NJ: Erlbaum.

Kearins, J. M. (1981). Visual spatial memory in Australian Aboriginal children of desert regions. *Cognitive Psychology, 13,* 434–460.

Keil, F. C. (1984). Transition mechanisms in cognitive development and the structure of knowledge. In R. J. Sternberg (Ed.), *Mechanisms of cognitive development* (pp. 81–99). San Francisco: Freeman.

Kosslyn, S. M., & Koenig, O. (1995). *Wet mind: The new cognitive neuroscience.* New York: Free Press.

Lemann, N. (1999). *The big test: The secret history of the American meritocracy.* New York: Farrar, Straus & Giroux.

MacLeod, C. M., Hunt, E. B., & Mathews, N. N. (1978). Individual differences in the verification of sentence–picture relationships. *Journal of Verbal Learning and Verbal Behavior, 17,* 493–507.

Mayer, R. E., & Greeno, J. G. (1972). Structural differences between learning outcomes produces by different instructional methods. *Journal of Educational Psychology, 63,* 165–173.

Milgram, S. (1974). *Obedience to authority.* New York: Harper & Row.

Mulholland, T. M., Pellegrino, J. W., & Glaser, R. (1980). Components of geometric analogy solution. *Cognitive Psychology, 12*, 252–284.

Neisser, U. (1982). *Memory observed.* New York: Freeman.

Newell, A., & Simon, H. A. (1972). *Human problem solving.* Englewood Cliffs, NJ: Prentice-Hall.

Pellegrino, J. W., & Glaser, R. (1979). Cognitive correlates and components in the analysis of individual differences. In R. J. Sternberg & D. K. Detterman (Eds.), *Human intelligence: Perspectives on its theory and measurement* (pp. 61–88). Norwood, NJ: Ablex.

Pellegrino, J. W., & Kail, R. (1982). Process analyses of spatial aptitude. In R. J. Sternberg (Ed.), *Advances in the psychology of human intelligence* (Vol. 1, pp. 311–365). Hillsdale, NJ: Erlbaum.

Raaheim, K. (1974). *Problem solving and intelligence.* Oslo: Universitetsforlaget.

Resnick, L. B., & Glaser, R. (1976). Problem solving and intelligence. In L. B. Resnick (Ed.), *The nature of intelligence* (pp. 205–230). Hillsdale, NJ: Erlbaum.

Rushton, J. P., & Jensen, A. R. (2005). Thirty years of research on race differences in cognitive ability. *Psychology, Public Policy, and Law, 11*, 235–294.

Schank, R. C. (1980). How much intelligence is there in artificial intelligence? *Intelligence, 4*, 1–14.

Schank, R. C., & Abelson, R. P. (1977). *Scripts, plans, goals, and understanding.* Hillsdale, NJ: Erlbaum.

Schmidt, F. L., & Hunter, J. E. (1998). The validity and utility of selection methods in personnel psychology: Practical and theoretical implications of 85 years of research findings. *Psychological Bulletin, 124*, 262–274.

Siegler, R. S. (1986). Unities across domains in children's strategy choices. In M. Perlmutter (Ed.), *The Minnesota Symposia on Child Psychology: Vol. 19. Perspectives on intellectual development* (pp. 1–48). Hillsdale, NJ: Erlbaum.

Simon, H. A., & Reed, S. K. (1976). Modeling strategy shifts in a problem solving task. *Cognitive Psychology, 8*, 86–97.

Snow, R. E. (1980). Aptitude processes. In R. E. Snow, P. A. Frederico, & W. E. Montague (Eds.), *Aptitude, learning, and instruction: Cognitive process analyses of aptitude* (Vol. 1, pp. 27–63). Hillsdale, NJ: Erlbaum.

Snow, R. E., Kyllonen, P. C., & Marshalek, B. (1984). The topography of ability and learning correlations. In R. J. Sternberg (Ed.), *Advances in the psychology of human intelligence* (Vol. 2, pp. 47–103). Hillsdale, NJ: Erlbaum.

Snow, R. E., & Lohman, D. F. (1984). Toward a theory of cognitive aptitude for learning from instruction. *Journal of Educational Psychology, 76*, 347–376.

Stemler, S., Sternberg, R. J., Grigorenko, E. L., Jarvin, L., & Sharpes, D. K. (2009). Using the theory of successful intelligence as a framework for developing assessments in AP Physics. *Contemporary Educational Psychology, 34*, 195–209.

Stemler, S. E., Grigorenko, E. L., Jarvin, L., & Sternberg, R. J. (2006). Using the theory of successful intelligence as a basis for augmenting AP exams in psychology and statistics. *Contemporary Educational Psychology, 31*(2), 344–376.

Sternberg, R. J. (1977). *Intelligence, information processing, and analogical reasoning: The componential analysis of human abilities.* Hillsdale, NJ: Erlbaum.

Sternberg, R. J. (1979). The nature of mental abilities. *American Psychologist, 34*, 214–230.

Sternberg, R. J. (1981). Intelligence and nonentrenchment. *Journal of Educational Psychology, 73*, 1–16.

Sternberg, R. J. (1982). Reasoning, problem solving, and intelligence. In R. J. Sternberg (Ed.), *Handbook of human intelligence* (pp. 225–307). New York: Cambridge University Press.

Sternberg, R. J. (1983). Components of human intelligence. *Cognition, 15*, 1–48.

Sternberg, R. J. (1985a). *Beyond IQ: A triarchic theory of human intelligence.* New York: Cambridge University Press.

Sternberg, R. J. (1985b). Implicit theories of intelligence, creativity, and wisdom. *Journal of Personality and Social Psychology, 49*, 607–627.

Sternberg, R. J. (1987). Most vocabulary is learned from context. In M. G. McKeown & M. E. Curtis (Eds.), *The nature of vocabulary acquisition* (pp. 89–105). Hillsdale, NJ: Erlbaum.

Sternberg, R. J. (1988). *The triarchic mind: A new theory of human intelligence.* New York: Viking.

Sternberg, R. J. (1990). *Metaphors of mind.* New York: Cambridge University Press.

Sternberg, R. J. (1993). *Sternberg Triarchic Abilities Test.* Unpublished test.

Sternberg, R. J. (1995). *In search of the human mind.* Fort Worth, TX: Harcourt Brace.

Sternberg, R. J. (1997). *Successful intelligence.* New York: Plume.

Sternberg, R. J. (1998). Abilities are forms of developing expertise. *Educational Researcher, 27*(3), 17–20.

Sternberg, R. J. (1999). The theory of successful intelligence. *Review of General Psychology, 3*, 292–316.

Sternberg, R. J. (Ed.). (2000). *Handbook of intelligence.* New York: Cambridge University Press.

Sternberg, R. J. (2003a). Construct validity of the theory of successful intelligence. In R. J. Sternberg, J. Lautrey, & T. I. Lubart (Eds.), *Models of intelligence: International perspectives* (pp. 55–80). Washington, DC: American Psychological Association.

Sternberg, R. J. (2003b). *Wisdom, intelligence, and cre-*

ativity synthesized. New York: Cambridge University Press.

Sternberg, R. J. (2004). Culture and intelligence. *American Psychologist, 59*(5), 325–338.

Sternberg, R. J. (2005a). The theory of successful intelligence. *Interamerican Journal of Psychology, 39*(2), 189–202.

Sternberg, R. J. (2005b). The triarchic theory of successful intelligence. In D. P. Flanagan & P. L. Harrison (Eds.), *Contemporary intellectual assessment* (2nd ed., pp. 103–119). New York: Guilford Press.

Sternberg, R. J. (2007). Finding students who are wise, practical, and creative. *Chronicle of Higher Education, 53*(44), B11.

Sternberg, R. J. (2008). Successful intelligence as a framework for understanding cultural adaptation. In S. Ang & L. Van Dyne (Eds.), *Handbook on cultural intelligence* (pp. 306–317). New York: Sharpe.

Sternberg, R. J. (2009). The theory of successful intelligence as a basis for new forms of ability testing at the high school, college, and graduate school levels. In J. C. Kaufman (Ed.), *Intelligent testing: Integrating psychological theory and clinical practice* (pp. 113–147). New York: Cambridge University Press.

Sternberg, R. J. (2010a). *College admissions for the 21st century*. Cambridge, MA: Harvard University Press.

Sternberg, R. J. (2010b). WICS: A new model for cognitive education. *Journal of Cognitive Education and Psychology, 9*, 34–46.

Sternberg, R. J. (2010c). WICS: A new model for school psychology. *School Psychology International, 31*(6), 599–616.

Sternberg, R. J., & Clinkenbeard, P. R. (1995). The triarchic model applied to identifying, teaching, and assessing gifted children. *Roeper Review, 17*(4), 255–260.

Sternberg, R. J., & Davidson, J. E. (1982, June). The mind of the puzzler. *Psychology Today*, pp. 37–44.

Sternberg, R. J., Ferrari, M., Clinkenbeard, P. R., & Grigorenko, E. L. (1996). Identification, instruction, and assessment of gifted children: A construct validation of a triarchic model. *Gifted Child Quarterly, 40*, 129–137.

Sternberg, R. J., Forsythe, G. B., Hedlund, J., Horvath, J., Snook, S, Williams, W. M., et al. (2000). *Practical intelligence in everyday life*. New York: Cambridge University Press.

Sternberg, R. J., & Gardner, M. K. (1982). A componential interpretation of the general factor in human intelligence. In H. J. Eysenck (Ed.), *A model for intelligence* (pp. 231–254). Berlin: Springer-Verlag.

Sternberg, R. J., & Grigorenko, E. L. (Eds.). (2002). *The general factor of intelligence: How general is it?* Mahwah, NJ: Erlbaum.

Sternberg, R. J., & Grigorenko, E. L. (2004). Successful intelligence in the classroom. *Theory into Practice, 43*(4), 274–280.

Sternberg, R. J., & Grigorenko, E. L. (2007). *Teaching for successful intelligence* (2nd ed.). Thousand Oaks, CA: Corwin Press.

Sternberg, R. J., Grigorenko, E. L., Ferrari, M., & Clinkenbeard, P. (1999). A triarchic analysis of an aptitude–treatment interaction. *European Journal of Psychological Assessment, 15*, 1–11.

Sternberg, R. J., Grigorenko, E. L., & Kidd, K. K. (2005). Intelligence, race, and genetics. *American Psychologist, 60*(1), 46–59.

Sternberg, R. J., Grigorenko, E. L., & Zhang, L.-F. (2008). Styles of learning and thinking matter in instruction and assessment. *Perspectives on Psychological Science, 3*(6), 486–506.

Sternberg, R. J., Jarvin, L., & Grigorenko, E. L. (2009). *Teaching for wisdom, intelligence, creativity, and success*. Thousand Oaks, CA: Corwin Press.

Sternberg, R. J., Jarvin, L., & Grigorenko, E. L. (2011). *Explorations of giftedness*. New York: Cambridge University Press.

Sternberg, R. J., & Ketron, J. L. (1982). Selection and implementation of strategies in reasoning by analogy. *Journal of Educational Psychology, 74*, 399–413.

Sternberg, R. J., Nokes, K., Geissler, P. W., Prince, R., Okatcha, F., Bundy, D. A., et al. (2001). The relationship between academic and practical intelligence: A case study in Kenya. *Intelligence, 29*, 401–418.

Sternberg, R. J., Okagaki, L., & Jackson, A. (1990). Practical intelligence for success in school. *Educational Leadership, 48*, 35–39.

Sternberg, R. J., & Powell, J. S. (1983). Comprehending verbal comprehension. *American Psychologist, 38*, 878–893.

Sternberg, R. J., & the Rainbow Project Collaborators. (2005). Augmenting the SAT through assessments of analytical, practical, and creative skills. In W. Camara & E. Kimmel (Eds.). *Choosing students: Higher education admission tools for the 21st century* (pp. 159–176). Mahwah, NJ: Erlbaum.

Sternberg, R. J., & the Rainbow Project Collaborators. (2006). The Rainbow Project: Enhancing the SAT through assessments of analytical, practical and creative skills. *Intelligence, 34*(4), 321–350.

Sternberg, R. J., & Rifkin, B. (1979). The development of analogical reasoning processes. *Journal of Experimental Child Psychology, 27*, 195–232.

Sternberg, R. J., Torff, B., & Grigorenko, E. L. (1998). Teaching triarchically improves school achievement. *Journal of Educational Psychology, 90*, 374–384.

Sternberg, R. J., & Weil, E. M. (1980). An aptitude–strategy interaction in linear syllogistic reasoning. *Journal of Educational Psychology, 72*, 226–234.

Super, C. M., & Harkness, S. (1982). The infants' niche in rural Kenya and metropolitan America. In L. L. Adler (Ed.), *Cross-cultural research at issue* (pp. 47–55). New York: Academic Press.

Turkheimer, E., Haley, A., Waldron, M., D'Onofrio, B., & Gottesman, I. I. (2003). Socioeconomic status modifies heritability of IQ in young children. *Psychological Science, 14*(6), 623–628.

Vernon, P. E. (1971). *The structure of human abilities.* London: Methuen.

Vygotsky, L. S. (1978). *Mind in society: The development of higher psychological processes* (M. Cole, V. John-Steiner, S. Scribner, & E. Souberman, Eds. & Trans.). Cambridge, MA: Harvard University Press.

Wagner, R. K., & Sternberg, R. J. (1987). Executive control in reading comprehension. In B. K. Britton & S. M. Glynn (Eds.), *Executive control processes in reading* (pp. 1–21). Hillsdale, NJ: Erlbaum.

Williams, W. M., Blythe, T., White, N., Li, J., Gardner, H., & Sternberg, R. J. (2002). Practical intelligence for school: Developing metacognitive sources of achievement in adolescence. *Developmental Review, 22*, 162–210.

CHAPTER 7

Planning, Attention, Simultaneous, Successive
A Cognitive-Processing-Based Theory of Intelligence

Jack A. Naglieri
J. P. Das
Sam Goldstein

Practitioners and test authors have become increasingly conscious of the need for theory-based intelligence tests (Lidz, 1991). There is also an increasing recognition that psychological processes should be measured especially in order to make better diagnostic and instructional decisions (Naglieri & Otero, 2011). The Planning, Attention, Simultaneous, and Successive (PASS) cognitive-processing-based theory of intelligence as measured by the Cognitive Assessment System (CAS; Naglieri & Das, 1997a) fulfills that need.

The development of processing-based intelligence tests began with the original Kaufman Assessment Battery for Children (K-ABC; Kaufman & Kaufman, 1983). Alan and Nadeen Kaufman published the first measure of intelligence that was conceptualized and well developed with an emphasis on cognitive processing rather than traditional general ability. The second intelligence test to be specifically developed from a neuropsychological perspective on ability was the CAS (Naglieri & Das, 1997a; see Naglieri & Otero, 2011). These tests marked a change from the traditional verbal–nonverbal organizational approach used since the Army mental testing program described by Yoakum and Yerkes (1920) nearly 100 years ago. The K-ABC and CAS brought about an evolution

in the field of intelligence testing by emphasizing (1) that a *test* of intelligence should be based on a *theory* of intelligence; and (2) that the test should measure basic psychological processes defined by the intellectual demands of the test, not the content of the questions (e.g., verbal or nonverbal). This raises two important issues: What is a theory, and what is a cognitive process?

IQ tests have been devoid of a theoretical foundation since they were first introduced more than 100 years ago (Naglieri & Kaufman, 2008). In recent years, considerable efforts have been made to reconceptualize already published tests within some theoretical framework. For example, both the Stanford–Binet Intelligence Scales, Fifth Edition (Roid, 2003) and the Differential Ability Scales—Second Edition (Elliott, 2007) have been linked to the Cattell–Horn–Carroll (CHC) view of intelligence. Luria's neuropsychological theory provided the foundation of the PASS theory used for the CAS, and the KABC-II is based on both theoretical models (Luria's theory and the CHC model). Clearly, in recent years, test authors have been making efforts either to build tests on a theory of intelligence or to attach a theory to a test. In either case, the field of IQ testing has evolved considerably in the past 30 years.

ORIGINS OF THE PASS THEORY

The PASS theory (Naglieri & Das, 1997a) is rooted in the work of A. R. Luria (1966, 1973a, 1973b, 1980) on the functional aspects of brain structures. Naglieri and Das used Luria's work as a blueprint for defining the important components of human intelligence (Das, Naglieri, & Kirby, 1994; Naglieri & Das, 1997a) because they strongly believed that a test of intelligence should be based on a theory of intelligence, and that a theory of intelligence should be based on an understanding of basic psychological processes. Their efforts represented the first time that a specific researched neuropsychological theory was used to reconceptualize the concept of human intelligence and provide a specific tool to measure that theory.

Luria theorized that human cognitive functions can be conceptualized within a framework of three separate but related "functional units" that provide four basic psychological processes. The three brain systems are referred to as *functional units* because the neuropsychological mechanisms work in separate but interrelated systems. Luria (1973b) stated that "each form of conscious activity is always a complex functional system and takes place through the combined working of all three brain units, each of which makes its own contribution" (p. 99). The four processes form a "working constellation" (Luria, 1966, p. 70) of cognitive activity. A person may therefore perform the same task with different contributions of the PASS processes, along with the application of the person's knowledge and skills.

Although effective functioning is accomplished through the integration of all processes as demanded by the particular task, not every process is equally involved in every task. For example, tasks like math calculation may be dominated by a single process (e.g., planning), while tasks such as reading decoding may be strongly related to another process (e.g., successive). Effective functioning—for example, processing of visual information—also involves three hierarchical levels of the brain. Consistent with structural topography, these can be described in the following manner. First, there is the *projection area*, where the modality characteristic of the information is important. Above the projection area is the *association area*, where information loses part of its association with a particular modality. Above the association area is the *overlapping zone*, where information is no longer modality-specific. This enables information to be integrated from various senses and processed at a

higher level. Thus modality is most important at the level of initial reception, and less important at the level where information is integrated.

Description of the Three Functional Units

The function of the first unit provides regulation of cortical arousal and attention; the second codes information using simultaneous and successive processes; and the third provides for strategy development, strategy use, self-monitoring, and control of cognitive activities.

According to Luria (1973b), the first of these three functional units of the brain, the attention–arousal system, is located primarily in the brainstem, the diencephalon, and the medial regions of the cortex. This unit provides the brain with the appropriate level of arousal or cortical tone, as well as directive and selective attention. When many stimuli are presented to a person who is then required to pay attention to only one stimulus, the inhibition of responding to other (often more salient) stimuli and the focus of attention to the target stimulus, depends on the first functional unit. Luria stated that optimal conditions of arousal are needed before the more complex forms of attention, involving "selective recognition of a particular stimulus and inhibition of responses to irrelevant stimuli" (p. 271), can occur. Moreover, only when individuals are sufficiently aroused and their attention is adequately focused can they utilize processes in the second and third functional units.

The second functional unit is associated with the occipital, parietal, and temporal lobes posterior to the central sulcus of the brain. This unit is responsible for receiving, processing, and retaining information the person obtains from the external world. This unit involves simultaneous processing and successive processes. Simultaneous processing involves integrating stimuli into groups so that the interrelationships among the components are understood. For example, in order for a person to produce a diagram correctly when given the instruction "Draw a triangle above a square that is to the left of a circle under a cross," the relationships among the different shapes must be correctly comprehended. Whereas simultaneous processing involves working with stimuli that are interrelated, successive processing involves information that is linearly organized and integrated into a chain-like progression. For example, successive processing is involved in the production of sequences of sounds used to make words, decoding of unfamiliar words, production of syntactic aspects of language, and speech articulation. Following a sequence such as the order of operations in a math problem is another example of successive processing. In contrast, simultaneous processing involves integration of separate elements into groups.

The third functional unit is associated with the prefrontal areas of the frontal lobes of the brain (Luria, 1980). Luria stated that "the frontal lobes synthesize the information about the outside world . . . and are the means whereby the behavior of the organism is regulated in conformity with the effect produced by its actions" (1980, p. 263). This unit provides for the programming, regulation, and verification of behavior, and is responsible for behaviors such as asking questions, solving problems, and self-monitoring (Luria, 1973b). Other responsibilities of the third functional unit include the regulation of voluntary activity, conscious impulse control, and various linguistic skills such as spontaneous conversation. The third functional unit provides for the most complex aspects of human behavior, including personality and consciousness (Das, 1980).

Functional Units: Influences and Issues

Luria's organization of the brain into functional units accounts for cultural influences on higher cognition as well as biological factors. He stated that "perception and memorizing, gnosis and praxis, speech and thinking, writing, reading and arithmetic, cannot be regarded as isolated or even indivisible 'faculties'" (1973b, p. 29). That is, we cannot, as phrenologists attempted to do, identify a "writing" spot in the brain; instead, we must consider the concept of units of the brain that provide a function. Luria (1973b) described the advantage of this approach:

> It is accordingly our fundamental task not to "localize" higher human psychological processes in limited areas of the cortex, but to ascertain by careful analysis which groups of concertedly working zones of the brain are responsible for the performance of complex mental activity; when contributions made by each of these zones to the complex functional system; and how the relationship between these concertedly working parts of the brain in the performance of complex mental activity changes in the various stages of its development. (p. 34)

Activities such as reading and writing can be analyzed and linked as constellations of activities

to specific working zones of the brain that support them (Luria, 1979, p. 141). Because the brain operates as an integrated functional system, however, even a small disturbance in an area can cause disorganization in the entire functional system (Das & Varnhagen, 1986).

Luria's concept of dynamic functional units provides the foundation for PASS processes. These basic psychological processes are firmly based on biological correlates, yet develop within a sociocultural milieu. In other words, they are influenced in part by a person's cultural experiences. Luria (1979) noted that "the child learns to organize his memory and to bring it under voluntary control through the use of the mental tools of his culture" (p. 83). Kolb, Gibb, and Robinson (2003) have also noted that although "the brain was once seen as a rather static organ, it is now clear that the organization of brain circuitry is constantly changing as a function of experience" (p. 1). Similarly, Stuss and Benson (1990) recognize this interplay and especially the use of speech as a regulatory function when they state:

> The adult regulates the child's behavior by command, inhibiting irrelevant responses. The child learns to speak, the spoken instruction shared between the child and adult are taken over by the child, who uses externally stated and often detailed instructions to guide his or her own behavior. By the age of 4 to 4½, a trend towards internal and contract speech (inner speech) gradually appears. The child begins to regulate and subordinate his behavior according to his/ her speech. Speech, in addition to serving communication thought, becomes a major self-regulatory force, creating systems of connections for organizing active behavior inhibiting actions irrelevant to the task at hand. (p. 34)

Luria stressed the role of the frontal lobes in language, organization, and direction of behavior and speech as a cultural tool that furthers the development of the frontal lobes and self-regulation. Cultural experiences thus actually help to accelerate the utilization of planning and self-regulation, as well as the other cognitive processes.

Luria (1979) also points out that abstraction and generalizations are themselves products of the cultural environment. Children learn, for example, to attend selectively to relevant objects through playful experiences and conversations with adults. Even simultaneous and successive processes are influenced by cultural experiences (e.g., learning songs, poems, rules of games, etc.). Naglieri (2003) has summarized the influence of social interaction on children's use of plans and strategies, and the resulting changes in performance on classroom tasks.

The relationship between the third and first functional units is particularly strong. The first functional unit works in cooperation with, and is regulated by, higher systems of the cerebral cortex, which receive and process information from the external world and determine an individual's dynamic activity (Luria, 1973b). In other words, this unit has a reciprocal relationship with the cortex. It influences the tone of the cortex and is itself influenced by the regulatory effects of the cortex. This is possible through the ascending and descending systems of the reticular formation, which transmit impulses from lower parts of the brain to the cortex and vice versa (Luria, 1973b). For the PASS theory, this means that attention and planning are necessarily strongly related because attention is often under the conscious control of planning. That is, our planning of behavior dictates the allocation of our limited attentional resources. This also helps explain how these two components of the theory can be related to the concept of *executive function*.

Although there is not yet a consensus-based definition of executive function, most theorists agree that this is an ability that is necessary for purposeful behavior so that goals are achieved. The frontal lobes (especially the dorsolateral and the ventromedial regions), in combination with midbrain structures in the basal ganglia and the cerebellum, are a key to efficient executive functioning. Tasks that measure this cognitive process should be relatively unfamiliar, so that the examinee has to develop a way to solve the problem; should call for self-monitoring and error correction; could involve selective attention in settings where a highly learned response has to be inhibited; and should draw upon methods of working with information that needs to be remembered over a short period of time. All these attributes are contained in the planning and attention constructs of PASS theory as measured by the CAS Planning and Attention scales.

The Three Functional Units and PASS Theory

Luria's concept of the three functional units as the basis of PASS theory is diagrammatically shown in Figure 7.1. Although rendering a complex functional system in two-dimensional space has its limitations, the diagram illustrates some of the im-

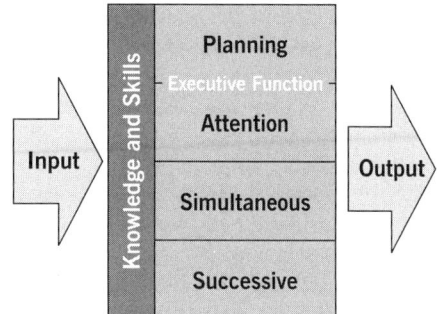

FIGURE 7.1. Diagram of the PASS theory of intelligence. Copyright 2011 by Jack A. Naglieri.

portant characteristics of the PASS theory. First, an important component of the theory is the role of a person's fund of information. Knowledge and skills are a part of each of the processes because past experiences, learning, emotions, and motivations provide the background as well as the sources for the information to be processed. This information is received from external sources through the sense organs. The information may involve memory, or perception, or thinking (Das, Kirby, Jarman, 1975, 1979), but all will be analyzed according to the processing demand(s) of the task. When that sensory information is sent to the brain for analysis, central processes become active. However, internal cognitive information in the form of images, memory, and thoughts becomes part of the input as well. Thus the four processes operate within the context of an individual's knowledge base and cannot operate outside the context of knowledge. "Cognitive processes rely on (and influence) the base of knowledge, which may be temporary (as in immediate memory) or more long term (that is, knowledge that is well learned)" (Naglieri & Das, 1997c, p. 145). Cognitive processing also influences knowledge acquisition, and learning can influence cognitive processing. Both are also influenced by membership in particular social and cultural milieus (Das & Abbott, 1995, p. 158). The importance of knowledge is therefore integral to the PASS theory. A person may read English very well and have good PASS processes, but may falter when required to read Japanese text—due to a deficient knowledge of Japanese, rather than a processing deficit.

A cognitive process is described by Naglieri (2011) as a "foundational, neuropsychologically identified ability that provides the means by which an individual functions in this world" (p. 147). He goes on to clarify that cognitive processes underlie all mental and physical activity, and that the application of cognitive processes allows for the acquisition of all types of knowledge and skills. However, it is very important to recognize that knowledge and skills are not examples of basic psychological processes, but instead the results of the application of these processing abilities. It is also important to recognize that cognitive processes should be defined on the basis of a coherent theory that has been proposed, operationalized, tested, and shown to have reliability and validity. In the next section we describe a theory of intelligence grounded in cognitive and neuropsychological psychology and to demonstrate its validity.

Planning is a frontal lobe function. More specifically, it is associated with the prefrontal cortex and is one of the main abilities that distinguishes humans from other primates. The prefrontal cortex

> plays a central role in forming goals and objectives, and then in devising plans of action required to attain these goals. It selects the cognitive skills required to implement the plans, coordinates these skills, and applies them in a correct order. Finally, the prefrontal cortex is responsible for evaluating our actions as success or failure relative to our intentions. (Goldberg, 2001, p. 24)

Planning therefore helps us select or develop the plans or strategies needed to complete tasks for which a solution is needed, and is critical to all activities where a child or adult has to determine how to solve a problem. It includes generation, evaluation, and execution of a plan, as well as self-monitoring and impulse control. Thus planning allows for the solution of problems; the control of attention, simultaneous, and successive processes; and selective utilization of knowledge and skills (Das, Kar, & Parrila, 1996).

Attention is a mental process that is closely related to the orienting response. The base of the brain allows the organism to direct focused, selective attention toward a stimulus over time and to resist loss of attention to other stimuli. The longer attention is required, the more the activity is one that demands vigilance. Attention is controlled by intentions and goals, and involves knowledge and skills as well as the other PASS processes.

Simultaneous processing is essential for organization of information into groups or a coherent whole. The parietal, occipital, and temporal brain regions provide a critical "ability" to see patterns as interrelated elements. Because of the strong spatial characteristics of most simultaneous tasks, there is a strong visual–spatial dimension to activities that demand this type of processing. Simultaneous processing, however, is not limited to nonverbal content, as illustrated by the important role it plays in the grammatical components of language and comprehension of word relationships, prepositions, and inflections.

Successive processing is involved in the use of stimuli arranged in a specific serial order. Whenever information must be remembered or completed in a specific order, successive processing will be involved. Importantly, however, the information must not be able to be organized into a pattern (e.g., the number 9933811 organized into 99-33-8-11); instead, each element can only be related to those that precede it. Successive processing is usually involved with the serial organization of sounds and movements in order. It is therefore integral to, for example, working with sounds in sequence and early reading.

The PASS theory is an alternative to approaches to intelligence that have traditionally included verbal, nonverbal, and quantitative tests. Not only does this theory expand the view of what "abilities" should be measured, but it also puts emphasis on basic psychological processes and precludes the use of verbal achievement-like tests such as vocabulary. In addition, the PASS theory is an alternative to the notion of a general intelligence. Instead, the functions of the brain are considered the building blocks of ability conceptualized within a cognitive processing framework. Although the theory may have its roots in neuropsychology, "its branches are spread over developmental and educational psychology" (Das & Varnhagen, 1986, p. 130), as well as over neurological dysfunctions. Thus the PASS theory of cognitive processing, with its links to developmental and neuropsychology, provides an advantage in explanatory power over the notion of general intelligence (Naglieri & Das, 2002).

OPERATIONALIZATION AND APPLICATION OF THE THEORY

The PASS theory is operationalized by the CAS (Naglieri & Das, 1997a) and the forthcoming CAS-2 (Naglieri, Das, & Goldstein, 2012). This instrument is amply described in the CAS interpretive handbook (Naglieri & Das, 1997b) and by Naglieri and Otero in Chapter 15 of the present book.

Naglieri and Das (1997a) generated tests to measure the theory, following a systematic and empirically based test development program designed to obtain efficient measures of the processes that could be individually administered. The PASS theory was used as the foundation of the CAS, so the content of the test was determined by the theory and not influenced by previous views of ability. This is further elaborated in Chapter 15 of this book.

EMPIRICAL SUPPORT FOR THE THEORY

Dillon (1986) suggested six criteria (validity, diagnosis, prescription, comparability, replicability/standardizability, and psychodiagnostic utility) for evaluation of a theory of cognitive processing. Naglieri (1989) evaluated the PASS model on these criteria, using the information available at that time; in this chapter, we use the same criteria to evaluate the current status of the PASS theory as operationalized by the CAS. This section includes summaries of research due to space limitations, but additional information is provided in Chapter 15 of this text and in other resources (Naglieri, 1999, 2003; Naglieri & Das, 1997b).

Validity

The fundamental validity of the PASS theory is rooted in the neuropsychological work of Luria (1966, 1973a, 1973b, 1980, 1982), who associated areas of the brain with basic psychological processes as described earlier in this chapter. Luria's research was based on an extensive combination of his and other researchers' understanding of brain functions, amply documented in his book *The Working Brain* (1973b). Using Luria's three functional units as a backdrop, Das and colleagues (Das, 1972; Das et al., 1975, 1979; Das, Naglieri, & Kirby, 1994) initiated the task of finding ways to measure the PASS processes. These efforts included extensive analysis of the methods used by Luria, related procedures used within neuropsychology, experimental research in cognitive and educational psychology, and related areas. This work, subsequently summarized in several books (e.g., Das, Naglieri, & Kirby, 1994; Kirby, 1984; Kirby & Williams, 1991; Naglieri, 1999; Naglieri & Das, 1997b), demonstrated that the PASS processes associated with Luria's concept of the three functional units could be measured. This work

also illustrated that the theoretical conceptualization of basic psychological processes had considerable potential for application.

Initial studies of the validity of the PASS theory included basic and essential elements for a test of children's cognitive competence, such as developmental changes. Researchers found that performance on early versions of tests of these processes showed evidence of developmental differences by age for children of elementary and middle school ages (Das, 1972; Das & Molloy, 1975; Garofalo, 1986; Jarman & Das, 1977; Kirby & Das, 1978; Kirby & Robinson, 1987; Naglieri & Das, 1988, 1997b) and for high school and college samples (Ashman, 1982; Das & Heemsbergen, 1983; Naglieri & Das, 1988).

Naglieri, Das, and their colleagues have also demonstrated that the constructs represented in the PASS theory are strongly related to achievement. A full discussion of those results is provided by Naglieri and Otero in Chapter 15 of this book. The results demonstrate that the PASS constructs are strongly related to achievement, and the evidence thus far suggests that the theory is more strongly related to achievement than are other measures of ability. Importantly, despite the fact that the measures of PASS processes do not include achievement-like subtests (e.g., vocabulary and arithmetic), the evidence demonstrates the utility of the PASS theory as operationalized by the CAS for predication of academic performance. Because one purpose of the CAS is to anticipate levels of academic performance on the basis of levels of cognitive functioning, these results provide critical support for the theory.

Support for the theory's validity from a neuropsychological perspective is provided by research examining the PASS processes and brain function. For example, Luria initially described simultaneous processing as a function of the occipitoparietal region, whereas he described successive processing as a function of a frontotemporal region (each had a bilateral location). A recent experiment from Japan (Okuhata, Okazaki, & Maekawa, 2009) studied the two processes via electroencephalography. The researchers investigated patterns during six tasks of the CAS (Naglieri & Das, 1997a), three from the Simultaneous scale and three from the Successive scale. The results showed two significantly distinguishable coherence patterns corresponding to the two types of processing. Both processes are localized in the posterior part of the brain, as Luria suggested. Similarly, McCrea (2007) showed that simultaneous processing is strongly dependent on occipitoparietal activity, whereas successive processing shows frontotemporal specificity, with some evidence of interhemispheric coordination across the prefrontal cortex. McCrea's results provide support for the validity of the PASS composite scales. In addition, Christensen, Goldberg, and Bougakov (2009) have provided a substantive summary of brain imaging research that supports both Luria's conceptualizations and PASS theory.

Diagnosis

There are two important aims of diagnosis: first, to determine whether variations in characteristics help distinguish one group of children from another; and second, to determine whether these data help with intervention decisions. Prescription is discussed in the next section; the question of diagnosis is addressed here. One way to examine the utility of PASS cognitive profiles is by analysis of the frequency of PASS cognitive weaknesses for children in regular and special educational settings. It is important to note, however, that these studies look at PASS *scale* profiles—not *subtest* profiles, which have been the focus of profile analysis research in the past. A second way is to examine diagnostic utility is by examination of specific populations (e.g., children with attention-deficit/hyperactivity disorder [ADHD], autism, or learning disabilities). We summarize the relevant research in both areas below, beginning with discussion of specific populations.

Special Populations

Children with Reading Disabilities

The application of PASS theory and the CAS to understanding reading disabilities has important implications for diagnosing (and treating) reading disabilities (see Das, 2009, for a more complete discussion). Essentially, reading researchers generally agree that phonological skills play an important role in early reading, and some have suggested this to be the major cause of reading disability for children (Stanovich, 1988; Wagner, Torgesen, & Rashotte, 1994). One of the most frequently cited articles in the field, by Torgesen, Wagner, and Rashotte (1994), proposes that phonological skills are causally related to normal acquisition of reading skills. Support for this claim can also be found in the relationship between prereaders' phonological scores and their reading development 1–3 years

later (e.g., Bradley & Bryant, 1985). Moreover, Share and Stanovich (1995) concluded that there is strong evidence that poor readers, as a group, are impaired in a very wide range of basic tasks in the phonological domain. Das, Naglieri, and Kirby (1994) have suggested, however, that underlying a phonological skills deficit is a specific deficit in successive processing that leads to word-reading deficits.

Das, Mishra, and Kirby (1994) found that Successive scale scores from the CAS were better than a test of phonemic segmentation at distinguishing normal readers from children with dyslexia. Additional studies have since supported the hypothesis that in predicting reading disabilities, PASS processes are as important as phonological skills (Das, Parrila, & Papadopoulos, 2000). Several recent studies of Canadian First Nations children are particularly important. Das, Janzen, and Georgiou (2007) reported that successive processing made a unique contribution to predicting both word identification and reading pseudowords (word attack). Furthermore, the poor readers demonstrated a significant weakness on the CAS Successive scale, both in relation to the norm and in relation to their scores on the other three CAS scales. Similarly, Naglieri, Otero, DeLauder, and Matto (2007) reported Successive scale deficits for bilingual children with reading disabilities who were administered the CAS in English and Spanish. In addition, 90% of the children with reading disabilities had a cognitive weakness on both the English and Spanish versions of the CAS.

In contrast to the relationship between reading decoding and successive processing, disability in comprehension has been shown to be primarily related to deficits in simultaneous processing (Das et al., 1996; Das, Naglieri, & Kirby, 1994; Naglieri & Das, 1997c). In a recent study conducted with English-speaking children in India, Mahapatra, Das, Stack-Cutler, and Parrila (2010) found that children with comprehension problems had a substantially lower mean score on the CAS Simultaneous scale. These studies further suggest that PASS profiles could have utility for diagnosis of reading disabilities, as suggested by Naglieri (1999, 2000, 2011).

Children with ADHD

A deficit on the CAS Planning, not Attention, scale has been found for groups of children with a diagnosis of ADHD. This finding is consistent with Barkley's (1997) view that ADHD is actually a failure of self-control (i.e., planning in the PASS theory) rather than a failure of attention. The research in this area clearly confirms Barkley's view. For example, Naglieri, Goldstein, Iseman, and Schwebach (2003) examined CAS and Wechsler Intelligence Scale for Children—Third Edition (WISC-III) scores for children with ADHD. The results showed a large effect size for the Planning scale between the children with ADHD and the standardization sample, and a small effect size was found for the Attention scale. The differences between the two samples on the CAS Simultaneous and Successive scales were not significant. In regard to the WISC-III, the only difference that had a significant but small effect size was on the Processing Speed Index.

Naglieri, Salter, and Edwards (2004) confirmed the weakness of planning, but not attention, among children with ADHD. Participants in their study were 48 children (38 males and 10 females) referred to an ADHD clinic. The contrast group consisted of 48 children (38 males and 10 females) in regular education. The results indicated that the children in regular education settings earned mean PASS scale scores on the CAS that were all above average, ranging from 98.6 to 103.6. In contrast, the experimental group earned mean scores close to the norm on the CAS Attention, Simultaneous, and Successive scales (ranging from 97.4 to 104.0), but a significantly lower mean score on the Planning scale (90.3).

The low mean Planning score for the children with ADHD in these studies is consistent with the poor Planning performance reported in the previous research (Dehn, 2000; Naglieri et al., 2003; Paolitto, 1999) for children identified as having ADHD of the hyperactive–impulsive or combined types (Barkley, 1997). The consistency across these various studies suggests that some of these children have difficulty with planning rather than attention as measured by the CAS. Importantly, the PASS profiles of children with ADHD are different from those with reading decoding failure (low successive) and anxiety disorders (no distinctive PASS profile) (Naglieri & Conway, 2009). In addition, these findings suggest that determining whether a child with ADHD has a deficit in planning as measured by the CAS may be important for both diagnosis and intervention planning (Goldstein & Naglieri, 2006; Naglieri & Pickering, 2010).

These findings suggest that the PASS theory as operationalized by the CAS may have utility for differential diagnosis in reading disabilities and ADHD. The brain-related studies described in an earlier section go a step further in providing evidence for the validity of PASS constructs. Both kinds of research have implications for prescription that includes constructing intervention programs. We discuss prescription in a subsequent section.

PASS Profiles

Glutting, McDermott, Konold, Snelbaker, and Watkins (1998) have suggested that research concerning profiles for specific children is typically confounded because the "use of subtest profiles for both the initial formation of diagnostic groups and the subsequent search for profiles that might inherently define or distinguish those groups" (p. 601) results in methodological problems. They further suggested that researchers should "begin with unselected cohorts (i.e., representative samples, a proportion of which may be receiving special education), identify children with and without unusual subtest profiles, and subsequently compare their performance on external criteria" (p. 601). Naglieri (2000) has followed this research methodology, using the PASS theory and his (Naglieri, 1999) concepts of *relative weakness* and *cognitive weakness*.

Naglieri (1999) describes how to find disorders in one or more of the basic PASS processes as follows. A *relative weakness* is a significant weakness in relation to the child's mean PASS score, determined using the ipsative methodology originally proposed by Davis (1959) and modified by Silverstein (1982, 1993). A problem with this approach is that a child may have a significant weakness that falls within the average range if the majority of scores are above average. In contrast, a *cognitive weakness* is found when a child has a significant intraindividual difference on the PASS scale scores of the CAS (according to the ipsative method), and the lowest score *also* falls below some cutoff designed to indicate what is typical or average. The difference between a relative weakness and a cognitive weakness, therefore, is that the determination of a cognitive weakness is based on dual criteria (a low score relative to the child's mean and a low score relative to the norm group). Naglieri has further suggested that a cognitive weakness should be accompanied by an achievement test weakness comparable to the level of the PASS scale cognitive weakness. Children who have both a cognitive and an achievement test weakness should be considered candidates for special educational services if other appropriate conditions are also met (especially that the children's academic needs cannot be met in the regular educational environment).

Naglieri (2000) found that the relative-weakness method (the approach more commonly used in school psychology) identified children who earned average scores on the CAS as well as on achievement, and that approximately equal percentages of children from regular and special education classes had a relative weakness. Thus the concept of relative weakness did not identify children who achieved differently from children in regular education. By contrast, children with a cognitive weakness earned lower scores on achievement, and the more pronounced the cognitive weakness, the lower the achievement scores. Third, children with a PASS scale cognitive weakness were more likely to have been previously identified and placed in special education. Finally, the presence of a cognitive weakness was significantly related to achievement, whereas the presence of a relative weakness was not.

The findings for relative weakness partially support previous authors' arguments against the use of profile analysis for tests like the Wechsler scales (see Glutting et al., 1998, for a summary). The results for cognitive weakness support the PASS-theory-driven approach that includes the dual criteria of a significant profile and below-normal performance, called the *discrepancy–consistency model* (Naglieri, 1999, 2011). The approach is also different from the subtest analysis approach because the method uses the PASS-theory-based scales included in the CAS, rather than the traditional approach of analyzing a pattern of specific subtests. Finally, the approach is different because the focus is on cognitive, rather than relative, weaknesses (Naglieri, 1999).

The Discrepancy–Consistency Model

Naglieri's (2000) findings support the view that PASS theory can be used to identify children with cognitive and related academic difficulties for the purpose of eligibility determination and, by extension, instructional planning. Naglieri (2003, 2011) and Naglieri and Pickering (2010) provide theoretical and practical guidelines for how a child's PASS-based cognitive weakness and accompanying academic weakness may meet criteria for special educational programming. If a child has a cognitive weakness on one of the four PASS constructs and comparable scores in reading and spelling, along with other appropriate data, the child

may qualify for specific learning disability (SLD) services.

The example presented in Figure 7.2 illustrates how this theory can be used to identify a child as having an SLD. The 2004 Individuals with Disabilities Education Act define an SLD as "a disorder in one or more of the basic psychological processes [PASS processes are clearly consistent with this language] involved in understanding or in using language, spoken or written, that may manifest itself in an imperfect ability to listen, think, read, write, spell, or to do mathematical calculations" (p. 27). In the hypothetical case described here, there is a disorder in successive processing that is involved in the child's academic failure in reading and spelling. Assuming that the difficulty with successive processing has made attempts to teach the child ineffective, some type of special educational program may be appropriate.

The PASS theory provides a workable framework for determination of a disorder in basic psychological processes that can be integrated with academic performance and all other relevant information to help make a diagnosis. Of course, the determination of an SLD or any other disorder is not made solely on the basis of PASS constructs, but these play an important role in the identification process. The connections between PASS theory and academic instruction (discussed elsewhere in this chapter and in Chapter 15) have also led researchers to begin an examination of the diagnostic potential of PASS profiles.

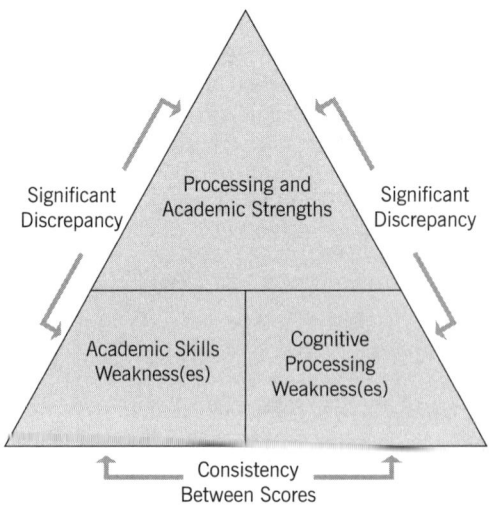

FIGURE 7.2. Discrepancy–consistency model for diagnosis. Copyright 2011 by Jack A. Naglieri.

It is important to note that emphasis is placed at the PASS theoretical level rather than the specific subtest level. Subtests are simply varying ways of measuring each of the four processes, and by themselves have less reliability than the composite scale score that represents each of the PASS processes. It is also important to recognize that profile analysis of the PASS constructs should not be made in isolation or without vital information about a child's academic performance. The procedure described here illustrates that PASS profile analysis must include achievement variation, which allows differential diagnosis based upon a configuration of variables across tests rather than simply within one test. Thus a child with a written language disorder may have a cognitive weakness in planning, with similarly poor performance on tests that measure skills in writing a story (Johnson, Bardos, & Tayebi, 2003). In contrast, a child with ADHD may have a cognitive weakness in planning, along with behavioral disorganization, impulsivity, and general loss of regulation (Naglieri & Conway, 2009). Planning weaknesses may be seen in both children, but the larger context of their problems is different.

Diagnosis: Summary

In concluding this section on the diagnostic uses of PASS theory, we have presented some samples of empirical studies on all four processes, especially successive and simultaneous processing in reading disabilities. A second aspect of our research has focused on PASS processes as these help in understanding the role of planning in ADHD. Moreover, PASS theory has had several applications in current areas of concern in education relating to diagnosis and placement, as Naglieri (1999, 2011) has discussed. Because of space limitations in this chapter, we cannot present them here. However, Chapter 15 of this book includes this discussion.

In summary, the research on PASS profiles has suggested that different homogeneous groups have distinctive weaknesses. Children with reading disabilities perform adequately on all PASS constructs except successive processing. This is consistent with the view of Das (see Das, 2009; Das, Naglieri, & Kirby, 1994) that reading failure results from a deficit in sequencing of information (successive processing). Those with the combined type of ADHD perform poorly in planning (they lack cognitive control), but adequately on the remaining PASS constructs (Dehn, 2000; Naglieri et al., 2003; Paolitto, 1999). Children with the inattentive type of ADHD have adequate PASS scores except on attention (Naglieri & Pickering, 2010). Finally, Naglieri and colleagues (2003) found that children with anxiety disorders had a different PASS profile from those with ADHD. These findings strongly support the view that PASS has relevance for understanding the cognitive processing components of these disorders.

Prescription

Dillon (1986) argued that the extent to which a theory of cognitive processing informs the user about interventions is an important dimension of validity. The PASS theory appears to have an advantage in this regard. There are several resources for applying the PASS theory to academic remediation and instruction, which we discuss briefly. The first consists of the PASS Reading Enhancement Program (PREP) and Cognition Enhancement Training (COGENT), developed by Das; the second is the Planning Facilitation Method, described by Naglieri; and the third is Naglieri and Pickering's book *Helping Children Learn: Intervention Handouts for Use in School and at Home* (2nd ed., 2010). The first two methods are based on empirical studies and discussed by Das (2009) in experiments on intervention (Das, Mishra, & Pool, 1995; Das et al., 2000; Hayward, Das, & Janzen, 2007), and summarized in *Reading Difficulties and Dyslexia: An Interpretation for Teachers* (Das, 2009). These references describe several approaches to academic interventions using PASS as the interpretive framework. The instructional methods typically use the inductive method and encourage discovery-based learning rather than direct instruction. The concepts behind the methods are more fully described below.

Description of the PREP and COGENT

The PREP was developed as a cognitively based remedial program based on the PASS theory of cognitive functioning (Das, Naglieri, & Kirby, 1994). It aims at improving the processing strategies—specifically, simultaneous and successive processing—that underlie reading, while at the same time avoiding the direct teaching of word-reading skills such as phoneme segmentation or blending. PREP is also founded on the premise that the transfer of principles is best facilitated through inductive, rather than deductive, inference (see Das, 1999 and 2009, for details). The program is therefore structured so that indirectly acquired strategies are likely to be used in appropriate ways.

The PREP is appropriate for poor readers in grades 2–5 who are experiencing reading problems. Each of the 10 PREP tasks involves both a cognitive processing component and a curriculum-related component. The cognitive processing components, which require the application of simultaneous or successive strategies, include structured nonreading tasks. These tasks also facilitate transfer by providing the opportunity for children to develop and internalize strategies in their own way (Das et al., 1995). The curriculum-related components involve the same cognitive demands as their matched cognitive processing components (e.g., simultaneous and successive processing). These cognitive processes have been closely linked to reading and spelling (Das, Naglieri, & Kirby, 1994). Several studies attest to the PREP's efficacy for enhancement of reading and comprehension (Boden & Kirby, 1995; Carlson & Das, 1997; Das et al., 1995; Parrila, Das, Kendrick, Papadopoulos, & Kirby, 1999).

The utility of the PREP was examined (Das, Hayward, Georgiou, Janzen, & Boora, 2008) with Canadian First Nations children. The effectiveness of two reading intervention programs (phonics-based and PREP) was investigated in study 1 with 63 First Nations children identified as poor readers in grades 3 and 4. In study 2, the efficacy of additional sessions for inductive learning was compared to that of PREP. Results of study 1 showed a significant improvement in word reading and pseudoword decoding reading tasks following PREP. The phonics-based program resulted in similar improvement in only one of the reading tasks, word decoding. In study 2, the important dependent variables were word reading and word decoding, as well as passage comprehension. Results showed that PREP participants evidenced continued improvements in their reading decoding and comprehension.

The next research on the PREP (Mahapatra et al., 2010) involved two groups of children selected from two English schools in India. The group receiving PREP consisted of 15 poor readers in grade 4 who experienced difficulty in comprehension; a comparison group of 15 normal readers in grade 4 did not receive PREP. Performance on tests of word reading and reading comprehension (Woodcock Reading Mastery Tests), and performance on tests of PASS cognitive processes, were recorded at pretest and posttest. Results showed a significant improvement in comprehension as well as in simultaneous processing scores in the PREP group, suggesting that this approach is effective even for

children whose first language is not English. This has obvious application possibilities for all children who learn English as a second language.

COGENT is a program designed to improve the cognitive development of children ages 4–7 or those who are beginning readers. It is designed for the enhancement of cognitive processes related to literacy and school learning. The main objective is to supplement children's literacy skills, and the program should benefit the cognitive development of normal children as well as children with special needs. COGENT consists of five distinct modules, each designed to activate different aspects of cognitive processes, language, and literacy. The tasks are also designed to enhance phonological awareness, working memory, and spatial relationships expressed in statements provided by the facilitator, for example. Further elaboration of the COGENT program is provided by Das (2004, 2009) and in a recent study by Hayward and colleagues (2007). This last study is important because it suggests that COGENT and PREP were effective in samples of First Nations children, which include a large proportion of children with reading difficulties.

Hayward and colleagues (2007) studied 45 grade 3 students from a reservation school in western Canada, who were divided into remedial groups and a no-risk control group. One remedial group was administered COGENT in the classroom throughout the school year. The second group received COGENT for the first half of the year, followed by PREP on a pull-out basis. Results showed significant improvements in word reading and comprehension for those exposed to COGENT.

Essentials of the Planning Facilitation Method

The effectiveness of teaching children to be more strategic when completing in-class math calculation problems is well illustrated by research that has examined the relationship between strategy instruction and CAS Planning scores. Four studies have focused on planning and math calculation (Hald, 1999; Naglieri & Gottling, 1995, 1997; Naglieri & Johnson, 2000). The methods used by these researchers were based on similar research by Cormier, Carlson, and Das (1990) and Kar, Dash, Das, and Carlson (1992). The researchers utilized methods designed to stimulate children's use of planning, which in turn had positive effects on problem solving on nonacademic as well as academic tasks. The method was based on the assumption that planning processes should be facilitated rather than directly taught, so that the children would discover the value of strategy use without being specifically told to do so.

The Planning Facilitation Method has been applied with individuals (Naglieri & Gottling, 1995) and groups of children (Iseman & Naglieri, 2011; Naglieri & Gottling, 1997; Naglieri & Johnson, 2000). Students completed mathematics worksheets that were developed according to the math curriculum in a series of baseline and intervention sessions over a 2-month period. During baseline and intervention phases, three-part sessions consisted of 10 minutes of math, followed by 10 minutes of discussion, followed by a further 10 minutes of math. During the baseline phase, discussion was irrelevant to the mathematics problems; in the intervention phase, however, a group discussion designed to encourage self-reflection was facilitated, so that the children would understand the need to plan and use efficient strategies.

The teachers provided questions or observations that facilitated discussion and encouraged the children to consider various ways to be more successful. Such questions included "How did you do the math?", "What could you do to get more [answers] correct?", or "What will you do next time?" The teachers made no direct statements such as "That is correct," or "Remember to use that same strategy." Teachers also did not provide feedback about the accuracy of previous math work completed, and they did not give mathematics instruction. The role of the teachers was to facilitate self-reflection and encourage the children to complete the worksheets in a planful manner. A description of this method, presented as a handout for teachers, is provided by Naglieri and Pickering (2010). The positive effects of this intervention have been consistent across research studies, as presented in Chapter 15 of this book.

Naglieri and Pickering's Approach

In *Helping Children Learn: Intervention Handouts for Use in School and at Home*, Naglieri and Pickering (2010) provide a way to apply PASS concepts across a wide variety of academic and nonacademic areas. The book contains chapters that explain, using case examples, how to select interventions on the basis of a child's PASS strengths and weaknesses. There are instructional handouts for the major academic areas (e.g., reading, writing, math), and general areas as well (e.g., test taking, memory); handouts are provided in both English and Spanish. The use of this tool is more fully described in Chapter 15 of this book.

Comparability

The extent to which cognitive processing constructs have relevance to some target task is an important criterion of validity for a theory, and one that is relevant to evaluation of the PASS theory. One example of the comparability of PASS theory and classroom performance can be found in the relationships between the attention portion of the theory and the actual in-class behaviors of children.

Attention Tests and Teachers' Ratings of Attention

The validity of the PASS theory can be assessed by examining the comparability of PASS scores with classroom performance.

Earlier in this chapter, we have discussed the relationship between PASS and academic achievement scores. In this section, we look at one particular issue: the relationship between attention measures and ratings of attention in the classroom. This is an environment where a child must selectively attend to some stimuli and ignore others. The selectivity aspect relates to intentional discrimination between stimuli. Ignoring irrelevant stimuli implies that the child is resisting distraction. In terms of the PASS theory, this means that attention involves at least three essential dimensions, which are selection, shifting, and resistance to distraction. One way to examine the comparability of the PASS theory to classroom attention is therefore to look at the relationships between measures of attention and of actual attending in the classroom.

Das, Snyder, and Mishra (1992) examined the relationship between teachers' ratings of children's attentional behavior in the classroom and those children's performances on the CAS subtests of Expressive Attention and Receptive Attention. An additional test, Selective Auditory Attention, was included in this study; this test was taken from an earlier version of the CAS (Naglieri & Das, 1988). All three of these tasks had been shown to form a separate factor identified as Attention, which is independent of the three other PASS processes (Das et al., 1992).

Teachers' ratings of students' attention status in class were made with Das's Attention Checklist (ACL). This is a checklist containing 12 items that rate the degree to which attentional behavior is shown by a child. All the items on this checklist load on one factor that accounts for more than 70% of the variance, and the ACL has high reliability (alpha of .94; Das & Melnyk, 1989). In addition to the CAS and ACL, the children were given the Conners 28-item rating scale. Das and colleagues (1992) found that the ACL and Conners Inattention/Passivity items were strongly correlated ($r = .86$), but that the correlation between the ACL and the Conners Hyperactivity scale was substantially lower ($r = .54$). This is logical because the ACL is more a measure of inattention than of hyperactivity.

The correlations of ACL and the Attention subtest scores suggested that classroom behaviors and performance on measures of cognitive processing were related. The ACL correlated significantly ($p < .01$) with Expressive Attention ($r = .46$) and the Selective Auditory Attention false-detection score ($r = .37$). No other correlations with the ACL were significant. The relationship between the ACL and children's performance on the CAS was further examined via factor analysis. Two factors were obtained: One had high loadings on the CAS Attention subtest scores (Receptive Attention and a smaller loading on Expressive Attention) and the omission score on the Selective Auditory Attention task, whereas the other factor had high loadings on the ACL, the commission errors on the Selective Auditory Attention task (which reflects distractibility), and the Expressive Attention task. Thus it was clear that the ACL, which measures teachers' ratings of attention in the classroom, was associated with performance on objective tasks that require resistance to distraction. Their common link is most probably failure to inhibit attention to distracters. This was further supported in subsequent studies (Das, 2002). Therefore we suggest that attention as defined by the PASS theory is useful to explain why teachers' ratings of attention in the classroom correlated with performance on the two CAS tasks that require selectivity and resistance to distraction.

Replicability/Standardizability

The value of any theory of cognitive processing is ultimately related to the extent to which it can be uniformly applied across examiners and organized into a formal and standardized method to assure replication across practitioners. The availability of norms and interpretive guidelines provided the

basis for accurate, consistent, and reliable interpretation of PASS scores as operationalized by the CAS (Naglieri & Das, 1997a). The CAS is a reliable measure of PASS constructs normed on a large representative sample of children 5 through 17 years of age (see Naglieri & Otero, Chapter 15, this volume). In summary, we suggest that the CAS is acceptable as a reliable and valid assessment of the PASS processes, and that it can be used in a variety of settings for a number of different purposes, as shown in several books and the CAS interpretive handbook (Naglieri & Das, 1997b).

Psychodiagnostic Utility

Dillon's (1986) *psychodiagnostic utility* criterion deals with the ease with which a particular theory of cognitive processing can be used in practice. This criterion is linked to Messick's (1989) idea of *consequential validity* and emphasizes the transition from theory to practice, the extent to which the theory can be effectively applied. The best theory of intelligence, ability, or cognitive processing will ultimately have little impact on the lives of children unless the constructs (1) have been operationalized into a practical method that can be efficiently administered; (2) can be assessed in a reliable manner; and (3) yield scores that are interpretable within the context of some relevant comparison system. As we have mentioned here and in other publications, the PASS theory and the CAS appear to have sufficient applications for diagnosis and treatment. They have value in detecting the cognitive difficulties experienced by children in several diagnostic groups (children with dyslexia, ADHD/traumatic brain injury, and intellectual disabilities [including Down syndrome]), as well as in constructing programs for cognitive enhancement (Das, 2002; Naglieri, 2003).

CONCLUDING REMARKS

The field of intelligence and intelligence testing has been experiencing a healthy evolution in concept and practice. Researchers and practitioners have increased the attention they give to theory, and the importance of basing a test of intelligence upon a theory of intelligence is now widely acknowledged. It has been more than 90 years since Pintner (1925) noted that researchers who were studying ability were "attempting to define it more sharply and endow it with a stricter scientific connotation" (p. 53). Although tests representing the general intelligence perspective are still widely used today, tests based on newer conceptualizations of ability—and especially ability defined on the basis of basic psychological processes—are becoming more popular, particularly as the evidence for the process-based approach grows.

The most important difference between measures of general intelligence and PASS theory as operationalized by the CAS lies in the fact that the CAS represents a specific view of intelligence derived from a neuropsychological conceptualization of four distinct but interrelated abilities. We use the term *cognitive process* as a modern term for *ability* and choose a multidimensional, rather than unidimensional, view (Das & Naglieri, 1992). It is a theory for which research has increasingly demonstrated utility (as summarized in this chapter and in Chapter 15 and elsewhere (Naglieri, 2011; Naglieri & Conway, 2009). We suggest that PASS theory is a modern alternative to *g* and IQ, based on neuropsychology and cognitive psychology, and that it is well suited to meet the needs of school psychologists practicing in the 21st century.

REFERENCES

Ashman, A. F. (1982). Strategic behavior and linguistic functions of institutionalized moderately retarded persons. *International Journal of Rehabilitation Research, 5*, 203–214.

Barkley, R. A. (1997). *ADHD and the nature of self-control.* New York: Guilford Press.

Boden, C., & Kirby, J. R. (1995). Successive processing, phonological coding, and the remediation of reading. *Journal of Cognitive Education, 4*, 19–32.

Bradley, L., & Bryant, P. (1985). *Rhyme and reason in reading and spelling.* Ann Arbor: University of Michigan Press.

Carlson, J., & Das, J. P. (1997). A process approach to remediating word decoding deficiencies in Chapter 1 children. *Learning Disability Quarterly, 20*, 93–102.

Christensen, A., Goldberg, E., & Bougakov, D. (2009). *Luria's legacy in the 21st century.* New York: Oxford University Press.

Cormier, P., Carlson, J. S., & Das, J. P. (1990). Planning ability and cognitive performance: The compensatory effects of a dynamic assessment approach. *Learning and Individual Differences, 2*, 437–449.

Das, J. P. (1972). Patterns of cognitive ability in non-

retarded and retarded children. *American Journal of Mental Deficiency, 77*, 6–12.

Das, J. P. (1980). Planning: Theoretical considerations and empirical evidence. *Psychological Research* [W. Germany], *41*, 141–151.

Das, J. P. (1999). *PASS Reading Enhancement Program (PREP).* Edmonton: Developmental Disabilities Centre, University of Alberta.

Das, J. P. (2002). A better look at intelligence. *Current Directions in Psychology, 11*, 28–32.

Das, J. P. (2004). *The Cognitive Enhancement Training program (COGENT).* Edmonton: Developmental Disabilities Centre, University of Alberta.

Das, J. P. (2009). *Reading difficulties and dyslexia: An interpretation for teachers* (rev. ed.). Thousand Oaks, CA: Sage.

Das, J. P., & Abbott, J. (1995). PASS: An alternative approach to intelligence. *Psychology and Developing Societies, 7*(2), 155–184.

Das, J. P., Hayward, D., Georgiou, G., Janzen, T., & Boora, N. (2008). Comparing the effectiveness of two reading intervention programs for children with reading disabilities. *Journal of Cognitive Education and Psychology, 7*, 199–222.

Das, J. P., & Heemsbergen, D. (1983). Planning as a factor in the assessment of cognitive processes. *Journal of Psychoeducational Assessment, 1*, 1–16.

Das, J. P., Janzen, T., & Georgiou, G. (2007). Correlates of Canadian native children's reading performance: From cognitive styles to cognitive processes. *Journal of School Psychology, 45*, 589–602.

Das, J. P., Kar, B. C., & Parrila, R. K. (1996). *Cognitive planning: The psychological basis of intelligent behavior.* Thousand Oaks, CA: Sage.

Das, J. P., Kirby, J. R., & Jarman, R. F. (1975). Simultaneous and successive syntheses: An alternative model for cognitive abilities. *Psychological Bulletin, 82*, 87–103.

Das, J. P., Kirby, J. R., & Jarman, R. F. (1979). *Simultaneous and successive cognitive processes.* New York: Academic Press.

Das, J. P., & Melnyk, L. (1989). Attention Checklist: A rating scale for mildly mentally handicapped adolescents. *Psychological Reports, 64*, 1267–1274.

Das, J. P., Mishra, R. K., & Kirby, J. R. (1994). Cognitive patterns of dyslexics: Comparison between groups with high and average nonverbal intelligence. *Journal of Learning Disabilities, 27*, 235–242.

Das, J. P., Mishra, R. K., & Pool, J. E. (1995). An experiment on cognitive remediation or word-reading difficulty. *Journal of Learning Disabilities, 28*, 66–79.

Das, J. P., & Molloy, G. N. (1975). Varieties of simultaneous and successive processing in children. *Journal of Educational Psychology, 67*, 213–220.

Das, J. P., & Naglieri, J. A. (1992). Assessment of attention, simultaneous–successive coding and planning. In H. C. Haywood & D. Tzuriel (Eds.), *Interactive assessment* (pp. 207–232). New York: Springer-Verlag.

Das, J. P., Naglieri, J. A., & Kirby, J. R. (1994). *Assessment of cognitive processes*. Needham Heights, MA: Allyn & Bacon.

Das, J. P., Parrila, R. K., & Papadopoulos, T. C. (2000). Cognitive education and reading disability. In A. Kozulin & Y. Rand (Eds.), *Experience of mediated learning* (pp. 276–291). Amsterdam: Pergamon Press.

Das, J. P., Snyder, T. J., & Mishra, R. K. (1992). Assessment of attention: Teachers' rating scales and measures of selective attention. *Journal of Psychoeducational Assessment, 10*, 37–46.

Das, J. P., & Varnhagen, C. K. (1986). Neuropsychological functioning and cognitive processing. In J. E. Obrzut & G. W. Hynd (Eds.), *Child neuropsychology: Vol. 1. Theory and research* (pp. 117–140). New York: Academic Press.

Davis, F. B. (1959). Interpretation of differences among averages and individual test scores. *Journal of Educational Psychology, 50*, 162–170.

Dehn, M. J. (2000). *Cognitive Assessment System performance of ADHD children*. Paper presented at the annual convention of the National Association of School Psychologists, New Orleans, LA.

Dillon, R. F. (1986). Information processing and testing. *Educational Psychologist, 21*, 161–174.

Elliott, C. D. (2007). *Differential Ability Scales—Second Edition*. San Antonio, TX: Harcourt Assessment.

Garofalo, J. (1986). Simultaneous synthesis, regulation and arithmetical performance. *Journal of Psychoeducational Assessment, 4*, 229–238.

Glutting, J. J., McDermott, P. A., Konold, T. R., Snelbaker, A. J., & Watkins, M. L. (1998). More ups and downs of subtest analysis: Criterion validity of the DAS with an unselected cohort. *School Psychology Review, 27*, 599–612.

Goldberg, E. (2001). *The executive brain: Frontal lobes and the civilized mind*. New York: Oxford University Press.

Goldstein, S., & Naglieri, J. A. (2006). The role of intellectual processes in the DSM-V diagnosis of ADHD. *Journal of Attention Disorders, 10*, 3–8.

Hald, M. E. (1999). A PASS cognitive processes intervention study in mathematics. Unpublished doctoral dissertation, University of Northern Colorado.

Hayward, D., Das, J. P., & Janzen, T. (2007). Innovative programs for improvement in reading through cognitive enhancement: A remediation study of Canadian First Nations children. *Journal of Learning Disabilities, 40*, 443–457.

Iseman, J., & Naglieri, J. A. (2011). A cognitive strategy instruction to improve math calculation for children with ADHD: A randomized controlled study. *Journal of Learning Disabilities, 44*(2), 184–195.

Jarman, R. F., & Das, J. P. (1977). Simultaneous and successive synthesis and intelligence. *Intelligence, 1*, 151–169.

Johnson, J. A., Bardos, A. N., & Tayebi, K. A. (2003). Discriminant validity of the Cognitive Assessment System for students with written expression disabilities. *Journal of Psychoeducational Assessment, 21*, 180–195.

Kar, B. C., Dash, U. N., Das, J. P., & Carlson, J. S. (1992). Two experiments on the dynamic assessment of planning. *Learning and Individual Differences, 5*, 13–29.

Kaufman, A. S., & Kaufman, N. L. (1983). *Kaufman Assessment Battery for Children*. Circle Pines, MN: American Guidance Service.

Kirby, J. R. (1984). *Cognitive strategies and educational performance*. New York: Academic Press.

Kirby, J. R., & Das, J. P. (1978). Information processing and human abilities. *Journal of Educational Psychology, 70*, 58–66.

Kirby, J. R., & Robinson, G. L. (1987). Simultaneous and successive processing in reading disabled children. *Journal of Learning Disabilities, 20*, 243–252.

Kirby, J. R., & Williams, N. H. (1991). *Learning problems: A cognitive approach*. Toronto: Kagan & Woo.

Kolb, B., Gibb, R., & Robinson, T. E. (2003). Brain plasticity and behavior. *Current Directions in Psychological Science, 12*, 1–4.

Lidz, C. S. (1991). *Practitioner's guide to dynamic assessment*. New York: Guilford Press.

Luria, A. R. (1966). *Human brain and psychological processes*. New York: Harper & Row.

Luria, A. R. (1973a). The origin and cerebral organization of man's conscious action. In S. G. Sapir & A. C. Nitzburg (Eds.), *Children with learning problems* (pp. 109–130). New York: Brunner/Mazel.

Luria, A. R. (1973b). *The working brain*. New York: Basic Books.

Luria, A. R. (1979). *The making of mind: A personal account of Soviet psychology*. Cambridge, MA: Harvard University Press.

Luria, A. R. (1980). *Higher cortical functions in man* (2nd ed.). New York: Basic Books.

Mahapatra, S., Das, J. P., Stack-Cutler, H., & Parrila, R. (2010). Remediating reading comprehension difficulties: A cognitive processing approach. *Reading Psychology, 31*(5), 428–453.

McCrea, S. M. (2007). Measurement of recovery after traumatic brain injury: A cognitive-neuropsychological comparison of the WAIS-R with the Cognitive Assessment System (CAS) in a single case of atypical language lateralization. *Applied Neuropsychology, 14*, 296–304.

Messick, S. (1989). Validity. In R. L. Linn (Ed.), *Educational measurement* (pp. 13–103). New York: American Council of Education/Macmillan.

Naglieri, J. A. (1989). A cognitive processing theory for the measurement of intelligence. *Educational Psychologist, 24*, 185–206.

Naglieri, J. A. (1999). *Essentials of CAS assessment.* New York: Wiley.

Naglieri, J. A. (2000). Can profile analysis of ability test scores work?: An illustration using the PASS theory and CAS with an unselected cohort. *School Psychology Quarterly, 15*, 419–433.

Naglieri, J. A. (2003). Current advances in assessment and intervention for children with learning disabilities. In T. E. Scruggs M. A. Mastropieri (Eds.), *Advances in learning and behavioral disabilities: Vol. 16. Identification and assessment* (pp. 163–190). Greenwich, CT: JAI Press.

Naglieri, J. A. (2011). The discrepancy/consistency approach to SLD identification using the PASS theory. In D. P. Flanagan & V. C. Alfonso (Eds.), *Essentials of specific learning disability identification* (pp. 145–172). Hoboken, NJ: Wiley.

Naglieri, J. A., & Conway, C. (2009). The Cognitive Assessment System. In J. A. Naglieri & S. Goldstein (Eds.), *A practitioner's guide to assessment of intelligence and achievement* (pp. 3–10). New York: Wiley.

Naglieri, J. A., & Das, J. P. (1988). Planning–arousal–simultaneous–successive (PASS): A model for assessment. *Journal of School Psychology, 26*, 35–48.

Naglieri, J. A., & Das, J. P. (1997a). *Das–Naglieri Cognitive Assessment System.* Itasca, IL: Riverside.

Naglieri, J. A., & Das, J. P. (1997b). *Das–Naglieri Cognitive Assessment System: Interpretive handbook.* Itasca, IL: Riverside.

Naglieri, J. A., & Das, J. P. (1997c). Intelligence revised. In R. Dillon (Ed.), *Handbook on testing* (pp. 136–163). Westport, CT: Greenwood Press.

Naglieri, J. A., & Das, J. P. (2002). Practical implications of general intelligence and PASS cognitive processes. In R. J. Sternberg & E. L. Grigorenko (Eds.), *The general factor of intelligence: How general is it?* (pp. 855–884). New York: Erlbaum.

Naglieri, J. A., Das, J. P., & Goldstein, S. (2012). *Cognitive Assessment System—Second Edition.* Austin, TX: PRO-ED.

Naglieri, J. A., Goldstein, S., Iseman, J. S., & Schwebach, A. (2003). Performance of children with attention deficit hyperactivity disorder and anxiety/depression on the WISC-III and Cognitive Assessment System (CAS). *Journal of Psychoeducational Assessment, 21*, 32–42.

Naglieri, J. A., & Gottling, S. H. (1995). A cognitive education approach to math instruction for the learning disabled: An individual study. *Psychological Reports, 76*, 1343–1354.

Naglieri, J. A., & Gottling, S. H. (1997). Mathematics instruction and PASS cognitive processes: An intervention study. *Journal of Learning Disabilities, 30*, 513–520.

Naglieri, J. A., & Johnson, D. (2000). Effectiveness of a cognitive strategy intervention to improve math calculation based on the PASS theory. *Journal of Learning Disabilities, 33*, 591–597.

Naglieri, J. A., & Kaufman, A. S. (2008). IDEIA 2004 and specific learning disabilities: What role does intelligence play? In E. Grigorenko (Ed.), *Educating individuals with disabilities: IDEIA 2004 and beyond* (pp. 165–195). New York: Springer.

Naglieri, J. A., & Otero, T. (2011). Cognitive Assessment System: Redefining intelligence from a neuropsychological perspective. In A. Davis (Ed.), *The handbook of pediatric neuropsychology* (pp. 320–333). New York: Springer.

Naglieri, J. A., Otero, T., DeLauder, B., & Matto, H. (2007). Bilingual Hispanic children's performance on the English and Spanish versions of the Cognitive Assessment System. *School Psychology Quarterly, 22*, 432–448.

Naglieri, J. A., & Pickering, E. (2010). *Helping children learn: Intervention handouts for use in school and at home* (2nd ed.). Baltimore: Brookes.

Naglieri, J. A., Salter, C. J., & Edwards, G. (2004). Assessment of children with ADHD and reading disabilities using the PASS theory and Cognitive Assessment System. *Journal of Psychoeducational Assessment, 22*, 93–105.

Okuhata, S., Okazaki, S., & Maekawa, H. (2009). EEG coherence pattern during simultaneous and successive processing tasks. *International Journal of Psychophysiology, 72*(2), 89–96.

Paolitto, A. W. (1999). Clinical validation of the Cognitive Assessment System with children with ADHD. *ADHD Report, 7*, 1–5.

Parrila, R. K., Das, J. P., Kendrick, M., Papadopoulos, T., Kirby, J. (1999). Efficacy of a cognitive reading remediation program for at-risk children in grade 1. *Developmental Disabilities Bulletin, 27*, 1–31.

Pintner, R. (1925). *Intelligence testing.* New York: Henry Holt.

Roid, G. H. (2003). *Stanford–Binet Intelligence Scales, Fifth Edition.* Austin, TX: Pro-Ed.

Share, D. L., & Stanovich, K. E. (1995). Cognitive processes in early reading development: Accommodating individual differences into a model of acquisition. *Issues in Education, 1,* 1–57.

Silverstein, A. B. (1982). Pattern analysis as simultaneous statistical inference. *Journal of Consulting and Clinical Psychology, 50,* 234–240.

Silverstein, A. B. (1993). Type I, type II, and other types of errors in pattern analysis. *Psychological Assessment, 5,* 72–74.

Stanovich, K. E. (1988). Explaining the differences between the dyslexic and the garden-variety poor reader: The phonological–core variable–difference model. *Journal of Learning Disabilities, 21,* 590–604, 612.

Stuss, D. T., & Benson, D. F. (1990). The frontal lobes and language. In E. Goldberg (Ed.), *Contemporary psychology and the legacy of Luria* (pp. 29–50). Hillsdale, NJ: Erlbaum.

Torgesen, J. K., Wagner, R. K., & Rashotte, C. A. (1994). Longitudinal studies of phonological processing and reading. *Journal of Learning Disabilities, 27,* 276–286.

Wagner, R. K., Torgesen, J. K., & Rashotte, C. A. (1994). Development of reading-related phonological processing abilities: New evidence of bi-directional causality from a latent variable longitudinal study. *Developmental Psychology, 30,* 73–87.

Yoakum, C. S., & Yerkes, R. M (1920). *Army mental tests.* New York: Holt.

PART III

CONTEMPORARY INTELLIGENCE, COGNITIVE, AND NEUROPSYCHOLOGICAL BATTERIES (AND ASSOCIATED ACHIEVEMENT TESTS)

The Wechsler Adult Intelligence Scale— Fourth Edition and the Wechsler Memory Scale—Fourth Edition

Lisa Whipple Drozdick
Dustin Wahlstrom
Jianjun Zhu
Lawrence G. Weiss

The Wechsler Adult Intelligence Scale—Fourth Edition (WAIS-IV; Wechsler, 2008) is the most recent revision of the WAIS and incorporates numerous changes from previous editions while maintaining the integrity and tradition of the Wechsler scales. It is used to assess intellectual and cognitive functioning in adults and adolescents ages 16–90 and provides information on an individual's general intellectual ability, as well as abilities across various cognitive domains. Since the WAIS-IV provides an overall estimate of cognitive functioning, it is frequently used alongside other instruments in comprehensive evaluations.

Memory is frequently evaluated along with intellectual functioning or cognitive ability. The co-norming of the WAIS-IV and the Wechsler Memory Scale—Fourth Edition (WMS-IV; Wechsler, 2009) allows the direct comparison of performance across the two measures. A common referral suggesting the combined use of the WAIS-IV and WMS-IV involves poor or questionable cognitive or memory performance. When used together, the WAIS-IV provides a measure of general cognitive ability within which WMS-IV results can be interpreted.

This chapter presents an overview of the WAIS-IV and the WMS-IV, followed by guidelines on the use and interpretation of the instruments separately and in combination. Each overview presents a brief description of the theory and structure of the instrument, detailed descriptions of the subtests and composites, and information on psychometric properties. The section on interpretation provides general information regarding test interpretation, followed by specific interpretive information for each instrument and information on interpreting WMS-IV scores within the context of WAIS-IV scores. Finally, a case study is presented to illustrate the combined use of the WAIS-IV and WMS-IV.

THEORETICAL UNDERPINNINGS OF THE WAIS-IV

Although trained in statistics by Charles Spearman and Karl Pearson, David Wechsler was best known for his clinical acumen and developed his tests to be clinical instruments (Kaufman, 1992). However, Wechsler was influenced by two key theorists of intelligence at the time: the aforementioned Charles Spearman, as well as Edward Thorndike. Spearman's concept of g and general intelligence was an obvious influence (Kaufman & Lichtenberger, 1999; Tulsky, Zhu, & Prifitera, 2000; Weiss, Saklofske, Coalson, & Raiford, 2010), as Wechsler viewed intelligence as a global entity. However, Thorndike's influence was also evident, as Wechsler conceived of this global entity as consisting of elements that are qualitatively different (Wechsler, 1939, 1950, 1975). He articulated this view best in his initial Wechsler–Bellevue Intelligence Scale, where he described intelligence as

> the aggregate or global capacity of the individual to act purposefully, to think rationally, and to deal effectively with his [or her] environment. It is global because it characterizes the individual's behavior as a whole; it is aggregate because it is composed of elements or abilities which, though not entirely independent, are qualitatively differentiable. (Wechsler, 1939, p. 3)

It is important to note here that Wechsler's theory of intelligence also incorporated a number of abilities that are not assessed by modern IQ tests, but nevertheless affect an individual's ability to navigate his or her environment effectively. These include personality, emotional, and conative factors, such as drive, persistence, curiosity, and temperament (Wechsler, 1950). Although Wechsler was unsuccessful in developing a measure of these noncognitive intellective skills, his practical and clinically based overarching theory of intelligence resulted in a number of strengths that have made the Wechsler intelligence scales the most widely used in the world today (Archer, Buffington-Vollum, Stredny, & Handel, 2006; Stinnett, Havey, & Oehler-Stinnett, 1994). Perhaps most importantly, the Wechsler scales are considered valid and clinically useful instruments, providing clinicians with an accurate snapshot of an individual's functioning that is related to the person's behavior in real-world settings (Fergusson, Horwood, & Ridder, 2005; Groth-Marnat & Teal, 2000; Weiss, Gale, Batty, & Deary, 2009).

The broad nature of Wechsler's theory provides a framework that modern-day developers can use to guide revisions to his tests. Within this framework, current theories from the fields of intelligence, developmental psychology, neuropsychology, and cognitive neuroscience have been incorporated into past Wechsler scales to align revisions with updated scientific findings, while simultaneously maintaining those practical aspects of the scales that were most important to the original author. This ability to incorporate data from multiple fields of research and practice highlights one of the Wechsler scales' greatest strengths: flexibility. Having an instrument tied to a specific theory limits the ability of the test to evolve independently of the theory. Moreover, if the theory changes to accommodate new information, the test becomes

outdated. Because the Wechsler scales are not tied to a specific theory, the scales can be altered in response to data, findings in the field of intelligence, or other scientific advances.

It is within this context that the WAIS-IV was revised, and many of the revisions discussed later in this chapter are the result of recent advances in basic and clinical research. For example, a growing body of literature has emphasized the importance of fluid reasoning in general cognitive functioning (Carroll, Appendix, this volume; Sternberg, 2000), and Figure Weights, a measure of quantitative reasoning, was added to the WAIS-IV to enhance the measure of this construct. To reflect the increased emphasis of fluid reasoning on the WAIS-IV, the Perceptual Organization Index (POI) of the WAIS-III has been changed to the Perceptual Reasoning Index (PRI). Similarly, working memory has long been recognized as an important predictor of individual differences in learning and fluid reasoning (Conway, Cowan, Bunting, Therriault, & Minkoff, 2002; Fry & Hale, 1996; Perlow, Jattuso, & Moore, 1997), and recent work has indicated a very close association between working memory capacity and g (Colom, Rebollo, Palacios, Espinosa, & Kyllonen, 2004; Conway, Kane, & Engle, 2003). In addition, working memory training has been linked to improvements in fluid reasoning ability, suggesting a dynamic interplay between the two in the control of cognitive functioning (Jaeggi, Buschkuehl, Jonides, & Perrig, 2008). To address the growing importance of working memory, Digit Span Sequencing was added to the Digit Span subtest. This change increases the role of mental manipulation and results in greater demands on working memory, relative to previous versions of Digit Span. Arithmetic was also altered to more purely reflect working memory, as opposed to verbal comprehension skills or mathematical knowledge. For example, difficult items require several successive simple mathematical steps that have to be represented in working memory instead of the complex calculations included in earlier versions.

Processing speed is also a construct of recent interest in the intelligence literature, as research suggests that it interacts with working memory and fluid intelligence; processing speed mediates the relationship between working memory and reasoning (Fry & Hale, 1996, 2000; Jensen, 1998; Salthouse, 1996; but see Conway et al., 2002). Specifically, it has been proposed that rapid information processing may reduce working memory demands, which in turn releases cognitive resources for more complex forms of reasoning (Weiss et al., 2010).

Furthermore, factor-analytic research has identified processing speed as an important component of the Cattell–Horn–Carroll (CHC) model of intelligence (Carroll, 1993), and it has been shown to be sensitive to a number of clinical syndromes, including attention-deficit/hyperactivity disorder (ADHD) (Schwean & Saklofske, 2005), traumatic brain injury (TBI) (Kennedy, Clement, & Curtiss, 2003), epilepsy (Berg et al., 2008), and multiple sclerosis (Forn, Belenguer, Parcet-Ibars, & Ávila, 2008). The WAIS-IV includes both the Coding and Symbol Search subtests in the calculation of the Full Scale Intelligence Quotient (FSIQ). As a result, the contribution of processing speed subtests to the FSIQ increased from 9% in the WAIS-III to 20% in the WAIS-IV, reflecting the growing importance of this construct in intellectual assessment.

Overall, confounding variables have been reduced in the WAIS-IV, thereby increasing the test's ability to tap relatively pure cognitive functions. For example, to reduce the influence of declining processing speed on the scores of older adults (Lee, Gorsuch, Saklofske, & Patterson, 2008), time-bonus points were removed from Arithmetic and reduced on Block Design. Similarly, Cancellation was added as an alternative processing speed subtest with fewer fine motor demands than the Coding subtest, and Visual Puzzles demands less fine motor control than Object Assembly, which it replaces on the PRI. Despite these changes, care has been taken to ensure that the test retains its validity and clinical utility. A century of cognitive research has demonstrated that human cognitive functions form a dynamically unified entity, as evidenced by the above discussion of fluid reasoning, working memory, and processing speed. Wechsler himself noted the dynamic nature of intellectual abilities, noting that they "appear to behave differently when alone from what they do when operating in concert" (1975, p. 138). Therefore, while the measurement of pure cognitive functions is ideal from a theoretical and psychometric standpoint, it does not necessarily result in information that is clinically rich or practically useful in real-world applications (Weiss et al., 2010; Zachary, 1990). Thus the WAIS-IV reflects a balance between theoretically sound cognitive constructs and the need to maintain the predictive value and clinical utility characterizing past versions of the WAIS.

The Wechsler intelligence scales have been criticized for what some perceive as a lack of theoretical orientation (Beres, Kaufman, & Perlman, 2000; Kaufman & Lichtenberger, 1999; McGrew & Flanagan, 1997). Although Wechsler selected cognitive tasks for his intelligence battery that were clinically grounded rather than tied to a specific theory of intelligence, subsequent revisions have kept pace with modern advances in clinical and neuropsychological research, and the current editions align and correlate well with tests created more recently and based on specific theories of intelligence, such as the CHC and Luria models. For instance, after analyzing the factor structure of more than 450 datasets, Carroll (1993) revealed the presence of a general intelligence factor, and several studies have provided evidence suggesting that intelligence is composed of specific narrow abilities that appear to cluster into higher-order ability domains (Carroll, 1993; Cohen, 1952, 1957; Horn, 1994). With respect to the WAIS-IV, recent independent analyses of the standardization sample suggest that the cognitive domains measured by the test align closely with those specified by recent models of intelligence (Benson, Hulac, & Kranzler, 2010; Keith, as cited in Lichtenberger & Kaufman, 2009), which include crystallized ability, visual processing, fluid reasoning, short-term memory, and processing speed. These results suggest that the cognitive constructs measured by the WAIS-IV are similar to those of other tests that are designed around specific theories. This is also supported by the fact that the Wechsler scales correlate highly with theory-based intelligence measures, such as the Kaufman Adolescent and Adult Intelligence Test (KAIT; Kaufman & Kaufman, 1993) and the Differential Ability Scales (Elliott, 1990). The totality of this evidence has caused some to reconsider their stance regarding the theoretical nature of the Wechsler scales. For instance, Alan Kaufman has stated that "I have since reconsidered my stance on the lack of a theoretical framework for Wechsler's scales" (Kaufman, 2010, p. xvi), as "the WAIS-IV also was developed with specific theoretical foundations in mind. In fact, revisions were made purposely to reflect the latest knowledge from literature in the areas of intelligence theory, adult cognitive development, and cognitive neuroscience" (Lichtenberger & Kaufman, 2009, p. 20).

DESCRIPTION OF WAIS-IV SUBTESTS AND COMPOSITES

All Wechsler intelligence scales provide factor-based index scores that measure major cognitive domains identified in contemporary theories of intelligence. The primary advantage of the index scores is their measurement of relatively purer cognitive domains, which allows the clinician to evaluate specific aspects of cognitive functioning more clearly. For example, children with learning disorders may be expected to perform poorly on working memory tasks (Gathercole, Hitch, Service, & Martin, 1997; Wechsler, 2003), and individuals with TBI may exhibit poor processing speed skills (Mathias & Wheaton, 2007). The WAIS-IV provides four index scores: the Verbal Comprehension Index (VCI), the PRI, the Working Memory Index (WMI), and the Processing Speed Index (PSI). In addition to these four core indexes, the WAIS-IV also provides the optional General Ability Index (GAI), which consists of subtests from the VCI and PRI.

The WAIS-IV consists of 15 total subtests (10 core and 5 supplemental), three of which are new: Visual Puzzles, Figure Weights, and Cancellation. Table 8.1 lists the WAIS-IV subtests, as well as the IQ and index scales to which each contributes. Despite the changes made to the WAIS-IV, the correlations with the WAIS-III are high, suggesting that they measure closely related constructs. For example, the FSIQ correlation is .94, and the index scale correlations range between .84 for the PRI (correlated with the POI on WAIS-III) and .91 for the VCI (Wechsler, 2008). The WAIS-IV

is normed for individuals between the ages of 16 years, 0 months (16:0 years) and 90:11 years. The following sections describe each of the WAIS-IV index scores, as well as the core and supplemental subtests that contribute to each.

Full Scale Intelligence Quotient

The FSIQ estimates an individual's general level of intellectual functioning. It is the aggregate score derived from the core subtest scores. The FSIQ is usually considered the score most representative of *g*, or global intellectual functioning; this is important because it is a robust predictor of an array of important life outcomes, such as academic performance and occupational attainment, as well as accidental injury, chronic illness, medication adherence, and even premature death (Deary, 2009; Gottfredson, 1997; Gottfredson & Deary, 2004). Furthermore, general intelligence consistently emerges in factor-analytic studies—a finding that has been replicated in research using international adaptations of the Wechsler scales (Bowden, Lange, Weiss, & Saklofske, 2008; Georgas, Weiss, van de Vijver, & Saklofske, 2003). As depicted in Table 8.1, 10 subtests contribute to the WAIS-IV FSIQ: 3 from the VCI, 3 from the PRI, 2 from the WMI, and 2 from the PSI.

TABLE 8.1. Subtests and Related Composite Scores of the WAIS-IV

Subtest	Contribution to IQ and factor index scales					
	VCI	PRI	WMI	PSI	FSIQ	GAI
Vocabulary	✓				✓	✓
Similarities	✓				✓	✓
Information	✓				✓	✓
Comprehension	(✓)					
Digit Span			✓		✓	
Arithmetic			✓		✓	
Letter–Number Sequencing			(✓)			
Block Design		✓			✓	✓
Matrix Reasoning		✓			✓	✓
Visual Puzzles		✓			✓	✓
Figure Weights		(✓)				
Picture Completion		(✓)				
Coding				✓	✓	
Symbol Search				✓	✓	
Cancellation				(✓)		

Note. VCI, Verbal Comprehension Index; PRI, Perceptual Reasoning Index; WMI, Working Memory Index; PSI, Processing Speed Index; FSIQ, Full Scale IQ; GAI, General Ability Index. Check marks indicate the core subtests contributing to an index score. Supplemental subtests are designated by parentheses.

Verbal Comprehension Index

The VCI is a measure of verbal concept formation, verbal reasoning and comprehension, acquired knowledge, and attention to verbal stimuli. It is a measure of crystallized intelligence, and hence reflects an individual's ability to reason by using previously learned information (Lichtenberger & Kaufman, 2009). Because VCI subtests measure concepts such as vocabulary or factual knowledge, they require a certain level of exposure to cultural and educational opportunities. However, it would be incorrect to assume that the VCI is simply a reflection of learned facts or education, as individual differences in knowledge acquisition depend not only on opportunity, but also on the application of other cognitive abilities during those experiences in order to take advantage of opportunity (Weiss et al., 2010). As such, while VCI subtests measure an individual's understanding of verbal concepts, they also reflect the utilization of experience to learn these concepts and the ability to apply them in novel situations.

Vocabulary

The Vocabulary subtest consists of both picture-naming items and word definition items. For picture-naming items, the examinee names the object presented visually. For word definition items, the examinee defines words that are read aloud by the examiner and presented visually in the stimulus book (e.g., "What does *conceive* mean?"). Vocabulary measures an individual's verbal concept formation as expressed through recall of acquired knowledge. It also measures crystallized intelligence, fund of knowledge, verbal conceptualization, learning ability, long-term memory, and degree of language development (Kaufman & Lichtenberger, 2006; Sattler & Ryan, 2009). The Vocabulary subtest is a good measure of *g* and has adequate to ample specificity (Lichtenberger & Kaufman, 2009; Sattler & Ryan, 2009).

Similarities

For each Similarities item, the examinee is presented with two words that represent common concepts and asked to describe how they are alike (e.g., "In what way are fish and birds alike?"). The Similarities subtest measures verbal concept formation and reasoning. It also involves verbal comprehension, making distinctions between nonessential and essential features, and verbal expression and problem solving (Kaufman & Lichtenberger, 2006; Sattler & Ryan, 2009). This subtest is a fair to good measure of *g* and has an adequate amount of specificity (Lichtenberger & Kaufman, 2009; Sattler & Ryan, 2009).

Comprehension

The Comprehension subtest requires the examinee to answer questions based on his or her understanding of general principles and social situations (e.g., "What is the advantage of keeping money in a bank?"). The subtest measures practical reasoning and judgment. It also involves verbal comprehension and expression, crystallized knowledge, common sense, and verbal reasoning (Kaufman & Lichtenberger, 2006; Sattler & Ryan, 2009). Comprehension is a fair to good measure of *g* (Lichtenberger & Kaufman, 2009; Sattler & Ryan, 2009). Its specificity is adequate in a majority of the standardization sample age bands, but inadequate in the age ranges of 30–34 and 85–90 years (Sattler & Ryan, 2009).

Information

Information requires the examinee to answer questions that address a broad range of general knowledge topics (e.g., "Name the country that launched the first man-made satellite"). It measures an individual's ability to acquire, retain, and retrieve general factual knowledge. It involves crystallized intelligence, long-term memory, and verbal expressive ability (Kaufman & Lichtenberger, 2006; Sattler & Ryan, 2009). This subtest is a fair to good measure of *g* and has an adequate to ample amount of specificity (Lichtenberger & Kaufman, 2009; Sattler & Ryan, 2009).

Perceptual Reasoning Index

The PRI is a measure of fluid reasoning, spatial processing, attentiveness to detail, and visual–motor integration. It also reflects working memory and processing speed skills, based on evidence that these abilities are intertwined with fluid reasoning. As discussed previously, it replaces the POI from the WAIS-III. This updated nomenclature reflects the increased emphasis on fluid reasoning in the WAIS-IV, which results from the addition of Visual Puzzles and Figure Weights and the removal of Object Assembly and Picture Arrangement.

Block Design

The Block Design subtest requires the examinee to view a constructed model or a picture in the stimulus book and to use one-color or two-color blocks to recreate the design within a specified time limit (see Figure 8.1). This subtest measures the ability to analyze and synthesize abstract visual stimuli. It also involves visual perception and organization, visual–spatial problem solving, visual nonverbal reasoning, visual–motor coordination, learning, and the ability to separate figure and ground in visual stimuli (Kaufman & Lichtenberger, 2006; Sattler & Ryan, 2009). Block Design is a fair measure of *g* and has an adequate to ample amount of specificity (Lichtenberger & Kaufman, 2009; Sattler & Ryan, 2009).

Matrix Reasoning

For each Matrix Reasoning item, the examinee looks at an incomplete matrix and selects the missing portion from five response options (see Figure 8.2). This subtest is designed to measure fluid intelligence and inductive reasoning. It also measures spatial visualization, visual organization, visual-perceptual discrimination, and nonverbal reasoning (Kaufman & Lichtenberger, 2006; Sattler & Ryan, 2009). Matrix Reasoning is a fair to good measure of *g* and has an adequate to ample amount of specificity (Lichtenberger & Kaufman, 2009; Sattler & Ryan, 2009).

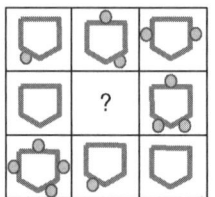

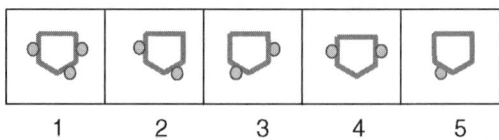

FIGURE 8.2. Example from the WAIS-IV Matrix Reasoning subtest.

Visual Puzzles

Visual Puzzles is a new core subtest. On Visual Puzzles, examinees reproduce a geometric image by choosing three response options that can be combined to form the image from six available options within a predetermined time limit (see Figure 8.3). It was designed to measure perceptual organization and reasoning. It also measures visual–spatial construction, analysis and synthesis, and simultaneous processing (Groth-Marnat, 2009; Lichtenberger & Kaufman, 2009; Sattler & Ryan, 2009). It is a fair measure of *g* and has adequate to ample specificity (Lichtenberger & Kaufman, 2009; Sattler & Ryan, 2009).

Picture Completion

Picture Completion requires the examinee to view a picture and then point to or name the important part missing within a specified time limit (see Figure 8.4). This subtest measures visual perception and organization. It also requires visual discrimination, visual recognition of essential details of objects, crystallized knowledge, reasoning, and visual long-term memory (Kaufman & Lichtenberger, 2006; Sattler & Ryan, 2009). It is a fair measure of *g* and has an adequate to ample amount of specificity (Lichtenberger & Kaufman, 2009; Sattler & Ryan, 2009).

Figure Weights

Figure Weights is a new subtest in the WAIS-IV. For each item, individuals must balance a scale by identifying the correct response option within a

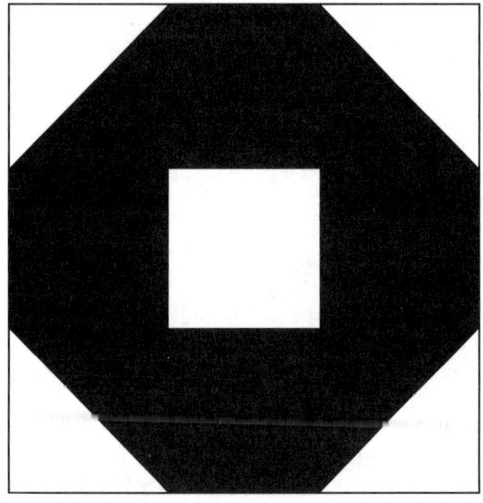

FIGURE 8.1. Example from the WAIS-IV Block Design subtest.

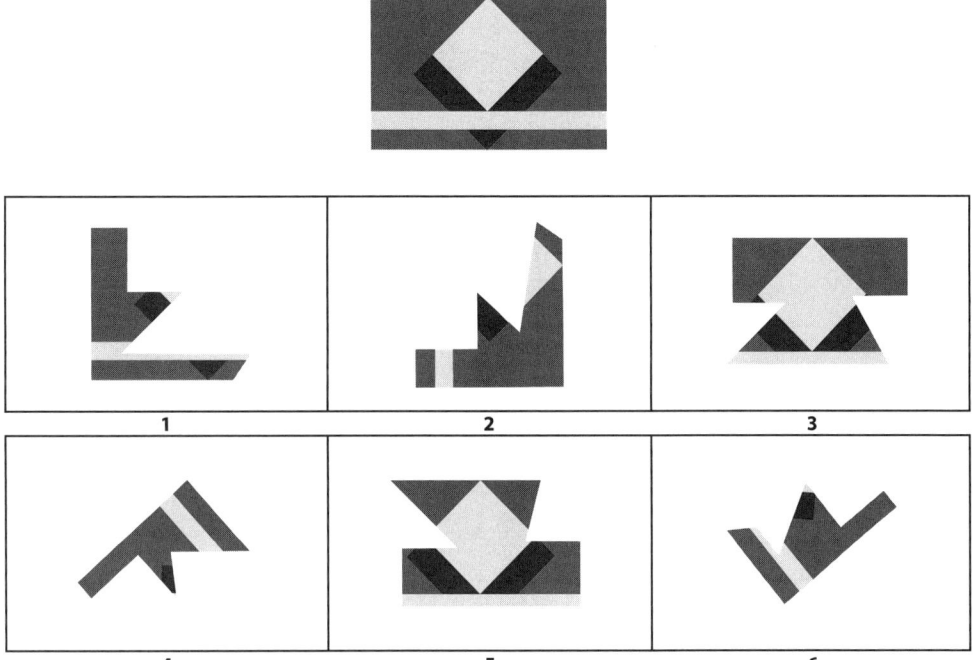

FIGURE 8.3. Example from the WAIS-IV Visual Puzzles subtest.

specified time limit (see Figure 8.5). In order to determine the correct response, the examinee must figure out the relationships between shapes that balanced a previous scale and apply these relationships to the incomplete scale. It measures quantitative and analogical reasoning. It also requires mental flexibility and set shifting (Lichtenberger & Kaufman, 2009; Weiss et al., 2010). Figure Weights is a good measure of *g* (Lichtenberger & Kaufman, 2009) and has adequate to ample specificity (Sattler & Ryan, 2009).

Working Memory Index

The WMI measures the capacity to store incoming auditory information temporarily, as well as

the ability to manipulate this information mentally and hold it in storage for later goal-directed use (Wechsler, 2008; Zhu, Weiss, Prifitera, & Coalson, 2003). Because working memory is a key component of learning, differences in working memory capacity may account for some of the variance in individual differences related to learning capacity and fluid reasoning (Conway et al., 2002; Fry & Hale; 1996; Sternberg, 1995).

Digit Span

The Digit Span subtest has traditionally been composed of two parts: Digit Span Forward and Digit Span Backward. Digit Span Forward requires the examinee to repeat numbers in the same order

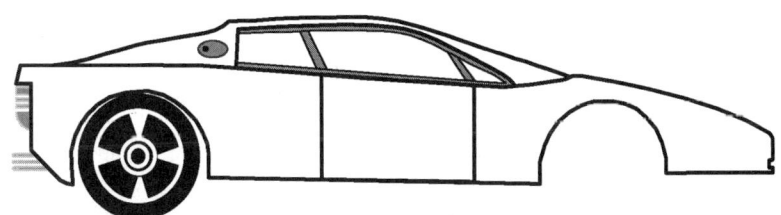

FIGURE 8.4. Example from the WAIS-IV Picture Completion subtest.

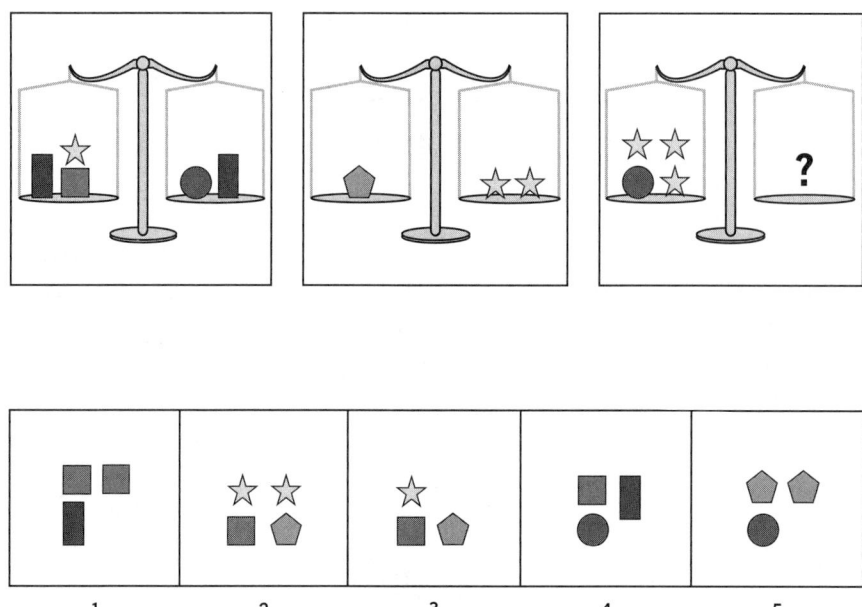

FIGURE 8.5. Example from the WAIS-IV Figure Weights subtest.

as read aloud by the examiner, and Digit Span Backward requires the examinee to repeat the numbers in the reverse order of that presented by the examiner. The WAIS-IV has added Digit Span Sequencing, which requires examinees to sequentially order the numbers presented by the examiner. This subtest measures working memory, in addition to auditory short-term memory, sequential processing, numerical ability, attention, and concentration (Kaufman & Lichtenberger, 2006; Lichtenberger & Kaufman, 2009; Sattler & Ryan, 2009). It is a fair to good measure of *g* and has adequate to ample specificity (Lichtenberger & Kaufman, 2009; Sattler & Ryan, 2009).

Arithmetic

In Arithmetic, the examinee mentally solves a series of orally presented arithmetic problems within a specified time limit (e.g., "Jim buys five stamps, and his mother gives him two more. He then uses one to mail a letter. How many stamps does he have left?"). In addition to auditory working memory, performing the Arithmetic task involves auditory verbal comprehension, mental computation, concentration, attention, long-term memory, numerical reasoning ability, sequential processing, and fluid reasoning (Benson et al., 2010; Kaufman

& Lichtenberger, 2006; Sattler & Ryan, 2009). Although the subtest loads mainly on the Working Memory factor, it shows a secondary loading on the Verbal Comprehension factor due to verbal comprehension demands (Wechsler, 2008). It is a good measure of *g* and has adequate to ample specificity (Lichtenberger & Kaufman, 2009; Sattler & Ryan, 2009).

Letter–Number Sequencing

In Letter–Number Sequencing, the examiner reads a sequence of numbers and letters to the examinee, who recalls the numbers in ascending order and the letters in alphabetical order. This subtest is based in part on the work of Gold, Carpenter, Randolph, Goldberg, and Weinberger (1997), who developed a similar task for individuals with schizophrenia. In addition to sequencing and working memory, the task involves auditory sequential processing, immediate auditory memory, attention, numerical ability, auditory working memory, visual–spatial imaging, and processing speed (Crowe, 2000; Kaufman & Lichtenberger, 2006; Sattler & Ryan, 2009). Letter–Number Sequencing is a fair measure of *g* and has adequate to ample specificity (Lichtenberger & Kaufman, 2009; Sattler & Ryan, 2009).

Processing Speed Index

Performance on the PSI is an indication of the rapidity with which an individual can process simple or routine information without making errors. Historically, cognitive research indicates that the speed of information processing correlates significantly with g (Jensen, 1982; Neisser et al., 1996; Neubauer & Knorr, 1998). Because learning often involves a combination of routine and complex information processing, a processing speed weakness may make comprehending novel information more time-consuming and difficult, and leave an individual with less mental energy for the complex task of understanding new material. The PSI is of specific interest on the WAIS, as it is especially sensitive to aging (Kaufman, 2001; Lichtenberger & Kaufman, 2009) and has been hypothesized to underlie age-related declines in other cognitive domains (Salthouse, 2004).

Coding

Coding requires the examinee to copy symbols that are paired with numbers. Using a key, the examinee draws a symbol in each numbered box within a specified time limit (see Figure 8.6). In addition to visual–motor processing speed, the subtest measures short-term memory, learning ability, visual perception, visual–motor coordination, visual scanning ability, sequential processing, and attention (Kaufman & Lichtenberger, 2006; Sattler & Ryan, 2009). It is a fair measure of g and has adequate to ample specificity (Lichtenberger & Kaufman, 2009; Sattler & Ryan, 2009).

Symbol Search

Symbol Search requires the examinee to scan a group of symbols and indicate whether the target symbols match any of the symbols in the group within a specified time limit (see Figure 8.7). In addition to visual–motor processing speed, the subtest also involves short-term visual memory, perceptual organization, learning ability, perceptual and psychomotor speed, visual–motor coordination, visual discrimination, and attention/concentration (Kaufman & Lichtenberger, 2006; Sattler & Ryan, 2009). Symbol Search is a fair measure of g (Lichtenberger & Kaufman, 2009) and has adequate to ample specificity for most age ranges, but inadequate specificity in the 30- to 54-year-old age band (Sattler & Ryan, 2009).

Cancellation

Cancellation is a new addition to the WAIS-IV. It originally appeared on the WISC-IV as a measure of processing speed that required fewer fine motor demands than subtests such as Coding. Traditionally, cancellation tasks are interpreted as measures of sustained attention, spatial neglect, and response inhibition (Lezak, Howieson, & Loring, 2004). On the WAIS-IV, examinees are required to identify and mark target stimuli that are interspersed among distracters. The stimuli are presented in a random array on the first trial and organized into rows on the second trial. Cancellation is a poor measure of g (Lichtenberger & Kaufman, 2009) but has adequate to ample specificity (Sattler & Ryan, 2009).

General Ability Index

The GAI is an optional index first described in reference to the WISC-III (Prifitera, Weiss, & Saklofske, 1998). It is an aggregate of subtests from the VCI and PRI, and provides an estimate of intellectual functioning with reduced influences of working memory and processing speed. The GAI

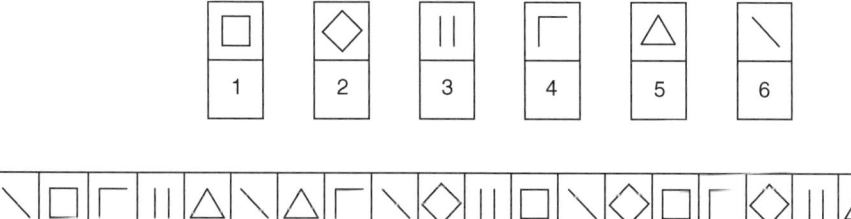

FIGURE 8.6. Example from the WAIS-IV Coding subtest.

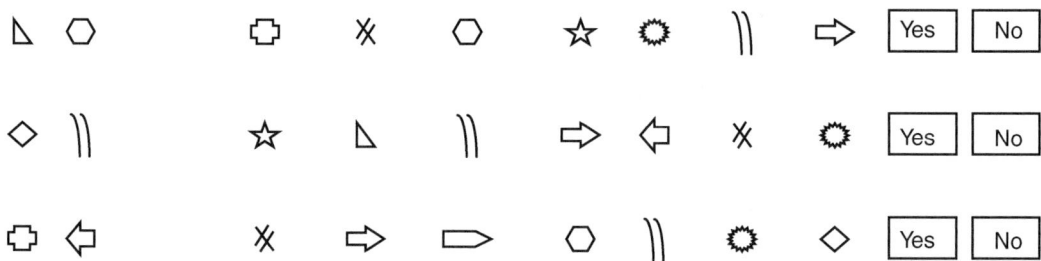

FIGURE 8.7. Example from the WAIS-IV Symbol Search subtest.

is utilized for all the ability–memory comparisons with the WMS-IV to increase the ability to detect discrepancies in individuals with processing speed and working memory deficits—commonly observed difficulties in individuals with memory deficits (see Glass, Bartels, & Ryan, 2009; Lange & Chelune, 2006; Lange, Chelune, & Tulsky, 2006). However, the GAI should not be used solely as a substitute for overall ability because the WMI and PSI are significantly lower than the VCI and PRI, as working memory and processing speed are important contributors to intelligence (Prifitera, Saklofske, & Weiss, 2005; Weiss et al., 2010).

PSYCHOMETRIC PROPERTIES OF THE WAIS-IV

Standardization Sample

The WAIS-IV has an excellent normative sample (Sattler & Ryan, 2009). It includes 2,200 individuals divided into 13 age bands (see Wechsler, 2008, for detailed descriptions of the age bands). Each age band below 70 years contains 200 examinees, whereas each age band from the ages of 70 to 90 years includes 100 examinees. The stratification of the normative sample matches 2005 U.S. census data closely on five key demographic variables: age, gender, race/ethnicity, educational level, and geographic region.

Reliability

The reliabilities for the WAIS-IV are strong (Wechsler, 2008). First, the overall internal-consistency reliability coefficients for the normative sample are in the .90s for all index scores and .98 for the FSIQ. At the subtest level, the overall internal-consistency reliability coefficients of the normative sample are in the .80s or .90s for all core subtests. In addition, Cancellation is the

only supplemental subtest with a reliability below .80, although it is still within the acceptable range (.78). The internal-consistency coefficients of the WAIS-IV subtests calculated from clinical samples are very consistent with those obtained from the normative group, with all subtest coefficients in the .80–.90 range. Second, the test–retest stability coefficients for the WAIS-IV index scores vary from .87 to .96, and the subtest stability coefficients range from .74 to .90. The test–retest stability of the FSIQ is .96. Finally, the interscorer agreement for most WAIS-IV subtests is .98–.99. Even the Verbal Comprehension subtests, which require greater judgment in scoring, have interscorer agreement above .90.

Validity

There is ample evidence to support the validity of the WAIS-IV. The exploratory and confirmatory factor-analytic studies reported in the test manual provide strong evidence of construct validity. These studies clearly demonstrate that in addition to measuring general intellectual ability, the Wechsler scales measure four cognitive domains: Verbal Comprehension, Perceptual Reasoning, Working Memory, and Processing Speed (Wechsler, 2008). Further evidence of construct validity has also been provided by independent examinations of the WAIS-IV data. For example, additional factor-analytic studies indicate that the basic factor structure of the WAIS-IV holds for individuals with clinical syndromes such as schizophrenia and TBI (Goldstein & Saklofske, 2010). Similarly, factor analyses in samples of individuals with autism spectrum disorders have revealed verbal comprehension, perceptual reasoning, and freedom from distractibility factors, as well as a social cognition factor (Goldstein et al., 2008; Goldstein & Saklofske, 2010). In addition, the WAIS-IV and its predecessors correlate highly with other measures of intelligence. As presented in the WAIS-IV technical and interpretive manual (Wechsler, 2008), the WAIS-IV FSIQ correlates .94 with the WAIS-III FSIQ, and correlations between index scores are all above .83. Moreover, previous versions of the WAIS correlate highly with other measures of intelligence, such as the KAIT and the Stanford–Binet Intelligence Scale: Fourth Edition (Wechsler, 1997). Finally, the WAIS-IV has good concurrent validity, as it correlates highly with composites from the Wechsler Individual Achievement Test—Second Edition (WIAT-II; Psychological Corporation, 2005), with correlation coefficients ranging from .34 to .88. It also correlates with the Delis–Kaplan Executive Function System (D-KEFS; Delis, Kaplan, & Kramer, 2001), the California Verbal Learning Test—Second Edition (CVLT-II; Delis, Kramer, Kaplan, & Ober, 2000), and the Repeatable Battery for the Assessment of Neuropsychological Status (RBANS; Randolph, 1998), with high correlations between similar constructs such as the WAIS-IV PRI and RBANS Visuospatial/Constructional scale, and lower correlations between dissimilar constructs such as WAIS-IV indexes and delayed memory scores on the CVLT-II and RBANS (Wechsler, 2008).

THEORETICAL UNDERPINNINGS OF THE WMS-IV

The assessment of memory is a key component of many evaluations of cognitive functioning. A classic example is the measurement of memory ability in evaluations for dementia or mild cognitive impairment. However, memory is affected by many other neurocognitive and learning disorders, including TBI, stroke, epilepsy, intellectual disabilities, learning disorders, and autism spectrum disorders (Bauer, 2008; Eichenbaum, 2008; Squire & Schacter, 2002). In addition, knowledge of an examinee's memory ability can be helpful in learning assessments to help tailor interventions or training programs to a student's learning ability.

The WMS is one of the most popular memory assessment instruments (Rabin, Barr, & Burton, 2005). It was first published in 1945 (Wechsler, 1945) and has undergone several revisions since the initial publication (e.g., Russell's WMS [Russell, 1975, 1988]; WMS-III [Wechsler, 1997]). The changes in the WMS across revisions reflect the growing research on and theories of learning and memory. Squire (1987) described *learning* as the process through which new information is ac-

quired, and *memory* as the persistence of learning so it can be recalled at a later time. The WMS-IV measures both learning and memory ability. Several key concepts are used across measures of learning and memory and are defined here. For more detailed descriptions of learning and memory processes, theories, and measurement, see Byrne (2001), Lezak and colleagues (2004), or Squire and Schacter (2002).

Learning and memory involve encoding, storage or consolidation, and retrieval of information. *Encoding* is the transformation of external information into mental representations or memories; it reflects the entry of information into the memory system. *Consolidation* is the process through which information in immediate memory is transferred and solidified into or stored in long-term memory stores, and *retrieval* involves recalling information from long-term memory stores into active conscious awareness. The WMS-IV measures all three of these concepts.

Many theories divide memory into short-term memory and long-term memory (e.g., Atkinson & Shiffrin, 1968). *Short-term memory* refers to brief, temporary storage of information, lasting from a few seconds to a few minutes. More permanent or long-term memories, lasting from hours to years, are considered *long-term memory*. The WMS-IV measures both short- and long-term memory with the immediate and delayed conditions of Logical Memory, Verbal Paired Associates, Designs, and Visual Reproduction.

Working memory has recently been included as a component of short-term memory. Working memory involves temporary storage and manipulation of information, and the amount of information that can be held in it is very limited. In Baddeley's model, the working memory system has multiple components (Baddeley, 2000, 2003). The *central executive* is a regulatory system that oversees two information activation/storage systems, the *phonological loop* and the *visuospatial sketchpad*. Auditory information is processed and temporarily stored in the phonological loop, and visual information is processed and temporarily stored in the visuospatial sketchpad. In addition to these processes, the *episodic buffer*, regulated by the central executive, transfers information into long-term memory and holds interrelated information in working memory. The central executive controls the flow of information and the attention system, and engages long-term memory as needed. This coordination of cognitive processes by the central executive facilitates learning and other complex cognitive tasks.

Long-term memory is often described as *implicit* (procedural) or *explicit* (declarative) memory. *Implicit* or procedural memory involves learning from experiences without being consciously aware of learning, such as learning to ride a bike or drive a car. *Explicit* or declarative memory involves the conscious storage and retrieval of information, such as personal or factual knowledge. Explicit memory consists of *semantic* and *episodic* memory. *Semantic memory* is the memory for facts and concepts, whereas *episodic memory* is the recollection of personal events and the contexts in which they occur. None of the information required for performance on the WMS-IV is learned prior to the testing session. Therefore, the WMS-IV is primarily a measure of explicit episodic memory as the "information presented is novel and contextually bound by the testing situation and requires the examinee to learn and retrieve information" (Wechsler, 2009, p. 2).

DESCRIPTION OF WMS-IV SUBTESTS AND INDEXES

Two batteries were developed for the WMS-IV: the Adult and Older Adult batteries. The Older Adult battery contains fewer subtests than the Adult battery and provides a shorter administration time. In addition, the content of the auditory memory subtests differs across the two batteries, with fewer stimuli in the Older Adult battery subtests. These changes have reduced the testing time and improved the subtest floors for older adults. The Adult battery can be used for ages 16–69, and the Older Adult battery is used for individuals ages 65–90. In the overlapping ages of 65–69, the examiner may select the battery that is more appropriate for the individual being tested.

The WMS-IV Adult battery contains seven subtests, including six primary subtests and one optional subtest. Four of the primary subtests have immediate-recall (I), delayed-recall (II), and delayed-recognition conditions. Scores from the primary subtests combine to create five index scores: the Auditory Memory Index (AMI), the Visual Memory Index (VMI), the Visual Working Memory Index (VWMI), the Immediate Memory Index (IMI), and the Delayed Memory Index (DMI). The WMS-IV Older Adult battery contains five subtests, including four primary subtests and one optional subtest. Three of the primary subtests have both immediate- and delayed-recall condi-

tions and a delayed-recognition condition, which are combined to form four index scores. The VWMI is not available in the Older Adult battery. Unlike the overall FSIQ in the WAIS-IV, there is not an overall memory ability score; index scores are related to specific domains of memory.

Table 8.2 lists the WMS-IV subtests, the conditions within each subtest, and (where applicable) the index scores to which each subtest contributes. For subtests that have both immediate and delayed conditions, the separate conditions are listed in this table. Note that a single subtest may contribute to more than one index. Some subtest conditions produce scores that are not used to derive index scores, but are considered process scores. These are also optional and denoted with parentheses in Table 8.2. Process scores assist in the interpretation of performance by describing specific skills or abilities required to perform the tasks on the WMS-IV. For example, the Visual Reproduction subtest requires the examinee to draw responses. In order to assess the impact of poor motor ability, a copy condition provides a measure of motor skills.

Subtest Descriptions

It is important to note that the factor analyses conducted with the WMS-IV standardization do not include the Brief Cognitive Status Exam (BCSE). In addition, they do not separate the immediate and delayed memory factors due to the high correlations between these factors (Hoelzle, Nelson, & Smith, 2011; Wechsler, 2009). Although the immediate and delayed factors cannot be separated in factor analyses, they are clinically meaningful and useful (Millis, Malina, Bowers, & Ricker, 1999; Tulsky, Ivnik, Price, & Wilkins, 2003).

Brief Cognitive Status Exam

The BCSE is new to the WMS-IV. It consists of multiple types of items designed to quickly assess various areas of cognitive functioning. The items included in the BCSE were derived from subtests included in the WMS-III (e.g., Mental Control) or from common mental status and neuropsychological measures (e.g., Inhibition). Items include orientation, mental control, incidental memory, clock drawing, inhibition control, and verbal production. Each section of items is used to create a weighted score representing that cognitive ability. The weighted scores are summed to provide an

TABLE 8.2. Subtests and Related Composite Scores of the WMS-IV

Subtest and condition	Contribution to index scales				
	AMI	VMI	VWMI*	IMI	DMI
(BCSE)					
Logical Memory I	✓			✓	
Logical Memory II	✓				✓
(Logical Memory Recognition)					
Verbal Paired Associates I	✓			✓	
Verbal Paired Associates II	✓				✓
(Verbal Paired Associates Recognition)					
(Verbal Paired Associates Word Recall)					
Designs I*		✓		✓	
Designs II*		✓			✓
(Designs Recognition)*					
Visual Reproduction I		✓		✓	
Visual Reproduction II		✓			✓
(Visual Reproduction Recognition)					
(Visual Reproduction Copy)					
Spatial Addition*			✓		
Symbol Span			✓		

Note. AMI, Auditory Memory Index; VMI, Visual Memory Index; VWMI, Visual Working Memory Index; IMI, Immediate Memory Index; DMI, Delayed Memory Index. Asterisks indicate subtests/conditions not included in the Older Adult battery. Check marks indicate primary subtests contributing to an index score. Optional subtests or conditions are in parentheses.

overall BCSE Total Raw Score, which is converted into a classification level indicating the examinee's general cognitive ability.

The BCSE is designed to measure an individual's basic cognitive ability across a variety of tasks. Unlike the comprehensive assessment of cognitive ability provided by the WAIS-IV, the BCSE is intended to provide a quick snapshot of an individual's cognitive status. When the WAIS-IV and WMS-IV are used together, it may not be necessary to administer the BCSE. However, the BCSE provides an opportunity for success early in an assessment session, as most examinees can answer some of the items on the BCSE. Individual items measure orientation to time, mental manipulation of information, incidental memory, planning and organization, the ability to inhibit an overlearned response, and verbal fluency. Other abilities that may be used during this task include confrontation naming, visual perception and attention, processing speed, working memory, planning, cognitive flexibility, auditory comprehension, and verbal expression (Drozdick, Holdnack, & Hilsabeck, 2011; Wechsler, 2009).

Logical Memory

In the Logical Memory subtest, the examinee is read two stories and asked to recall them immediately after presentation and after a 20- to 30-minute delay. Different stories are presented in the Adult and Older Adult batteries. One story in the Older Adult battery is presented twice, creating a multitrial learning task in this age range. Neither story is repeated in the Adult battery. In the recognition task, the examinee answers a series of yes–no questions about details from the stories. Logical Memory measures memory for information presented orally. It measures encoding, immediate and long-term retrieval, and recognition of organized, sequentially related auditory information. It also involves auditory comprehension, receptive and auditory language, auditory working memory, auditory attention and concentration, and hearing acuity (Drozdick et al., 2011; Groth-Marnat, 2009; Lichtenberger, Kaufman, & Lai, 2002). There is a long history of clinical and concurrent validity for Logical Memory (see Lezak et al., 2004, for a review). This subtest contributes to the AMI, IMI, and DMI.

Verbal Paired Associates

In Verbal Paired Associates, the examinee is read a series of paired words. The pairs are either related (e.g., *cat–dog*) or unrelated (*dog–pencil*). After being presented the list, the examinee is read the first word of each pair and asked to recall the second word. If the examinee misses an item, the correct word is given. Four learning trials are given during the immediate condition. Following a 20- to 30-minute delay, the examinee is asked to recall the second word in each pair again. In the recognition condition, the examinee is read a word pair and asked to indicate whether it is a pair from the list. In the word recall condition, the examinee is asked to recall the individual words from the word pairs; no cues are provided, and the examinee does not have to recall the words in pairs.

Verbal Paired Associates measures the ability to learn and retrieve associated words presented orally. It involves short-term auditory learning, long-term cued and recognition auditory memory, and associative memory. Other skills include auditory perception and comprehension, auditory working memory or rehearsal, expressive and receptive language, and hearing acuity (Groth-Marnat, 2009; Holdnack & Drozdick, 2010; Lichtenberger et al., 2002). Like Logical Memory, Verbal Paired Associates has a long history of clinical and concurrent validity studies (see Lezak et al., 2004, for a review). This subtest contributes to the AMI, IMI, and DMI.

Designs

Designs is a new subtest in the WMS-IV. It requires the examinee to view a 4 × 4 grid in the stimulus book (see Figure 8.8). The grid contains designs in some of the cells. Following exposure, the grid is removed from view, and the examinee uses a blank grid and design cards to reproduce the image from memory. Four grids are shown and recalled both immediately and following a 20- to 30-minute delay. A recognition condition may be given following delayed recall. This subtest measures the ability to recall details and spatial information for abstract visual designs. It involves memory for visual detail and spatial memory; encoding and immediate and long-term retrieval of visual and spatial information; visual perception and organization; self-monitoring; and auditory comprehension. It also involves visual acuity, visual working memory, and gross motor ability (Drozdick et al., 2011; Groth-Marnat, 2009; Holdnack & Drozdick, 2010). This subtest contributes to the VMI, IMI, and DMI in the Adult battery.

Visual Reproduction

For each Visual Reproduction item, the examinee is shown a design for 10 seconds and then asked to draw the design from memory (see Figure 8.9). A total of five designs are shown sequentially, with recall both immediately after presentation and following a 20- to 30-minute delay. Performance on Visual Reproduction is affected by motor-constructional abilities (Gfeller, Meldrum, & Jacobi, 1995; Larrabee & Curtiss, 1995). An optional copy condition is available to assess the influence of motor difficulties. No modifications to Visual Reproduction administration were made from the WMS-III; however, the scoring has been modified to focus on the memory aspects of recall instead of motor accuracy. Visual Reproduction is designed

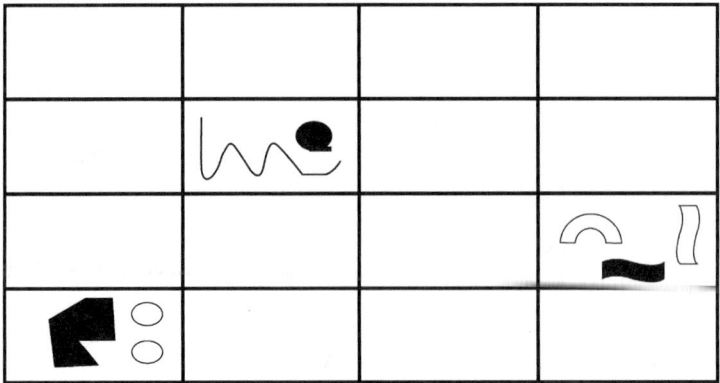

FIGURE 8.8. Example from the WAIS-IV Designs subtest.

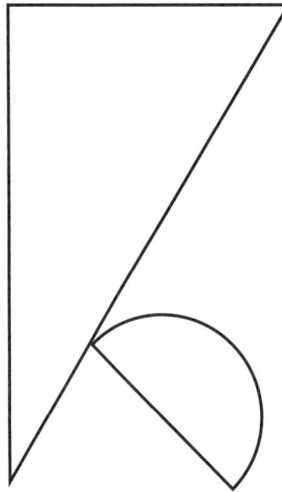

FIGURE 8.9. Example from the WAIS-IV Visual Reproduction subtest.

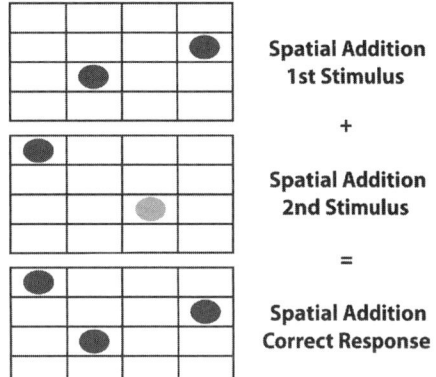

FIGURE 8.10. Example from the WAIS-IV Spatial Addition subtest.

to assess immediate and long-term visual memory for abstract designs. It also involves visual–motor coordination, visual–spatial construction, visual perception and organization, processing speed, planning, self-monitoring, and language ability (Drozdick et al., 2011; Groth-Marnat, 2009; Lezak et al., 2004). This subtest contributes to the VMI, IMI, and DMI.

Spatial Addition

Spatial Addition is a new subtest and requires the examinee to look at two grids presented sequentially and produce a new grid by combining the images across the two grids. Each presented grid contains blue and/or red circles. The examinee is instructed to remember the locations of the blue circles and to ignore the red circles. After being shown both grids, the examinee places cards in the grid based on a set of rules. Figure 8.10 presents an example of a Spatial Addition item. This subtest measures visual–spatial working memory. It also involves visual perception and organization, executive functions, and gross motor ability (Drozdick et al., 2011; Groth-Marnat, 2009). This subtest contributes to the VWMI in the Adult battery.

Symbol Span

For each Symbol Span item, the examinee is shown an array of abstract symbols. The array is

then removed, and the examinee is shown a second array of symbols containing both the symbols the examinee was shown previously and distracter symbols (see Figure 8.11). The examinee must select the correct symbols in the order presented in the original array. Partial credit is awarded for selecting the correct symbols in an incorrect order. Symbol Span is a new subtest. The task involves visual-sequencing working memory. It also involves mental manipulation of visual material, attention, mental flexibility, visual–spatial imaging, and visual perception and attention (Drozdick et al., 2011; Groth-Marnat, 2009). This subtest contributes to the VWMI in the Adult battery.

WMS-IV Index Descriptions

The WMS-IV index scores measure major domains of memory, whereas the subtest scores measure specific aspects of memory. For example, the AMI score summarizes an individual's performance across subtests designed to measure auditory memory, while Logical Memory and Verbal Paired

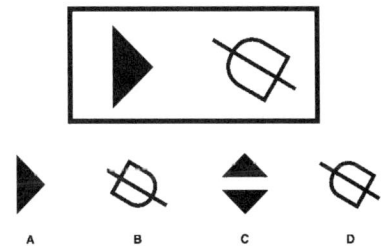

FIGURE 8.11. Example from the WAIS-IV Symbol Span subtest.

Associates measure more specific aspects of auditory memory. An individual can obtain an average AMI with multiple ranges of subtest scores—for example, average scores on all contributing subtests, or above-average scores on Logical Memory and below-average scores on Verbal Paired Associates. Therefore, it is important to evaluate performance on index scores in the context of the performance on the contributing subtests.

Auditory Memory Index

The AMI is a measure of memory for orally presented information, both immediately and following a delay. It requires auditory attention, comprehension, and retrieval (Groth-Marnat, 2009; Wechsler, 2009). It consists of the Logical Memory and Verbal Paired Associates immediate- and delayed-recall conditions. It is composed of the same subtests across both batteries.

Visual Memory Index

The VMI is a measure of memory for information presented visually—specifically, abstract visual designs and spatial information. It measures visual perception and organization, as well as immediate and delayed recall and recognition of visual and spatial details (Groth-Marnat, 2009; Wechsler, 2009). It consists of the Designs and Visual Reproduction immediate and delayed conditions in the Adult battery. For the Older Adult battery, it consists of the Visual Reproduction immediate and delayed conditions.

Visual Working Memory Index

The VWMI measures the ability to encode, manipulate and recall visual and spatial information. It is a visual analogue to the WAIS-IV WMI, which measures auditory working memory. It involves attending to, mentally manipulating, and organizing visual information (Groth-Marnat, 2009; Wechsler, 2009). It consists of the Spatial Addition and Symbol Span subtests and is only available in the Adult battery. The WAIS-IV WMI focuses solely on verbal working memory tasks, whereas the WMS-IV VWMI contains visual and spatial working memory tasks. The primary benefit of this structure is interpretive clarity, as some modern theories of working memory posit distinct systems underlying visual and auditory information processing (Baddeley, 2003).

Immediate Memory Index

Performance on the IMI is an indication of the examinee's ability to recall presented information immediately. It is a good indication of an examinee's ability to encode auditory and visual information. It consists of the immediate-recall conditions of Logical Memory, Verbal Paired Associates, Designs, and Visual Reproduction in the Adult battery, and the immediate-recall conditions of Logical Memory, Verbal Paired Associates, and Visual Reproduction in the Older Adult battery. Since it includes measures of auditory and visual memory, discrepancies between performance on these modalities will affect performance on this index.

Delayed Memory Index

Performance on the DMI is an indication of the examinee's ability to recall presented information following a delay in which other tasks are being completed. It is a good indication of an examinee's ability to consolidate and retrieve auditory and visual information. The DMI differs from the General Memory Index (GMI) of the WMS-III. The GMI included measures of both delayed recall and recognition. Although the Designs subtest includes aspects of recognition memory, recognition tasks are not included in the DMI. The DMI consists of the delayed-recall conditions of Logical Memory, Verbal Paired Associates, Designs, and Visual Reproduction in the Adult battery, and the delayed-recall conditions of Logical Memory, Verbal Paired Associates, and Visual Reproduction in the Older Adult battery. Since it includes measures of auditory and visual memory, discrepancies between performance on these modalities will affect performance on this index.

PSYCHOMETRIC PROPERTIES OF THE WMS-IV

Standardization Sample

The WMS-IV has excellent normative samples, with 900 individuals included in the Adult battery sample and 500 included in the Older Adult battery sample. The samples were divided into 14 age bands (9 in the Adult battery and 5 in the Older Adult battery), with 100 individuals in each age band (see Wechsler, 2009, for detailed descriptions of the age bands). The stratification of the normative sample matches 2005 U.S. census data closely on five key demographic variables: age, gender, race/ethnicity, educational level, and geographic region.

The co-collection of the WAIS-IV and WMS-IV normative samples provided the opportunity for the mean ability level for each WMS-IV age band to be set at a GAI of 100, without requiring weighting of the normative sample. This ensured that the norms for the WMS-IV were not biased due to a high- or low-ability sample. In addition, the normative sample was screened for cognitive impairment and suboptimal effort.

Reliability

The reliabilities for the WMS-IV are good to excellent (Groth-Marnat, 2009; Wechsler, 2009) as indicated by internal-consistency and test–retest reliability estimates and interscorer agreement rates. The overall internal-consistency reliability coefficients for the normative samples are in the .90s for all index scores. At the subtest level, the overall internal-consistency reliability coefficients of the normative samples are in the .80s or .90s for all of the primary subtest scores, with the exception of Verbal Paired Associates II in the Older Adult battery. The lower reliability (.74) in this subtest is due to the small range of scores available in this measure. The internal-reliability coefficients for the process scores are lower, ranging from .74 to .77. The internal-consistency coefficients calculated using clinical samples are generally higher but fairly consistent with those obtained from the normative group, with all subtest coefficients in the .86–.97 range. The test–retest stability coefficients for the WMS-IV tend to be lower than those observed in the WAIS-IV, due to ceiling effects, fluctuations in motivation, and practice effects, which are observed in most memory measures (Strauss, Sherman, & Spreen, 2006). Stability coefficients for the index scores range from .80 to .87, and the subtest stability coefficients range from .64 to .79. The test–retest stability of the process scores ranges from .59 to .76. Finally, the interscorer agreement for most WMS-IV subtests is .98–.99. Even the subtests involving more subjective scoring have interscorer agreement above .90.

Validity

There is strong evidence to support the validity of the WMS-IV (Drozdick et al., 2011; Groth-Marnat, 2009; Wechsler, 2009). The confirmatory factor-analytic studies reported in the WMS-IV technical and interpretive manual provide strong evidence of construct validity for the AMI, VMI, and VWMI. As described earlier, the IMI and DMI are not supported by factor-analytic studies, due to the high correlation of these indexes. Further evidence of construct validity has also been provided by independent examinations of the Adult battery normative sample. A series of exploratory principal component analyses conducted by Hoelzle and colleagues (2011) on each of the Adult battery normative age bands supported a two-factor structure for the WMS-IV, differentiating auditory and visual factors. This study failed to differentiate the VMI and VWMI, but confirmed the visual factor.

In addition to factor-analytic support, the WMS-IV correlates highly with its predecessor and other memory measures. The WMS-IV technical and interpretive manual (Wechsler, 2009) reports the correlations of the WMS-IV with the WMS-III, WMS-III Abbreviated, CVLT-II, and Children's Memory Scale (CMS; Cohen, 1997). In general, the correlations with the WMS-III are high, although they are lower in the visual memory domain because of the significant changes to visual memory measures in the WMS-IV. With regard to the other memory measures, the correlations are low to moderate, with higher correlations in measures assessing similar constructs (e.g., the AMI with Verbal Immediate Memory in CMS). Finally, the WMS-IV has good predictive validity, as it correlates highly with composites from the WIAT-II, with correlation coefficients ranging from .29 to .77. Correlations with the D-KEFS, RBANS, Texas Functional Living Scales (Cullum, Saines, & Weiner, 2009), and Independent Living Scales (Loeb, 1996) are also reported; these support the concurrent validity and structure of the WMS-IV (Cullum et al., 2009; Wechsler, 2009).

CLINICAL APPLICATIONS

Because the Wechsler intelligence scales are reliable and valid instruments for comprehensive assessment of general cognitive functioning, clinicians have found many clinical applications of these instruments. The WAIS-IV is one of several key instruments for the assessment or diagnosis of (1) psychoeducational and developmental disorders, such as developmental delay, developmental risk, intellectual disabilities, learning disabilities, ADHD, language disorders, motor impairment, and autism; (2) cognitive giftedness; (3) neuropsychological disorders, such as TBI, Alzheimer's disease, Huntington's disease, Parkinson's disease, multiple sclerosis, and temporal lobe epilepsy; and (4) alcohol-related disorders, such as chronic alcohol abuse and Korsakoff syndrome. In addition to the many clinical validation studies reported in the WAIS-IV technical and interpretive manual (Wechsler, 2008), please refer to Kaufman and Lichtenberger (1999), Prifitera and Saklofske (1998), Sattler (2008), and Tulsky, Saklofsky, and colleagues (2003) for more detailed discussions of the clinical utilities of the Wechsler scales.

The various editions of the WMS are among the mostly widely used assessments of memory functioning (Rabin et al., 2005). The WMS-IV can be an instrumental component of any evaluation involving memory functioning, including evaluations of (1) memory complaints, such as those seen with dementia, depression, and mild cognitive impairment; (2) neuropsychological disorders, such as brain injury or insult, temporal lobe epilepsy, or multiple sclerosis; (3) learning disorders; and (4) substance use disorders or exposure to toxic substances, such as Korsakoff syndrome or heavy metal exposure. See the WMS-IV technical and interpretive manual (Wechsler, 2009) for the clinical validation studies of the WMS-IV. In addition, see Groth-Marnat (2009), Lichtenberger and colleagues (2002), and Strauss and colleagues (2006) for more information on clinical utility of the WMS-IV and WMS-III.

A number of issues need to be considered when clinicians are administering the WAIS-IV and WMS-IV in conjunction with each other. First, the WMS-IV should be administered prior to the WAIS-IV if they are given during the same testing session. Zhu and Tulsky (2000) found small order effects on the WMS-III when it was administered following the WAIS-III but not vice versa. Second, as described previously, the GAI is used instead of the FSIQ for ability–memory comparisons. Finally, the WAIS-IV and WMS-IV both assess working memory. Although they measure different modalities, only one of the indexes needs to be administered if modality-specific weaknesses are not observed.

INTERPRETATION

In addition to the basic interpretation steps and procedures suggested in the technical manuals of the WAIS-IV and WMS-IV (Wechsler, 2008, 2009), many interpretation strategies, methods, and procedures developed by experienced clinicians and researchers for the previous and current versions of the Wechsler scales continue to be valid and useful (Groth-Marnat, 2009; Lichtenberger & Kaufman, 2009; Sattler, 2008). Although a detailed discussion of interpretation strategies, methods, and procedures is beyond the scope of this chapter, the following interpretive considerations may help readers understand the nature of clinical interpretation. However, these suggestions should not be used as a "cookbook" or comprehensive guideline for interpretation. Clinical interpretation is a very complicated hypothesis-testing process that varies across evaluations. Therefore, no single approach will work for all scenarios, and WAIS-IV and WMS-IV data should always be interpreted within the context of such information as medical and psychosocial history, behavioral observations, and referral questions.

Basic Interpretation of Wechsler Scores

Scores

The Wechsler scales utilize two types of *standard scores*: *scaled scores* and *composite scores* (i.e., IQ and index scores). The conversion of raw scores into standard scores allows clinicians to interpret scores within the Wechsler scales and between the Wechsler scales and other related measures. The scaled scores and composite scores are age-corrected standard scores that allow comparison of each individual's cognitive functioning with other individuals in the same age group.

Scaled scores are derived from the total raw scores on each subtest. They are scaled to a metric with a mean of 10 and a standard deviation (SD) of 3. A subtest scaled score of 10 reflects the average performance of a given age group. Scores of 7 and 13 correspond to 1 SD below and above the mean, respectively, and scaled scores of 4 and 16 deviate 2 SDs from the mean.

Composite scores (e.g., the FSIQ, PRI, and AMI) are standard scores derived from various combinations of subtest scaled scores. They are scaled to a metric with a mean of 100 and an SD of 15. A score of 100 on any composite defines an average performance. Scores of 85 and 115 correspond to 1 SD below and above the mean, respectively, and scores of 70 and 130 deviate 2 SDs from the mean.

In general, standard scores provide the most accurate descriptions of test data. However, for individuals unfamiliar with test interpretation, standard scores are often difficult to understand. Other methods, such as percentile ranks and verbal descriptive classifications, are often used in conjunction with standard scores to describe an examinee's performance. Scores on the Wechsler scales should be reported with confidence intervals, so that each score is evaluated in light of the score's reliability. Confidence intervals delineate a range of scores in which the examinee's true score is most likely to fall and remind the examiner that the observed score contains measurement error.

For several process scores on the WMS-IV, the majority of individuals in the normative sample obtained perfect or near-perfect scores, resulting in a skewed distribution of raw scores. Cumulative percentage ranges are used to describe performance for these scores (i.e., ≤2%, 3–9%, 10–16%, 17–25%, 26–50%, 51–75%, and >75%). Cumulative percentages describe the percentage of individuals who obtained the same or lower score on a task as the examinee. For example, a cumulative percentage range of 51–75 means the examinee scored as well as 51–75% of the normative sample.

Level of Performance

The IQ, index, and scaled scores can be characterized as falling within a certain level of performance (e.g., superior, high average, average, low average). The *level of performance* refers to the rank obtained by an individual on a given test, compared to the performance of an appropriate normative group. The descriptive classifications corresponding to scores on the WAIS-IV and WMS-IV are presented in Table 8.3. Descriptive classifications allow communication of results in

TABLE 8.3. Descriptive Classifications of WAIS-IV and WMS-IV Composite and Index Scores

Score	Classification	Percent included in theoretical normal curve
130 and above	Very superior	2.2
120–129	Superior	6.7
110–119	High average	16.1
90–109	Average	50.0
80–89	Low average	16.1
70–79	Borderline	6.7
69 and below	Extremely low	2.2

terms most individuals can comprehend. Test results can be described in a manner similar to the following example: "Compared to individuals of similar age, the examinee performed in the low average [descriptive classification] range on a measure of general intelligence [domain content]."

For clinical evaluations, the level of performance provides an estimate of the presence and severity of relative strengths or weaknesses in an individual's performance. This can help with clinical decisions for individuals whose level of performance is significantly lower than that of the normative group, either overall or within specific cognitive or memory domains. Alternatively, clinical decisions can be based on relative strengths and weaknesses within an individual's scores (e.g., a specific score is significantly lower than the individual's other scores, representing an intraindividual weakness).

Description of Composite Scores

For both the WAIS-IV and WMS-IV, the composite scores are more reliable than the subtest scaled scores, and in general they are the first scores examined by the practitioner. On the WAIS-IV, the FSIQ is typically the first score reported and described, as it is the most reliable score on the WAIS-IV and describes the examinee's general intellectual functioning. The FSIQ standard score is typically provided, as well as the percentile rank and the confidence interval surrounding the score. Although it is the best single-point predictor of cognitive ability, there are many cases in which additional scores are required to portray a person's cognitive ability accurately, especially those characterized by extreme discrepancies between index scores. See other recently released volumes for guidance on interpreting the FSIQ in cases with extreme index score variability (Lichtenberger & Kaufman, 2009; Weiss et al., 2010). However, note that extreme index score discrepancies do not invalidate the FSIQ; rather, interpretation of the FSIQ should account for the index discrepancies. Regardless of the presence of index discrepancies, the four index scores should always be included with the FSIQ in the first level of interpretation, as differences in index score profiles may yield important clinical information. For example, research using previous editions of the WAIS has demonstrated that several clinical syndromes are characterized by unique index score profiles, including schizophrenia, autism, and TBI (Goldstein & Saklofske, 2010).

Analysis of Discrepancies among Composite Scores

Given the clinical significance of index score differences on the WAIS and WMS (Dori & Chelune, 2004; Goldstein & Saklofske, 2010; Lange et al., 2006; Wilde et al., 2001) and the impact of extreme index score discrepancies on the interpretation of the FSIQ, index score discrepancy analyses are an important step in WAIS-IV and WMS-IV interpretation. The first step of the discrepancy analysis is to determine the statistical significance of the discrepancy between a pair of composite scores either within or between the WAIS-IV and WMS-IV. Discrepancy analyses can be derived by using three different methods: simple difference, predicted difference, and contrast scaled scores. The simple-difference method can be used to compare scores within the WAIS-IV or WMS-IV, and the contrast scaled score approach can be used for comparing scores within the WMS-IV. In addition, all three methods can be used to evaluate ability–memory discrepancies between the WAIS-IV and WMS-IV.

For the simple-difference and predicted-difference methods, statistical significance and clinical significance of score differences are important concepts to understand. A *statistically significant difference* between scores (e.g., between the VCI and the PRI scores) means that the likelihood of obtaining a similar difference by chance is very low (e.g., $p < .05$) if the true difference between the scores is zero. The level of significance reflects the level of confidence a clinician can have that the difference between the scores, called the *difference score*, is a true difference. Along with statistical significance, it is important to consider the base rate of various difference scores in the general population. Even a statistically significant difference may occur frequently in normally developing and aging individuals. Often the difference between an individual's composite scores is significant in the statistical sense, but occurs frequently among individuals in the general population. The statistical significance of discrepancies between scores and the frequency of the difference in the normative population are two separate issues and have different implications for test interpretation (Sattler, 2008). In order for a score difference to be considered clinically meaningful, it should be relatively rare. There are no strict guidelines to determine whether a significant difference is rare, and clinicians are advised to take into account medical history, cultural context, and other factors when making that decision. That being said, Sat-

tler (2008) advises that score differences occurring in fewer than 15% of the standardization sample should be considered unusual.

Simple- and Predicted-Difference Methods

The simple-difference method involves the subtraction of an obtained score from a second obtained score. In the predicted-difference method, the ability score is used in a regression equation to calculate a predicted score. The examinee's actual performance is then compared to the predicted score. These methods are easy to compute and to interpret. The score difference is identified as either a relative strength or a relative weakness, or no difference is observed between the variables. To determine whether the scores are statistically different, the difference score for each comparison is compared to the established cutoff required for statistical significance. The WAIS-IV and WMS-IV administration manuals provide clinicians with the minimum differences between index scores required for statistical significance at the .15 and .05 levels by age group. The manuals also provide base rates of the various index score discrepancies in the normative sample. The WMS-IV technical and interpretive manual also provides this information for the ability–memory discrepancies.

Contrast Scaled Score Method

The contrast scaled score methodology applies standard norming procedures to adjust a dependent measure by a control variable. These scores answer specific clinical questions, such as "Is the DMI above or below average, given the examinee's IMI score?". Tables for deriving the contrast scaled scores for the WMS-IV indexes are found in the WMS-IV administration and scoring manual. The tables for deriving the ability–memory contrast scaled scores are found in the WMS-IV technical and interpretive manual. A contrast scaled score is interpreted in the same manner as all scaled scores. For example, a 53-year-old examinee with a GAI of 87 and a DMI of 76 would obtain a contrast scaled score of 6, indicating borderline delayed memory ability given the examinee's general ability.

Evaluation of Subtest Strengths and Weaknesses

Cognitive profiles describe an examinee's relative strengths and weaknesses. It is very common for examinees to perform better on some subtests than on others, and for clinicians to want to interpret these differences as meaningful. The risk of overinterpretation is high, given the frequency of subtest variation; clinicians can minimize this risk by assessing subtest strengths and weaknesses in the context of referral questions, as well as all sources of corroborating and contradicting evidence. However, there are many situations in which subtest level differences are important (e.g., neuropsychological evaluation of individuals with focal brain damage), and the Wechsler scales provide three types of subtest score comparisons.

The three methods utilized to compare subtest scores are a comparison to the mean subtest score, difference scores, and contrast scaled scores. First, in order to identify subtest strengths or weaknesses, the WAIS-IV provides the minimum difference between a single subtest and the mean of all subtests required for statistical significance at the .15 and .05 levels, as well as the base rates of these differences. Second, for cases in which it is more appropriate to compare two subtest scores directly (e.g., Digit Span and Arithmetic within the context of interpreting the WMI), the WAIS-IV provides the difference between all possible pairs of subtests required for statistical significance at the .15 and .05 levels, as well as the base rate information for the differences; the WMS-IV provides the same information for specified subtest comparisons. Finally, contrast scaled scores are provided for several WMS-IV subtest comparisons.

BRIEF CASE STUDY

Examinee: Elizabeth H.
Report date: 6/13/2011
Age: 72 years
Date of birth: 2/18/1939
Gender: Female
Years of education: 14
Tests administered: WAIS-IV, WMS-IV

Reason for Referral

Mrs. H. was referred for an evaluation by her primary care physician, Dr. Jordan Lane, due to concerns about her memory and ability to manage her medications.

History

Mrs. H. is a 72-year-old widowed female who was born in the United States to parents who were first-generation immigrants from Mexico. She speaks English as her primary language and has 14 years of education in the United States. She attended college for 2 years before marrying and raising five children. She has good relationships with her children and grandchildren, and is active in several church and charity groups. She currently lives alone with some assistance from her children. Recently her children have noticed that she frequently misplaces items, repeats stories, and has trouble organizing her bills and calendar. Mrs. H. denies significant problems, but reports feeling more tired and admits forgetting where she places things. She also reports that it is harder for her to learn new things and that she is sometimes overwhelmed by preparing for meetings and appointments.

Behavioral Observations

Mrs. H. was well groomed and polite. She exhibited appropriate behavior throughout the assessment. She was alert and oriented to time and place. She appeared to give forth good effort and did not require redirection to the testing. She appeared to fatigue easily, however, and several breaks were given to allow her to rest and refocus on testing.

Test Results

Mrs. H. completed the 10 core subtests of the WAIS-IV (see Tables 8.4 and 8.5 for her compos-

TABLE 8.4. Mrs. H.'s WAIS-IV Composite Scores

Scale	Composite score	Percentile rank	Confidence interval (95%)	Qualitative description
Verbal Comprehension Index (VCI)	93	32	88–99	Average
Perceptual Reasoning Index (PRI)	100	50	94–106	Average
Working Memory Index (WMI)	80	9	74–88	Low average
Processing Speed Index (PSI)	84	14	77–94	Low average
General Ability Index (GAI)	96	39	91–101	Average
Full Scale IQ (FSIQ)	88	21	84–92	Low average

TABLE 8.5. Mrs. H.'s WAIS-IV Subtest Scores

Subtests	Scaled score	Percentile rank
Similarities	8	25
Vocabulary	8	25
Information	10	50
Block Design	8	25
Matrix Reasoning	14	91
Visual Puzzles	8	25
Digit Span	6	9
Arithmetic	7	16
Coding	8	25
Symbol Search	6	9

ite and subtest scores, respectively). She obtained an FSIQ of 88 (84–92 at the 95% confidence interval), indicating low average overall intellectual functioning in comparison to her same-age peers in the normative sample. Her performance across the index scores shows variability among the skills measured by the FSIQ. Specifically, she demonstrated average verbal comprehension (VCI = 91 [85–98]) and perceptual reasoning (PRI = 100 [94–106]) abilities. However, her auditory working memory (WMI = 80 [74–88]) and processing speed (PSI = 84 [77–94]) are in the low average range. The GAI was also computed in order to examine ability–memory discrepancies. Her GAI of 96 (91–101) indicates that her general verbal and nonverbal problem-solving ability is in the average range.

The WAIS-IV index comparisons for Mrs. H. show that verbal and perceptual reasoning abilities are significantly better than working memory. Similarly, processing speed is significantly lower than perceptual reasoning abilities. FSIQ is significantly lower than GAI. The score profile indicates relative weaknesses in both working memory and processing speed. Subsequently, FSIQ is lower

than GAI, due to the impact of significantly lower processing speed and working memory. Although significant index-level variability in performance was observed, significant variability in subtest performance was only observed in the perceptual reasoning domain.

Mrs. H.'s performance on the measures within the PRI was variable. On a task of nonverbal visual–spatial reasoning, she performed above average (Matrix Reasoning = 14); however, scores on measures of nonverbal concept formation and nonverbal reasoning were in the average range (Block Design = 8, Visual Puzzles = 8). It is interesting to note that there were no time constraints on the subtest on which Mrs. H. performed in the above-average range. Her lower performance on the other tests may have been influenced by time constraints. Outside of this relative strength, Mrs. H.'s performance was relatively consistent across subtests and domains.

Mrs. H. also completed the WMS-IV (see Tables 8.6 and 8.7 for her index and subtest scores, respectively) to examine her memory abilities. Her low average score on the BCSE is consistent with her performance on the WAIS-IV. Her performance across the WMS-IV index scores shows variability. Specifically, she has borderline auditory memory ability (AMI = 72 [67–80]) and low average visual and immediate memory abilities (VMI = 82 [78–87]; IMI = 80 [75–87], respectively). However, her delayed memory is extremely low (DMI = 67 [62–77]). Mrs. H. appears to be having fairly significant problems with her memory—in particular, her ability to recall information following a delay. On a measure of visual working memory, her performance was in the average range, suggesting relatively intact ability to encode and mentally manipulate visual information.

Mrs. H.'s DMI is significantly lower than her IMI (note that neither the IMI nor the DMI is compared to the AMI or VMI because they share common subtests). Contrast scores also indicate that delayed memory is extremely low, given her

TABLE 8.6. Mrs. H.'s WMS-IV Index Scores

Scale	Composite score	Percentile rank	Confidence interval (95%)	Qualitative description
Auditory Memory Index (AMI)	72	3	67–80	Borderline
Visual Memory Index (VMI)	82	12	78–87	Low average
Immediate Memory Index (IMI)	80	9	75–87	Low average
Delayed Memory Index (DMI)	67	1	62–77	Extremely low

TABLE 8.7. Mrs. H.'s WMS-IV Subtest Scores

Subtests	Scaled score	Percentile rank
Logical Memory I	6	9
Logical Memory II	3	1
Verbal Paired Associates I	6	9
Verbal Paired Associates II	6	9
Visual Reproduction I	8	25
Visual Reproduction II	5	5
Symbol Span	8	25
BCSE	—	Low average

immediate-recall ability. The AMI and VMI are not significantly different, suggesting that the memory problems Mrs. H. is experiencing are not specific to either auditory or visual memory.

Within the AMI, IMI, and DMI, none of the subtest scores were significantly different from the mean of the subtest scaled scores within the domain. However, a significant pairwise difference between Visual Reproduction I and II is evident. This suggests relatively stable performance within domains. The contrast scores for the primary subtest scores revealed relatively consistent performance on Verbal Paired Associates delayed-recall when immediate-recall abilities were considered. However, delayed-recall scores on both Logical Memory and Visual Reproduction were unexpectedly low, given her immediate-recall ability. Overall, Mrs. H. appears to be having difficulties with long-term memory. In addition, delayed memory appears to be a significant weakness compared to immediate memory.

In addition to the recall conditions, Mrs. H. also completed optional WMS-IV conditions, including the recognition trials for all three delayed memory conditions—Verbal Paired Associates Word Recall and Visual Reproduction Copy. The optional conditions provide additional information about Mrs. H.'s performance on specific subtests. For both verbal memory subtests, recall memory was slightly lower than expected, given the examinee's ability to recognize information. Her performance on Logical Memory II recognition was extremely low, suggesting that her memory does not improve with cueing and that her problems with delayed memory are due to an inability to encode and retain verbal information. On Verbal Paired Associates Recognition, she performed in

the low average range (17–25%) for delayed recognition and word recall (scaled score = 6). The Visual Reproduction optional conditions indicate that Mrs. H. has average recognition (26–50%) for the visual designs. Her ability to copy the designs is also in the average range (26–50%). The Recognition and Immediate Recall versus Delayed Recall contrast scaled scores indicate that delayed free recall is unexpectedly low compared to both recognition and immediate encoding ability, indicating difficulties with encoding and retrieval of visual details and spatial relations among the details. The Visual Reproduction Copy versus Immediate Recall scores show that her immediate memory performance was lower than expected, given her ability to directly copy the design. Thus the low scores on this subtest are not likely to be attributable to poor motor control.

The WAIS-IV and WMS-IV index comparisons were completed to determine whether Mrs. H.'s memory functioning is consistent with her general cognitive functioning. Table 8.8 displays Mrs. H.'s WAIS-IV/WMS-IV index comparisons, using the predicted-difference method and contrast scores. When the predicted-difference discrepancy model was applied with GAI as the predictor, significant differences were observed between GAI and AMI (base rate = 2–3%), VMI (base rate = 10%), IMI (base rate = 5–10%), and DMI (base rate > 1%). These results indicate that memory functioning is significantly lower than expected, considering Mrs. H.'s general problem-solving ability. Her low memory scores are not likely to be attributable to low general ability. The contrast scaled scores also suggest memory problems that are not consistent with her general cognitive abilities. When GAI was controlled for, her AMI, VMI, IMI, and DMI were all lower than expected.

Mrs. H. was referred for this evaluation due to reports of memory difficulties. Her profile supports the presence of significant memory problems, in addition to problems with processing speed and verbal working memory. Although her performance in most domains was relatively stable, a strength was noted on an untimed measure of nonverbal fluid reasoning.

Summary

Mrs. H. is a 72-year-old widowed female with a history of memory problems. She was administered the WAIS-IV and WMS-IV to determine her general cognitive and memory abilities. Her general intellectual ability is in the low average

TABLE 8.8. Mrs. H.'s Ability–Memory Discrepancy Analyses and Contrast Scores

	Predicted-difference method				
	Predicted WMS-IV index score	Actual WMS-IV index score	Difference	Critical value	Base rate
AMI	98	72	26	10.41	2–3
VMI	98	82	16	7.89	10
IMI	97	80	17	9.97	5–10
DMI	98	67	31	12.33	<1
	Contrast scaled score method				
	WAIS-IV composite	WMS-IV index score	Contrast score		
GAI vs. AMI	96	72	4		
GAI vs. VMI	96	82	6		
GAI vs. IMI	96	80	5		
GAI vs. DMI	96	67	3		
VCI vs. AMI	93	72	4		
PRI vs. VMI	100	82	5		
WMI vs. AMI	80	72	6		

range, with weaknesses observed in verbal working memory and processing speed. Her memory performance was lower than expected given her general problem-solving ability, with particular problems with delayed memory. Differences were not observed between auditory and verbal memory. It is very likely that Mrs. H. is experiencing mild cognitive impairment.

REFERENCES

Archer, R. P., Buffington-Vollum, J. K., Stredny, R. V., & Handel, R. W. (2006). A survey of psychological test use patterns among forensic psychologists. *Journal of Personality Assessment, 87*(1), 84–94.

Atkinson, R. C., & Shiffrin, R. M. (1968). A proposed system and its control processes. In K. W. Spence & J. T. Spence (Eds.), *The psychology of learning and motivation: Advances in research and theory* (Vol. 2, pp. 82–90). New York: Academic Press.

Baddeley, A. D. (2000). The episodic buffer: A new component of working memory? *Trends in Cognitive Sciences, 4,* 417–423.

Baddeley, A. D. (2003). Working memory: Looking back and looking forward. *Nature Reviews Neuroscience, 4*(10), 829–839.

Bauer, R. M. (2008). The three amnesias. In J. E. Morgan & J. H. Ricker (Eds.), *Textbook of clinical neuropsychology* (pp. 729–742). New York: Taylor & Francis.

Benson, N., Hulac, D. M., & Kranzler, J. H. (2010). Independent examination of the Wechsler Adult Intelligence Scale—Fourth Edition (WAIS-IV): What does the WAIS-IV measure? *Psychological Assessment, 22*(1), 121–130.

Beres, K. A., Kaufman, A. S., & Perlman, M. D. (2000). Assessment of child intelligence. In G. Goldstein & M. Hersen (Eds.), *Handbook of psychological assessment* (3rd ed., pp. 65–96). New York: Pergamon Press.

Berg, A. T., Langfitt, J. T., Testa, F. M., DiMario, F., Kulas, J., Westerveld, M., et al. (2008). Residual cognitive effects of uncomplicated idiopathic and cryptogenic epilepsy. *Epilepsy and Behavior, 13*(4), 614–619.

Bowden, S. C., Lange, R. T., Weiss, L. G., & Saklofske, D. H. (2008). Invariance of the measurement model underlying the WAIS-III in the United States and Canada. *Educational and Psychological Measurement, 68,* 1024–1040.

Byrne, B. M. (2001). Structural equation modeling: Perspectives on the present and the future. *International Journal of Testing, 1*(3–4), 327–334.

Carroll, J. B. (1993). *Human cognitive abilities: A survey of factor analytic studies.* New York: Cambridge University Press.

Cohen, J. (1952). A factor-analytically based rationale for the Wechsler–Bellevue. *Journal of Consulting Psychology, 16,* 272–277.

Cohen, J. (1957). A factor-analytically based rationale for the Wechsler Adult Intelligence Scale. *Journal of Consulting Psychology, 21,* 451–457.

Cohen, M. (1997). *Children's Memory Scale*. San Antonio, TX: Pearson.

Colom, R., Rebollo, I., Palacios, A., Espinosa, M. J., & Kyllonen, P. C. (2004). Working memory is (almost) perfectly predicted by *g*. *Intelligence*, *32*(3), 277–296.

Conway, A. R. A., Cowan, N., Bunting, M. F., Therriault, D. J., & Minkoff, S. R. B. (2002). A latent variable analysis of working memory capacity, short-term memory capacity, processing speed, and general fluid intelligence. *Intelligence*, *30*, 163–183.

Conway, A. R. A., Kane, M. J., & Engle, R. W. (2003). Working memory capacity and its relation to general intelligence. *Trends in Cognitive Sciences*, *7*(12), 547–552.

Crowe, S. F. (2000). Does the letter number sequencing task measure anything more than digit span? *Assessment*, *7*(2), 113–117.

Cullum, M., Saines, K., & Weiner, M. F. (2009). *Texas Functional Living Scales*. San Antonio, TX: Pearson.

Deary, I. J. (2009). Introduction to the special issue on cognitive epidemiology. *Intelligence*, *37*(6), 517–519.

Delis, D. C., Kaplan, E., & Kramer, J. H. (2001). *Delis–Kaplan Executive Function System*. San Antonio, TX: Pearson.

Delis, D. C., Kramer, J. H., Kaplan, E., & Ober, B. A. (2000). *California Verbal Learning Test—Second Edition*. San Antonio, TX: Pearson.

Dori, G. A., & Chelune, G. J. (2004). Education-stratified base-rate information on discrepancy scores within and between the Wechsler Adult Intelligence Scale—Third Edition and the Wechsler Memory Scale—Third Edition. *Psychological Assessment*, *16*, 146–154.

Drozdick, L. W., Holdnack, J. A., & Hilsabeck, R. (2011). *Essentials of WMS-IV assessment*. Hoboken, NJ: Wiley.

Eichenbaum, H. (2008). *Learning and memory*. New York: Norton.

Elliott, C. D. (1990). *Differential Ability Scales: Introductory and technical handbook*. San Antonio, TX: Psychological Corporation.

Fergusson, D. M., Horwood, L. J., & Ridder, E. M. (2005). Show me the child at seven II: Childhood intelligence and later outcomes in adolescence and young adulthood. *Journal of Child Psychology and Psychiatry*, *46*(8), 850–858.

Forn, C., Belenguer, A., Parcet-Ibars, M. A., & Ávila, C. (2008). Information-processing speed is the primary deficit underlying the poor performance of multiple sclerosis patients in the Paced Auditory Serial Addition Test (PASAT). *Journal of Clinical and Experimental Neuropsychology*, *30*(7), 789–796.

Fry, A. F., & Hale, S. (1996). Processing speed, working memory, and fluid intelligence: Evidence for a developmental cascade. *Psychological Science*, *7*, 237–241.

Fry, A. F., & Hale, S. (2000). Relationships among processing speed, working memory, and fluid intelligence in children. *Biological Psychology*, *54*, 1–34.

Gathercole, S. E., Hitch, G. J., Service, E., & Martin, A. J. (1997). Phonological short-term memory and new word learning in children. *Developmental Psychology*, *33*(6), 966–979.

Georgas, J., Weiss, L. G., van de Vijver, F. J. R., & Saklofske, D. H. (Eds.). (2003). *Culture and children's intelligence: Cross-cultural analysis of the WISC-III*. San Diego, CA: Academic Press.

Gfeller, J. D., Meldrum, D. L., & Jacobi, K. A. (1995). The impact of constructional impairment on the WMS-R visual reproduction subtests. *Journal of Clinical Psychology*, *51*, 58–63.

Glass, L. A., Bartels, J. M., & Ryan, J. J. (2009). WAIS-III FSIQ and GAI in ability-memory discrepancy analysis. *Applied Neuropsychology*, *16*, 19–22.

Gold, J. M., Carpenter, C., Randolph, C., Goldberg, T. E., & Weinberger, D. R. (1997). Auditory working memory and Wisconsin Card Sorting Test performance in schizophrenia. *Archives of General Psychiatry*, *54*, 159–165.

Goldstein, G., Allen, D. N., Minshew, N. J., Williams, D. L., Volkmar, F., Klin, A., et al. (2008). The structure of intelligence in children and adults with high functioning autism. *Neuropsychology*, *22*, 301–312.

Goldstein, G., & Saklofske, D. H. (2010). The Wechsler intelligence scales in the assessment of psychopathology. In L. G. Weiss, D. H. Saklofske, D. Coalson, & S. E. Raiford, (Eds.), *WAIS-IV clinical use and interpretation: Scientist-practitioner perspectives* (pp. 189–216). London: Elsevier.

Gottfredson, L. S. (1997). Mainstream science on intelligence: An editorial with 52 signatories, history, and bibliography. *Intelligence*, *24*, 13–23.

Gottfredson, L. S., & Deary, I. J. (2004). Intelligence predicts health and longevity, but why? *Current Directions in Psychological Science*, *13*(1), 1–4.

Groth-Marnat, G. (2009). *Handbook of psychological assessment* (5th ed.). Hoboken, NJ: Wiley.

Groth-Marnat, G., & Teal, M. (2000). Block Design as a measure of everyday spatial abilities: A study of ecological validity. *Perceptual and Motor Skills*, *90*(2), 522–426.

Hoelzle, J. B., Nelson, N. W., & Smith, C. A. (2011). Comparison of Wechsler Memory Scale—Fourth Edition (WMS-IV) and Third Edition (WMS-III) dimensional structures: Improved ability to evaluate auditory and visual constructs. *Journal of Clinical and Experimental Neuropsychology*, *33*(3), 283–291.

Holdnack, J. A., & Drozdick, L. W. (2010). Using WAIS-

IV with WMS-IV. In L. G. Weiss, D. H. Saklofske, D. Coalson, & S. E. Raiford (Eds.), *WAIS-IV clinical use and interpretation: Scientist-practitioner perspectives* (pp. 237–283). London: Elsevier.

Horn, J. L. (1994). Theory of fluid and crystallized intelligence. In R. J. Sternberg (Ed.), *Encyclopedia of human intelligence* (pp. 443–451). New York: Macmillan.

Jaeggi, S. M., Buschkuehl, M., Jonides, J., & Perrig, W. J. (2008). Improving fluid intelligence with training on working memory. *Proceedings of the National Academy of Sciences USA, 105*(19), 6829–6833.

Jensen, A. R. (1982). Reaction time and psychometric g. In H. J. Eysenck (Ed.), *A model for intelligence* (pp. 93–132). New York: Springer-Verlag.

Jensen, A. R. (1998). *The g factor: The science of mental ability.* Westport, CT: Praeger.

Kaufman, A. S. (1992). Dr. Wechsler remembered. *The School Psychologist, 46*(2), 4–5.

Kaufman, A. S. (2001). WAIS-III IQs, Horn's theory, and generational changes from young adulthood to old age. *Intelligence, 29,* 131–167.

Kaufman, A. S. (2010). Foreword. In L. G. Weiss, D. H. Saklofske, D. Coalson, & S. E. Raiford (Eds.), *WAIS-IV clinical use and interpretation: Scientist-practitioner perspectives* (pp. xiii–xxii). London: Elsevier.

Kaufman, A. S., & Kaufman, N. L. (1993). *Kaufman Adolescent and Adult Intelligence Test.* Circle Pines, MN: American Guidance Service.

Kaufman, A. S., & Lichtenberger, E. O. (1999). *Essentials of WAIS-III assessment.* New York: Wiley.

Kaufman, A. S., & Lichtenberger, E. O. (2006). *Assessing adolescent and adult intelligence* (3rd ed.). Hoboken, NJ: Wiley.

Kennedy, J. E., Clement, P. F., & Curtiss, G. (2003). WAIS-III Processing Speed Index scores after TBI: The influence of working memory, psychomotor speed and perceptual processing. *Clinical Neuropsychologist, 17*(3), 303–307.

Lange, R. T., & Chelune, G. J. (2006). Application of new WAIS-III/WMS-III discrepancy scores for evaluating memory functioning: Relationship between intellectual and memory ability. *Journal of Clinical and Experimental Neuropsychology, 28,* 592–604.

Lange, R. T., Chelune, G. J., & Tulsky, D. S. (2006). Development of WAIS-III General Ability Index minus WMS-III memory discrepancy scores. *The Clinical Neuropsychologist, 20,* 382–395.

Larrabee, G. J., & Curtiss, J. (1995). Construct validity of various verbal and visual memory tests. *Journal of Clinical and Experimental Neuropsychology, 17,* 536–547.

Lee, H. F., Gorsuch, R., Saklofske, D. H., & Patterson, C. (2008). Cognitive differences for ages 16 to 89 (Canadian WAIS-III): Curvilinear with Flynn and processing speed corrections. *Journal of Psychoeducational Assessment, 26*(4), 382–394.

Lezak, M. D., Howieson, D. B., & Loring, D. W. (2004). *Neuropsychological assessment* (4th ed.). New York: Oxford University Press.

Lichtenberger, E. O., & Kaufman, A. S. (2009). *Essentials of WAIS-IV assessment.* Hoboken, NJ: Wiley.

Lichtenberger, E. O., Kaufman, A. S., & Lai, Z. C. (2002). *Essentials of WMS-III assessment.* New York: Wiley.

Loeb, P. A. (1996). *Independent Living Scales.* San Antonio, TX: Pearson.

Mathias, J. L., & Wheaton, P. (2007). Changes in attention and information-processing speed following severe traumatic brain injury: A meta-analytic review. *Neuropsychology, 21*(2), 212–223.

McGrew, K. S., & Flanagan, D. P. (1997). Beyond g: The impact of Gf-Gc specific cognitive abilities research on the future use and interpretation of intelligence tests in the schools. *School Psychology Review, 26*(2), 189–210.

Millis, S. R., Malina, A. C., Bowers, D. A., & Ricker, J. H. (1999). Confirmatory factor analysis of the WMS-III. *Journal of Clinical and Experimental Neuropsychology, 21,* 87–93.

Neisser, U., Boodoo, G., Bouchard, T. J., Boykin, A. W., Brody, N., Ceci, S. J., et al. (1996). Intelligence: Knowns and unknowns. *American Psychologist, 51*(2), 77–101.

Neubauer, A. C., & Knorr, E. (1998). Three paper-and-pencil tests for speed of information processing: Psychometric properties and correlations with intelligence. *Intelligence, 26*(2), 123–151.

Perlow, R., Jattuso, M., & Moore, D. D. (1997). Role of verbal working memory in complex skill acquisition. *Human Performance, 10*(3), 283–302.

Prifitera, A., & Saklofske, D. H. (Eds.). (1998). *WISC-III clinical use and interpretation: Scientist-practitioner perspectives.* San Diego, CA: Academic Press.

Prifitera, A., Saklofske, D. H., & Weiss, L. G. (Eds.). (2005). *WISC-IV clinical use and interpretation: Scientist-practitioner perspectives.* Amsterdam: Elsevier Academic Press.

Prifitera, A., Weiss, L. G., & Saklofske, D. H. (1998). The WISC-III in context. In A. Prifitera & D. H. Saklofske (Eds.), *WISC-III clinical use and interpretation: Scientist-practitioner perspectives* (pp. 1–38). San Diego, CA: Academic Press.

Psychological Corporation. (2005). *Wechsler Individual Achievement Test—Second Edition: Update 2005.* San Antonio, TX: Author.

Rabin, L. A., Barr, W. B., & Burton, L. A. (2005). Assessment practices of clinical neuropsychologists in the United States and Canada: A survey of INS, NAN, and APA division 40 members. *Archives of Clinical Neuropsychology, 20,* 33–65.

Randolph, C. (1998). *Repeatable battery for the Assessment of Neuropsychological Status.* San Antonio, TX: Pearson.

Russell, E. W. (1975). A multiple scoring method for the assessment of complex memory functions. *Journal of Consulting and Clinical Psychology, 43,* 800–809.

Russell, E. W. (1988). Renorming Russell's version of the Wechsler Memory Scale. *Journal of Clinical and Experimental Neuropsychology, 10,* 235–249.

Salthouse, T. A. (1996). The processing-speed theory of adult age differences in cognition. *Psychological Review, 103,* 403–428.

Salthouse, T. A. (2004). Localizing age-related individual differences in a hierarchical structure. *Intelligence, 32,* 541–561.

Sattler, J. M. (2008). *Assessment of children: Cognitive foundations* (5th ed.). San Diego, CA: Jerome M. Sattler.

Sattler, J. M., & Ryan, J. J. (2009). Assessment with the *WAIS-IV.* San Diego, CA: Jerome M. Sattler.

Schwean, V., & Saklofske, D. H. (2005). Assessment of attention deficit hyperactivity disorder with the WISC-IV. In A. Prifitera, D. Saklofske, & L. G. Weiss (Eds.), *WISC-IV clinical use and interpretation: Scientist–practitioner perspectives* (pp. 235–280). Amsterdam: Elsevier Academic Press.

Squire, L. R. (1987). *Memory and brain.* New York: Oxford University Press.

Squire, L. R., & Schacter, D. L. (2002). *Neuropsychology of memory* (3rd ed.). New York: Guilford Press.

Sternberg, R. J. (1995). *In search of the human mind.* Fort Worth, TX: Harcourt Brace.

Sternberg, R. J. (Ed.). (2000). *Handbook of intelligence.* New York: Cambridge University Press.

Stinnett, T. A., Havey, J. M., & Oehler-Stinnett, J. (1994). Current test usage by practicing school psychologists: A national survey. *Journal of Psychoeducational Assessment, 12*(4), 331–350.

Strauss, E., Sherman, E. M. S., & Spreen, O. (2006). *A compendium of neuropsychological tests: Administration, norms, and commentary* (3rd ed.). New York: Oxford University Press.

Tulsky, D. S., Ivnik, R. J., Price, L. R., & Wilkins, C. (2003). Assessment of cognitive functioning with the WAIS-III and WMS-III: Development of a 6-factor model. In D. S. Tulsky, D. H. Saklofsky, G. J. Chelune, R. K. Heaton, R. J. Ivnik, R. Bornstein, et al. (Eds.), *Clinical interpretation of the WAIS-III and WMS-III* (pp. 147–179). San Diego, CA: Academic Press.

Tulsky, D. S., Saklofsky, D. H., Chelune, G. J., Heaton, R. K., Ivnik, R. J., Bornstein, R., et al. (Eds.). (2003). *Clinical interpretation of the WAIS-III and WMS-III.* San Diego, CA: Academic Press.

Tulsky, D. S., Zhu, J., & Prifitera, A. (2000). Assessing adult intelligence with the WAIS-III. In G. Goldstein & M. Hersen (Eds.), *Handbook of psychological assessment* (3rd ed.). New York: Pergamon Press.

Wechsler, D. (1939). *The measurement of adult intelligence.* Baltimore: Williams & Wilkins.

Wechsler, D. (1945). A standardized memory scale for clinical use. *Journal of Psychology, 19,* 87–95.

Wechsler, D. (1950). Cognition, conative, and non-intellective intelligence. *American Psychologist, 5,* 78–83.

Wechsler, D. (1975). Intelligence defined and undefined: A relativistic appraisal. *American Psychologist, 30,* 135–139.

Wechsler, D. (1997). *WAIS-III–WMS-III technical manual.* San Antonio, TX: Psychological Corporation.

Wechsler, D. (2003). *Wechsler Intelligence Scale for Children—Fourth Edition.* San Antonio, TX: Psychological Corporation.

Wechsler, D. (2008). *Wechsler Adult Intelligence Scale—Fourth Edition.* San Antonio, TX: Pearson.

Wechsler, D. (2009). *Wechsler Memory Scale—Fourth Edition.* San Antonio, TX: Pearson.

Weiss, A., Gale, C. R., Batty, D., & Deary, I. J. (2009). Emotionally stable, intelligent men live longer: The Vietnam experience study cohort. *Psychosomatic Medicine, 71,* 385–394.

Weiss, L. G., Saklofske, D. H., Coalson, D., & Raiford, S. E. (Eds.). (2010). *WAIS-IV clinical use and interpretation: Scientist-practitioner perspectives.* London: Elsevier.

Wilde, N. J., Strauss, E., Chelune, G. J., Loring, D. W., Martin, R. C., Hermann, B. P., et al. (2001). WMS-III performance in patients with temporal lobe epilepsy: Group differences and individual classification. *Journal of the International Neuropsychological Society, 7,* 881–891.

Zachary, R. A. (1990). Wechsler's intelligence scales: Theoretical and practical considerations. *Journal of Psychoeducational Assessment, 8,* 276–289.

Zhu, J., & Tulsky, D. S. (2000). Co-norming of the WAIS-III and WMS-III: Is there a test order effect on IQ and memory scores? *Clinical Neuropsychologist, 14*(4), 461–467.

Zhu, J., Weiss, L. G., Prifitera, A., & Coalson, D. (2003). The Wechsler intelligence scales for children and adults. In M. Hersen (Series Ed.) & G. Goldstein & S. R. Beers (Vol. Eds.), *Comprehensive handbook of psychological assessment: Vol. 1. Intellectual and neuropsychological assessment* (pp. 51–75). New York: Wiley.

CHAPTER 9

The Wechsler Preschool and Primary Scale of Intelligence—Third Edition, the Wechsler Intelligence Scale for Children—Fourth Edition, and the Wechsler Individual Achievement Test—Third Edition

Dustin Wahlstrom
Kristina C. Breaux
Jianjun Zhu
Lawrence G. Weiss

The Wechsler intelligence scales are a family of individually administered instruments for assessing the intellectual functioning of children and adults across the lifespan continuum. Of these tests, two are currently designed specifically for the assessment of children: the Wechsler Preschool and Primary Scale of Intelligence—Third Edition (WPPSI-III; Wechsler, 2002a), for children between the ages of 2 years, 6 months (2:6 years) and 7:3 years, and the Wechsler Intelligence Scale for Children—Fourth Edition (WISC-IV) (Wechsler, 2003a), for children between the ages of 6:0 and 16:11 years. Since the original publication of the Wechsler–Bellevue Intelligence Scale in 1939, the Wechsler scales have had a tremendous influence on the field of psychological assessment. They represent the most widely used and researched intelligence tests in the field today, due in large part to their comprehensiveness, clinical utility, ecological validity, and theoretical soundness (Kamphaus, 1993; Kaplan & Saccuzzo, 2005; Sattler, 2008; Wasserman & Maccubbin, 2002).

The Wechsler family of tests has expanded over the years to include measures outside the intelligence domain. One of the more widely used is the Wechsler Individual Achievement Test—Third Edition (WIAT-III; Pearson, 2009), which was de-veloped to address the growing demand for standardized achievement testing in special education and clinical settings. Intelligence and achievement tests are frequently used in conjunction with each other, whether to identify learning disabilities or to assess the impact of clinical syndromes, acquired injury, or delays in other cognitive domains on learning and academic potential. The Wechsler family of assessment instruments facilitates this process by providing statistical linkage between the intelligence and academic measures, which supplies practitioners with an important tool to support their clinical interpretations and conclusions. The current chapter provides an overview of all three measures, beginning with the intelligence tests, and concluding with a joint interpretive section and clinical case example to illustrate how results from intelligence and achievement measures can be integrated to provide richer clinical information than either type of test provides alone.

HISTORY AND THEORY BEHIND THE WPPSI-III AND WISC-IV

For a more comprehensive review of the theory underlying the Wechsler scales and the history of their development, see Drozdick, Wahlstrom, Zhu, & Weiss (Chapter 8, this volume), as well as Tulsky and colleagues (2003) and Weiss, Saklofske, Coalson, and Raiford (2010). Briefly, the Wechsler scales have been described as atheoretical relative to other tests (Beres, Kaufman, & Perlman, 2000; Kaufman & Lichtenberger, 1999; Shaw, Swerdlik, & Laurent, 1993)—a claim that probably stems from David Wechsler's reputation as an astute clinician and his inclusion of existing measures with proven clinical and practical utility during construction of the original Wechsler–Bellevue. Nonetheless, to describe them as atheoretical is inaccurate. Wechsler was inspired by Charles Spearman's and Edward Thorndike's theories of intelligence at the time, and the Wechsler scales have undergone numerous revisions that have been guided by shifts in our theoretical conceptualization of IQ (which have in turn been influenced by advances in sociology, clinical and developmental psychology, and cognitive neuroscience).

Modern editions of Wechsler's tests have changed dramatically from their original versions. This is evidenced by the fact that 40% of the WISC-IV subtests have been developed since the publication of the original WISC in 1949, and only 24% of the original items on the retained subtests have yet to be replaced. Similarly, 57% of the current WPPSI-III subtests have been developed since the publication of the original WPPSI in 1967. Of the WPPSI subtests that have been retained, only 23% of the original item content remains. Reflected in these changes is the updated theoretical structure of the Wechsler scales, which results from added subtests of fluid reasoning (Picture Concepts and Matrix Reasoning), increased contribution of working memory and processing speed to the measure of general intelligence, and improved measurement of relatively pure cognitive functions by reducing confounds such as time bonuses and fine motor demands. These constructs are increasingly recognized as critical contributors to general intellectual ability, as well as to our understanding of intelligence as a dynamic construct that involves the interaction of working memory, processing speed, and fluid reasoning with other cognitive variables (Colom, Rebollo, Palacios, Espinosa, & Kyllonen, 2004; Conway, Cowan, Bunting, Therriault, & Minkoff, 2002; Fry & Hale, 1996, 2000; Jaeggi, Buschkuehl, Jonides, & Perrig, 2008; Salthouse, 1996; Weiss et al., 2010).

The importance of working memory and processing speed are especially relevant to the childhood populations served by the WPPSI-III and WISC-IV, as the development of processing speed and working memory skills may underlie the development of fluid reasoning, with processing speed mediating developmental gains in working memory as well (Fry & Hale, 1996). Furthermore, the Working Memory Index (WMI) is second only to the Verbal Comprehension Index (VCI) in the prediction of reading, writing, and math as measured by standardized achievement tests (Hale, Fiorello, Kavanagh, Hoeppner, & Gaither, 2001; Konold, 1999); working memory is related as well to other academic tasks, such as spelling, reading comprehension, note taking, and following instructions (Daneman & Merikle, 1996; Engle, Carullo, & Collins, 1991; Kiewra & Benton, 1988; Ormrod & Cochran, 1988).

Although many of these advances have been developed by clinical researchers since Wechsler's death in 1981, he recognized the importance of the processes that underlie working memory, processing speed, and fluid reasoning (even before they were named as such) and utilized subtests measuring these processes in his early intelligence batteries. For example, Digit Span and Arithmetic, which were initially part of Wechsler's Verbal IQ (VIQ), are now considered to be primarily tests of working memory. Similarly, Digit–Symbol Coding originally contributed to Performance IQ (PIQ) but is currently understood as a measure of processing speed, and a number of original Wechsler subtests measured fluid reasoning in addition to other cognitive constructs.

The ultimate result of Wechsler's foresight and the changes made since his death is a family of tests that, despite being criticized as atheoretical, yield constructs that align very closely with recent models of intelligence. In addition to the four-factor model reported in test manuals (see below), independent examinations of the WISC-IV indicate that it measures several constructs central to Cattell–Horn–Carroll (CHC)–based models of intelligence, including crystallized ability, visual processing, fluid reasoning, short-term memory, and processing speed (Keith, Goldenring Fine, Taub, Reynolds, & Kranzler, 2006). Furthermore, these factor loadings are similar for all age bands in the standardization sample, indicating that the test measures similar psychological constructs regardless of age. These findings, as well as the four-factor model, have been replicated by groups using standardization samples from other countries (Chen, Keith, Chen, & Chang, 2009; Georgas, van de Vijver, Weiss, & Saklofske, 2003). Finally, the WISC-IV and WPPSI-III correlate highly with other intelligence tests that were created to assess particular neurocognitive theories, such as the Kaufman Assessment Battery for Children— Second Edition (KABC-II; Kaufman & Kaufman, 2004) and the Differential Ability Scales—Second Edition (DAS-II; Elliott, 2007).

DESCRIPTION OF WISC-IV AND WPPSI-III SUBTESTS AND COMPOSITES

As all the Wechsler scales do, the WISC-IV and WPPSI-III yield subtest scores, as well as composite index scores and a general intelligence score. General descriptions of the Wechsler Full Scale IQ (FSIQ), index scores, and subtests are provided in Chapter 8 of this volume; thus, rather than focusing on the general nature of the subtests and index scores that constitute the WPPSI-III and WISC-IV, this chapter instead focuses on issues specific to these two tests. Some subtests, however, were not described in Chapter 8 and are mentioned here in greater detail.

Table 9.1 contains the WISC-IV and WPPSI-III subtests, as well as the index scores to which each contributes. Due to the rapid development of cognitive skills during early childhood, the WPPSI-III is divided into two batteries for children ages 2:6–3:11 and 4:0–7:3 years. The battery for younger children consists of four core subtests and one supplemental subtest, whereas the battery for older children is composed of seven core subtests and seven supplemental subtests. Children in the younger age band take fewer tests with expressive language and sustained attention demands, thus reducing these confounds during an age at which the acquisition of these skills varies widely. The WISC-IV consists of 10 core subtests and 5 supplemental subtests, all of which can be administered to the full age range of the test. The WISC-IV yields an FSIQ, as well as four composite scores: the VCI, Perceptual Reasoning Index (PRI), WMI, and Processing Speed Index (PSI). Although not provided in the test manual, clinicians can also calculate the General Ability Index (GAI) and Cognitive Proficiency Index (CPI). In addition to the FSIQ, the WPPSI-III yields a VIQ, a PIQ, and an optional General Language Composite (GLC) in the battery for younger children. It provides the FSIQ, VIQ, and PIQ as core index scores, as well as an optional Processing Speed Quotient (PSQ) and the optional GLC in the battery for older children. Five new subtests are included in the WISC-IV:

Picture Concepts, Matrix Reasoning, Word Reasoning, Letter–Number Sequencing, and Cancellation. Seven new subtests were added to the WPPSI-III: Matrix Reasoning, Picture Concepts, Symbol Search, Word Reasoning, Coding, Receptive Vocabulary, and Picture Naming.

Descriptions of Composite Scores

Full Scale Intelligence Quotient (WISC-IV and WPPSI-III)

The WISC-IV FSIQ is a measure of general cognitive ability derived from the 10 core subtests that make up the four index scores. Relative to its predecessors, the WISC-IV FSIQ places greater emphasis on fluid reasoning, working memory, and processing speed. Similarly, the WPPSI-III FSIQ contains greater contributions from subtests measuring fluid reasoning and processing speed. Overall, general cognitive ability is a robust predictor of important life outcomes (Gottfredson, 1997). Perhaps most important considering the age ranges covered by the WPPSI-III and WISC-IV, the FSIQ is a good predictor of academic achievement— a relationship that has been replicated in both normal and clinical populations (Watkins, Glutting, & Lei, 2007; Watkins, Lei, & Canivez, 2007; Wechsler, 2002b, 2003b). This may hold true even when there is variable performance across index scores (Daniel, 2007; Watkins, Glutting, et al., 2007), though others have suggested that the FSIQ is a less reliable predictor than the index scores in these situations (Fiorello et al., 2007; Hale, Fiorello, Kavanaugh, Holdnack, & Aloe, 2007).

Verbal Comprehension Index/Verbal IQ (WISC-IV and WPPSI-III)

The WISC-IV VCI and WPPSI-III VIQ are indexes of crystallized intelligence that are intended to measure verbal concept formation, verbal reasoning and comprehension, acquired knowledge, and attention to verbal stimuli. Research using the WISC-IV and WIAT-II suggests that the VCI is the best predictor of academic achievement after g (Glutting, Watkins, Konold, & McDermott, 2006). As might be expected from this finding, Verbal Comprehension subtests have the highest g loadings on Wechsler tests. Vocabulary, Information, Similarities, Comprehension, and Word Reasoning are all good measures of g on both the WISC-IV and WPPSI-III (Sattler, 2008). They have specificities that range from ample to inad-

TABLE 9.1. Subtests and Related Composite Scores of the WISC-IV and WPPSI-III

WISC-IV subtests	Contribution to IQ and factor index scales					
	VCI	PRI	WMI	PSI	FSIQ	GAI
Vocabulary	✓				✓	✓
Similarities	✓				✓	✓
Comprehension	✓				✓	✓
Information	(✓)				(✓)	
Word Reasoning	(✓)				(✓)	
Letter–Number Sequencing			✓		✓	
Digit Span			✓		✓	
Arithmetic			(✓)		(✓)	
Block Design		✓			✓	✓
Matrix Reasoning		✓			✓	✓
Picture Concepts		✓			✓	✓
Picture Completion		(✓)			(✓)	
Coding				✓	✓	
Symbol Search				✓	✓	
Cancellation				(✓)	(✓)	

WPPSI-III subtests	Contribution to IQ and factor index scales				
	VIQ	PIQ	PSQ	FSIQ	GLC
Ages 2:6–3:11					
Information	✓			✓	
Block Design		✓		✓	
Object Assembly		✓		✓	
Receptive Vocabulary	✓			✓	✓
Picture Naming	(✓)			(✓)	✓
Ages 4:0–7:3					
Vocabulary	✓			✓	
Information	✓			✓	
Word Reasoning	✓			✓	
Similarities	(✓)			(✓)	
Comprehension	(✓)			(✓)	
Block Design		✓		✓	
Matrix Reasoning		✓		✓	
Picture Concepts		✓		✓	
Picture Completion		(✓)		(✓)	
Object Assembly		(✓)		(✓)	
Coding			✓	✓	
Symbol Search			✓	(✓)	
Receptive Vocabulary	✓*				*
Picture Naming	*				*

Note. VCI, Verbal Comprehension Index; PRI, Perceptual Reasoning Index; WMI, Working Memory Index; PSQ, Processing Speed Quotient; FSIQ, Full Scale IQ; GAI, General Ability Index; VIQ, Verbal IQ; PIQ, Performance IQ; GLC, General Language Composite. Check marks indicate the core subtests contributing to a composite score. Supplemental subtests are designated by parentheses. Subtests denoted with an asterisk are optional.

equate, depending on the age range (see Sattler, 2008, for more details).

Perceptual Reasoning Index/Performance IQ (WISC-IV and WPPSI-III)

The PRI and PIQ are designed to measure fluid reasoning, spatial processing, attentiveness to detail, and visual–motor integration. Furthermore, the PRI measures working memory and processing speed, given the relationship between these skills and fluid reasoning. Block Design, Matrix Reasoning, and Picture Completion are fair measures of g on the WISC-IV and WPPSI-III (Sattler, 2008). They also have ample specificity, with the exception of Picture Completion, which has adequate specificity in one age group (Sattler, 2008).

Working Memory Index (WISC-IV)

The WMI is intended to measure the capacity to store and utilize information temporarily in the pursuit of a goal-directed action (Wechsler, 2008; Zhu, Weiss, Prifitera, & Coalson, 2003). It has been recognized as an important higher-order cognitive process and is closely related to fluid reasoning and the ability to learn new information (Conway et al., 2002; Fry & Hale, 1996). Digit Span and Letter–Number Sequencing are fair measures of g on the WISC-IV. Arithmetic is a good measure of g. Digit Span and Letter–Number Sequencing have ample specificity, whereas Arithmetic's specificity is adequate to ample (Sattler, 2008).

Processing Speed Index/Quotient (WISC-IV and WPPSI-III)

The PSI and PSQ measure simple visual–motor processing. Though concerned with the processing of "simple" information, processing speed is highly related to general cognitive ability, working memory, and fluid reasoning (Fry & Hale, 1996, 2000; Salthouse, 1996). Coding and Symbol Search are fair measures of g on the WISC-IV and WPPSI-III. Both have mostly ample specificity, with the exception of WPPSI-III Coding, which has adequate specificity in the 6:0–6:11 age range (Sattler, 2008). Cancellation is a poor measure of g and has ample specificity (Sattler, 2008).

General Language Composite (WPPSI-III)

The GLC consists of the Receptive Vocabulary and Picture Naming subtests. It is intended to provide a measure of language competence, including both receptive and expressive vocabulary, for children between the ages of 2:6 and 3:11. Although it is optional for the older age band, the GLC may be used as a measure of language ability for children suspected of having language delays, as the complexity of receptive and expressive processing demands is lower for GLC subtests than for VIQ subtests. When combined with other sources of information, such as parent report and behavioral observations, low scores on the GLC may warrant further evaluation with a language specialist.

General Ability and Cognitive Proficiency Indexes (WISC-IV)

The GAI and CPI are optional indexes on the WISC-IV. They are not provided in the test manual, but rather in technical reports that were released after the test's publication (Raiford, Weiss, Rolfhus, & Coalson, 2005; Weiss & Gabel, 2008). The GAI is derived from an aggregate of subtests constituting the VCI and PRI; conversely, the CPI is derived from subtests of the WMI and PRI. Thus the GAI measures a subset of intellectual functioning with reduced influences of working memory and processing speed, and the CPI represents an index of cognitive processing proficiency that reduces crystallized knowledge, verbal reasoning, and fluid reasoning demands.

Information from the GAI and CPI may be especially useful in the context of special education evaluations. First, discrepancies between ability and achievement continue to be used to assist the identification of learning disabilities, and the GAI may provide an alternative index of intellectual functioning in cases where the WMI and/or PSI are significantly discrepant from the VCI and/or PRI. Second, difficulties with information processing interfere with learning, and the CPI, which indexes a student's abilities in this area, may provide insight into his or her academic struggles (Weiss & Gabel, 2008; Weiss, Saklofske, Prifitera, & Holdnack, 2006). Evidence from the WISC-IV standardization sample indicates that these two scales may be uniquely informative when interpreted in concert (Weiss & Gabel, 2008); the GAI–CPI discrepancy identified up to 50% of individuals in the reading and writing disorder samples. Thus these indexes may provide additional insight into the processing strengths and weaknesses of at-risk students, and may help tailor specific cognitive interventions when ability–achievement discrepancies are present (Weiss, Beal, Saklofske, Alloway,

& Prifitera, 2008). It should be noted that the use of the GAI and CPI is not limited to learning disability evaluations. Discrepancies in which the GAI is higher than the CPI are also implicated in traumatic brain injury and Asperger disorder, and the GAI is discrepant from the FSIQ in a multitude of clinical populations, including children with intellectual disability, traumatic brain injury, attention-deficit/hyperactivity disorder (ADHD), autism, and Asperger disorder (Saklofske, Weiss, Raiford, & Prifitera, 2006; Strauss, Sherman, & Spreen, 2006). However, the GAI should not be used as a substitute for FSIQ solely because the WMI or PSI is low, as working memory and processing speed represent important aspects of general cognitive ability.

Subtest Descriptions

As stated above, this chapter only includes descriptions of the Wechsler subtests that are not provided in Chapter 8 of this volume. See Table 9.2 for abbreviated descriptions of all subtests included in the WISC-IV and WPPSI-III, as well as Chapter 8 for a detailed discussion of the subtests excluded from this section.

Picture Concepts (WISC-IV and WPPSI-III)

Picture Concepts loads on the WISC-IV PRI and the WPPSI-III PIQ. For each Picture Concepts item, the examinee is presented with two or three rows of pictures and chooses one picture from each row to form a group with a common characteristic (Figure 9.1). This is a new core subtest for the WPPSI-III and WISC-IV. Although verbal mediation may be involved, Picture Concepts is considered the nonverbal counterpart of Similarities (Wechsler, 2002a, 2003a). It is designed to measure abstract, categorical reasoning ability. It is a fair measure of *g* on the WISC-IV and WPPSI-III and has ample specificity on both (Sattler, 2008).

Word Reasoning (WISC-IV and WPPSI-III)

Word Reasoning contributes to the WISC-IV VCI and the WPPSI-III VIQ. In Word Reasoning, the examinee is asked to identify the common concept being described in a series of clues. A new subtest for the WPPSI-III and WISC-IV, Word Reasoning is a task of verbal reasoning similar to the Word Context subtest of the Delis–Kaplan Executive Function System (Delis, Kaplan, & Kramer, 2001), the Riddles subtest of the Kauf-

man Assessment Battery for Children (Kaufman & Kaufman, 1983), and cloze tasks (i.e., tasks requiring the child to complete missing portions of a sentence). An example of a Word Reasoning item is "It is used for transportation, and it goes on water. What is it?" In addition to verbal reasoning, these tasks have been shown to measure verbal comprehension, analogical and general reasoning ability, verbal abstraction, domain knowledge, the ability to integrate and synthesize different types of information, and the ability to generate alternative concepts (Ackerman, Beier, & Bowen, 2000; Alexander & Kulikowich, 1991; Delis et al., 2001; DeSanti, 1989; McKenna & Layton, 1990; Newstead, Thompson, & Handley, 2002; Ridgeway, 1995). Word Reasoning is a good measure of *g* on both the WPPSI-III and WISC-IV and has specificity that ranges from ample to inadequate, depending on the age band (see Sattler, 2008, for more details).

Object Assembly (WPPSI-III)

Object Assembly contributes to the WPPSI-III PIQ. For all items in Object Assembly, the examinee fits the pieces of a puzzle together to form a meaningful whole within specified time limits. It is designed to assess perceptual organization. It also measures perceptual integration and synthesis of part–whole relationships, use of sensory motor feedback, spatial ability, fluid ability, visual–motor reasoning, trial-and-error learning, visual–motor coordination, cognitive flexibility, persistence, and motor coordination and dexterity (Cooper, 1995; Politano & Finch, 1996; Ryan & Smith, 2003; Sattler, 2008; Wechsler, 1991). Scores on this subtest may be influenced by a child's experience with puzzles, visual-perceptual problems, or response to time pressures (Kaufman, 1994; Kaufman & Lichtenberger, 1999; Lichtenberger & Kaufman, 2003). It is a fair measure of *g* on the WPPSI-III and has an ample amount of specificity (Sattler, 2008).

Receptive Vocabulary (WPPSI-III)

Receptive Vocabulary loads on the WPPSI-III VIQ but also contributes to the GLC. For each item, the child looks at a group of four pictures and points to the one the examiner names aloud. It is a receptive language measure of concept formation. It also measures auditory and visual discrimination, auditory processing, auditory memory, integration of visual perception and auditory input, and receptive language ability (Brownell, 2000; Semel,

TABLE 9.2. Descriptions of WISC-IV and WPPSI-III Subtests

Subtest	Test	Description
Verbal Comprehension Index/VIQ		
Comprehension*	WISC-IV/WPPSI-III	The child answers questions based on his or her understanding of general principles and social situations.
Information*	WISC-IV/WPPSI-III	The child answers questions about a broad range of general-knowledge topics.
Similarities*	WISC-IV/WPPSI-III	The child is read two words that represent common concepts and describes how they are similar.
Vocabulary*	WISC-IV/WPPSI-III	The child defines words that are read out loud by the examiner.
Word Reasoning	WISC-IV/WPPSI-III	The child identifies the common concept being described by the examiner in a series of clues.
Perceptual Reasoning Index/PIQ		
Block Design*	WISC-IV/WPPSI-III	Working within a specified time limit, the child views a model and/or picture and recreates it, using blocks.
Matrix Reasoning*	WISC-IV/WPPSI-III	The child views an incomplete matrix and chooses the response option that completes the matrix.
Object Assembly	WPPSI-III	Within a specified time limit, the child is presented with pieces of a puzzle and fits them together to form a meaningful whole.
Picture Completion*	WISC-IV	Working within a specified time limit, the child looks at a picture and identifies the important part missing.
Picture Concepts	WISC-IV/WPPSI-III	The child is presented with rows of pictures and chooses one picture from each row to form a group with a common characteristic.
Working Memory Index		
Arithmetic*	WISC-IV	Working within a specified time limit, the child mentally solves orally presented arithmetic problems.
Digit Span*	WISC-IV	The child is read a sequence of numbers and recalls the numbers in either forward or backward order.
Letter–Number Sequencing*	WISC-IV	The child hears a sequence of letters and numbers and recalls them in numerical and alphabetical order.
Processing Speed Index		
Cancellation*	WISC-IV	Working within a specified time limit, the child scans both a structured and a random array of objects and marks target objects.
Coding*	WISC-IV/WPPSI-III	Working within a specified time limit, the child uses a key to draw symbols that match corresponding shapes or numbers.
Symbol Search*	WISC-IV/WPPSI-III	Working within a specified time limit, the child marks whether target symbol(s) matches symbols in a search group.
General Learning Composite		
Picture Naming	WPPSI-III	The child names pictures that are displayed in a stimulus book.
Receptive Vocabulary	WPPSI-III	The child looks at four pictures and points to the one that matches the word the examiner speaks aloud.

*A full description of task demands and an example item can be found in Chapter 8 of this volume.

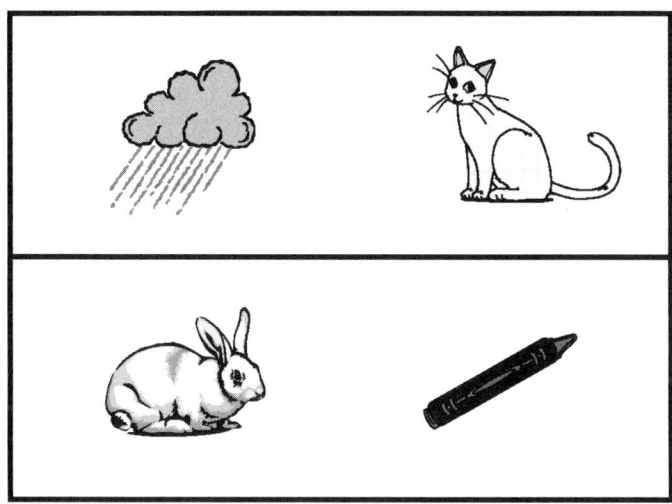

FIGURE 9.1. Example of a WISC-IV/WPPSI-III Picture Concepts item.

Wiig, & Secord, 1995; Wechsler, 2002a). Receptive Vocabulary is a good measure of *g* and has an ample amount of specificity (Sattler, 2008).

Picture Naming (WPPSI-III)

Picture Naming contributes to the WPPSI-III GLC. For each item, the child names a picture that is displayed in the stimulus book. This subtest is an expressive language test of concept formation. It also measures word retrieval from long-term memory, as well as association of visual stimuli with language (Brownell, 2000; German, 1989; Sattler, 2008; Wechsler, 2002a). This subtest is a good measure of *g* and has an adequate to ample amount of specificity (Sattler, 2008).

PSYCHOMETRIC PROPERTIES OF THE WISC-IV AND WPPSI-III

According to the criteria proposed by Flanagan and Alfonso (1995) and Bracken (1987), both the WPPSI-III and WISC-IV have outstanding psychometric properties.

Standardization Samples

The WPPSI-III and WISC-IV have excellent standardization samples (Sattler, 2008). The sizes of the normative samples are 1,700 and 2,200 for the WPPSI-III and WISC-IV, respectively (with the exception of WISC-IV Arithmetic, which was normed on 1,100 individuals). The sample size for most norming age groups is 200 cases. The stratification of the normative samples was closely matched to contemporary U.S. census data for five key demographic variables: age, gender, race/ethnicity, educational level, and geographic region.

Reliability

The WPPSI-III and WISC-IV composite scores have strong reliabilities (Wechsler, 2002b, 2003b). The overall internal-consistency reliability coefficients for the normative sample are in the .90s for all IQ and index scores except the PSI, which are not reported because they are speeded tests. At the subtest level, the overall internal-consistency reliability coefficients of the normative sample are in the .80s or .90s for all of the WPPSI-III subtests. Cancellation and Symbol Search have overall reliability coefficients of .79 on the WISC-IV, but with this exception, all other WISC-IV reliability coefficients are in the .80 and .90 range. Overall, the reliability of the WPPSI-III and WISC-IV for clinical samples is consistent with reliability estimates for the normative samples (Wechsler, 2002b, 2003b). The test–retest stability coefficients of the WPPSI-III and WISC-IV FSIQ scores are .92 and .93, respectively. The test–retest coefficients of the index scores range from .84 to .93, and the subtest coefficients range from .74 to .92. Finally, the interscorer agreement of the WPPSI-III and WISC-IV subtests are all in the high .90s for the nonverbal subtests and above .90 for the verbal subtests, which require more subjective scoring techniques.

Validity

There is ample evidence to support the validity of the WPPSI-III and WISC-IV. A long history of factor-analytic research provides converging evidence suggesting that the Wechsler scales measure the four primary domains mentioned above: Verbal Comprehension, Perceptual Organization/Perceptual Reasoning, Working Memory, and Processing Speed. This evidence comes from the test manuals of the WPPSI-III, the WISC-IV, and their predecessors (Wechsler, 1991, 1997, 2002b, 2003b, 2008), as well as additional examination of the standardization samples (Kamphaus, Benson, Hutchinson, & Platt, 1994) and other independent samples (Roid, Prifitera, & Weiss, 1993). Importantly, these findings can be replicated across major ethnic groups (Kamphaus et al., 1994), as well as across clinical populations that include psychiatric inpatients (Tupa, Write, & Fristad, 1997), children with traumatic brain injuries (Donders & Warschausky, 1997), and students referred for special education evaluations (Watkins, Wilson, Kotz, Carbone, & Babula, 2006). Furthermore, subsequent adaptations in different countries have provided additional evidence supporting the construct validity of the Wechsler scales. For example, the four-factor solution has been replicated in Canada (Wechsler, 1995b), Australia (Wechsler, 1995a), Taiwan (Chen et al., 2009; Wechsler, 1997), and Japan (Wechsler, 1998). In a factor analysis of WISC-III data from 15 nations ($N = 15,999$), Georgas and colleagues (2003) replicated the four-factor structure, although in some countries Arithmetic loaded mostly on the Verbal Comprehension factor, producing a three-factor structure. Taken together, results from these studies indicate that the latent traits measured by the Wechsler scales appear consistently across different ages, ethnicities, cultures, and specific clinical populations. Furthermore, they support the updated theoretical foundations of the Wechsler scales, as converging evidence suggests that the tests measure working memory, processing speed, and fluid reasoning, among other cognitive abilities recently identified as critical to the construct of intelligence.

In addition to the factor-analytic work supporting the construct validity of the WISC-IV and WPPSI-III, a multitude of evidence also supports their utility as clinical tools. This is consistent with David Wechsler's original intent of developing an intelligence battery that was, above all else, a clinically useful instrument. Numerous studies demonstrate that several special groups (e.g., children with ADHD, autism, Asperger disorder, learning disability, traumatic brain injury, giftedness, etc.) demonstrate patterns of index score strengths and weakness that are unique relative to the normative sample (Calhoun & Mayes, 2005; Ghaziuddin & Mountain-Kimchi, 2004; Harrison, DeLisle, & Parker, 2008; Prifitera et al., 2005; Sweetland, Reina, & Tatti, 2006; Wechsler, 2002b, 2003b; Weiss et al., 2006). In addition, the Wechsler scales provide important information regarding cognitive strengths and weaknesses in the context of special education evaluations, making it a useful tool in this context as well. Overall, this evidence provides further support of validity for the WISC-IV and WPPSI-III, as they are sensitive to a number of clinical disorders that are known to affect cognitive functioning.

Finally, the Wechsler scales also correlate highly with other measures of intelligence. Table 9.3 presents the correlation coefficients between the WPPSI-III/WISC-IV and two other well-known contemporary measures of intelligence: the KABC-II and DAS-II. The magnitude of these correlations is high and provides evidence of concurrent validity, as the Wechsler scales appear to measure very similar constructs relative to other modern intelligence batteries. Similarly, the WPPSI-III and WISC-IV correlate strongly with academic achievement as measured by the WIAT-III (discussed below; Pearson, 2009). Correlations between the WPPSI-III FSIQ and WIAT-III indexes range from .43 to .78, and correlations between the WISC-IV and WIAT-III composites range from .53 to .82.

TABLE 9.3. Correlations between the WPPSI-III/WISC-IV and Other Intelligence Scales

	KABC-II FCI[a]	KABC-II MPI[a]	DAS-II GCA[b]
WPPSI-III FSIQ (ages 3–4)	.81	.76	—
WPPSI-III FSIQ (ages 5–6)	.81	.73	—
WPPSI-III FSIQ (all ages)	—	—	.87
WISC-IV FSIQ	.89	.88	.84

Note. FCI, Fluid–Crystallized Index; MPI, Mental Processing Index; GCA, General Conceptual Ability.
[a]Kaufman and Kaufman (2004).
[b]Elliott (2007).

BACKGROUND AND HISTORY OF THE WIAT-III

The WIAT-III is a comprehensive, individually administered achievement test of listening, speaking, reading, writing, and mathematics skills. Both grade and age norms are provided for testing individuals who are in prekindergarten (PreK) through grade 12 or ages 4:0 through 50:11 years. Separate norms are provided for fall, winter, and spring for grades PreK–12. Administration time varies based upon a number of factors such as the grade and skill level of the examinee and the number of subtests administered; however, subtest administration time is typically between 1 and 15 minutes, depending upon the subtest.

The original WIAT (Wechsler, 1992) was designed to measure the academic achievement of students in kindergarten through high school, ages 5:0–19:11. The WIAT provided eight subtests to correspond to each of the areas of learning disability identification specified by the Education for All Handicapped Children Act of 1975, and was the first test of its kind to be linked with the Wechsler ability scales for conducting ability–achievement discrepancy analyses. Nine years later, the WIAT-II (Psychological Corporation, 2001) was published

with one new subtest (Pseudoword Decoding) and significant revisions to the existing subtests. Subsequently, updated scoring and normative materials were released in 2002 and 2005. The WIAT-II was designed for children, adolescents, college students, and adults ages 4:0 through 85:11 years. The WIAT-III retains updated versions of the subtests included in the previous editions and adds five new subtests: Early Reading Skills, Oral Reading Fluency, Math Fluency—Addition, Math Fluency—Subtraction, and Math Fluency—Multiplication. In addition, the former Written Expression subtest was split into three distinct subtests: Alphabet Writing Fluency, Sentence Composition, and Essay Composition. It is normed for individuals between the ages of 4:0 and 50:11 years.

DESCRIPTION OF WIAT-III SUBTESTS AND COMPOSITES

As shown in Table 9.4, the WIAT-III covers all eight areas specified by the Individuals with Disabilities Education Improvement Act of 2004 (IDEA 2004), with 16 subtests and 8 composite scores (7 achievement area composites and a Total Achievement composite). With the exception of

TABLE 9.4. Alignment of WIAT-III with IDEA 2004

IDEA 2004 areas of achievement	WIAT-III subtests	WIAT-III composites	
Oral expression	Oral Expression	Oral Language	
Listening comprehension	Listening Comprehension		
Written expression	Alphabet Writing Fluency Sentence Composition Essay Composition Spelling	Written Expression	
Basic reading skills	Early Reading Skills[a] Word Reading Pseudoword Decoding	Basic Reading	Total Reading
Reading fluency skills	Oral Reading Fluency	Reading Comprehension and Fluency	
Reading comprehension	Reading Comprehension		
Mathematics calculation	Numerical Operations	Mathematics	
Mathematics problem solving	Math Problem Solving		
	Math Fluency—Addition Math Fluency—Subtraction Math Fluency—Multiplication	Math Fluency	

[a]Early Reading Skills does not contribute to either the Basic Reading or Total Reading composite.

the three Math Fluency subtests, each subtest contributes to the Total Achievement composite to provide an estimate of overall academic achievement. An examiner may choose to administer as many or as few subtests as he or she deems appropriate for the purpose of the evaluation, the types of scores required, and the grade level of the student.

Subtest Descriptions

Listening Comprehension, administered to examinees ages 4–50 (grades PreK–12+), contains two components, Receptive Vocabulary and Oral Discourse Comprehension. For Receptive Vocabulary, the examinee points to the picture that best illustrates the meaning of each word he or she hears. For Oral Discourse Comprehension, the examinee listens to sentences and passages and orally responds to comprehension questions.

Early Reading Skills, administered to examinees ages 4–9 (grades PreK–3), requires the examinee to name letters, identify and generate rhyming words, identify words with the same beginning and ending sounds, blend sounds, match sounds with letters and letter blends, and match written words with pictures that illustrate their meaning.

Reading Comprehension, administered to examinees ages 6–50 (grades 1–12+), requires the examinee to read narrative and expository passages (either aloud or silently), and then orally respond to literal and inferential comprehension questions read aloud by the examiner.

Math Problem Solving, administered to examinees ages 4–50 (grades PreK–12+), measures untimed math problem-solving skills in the areas of basic concepts, everyday applications, geometry, and algebra. The items require oral or pointing responses.

Alphabet Writing Fluency, administered to examinees ages 4–9 (grades PreK–3), measures the ability to write letters of the alphabet within a 30-second time limit. The examinee may write letters in any order, in cursive or print, in uppercase or lowercase.

Sentence Composition, administered to examinees ages 6–50 (grades 1–12+), contains two components: Sentence Combining and Sentence Building. Sentence Combining requires the examinee to combine two or three sentences into one sentence that preserves the meaning of the original sentences. Sentence Building requires the

examinee to write sentences that include a target word.

Word Reading, administered to examinees ages 6–50 (grades 1–12+), measures speed and accuracy of oral single-word reading. The examiner records the item reached at 30 seconds to measure reading speed; however, the examinee continues reading the list of words without a time limit until the discontinue rule is met or the last item is read.

Essay Composition, administered to examinees ages 8–50 (grades 3–12+), measures spontaneous, compositional writing skills. The examinee is given 10 minutes to respond to one essay prompt.

Pseudoword Decoding, administered to examinees ages 6–50 (grades 1–12+), requires the examinee to read aloud from a list of pseudowords. As in the Word Reading subtest, the examiner records the item reached at 30 seconds to measure reading speed; however, the examinee continues reading the list of words without a time limit until the discontinue rule is met or the last item is read.

Numerical Operations, administered to examinees ages 5–50 (grades K–12+), measures untimed, written math calculation skills in the areas of basic skills, basic operations with integers, geometry, algebra, and calculus.

Oral Expression, administered to examinees ages 4–50 (grades PreK–12+), contains three components: Expressive Vocabulary, Oral Word Fluency, and Sentence Repetition. Expressive Vocabulary measures speaking vocabulary and word retrieval ability by requiring the examinee to say the word that best corresponds to a given picture and definition. Oral Word Fluency measures how quickly and easily the examinee can name things belonging to a given category within 60 seconds. Sentence Repetition measures oral syntactic knowledge and short-term memory by asking the examinee to repeat sentences verbatim.

Oral Reading Fluency, administered to examinees ages 6–50 (grades 1–12+), measures oral reading speed, accuracy, fluency, and prosody by requiring the examinee to read passages aloud. Fluency is calculated as the average number of words read correctly per minute. A qualitative scale is used to assess reading prosody.

Spelling, administered to examinees ages 5–50 (grades K–12+), requires the examinee to spell (write) letter sounds or words, depending upon grade level. The examinee hears each letter sound within the context of a word, and each word within the context of a sentence.

Math Fluency—Addition, administered to examinees ages 6–50 (grades 1–12+), requires the examinee to solve written addition problems within a 60-second time limit.

Math Fluency—Subtraction, administered to examinees ages 6–50 (grades 1–12+), requires the examinee to solve written subtraction problems within a 60-second time limit.

Math Fluency—Multiplication, administered to examinees ages 8–50 (grades 3–12+), requires the examinee to solve written multiplication problems within a 60-second time limit.

PSYCHOMETRIC PROPERTIES OF THE WIAT-III

The standardization sample of the WIAT-III meets or exceeds current practice recommendations, and the psychometric properties are generally strong (see Dumont & Willis, 2010).

Standardization Samples

The WIAT-III was standardized on nationally stratified samples of 2,775 students in the grade-norm sample (grades PreK–12), 1,826 students in the age-norm sample (ages 4:0–19:11), and 225 individuals in the adult age-norm sample (ages 20:0–50:11). The stratification of the normative samples matches recent U.S. census data closely on the following key demographic variables: grade/age, sex, race/ethnicity, parental educational level, and geographic region. Approximately 8% of the school-age normative samples included individuals with diagnosed clinical disorders, and approximately 2% were identified as academically gifted.

Reliability

The reliability coefficients for the school-age and adult samples are generally consistent. Across these samples, the average internal-consistency (split-half) reliability coefficients for the composite scores and for Math Problem Solving, Word Reading, Pseudoword Decoding, Numerical Operations, Spelling (and Math Fluency—Subtraction and Math Fluency—Multiplication for the adult sample only) are in the .90s. The average split-half reliability coefficients for Listening Comprehension, Early Reading Skills (school-age sample only), Reading Comprehension, Sentence Composition, Essay Composition, Essay Composition: Grammar and Mechanics, Oral Expression, and select Math Fluency subtests are predominantly in the .80s and .90s.

The split-half reliability method is not appropriate for measuring the reliability of subtests without item-level data or subtests that are speeded; rather, test–retest stability coefficients are used as the reliability estimates for these subtests. The WIAT-III subtest and composite scores possess adequate stability across time. Average test–retest gains are larger for the Listening Comprehension, Reading Comprehension, and Oral Expression subtests, and smaller for the Written Expression subtests than for the other subtests. For the school-age sample, the average corrected stability coefficients are excellent (.87–.96) for the composite scores; excellent (.90–.94) for Reading Comprehension, Word Reading, Pseudoword Decoding, Oral Reading Fluency, Oral Reading Rate, and Spelling; good (.82–.89) for Early Reading Skills, Math Problem Solving, Essay Composition, Essay Composition: Grammar and Mechanics, Numerical Operations, Oral Expression, Oral Reading Accuracy, Math Fluency—Addition, Math Fluency—Subtraction, and Math Fluency—Multiplication; and adequate (.75 and .79, respectively) for Listening Comprehension and Sentence Composition. Alphabet Writing Fluency is a speeded subtest with a restricted raw score range, so a lower average stability coefficient (.69) is expected. For the adult sample, the average corrected stability coefficients are excellent (.90–.97) for the composite scores; excellent (.90–.97) for Math Problem Solving, Word Reading, Pseudoword Decoding, Numerical Operations, Oral Expression, Oral Reading Fluency, Oral Reading Rate, Spelling, Math Fluency—Subtraction, and Math Fluency—Multiplication; good (.81–.87) for Listening Comprehension, Reading Comprehension, Sentence Composition, Essay Composition: Grammar and Mechanics, and Math Fluency—Addition; and adequate (.78 and .74, respectively) for Essay Composition and Oral Reading Accuracy.

Validity

The validity of the WIAT-III has been demonstrated via intercorrelation data, correlations with other measures, and clinical studies. The subtests that make up each composite are generally moderately correlated with one another and show expected relationships (e.g., strong correlations between Math Problem Solving and Numerical Operations, and between Word Reading and Pseudoword Decoding) and discriminant evidence of validity (e.g., the mathematics subtests correlate more highly with each other than with other subtests). Correlations among the composite scores range from .45 to .93, with stronger correlations among the reading composites, and weaker correlations between the Math Fluency composites and other composites. Construct validity has been established by correlating the WIAT-III with other tests. Correlations with the WIAT-II indicate that the two are measuring similar constructs. The corrected correlations between the composite scores for the two tests range from .76 (Oral Language) to .93 (Total Achievement), and correlations between the common subtests range from .62 (Oral Expression) to .86 (Spelling). Consistent with expectations, the corrected correlations are high for subtests that are highly similar in content and structure, and relatively low for subtests in which content and structure were modified considerably for the WIAT-III.

Correlations between the WIAT-III and the Wechsler intelligence scales (WPPSI-III, WISC-IV, WAIS-IV, and the Wechsler Nonverbal Scale of Ability [WNV]), and between the WIAT-III and the DAS-II, are consistent with expectations regarding typical correlations between cognitive ability and achievement measures. The correlations between the WIAT-III and the overall cognitive ability scores range from .60 to .82. These correlations provide divergent evidence of validity, suggesting that the WIAT-III and the cognitive ability tests are measuring different constructs with varying degrees of overlap in the cognitive skills required.

To establish the validity and clinical utility of the WIAT-III, clinical studies were conducted with students identified as academically gifted and talented, students with mild intellectual disability, students with expressive language disorder, and students with learning disabilities in the areas of reading, written expression, and mathematics. Results showed expected patterns of performance in each study. Students identified as gifted/talented scored consistently higher than a matched control group across all subtests and composites except Early Reading Skills and Alphabet Writing Fluency. Students with mild intellectual disability scored significantly lower than a matched control group across all subtests and composites. Results from the study of expressive language disorder confirmed that the oral language subtests and several other subtests and composites requiring expressive language and related skills reliably differentiate between students with this disorder and their age-matched peers. Students with reading disabilities (approximately 10% diagnosed with comorbid

writing disabilities) scored significantly lower than a matched control group on all reading-related subtests and composites, in addition to the Total Achievement composite, the Spelling subtest, and the Written Expression composites. Students with writing disabilities (approximately 18% diagnosed with comorbid reading disabilities) scored significantly lower than a matched control group on all writing-related subtests and composites (except the Alphabet Writing Fluency subtest), in addition to the Total Achievement composite and some reading-related subtests and composites. Students with mathematics disabilities performed significantly lower than a matched control group on all math-related subtests and composites. These results provide evidence that the WIAT-III reliably differentiates between students in these special groups and their age-matched peers.

INTERPRETATION

The WPPSI-III, WISC-IV, and WIAT-III technical manuals provide basic instruction regarding their interpretation (Breaux, 2009; Wechsler, 2002b, 2003b). Leading clinicians and researchers have developed more in-depth and alternative interpretive strategies for these tests, all of which represent valid and useful approaches to test interpretation (Flanagan & Kaufman, 2009; Lichtenberger & Kaufman, 2003; Prifitera, Saklofske, & Weiss, 2008; Sattler, 2008; Weiss et al., 2006). A detailed guide to interpretation is outside the scope of this chapter, and we refer the reader to these other outstanding volumes, as well as the technical and interpretive guides, for further information. Instead, we provide basic information illustrating how the WPPSI-III, WISC-IV, and WIAT-III can be utilized by practitioners. In addition, we include guidance for how these measures can be integrated within the context of learning disability evaluations. When reading this section, the reader is encouraged to note that psychological assessment is a complex problem-solving process (Prifitera, Saklofske, & Weiss, 2005), and test results should always be interpreted in conjunction with a thorough history and careful clinical observations of the individual.

Common Wechsler Scores

The WPPSI-III and WISC-IV utilize two types of standard scores: *scaled scores* and *composite scores* (i.e., IQ and index scores). These scores are age-referenced standard scores computed by comparing an examinee's raw scores to others within his or her age group. The WIAT-III provides both age-based and grade-based subtest and composite standard scores, which are computed by comparing an examinee's raw scores to others within his or her age or grade group. Not only do these scores allow clinicians to compare an individual's performance to the standardization sample, but because they are based on a similar metric, they allow for comparisons within and across Wechsler scales, as well as between Wechsler tests and other commonly used assessment batteries.

For the intelligence tests, scaled scores are derived from the total raw scores on each subtest and have a mean of 10 and a standard deviation (*SD*) of 3. Composite scores (e.g., FSIQ, VCI, etc.) are standard scores based on the sum of various subtest scaled scores. They have a mean of 100 and an *SD* of 15. On the WIAT-III, both the subtest and composite standard scores have a mean of 100 and an *SD* of 15.

Standard scores are typically the most accurate descriptions of test data. For those without formal training in psychometrics (examinees, parents, educators, etc.), the concept of standard scores is often difficult to understand. Thus the Wechsler scales provide a number of other metrics to help communicate test results, which include percentile ranks and test age equivalents (and grade equivalents for the WIAT-III), both of which should be provided when appropriate on the WPPSI-III, WISC-IV, and WIAT-III. A *percentile rank* is the percentage of individuals within the examinee's age range obtaining a score below or equivalent to the examinee, whereas an *age equivalent* is the age of individuals who, on average, obtain the examinee's raw score. Standard scores on the Wechsler scales should always be accompanied by a confidence interval, which is based on the scales' reliability and expresses the likelihood that an examinee's true score (i.e., the score he or she would obtain if there was no error in the test) falls within a specified range around the actual score that he or she obtained. The confidence interval is important because it communicates the error that is inherent in all psychological tests.

Levels of Performance

Wechsler standard scores can also be communicated by describing a range of performance within which each score falls (e.g., superior, average, extremely low, etc.), which corresponds to the rela-

TABLE 9.5. Qualitative Descriptions of WIAT-III Standard Scores

Standard score	Classification	Percent included in theoretical normal curve
146 and above	Very superior	> 99
131–145	Superior	98–99
116–130	Above average	86–98
85–115	Average	16–84
70–84	Below average	2–14
55–69	Low	1–2
54 and below	Very low	< 1

tionship of the examinee's score to that of his or her normative group. See Table 9.5 for the descriptive classifications corresponding to various standard scores obtained on the WIAT-III (descriptive classifications for the WISC-IV and WPPSI-III are the same as those for the adult Wechsler scales and can be found in Chapter 8 of this volume, as well as the test manuals). The level of performance is important for determining whether an examinee demonstrates any cognitive strengths or weaknesses, which can be defined in one of two ways. In the normative approach, an individual's scores can be defined as strong (e.g., superior, etc.) or weak (e.g., extremely low, etc.) relative to the normative group that the standard scores are based on. Conversely, in the intraindividual approach, scores can be characterized as strong or weak relative to the examinee's own performance on other subtests or indexes within the test battery. Both scores yield information that can be used in different ways to inform diagnostic formulation or targeted intervention planning. For example, a normative approach may be used to identify cognitive impairment that qualifies a child for disability services, whereas an intraindividual approach may identify cognitive and academic strengths and weaknesses to target as part of a learning disability intervention program.

Basic Interpretation of the WISC-IV and WPPSI-III

Reporting and Describing Index Scores

The IQ and index scores are much more reliable measures than the subtest scaled scores, and in general they are the first scores examined by the practitioner. FSIQ often represents the primary level of interpretation in most testing sessions. Some controversy exists in the literature regarding the interpretability and clinical utility of the FSIQ in children, especially in clinical samples characterized by significant variation in index scores (for an example, see the 2007 special issue of *Applied Neuropsychology*, Volume 14, No. 1). However, the FSIQ is the best single point predictor of achievement and important life outcomes, and evidence suggests that it remains valid and predictive even in cases characterized by extreme index score discrepancies (Daniel, 2007; Watkins, Lei, et al., 2007). Thus, although interpretation should always begin with consideration of the FSIQ, interpretation should also be augmented by examination of index score patterns. This is especially important when there are index score discrepancies, as index-level strengths and weaknesses can provide important insight into a child's world that cannot be obtained from the FSIQ alone. For example, many clinical disorders are characterized by unique index score discrepancies, though we should note that there is enough overlap of profile patterns across disorders for us to caution against the use of profile patterns for diagnostic purposes in the absence of additional information.

Assessing for Discrepancies among Index Scores

As noted above, analyzing index score discrepancies is important because they may yield important clinical information and augment the interpretation of the FSIQ. In order for two indexes to be considered discrepant, the difference between them must be statistically significant. This means that the likelihood of obtaining the observed difference by chance is very low ($p < .05$) and indicates that the clinician can conclude with relative certainty that the difference between the scores is a true difference. The Wechsler scales provide critical values at which differences between index scores can be deemed statistically significant. Alternatively, clinicians with no a priori hypotheses may be interested in evaluating index-level strengths and weaknesses by comparing index scores to the mean of all index scores, which reduces the error rate resulting from multiple comparisons (e.g., comparing multiple index scores to each other). Information regarding these comparisons is not provided in test manuals, but can be found in other references (Flanagan & Kaufman, 2009; Grégoire, Coalson, & Zhu, 2011).

Determining whether the difference between index scores is statistically significant is the first step in this level of interpretation; however, not all statistically significant differences are clinically meaningful. Many statistically significant index score discrepancies are commonly found among individuals in the general population, whereas others are relatively rare. Thus the significance and frequency of a difference have different implications for test interpretation (Matarazzo & Herman, 1985; Payne & Jones, 1957; Sattler, 2008; Silverstein, 1981). To assist clinicians in determining whether differences are rare or not, the Wechsler scales provide base rate data for various index score discrepancies. Because the discrepancies among index scores are related to ability level, the base rate data are also provided for five ability levels. In addition, the base rates are provided by the direction of the discrepancy because previous research has revealed that the frequencies of score differences vary with the direction of the difference (Sattler, 2008). For instance, the percentage of the WISC-IV normative sample with VCI scores greater than their PRI scores is not the same percentage of the normative sample with PRI scores greater than their VCI scores. Clinically speaking, the direction of VCI–PRI discrepancy is related to different patterns of cognitive strengths and weaknesses that may be unique to particular clinical disorders (Rourke, 1998).

Examining Subtest Scatter, as well as Strengths and Weaknesses

IQ and index scores are estimates of overall functioning in their respective areas and should always be evaluated within the context of the subtests that contribute to them (Flanagan & Kaufman, 2009; Wechsler, 2002b, 2003b). It is good practice to evaluate the level of score consistency or variability among subtest scaled scores before interpreting composite scores. In a case characterized by extreme subtest score variability, consideration of this variability augments the interpretation of the index score and may yield a more complete picture of the child's cognitive strengths and weaknesses relative to the index score alone. The Wechsler scales provide two ways of reporting subtest variability: (1) subtest scatter and (2) subtest strengths and weaknesses. The scatter score is calculated by subtracting the lowest score from the highest one. The Wechsler scales provide base rate data in the manuals for evaluating how frequently such a scatter occurred in the normative sample.

If the subtest scaled scores demonstrate significant variability, it is a good practice to conduct an analysis of subtest strengths and weaknesses. Such an analysis is usually hypothesis-driven and focused on certain cognitive domains associated to the referral question (Kamphaus, 1993). The first step of a strengths-and-weaknesses analysis is to determine whether or not the differences between each scaled score and the average of all scaled scores are statistically significant (the mean of just PRI or VCI subtests can also be used). The clinician should then examine whether such differences occur rarely. Score differences can be statistically significant yet occur frequently within a general population. All the latest versions of the Wechsler intelligence scales provide tables of critical values and base rates that can be referred to for a strengths-and-weaknesses analysis.

Basic Interpretation of the WIAT-III

Interpretation of WIAT-III results should be guided by the referral question or the purpose of the evaluation. Within this framework, the test results may be used to support or disconfirm hypotheses. Clinicians begin by interpreting the composite scores to determine whether the scores are consistent with the Total Achievement composite and with the other composite scores. The Total Achievement composite may also be compared with the FSIQ score from a cognitive ability test such as the WPPSI-III or WISC-IV. Next, clinicians identify academic strengths and weaknesses by evaluating the pattern of subtest and composite scores, and consider both the statistical significance and base rate of score discrepancies to determine whether differences are clinically meaningful. In addition, interpretation of subtest skills analysis data provides more in-depth information about the student's skill strengths and weaknesses. Goal statements are provided to assist practitioners in formulating individualized education programs.

For comparing performance across test sessions and measuring change over time, growth scale values (GSVs) are provided at the subtest level. Unlike standard scores and percentile ranks, GSVs do not compare performance to a normative sample. Rather, the pattern of GSVs over time indicates whether the examinee's skill level has changed relative to his or her own previous skill level. Finally, the results of the WIAT-III may be incorporated into an analysis for the identification of a specific learning disability. The WIAT-III provides data and interpretation information for calculating a traditional *ability–achievement discrepancy* (AAD) analysis or a *pattern of strengths and weaknesses* (PSW) analysis.

Integration of IQ and Achievement Results in Learning Disability Assessments

IDEA 2004 provides clinicians with greater flexibility in determining the methods that should be used for learning disability identification. The WIAT-III includes two of the more commonly used analyses in the field: AAD analysis and PSW analysis. Both of these analyses require the integration of standardized achievement and ability measures, and the WIAT-III manual and Scoring Assistant provide links to both the WPPSI-III and WISC-IV. It should be noted at the outset that significant discrepancies as described by either the AAD or PSW approach are often used as administrative criteria to determine eligibility for special education services in public school systems, but they are never sufficient for clinical diagnosis of a learning disability. Although they are important empirical sources of information, they must be interpreted as part of a larger evaluation that includes educational records, medical history, social and emotional functioning, and other information.

AAD Analysis

An AAD is characterized by performance on an academic achievement test that is significantly lower than what would be expected from an examinee's performance on a cognitive ability measure. Although discrepancies of this sort sometimes indicate the presence of a learning disability, many other factors may cause academic achievement to be discordant with cognitive ability. For example, children who struggle with extreme inattention or anxiety may be at a disadvantage relative to peers with respect to knowledge acquisition. Similarly, bright and motivated children with learning disabilities may compensate for their learning difficulties through the use of executive compensatory strategies, hard work, or external support. In other words, although the presence of an AAD indicates that a child is not achieving at his or her potential, the reason for underachievement requires further investigation and cannot be inferred from the presence of the discrepancy alone. For this reason, an AAD analysis should be accompanied by other sources of information (Berninger & O'Donnell,

2005; Shinn, 2007; Siegel, 2003) when it is used to identify a learning disability.

The WIAT-III provides two methods for calculating AAD: the simple-difference method and the predicted-achievement method (formulas to calculate simple-difference critical values and base rates, as well as those for the predicted-achievement method, can be found in Rust & Golombok, 1999). The predicted-achievement method is typically preferred because it accounts for regression to the mean, as well as the correlations between the two tests used in the analysis. To assist in predicted-achievement calculations, the WIAT-III provides subtest and standard scores predicted from a number of cognitive batteries, including the WISC-IV and WPPSI-III. The FSIQ is typically used to predict achievement scores, though other index scores may be substituted for cases in which the FSIQ is an inadequate estimate of cognitive abilities.

PSW Analysis

IDEA 2004 allows clinicians to consider a child's "pattern of strengths and weaknesses" in determining eligibility for learning disability services. The WIAT-III offers the capability of conducting a PSW analysis based on the concordance–discordance model developed by Hale and Fiorello (2004), utilizing scores from the WIAT-III and another cognitive ability measure such as the WISC-IV or WPPSI-III. The PSW model is often preferred because it requires the identification of a relative processing weakness, which helps to clarify the factors underlying academic difficulties (e.g., a cognitive processing deficit as opposed to emotional factors, poor instruction, etc.). Doing so can facilitate differential diagnosis and treatment planning, which is often difficult, given that students with learning problems are a heterogeneous group (Hale, Fiorello, et al., 2008).

The PSW analysis provided by the WIAT-III Scoring Assistant conducts two score comparisons, each of which must be significantly different to meet the model's criteria for learning disability identification: (1) processing strength versus achievement weakness and (2) processing strength versus processing weakness. In order to calculate the PSW analysis with the WIAT-III and either the WISC-IV or WPPSI-III, the following steps are necessary. First, the WIAT-III subtest or composite score that reflects the student's achievement weakness should be identified; the examiner must check first to make sure that the composite score is unitary

(i.e., subtest scores do not show significant scatter). Scores below 85 are typically chosen, though scores above 85 may be acceptable in some cases (e.g., gifted students). Second, the cognitive weakness is identified; again, the examiner must make sure that the index is interpretable and theoretically related to the achievement weakness (see Hale et al., 2001; Hale, Fiorello, Bertin, & Sherman, 2003). Finally, a cognitive strength is identified that is interpretable and is not related to the academic weakness identified in step 1. The WIAT-III manual advises against the use of the WMI or PSI as indicators of cognitive strengths because they have lower g loadings (Pearson, 2009).

ILLUSTRATIVE CASE STUDY

Examinee: Andy Ford
Report date: 11/18/2009
Age: 12 years
Date of birth: 11/13/97
Gender: Male
Grade: 6
Tests administered: WISC-IV, WIAT-III

Reason for Referral

Andy is a 12-year-old male referred for evaluation at the recommendation of his pediatrician. He has a history of school underachievement, and the purpose of the current evaluation is to clarify the factors underlying his academic difficulties.

Family History

Andy lives with his parents and two older sisters, with whom he has lived since birth. Andy comes from a culturally diverse family background. His father is European American. His mother was born in the United States, and her parents were first-generation immigrants from Brazil. Andy's mother obtained her master's degree and is employed as a nurse. His father graduated from college and works in sales. No significant stressors were reported at home.

Language Development

Andy's dominant language is English, and his parents and siblings speak English at home. Andy's maternal grandmother, who lives nearby and sees Andy several times a month, speaks to him in Portuguese. Andy's mother reported that Andy understands Portuguese and speaks some Portuguese to his grandmother, but prefers speaking in English. No history of speech or language delays was reported, although he spoke his first words and used short sentences slightly later than expected.

Medical and Developmental History

Mrs. Ford reported that Andy was born following a full-term pregnancy free of complications. With the exception of his language development, Andy met all major developmental milestones within normal limits. Medical history is significant for frequent ear infections at the age of 2 years, which were treated with the placement of pressure equalizer tubes. No other hospitalizations, surgeries, or chronic illnesses were reported. A recent physical exam revealed normal hearing and vision. Andy is not currently on medication.

Educational History

Andy is in the sixth grade, his first year in middle school. Andy attends a general education classroom and has never been evaluated for special education services. However, Andy received a speech and language screening, which indicated his oral language abilities are within normal limits. Mrs. Ford noted that he has generally struggled with reading and writing tasks, but has compensated for these difficulties by spending more time studying the subjects with his parents. As the coursework became more complex in middle school, Andy struggled to keep up in class and earned below-average grades in English language arts his first semester. He was assigned a small-group tutoring service and support from a classroom aide, neither of which was effective in improving his test scores.

Mrs. Ford reported that Andy is motivated to do well in school but frustrated by his lack of success. His attendance record is excellent, and he has no reported disciplinary problems. Andy spends approximately 1 hour per night completing his homework. Mrs. Ford reported that Andy rarely forgets to bring assignments home or turn in completed work.

Behavioral Observations

Andy appeared alert and motivated. He appeared shy at the beginning of testing, but rapport was established quickly and maintained throughout testing. His speech was goal-directed and fluent, without errors of articulation, and his receptive language appeared adequate for testing purposes. Andy was cooperative on all tasks.

Interpretation of WISC-IV Results

Index Score Descriptions

Andy was administered 10 subtests of the WISC-IV (see Tables 9.6 and 9.7 for his composite and subtest scores, respectively). Andy's general cognitive ability is within the average range of intellectual functioning, as measured by the FSIQ. His overall thinking and reasoning abilities exceed those of approximately 25% of children his age (FSIQ = 90; 95% confidence interval = 85–95), indicating well-developed overall cognitive functioning.

Andy's verbal reasoning abilities, as measured by the VCI, are in the low average range and above those of approximately 16% in the normative sample (VCI = 85; 95% confidence interval = 79–93). The VCI is designed to measure verbal reasoning and concept formation. Andy performed comparably on the verbal subtests contributing to the VCI, suggesting that these verbal cognitive abilities are similarly developed.

Andy's low average performance on the VCI was significantly lower than his average performance on the PRI and WMI, by 15 and 12 points, respectively. The discrepancies indicate that Andy's skills in the areas of nonverbal reasoning, sus-

TABLE 9.6. Andy's WISC-IV Composite Scores

Composite	Sum of scaled scores	Composite score	Percentile rank	95% confidence interval	Qualitative description
Verbal Comprehension Index (VCI)	22	85	16	79–93	Low average
Perceptual Reasoning Index (PRI)	30	100	50	92–108	Average
Working Memory Index (WMI)	19	97	42	90–105	Average
Processing Speed Index (PSI)	17	91	27	83–101	Average
Full Scale IQ (FSIQ)	88	90	25	85–95	Average

TABLE 9.7. Andy's WISC-IV Subtest Scores

Subtest	Raw score	Scaled score	Age equivalent
Similarities	17	7	9:2
Vocabulary	31	7	9:6
Comprehension	22	8	10:6
Block Design	30	8	9:10
Picture Concepts	21	12	16:6
Matrix Reasoning	24	10	12:10
Digit Span	17	10	13:6
Letter–Number Sequencing	16	9	9:6
Coding	42	7	9:10
Symbol Search	27	10	12:2

tained attention, and effortful mental control are better developed than his verbal reasoning skills, and suggest a relative weakness for Andy in complex verbal information processing. In addition, only 13% of children with overall cognitive skills similar to Andy score higher on the PRI than on the VCI, indicating that Andy's relatively rare discrepancy of 15 points may be of clinical importance. Conversely, nearly 20% of children with similar overall cognitive function score 12 points higher on the WMI than on the VCI, indicating that it is a more common discrepancy in the general population.

Andy's nonverbal reasoning abilities, as measured by the PRI, are in the average range and above those of approximately 50% of children his age (PRI = 100; 95% confidence interval = 92–108). The PRI is designed to measure fluid reasoning in the perceptual domain with tasks that assess nonverbal concept formation, visual perception and organization, simultaneous processing, visual–motor coordination, learning, and the ability to separate figure and ground in visual stimuli. Andy's performance on the Picture Concepts subtest was significantly better than his own mean score on the PRI (Picture Concepts scaled score = 12). This subtest is designed to measure fluid reasoning and abstract categorical reasoning ability. The task invokes verbal concepts, but does not require verbal responses. These results suggest that Andy demonstrates a relative strength in these areas, though it should be noted that 25% of children exhibit a similar strength on the Picture Concepts subtest.

Andy's abilities to sustain attention, concentrate, and exert mental control, as measured by the WMI, are in the average range. He performed better than approximately 42% of children his age

in the standardization sample (WMI = 97; 95% confidence interval = 90–105). These results suggest that relative to other children his age, Andy demonstrates the mental control and attentional skills necessary to facilitate learning and support more complex information processing. Andy performed comparably on working memory subtests.

Finally, Andy's abilities to process simple or routine visual material without making errors, as measured by the PSI, are in the average range compared to those in the standardization sample. He performed better than approximately 27% of children his age on these tasks (PSI = 91; 95% confidence interval = 83–101). Learning often involves both routine and complex information processing, and Andy's performance on the PSI suggests that he demonstrates the basic processing abilities necessary to acquire new information.

In summary, Andy demonstrates overall cognitive skills in the average range. His nonverbal reasoning, sustained attention, mental control, and ability to process simple or routine information are average. His verbal reasoning skills are low average and significantly lower than his nonverbal reasoning, sustained attention, and mental control, indicating a weakness in this area relative to his other cognitive skills.

Interpretation of WIAT-III Results

Given Andy's history of difficulties in reading and writing, he was administered the WIAT-III subtests of Word Reading, Pseudoword Decoding, Reading Comprehension, and Written Expression. To evaluate a possible area of strength, the Math Problem Solving subtest was administered. Results were interpreted using age-based norms.

Results are presented in Table 9.8. Andy demonstrated overall reading skills in the below-average range, performing better than only about 7% of others in the standardization sample (Basic Reading composite = 78, 95% confidence interval = 74–82). His ability to read single words aloud was below average for children his age. He read 18 words in 30 seconds, which was better than approximately 5% of children his age (Word Reading = 75, 95% confidence interval = 70–80). His pseudoword decoding (i.e., the ability to sound out made up words) was below average and above that of 10% of children his age (Pseudoword Decoding = 81, 95% confidence interval = 76–86). He was able to sound out 13 pseudowords in 30 seconds. An evaluation of the skills analysis data for Word Reading and Pseudoword Decoding revealed specific weaknesses in recognizing more advanced vowel types (e.g., vowel digraphs and diphthongs), consonant blends, and common suffixes. Finally, Andy's reading comprehension was average (Reading Comprehension = 98, 95% confidence interval = 86–110). His ability to read passages and provide oral responses to open-ended comprehension questions was better than that of 45% of his peers.

Andy was assessed with two Written Expression subtests. His ability to spell single words read aloud by the examiner was at the low end of average and better than that of 18% of his peers (Spelling = 86, 95% confidence interval = 80–92). A skills analysis revealed particular difficulty spelling irregular vowels and certain suffixes (e.g., *-ous, -ious*), suggesting greater difficulty with orthography than with phonology. His written productivity, theme development, and text organization were also at the low end of average and better than those of approximately 23% of children his age (Essay Composition = 83, 95% confidence interval = 73–93). His one-paragraph essay included a simple introduction and two clearly stated reasons; however, he did not include elaborations, transition words, or a conclusion.

Finally, Andy's math problem-solving skills were average (Math Problem Solving = 105, 95% confidence interval = 97–113). His ability to complete math calculations quickly and accurately, as well as solve word problems, was better than that of 63% of the standardization sample.

Overall, the results of academic testing with the WIAT-III reveal relative weaknesses in the areas of single-word recognition and decoding. Despite these weaknesses, Andy demonstrates average reading comprehension skills. Consistent with his average overall cognitive functioning, he seems to effectively utilize compensatory strategies and context cues to circumvent his word recognition difficulties while reading in context. Andy's written expression skills are below average. His highest score was in the area of math problem solving, which represents a relative strength for Andy.

AAD Analysis

With Andy's FSIQ from the WISC-IV as the basis, the predicted-difference method was utilized to assess for discrepancies between his predicted and actual achievement on the Basic Reading composite, as well as the Spelling and Essay Composition subtests. This analysis revealed that Andy's performance on the Basic Reading composite was significantly below what would be predicted from his FSIQ ($p < .01$). This level of discrepancy was evident in only 10% of children in the normative sample; as such, it is a relatively rare occurrence. No discrepancies were revealed between Andy's

TABLE 9.8. Andy's WIAT-III Composite and Subtest Scores

Composite/subtest	Raw score	Standard score	95% confidence interval	Percentile	Age equivalent	Qualitative descriptor
Basic Reading	—	78	74–82	7		*Below average*
Word Reading	31	75	70–80	5	8:4	Below average
Pseudoword Decoding	19	81	76–86	10	7:8	Below average
Reading Comprehension	32*	98	86–110	45	11:4	Average
Spelling	24	86	80–92	18	9:4	Average
Essay Composition	—	83	73–93	23	8:6	Below average
Math Problem Solving	54	105	97–113	63	13:4	Average

*Raw score was converted to weighted raw score before standard score was calculated.

cognitive functioning and written expression skills. This analysis suggests that relative to his overall cognitive functioning, Andy is demonstrating significant underachievement in the area of basic reading skills—a necessary but insufficient condition for identifying a learning disability.

PSW Analysis

To further evaluate for the presence of a learning disability, a PSW analysis was conducted. Andy's score on the Basic Reading composite was used as the academic weakness. His VCI on the WISC-IV was identified as his cognitive weakness, as verbal comprehension is related to basic reading skills and his VCI score was significantly lower than his scores in other cognitive domains. Andy's PRI score was identified as his cognitive strength, as his skills in this area are average, and perceptual reasoning is not thought to be theoretically related to basic reading skills. This analysis revealed that Andy's academic and cognitive weaknesses were significantly lower relative to his cognitive strength ($p < .01$ for both the Basic Reading composite and the VCI compared to the PRI). Like the results of the AAD analysis, these results support a possible diagnosis of a learning disability in the area of reading.

Conclusions and Recommendations

Andy is a 12-year-old male with a history of difficulties in reading and spelling. The results of the current evaluation revealed overall cognitive skills in the average range, with his verbal comprehension abilities underdeveloped relative to his perceptual reasoning and working memory abilities. Andy's reading is below average and a relative weakness for him; his written expression skills are below average, and his math problem-solving skills are average. Analyses revealed a pattern of strengths and weaknesses consistent with a learning disability in the area of basic reading: Andy's academic weakness (basic reading) and cognitive weakness (VCI) are significantly lower than his cognitive strength (PRI). These results are consistent with parent and teacher reports.

Andy's present level of reading achievement, as well as the interventions already implemented, suggests that he may benefit from reading instruction that integrates reading and spelling to reinforce what is taught and incorporates single-word reading of both real words and nonwords. He may benefit most from instruction that is explicit and

systematic, offering repetition and opportunities to practice and reinforce skills in a variety of contexts to develop automaticity. Specifically, Andy needs work in the areas of phoneme–grapheme relationships, sight words, and structural analysis. Given Andy's strength in perceptual reasoning and math, he may enjoy opportunities to track and chart his progress over time. Decisions regarding classroom accommodations and modifications will be made in collaboration with Andy's parents and teachers.

REFERENCES

Ackerman, P. L., Beier, M. E., & Bowen, K. R. (2000). Explorations of crystallized intelligence: Completion tests, cloze tests, and knowledge. *Learning and Individual Differences, 12*(1), 105–121.

Alexander, P. A., & Kulikowich, J. M. (1991). Domain knowledge and analogic reasoning ability as predictors of expository text comprehension. *Journal of Reading Behavior, 23*(2), 165–190.

Beres, K. A., Kaufman, A. S., & Perlman, M. D. (2000). Assessment of child intelligence. In G. Goldstein & M. Hersen (Eds.), *Handbook of psychological assessment* (3rd ed., pp. 65–96). New York: Pergamon Press.

Berninger, V. W., & O'Donnell, L. (2005). Research-supported differential diagnosis of specific learning disabilities. In A. Prifitera, D. H. Saklofske, & L. G. Weiss (Eds.), *WISC-IV clinical use and interpretation: Scientist-practitioner perspectives* (pp. 189–233). New York: Academic Press.

Bracken, B. A. (1987). Limitations of preschool instruments and standards for minimal level of technical adequacy. *Journal of Psychoeducational Assessment, 4*, 313–326.

Breaux, K. C. (2009). *WIAT-III technical manual.* San Antonio, TX: Pearson.

Brownell, R. (Ed.). (2000). *Expressive One-Word Picture Vocabulary Test—Third Edition.* Novato, CA: Academic Therapy Press.

Calhoun, S. L., & Mayes, S. D. (2005). Processing speed in children with clinical disorders. *Psychology in the Schools, 42*(4), 333–343.

Chen, H. Y., Keith, T. Z., Chen, Y. H., & Chang, B. S. (2009). What does the WISC-IV measure?: Validation of the scoring and CHC-based interpretative approaches. *Journal of Research in Education Studies, 54*(3), 85–108.

Colom, R., Rebollo, I., Palacios, A., Espinosa, M. J., & Kyllonen, P. C. (2004). Working memory is (almost) perfectly predicted by g. *Intelligence, 32*(3), 277–296.

Conway, A. R. A., Cowan, N., Bunting, M. F., Therri-ault, D. J., & Minkoff, S. R. B. (2002). A latent vari-able analysis of working memory capacity, short-term memory capacity, processing speed, and general fluid intelligence. *Intelligence, 30,* 163–183.

Cooper, S. (1995). *The clinical use and interpretation of the Wechsler Intelligence Scale for Children* (3rd ed.). Springfield, IL: Thomas.

Daneman, M., & Merikle, M. (1996). Working memory and language comprehension: A meta-analysis. *Psy-chonomic Bulletin Review, 3,* 422–433.

Daniel, M. H. (2007). Scatter and the construct validity of FSIQ: Comment on Fiorello et al. (2007). *Applied Neuropsychology, 14*(4), 291–295.

Delis, D. C., Kaplan, E., & Kramer, J. H. (2001). *Delis–Kaplan Executive Function System.* San Antonio, TX: Psychological Corporation.

DeSanti, R. J. (1989). Concurrent and predictive valid-ity of a semantically and syntactically sensitive cloze scoring system. *Reading, Research, and Instruction, 28*(2), 29–40.

Donders, J., & Warschausky, S. (1997). WISC-III factor index score patterns after traumatic head injury in children. *Child Neuropsychology, 3,* 71–78.

Dumont, R., & Willis, J. O. (2010). Strengths and weak-nesses of the WIAT-III and KTEA-II. In E. O. Lich-tenberger & K. C. Breaux, *Essentials of WIAT-III and KTEA-II assessment.* Hoboken, NJ: Wiley.

Elliott, C. D. (2007). *Differential Ability Scales—Second Edition: Introductory and technical handbook.* San An-tonio, TX: Harcourt Assessment.

Engle, R. W., Carullo, J. J., & Collins, K. W. (1991). Individual differences in working memory for com-prehension and following directions. *Journal of Edu-cational Research, 84,* 253–262.

Fiorello, C. A., Hale, J. B., Holdnack, J. A., Kavanaugh, J. A., Terrell, J., & Long, L. (2007). Interpreting in-telligence test results for children with disabilities: Is global intelligence relevant? *Applied Neuropsychology, 14*(1), 2–12.

Flanagan, D. P., & Alfonso, V. C. (1995). A critical re-view of the technical characteristics of new and re-cently revised intelligence test for preschool children. *Journal of Psychoeducational Assessment, 13,* 66–90.

Flanagan, D. P., & Kaufman, A. S. (2009). *Essentials of WISC-IV assessment* (2nd ed.). Hoboken, NJ: Wiley.

Fry, A. F., & Hale, S. (1996). Processing speed, working memory, and fluid intelligence: Evidence for a devel-opmental cascade. *Psychological Science, 7,* 237–241.

Fry, A. F., & Hale, S. (2000). Relationships among pro-cessing speed, working memory, and fluid intelligence in children. *Biological Psychology, 54,* 1–34.

Georgas, J., van de Vijver, F. J. R. , Weiss, L. G., & Saklofske, D. H. (2003). A cross-cultural analysis of the WISC-III. In J. Georgas, L. G. Weiss, F. J. R. van de Vijver, & D. H. Saklofske (Eds.), *Culture and chil-dren's intelligence: Cross-cultural analysis of the WISC-III* (pp. 277–313). San Diego, CA: Academic Press.

German, D. J. (1989). *Test of Word Finding.* Austin, TX: Pro-Ed.

Ghaziuddin, M., & Mountain-Kimchi, K. (2004). De-fining the intellectual profile of Asperger syndrome: Comparison with high-functioning autism. *Journal of Autism and Developmental Disorders, 34*(3), 279–284.

Gottfredson, L. S. (1997). Why g matters: The complex-ity of everyday life. *Intelligence, 24*(1), 79–132.

Glutting, J. J., Watkins, M. W., Konold, T. R., & McDer-mott, P. A. (2006). Distinctions without a difference: The utility of observed versus latent factors from the WISC-IV in estimating reading and math achieve-ment on the WIAT-II. *Journal of Special Education, 40*(2), 103–114.

Grégoire, J., Coalson, D. L., & Zhu, J. J. (2011). Analysis of WAIS-IV index score scatter using significant de-viation from the mean index score. *Assessment, 18,* 168–177.

Hale, J. B., & Fiorello, C. A. (2004). *School neuropsy-chology: A practitioner's handbook.* New York: Guil-ford Press.

Hale, J. B., Fiorello, C. A., Bertin, M., & Sherman, R. (2003). Predicting math achievement through neu-ropsychological interpretation of WISC-III variance components. *Journal of Psychoeducational Assessment, 21,* 358–380.

Hale, J. B., Fiorello, C. A., Kavanagh, J. A., Hoeppner, J. B., & Gaither, R. A. (2001). WISC-III predictors of academic achievement for children with learning disabilities: Are global and factor scores comparable? *School Psychology Quarterly* [Special issue], *16*(1), 31–55.

Hale, J. B., Fiorello, C. A., Kavanaugh, J. A., Holdnack, J. A., & Aloe, A. M. (2007). Is the demise of IQ in-terpretation justified?: A response to special issue au-thors. *Applied Neuropsychology, 14*(1), 37–51.

Hale, J. B., Fiorello, C. A., Miller, J. A., Wenrich, K., Teodori, A., & Henzel, J. N. (2008). WISC-IV in-terpretation for specific learning disabilities iden-tification and intervention: A cognitive hypothesis testing approach. In A. Prifitera, D. H. Saklofske, & L. G. Weiss (Eds.), *WISC-IV clinical assessment and intervention* (2nd ed., pp. 109–171). San Diego, CA: Academic Press.

Harrison, A. G., DeLisle, M. M., & Parker, K. C. H. (2008). An investigation of the General Abilities Index in a group of diagnostically mixed patients. *Journal of Psychoeducational Assessment, 26*(3), 247–259.

Individuals with Disabilities Education Improvement

Act of 2004 (IDEA 2004), Pub. L. 108–446, 118 Stat. 2647 (2004).

Jaeggi, S. M., Buschkuehl, M., Jonides, J., & Perrig, W. J. (2008). Improving fluid intelligence with training on working memory. *Proceedings of the National Academy of Sciences USA, 105*(19), 6829–6833.

Kamphaus, R. W. (1993). *Clinical assessment of children's intelligence.* Needham Heights, MA: Allyn & Bacon.

Kamphaus, R. W., Benson, J., Hutchinson, S., & Platt, L. O. (1994). Identification of factor models for the WISC-III. *Educational and Psychological Measurement, 54*(1), 174–186.

Kaplan, R. M., & Saccuzzo, D. P. (2005). *Psychological testing: Principles, applications, and issues.* Belmont, CA: Thomson Wadsworth.

Kaufman, A. S. (1994). *Intelligent testing with the WISC-III.* New York: Wiley.

Kaufman, A. S., & Kaufman, N. L. (1983). *Kaufman Assessment Battery for Children.* Circle Pines, MN: American Guidance Service.

Kaufman, A. S., & Kaufman, N. L. (2004). *Kaufman Assessment Battery for Children—Second Edition.* Bloomington, MN: Pearson.

Kaufman, A. S., & Lichtenberger, E. O. (1999). *Essentials of WAIS-III assessment.* New York: Wiley.

Keith, T. Z., Goldenring Fine, J., Taub, G. E., Reynolds, M. R., & Kranzler, J. H. (2006). Higher order, multisample, confirmatory factor analysis of the Wechsler Intelligence Scale for Children—Fourth Edition: What does it measure? *School Psychology Review, 35*(1), 108–127.

Kiewra, K. A., & Benton, S. L. (1988). The relationship between information processing ability and note taking. *Contemporary Educational Psychology, 13,* 3–44.

Konold, T. R. (1999). Evaluating discrepancy analysis with the WISC-III and WIAT. *Journal of Psychoeducational Assessment, 17,* 24–35.

Lichtenberger, E. O., & Kaufman, A. S. (2003). *Essentials of WPPSI-III assessment.* Hoboken, NJ: Wiley.

Matarazzo, J. D., & Herman, D. O. (1985). Clinical uses of the WAIS-R: Base rates of differences between VIQ and PIQ in the WAIS-R standardization sample. In B. B. Wolman (Ed.), *Handbook of intelligence: Theories, measurements, and applications* (pp. 899–932). New York: Wiley.

McKenna, M. C., & Layton, K. (1990). Concurrent validity of cloze as a measure of intersentential comprehension. *Journal of Educational Psychology, 82*(2), 372–377.

Newstead, S. E., Thompson, V., & Handley, S. J. (2002). Generating alternatives: A key component in human reasoning? *Memory and Cognition, 30*(1), 129–137.

Ormrod, J. E., & Cochran, K. F. (1988). Relationship of verbal ability and working memory to spelling achievement and learning to spell. *Reading Research Instruction, 28,* 33–43.

Payne, R. W., & Jones, H. G. (1957). Statistics for the investigation of individual cases. *Journal of Clinical Psychology, 13,* 115–121.

Pearson. (2009). *Wechsler Individual Achievement Test—Third Edition.* San Antonio, TX: Author.

Politano, P. M., & Finch, A. J. (1996). The Wechsler Intelligence Scale for Children—Third Edition. In C. S. Newmark (Ed.), *Major psychological assessment instruments* (pp. 294–319). Boston: Allyn & Bacon.

Prifitera, A., Saklofske, D. H., & Weiss, L. G. (Eds.). (2005). *WISC-IV clinical use and interpretation: Scientist-practitioner perspectives.* Amsterdam: Elsevier Academic Press.

Prifitera, A., Saklofske, D. H., & Weiss, L. G. (Eds.). (2008). *WISC-IV clinical assessment and intervention* (2nd ed.). Amsterdam: Elsevier.

Psychological Corporation. (2001). *Wechsler Individual Achievement Test—Second Edition.* San Antonio, TX: Author.

Raiford, S. E., Weiss, L. G., Rolfhus, E., & Coalson, D. (2005). General Ability Index (WISC-IV Technical Report No. 4). Retrieved August 30, 2010, from *www.pearsonassessments.com/NR/rdonlyres/1439CDFE-6980-435F-93DA-05888C7CC082/0/80720_WISCIV_Hr_r4.pdf.*

Ridgeway, V. (1995). The use of cloze as a measure of the interactive use of prior knowledge and comprehension strategies. In W. M. Linek & E. G. Sturtevant (Eds.), *Generations of literacy: The seventeenth yearbook of the College Reading Association, 1995* (pp. 26–34). Commerce: East Texas State University.

Roid, G. H., Prifitera, A., & Weiss, L. G. (1993). Replication of the WISC-III factor structure in an independent sample. In B. A. Bracken & R. S. McCallum (Eds.), *Advances in psychological assessment: Wechsler Intelligence Scale for Children—Third Edition* (pp. 6–21). Brandon, VT: Clinical Psychology.

Rourke, B. P. (1998). Significance of Verbal–Performance discrepancies for subtypes of children with learning disabilities: Opportunities for the WISC-III. In A. Prifitera & D. Saklofske (Eds.), *WISC-III clinical use and interpretation: Scientist-practitioner perspectives* (pp. 139–156). San Diego, CA: Academic Press.

Rust, J., & Golombok, S. (1999). *Modern psychometrics: The science of psychological assessment* (2nd ed.). New York: Routledge.

Ryan, J. J., & Smith, J. W. (2003). Assessing the intelligence of adolescents with the Wechsler Adult Intelligence Scale—Third Edition. In C. R. Reynolds

& R. W. Kamphaus (Eds.), *Handbook of psychological and educational assessment of children: Intelligence, aptitude, and achievement* (2nd ed., pp. 147–173). New York: Guilford Press.

Saklofske, D. H., Weiss, L. G., Raiford, S. E., & Prifitera, A. (2006). Advanced clinical interpretation of WISC-IV index scores. In L. G. Weiss, D. H. Saklofske, A. Prifitera, & J. Holdnack (Eds.), *WISC-IV advanced clinical interpretation* (pp. 139–179). Amsterdam: Elsevier.

Salthouse, T. A. (1996). The processing-speed theory of adult age differences in cognition. *Psychological Review, 103*, 403–428.

Sattler, J. M. (2008). *Assessment of children: Cognitive foundations* (5th ed.). San Diego, CA: Jerome M. Sattler.

Semel, E., Wiig, E. H., & Secord, W. A. (1995). *Clinical Education of Language Fundamentals—Third Edition.* San Antonio, TX: Psychological Corporation.

Shaw, S. R., Swerdlik, M. E., & Laurent, J. (1993). Review of the Wechsler Intelligence Scale for Children (3rd ed.). In B. A. Bracken & R. S. McCallum (Eds.), *Advances in psychological assessment: Wechsler Intelligence Scale for Children—Third Edition* (pp. 151–160). Brandon, VT: Clinical Psychology.

Shinn, M. R. (2007). Identifying students at risk, monitoring performance, and determining eligibility within response to intervention: Research on educational need and benefit from academic intervention. *School Psychology Review, 36*(4), 601–617.

Siegel, L. S. (2003). IQ-discrepancy definitions and the diagnosis of LD: Introduction to the special issue. *Journal of Learning Disabilities, 36*, 2–3.

Silverstein, A. B. (1981). Reliability and abnormality of test score differences. *Journal of Clinical Psychology, 37*(2), 392–394.

Strauss, E., Sherman, E. M. S., & Spreen, O. (2006). *A compendium of neuropsychological tests: Administration, norms, and commentary* (3rd ed.). New York: Oxford University Press.

Sweetland, J. D., Reina, J. M., & Tatti, A. F. (2006). WISC-III Verbal/Performance discrepancies among a sample of gifted children. *Gifted Child Quarterly, 50*(1), 7–10.

Tulsky, D. S., Saklofsky, D. H., Chelune, G. J., Heaton, R. K., Ivnik, R. J., Bornstein, R., et al. (Eds.). (2003). *Clinical interpretation of the WAIS-III and WMS-III.* San Diego, CA: Academic Press.

Tupa, D. J., Write, M. O., & Fristad, M. A. (1997). Confirmatory factor analysis of the WISC-III with child psychiatric inpatients. *Psychological Assessment, 9*(3), 302–306.

Wasserman, J. D., & Maccubbin, E. M. (2002, August). *Wechsler at The Psychological Corporation: Chorus girls and taxi drivers.* Paper presented at the 110th Annual Convention of the American Psychological Association, Chicago.

Watkins, M. W., Glutting, J. J., & Lei, P. (2007). Validity of the Full Scale IQ when there is significant variability among WISC-III and WISC-IV factor scores. *Applied Neuropsychology, 14*(1), 13–20.

Watkins, M. W., Lei, P., & Canivez, G. L. (2007). Psychometric intelligence and achievement: A cross-lagged panel analysis. *Intelligence, 35*, 59–68.

Watkins, M. W., Wilson, S. M., Kotz, K. M., Carbone, M. C., & Babula, T. (2006). Factor structure of the Wechsler Intelligence Scale for Children—Fourth Edition among referred students. *Educational and Psychological Measurement, 66*, 975–983.

Wechsler, D. (1949). *Wechsler Intelligence Scale for Children.* New York: Psychological Corporation.

Wechsler, D. (1967). *Wechsler Preschool and Primary Scale of Intelligence.* New York: Psychological Corporation.

Wechsler, D. (1991). *Wechsler Intelligence Scale for Children—Third Edition.* San Antonio, TX: Psychological Corporation.

Wechsler, D. (1992). *Wechsler Individual Achievement Test.* New York: Psychological Corporation.

Wechsler, D. (1995a). *Manual for the Wechsler Intelligence Scale for Children—Third Edition: Australian edition.* Marrickville, Australia: Psychological Corporation.

Wechsler, D. (1995b). *Manual for the Wechsler Intelligence Scale for Children—Third Edition: Canadian edition.* Toronto: Psychological Corporation.

Wechsler, D. (1997). *WAIS-III–WMS-III technical manual.* San Antonio, TX: Psychological Corporation.

Wechsler, D. (1998). *Manual for the Wechsler Intelligence Scale for Children—Third Edition: Japanese edition.* Tokyo: Psychological Corporation.

Wechsler, D. (2002a). *Wechsler Preschool and Primary Scale of Intelligence—Third Edition.* San Antonio, TX: Psychological Corporation.

Wechsler, D. (2002b). *WPPSI-III technical and interpretive manual.* San Antonio, TX: Psychological Corporation.

Wechsler, D. (2003a). *Wechsler Intelligence Scale for Children—Fourth Edition.* San Antonio, TX: Psychological Corporation.

Wechsler, D. (2003b). *WISC-IV technical and interpretive manual.* San Antonio, TX: Psychological Corporation.

Wechsler, D. (2008). *WAIS-IV technical and interpretive manual.* San Antonio, TX: Pearson.

Weiss, L. G., Beal, A. L., Saklofske, D. H., Alloway, T. P., & Prifitera, A. (2008). Interpretation and intervention with WISC-IV in the clinical assessment context. In A. Prifitera, D. H. Saklofske, & L. G. Weiss (Eds.), *WISC-IV clinical assessment and intervention* (2nd ed., pp. 3–68). London: Elsevier.

Weiss, L. G., & Gabel, A. D. (2008). Using the Cognitive Proficiency Index in psychoeducational assessment (WISC-IV Technical Report No. 6). Retrieved August 30, 2010, from *www.pearsonassessments.com/NR/rdonlyres/E15   367FE   -D287-46B4-989A-609160D94DA8/0/WISCIVTechReport6.pdf.*

Weiss, L. G., Saklofske, D. H., Coalson, D., & Raiford, S. E. (2010). *WAIS-IV clinical use and interpretation: Scientist-practitioner perspectives.* London: Elsevier.

Weiss, L. G., Saklofske, D. H., Prifitera, A., & Holdnack, J. A. (2006). *WISC-IV advanced clinical interpretation.* London: Elsevier.

Zhu, J. J., Weiss, L. G., Prifitera, A., & Coalson, D. (2003). The Wechsler intelligence scales for children and adults. In M. Hersen (Series Ed.) & G. Goldstein & S. R. Beers (Vol. Eds.), *Comprehensive handbook of psychological assessment: Vol. 1. Intellectual and neuropsychological assessment* (pp. 51–75). New York: Wiley.

The Stanford–Binet Intelligence Scales, Fifth Edition

Gale H. Roid
Mark Pomplun

The Stanford–Binet Intelligence Scales, Fifth Edition (SB5; Roid, 2003a) battery consists of 10 cognitive ability subtests that are individually administered for the age range of 2–85+ years. The SB5 is now distributed in two forms: (1) the standard full-range battery covering all ability levels for ages 2 through 85+ and (2) an alternative kit for early childhood assessment (ages 2–7) that includes a narrower range of ability. The early childhood version was derived directly from the full-range version and packaged as an economical alternative designed for younger children (Roid, 2005b) for use by professionals working with preschool children. This early childhood version can also be used for low-functioning individuals (e.g., those with IQ below 80), regardless of chronological age.

Several features were added to the SB5 to increase the age and content range of the scales, including the following features:

- The SB5 is the first intellectual assessment battery to measure five cognitive factors in both the nonverbal (reduced-vocal-language) domain and the verbal (vocal-language-required) domain. The battery was constructed on a five-factor hierarchical model similar to the four-factor model of the Fourth Edition. The five

cognitive factors are Fluid Reasoning, Knowledge, Quantitative Reasoning, Visual–Spatial Processing, and Working Memory. A full half of the SB5 battery is devoted to the reduced-language (Nonverbal) section. The Nonverbal section uses "hands-on" tasks involving brightly colored pictures, toys, and other objects that engage examinees, particularly young children and individuals with low cognitive functioning.[1]

- Brightly colored toys, blocks, and pictures have been restored in the SB5.
- Extended low-end and high-end items allow for early childhood and giftedness assessment.
- New composite scores have a mean of 100 and a standard deviation of 15, including Full Scale IQ (FSIQ), Nonverbal IQ (NVIQ), Verbal IQ (VIQ), and the five factor index scores.
- The SB5 follows the long tradition begun by Binet and Simon (1908) and Terman (1916) by combining the point scale format of the Fourth Edition (Thorndike, Hagen, & Sattler, 1986) with the age-level format of the Terman and Merrill (1937, 1960) editions. Instead of levels defined by chronological age, however, the SB5 employs two point scale subtests as an abbreviated IQ to estimate the functional level of the examinee. These two subtests are called *routing subtests* because they route the examinee to the

appropriate level in the remaining nonverbal and verbal parts of the test. The functional levels were based on item difficulty estimates from item response theory (IRT; Rasch, 1980). One of the routing subtests, Vocabulary, has been used in all editions to tailor the remainder of the testing to the functional level of the examinee. For the SB5, a nonverbal subtest, Object-Series/Matrices, was added as a second routing test.

- An Abbreviated Battery IQ (ABIQ) is formed from the routing tests.
- IRT-based *change-sensitive scores* (CSSs) are optional for criterion-referenced interpretation.
- The SB5 Verbal and Nonverbal Working Memory subtests require two of the subsystems of short-term memory defined by Baddeley (1986), one for language and one for visual–spatial information. A nonverbal block-tapping task also requires the planning and motor control abilities within executive processing, in which the individual guides his or her own thinking processes (Lezak, 1995). These new subtests provide new tools for the assessment of elderly individuals, persons with neuropsychological disorders, and persons with learning disabilities (LDs).
- The SB5 is linked to the Woodcock–Johnson III (WJ III) Tests of Achievement (Woodcock, McGrew, & Mather, 2001a) for assessment of persons with LDs.

THEORY AND STRUCTURE

Based on the important research of Carroll (1993), the SB5 was constructed on a five-factor hierarchical cognitive model. The five factors were derived from the combined model of Carroll (1993), Cattell (1943), and Horn (1965, 1994). The combination of models, now called the *Cattell–Horn–Carroll* (CHC) theory (see Schneider & McGrew, Chapter 4, this volume, for a detailed discussion), normally lists 8–10 factors. Many of the supplemental factors, such as processing speed, auditory processing, and long-term retrieval, require specialized timing or test apparatus (e.g., tape recorders). However, the selection of the SB5's five cognitive factors (see Figure 10.1) was based on research on school achievement and on expert ratings of the importance of these factors in the assessment of reasoning, especially in giftedness assessment. Expert ratings were obtained from several sources. First, an advisory panel of prominent researchers, practitioners; and contracted consultants provided ratings. Next, ratings were obtained from a workshop on assessment of gifted individuals, held in Denver, Colorado. And, finally, input was obtained from key advisors such as John Carroll (1993), John Horn (1994), Richard Woodcock, and Kevin McGrew (Woodcock et al., 2001a), at meetings in which all four of these experts were present. Also, the memory factor was shifted from an emphasis on short-term memory only, as in the Fourth Edition of the Stanford–Binet, to an emphasis on working memory.

Some expert consultants and advisors disagreed about the role of a hierarchical general factor (*g*) in CHC theory and the five-factor version in SB5. The consensus of the SB5 development staff and its author, Gale H. Roid, was to emphasize the importance of the empirical studies of Carroll (1993) and the tradition of hierarchical models in previous versions of the Stanford–Binet. Therefore, the overall model shown in Figure 10.1 is a hierarchi-

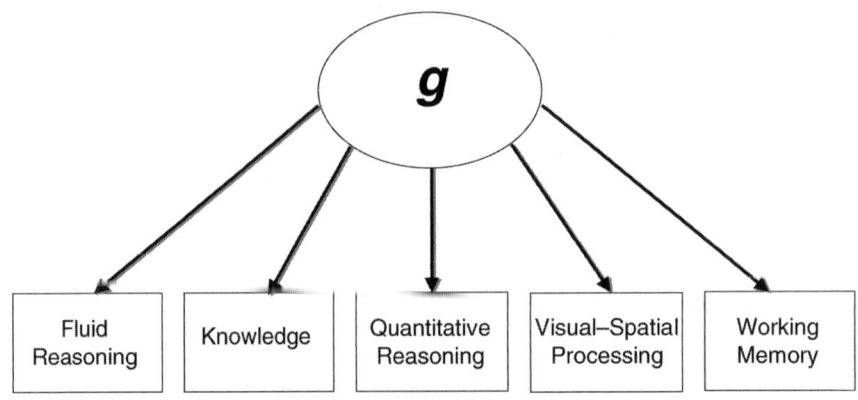

FIGURE 10.1. Theoretical model of SB5 cognitive factors.

cal *g* model, with five factors emphasizing reasoning abilities that can be easily administered within a 1-hour assessment.

The types of item content measured by the SB5 are shown in Table 10.1. The Verbal and Nonverbal domains include 5 subtests each, for a total of 10 subtests. The subtests each have raw score totals that are converted to various derived scores, such as the normalized scaled scores (mean = 10, standard deviation = 3) used to form the profile of 10 subtest scores used in the interpretation of the SB5. The Nonverbal subtests require a small degree of receptive language and allow for nonverbal responses such as pointing, moving blocks, or assembling pieces to indicate correct answers to problems presented in pictures, designs, or other illustrations. The Verbal subtests require facility with words and printed material (reading or speaking) to solve problems or indicate knowledge for each of the five cognitive factors covered by the test.

DESCRIPTION OF SUBTESTS

Table 10.1 shows contents of the SB5 subtests as reflected in the activities (tasks and types of items) that constitute each subtest. Testing begins with two subtests located in the first of three item books. Each item book (a spiral-bound book with a built-in easel) contains both the actual pictures and items of the test on one side of the page and examiner directions on the other side of the page.

The Nonverbal Fluid Reasoning subtest is Object-Series/Matrices, an extension of the Matrices subtest of the Fourth Edition, which is one of the routing subtests presented in a point scale format in item book 1. The Verbal Knowledge subtest is Vocabulary—also a routing subtest in the point scale format in item book 1. These two subtests are administered first and are used to route the examinees to the proper functional ability level on the remaining subtests. The remaining subtests are organized into sets of three to six items (called *testlets*), organized into functional ability levels based on the difficulty of the items. This structure of levels is similar to the classic design of the early editions of the Stanford–Binet. Item book 2 contains the four Nonverbal subtests—Knowledge, Quantitative Reasoning, Visual–Spatial Processing, and Working Memory. Nonverbal Knowledge includes an activity called Procedural Knowledge, in which the examinee expresses knowledge of objects shown in pictures by using gestures. Also, the classic Picture Absurdities (pointing and briefly explaining what is silly or unusual about a picture) is included in the more difficult levels of Nonverbal Knowledge.

Nonverbal Quantitative Reasoning includes items measuring numerical concepts and problems shown with counting rods (red plastic pieces designed as miniature rulers), blocks, or pictures. Nonverbal Visual–Spatial Processing tasks include the classic Form Board (a simple structured puzzle) and the new Form Patterns, in which pieces are used to form designs of animals, people, and ob-

TABLE 10.1. The Contents of SB5: The Activities That Compose the 10 Subtests (5 Nonverbal and 5 Verbal Subtests)

Cognitive factor	Nonverbal subtest activities	Verbal subtest activities
Fluid Reasoning	*Object-Series/Matrices	Early Reasoning Verbal Absurdities Verbal Analogies
Knowledge	Procedural Knowledge Picture Absurdities	*Vocabulary
Quantitative Reasoning	Nonverbal Quantitative Reasoning	Verbal Quantitative Reasoning
Visual–Spatial Processing	Form Board Form Patterns	Position and Direction
Working Memory	Delayed Response Block Span	Memory for Sentences Last Word

Note. Activities marked with an asterisk (*) are the initial routing tests used to tailor the assessment to the functional ability of the examinee.

jects. Nonverbal Working Memory is composed of an activity with plastic cups used to hide toys (Delayed Response) and a block-tapping task (Block Span).

Verbal Fluid Reasoning includes three types of tasks. Children and lower-functioning individuals begin with early reasoning tasks, such as identifying cause-and-effect relationships in pictures. Advanced examinees and adolescents progress to the Verbal Absurdities items (sentences expressing absurd contradictions), and finally, at the highest level, to difficult Verbal Analogy items ("A is to B as C is to D"). Verbal Quantitative Reasoning contains items containing numerical concepts and increasingly difficult word problems. The innovative Verbal Visual–Spatial Processing subtest employs some classic Binet items requiring understanding of verbal descriptions of spatial orientations ("Heading south, turn left, then right . . . ") and the explanation of directions on map-like displays. Finally, the Verbal Working Memory subtest includes the classic Binet task of remembering all the words in a given sentence, followed at the higher levels by a new task requiring memory of the last word in a series of sentences.

Two subtests (one Nonverbal and one Verbal) combine to form scores for each cognitive factor. Definitions of each of the factors are as follows:

• *Fluid Reasoning* is the ability to solve novel problems, whether with visual material in the Nonverbal domain or with words and print material in the Verbal domain.

• *Knowledge* is the fund of general information that is accumulated over time by the individual from experiences at home, in school, at work, or in the environment.

• *Quantitative Reasoning* is the ability to solve numerical problems, deal with fundamental number concepts, and solve word problems. The emphasis is on general logical, numerical thinking, with reduced dependency on academic mathematical knowledge (such as the ability to solve specific algebraic equations).

• *Visual–Spatial Processing* is the ability to see relationships among figural objects, describe or recognize spatial orientation, identify the "whole" among a diverse set of parts, and generally see patterns in visual material.

• *Working Memory* is the ability to hold both visual and verbal information in short-term memory and then transform it or "sort it out." An example of a working memory task was studied by Baddeley,

Logie, Nimmo-Smith, and Brereton (1985). They used a series of two, three, or more sentences presented one after the other. Some of the sentences made sense ("People eat food"), and some did not ("Cats sing water"). The examinee had to respond to each sentence, identifying the absurd sentences. Then, after all sentences were presented, the examinee had to recall key words from the sentences (in the preceding examples, *food* and *water*). Thus the task required the examinee to overcome the interference of responding to each sentence so that the key words could be sorted out and recalled. In the SB5, a similar (but less complex) task is used, in which a series of sentences (in the form of questions, answered "yes" or "no") is presented, and the examinee must recall the last word in each sentence; hence the subtest name, Last Word. Working memory is a very important clinical indicator of brain functioning, and difficulty with working memory is highly related to cognitive process deficits underlying LDs (Reid, Hresko, & Swanson, 1996). Some researchers believe that working memory is a central part of reasoning ability (e.g., Kyllonen & Christal, 1990).

TEST ADMINISTRATION AND SCORING

Background of the Examinee

The classic description of the role of the assessment professional given by Matarazzo (1990) is still highly relevant today. Matarazzo argued that assessment is quite different from measurement, and that intellectual assessment in particular requires experienced examiners who carefully evaluate the match between the instruments and the examinee. In administering the SB5, the examiner should reflect on the cultural and linguistic background of the examinee. In particular, if the examinee has communication difficulties, has a hearing difficulty, comes from a nonmajority culture, or has a dominant language other than English, great caution should be taken in administering the SB5 and interpreting results. Half of the SB5 consists of Nonverbal tasks and can be considered for administration as a separate battery from the Verbal subtests. The Verbal subtests of the SB5 do require English-language expression and word knowledge. The Nonverbal subtests require only pointing responses or a small degree of receptive language in most subtests, or brief gestures and expressive language in Nonverbal Knowledge (Picture Absurdities).

The examiner not only should reflect on the cultural and linguistic background or disability of the examinee, but should also look at acculturation (Dana, 1993). In the United States and Canada, *acculturation* is the degree to which an individual has learned, adopted, or possibly rejected elements of mainstream North American culture. If there is a question about acculturation, perhaps one of the various questionnaires developed for this purpose should be employed (Paniagua, 1994). Issues include whether the examinee and his or her family read in English, socialize outside their own linguistic culture, attend school, or attended school before coming to North America.

Preparation for Administration

Because the SB5 is a standardized instrument, careful attention should be given to the exact directions detailed in the examiner's manual (Roid, 2003b). Conveniently for the examiner, all directions for the instrument are printed on the examiner pages of the easel booklets, called *item books* in the SB5. As always, best practices should be followed; these include establishing rapport with the examinee prior to testing, practicing the administration of SB5 before using it in a clinical setting, and preparing all materials before testing. Also, the test environment should be controlled to minimize distractions. Variations in the order of administration, or various adaptations of the test

or accommodations due to disabilities, need to be documented carefully. When accommodations are allowed, they should be described in the report, and normative scores based on the national standardization of the SB5 should be interpreted with caution. In these cases, the SB5 offers the possibility of qualitative interpretation or use of the alternative criterion-referenced scoring system.

Administration

Figure 10.2 shows the standard administration procedure for the SB5. Testing begins with the first section of item book 1. This Nonverbal section of item book 1 presents the Object-Series/Matrices subtest, which is one of the routing subtests, provided in a point scale format. Unless there is a nonstandard administration emphasizing only nonverbal subtests, the next step is to administer a Verbal subtest, Vocabulary, the second routing subtest in item book 1. Following the administration of these routing subtests, point scale scores from these subtests are then used to determine the proper functioning level where testing will continue in item book 2 (Nonverbal) and item book 3 (Verbal). Therefore, the third step in the standard administration is to enter item book 2 at the proper level, indicated by the score on the Object-Series/Matrices subtest. The final step (step 4) is to route the subject to the proper Verbal level in item book 3, based on the score on the Vocabulary

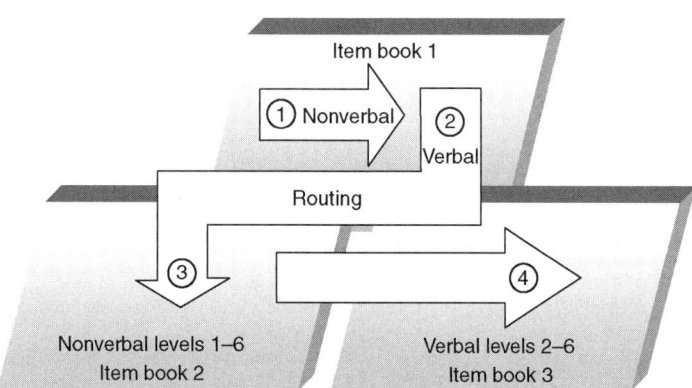

① Administer Object-Series/Matrices (Nonverbal Fluid Reasoning) routing subtest.

② Administer Vocabulary (Verbal Knowledge) routing subtest.

③ Route to Nonverbal levels section based on Object-Series/Matrices score.

④ Route to Verbal levels section based on Vocabulary score.

FIGURE 10.2. Standard administration of the SB5.

subtest. In both item books 2 and 3 (steps 3 and 4), the examiner should employ the basal and ceiling rules that are clearly marked on each page of the record form. Most examiners find that they will begin at the starting level indicated by the routing tests and test two levels (two pages in the record form for each domain—Nonverbal and Verbal).

Several important features of the SB5 test administration should be highlighted. First, the SB5 employs routing subtests in item book 1 to define the level at which the examinee will continue the assessment. This routing procedure adds precision to the measurement by tailoring the level of difficulty of the items to the examinee's ability level. Second, the SB5 employs different basal and ceiling rules for the routing subtests in comparison to the level subtests. In item book 1 for the routing subtest, the basal and ceiling rules are the typical ones found in point scales, with an age-estimated start point and a ceiling at a certain number of consecutive errors. Within the level subtests, the basal and ceiling rules are different from those in other batteries because they are based on sufficient (basal) or insufficient (ceiling) performance within a given level and subtest.

A second feature of the SB5 is that the level subtest sections in item books 2 and 3 are organized into smaller sections called *testlets*, as discussed previously. These testlets are designed to produce a maximum of 6 raw score points.[2] For example, the set of three Verbal Absurdity items (scored 0, 1, or 2 for different degrees of correctness) form a testlet for the Verbal Fluid Reasoning subtest, producing a maximum of 6 points. As the examinee is administered a series of testlets, the scores are accumulated to provide the total raw score for each subtest. When the examinee achieves too few points on a testlet, testing is stopped for that subtest, whereas testing of other subtests continues. Each subtest is consistently located in one of the four corners of the record form. So, to continue testing for an individual subtest, the examiner should simply turn to the next page of the record form and continue by administering the testlet located in the appropriate corner for that subtest.

In the third feature to be highlighted, the SB5 employs very few time limits and does not use time bonuses. However, in order to encourage a quick and efficient assessment, a system of examiner prompts is also employed on the most difficult items. For the most difficult items in Object-Series/Matrices, Quantitative Reasoning, and Verbal Analogies, for example, an examiner prompt rule employs a liberal 3-minute signal to encourage the examinee to move forward. This should not be a rigid time limit, but rather used as a method of moving examinees forward when they are stymied.

One of the final features of the SB5 is the use of teaching items. At the beginning of testlets that contain a new type of task for the examinee, the first item is employed not only as a sample item, but also as a teaching task in which feedback is given to the examinee. For certain unique tasks that are administered to lower-functioning examinees, these teaching items reveal the correct answer to the examinees for purposes of fairness.

Record Form

The record form for the SB5 has a familiar format. The first page includes a section for converting raw scores to normative scores and includes various profile graphs. Additional pages present one of the routing subtests or the levels subtest. For subtests requiring a verbal response, such as Vocabulary or Verbal Absurdities, spaces are provided for the examiner to write verbatim answers given by the examinee. Most of the items of the SB5 are scored according to a dichotomous format—that is, 0 or 1. However, some items have multiple score points. For example, Vocabulary items are scored 0, 1, or 2 to allow for partially correct answers.

After completing the identifying information about the examinee, the examiner begins with the routing subtests in item book 1 and records responses on pages 3 through 5 of the record form. Once the raw scores for each routing subtest are obtained, the examiner uses the Nonverbal routing table on page 6 to identify the recommended starting level for the examinee in the record form. The examiner then finds the same level in item book 2 by noting the color-printed stripes at the bottom of each page that identify the levels. For example, if the raw score on the Object-Series/Matrices routing subtest is 20 points, the routing table tells the examiner to start at level 3 on page 8 of the record form. The examiner proceeds to page 8 and begins with the instructions for level 3 in item book 2 (page 26). The next page of the item book (page 27) presents the first item in the Nonverbal Knowledge subtest (the Procedural Knowledge activity). This testlet has six items in which the examinee demonstrates the motions characteristic of people, using the pictured object shown on the examinee's side of the item book. The examiner sums the number correct for that testlet, and continues with the other three testlets on that page (next will be Quantitative Reasoning, in the bottom left corner of the record form).

Observing the basal and ceiling rules, the examiner continues on page 9 and beyond as needed in the Nonverbal section of the record form. Then the examiner goes to the level recommended by the Verbal routing table (on page 5), and administers the Verbal testlets indicated until the ceiling is reached for each of the four subtests being measured. In the case of a child or adult who does not speak English, or who has a documented, severe verbal communication disorder, a nonverbal administration may be chosen. This type of administration requires the examiner to begin with the Nonverbal routing subtest and complete the recommended Nonverbal testlets separately from the Verbal portions of the test to obtain the NVIQ and a profile of Nonverbal subtests.

Scoring

Once all the required subtests and testlets have been completed, the examiner copies all raw scores from the various pages of the record form to the summary tables on the front cover of the record form. First, the raw score totals for the routing subtests are entered in the section located in the upper left of the front cover of the record form. The routing subtests are each marked with a colored arrow labeled "Routing." For the testlet scores, the examiner begins entering the raw scores for testlets at the starting level and continues entering testlet scores until the ceiling is reached. All levels above the ceiling can be marked with a dash or zero. Credit is given for testlet scores below the starting level by tracing over the lightly printed numbers printed in the boxes for the lower-level testlets. The examiner sums the testlet scores (including credit for lower-level testlets not administered) down each column and places the sum in the boxes provided. Then the examiner uses the norm tables in the appendix of the examiner's manual (Roid, 2003b) to convert raw scores to derived scores used in interpretation of results.

Two systems of scoring are provided in the SB5: *norm-referenced* and *criterion-referenced*. First, the traditional normative standard scores are used to compare the examinee's performance to age-level peers from the nationally representative norm sample. As noted earlier, IQ scores (mean of 100, standard deviation of 15) include the NVIQ, VIQ, and FSIQ. Also, an optional ABIQ is available from the two routing subtests (Object-Series/Matrices plus Vocabulary). Factor index scores are

each composed of two subtests (one Nonverbal and one Verbal) and contrast performance on each of the five cognitive factors. For example, the Nonverbal Knowledge subtest scaled score is added to the Vocabulary (Verbal Knowledge) scaled score, and this sum is converted to the Knowledge factor index score. Because the factor index scores are expressed in the same metric as IQ scores (mean of 100, standard deviation of 15), they can be entered on the same type of profile as the IQ scores for visual comparison (located on the lower right of the front cover of the record form). The final set of normative scores is the set of 10 subtest profile scores (mean of 10, standard deviation of 3), including 5 Nonverbal and 5 Verbal subtests.

Also as noted earlier, a supplementary and optional scoring system employs CSSs, which convert raw scores into ability-level estimates from IRT analysis. Raw scores for each of the five factors and the three IQ scores are converted to Rasch-based scores (Rasch, 1980; Wright & Lineacre, 1999), in the same metric as the W scores of the WJ III Tests of Cognitive Abilities (Woodcock, McGrew, & Mather, 2001b). The average CSSs from the SB5 and W scores from the WJ III tests range from approximately 425 for 2-year-olds to 525 for high-functioning adults. These scores, along with the *growth scores* of the Leiter International Performance Scale—Revised (Roid & Miller, 1997), are centered at 500—the average score for examinees who are 10 years, 0 months of age. The interpretive manual for the SB5 (Roid, 2003c) explains the CSS scale. For example, the CSS for the Quantitative Reasoning factor can be related to increasingly complex mathematical concepts as the scores progress from 425 to 525.[3] Thus the CSSs can be "anchored" to the criterion of developmental age level as well as to the level of task difficulty, demonstrating their criterion-referenced characteristics. Also, CSS measures can be recorded across multiple tests and retests to measure change across time, whether that change is improvement or decline in cognitive function. Such scores are highly useful in clinical intervention research and in documenting the improvement of individuals in special education programs.

PSYCHOMETRIC PROPERTIES

Extensive studies of reliability, validity, and fairness were conducted as part of the SB5 standardization. These studies are detailed in the technical manual (Roid, 2003e). The main technical features of the

SB5 are briefly outlined here. Additional statistical analyses, useful tables, and case studies are presented in the interpretive manual (Roid, 2003c) and in Roid and Barram (2004).

The normative sample for the SB5 included 4,800 subjects, ages 2–96 years. The highest age grouping employed in the norm tables was 85+. The composition of the normative sample closely approximated the stratification percentages reported by the U.S. Bureau of the Census (2001). Stratification variables included sex, geographic region, ethnicity (African American, Asian American, European American, Hispanic, Native American, and other), and socioeconomic level (years of education completed or parents' educational attainment). In addition, subjects were tested (N = 1,365) from officially documented special groups, such as individuals with intellectual disabilities, LDs, attention-deficit/hyperactivity disorder (ADHD), and speech or hearing impairments. Details of these special studies are provided in Roid (2003e).

Internal-consistency reliability ranged from .95 to .98 for IQ scores and from .90 to .92 for the five factor index scores.[4] For the 10 subtests, average reliabilities ranged from .84 to .89, providing a strong basis for profile interpretation. Test–retest and interexaminer reliability studies were also conducted and showed the stability and consistency of SB5 scoring (Roid, 2003e). Test–retest data were collected on more than 80 subjects at four age levels: 2–5, 6–20, 21–59, and 60 years or older. Correlations between test and retest scores (stability coefficients) showed medians of .93 to .95 for IQ scores, .88 for factor index scores, and .82 for subtest scaled scores. The practice effect on scores, as measured by the size of the mean difference between test and retest scores, was smaller than expected, ranging from 2 to 5 points for IQ scores (with NVIQ shifting more than VIQ). However, the NVIQ practice effects on SB5 were small (2–5 points), compared to those for other prominent batteries such as the Wechsler Intelligence Scale for Children—Third Edition (WISC-III; Wechsler, 1991), where mean differences are often as high as 11–13 points on Performance IQ. Perhaps the stability of SB5 IQ scores is due to the complexity of tasks and the lack of time limits for most subtests.

IRT (Rasch, 1980; Wright & Lineacre, 1999) was used to design the routing procedure and levels, and to check the consistency among the items and tasks within each subtest. Thus the routing subtests (Object-Series/Matrices and Vocabulary in item book 1) are the first stage of a two-stage adaptive testing design. Ability is estimated from the Rasch-calibrated difficulties of the routing subtest items in order to place the examinee in the matching range of estimated ability in both the Nonverbal and Verbal levels. The levels sections of SB5 (item books 2 and 3) form the second stage of the two-stage assessment. For the subtests in this stage, testlets were chosen to create a stairstep design, with each testlet made increasingly difficult at each ascending level from level 1 to level 6. The Rasch analyses provide a verification that all items in a subtest, regardless of level or type of task, share communality with the underlying latent trait being measured collectively by the subtest items. Various indices of fit to the Rasch model were used to quantitatively verify fit to the unidimensional, underlying cognitive trait (Wright & Lineacre, 1999).

Evidence for content-, criterion-, and construct-related validity of SB5 is detailed in Roid (2003e), including extensive studies of concurrent, predictive, and factorial validity. Also, consequential validity and fairness of predicting achievement scores are reported in Roid (2003c). Examples of validity include correlations with other assessment batteries, as shown in Table 10.2. The technical manual for SB5 (Roid, 2003e) provides the details of these correlation studies, but some key descriptors of the samples employed are included in Table 10.2. The correlations shown in Table 10.2 are quite substantial and similar in magnitude to the concurrent correlations observed for other major intelligence batteries. The substantial predictive correlations between SB5 and two major achievement batteries (WJ III and the Wechsler Individual Achievement Test—Second Edition [WIAT-II]) provide a strong basis for comparing individuals' intellectual and achievement scores.

Extensive studies of the factor structure of SB5 were conducted and are summarized in Roid (2003e). Confirmatory factor analyses (CFAs) using LISREL 8.3 (Joreskog & Sorbom, 1999) were calculated for five successive age groups (2–5, 6–10, 11–16, 17–50, and 51+), and factor models with one, two, three, four, and five factors were compared. Split-half scores (scores for odd- and even-numbered items in each of the 10 subtests) were employed to provide more stable estimates of each factor in the maximum-likelihood analyses. The five-factor models showed superior fit, including a non-normed fit index ranging from .89 to .93, a comparative fit index ranging from .91 to .93, and a root mean square error of approximation ranging from .076 to .088. A second series of CFAs was

TABLE 10.2. Correlations of SB5 FSIQ Scores with Full-Scale Scores on Other Intelligence Tests and with Multiple Subtests in Achievement Batteries

Test	N	Age range	% Minority	Correlations
Stanford–Binet Fourth Edition	104	3–20	35%	.90
Stanford–Binet L-M Edition	80	3–19	17%	.85
Wechsler scales: WISC-III	66	6–16	47%	.84
Wechsler scales: WAIS-III	87	16–84	7%	.82
Wechsler scales: WIAT-II	80	6–15	19%	.53 to .80
WJ III Cognitive	145	4–11	25%	.90*
WJ III Achievement	472	6–19	29%	.66 to .84

Note. N, number of subjects; % Minority, percentage of the sample that was Asian American, African American, Native American (Indian), multiple-ethnicity, or other nonwhite/non-European American ethnicity; WISC-III, Wechsler Intelligence Scale for Children—Third Edition; WAIS-III, Wechsler Adult Intelligence Scale—Third Edition; WIAT-II, Wechsler Individual Achievement Test—Second Edition; WJ III, Woodcock–Johnson III. Correlations are product–moment coefficients, and the correlation marked with an asterisk (*) is based on a special WJ III composite score consisting of the five cognitive factors measured by the SB5. Correlation of the SB5 FSIQ with the multifactor General Intellectual Ability index of the WJ III was .78.

conducted with LISREL, using conventional full-length subtests across two batteries: the SB5 and the WJ III (Woodcock et al., 2001b). Again, the five-factor model showed the best fit, with all five factors aligning across the SB5 and WJ III as predicted.

RECENT USE OF THE SB5 IN RESEARCH AND PRACTICE

Roid and Barram (2004) presented data on the prediction of LDs from indexes that combined Knowledge and Working Memory subtests of the SB5. They also presented *shared ability composites* (combinations of subtests based on content or type of intellectual skill) for detailed interpretation of test results.

DiStefano and Dombrowski (2006) conducted exploratory factor analyses and CFAs on the SB5, using the published correlation matrices in the SB5 technical manual (Roid, 2003e). They concluded that the data showed strong confirmation of the overall general ability measured by the SB5, but did not confirm the five-factor structure from the subtest intercorrelation matrix data except for the 2- to 5-year age group. However, Roid (2003e) used split-half subtests (20 in total) and confirmed the five-factor structure based on a number of CFA fix statistics. The methodological differences between

these studies are important because CFA computer programs usually require two or more measures of each dimension to achieve proper estimation accuracy, and the DiStefano and Dombrowski study relied on only the existing 10 subtests.

Tippin (2007) presented a study of children with LDs in comparison to normative control children (ages 5–13 years), using the 10 subtests of the SB5. The study was summarized in Roid and Tippin (2009). The research contrasted a sample of 129 students who were diagnosed with a reading LD by school districts with 292 normative participants from the SB5 standardization sample, matched in terms of demographics to the LD group. The study found highly significant differences between the groups on many of the SB5 subtests, with effect sizes (standardized mean differences; Cohen, 1988) ranging from .46 to .81. The largest differences were for Nonverbal Quantitative Reasoning, and three Verbal subtests—Knowledge, Quantitative Reasoning, and Working Memory.

With the increasing need for nonverbal assessment, as indicated by the number of languages spoken in U.S. public schools (Reynolds & Kamphaus, 2003), the comprehensive, five-factor NVIQ of the SB5 has drawn more recent attention. Assessment professionals in some children's hospitals have adopted the SB5 (e.g., the Child Development and Rehabilitation Center in Portland, Oregon), and the NVIQ section was recently included as an intake test by autism research centers in the United States (C. Mazefsky, Children's Hospital of Pittsburgh, personal communication, August 2009).

Harlow (2010) studied the ethnic fairness of items and testlets from the SB5 nonverbal subtest on a Hispanic sample matched to a sample of white non-Hispanic, normative control subjects. Using indices of differential item functioning, Harlow found that the scores, the testlet scores, and the majority of items were free from evidence of potential bias. A few items showed favor to either the white non-Hispanic or Hispanic subjects, but the effects of ethnic difference were balanced out by the small effects favoring each group.

Roid and Edwards (2011) presented a detailed case study with brain scan data for a young adult woman who had sustained a severe traumatic brain injury in a car accident. The SB5 results for the young woman showed evidence of her improvement in function over a 7-year recovery period (as compared to previous Wechsler test data). Also, the Working Memory subtests showed continuing deficits in memory function, which were confirmed by other memory measures.

GENERAL INTERPRETATION OF SB5 TEST SCORES

Roid (2003b, 2003c) has recommended a seven-step interpretive strategy for the SB5. Each step is briefly described as follows. First, in steps 1 and 2, the purpose of the assessment and the context of the examinee are evaluated in terms of language and cultural factors to assure that the SB5 is the appropriate instrument for the individual and the assessment purpose. For example, if the examinee is a recent immigrant to the United States and does not speak or read English well, the individual's language context must be taken into account. In such a case, either accommodations in test administration (e.g., translation of items) or use of the nonverbal sections of SB5 alone may be necessary.

In the third step, the domains of Verbal and Nonverbal abilities, represented by VIQ and NVIQ, are contrasted and significant differences are noted. Given the high reliability and five-factor comprehensiveness of each domain in the SB5, the contrast between VIQ and NVIQ becomes much more important for interpretation than the same distinction in other intellectual batteries. Thus the fourth step of evaluating the overall level of cognitive performance, reflected in the FSIQ, may

have to be tempered when VIQ and NVIQ differ significantly. For example, for an examinee who is a recent immigrant to the United States and has Spanish as his or her dominant language, the VIQ may be only 85 while the NVIQ is 105, resulting in a difference that is both statistically significant and relatively rare in the normative sample (only 3.7% obtain a 20-point difference or greater). For these reasons, the NVIQ of 105 may be closer to the examinee's latent global ability than an FSIQ of 95, for example.

In the fifth step of interpretation, differences among the five factor index scores are evaluated through the use of tables provided in Roid (2003e) or Roid (2005a, included in Table 10.3). *Ipsative* comparisons (those made within an individual's own set of five factor index scores) can be made by looking at the numerical differences between each pair of scores (Roid, 2003e) or between the score and the average of the factor index scores (Table 10.3). Generally, differences of approximately 18–19 points are needed, pairwise, to show significance both statistically and practically (i.e., significance at the .05 level and rarity in the normative population). Because the five factors of SB5 were developed on the strong theoretical framework of the CHC model, the factor index profile should be valuable for cross-battery interpretation when other cognitive batteries have been administered to the examinee (Flanagan, Alfonso, & Ortiz, Chapter 19, this volume; Flanagan & Ortiz, 2001; McGrew & Flanagan, 1998). Table 10.3 presents the significance level and percentages of the population for differences between factor scores and the mean factor score for ages 2–5 or ages 6–85+ separately. The significance level is based on the method originally suggested by Davis (1959) and refined by Silverstein (1982), widely used in other cognitive tests. The procedure corrects for the multiple comparisons on the same person (it is called the *Bonferroni correction*).

In the sixth step of interpretation, the individual subtests (five Nonverbal and five Verbal) are compared and contrasted. Again, the statistical significance of score differences and the frequency of various magnitudes of difference in the normative population are examined. Several types of interpretive tables are provided in the technical manual (Roid, 2003e) and in the computer scoring software (Roid, 2003d). Subtest differences can be compared to the mean scaled score among all 10 subtests (the generally recommended procedure). Subtests should be compared to the mean of only the five Nonverbal subtests or only the Verbal sub-

TABLE 10.3. Differences between SB5 (or Early Childhood SB5) Factor Index Scores and the Average Score among the Five Factor Index Scores in an Examinee's Profile: Critical Values for Statistically Significant Differences and Various Percentages of the Standardization Population

Factor index score	Critical values of significance at .05	Differences obtained by 1% of population	Differences obtained by 2% of population	Differences obtained by 5% of population	Differences obtained by 10% of population	Differences obtained by 15% of population	Differences obtained by 25% of population
Ages 2–5							
Fluid Reasoning	9.0	29.3	24.1	20.0	16.2	14.4	11.6
Knowledge	8.8	26.8	23.7	18.9	16.0	13.6	10.6
Quantitative Reasoning	9.5	26.2	22.5	19.2	15.4	13.3	10.2
Visual–Spatial Processing	10.0	24.5	21.7	18.5	14.4	12.4	9.4
Working Memory	9.2	21.0	19.6	16.2	13.4	12.0	9.0
Ages 6–85+							
Fluid Reasoning	10.2	20.0	18.2	15.2	12.6	11.2	8.6
Knowledge	8.8	19.6	17.2	14.4	12.2	10.6	8.6
Quantitative Reasoning	9.5	17.8	15.9	13.2	11.0	9.6	7.6
Visual–Spatial Processing	10.0	19.2	17.4	14.0	11.4	9.8	7.6
Working Memory	9.2	21.6	18.6	15.4	12.8	11.0	8.8

Note. Significant differences should equal or exceed the values shown in column 2. Notable differences based on percentage of the population should equal or exceed the values shown in columns 3–8.

tests when there is a significant difference between NVIQ and VIQ. Tables to evaluate the differences between each pair of subtests within each factor (e.g., Nonverbal and Verbal Working Memory) are also provided, and are recommended especially for neuropsychological evaluations. Caution should be taken in comparing all possible pairwise combinations of subtests because the repetition of repeated statistical tests multiplies the likelihood of chance differences' being overemphasized. Fortunately, because the subtest reliability on SB5 is high (median internal consistency of .84 to .89), ipsative profile analysis on the SB5 (except as stated above) is on firmer ground than with tests having lower subtest reliability. Professional assessment practices always dictate, however, that multiple sources of information should be used to make diagnostic decisions about individuals. Therefore, diagnoses should not be made solely on the basis of a given individual's SB5 profile patterns.

In the final step of interpretation, various qualitative indicators of the examinee's performance should be considered. These include patterns of errors in the examinee's item responses (as seen in the record form). In addition, patterns of inattention or distractibility may be found because all items are arranged in order of increasing difficulty within each subtest and testlet. Alternatively, "testing the limits" can be employed after the standardized administration is completed. For example, school-age children can be asked to explain their thinking or strategies for solving quantitative problems, or elderly examinees can be given more time on working memory tasks (e.g., repetition of the last word in a series of sentences) to test the limits of their memory capacity.

CLINICAL INTERPRETATIONS BASED ON GROUP DIFFERENCES

Professionals who work with children are sometimes faced with difficult clinical decisions. These difficult decisions include cases where a child displays behavioral and cognitive indicators that are diagnostic indicators for more than one clinical classification. Examples of these include distinguishing between low-functioning autism and intellectual disabilities, or determining whether the weaknesses in the score profile of a student enrolled in an English-language learner (ELL) program are primarily due to a language deficit or to second-language status.

Discriminant-function analyses were used in a study conducted specifically for this chapter. The goal of the discriminant analyses was to distinguish group membership on the basis of factor index scores from the SB5 to aid in making difficult clinical decisions. After the discriminant functions were derived by the computer, any individual with a discriminant score above zero was assigned to one group, while an individual with a score below zero was assigned to the contrasting group.

Table 10.4 displays the group comparisons, including the number of subjects in each group, the SB5 FSIQ for each group, the variables in the prediction equation, the prediction coefficients (including the constant), and the classification percentage. The tough clinical distinctions studied here were as follows: ADHD versus average-IQ au-

tism, intellectual disabilities versus low-IQ autism, ELL status versus speech–language impairment, and mild intellectual disabilities versus all autism. The second column of Table 10.4 shows the number of subjects in each group, and the next column shows the average SB5 FSIQ for these groups. Each pair of contrasting groups had very similar average FSIQ values, indicating one of the difficulties in making clinical distinctions between these categories. The results displayed for each pair of groups include the coefficients (weights applied to each factor index score) and the constant derived for the best-fitting prediction equation. In addition, the results include a measure of the accuracy of the function (i.e., the classification percentage). This statistic shows the percentage of the original cases that were correctly classified with the linear prediction equation provided.

For the ADHD versus average-IQ autism comparison, the Fluid Reasoning and Quantitative Reasoning factor index scores were the best predictor scores. For the original groups, this equation correctly classified 61% of the students. For the intellectual disabilities versus low-IQ autism comparison, the Working Memory factor index score

TABLE 10.4. Descriptive Statistics for Each Group, Prediction Variables, Discriminant Functions, and Classification Percentages for Four Comparisons with SB5 Factors as Predictors

Group comparison	Number in group	SB5 FSIQ	Prediction variables	Coefficients of discriminant function	Classification percentage
ADHD vs. average- IQ autism	94 (ADHD), 41 (autism)	93 (ADHD), 89 (autism)	Fluid Reasoning	−.065	
			Quantitative Reasoning	.099	
			Constant	−3.235	61%
ID vs. low-IQ autism	119 (ID), 42 (autism)	56 (ID), 53 (autism)	Working Memory	.081	
			Constant	−4.991	58%
ELL status vs. SLI	66 (ELL), 108 (SLI)	91 (ELL), 85 (SLI)	Knowledge	−.062	
			Quantitative Reasoning	.091	
			Constant	−2.819	64%
Mild ID vs. all autism	73 (ID), 83 (autism)	66 (ID), 70 (autism)	Knowledge	.087	
			Working Memory	.065	
			Constant	−1.654	59%

Note. ADHD, attention-deficit/hyperactivity disorder; ID, intellectual disabilities; ELL, English-language learner; SLI, speech–language impairment.

was the best predictor score, and the equation correctly classified 58% of the original students. For the ELL status versus speech–language impairment comparison, the Knowledge and Quantitative Reasoning factor index scores were the best predictor scores, and the equation correctly classified 64% of the students. A subset of 73 individuals with intellectual disabilities had mild delays (e.g., IQ in the range of 60–69), and these persons were compared to all the individuals with autism. For this final comparison, the Knowledge and Working Memory factor index scores were the best predictor scores. For the original groups, this equation correctly classified 59% of the students.

The results of these analyses may provide guidance for difficult clinical decisions in the following way. If the values in Table 10.4 are used to determine diagnostic classification, each factor index score should be multiplied by the coefficient listed. Then the results must be summed for all the factor index scores included in the prediction, and the constant must be added (or subtracted if it has a minus sign). If the grand total is a positive number, the examiner can then form a clinical hypothesis that this individual's score pattern is more similar to that for people in the first group listed in the comparison. Similarly, if the grand total is a

negative number, the individual's score pattern is more similar to that for the second group in the comparison. The more the grand total differs from zero, the more confidence the clinician can have in the hypothesis.

INTERPRETATION BASED ON STUDIES OF ACHIEVEMENT PREDICTION

Another method of interpreting SB5 scores for school-age children and adolescents is to closely examine any scores related to academic achievement. School psychologists may find these achievement-related scores helpful in making recommendations to teachers and other school personnel who provide services to examinees.

The results presented in Table 10.5 are from a larger study of the predictive power of the SB5 Working Memory factor for reading and mathematics achievement (Pomplun, 2004). Establishing the nature of this relationship is important for the following reasons: (1) many modern theories of intelligence delineate specific cognitive abilities and school achievement variables (Carroll, 1993; Horn, 1994); (2) much of past research on specific abilities was based on tests with incomplete

TABLE 10.5. The Prediction of WJ III Mathematics Achievement by SB5 Quantitative Reasoning and Working Memory

WJ III criterion	SB5 predictors	Adjusted R^2	R^2 increase	Statistical significance
Calculation	Quantitative Reasoning	.370	—	.000
	+ Working Memory	.392	.022	.000
	+ Interaction	.391	.000	.623
Math Fluency	Quantitative Reasoning	.149	—	.000
	+ Working Memory	.191	.042	.000
	+ Interaction	.196	.005	.054
Applied Problems	Quantitative Reasoning	.361		.000
	+ Working Memory	.384	.023	.000
	+ Interaction	.385	.001	.128
Quantitative Concepts	Quantitative Reasoning	.421	—	.000
	+ Working Memory	.457	.036	.000
	+ Interaction	.461	.004	.028
Math Reasoning	Quantitative Reasoning	.448		.000
	+ Working Memory	.481	.033	.000
	+ Interaction	.489	.008	.003

Note. Data from Pomplun (2004).

factorial coverage (McGrew, Flanagan, Keith, & Vanderwood, 1997); and (3) current models of cognitive processes involved in achievement deficits postulate specific abilities, such as working memory (Felton & Pepper, 1995).

Some researchers believe that working memory is a central part of reasoning ability (Jensen, 1998). Wilson and Swanson (2001) concluded that deficits in mathematics were mediated by both a domain-general and a domain-specific working memory system. The Pomplun and Custer (2005) study extended this research by using a working memory measure consisting of both verbal and nonverbal measures, and also testing the interaction of this measure with other important predictors of mathematics achievement.

Three hundred and thirty-eight students ages 6–19 (median age = 10) were administered the SB5 and the WJ III Tests of Achievement (Woodcock et al., 2001a). The score for the SB5 Quantitative Reasoning factor was used as the primary predictor of mathematics achievement. The score for the SB5 Working Memory factor was used as the second predictor of mathematics achievement.

Specifically, the achievement tests from WJ III were Calculation, a test of basic math computation skills; Math Fluency, a timed test of basic computation skills; Applied Problems, a test of the proper selection and completion of computations for problems; Quantitative Concepts, a test of math concepts, symbols, and vocabulary through concepts and number series; and Math Reasoning, a composite of Quantitative Concepts and Applied Problems (McGrew & Woodcock, 2001).

The predictive power of the Working Memory factor was studied through a series of three hierarchical least-squares regression models, with each WJ III achievement test score as a criterion. For the prediction of each achievement test score, the first regression model had three predictors: the score for the Quantitative Reasoning factor, the score for the Working Memory factor, and a term for the interaction between Quantitative Reasoning and Working Memory (i.e., created by multiplying Quantitative Reasoning and Working Memory together). If the interaction term in this model was statistically significant, the sum of the two factors was conditional on the other predictor's score level. If the interaction term was nonsignificant, a second regression model (with two predictors, Quantitative Reasoning and Working Memory) was investigated. If the Working Memory variable was statistically significant, this indicated that the additivity of the two factors was constant across

score levels for each predictor. A probability level of .05 was used for statistical significance for each term in these models.

Table 10.5 contains results from the hierarchical prediction models with the different achievement criterion variables for the mathematics tests. These tables show the WJ III criterion variables, the SB5 predictors, the adjusted R^2, the increase in R^2 when variables were added, and the statistical significance of the increase in R^2. In Table 10.5, the Quantitative Reasoning score predicted from 15% to 45% of the variance (estimated from R^2) in the mathematics achievement test scores. Two of the five interaction terms were statistically significant at the .05 level, and another interaction term was nearly significant (.054). The interaction terms were statistically significant in the models for the prediction of Quantitative Concepts and Math Reasoning, and near significance for the prediction of Math Fluency. For the prediction of Math Reasoning achievement scores, the interaction was disordinal, with the regression lines crossing in the region of 130. The differences became larger as the predictor scores decreased. For example at a Quantitative Reasoning score of 70, a Working Memory score difference of 40 points translated into a predicted Math Reasoning score difference of more than 15 points. In contrast, at a Quantitative Reasoning score of 130, a Working Memory score difference of 40 points translated into a predicted Math Reasoning score difference of only 1 point.

Across the five WJ III mathematics achievement scores, Working Memory added from 2% to 4% to the prediction over and above the contribution of Quantitative Reasoning, based on the increases in R^2. Also, Working Memory added significantly to the interaction term for three achievement scores. The nature of the significant interaction terms suggests that using Working Memory to predict Math Reasoning translates into practically significant score differences in Math Reasoning only for those with below-average Quantitative Reasoning scores. For those with average or above-average Quantitative Reasoning scores, Working Memory does not add much to the predicted Math Reasoning scores. The results demonstrate the predictive validity of the unique SB5 measure of Working Memory based on Verbal and Nonverbal subtests. These results suggest that the interpretation of Working Memory scores along with Quantitative Reasoning scores may need to go beyond simply adding these scores (i.e., in a composite). Instead, Working Memory should be used to predict Math

Reasoning scores only for the students with below-average Quantitative Reasoning scores.

INTERPRETATION OF SB5 PROFILE PATTERNS USING SUBTEST SPECIFICITY

Several methods of interpreting the 10-subtest profile of the SB5 have been described in the section "General Interpretation of SB5 Test Scores" above. These include the analysis of subtest score differences by the methods of (1) examining statistical significance of differences, (2) comparing the magnitude of the differences to those found in the normative populations, (3) comparing the subtest scores to the mean of all 10 subtest scores in the individual's profile, and (4) comparing the individual's Nonverbal versus Verbal subtest scores for a given cognitive factor. To supplement these methods, a further analysis of the SB5 subtest specificity was completed for this chapter. Subtest specificity is derived from factor analysis of the subtest scores by separating profile score variance into common, specific, and error variance. Cohen (1957, 1959) originally studied the specificity of the Wechsler

scales, and nearly every major test battery has since been analyzed for specificity, including the Fourth Edition of the Stanford–Binet (Reynolds, Kamphaus, & Rosenthal, 1988). When clinicians assess the cognitive strengths and weaknesses of individuals based on individual profile scores, the implicit assumption is that each subtest has reliable specific variance.

Table 10.6 presents the common, specific, and error variance for each of the SB5 subtests in each of five age groups (2–5, 6–10, 11–16, 17–50, and 51+ years). The values in Table 10.6 were derived as follows. First, the internal-consistency reliability coefficients from Roid (2003e), averaged for each age group, were used to define error variance (the quantity of 1.0 minus the reliability). Second, the common variance was obtained from factor analysis of the subtest scores at each age level and was the communality (degree of shared variance across all subtests) of each subtest score. The difference between common variance and true variance was the specific variance. Analyses for Table 10.6 were conducted on the SB5 standardization sample (*N* = 4,800).

The bottom right corner of Table 10.6 shows the overall averages of 64% common, 22% specific,

TABLE 10.6. Percentages of Common, Specific, and Error Variance Derived from Factor Analysis for Each of the 10 SB5 Subtest Scaled Scores in Each of Five Age Groups

Subtest	Ages 2–5			Ages 6–10			Ages 11–16			Ages 17–50			Ages 51+			Average		
	C	S	E	C	S	E	C	S	E	C	S	E	C	S	E	C	S	E
NVFR	38	47	15	48	37	15	41	41	18	60	21	19	72	20	8	52	33	15
NVKN	59	27	14	64	15	21	63	21	16	73	15	12	75	12	13	67	18	15
NVQR	68	18	14	73	9	18	75	11	14	78	10	12	78	9	13	74	12	14
NVVS	54	34	12	60	23	17	45	36	19	66	23	11	68	24	8	59	28	13
NVWM	56	34	10	50	33	17	60	28	12	53	37	10	70	17	13	58	30	12
Nonverbal average	55	32	13	59	23	18	57	27	16	66	21	13	73	16	11	62	24	14
VFR	57	35	8	60	29	11	62	19	19	66	11	23	66	18	16	62	23	15
VKN	61	27	12	59	28	13	56	31	13	68	23	9	63	30	7	61	28	11
VQR	66	18	16	68	14	18	73	13	14	83	7	10	77	15	8	73	14	13
VVS	67	14	19	72	15	13	71	17	12	76	15	9	66	23	11	70	17	13
VWM	62	23	15	51	34	15	49	31	20	80	4	16	58	29	13	60	24	16
Verbal average	63	23	14	62	24	14	62	22	16	75	12	13	66	23	11	65	21	14
Overall average	59	28	13	60	24	16	59	25	16	70	17	13	69	20	11	64	22	14

Note. Based on *N* = 4,800. C, common; S, specific; E, error; NV, Nonverbal; V, Verbal; FR, Fluid Reasoning; KN, Knowledge; QR, Quantitative Reasoning; VS, Visual–Spatial Processing; WM, Working Memory.

and 14% error variance—a classic pattern of common variance > specific variance > error variance, meaning that the unique specificity of subtest variation is higher than error (Cohen, 1959). Also, the overall average common variance of 64% is similar to that for adult intelligence batteries (e.g., Wechsler Adult Intelligence Scale [WAIS], 66%; WAIS-R, 57%; see Roid & Gyurke, 1991). The age trend of increasing common variance across the preschool, school-age, and adult Wechsler scales can also be observed in Table 10.6. As shown in the bottom row of Table 10.6, average common variance ranged from 59% at ages 2–5 to 70% and 69% in the adult ranges. Presence of a substantial percentage of common variance provides evidence of construct validity for the composite IQ scores of the SB5, which summarize the overall level of cognitive ability across subtests.

Clinicians look for good specificity among subtests of a cognitive battery, in order to justify the interpretation of profile patterns and strengths and weaknesses. Cohen (1959) suggested 25% specificity that exceeds error variance as an ideal. As shown in the right column of Table 10.6, average specificity for the SB5 subtests ranged from 12% to 33% across age groups (overall average 22%). All subtests except Nonverbal Quantitative Reasoning had specificity higher than error variance. The bottom row of Table 10.6 shows that average specificity was greater and in the ideal range for preschool and school-age ranges (28% for 2–5, 24% for 6–10, and 25% for 11–17), as compared to the adult age levels (17% and 20%). Because common variance increases in the adult range due to an apparent globalization of abilities, specificity naturally decreases from that of the younger age ranges (Roid & Gyurke, 1991).

In terms of profile analysis of strengths and weaknesses in individuals, Table 10.6 indicates that an excellent level of average specificity was found for four subtests: Nonverbal Fluid Reasoning (33%), Nonverbal Visual–Spatial Processing (28%), Nonverbal Working Memory (30%), and Verbal Knowledge (28%). Clinicians should exercise some caution in interpretation of individual profile scores for Quantitative Reasoning due to their lower specificity, which is similar to the level of their error variance. However, Quantitative Reasoning is lower in specificity because of its excellent contribution to common variance (74% Nonverbal, 73% Verbal), and thus to overall IQ. Nonverbal Knowledge and Verbal Visual–Spatial Processing are also similar in their high common

variance and somewhat lower specificity than other subtests.

Examiners who make decisions about individuals (especially decisions that attach a label such as *intellectual disability* to individuals) should be cautious in the interpretation of differences among subtest scores of SB5, given that some degree of difference is due to measurement error. Also, error of measurement is compounded in the subtraction of two scores and in the comparison of all possible pairs of scores. The number of pairwise comparisons among 10 subtests is 45 (a large number for one individual), increasing the possibilities of chance differences. Profile patterns of individuals should be used cautiously in diagnosis unless there are several sources of information showing consistency among diagnostic signs in an individual's cumulative folder of background information.

Also, some researchers have questioned the wisdom of profile analysis that compares scores within one individual (ipsative analysis) in tests of cognitive ability. For example, McDermott, Fantuzzo, and Glutting (1990) concluded that most of the variance in intelligence tests such as the Wechsler scales was due to general ability (g) reflected in the Wechsler FSIQ because they were unable to identify differentiated profiles patterns from cluster analysis of normative data. They claimed that most of the profile patterns were "flat" (all scores low or all scores high), rather than differentiated profiles with scattered high and low scores. However, Roid (1994, 2003c), drawing on the recommendations of Aldenderfer and Blashfield (1984), showed that differentiated profile patterns can be found in 40–50% of individual profiles in large samples when sensitive cluster analysis methods are employed. Roid (1994) showed that the use of Pearson product–moment correlations (R. K. Blashfield, personal communication, February 22, 1992), rather than Euclidean distance, as a measure of profile similarity allowed differentiated profiles to emerge more clearly in large samples.

For these reasons, although interpretive caution is always recommended, clinicians should be encouraged that the subtest scores of the SB5 have good specificity for individual profile interpretation. The exceptions are profile patterns involving low or high scores for Quantitative Reasoning, for which more caution is needed. Also, the generally high level of subtest reliability in the SB5, as compared to many other cognitive batteries (average subtest reliabilities ranging from .84 to .89; Roid, 2003e), results in low error variance for all subtests throughout the age range and supports profile interpretation.

BRIEF CASE STUDY

Table 10.7 shows the SB5 subtest scores and composite IQ and factor index scores for a 7-year-old boy. Eduardo is from the southern region of the United States; his parents have some post-high school education. Although Eduardo has a Hispanic background, he was born in the United States and speaks English fluently; he is also being exposed to Spanish in his home environment. He has been identified as having documented LDs in writing and oral expression and shows some delays in reading. His LDs were identified with the WJ III (both cognitive and achievement tests), using the school district's regression discrepancy formulas. As was documented in research conducted by Roid (2003c, 2003e) and in this chapter (see "Interpretation Based on Studies of Achievement Prediction," above), the Working Memory factor index and the Working Memory subtests show significantly lower scores than other scores within his profile. The Working Memory score of 74 is significantly different from the other factor index scores, and this difference is relatively rare in the normative population (e.g., only 10.5% of subjects have a difference of 20 points or more between the

Working Memory and Quantitative Reasoning factor index scores). Also, according to Table 10.3, the Working Memory score of 74 is significantly different from the average of all the factor index scores (91.2). This 17.2 difference between 74 and 91.2 is found in less than 5% of the population (see critical value of 15.4 for the 5% percentage level in Table 10.3 for ages 6–85+, column 5).

At the individual subtest level, both the Nonverbal and the Verbal Working Memory scores are considerably lower than other scores in the profile (scores of 6 and 5 compared to the other subtests, which vary between 8 and 11; a 3-point difference between pairs of subtest scores is statistically significant). Not only are the low Working Memory factor and subtest scores lower than other scores, but they also reflect normative weaknesses of the individual in relation to the normative sample.

For these reasons, Eduardo's SB5 profile shows a pattern similar to that of other children with LDs (Roid, 2003c). Also, research on working memory has shown that deficits in the ability to process and transform information in short-term memory are connected to deficits in learning (Reid et al., 1996). This case study demonstrates the possibility that the Working Memory factor index and subtest scores of the SB5, when they are significantly lower than other scores in the profile, can be used with other data to support or refute hypotheses that LDs are present in an individual. For exam-

TABLE 10.7. SB5 Scores for the Case of a 7-Year-Old Male (Eduardo) with LD

IQ scores		Factor index scores		Subtest scaled scores[a]	
NVIQ	93	Fluid Reasoning	100	Nonverbal FR	11
VIQ	87			Verbal FR	9
FSIQ	90				
		Knowledge	97	Nonverbal KN	9
				Verbal KN	10
		Quantitative Reasoning	94	Nonverbal QR	10
				Verbal QR	8
		Visual–Spatial Processing	91	Nonverbal VS	9
				Verbal VS	8
		Working Memory	74	Nonverbal WM	6
				Verbal WM	5

Note. All scores are normalized standard scores. IQ and factor index scores have a mean of 100 based on the normative sample of 4,800 examinees, with a standard deviation of 15. Subtest scaled scores have a mean of 10 and a standard deviation of 3.
[a]FR, Fluid Reasoning; KN, Knowledge; QR, Quantitative Reasoning; VS, Visual–Spatial Processing; WM, Working Memory.

ple, in empirical studies comparing verified cases of LDs with normative cases, Roid (2003c) used composites of SB5 Working Memory and Knowledge subtest scores to classify individual cases of documented LDs in reading achievement. Sums of the two Nonverbal and the two Verbal Working Memory and Knowledge subtests were calculated and transformed into an IQ metric (mean of 100, standard deviation of 15) based on the SB5 norm sample for ages 5–7 years. To calculate the composite, the weight of 1.875 was multiplied by the sum of the four subtest scaled scores, and 25 points were added. For Eduardo, the rounded result for this composite was 81. When a cutoff score of 89 was used (designating LD cases as those with scores less than 89 on the new composite), 67% of the LD cases were correctly identified, although 17% of normative cases were falsely identified as LD cases. Thus the composite of Working Memory and Knowledge scores was accurate in about two-thirds of LD cases—high enough for clinical hypothesis testing, but too low for LD identification purposes. Such composites should only be used when further data on an individual, collected from classroom teachers, parents, other tests, and observations in multiple settings, are consistent with a diagnosis of an LD. For older students (age 8 years and older) and adults, the LD reading achievement composite should be calculated with a slightly different formula derived from an analysis of the SB5 norm sample (Roid & Barram, 2004). The composite should be calculated by multiplying the sum of the scaled scores (Working Memory and Knowledge) by 1.56 (instead of 1.875) and then adding 37.9 points (instead of 25) to the result. The adjustment to the formula will provide more predictive accuracy for older students and adults.

CONCLUSION: INNOVATIONS IN COGNITIVE ASSESSMENT

The most recent edition of the Stanford–Binet, the SB5, provides some intriguing new innovations in cognitive assessment. Foremost is the development of a factorially comprehensive Nonverbal domain of subtests, measuring five cognitive factors. The SB5 NVIQ is quite innovative among IQ measures because of its coverage of five factors from the work of Cattell (1943), Horn (1994), and Carroll (1993). Second, the innovative use of IRT in the SB5 is notable. Rasch analysis (Rasch, 1980; Wright & Lineacre, 1999) was employed throughout the development of items and subtest scales, and in the

design of the routing procedure. In the routing procedure, Rasch ability scores are estimated from two initial subtests used to assign a functional level for the remainder of the assessment. Also notable is the development of the criterion-referenced CSSs. The CSSs provide an innovative method of interpreting SB5 results and for tracking cognitive change (growth or decline) across time. Finally, the SB5 combines the classic age-level (now called functional-level) format of earlier editions with the point scale format used in the Fourth Edition, preserves many classic toys and tasks, enhances the cognitive factor composition of the battery, and continues the long tradition (beginning with Terman, 1916) of the Stanford–Binet.

NOTES

1. Note that the Nonverbal section requires a small degree of receptive language for the examinee to understand brief instructions by the examiner and does not rely solely on pantomime instructions.
2. The exception is level 1 of Nonverbal item book 2, which has two testlets with a maximum of 4 points each.
3. Quantitative items, as well as other items on the SB5, are also scaled in the CSS metric, allowing the items of the test to be related to the ability level of the examinees. For example, according to the calibration procedures of Wright and Lineacre (1999), a math item with difficulty 500 has a 50% probability of being mastered by the average 10-year-old, whereas a math item with difficulty 480 has a 90% probability of being answered correctly by the average 10-year-old.
4. See Roid (2003e) for more details. Split-half reliability formulas were used for subtests and composite reliabilities for IQ and factor scores. Coefficients reported in the text are the overall average reliabilities across age groups.

REFERENCES

Aldenderfer, M. S., & Blashfield, R. K. (1984). *Cluster analysis.* Beverly Hills, CA: Sage.

Baddeley, A. D. (1986). *Working memory.* Oxford: Clarendon Press.

Baddeley, A. D., Logie, R., Nimmo-Smith, I., & Brereton, N. (1985). Components of fluent reading. *Journal of Memory and Language, 24,* 119–131.

Binet, A., & Simon, T. (1908). Le développement de l'intelligence chez les enfants. *L'Année Psychologique, 14,* 1–94.

Carroll, J. B. (1993). *Human cognitive abilities: A survey*

of factor-analytic studies. New York: Cambridge University Press.

Cattell, R. B. (1943). The measurement of intelligence. *Psychological Bulletin, 40,* 153–193.

Cohen, J. (1957). The factorial structure of the WAIS between early adulthood and old age. *Journal of Consulting Psychology, 21,* 283–290.

Cohen, J. (1959). The factorial structure of the WISC at ages 7–6, 10–6, and 13–6. *Journal of Consulting Psychology, 23,* 285–299.

Cohen, J. (1988). *Statistical power analysis for the behavioral sciences* (2nd ed.). Hillsdale, NJ: Erlbaum.

Dana, R. H. (1993). *Multicultural assessment perspectives for professional psychology.* Boston: Allyn & Bacon.

Davis, F. B. (1959). Interpretation of differences among averages and individual test scores. *Journal of Educational Psychology, 50,* 162–170.

DiStefano, C., & Dombrowski, S. C. (2006). Investigating the theoretical structure of SB5. *Journal of Psychoeducational Assessment, 24,* 123–136.

Felton, R. H., & Pepper, P. P. (1995). Early identification and intervention of phonological deficits in kindergarten and early elementary children at risk for reading disability. *School Psychology Review, 24,* 405–414.

Flanagan, D. P., & Ortiz, S. O. (2001). *Essentials of cross-battery assessment.* New York: Wiley.

Harlow, S. C. (2010). *Item fairness of nonverbal subtests of SB5 in a Latino sample.* Unpublished doctoral dissertation, George Fox University.

Horn, J. L. (1965). *Fluid and crystallized intelligence.* Unpublished doctoral dissertation, University of Illinois, Urbana–Champaign.

Horn, J. L. (1994). Theory of fluid and crystallized intelligence. In R. J. Sternberg (Ed.), *Encyclopedia of human intelligence* (pp. 443–451). New York: Macmillan.

Jensen, A. R. (1998). *The g factor: The science of mental ability.* Westport, CT: Praeger.

Joreskog, K. G., & Sorbom, D. (1999). *LISREL 8: User's reference guide.* Chicago: Scientific Software.

Kyllonen, P. C., & Christal, R. E. (1990). Reasoning ability is (little more than) working-memory capacity. *Intelligence, 14*(4), 389–433.

Lezak, M. D. (1995). *Neuropsychological assessment* (3rd ed.). New York: Oxford University Press.

Matarazzo, J. D. (1990). Psychological assessment versus psychological testing: Validation from Binet to the school, clinic, and courtroom. *American Psychologist, 45*(9), 999–1017.

McDermott, P. A., Fantuzzo, J. W., & Glutting, J. J. (1990). Just say no to subtest analysis: A critique on Wechsler theory and practice. *Journal of Psychoeducational Assessment, 8,* 290–302.

McGrew, K. S., & Flanagan, D. P. (1998). *The intelli-gence test desk reference (ITDR): Gf-Gc cross-battery assessment.* Boston: Allyn & Bacon.

McGrew, K. S., Flanagan, D. P., Keith, T. Z., & Vanderwood, M. (1997). Beyond g: The impact of Gf-Gc specific abilities research on the future use and interpretation of intelligence test batteries in schools. *School Psychology Review, 26,* 189–210.

McGrew, K. S., & Woodcock, R. W. (2001). *Woodcock–Johnson III technical manual.* Itasca, IL: Riverside.

Paniagua, F. A. (1994). *Assessing and treating culturally diverse clients: A practical guide.* Thousand Oaks, CA: Sage.

Pomplun, M. (2004, August). *The importance of working memory in the prediction of academic achievement.* Paper presented at the annual meeting of the American Psychological Association, Honolulu.

Pomplun, M., & Custer, M. (2005). The construct validity of the Stanford–Binet 5 measures of working memory. *Assessment, 10*(10), 1–9.

Rasch, G. (1980). *Probabilistic models for some intelligence and attainment tests.* Chicago: University of Chicago Press.

Reid, D. K., Hresko, W. P., & Swanson, H. L. (Eds.). (1996). *Cognitive approaches to learning disabilities* (3rd ed.). Austin, TX: PRO-ED.

Reynolds, C. R., & Kamphaus, R. W. (2003). *Reynolds Intellectual Assessment Scales.* Lutz, FL: Psychological Assessment Resources.

Reynolds, C. R., Kamphaus, R. W., & Rosenthal, B. L. (1988). Factor analysis of the Stanford–Binet Fourth Edition for ages 2 through 23 years. *Measurement and Evaluation in Counseling and Development, 21,* 52–63.

Roid, G. H. (1994). Patterns of writing skills derived from cluster analysis of direct-writing assessments. *Applied Measurement in Education, 7*(2), 159–170.

Roid, G. H. (2003a). *Stanford–Binet Intelligence Scales, Fifth Edition.* Austin, TX: Pro-Ed.

Roid, G. H. (2003b). *Stanford–Binet Intelligence Scales, Fifth Edition: Examiner's manual.* Austin, TX: Pro-Ed.

Roid, G. H. (2003c). *Stanford–Binet Intelligence Scales, Fifth Edition: Interpretive manual.* Austin, TX: Pro-Ed.

Roid, G. H. (2003d). *Stanford–Binet Intelligence Scales, Fifth Edition: Scoring Pro* [Computer software]. Austin, TX: Pro-Ed.

Roid, G. H. (2003e). *Stanford–Binet Intelligence Scales, Fifth Edition: Technical manual.* Austin, TX: Pro-Ed.

Roid, G. H. (2005a). *Interpretation of SB5/Early SB5 factor index scores: Technical note.* Austin, TX: PRO-ED.

Roid, G. H. (2005b). *Stanford–Binet Intelligence Scales for Early Childhood, Fifth Edition.* Austin, TX: PRO-ED.

Roid, G. H., & Barram, A. (2004). *Essentials of Stan-*

ford–Binet Intelligence Scales (SB5) assessment. New York: Wiley.

Roid, G. H., & Edwards, K. (2011). Use of the Stanford–Binet Fifth Edition in a brain injury case. In N. Mather & L. Jaffe (Eds.), Comprehensive evaluations: Case reports for psychologists, diagnosticians, and special educators (pp. 600–609). Hoboken, NJ: Wiley.

Roid, G. H., & Gyurke, J. (1991). General-factor and specific variance in the WPPSI-R. Journal of Psychoeducational Assessment, 9, 209–223.

Roid, G. H., & Miller, L. J. (1997). Leiter International Performance Scale—Revised. Wood Dale, IL: Stoelting.

Roid, G. H., & Tippin, S. (2009). Assessment of intellectual strengths and weaknesses with the SB5. In J. Naglieri & S. Goldstein (Eds.), Practitioner's guide to assessing intelligence and achievement (pp. 127–152). Hoboken, NJ: Wiley.

Silverstein, A. B. (1982). Pattern analysis as simultaneous statistical inference. Journal of Consulting and Clinical Psychology, 50, 234–240.

Terman, L. M. (1916). The measurement of intelligence: An explanation of and a complete guide for the use of the Stanford revision and extension of the Binet–Simon Scale. Boston: Houghton Mifflin.

Terman, L. M., & Merrill, M. A. (1937). Measuring intelligence. Boston: Houghton Mifflin.

Terman, L. M., & Merrill, M. A. (Eds.). (1960). Stanford–Binet Intelligence Scale: Manual for the Third Revision Form L-M. Boston: Houghton Mifflin.

Thorndike, R. L., Hagen, E. P., & Sattler, J. M. (1986). The Stanford–Binet Intelligence Scale: Fourth Edition. Guide for administering and scoring. Chicago: Riverside.

Tippin, S. M. (2007). Stanford–Binet profile differences between normative children and those with learning disabilities or ADHD. Unpublished doctoral dissertation, George Fox University.

U.S. Bureau of the Census. (2001). Census 2000 summary file 1: United States. Washington, DC: Author.

Wechsler, D. (1991). Wechsler Intelligence Scale for Children—Third Edition. San Antonio, TX: Psychological Corporation.

Wilson, K. M., & Swanson, H. L. (2001). Are mathematics disabilities due to a domain-general or a domain-specific working memory deficit? Journal of Learning Disabilities, 34(3), 237–248.

Woodcock, R. W., McGrew, K. S., & Mather, N. (2001a). Woodcock–Johnson III Tests of Achievement. Itasca, IL: Riverside.

Woodcock, R. W., McGrew, K. S., & Mather, N. (2001b). Woodcock–Johnson III Tests of Cognitive Abilities. Itasca, IL: Riverside.

Wright, B. D., & Lineacre, J. M. (1999). WINSTEPS: Rasch analysis for all two-facet models. Chicago: MESA Press.

CHAPTER 11

The Kaufman Assessment Battery for Children— Second Edition and the Kaufman Test of Educational Achievement—Second Edition

Jennie Kaufman Singer
Elizabeth O. Lichtenberger
James C. Kaufman
Alan S. Kaufman
Nadeen L. Kaufman

This chapter provides an overview of two comprehensive, individually administered Kaufman tests: the second edition of the Kaufman Assessment Battery for Children (KABC-II; Kaufman & Kaufman, 2004a), and the second edition of the Kaufman Test of Educational Achievement (KTEA-II; Kaufman & Kaufman, 2004c). The KABC-II is discussed first, followed by the KTEA-II, with the following topics featured for each of these multisubtest batteries: theory and structure, description of subtests, administration and scoring, psychometric properties, interpretation, and clinical applications. A special section on the innovations in measures of cognitive assessment is also provided for the KABC-II. An illustrative case report is presented as well, to exemplify the KABC-II and KTEA-II in practice.

KAUFMAN ASSESSMENT BATTERY FOR CHILDREN—SECOND EDITION

Theory and Structure

Structure and Organization

The KABC-II (Kaufman & Kaufman, 2004a) measures the processing and cognitive abilities of children and adolescents between the ages of

3 years, 0 months and 18 years, 11 months (3:0 and 18:11). Like the original K-ABC (Kaufman & Kaufman, 1983), the second edition is an individually administered, theory-based, clinical instrument that is used worldwide (e.g., Malda, van de Vijver, Srinivasan, Transler, & Sukumar, 2010; Vannetzel, 2010). However, the KABC-II represents a substantial revision of the K-ABC, with a greatly expanded age range (3:0–18:11 instead of 2:6–12:6) and the addition of 8 new subtests (plus a Delayed Recall scale) to the battery. Of the original 16 K-ABC subtests, 8 were eliminated and 8 were retained. Like the K-ABC, the revised battery provides examiners with a Nonverbal scale, composed of subtests that may be administered in pantomime and responded to motorically, to permit valid assessment of children who have hearing impairments, limited English proficiency, and so forth.

The KABC-II is grounded in a dual theoretical foundation: Luria's (1966, 1970, 1973) neuropsychological model, featuring three blocks or functional units, and the Cattell–Horn–Carroll (CHC) approach to categorizing specific cognitive abilities (Carroll, 1993; Flanagan, McGrew, & Ortiz, 2000; Horn & Noll, 1997; see also Horn & Blankson, Chapter 3, this volume, and Schneider & McGrew, Chapter 4, this volume). In contrast, the K-ABC had a single theoretical foundation: the distinction between sequential and simultaneous processing. The dual theoretical model has been seen as a notable strength of the KABC-II in one review of the battery (Bain & Gray, 2008), but, interestingly, it has been perceived as both an asset and a limitation by a reviewer of the French KABC-II: Vannetzel (2010) states that

the use of multifold perspectives is an essential point from the view of epistemology of the psychological assessment and of precision in terms of practice and level of formation. This plural paradigm, very risky in regards to the theoretical pertinence that it demands from the practitioner, illustrates rather well the "new world" in which psychometrics entered at the turn of the twenty-first century. (p. 233)

The KABC-II includes both Core and Expanded Batteries, with only the Core Battery needed to yield a child's scale profile. The KABC-II Expanded Battery offers supplementary subtests to increase the breadth of the constructs measured by the Core Battery and to follow up hypotheses. Administration time for the Core Battery takes about 30–70 minutes, depending on the child's age and whether the examiner administers the CHC model of the KABC-II or the Luria model. One of the features of the KABC-II is the flexibility it affords the examiner in determining the theoretical model to administer to each child.

When interpreted from the Luria model, the KABC-II focuses on mental processing, excludes acquired knowledge to the extent possible, and yields a global standard score called the Mental Processing Index (MPI) with a mean of 100 and a standard deviation (SD) of 15. Like the original K-ABC, the Luria model measures *sequential processing* and *simultaneous processing*, but the KABC-II goes beyond this dichotomy to measure two additional constructs: *learning ability* and *planning ability*.

From the vantage point of the CHC model, the KABC-II Core Battery includes all scales in the Luria system, but they are interpreted from an alternative perspective; for example, the scale that measures sequential processing from the Luria perspective is seen as measuring the CHC ability of *short-term memory* (Gsm), and the scale that measures planning ability (Luria interpretation) aligns with Gf or *fluid reasoning* (CHC interpretation). The CHC model includes one extra scale that is *not* in the Luria model—namely, a measure of *crystallized ability* (Gc), which is labeled Knowledge/Gc. The global standard score yielded by the CHC model is labeled the Fluid–Crystallized Index (FCI), also with a mean of 100 and SD of 15.

Table 11.1 summarizes the dual-model approach, showing the Luria process and the corresponding CHC ability measured by each scale. The use of two theoretical models allows examiners to choose the model that best meets the needs of the child or adolescent being evaluated. The dual labels for the scales reflect the complexity of what the cognitive tasks measure and how their scores are interpreted. Examiners must select either the Luria or CHC model *before* they administer the test, thereby determining which global score should be used—the MPI (Luria model) or FCI (CHC model).

TABLE 11.1. The Dual Theoretical Foundations of the KABC-II

	Interpretation of scale from Luria theory	Interpretation of scale from CHC theory	Name of KABC-II scale
	Learning ability	Long-term storage and retrieval (Glr)	Learning/Glr
	Sequential processing	Short-term memory (Gsm)	Memory/Gsm
	Simultaneous processing	Visual processing (Gv)	Simultaneous/Gv
	Planning ability	Fluid reasoning (Gf)	Planning/Gf
		Crystallized ability (Gc)	Knowledge/Gc
Name of global score	Mental Processing Index (MPI)	Fluid–Crystallized Index (FCI)	

Note. Knowledge/Gc is included in the CHC system for the computation of the FCI, but it is excluded from the Luria system for the computation of the MPI. The Planning/Gf scale is for ages 7–18 only. All other scales are for ages 4–18. Only the MPI and FCI are offered for 3-year-olds.

- The CHC model is the model of choice—except in cases where including measures of acquired knowledge (crystallized ability) is believed by the examiner to compromise the validity of the FCI. In those cases, the Luria-based global score (MPI) is preferred.
- The CHC model is given priority over the Luria model because we believe that knowledge/Gc is, in principle, an important aspect of cognitive functioning. Therefore, the CHC model (FCI) is preferred for children with known or suspected disabilities in reading, written expression, or mathematics; for children assessed for giftedness or intellectual disabilities; for children assessed for emotional or behavioral disorders; and for children assessed for attentional disorders such as attention-deficit/hyperactivity disorder (ADHD).
- Situations in which the Luria model (MPI) is preferred include, but are not limited to, the following:
  - A child from a bilingual background.
  - A child from any nonmainstream cultural background that may have affected knowledge acquisition and verbal development.
  - A child with known or suspected language disorders, whether expressive, receptive, or mixed receptive–expressive.
  - A child with known or suspected autism.
  - An examiner with a firm commitment to the Luria processing approach who believes that acquired knowledge should be excluded from any global cognitive score (regardless of reason for referral).

This set of recommendations does not imply that we consider one model to be theoretically superior to the other. Both theories are equally important as foundations of the KABC-II. The CHC psychometric theory emphasizes specific cognitive abilities, whereas the Luria neuropsychological theory emphasizes *processes*—namely, the way children process information when solving problems. Both approaches are valid for understanding how children learn and solve new problems, which is why each scale has two names, one from Luria theory and the other from CHC theory. Regardless of the model of the KABC-II that is *administered* (Luria or CHC), the way in which psychologists *interpret* the scales will undoubtedly be influenced by their theoretical preference.

On the original K-ABC, the Sequential and Simultaneous Processing scales were joined by a separate Achievement scale. That concept is continued with the Luria model of the KABC-II, although conventional kinds of achievement (reading, arithmetic) are excluded from the KABC-II Knowledge/Gc scale.

At age 3, only a global score is offered, either the MPI or FCI. For ages 4–18, the global scale is joined by an array of scales (see Table 11.1). The Planning/Gf scale is included only at ages 7–18 because a factor corresponding to the high-level set of abilities did not emerge for younger children. All KABC-II scales have a mean of 100 and *SD* of 15.

Theory: Luria and CHC

Luria (1970) perceived the brain's basic functions to be represented by three main blocks or functional systems, which are responsible for arousal and attention (block 1); the use of one's senses to analyze, code, and store information (block 2); and the application of executive functions for formulating plans and programming behavior (block 3). Within block 2, Luria (1966) distinguished between "two basic forms of integrative activity of the cerebral cortex" (p. 74), which he labeled *successive* and *simultaneous*. Despite Luria's interpretation of three blocks, each with separate functions, his focus was on *integration* among the blocks to be capable of complex behavior. Block 3 is very closely related to the functions of block 1, as both blocks are concerned with overall efficiency of brain functions; part of the role of block 2 is to establish connections with block 3 (Reitan, 1988). Indeed, "integration of these systems constitutes the real key to understanding how the brain mediates complex behavior" (Reitan, 1988, p. 333).

In the development of the KABC-II, the test authors emphasized the integration of the three blocks, not the measurement of each block in isolation. The block 1 arousal functions are key aspects of successful test performance on any cognitive task, but attention and concentration per se do not fit Kaufman and Kaufman's definition of high-level, complex, intelligent behavior. The Learning/Glr scale requires much sustained attention and concentration (block 1), but depends more on the integration of the three blocks than on any one in isolation. The Sequential/Gsm and Simultaneous/Gv scales are deliberately targeted to measure the block 2 successive and simultaneous functions, respectively, but again the test authors have striven for complexity. Luria (1966) defined the block 2 functions of analysis and storage of incoming stimuli via successive and simultaneous processing as *coding* functions, not problem-solving functions. But because block 2 is responsible for establishing connections with block 3, the KABC-II measures of simultaneous processing require not just the analysis, coding, and storage of incoming stimuli, but also the block 3 executive functioning processes for success. In addition, block 2 requires the integration of the incoming stimuli; hence subtests like Word Order and Rover require synthesis of auditory and visual stimuli. Planning/Gf is intended to measure Luria's block 3; again, however, success on these complex tasks requires not just executive functioning, but also focused attention (block 1) and the coding and storage of incoming stimuli (block 2).

The CHC model is a psychometric theory that rests on a large body of research, especially factor-analytic investigations, accumulated over decades. The CHC theory represents a data-driven theory, in contrast to Luria's clinically driven theory. CHC theory has two separate psychometric lineages: (1) Raymond Cattell's (1941) original Gf-Gc theory, which was expanded and refined by Horn (1968, 1985, 1989) to include an array of abilities (not just Gf and Gc); and (2) John Carroll's (1943, 1993) half-century of rigorous efforts to summarize and integrate the voluminous literature on the factor analysis of cognitive abilities. Ultimately, Horn and Carroll agreed to merge their separate but overlapping models into the unified CHC theory. This merger was done in a personal communication to Richard Woodcock in July 1999; the specifics of CHC theory and its applications have been articulated by Dawn Flanagan, Kevin McGrew, and their colleagues (Flanagan et al., 2000; Flanagan & Ortiz, 2001; see also Schneider & McGrew, Chapter 4, this volume).

Both the Cattell–Horn and Carroll models essentially started from the same point—Spearman's (1904) *g* factor theory. Though they took different paths, they ended up with remarkably consistent conclusions about the spectrum of broad cognitive abilities. Cattell built upon Spearman's *g* to posit two kinds of *g*: *fluid intelligence* (Gf), the ability to solve novel problems by using reasoning (believed by Cattell to be largely a function of biological and neurological factors), and *crystallized intelligence* (Gc), a knowledge-based ability that is highly dependent on education and acculturation.

Almost from the beginning of his collaboration with Cattell, Horn believed that the psychometric data, as well as neurocognitive and developmental data, were suggesting more than just these two general abilities. Horn (1968) quickly identified

four additional abilities; by the mid-1990s, his model included 9–10 *broad abilities* (Horn, 1989; Horn & Hofer, 1992; Horn & Noll, 1997). The initial dichotomy had grown, but not in a hierarchy. Horn retained the name of Gf-Gc theory, but the diverse broad abilities were treated as equals, not as part of any hierarchy.

Carroll (1993) developed a hierarchical theory based on his in-depth survey of factor-analytic studies composed of three levels or strata of abilities: *stratum III (general)*, a Spearman-like *g*, which Carroll considered to be a valid construct based on overwhelming evidence from factor analysis; *stratum II (broad)*, composed of eight broad factors that correspond reasonably closely to Horn's broad abilities; and *stratum I (narrow)*, composed of numerous fairly specific abilities, organized by the broad factor with which each is most closely associated (many relate to level of mastery, response speed, or rate of learning).

To Horn, the *g* construct had no place in his Gf-Gc theory; consequently, Carroll's stratum III is not usually considered part of CHC theory. Nonetheless, the KABC-II incorporates stratum III in its theoretical model because it corresponds to the global measure of general cognitive ability, the FCI. However, the *g* level is intended more as a practical than a theoretical construct. The KABC-II scales correspond to 5 of the 10 broad abilities that make up CHC stratum II—Glr, Gsm, Gv, Gf, and Gc. The test authors chose not to include separate measures of Gq (*quantitative knowledge*) or Grw (*reading and writing*) because they believe that reading, writing, and mathematics fit in better with tests of academic achievement, like the KTEA-II (Kaufman & Kaufman, 2004c); however, Gq is present in some KABC-II tasks. The Gq ability measured, though, is considered secondary to other abilities measured by these subtests.

The KABC-II assesses 15 of the approximately 70 CHC narrow abilities. Table 11.2 shows the relationship of the KABC-II scales and subtests to the three strata. For the KABC-II, the broad abilities are of primary importance for interpreting the child's cognitive profile. In developing the KABC-II, the test authors did not strive to develop "pure" tasks for measuring the five CHC broad abilities. In theory, for example, Gv tasks should exclude Gf or Gs. In practice, however, the goal of comprehensive tests of cognitive ability is to measure problem solving in different contexts and under different conditions, with complexity being necessary to assess high-level functioning. Consequently, the test authors constructed measures that featured a par-

TABLE 11.2. General (Stratum III), Broad (Stratum II), and Narrow (Stratum I) CHC Abilities Measured by the KABC-II

CHC ability	Measured on KABC-II by:
General ability (stratum III in Carroll's theory)	**Mental Processing Index (MPI)**—Luria model of KABC-II (excludes acquired knowledge), ages 3–18
	Fluid–Crystallized Index (FCI)—CHC model of KABC-II (includes acquired knowledge), ages 3–18
Broad ability (stratum II in CHC theory)	
Long-term storage and retrieval (Glr)	**Learning/Glr Index** (ages 4–18)
Short-term memory (Gsm)	**Sequential/Gsm Index** (ages 4–18)
Visual processing (Gv)	**Simultaneous/Gv Index** (ages 4–18)
Fluid reasoning (Gf)	**Planning/Gf Index** (ages 7–18)
Crystallized ability (Gc)	**Knowledge/Gc Index** (ages 4–18)
Narrow ability (stratum I in CHC theory)	
Glr: Associative memory (MA)	*Atlantis, Rebus, Delayed Recall scale*
Glr: Learning abilities (L1)	*Delayed Recall scale*
Gsm: Memory span (MS)	*Word Order* (without color interference), *Number Recall, Hand Movements*
Gsm: Working memory (WM)	*Word Order* (with color interference)
Gv: Visual memory (MV)	*Face Recognition, Hand Movements*
Gv: Spatial relations (SR)	*Triangles*
Gv: Visualization (VZ)	*Triangles, Conceptual Thinking, Block Counting, Story Completion*
Gv: Spatial scanning (SS)	*Rover*
Gv: Closure speed (CS)	*Gestalt Closure*
Gf: Induction (I)	*Conceptual Thinking, Pattern Reasoning, Story Completion*
Gf: General sequential reasoning (RG)	*Rover, Riddles*
Gc: General information (K0)	*Verbal Knowledge, Story Completion*
Gc: Language development (LD)	*Riddles*
Gc: Lexical knowledge (VL)	*Riddles, Verbal Knowledge, Expressive Vocabulary*
Gq: Math achievement (A3)	*Rover, Block Counting*

Note. Gq, quantitative ability. KABC-II scales are in **bold**, and KABC-II subtests are in *italics*. All KABC-II subtests are included, both Core and supplementary. CHC stratum I categorizations are courtesy of D. P. Flanagan (personal communication, October 2, 2003).

ticular ability while incorporating aspects of other abilities. To illustrate, Rover is primarily a measure of Gv because of its visualization component, but it also involves Gf; Story Completion emphasizes Gf, but Gc is also required to interpret the social situations that are depicted.

Description of KABC-II Subtests

Sequential/Gsm Scale

• *Word Order (Core for ages 3:0–18:11).* The child touches a series of silhouettes of common objects in the same order as the examiner has said the names of the objects; more difficult items in-

clude an interference task (color naming) between the stimulus and response.

• *Number Recall (supplementary for ages 3:0–3:11; Core for ages 4:0–18:11).* The child repeats a series of numbers in the same sequence as the examiner has said them, with series ranging in length from two to nine numbers; the numbers are digits, except that 10 is used instead of 7 to ensure that all numbers are one syllable.

• *Hand Movements (supplementary for ages 4:0–18:11; Nonverbal scale for ages 4:0–18:11).* The child copies the examiner's precise sequence of taps on the table with the fist, palm, or side of the hand.

Simultaneous/Gv Scale

• *Triangles (Core for ages 3:0–12:11; supplementary for ages 13:0–18:11; Nonverbal scale for ages 3:0–18:11)*. For most items, the child assembles several identical rubber triangles (blue on one side, yellow on the other) to match a picture of an abstract design; for easier items, the child assembles a different set of colorful rubber shapes to match a model constructed by the examiner.

• *Face Recognition (Core for ages 3:0–4:11; supplementary for ages 5:0–5:11; nonverbal scale for ages 3:0–5:11)*. The child attends closely to photographs of one or two faces that are exposed briefly, and then selects the correct face or faces, shown in a different pose, from a group photograph.

• *Conceptual Thinking (Core for ages 3:0–6:11; Nonverbal scale for ages 3:0–6:11)*. The child views a set of four or five pictures and then identifies the one picture that does not belong with the others; some items present meaningful stimuli, and others use abstract stimuli.

• *Rover (Core for ages 6:0–18:11)*. The child moves a toy dog to a bone on a checkerboard-like grid that contains obstacles (rocks and weeds), and tries to find the "quickest" path—the one that takes the fewest moves.

• *Block Counting (supplementary for ages 5:0–12:11; Core for ages 13:0–18:11; Nonverbal scale for ages 7:0–18:11)*. The child counts the exact number of blocks in various pictures of stacks of blocks; the stacks are configured so that one or more blocks are hidden or partially hidden from view.

• *Gestalt Closure (supplementary for ages 3:0–18:11)*. The child mentally "fills in the gaps" in a partially completed "inkblot" drawing, and names (or describes) the object or action depicted in the drawing.

Planning/Gf Scale (Ages 7–18 Only)

• *Pattern Reasoning (Core for ages 7:0–18:11; Nonverbal scale for ages 5:0–18:11; Core for ages 5:0–6:11, but on the Simultaneous/Gv scale)*. The child is shown a series of stimuli that form a logical, linear pattern, but one stimulus is missing; the child completes the pattern by selecting the correct stimulus from an array of four to six options at the bottom of the page (most stimuli are abstract, geometric shapes, but some easy items use meaningful shapes).

• *Story Completion (Core for ages 7:0–18:11; Nonverbal scale for ages 6:0–18:11; supplementary for ages 6:0–6:11, but on the Simultaneous/Gv scale)*. The child is shown a row of pictures that tell a story, but some of the pictures are missing. The child is given a set of pictures, selects only the ones that are needed to complete the story, and places the missing pictures in their correct locations.

Learning/Glr Scale

• *Atlantis (Core for ages 3:0–18:11)*. The examiner teaches the child the nonsense names for fanciful pictures of fish, plants, and shells; the child demonstrates learning by pointing to each picture (out of an array of pictures) when it is named.

• *Rebus (Core for ages 3:0–18:11)*. The examiner teaches the child the word or concept associated with each particular rebus (drawing), and the child then "reads" aloud phrases and sentences composed of these rebuses.

• *Delayed Recall (supplementary scale for ages 5:0–18:11)*. The child demonstrates delayed recall of paired associations learned about 20 minutes earlier during the Atlantis and Rebus subtests (this requires the examiner to administer the Atlantis—Delayed and Rebus—Delayed tasks).

Knowledge/Gc Scale (CHC Model Only)

• *Riddles (Core for ages 3:0–18:11)*. The examiner provides several characteristics of a concrete or abstract verbal concept, and the child has to point to it (early items) or name it (later items).

• *Expressive Vocabulary (Core for ages 3:0–6:11; supplementary for ages 7:0–18:11)*. The child provides the name of a pictured object.

• *Verbal Knowledge (supplementary for ages 3:0–6:11; Core for ages 7:0–18:11)*. The child selects from an array of six pictures the one that corresponds to a vocabulary word or answers a general information question.

Administration and Scoring

For the KABC-II, the Core Battery for the Luria model comprises five subtests for 3-year-olds, seven subtests for 4- and 5-year-olds, and eight subtests for ages 6–18. The CHC Core Battery includes two additional subtests at each age, both measures of crystallized ability. Approximate average administration times for the Core Battery, by age, are given in Table 11.3. For the CHC test battery, the additional two Core subtests add about 10 minutes to the testing time for ages 3–6 and about 15 minutes for ages 7–18 years.

TABLE 11.3. Average Administration Times (in Minutes) for the KABC-II Core Battery

Ages =	MPI (Luria model)	FCI (CHC model)
3–4	30	40
5	40	50
6	50	60
7–18	55	70

Examiners who choose to administer the entire Expanded Battery—all Core and supplementary subtests, the Delayed Recall scale, and all measures of crystallized ability—can expect to spend just under 60 minutes for 3- and 4-year-olds, about 90 minutes for ages 5 and 6, and about 100 minutes for ages 7–18. However, examiners who choose to administer supplementary subtests need not give all of the available subtests to a given child or adolescent—just the ones that are most pertinent to the reasons for referral.

Sample and teaching items are included for all subtests, except those that measure acquired knowledge, to ensure that children understand what is expected of them to meet the demands of each subtest. Scoring of all subtests is objective. Even the Knowledge/Gc subtests require pointing or one word responses rather than longer verbal responses, which often introduce subjectivity into the scoring process.

In their KABC-II review, Bain and Gray (2008) state that "generally, the KABC-II is easy to administer with practice and is inherently interesting for children, with several manipulative opportunities and brightly colored, well-designed stimuli. Some of the newly developed subtests are particularly attractive" (p. 100). They do note, however, that the numerous test materials "plus the manual make up a kit that is far from the lightest, most compact kit in the typical examiner's repertoire" (p. 100).

Psychometric Properties

The KABC-II is a psychometrically sound instrument. A brief review of the instrument's standardization sample, reliability, and validity is provided in this chapter. For a thorough description of the normative sample and reliability, stability, and validity data, see the KABC-II manual (Kaufman & Kaufman, 2004a) and *Essentials of KABC-II Assessment* (Kaufman, Lichtenberger, Fletcher-Janzen, & Kaufman, 2005).

Standardization Sample

The KABC-II standardization sample was composed of 3,025 children and adolescents. The sample matched the U.S. population on the stratification variables of gender, race/ethnicity, socioeconomic status (SES—parental education), region, and special education status. Each year of age between 3 and 18 was represented by 125–250 children, about equally divided between males and females, with most age groups consisting of exactly 200 children.

Reliability

KABC-II global scale (MPI and FCI) split-half reliability coefficients were in the mid-.90s for all age groups (only the value of .90 for the MPI at age 3 was below .94). The mean MPI coefficient was .95 for ages 3–6 and ages 7–18; the mean values for FCI were .96 (ages 3–6) and .97 (ages 7–18). Mean split-half reliability coefficients for the separate scales (e.g., Learning/Glr, Simultaneous/Gv) averaged .91–.92 for ages 3–6 and ranged from .88 to .93 (mean = .90) for ages 7–18. Similarly, the Nonverbal Index—the alternative global score for children and adolescents with hearing impairments, limited English proficiency, and the like—had an average coefficient of .90 for 3- to 6-year-olds and .92 for those ages 7–18. Mean split-half values for Core subtests across the age range were .82 (age 3), .84 (age 4), .86 (ages 5–6), and .85 (ages 7–18). Nearly all Core subtests had mean coefficients of .80 or greater at ages 3–6 and 7–18. Stability data over an interval of about 1 month for three age groups (total N = 203) yielded coefficients of .86–.91 for the MPI and .90–.94 for the FCI. Stability coefficients for the separate scales averaged .81 for ages 3–6 (range = .74–.93), .80 for ages 7–12 (range = .76–.88), and .83 for ages 13–18 (range = .78–.95). Bain and Gray (2008) have concluded that "the reliability coefficients are consistently high" (p. 100).

Validity

Construct validity was given strong support by the results of confirmatory factor analysis (CFA). The CFA supported four factors for ages 4 and 5–6, and five factors for ages 7–12 and 13–18, with the factor structure supporting the scale structure for these broad age groups. The fit was excellent for all age groups; for ages 7–12 and 13–18, the five-factor solution provided a significantly better fit than the four-factor solution. In addition to the CFA evidence provided in the KABC-II manual, strong independent support for the theory-based structure of the KABC-II was provided in a reanalysis of standardization data for all age groups (Reynolds, Keith, Fine, Fisher, & Low, 2007), and for a new sample of 200 preschool children ages 4–5 years (Hunt, 2008; Morgan, Rothlisberg, McIntosh, & Hunt, 2009). In addition, Reynolds and Keith (2007) demonstrated that the factor structure was invariant for high- and low-ability groups, and the construct validity of the KABC-II has also been demonstrated cross-culturally—for example, for 598 low-SES Kannada-speaking children ages 6–10 years in Bangalore, South India (Malda et al., 2010).

Correlation coefficients between the FCI and the Wechsler Intelligence Scale for Children (WISC; Wechsler, 1991, 2003) Full Scale IQ (FSIQ), corrected for the variability of the norms sample, were .89 for the WISC-IV (N = 56, ages 7–16) and 77 for the WISC-III (N = 119, ages 8–13). The FCI also correlated .78 with Woodcock–Johnson III (WJ III; Woodcock, McGrew, & Mather, 2001) General Intellectual Ability (GIA) (N = 86, ages 7–16), .72 with the K-ABC Mental Processing Composite (MPC) for preschool children (N = 67), and 84 with the K-ABC MPC for school-age children (N = 48). Correlations with the MPI were generally slightly lower (by an average of .05).

Fletcher-Janzen (2003) conducted a correlational study with the WISC-IV for 30 Native American children from Taos, New Mexico, who were tested on the KABC-II at an average age of 7:8 (range = 5–14) and on the WISC-IV at an average age of 9:3. As shown in Table 11.4, the two global scores correlated about .85 with the WISC-IV FSIQ. This strong relationship indicates that the KABC-II global scores and the WISC-IV global score measure the same construct; nevertheless, the KABC-II yielded global scores that were about 0.5 SD higher than the FSIQ for this Native American sample.

Correlations were obtained between the KABC-II and achievement on the WJ III, the Wechsler Individual Achievement Test—Second Edition (WIAT-II; Psychological Corporation, 2001), and the Peabody Individual Achievement Test—Revised/Normative Update (PIAT-R/NU; Markwardt, 1998) for six samples with a total N of 401. Coefficients between the FCI and total achievement for the six samples, corrected for the variability of the norms sample, ranged from .67 on the PIAT-R/NU for grades 1–4 to .87 on the WIAT-II for grades 6–10 (mean r = .75). For these same samples, the MPI correlated .63 to .83 (mean r = .71). In addition, the KABC-II FCI correlated .79 (and the MPI correlated .74) with total achievement on the KABC-II Comprehensive Form for 2,475 individuals ages 4½ through 18 years (Kaufman & Kaufman, 2004c, Table 7.25). Correlations with KTEA-II Brief Form total achievement were as follows: FCI = .60 for ages 4½–6 (N = 324), .71 for ages 7–12 (N = 526), and .76 for ages 13–18 (N = 418) (Kaufman & Kaufman, 2005, Tables 6.20–6.22). (Corresponding values for the MPI were .60, .67, and .71, respectively.)

Interpretation

What the Scales Measure

Sequential/Gsm (Ages 4–18)

• *CHC interpretation.* Short-term memory (Gsm) is the ability to apprehend and hold information in immediate awareness briefly, and then use that information within a few seconds, before it is forgotten.

TABLE 11.4. Means, *SD*s, and Correlations between KABC-II and WISC-IV Global Scores for 30 Native American Children and Adolescents from Taos, New Mexico

KABC-II and WISC-IV global scores	Mean	SD	r with WISC-IV FSIQ	Mean difference MPI vs. FSIQ	Mean difference FCI vs. FSIQ
KABC-II					
Mental Processing Index (MPI)	95.1	13.3	.86	+8.4	—
Fluid–Crystallized Index (FCI)	94.1	12.5	84	—	+7.4
WISC-IV					
Full Scale IQ (FSIQ)	86.7	12.3	—	—	—

Note. Children were tested first on the KABC-II (age range = 5–14, mean = 7:8) and second on the WISC-IV (age range = 6–15, mean = 9:3). Data from Fletcher-Janzen (2003).

- *Luria interpretation.* Sequential processing is used to solve problems, where the emphasis is on the serial or temporal order of stimuli. For each problem, the input must be arranged in a strictly defined order to form a chain-like progression; each idea is linearly and temporally related only to the preceding one.

Simultaneous/Gv (Ages 4–18)

- *CHC interpretation.* Visual processing (Gv) is the ability to perceive, manipulate, and think with visual patterns and stimuli, and to mentally rotate objects in space.

- *Luria interpretation.* Simultaneous processing demands a Gestalt-like, frequently spatial, integration of stimuli. The input has to be synthesized simultaneously, so that the separate stimuli are integrated into a group or conceptualized as a whole.

Learning/Glr (Ages 4–18)

- *CHC interpretation.* Long-term storage and retrieval (Glr) is the ability both to store information in long-term memory and to retrieve that information fluently and efficiently. The emphasis of Glr is on the *efficiency* of the storage and retrieval, not on the specific nature of the information stored.

- *Luria interpretation.* Learning ability requires an integration of the processes associated with all three of Luria's functional units. The attentional requirements for the learning tasks are considerable, as focused, sustained, and selective attention are requisites for success. However, for effective paired-associate learning, children need to apply both block 2 processes, sequential and simultaneous. Block 3 planning abilities help them generate strategies for storing and retrieving the new learning.

Planning/Gf (Ages 7–18)

- *CHC interpretation.* Fluid reasoning (Gf) refers to a variety of mental operations that a person can use to solve a novel problem with adaptability and flexibility—operations such as drawing inferences and applying inductive or deductive reasoning. Verbal mediation also plays a key role in applying fluid reasoning effectively.

- *Luria interpretation.* Planning ability requires hypothesis generation, revising one's plan of action, monitoring and evaluating the best hypothesis for a given problem (decision making), flexibility, and impulse control. This set of high-level skills is associated with executive functioning.

Knowledge/Gc (Ages 4–18)—CHC Model Only

- *CHC interpretation.* Crystallized ability (Gc) reflects a person's specific knowledge acquired within a culture, as well as the person's ability to apply this knowledge effectively. Gc emphasizes the *breadth* and *depth* of the specific information that has been stored.

- *Luria interpretation.* The Knowledge/Gc scale is not included in the MPI, but may be administered as a supplement if the examiner seeks a measure of the child's acquired knowledge. From a Luria perspective, Knowledge/Gc measures a person's knowledge base, developed over time by applying block 1, block 2, and block 3 processes to the acquisition of factual information and verbal concepts. Like Learning/Glr, this scale requires an integration of the key processes, but unlike learning ability, acquired knowledge emphasizes the *content* more than the *process*.

Gender Differences

Analysis of KABC-II standardization data explored gender differences at four different age ranges: 3–4 years, 5–6 years, 7–12 years, and 13–18 years. At ages 3–4, females significantly outperformed males on the MPI, FCI, and Nonverbal Index by about 5 points (0.33 *SD*), but there were no other significant differences on the global scales at any age level (J. C. Kaufman, 2003). Consistent with the literature on gender differences, females tended to score higher than males at preschool levels. Females scored significantly higher than males at ages 3 and 4 years by about 3–4 points, with significant differences emerging on Learning/Glr (0.27 *SD*) and Simultaneous/Gv (0.34 *SD*). Also consistent with previous findings, males scored significantly higher than females on the Simultaneous/Gv scale at ages 7–12 (0.24 *SD*) and 13–18 (0.29 *SD*). Females earned significantly higher scores than males at ages 5–6 on the Sequential/Gsm scale (0.22 *SD*) and at ages 13–18 on the Planning/Gf scale (0.13 *SD*).

In a subsequent study of gender differences on the KABC-II at ages 6–18 years, also based on standardization data, Reynolds, Ridley, and Patel (2008) applied multigroup higher-order analysis of mean and covariance structures and of multiple-indicator/multiple-cause models. They found that males consistently demonstrated a significant mean advantage on the latent visual–spatial ability (Gv) factor, even when g was controlled for, and the same finding held true for the latent crystallized ability (Gc) factor at all ages except 17–18. Females scored higher on the latent higher-order g factor at all ages, although the difference was significant at only two ages. No significant age × gender interaction effect was identified (Reynolds et al., 2008). In a study of 137 Mexican American children ages 7–12 years, Gomez (2008) found a slight superiority of males over females on the MPI. In general, in all studies, gender differences on the KABC-II are small; even when significant, they tend to be small in effect size (McLean, 1995).

Ethnicity Differences

Because the original K-ABC yielded considerably smaller ethnic differences than conventional IQ tests did, it was especially important to determine the magnitude of ethnic differences for the substantially revised and reconceptualized KABC-II. On the original K-ABC, the mean MPC for African American children ages 5:0–12:6 was 93.7 (Kaufman & Kaufman, 1983, Table 4.35). On the KABC-II, the mean MPI for African American children ages 7–18 in the standardization sample (N = 315) was 94.8, and the mean FCI was 94.0. On the two new KABC-II scales, African American children ages 7–18 averaged 94.3 (Planning/Gf) and 98.6 (Learning/Glr). At ages 3–6, African American children averaged 98.2 on Learning/Glr.

When standard scores were adjusted for SES and gender, European Americans scored 4.4 points higher than African Americans at 7–12 years on the MPI—smaller than an adjusted difference of 8.6 points on WISC-III FSIQ at ages 6–11 (J. C. Kaufman, 2003), and smaller than the 6-point difference at ages 6–11 on the WISC-IV. At the 13- to 18-year level, European Americans scored 7.7 points higher than African Americans on the adjusted MPI (J. C. Kaufman, 2003)—substantially smaller than the 14.1-point discrepancy on adjusted WISC-III FSIQ for ages 12–16, and also smaller than the 11.8-point difference at ages 12–16 on the WISC-IV. (WISC-III data are from Prifitera, Weiss, & Saklofske, 1998; WISC-IV data are from Prifitera, Weiss, Saklofske, & Rolfhus, 2005.) The adjusted discrepancies of 6.2 points (ages 7–12) and 8.6 points (ages 13–18) on the FCI, which includes measures of acquired knowledge, were also

smaller than WISC-III and WISC-IV FSIQ differences. The KABC-II thus seems to continue in the K-ABC tradition of yielding higher standard scores for African Americans than are typically yielded on other instruments. In addition, as shown in Table 11.4, the mean MPI and FCI earned by the 30 Native American children in Taos are about 7–8 points higher than this sample's mean WISC-IV FSIQ.

Further ethnicity analyses of KABC-II standardization data were conducted for the entire age range of 3–18 years, which included 1,861 European Americans, 545 Hispanics, 465 African Americans, 75 Asian Americans, and 68 Native Americans. When adjusted for SES and gender, mean MPIs were 101.7 for European Americans, 97.1 for Hispanics, 96.0 for African Americans, 103.4 for Asian Americans, and 97.6 for Native Americans. Mean adjusted FCIs were about 1 point lower than the mean MPIs for all groups except European Americans (who had a slightly higher FCI) (J. C. Kaufman, 2003).

A recent doctoral dissertation examined ethnic differences for 49 African American and 49 European American preschool children from a U.S. Midwestern city (mean age = 5 years), who were matched on age, sex, and level of parental education (Dale, 2009). African American and European American preschool children had similar patterns of highs and lows in their profiles of scores and performed comparably on the different scales. Differences on the FCI (European American mean = 97.06, African American mean = 95.59) were a trivial and nonsignificant 1.47 points, "the smallest gap seen in the literature" (Dale, 2009, p. viii).

Clinical Applications

Like the original K-ABC, the KABC-II was designed to be a clinical and psychological instrument, not merely a psychometric tool. It has a variety of clinical benefits and uses:

1. The identification of process integrities and deficits for assessment of individuals with specific learning disabilities.
2. The evaluation of individuals with known or suspected neurological disorders, when the KABC-II is used along with other tests as part of a comprehensive neuropsychological battery.
3. The integration of the individual's profile of KABC-II scores with clinical behaviors observed during the administration of each subtest (Fletcher-Janzen, 2003)—identified as

Qualitative Indicators (QIs) on the KABC-II record form (see Kaufman & Kaufman, 2004a; Kaufman et al., 2005).

4. The selection of the MPI to promote the fair assessment of children and adolescents from African American, Hispanic, Native American, and Asian American backgrounds (an application that has empirical support, as summarized briefly in the previous section on "Ethnicity Differences" and in Table 11.4).

5. Evaluation of individuals with known or suspected ADHD, intellectual disabilities/developmental delays, speech–language difficulties, emotional/behavioral disorders, autism, reading/math disabilities, intellectual giftedness, and hearing impairment (KABC-II data on all of these clinical samples are presented and discussed in the KABC-II manual).

We believe that whenever possible, clinical tests such as the KABC-II should be interpreted by the same person who administered them—an approach that enhances the clinical benefits of the instrument and its clinical applications. The main goal of any evaluation should be to *effect change* in the person who was referred. Extremely competent and well-trained examiners are needed to best accomplish that goal; we feel more confident in a report writer's ability to effect change and to derive clinical benefits from an administration of the KABC-II when the professional who interprets the test data and writes the case report has also administered the test and directly observed the individual's test behaviors.

Innovations in Measures of Cognitive Assessment

Several of the features described here for the KABC-II are innovative in comparison to the Wechsler and Stanford–Binet tradition of intellectual assessment, which has century-old roots. However, some of these innovations are not unique to the KABC-II; rather, several of these innovations are shared by other contemporary instruments, such as the WJ III (Woodcock et al., 2001), the Cognitive Assessment System (CAS; Naglieri & Das, 1997), and the most recent revisions of the Wechsler scales (Wechsler, 2002, 2003, 2008).

Integrates Two Theoretical Approaches

As discussed previously, the KABC-II utilizes a dual theoretical approach—Luria's neuropsycho-

logical theory and CHC theory. This dual model permits alternative interpretations of the scales, based on the examiner's personal orientation or based on the specific individual being evaluated. One of the criticisms of the original K-ABC was that the mental processing scales were interpreted solely from the sequential–simultaneous perspective, despite the fact that alternative interpretations are feasible (Keith, 1985). The KABC-II has addressed that criticism and has provided a strong theoretical foundation for the test by building the test on a dual theoretical model. In their review of the KABC-II, Bain and Gray (2008) have praised the theoretical model:

> In terms of construct validity, Kaufman and Kaufman's efforts to combine the two theoretical models, the Luria model and the CHC model, into one instrument is particularly attractive to those of us who favored the use of the original K-ABC for younger children but found ourselves scrambling for variations on subtests measuring broad and narrow abilities for cross-battery assessment. (p. 100)

(For a comprehensive review of cross-battery assessment, see Flanagan, Alfonso, & Ortiz, Chapter 19, this volume.)

Provides the Examiner with Optimal Flexibility

The two theoretical models that underlie the KABC-II not only provide alternative interpretations of the scales, but also give the examiner the flexibility to select the model (and hence the global score) that is better suited to the individual's background and reason for referral. As mentioned earlier, the CHC model is ordinarily the model of choice, but examiners can choose to administer the Luria model when excluding measures of acquired knowledge from the global score promotes fairer assessment of a child's general cognitive ability. The MPI that results is an especially pertinent global score, for example, for individuals who have a receptive or expressive language disability or who are from a bilingual background. This flexibility of choice permits fairer assessment for anyone referred for an evaluation.

The examiner's flexibility is enhanced as well by the inclusion of supplementary subtests for most scales, including a supplementary Delayed Recall scale to permit the evaluation of a child's recall of paired associations that were learned about 20 minutes earlier. Hand Movements is a supplementary Sequential/Gsm subtest for ages 4–18, and Gestalt Closure is a supplementary task across the entire 3–18 range. Supplementary subtests are not included in the computation of standard scores on any KABC-II scales, but they do permit the examiner to follow up hypotheses suggested by the profile of scores on the Core Battery, to generate new hypotheses, and to increase the breadth of measurement on the KABC-II constructs.

Promotes Fairer Assessment of Minority Children

As mentioned earlier, children and adolescents from minority backgrounds—African American, Hispanic, Asian American, and Native American—earned mean MPIs that were close to the normative mean of 100, even prior to adjustment for SES and gender. In addition, there is some evidence that the discrepancies between European Americans and African Americans are smaller on the KABC-II than on the WISC-IV, and that Native Americans score higher on the KABC-II than the WISC-IV (see Table 11.4). These data, as well as additional data (Dale, 2009), suggest that the KABC-II, like the original K-ABC, will be useful for promoting fairer assessment of children and adolescents from minority backgrounds.

Offers a Separate Nonverbal Scale

Like the K-ABC, the KABC-II offers a reliable, separate Nonverbal scale composed of subtests that can be administered in pantomime and responded to nonverbally. This special global scale, for the entire 3–18 age range, permits valid assessment of children and adolescents with hearing impairments, moderate to severe speech–language disorders, limited English proficiency, and so forth.

Permits Direct Evaluation of a Child's Learning Ability

The KABC-II Learning/Glr scale allows direct measurement of a child's ability to learn new information under standardized conditions. These tasks also permit examiners to observe the child's ability to learn under different conditions; for example, Atlantis gives the child feedback after each error, but Rebus does not offer feedback. In addition, Rebus involves meaningful verbal labels for symbolic visual stimuli, whereas Atlantis involves nonsensical verbal labels for meaningful visual

stimuli. When examiners choose to administer the supplementary Delayed Recall scale to children ages 5–18, they are then able to assess the children's ability to retain information that was taught earlier in the evaluation. The inclusion of learning tasks on the KABC-II (and on the WJ III and the Kaufman Adolescent and Adult Intelligence Test [KAIT; Kaufman & Kaufman, 1993]) reflects an advantage over the Wechsler scales, which do not directly measure learning ability.

KAUFMAN TEST OF EDUCATIONAL ACHIEVEMENT—SECOND EDITION (KTEA-II)

Test Development and Structure

The KTEA-II (Kaufman & Kaufman, 2004c) was developed to assess the academic achievement of children, adolescents, and adults. The KTEA-II has two versions: the Brief Form for ages 4½–90 years (Kaufman & Kaufman, 2005), and the Comprehensive Form for ages 4½ through 25. The Comprehensive Form assesses four academic domains (Reading, Math, Written Language, and Oral Language), and the Brief Form assesses three of those four domains (all except Oral Language). Although the Brief and Comprehensive Forms cover three of the same academic domains, there is no overlap in items between the two forms of the test. In addition, the Comprehensive Form consists of two independent parallel forms, A and B. This section of this chapter focuses mostly on the KTEA-II Comprehensive Form.

The content development for each KTEA-II subtest is described in depth in Chapter 5 of the KTEA-II Comprehensive Form manual (Kaufman & Kaufman, 2004c). Generally, the test developers first defined at a conceptual level which skills should be measured for a particular academic domain. To determine what should be measured within each academic domain, both literature reviews and expert opinion were used. The original K-TEA items were reviewed to determine which item formats should be retained and which should be modified. Expert advisors contributed suggestions for content and item formats for written expression, oral expression, listening comprehension, and reading related skills because these were the four new achievement areas to be added to the previous edition of the test. The test developers also made sure that certain skills were systematically represented in the content for each subtest. Creating an informative error analysis, with a more fine-grained approach to classifying errors on some subtests, was also a key part of the subtest content development.

Description of Composite Domains

The 14 subtests of the KTEA-II Comprehensive Form are grouped into four domain composites and four Reading-Related composites. The four KTEA-II Comprehensive domain composites are Reading, Mathematics, Written Language, and Oral Language, and the four Reading-Related composites are Sound–Symbol, Decoding, Oral Fluency, and Reading Fluency. The composition of the KTEA-II Comprehensive Form varies slightly according to grade level (or age). For example, for grade 1 through age 25, six of the eight subtests contribute to the Comprehensive Achievement Composite (CAC), but for ages 4½ through kindergarten, four of the eight subtests come together to yield the CAC.

For children and adolescents in grades 1–12 and above, the four aforementioned domain composites are calculated on the basis of scores yielded from eight KTEA-II Comprehensive Form subtests. From grade 1 to grade 12 and up, two of the Reading-Related composites are calculated for the entire age range: Decoding and Oral Fluency. However, Sound–Symbol is calculated only for grades 1–6, and Reading Fluency is calculated only for grades 3–12 and above.

At the kindergarten level, eight subtests can be administered in total, and the KTEA-II Comprehensive Form yields three domain composites: Math, Written Language, and Oral Language. No domain composite for Reading is obtained for kindergarteners, but three Reading-Related subtests are administered: Letter and Word Recognition, Associational Fluency, and Naming Facility. One Reading-Related Composite may be calculated for kindergarteners: Oral Fluency.

Children who have not yet begun kindergarten (PreK) are administered seven subtests on the KTEA-II Comprehensive Form. The test yields two domain composites: Written Language and Oral Language. Although no domain composite for Math is calculated at the PreK level, Math Concepts and Applications (a math subtest) is administered to these children. In addition, three Reading-Related subtests are administered to PreK children: Letter and Word Recognition, Associational Fluency, and Naming Facility. One

Reading-Related Composite may be calculated for PreK children: Oral Fluency.

Description of KTEA-II Subtests

The following brief descriptions of each of the KTEA-II Comprehensive Form subtests are organized by content area. They also indicate the age and grade range at which each subtest may be administered, since the age range for each subtest varies.

Reading and Reading-Related Subtests

- *Letter and Word Recognition (ages 4:6–25:11).* The student identifies letters and pronounces words of gradually increasing difficulty. Most words are irregular, to ensure that the subtest measures word recognition (reading vocabulary) rather than decoding ability.

- *Reading Comprehension (grade 1–age 25:11).* For the easiest items, the student reads a word and points to its corresponding picture. In following items, the student reads a simple instruction and responds by performing the action. In later items, the student reads passages of increasing difficulty and answers literal or inferential questions about them. Finally, the student rearranges five sentences into a coherent paragraph and then answers questions about the paragraph.

- *Phonological Awareness (grades 1–6).* The student responds orally to items that require manipulation of sounds. Tasks include rhyming, matching sounds, blending sounds, segmenting sounds, and deleting sounds.

- *Nonsense Word Decoding (grade 1–age 25:11).* The student applies phonics and structural analysis skills to decode invented words of increasing difficulty.

- *Word Recognition Fluency (grade 3–age 25:11).* The student reads isolated words as quickly as possible for 1 minute.

- *Decoding Fluency (grade 3–age 25:11).* The student applies decoding skills to pronounce as many nonsense words as possible in 1 minute.

- *Associational Fluency (ages 4:6–25:11).* The student says as many words as possible in 30 seconds that belong to a semantic category or have a specified beginning sound.

- *Naming Facility (RAN) (ages 4:6–25:11).* The student names objects, colors, and letters as quickly as possible.

Math Subtests

• *Math Concepts and Applications (ages 4:6–25:11)*. The student responds orally to test items that focus on the application of mathematical principles to real-life situations. Skill categories include number concepts, operation concepts, rational numbers, measurement, shape and space, data investigations, and higher math concepts.

• *Math Computation (grade K–age 25:11)*. The student computes solutions to math problems printed in a student response booklet. Skills assessed include addition, subtraction, multiplication, and division operations; fractions and decimals; and square roots, exponents, signed numbers, and algebra.

Written Language Subtests

• *Written Expression (ages 4:6–25:11)*. Kindergarten and PreK children trace and copy letters and write letters from dictation. At grades 1 and higher, the student completes writing tasks in the context of an age-appropriate storybook format. Tasks at those levels include writing sentences from dictation, adding punctuation and capitalization, filling in missing words, completing sentences, combining sentences, writing compound and complex sentences, and (starting at spring of grade 1) writing an essay based on the story the student has helped complete.

• *Spelling (grade 1–age 25:11)*. The student writes words dictated by the examiner from a steeply graded word list. Words have been selected to match acquired spelling skills at each grade level, and for their potential for error analysis. Early items require students to write single letters that represent sounds. The remaining items require students to spell orthographically regular and irregular words of increasing complexity.

Oral Language Subtests

• *Listening Comprehension (ages 4:6–25:11)*. The student listens to passages played on a CD and then responds orally to questions asked by the examiner. Questions measure literal and inferential comprehension.

• *Oral Expression (ages 4:6–25:11)*. The student performs specific speaking tasks in the context of a real-life scenario. Tasks assess pragmatics, syntax, semantics, and grammar.

Administration and Scoring

The KTEA-II Comprehensive Form provides much flexibility for examiners. If only one particular domain of academic functioning is of concern, an examiner may choose to administer a single subtest or any combination of subtests in that domain in order to assess a student's academic achievement. If multiple domains need to be measured, then all of the age-appropriate subtests can be administered to obtain the desired composite score(s). As in most standardized tests of individual achievement, the KTEA-II items are ordered by difficulty, with the easiest items being administered first. Grade-based starting points are listed in the record form and on the first page of a subtest's directions in the easel. A difference from many cognitive tests, such as the KABC-II, is that very few KTEA-II subtests include sample or teaching items. Most subtests on the KTEA-II are not timed (however, timing is required on Word Recognition Fluency, Decoding Fluency, Associational Fluency, and Naming Facility). Lichtenberger and Breaux (2010) provide subtest-by-subtest notes on KTEA-II administration and scoring that highlight pertinent information for each of the subtests, and that point out common errors in administration and scoring.

The KTEA-II yields several types of scores: raw scores, standard scores (subtests, domain composites, and CAC), grade equivalents, age equivalents, percentile ranks, and growth scale values. After scoring the subtests, error analysis procedures provide an examiner with more specific information about a student's performance than can be obtained from composite or subtest standard scores or comparisons. These error analysis procedures use information documented on the record form during KTEA-II administration to identify specific areas in which the student demonstrates strong, weak, or average skill development, as defined by the performance of the standardization sample.

Psychometric Properties

Standardization Sample

Standardization of the KTEA-II Comprehensive Form was conducted with an age-norm sample of 3,000 examinees ages 4.5 through 25, and a grade-norm sample of 2,400 students in grades K–12. For each grade level, the sample size ranged from 140 to 220 students, with more examinees contributing to the earlier grades. For each age level, the sample sizes ranged from 100 to 220 students (with the exception of age 19, which had a sample of only 18 examinees). As noted earlier, the KTEA-II Comprehensive Form contains two parallel forms (A and B), so approximately half of the norm sample was administered Form A and the other half was administered Form B. Corresponding to data from the 2001 Current Population Survey of the U.S. Bureau of the Census, the standardization sample closely matched the U.S. population on the variables of gender, ethnicity, parental education, geographic region, and special education or gifted placement.

Reliability

For both Forms A and B, the internal-consistency reliability of the KTEA-II Comprehensive Form is strong. The average internal-consistency reliability value across grades and forms for the CAC was .97. The averages for the Reading, Math, and Decoding Composites were .96, .96, and .97, respectively. For the Written Language and Sound–Symbol Composites, the average reliability values were .93. For the Oral Language and Oral Fluency Composites, the average reliabilities were .87 and .85, respectively. Reliability values based on age groups were very similar to what was reported for the reliability values found with the grade-level samples.

The two versions of the KTEA-II Comprehensive Form were administered to a sample of 221 children to calculate the alternate-form reliability values. On average, the forms were administered approximately 3½–4 weeks apart. The values for the alternate-form reliability were comparable to the high internal-consistency reliability values. The CAC showed very high consistency across time and forms (low to mid-90s). The Reading, Math, Written Language, Decoding, and Reading Fluency Composites had alternate-form reliabilities in the high .80s to mid-90s. These strong values indicate that the alternate forms of the KTEA-II will be useful for reducing practice effects when the test is administered more than once.

Validity

CFA gave strong construct validity support for the KTEA-II Comprehensive Form subtests and composites. The factor analysis proceeded in a stepwise fashion, with the eight primary subtests yielding a final model consisting of four factors. The final model had good fit statistics, and all subtests had high loadings on their factors, showing that the structure of the test was empirically grounded.

Correlations with other instruments were also conducted to evaluate the construct validity of the test. Correlations were calculated between the KTEA-II Comprehensive and Brief Forms and showed strong correspondence between the instruments. Coefficients were .85, .86, .78, and .89, respectively, for the Reading, Math, and Written Language Composites and the CAC. Further correlations were calculated between the KTEA-II Comprehensive Form and the following achievement tests: the WIAT-II, the WJ III Tests of Achievement (WJ III ACH; Woodcock et al., 2001), the PIAT-R/NU (Markwardt, 1998), and the Oral and Written Language Scales (OWLS; Carrow-Woolfolk, 1996). The results of the studies with the WIAT-II and WJ III ACH showed that most correlations between like-named composites were in the mid- to high .80s, and correlations between most of the total achievement scores hovered around .90. The correlations with the PIAT-R/NU overall composite score were .86 for both grades K–5 and grades 6–9. For domain composites, the PIAT-R/NU's highest correlations were for reading, ranging from .89 to .78, and lower correlations were found for mathematics and spelling (ranging from .67 to .70). The OWLS has three subtests, and the highest correlation with the KTEA-II was between the tests of Written Expression (.75); the instruments' measures of Oral Expression and Listening Comprehension correlated only at a modest level (in the .40s).

The KTEA-II Comprehensive Form manual also provides data showing the correlations between the KTEA-II and three tests of cognitive ability: the KABC-II, the WISC-III (Wechsler, 1991), and the WJ III Tests of Cognitive Abilities (WJ III COG; Woodcock et al., 2001). A very large sample (N = 2,520) was used in the study with the KABC-II, as this test was conormed with the KTEA-II. Sample sizes were 97 and 51 for the studies with the WISC-III and WJ III COG, respectively.

The KTEA-II CAC correlated .79 with the KABC-II FCI, .74 with the KABC-II MPI, and .69 with the KABC-II Nonverbal Index for the total sample. Very similar correlations were found between the CAC and global cognitive scores on the WISC-III and WJ III COG. The CAC correlated .79 with the WISC-III FSIQ and .82 with WJ III COG GIA. For all three tests of cognitive ability, the KTEA-II's Reading and Math Composites had the strongest relationships to overall cognitive ability. For the KABC-II FCI, WISC-III FSIQ, and WJ III GIA, correlations with the Reading Composite were .74, .69, and .72, respectively. Correlations with the Math Composite were .71, .65, and .76 for the KABC-II FCI, WISC-III FSIQ, and WJ III GIA, respectively. The other academic domains measured by the KTEA-II did not correlate as strongly with overall cognitive ability. For example, the KABC-II FCI correlations with the Written Language and Oral Language Composites were .66 and .67, respectively.

Interpretation

KTEA-II interpretation can help identify and promote understanding of a student's strong and weak areas of academic functioning, from both *normative* (age-based or grade-based) and *ipsative* (person-based) perspectives. Following the interpretive approaches advocated in the manual and other sources (Lichtenberger & Breaux, 2010), interpretation of the Comprehensive Form begins at the global level with looking at the CAC and domain composites, then moves to subtests, and finally to specific patterns of errors. Similar to how many good teachers intuitively apply error analysis skills in their everyday teaching, the KTEA-II authors believe that understanding test performance by studying a student's incorrect responses is a profitable method of helping the student progress (Kaufman & Kaufman, 2004c). Thus, when interpreting the KTEA-II Comprehensive Form from its most global scores to its most detailed level of error analysis, examiners can obtain data beyond an examinee's subtest and composite scores to provide specific information that becomes a basis for intervention.

Interpreting Reading Comprehension and Listening Comprehension

By reflecting on what is read, a person derives meaning from text during the process of reading comprehension. On the KTEA-II, items from the Reading Comprehension and Listening Comprehension subtests are divided into *literal* and *inferential* comprehension. Literal comprehension requires recognizing or recalling ideas, information or events that are explicitly stated in an oral or written text. In contrast, inferential comprehension requires the generation of new ideas from those stated in the text.

Interpreting Written Expression and Oral Expression

Communicating orally requires similar skills to those needed to communicate in written form. However, writing is more deliberate and structured, whereas oral communication is typically more spontaneous and natural. Difficulty in communicating orally and in written form can occur in many different areas:

- *Pragmatics*: how well the writing or speech adheres to the task demands to communicate in a comprehensible and functional manner.
- *Syntax*: how well constructed the student's sentences are.
- *Grammar*: appropriateness of the word forms.
- *Semantics*: correct use of words.
- *Mechanics*: capitalization and punctuation for written expression.

Interpreting Phonological Awareness

The Phonological Awareness subtest can reveal whether a child has mastered particular aspects of sound awareness and manipulation. Abilities that are important precursors to reading are tapped in this subtest: rhyming, sound matching, blending, segmenting, and deleting sounds. Information about deficits in certain areas of phonological awareness can be used in teaching early reading skills.

Interpreting Math Concepts and Applications

Math concepts and math applications are two related sets of abilities. The basic ideas and relationships on which the systems of mathematics are built are labeled *concepts*. Acquisition of math concepts requires students to master basic concepts before more advanced concepts can be learned. *Applications* involve using these concepts and skills to solve actual and hypothetical problems (e.g., reading graphs, balancing a checkbook). If a child has not yet mastered a certain concept or skill, he or she will not be able to apply that concept to solve an actual or hypothetical problem.

Interpreting Math Computation

The Math Computation subtest gives information about nine skill areas: addition, subtraction, multiplication, division, fractions, decimals, exponents, and algebra. Additional information is provided about 10 specific mathematical processes (such as regrouping, converting to common denominators, or placing decimal points). Interpretive information is gleaned from understanding a student's skill deficits, but even more instructionally relevant information may be revealed from the process errors that the student makes. Understanding why a child missed an item (e.g., adding when the child should have subtracted, or making an error when regrouping) can help determine how and where to provide additional remedial instruction for the child.

Interpreting Letter and Word Recognition, Nonsense Word Decoding, and Spelling

Students connect speech sounds to letter patterns during the process of decoding words. Three KTEA-II subtests tap this important skill:

- Nonsense Word Decoding assesses a student's ability to apply decoding and structural analysis skills to typically occurring letter patterns.
- Spelling requires students to relate speech sounds that they hear to letter patterns that they write.
- Letter and Word Recognition taps a student's ability to read words with unpredictable letter patterns.

Interpretation of performance on Letter and Word Recognition, Nonsense Word Decoding, and Spelling involves examining errors made across "categories corresponding to letters and letter combinations that have a predictable relationship to their sound. Errors involving unpredictable letter–sound relationships are qualitatively different from the other error categories because by definition those errors are not generalizable to other words" (Kaufman & Kaufman, 2004c, p. 46). Words with unpredictable patterns are categorized separately, which allows examiners to determine whether students' problem areas are in the decoding or spelling of predictable patterns.

Clinical Applications

Like the KABC-II, the KTEA-II has many clinical benefits and uses. The KTEA-II can be applied in the assessment of special populations, including students with learning disabilities, ADHD, intellectual/developmental disabilities, and giftedness. Special population studies are discussed in the test manual, as well as in books by Lichten-

berger and colleagues (Lichtenberger & Breaux, 2010; Lichtenberger & Smith, 2005). One of the primary benefits of the KTEA-II is that it can be used in tandem with the KABC-II to identify skill deficits and potential process deficits in children with learning difficulties. When an achievement measure like the KTEA-II is linked with a cognitive measure like the KABC-II, examiners can efficiently collect in-depth data that can help them test hypotheses, formulate a diagnosis, and make decisions about eligibility, as well as bridge the gap between assessment and intervention. The KTEA-II and the KABC-II were co-normed, and provide a cohesive theoretical basis for interpreting a comprehensive assessment battery.

Thus, to glean information about a wide spectrum of abilities within the CHC framework, examiners can integrate findings from the KTEA-II and KABC-II. As described earlier in the chapter, the KABC-II addresses five of the CHC broad abilities: short-term memory (Gsm), visual processing (Gv), long-term storage and retrieval (Glr), fluid reasoning (Gf), and crystallized ability (Gc). The KTEA-II Comprehensive Form measures three additional broad abilities: auditory processing (Ga), reading and writing (Grw), and quantitative knowledge (Gq). It also measures Glr narrow abilities that increase the breadth of the Glr narrow abilities measured by the KABC-II when the two batteries are administered together. Moreover, the KABC-II indirectly measures one of the Gq narrow abilities (i.e., mathematics achievement, by virtue of the fact that Rover and Block Counting each require a child to count). Publications by Flanagan and her colleagues describe CHC theory in depth, and provide more detail in test interpretation from that theoretical perspective (Flanagan, Ortiz, & Alfonso, 2007). Lichtenberger and Breaux (2010) provide a CHC-based analysis of each KABC-II and KTEA-II subtest that outlines the narrow CHC abilities measured by these tasks. This analysis is summarized below.

CHC Abilities Measured by KTEA-II and KABC-II Subtests

Long-Term Storage and Retrieval (Glr) Narrow Ability

Associative Memory

- KABC-II Atlantis
- KABC-II Rebus
- KABC-II Atlantis—Delayed
- KABC-II Rebus—Delayed

Learning Abilities

- KABC-II Atlantis—Delayed
- KABC-II Rebus—Delayed

Naming Facility

- KTEA-II Naming Facility (RAN)

Associational Fluency

- KTEA-II Associational Fluency (category items—e.g., foods, animals)

Word Fluency

- KTEA-II Associational Fluency (category items—e.g., words that start with the /d/ sound)

Meaningful Memory

- KTEA-II Listening Comprehension

Short-Term Memory (Gsm) Narrow Ability

Memory Span

- KABC-II Word Order (without color interference)
- KABC-II Number Recall
- KABC-II Hand Movements

Working Memory

- KABC-II Word Order (with color interference)

Note. Success on KTEA-II Phonological Awareness and Listening Comprehension is also dependent, to some extent, on Gsm.

Visual Processing (Gv) Narrow Ability

Visual Memory

- KABC-II Face Recognition
- KABC-II Hand Movements

Spatial Relations

- KABC-II Triangles

Visualization

- KABC-II Triangles
- KABC-II Conceptual Thinking
- KABC-II Block Counting

- KABC-II Pattern Reasoning
- KABC-II Story Completion

Spatial Scanning

- KABC-II Rover

Closure Speed

- KABC-II Gestalt Closure

Note. Success on KTEA-II Written Expression is also dependent, to some extent, on Visual Processing.

Fluid Reasoning (Gf) Narrow Ability

Induction

- KABC-II Conceptual Thinking
- KABC-II Pattern Reasoning
- KABC-II Story Completion

General Sequential Reasoning

- KABC-II Story Completion
- KABC-II Rover
- KABC-II Riddles

Quantitative Reasoning

- KTEA-II Math Concepts and Applications

Note. Success on KABC-II Rebus and four KTEA-II subtests (Reading Comprehension, Listening Comprehension, Oral Expression, and Written Expression) is also dependent, to some extent, on Fluid Reasoning.

Crystallized Ability (Gc) Narrow Ability

General Information

- KABC-II Verbal Knowledge (items that measure general information)
- KABC-II Story Completion

Language Development

- KABC-II Riddles

Lexical Knowledge

- KABC-II Riddles
- KABC-II Verbal Knowledge (items that measure vocabulary)

- KABC-II Expressive Vocabulary

Listening Ability

- KTEA-II Listening Comprehension

Oral Production and Fluency

- KTEA-II Oral Expression

Grammatical Sensitivity

- KTEA-II Oral Expression
- KTEA-II Written Expression

Note. Success on KABC-II Rebus is also dependent, to some extent, on Grammatical Sensitivity.

Auditory Processing (Ga) Narrow Ability

Phonetic Coding—Analysis

- KTEA-II Phonological Awareness (section 1, Rhyming; section 2, Sound Matching; section 4, Segmenting; section 5, Deleting Sounds)

Phonetic Coding—Synthesis

- KTEA-II Phonological Awareness (section 3, Blending)

Note. Deficits in certain Ga narrow abilities, such as Speech Sound Discrimination (US), may affect performance negatively on such tests as KABC-II Riddles, Word Order, and Number Recall, and KTEA-II Listening Comprehension.

Quantitative Knowledge (Gq) Narrow Ability

Mathematical Knowledge

- KTEA-II Math Concepts and Applications

Mathematical Achievement

- KTEA-II Math Computation
- KABC-II Rover
- KABC-II Block Counting

Reading and Writing (Grw) Narrow Ability

Reading Decoding

- KTEA-II Letter and Word Reading
- KTEA-II Nonsense Word Decoding

Reading Comprehension

- KTEA-II Reading Comprehension (paragraph items)

Verbal (Printed) Language Comprehension

- KTEA-II Reading Comprehension (items requiring student to do what a sentence says to do)

Spelling Ability

- KTEA-II Spelling

Writing Ability

- KTEA-II Written Expression

English Usage Knowledge

- KTEA-II Written Expression

Reading Speed

- KTEA-II Word Recognition Fluency
- KTEA-II Decoding Fluency

Recent Additional Research on the KTEA-II

A few recent investigations by Alan Kaufman, Xin Liu, and their colleagues with the KTEA-II provide additional information about the interpretation and clinical application of the KTEA-II.

- S. B. Kaufman, Liu, McGrew, and Kaufman (2010) conducted a study on *g*, or general intelligence, that examined the relationship between the well-known cognitive *g* and the *g* underlying achievement tests in the areas of reading, writing, and math. The KABC-II, KTEA-II Comprehensive Form, and WJ III (both COG and ACH) were studied for children, adolescents, and adults. Results for both the Kaufman tests and the WJ III indicated that the cognitive *g* and the achievement *g* correlated substantially, with the correlations generally increasing with increasing age (range of .78–.97). The two types of *g* were strongly related (but still distinct) in childhood, but demonstrated an especially close correspondence during the adolescent years of 13–19.

- Kaufman, Kaufman, Liu, and Johnson (2009) analyzed data from the adult portions of the

KTEA-II Brief Form and the Kaufman Brief Intelligence Test—Second Edition (KBIT-2; Kaufman & Kaufman, 2004b) for examinees ages 22–90 who were tested on both instruments (N = 555). They studied gender and education differences. In regard to gender, they found that females significantly outperformed males on the writing test (by 7.6 points), and that the reverse was true for the math test (4.2-point advantage for males), but no significant gender differences emerged for reading ability (or for fluid and crystallized intelligence as measured by the KBIT-2). Among academic skill areas, math had a significantly higher correlation with years of formal schooling (.63) than did either reading (.48) or writing (.49). As Kaufman and colleagues note, this finding makes sense because for reading and writing the skills needed to read and write efficiently are taught long before the end of high school. Math, however, is dependent on specific facts and concepts taught throughout one's formal schooling, including in the last few years of high school or in college.

• Using the same sample of 555 adults tested on the KTEA-II Brief Form and the KBIT-2, Kaufman, Johnson, and Liu (2008) studied age differences for nine age groups between 22–25 and 81–90 years, covarying educational attainment. Using multiple analysis of covariance, they found that reading ability was maintained through old age, but that math and writing were vulnerable to the effects of normal aging. (On the KBIT-2, consistent with previous research, crystallized intelligence was maintained and fluid intelligence was vulnerable.) Interestingly, when the reading decoding and reading comprehension portions of the KTEA-II Reading subtest were analyzed separately, the ability to read words was maintained through old age, but the ability to comprehend what one reads was vulnerable, decreasing with advancing age. Kaufman and colleagues point out an important clinical application of these findings—namely, that the maintenance of basic reading skills through old age supports the common practice of using word-reading tests to estimate premorbid ability in patients with neurological impairment, such as brain damage due to stroke or head injury.

KABC-II/KTEA-II ILLUSTRATIVE CASE STUDY

Name: Jessica T.
Age: 12 years, 3 months

Grade in school: 7
Evaluator: Jennie Kaufman Singer, PhD

Reason for Referral

Jessica was referred for a psychological evaluation by her mother, Mrs. T., who stated that Jessica has been struggling at school; she appears to have particular problems with reading comprehension. Jessica also exhibits difficulty following instructions at home and acts in an oppositional manner at times. In addition, Mrs. T. is concerned that Jessica tends to act angry and irritable much of the time, and seems to be depressed.

Evaluation Procedures

• Clinical interview with Jessica
• Collateral interview with Mrs. T.
• KABC-II
• KTEA-II, Comprehensive Form (Form A)
• Review of school records

Background Information

Mrs. T., a single mother, adopted Jessica when Jessica was 6 years old. Jessica's biological mother had a drug addiction; both Jessica and Jessica's younger sister (now age 9) were removed from the home by the Department of Social Services when the girls were ages 5 and 2. Jessica was living in a foster home when Mrs. T. adopted her. Jessica's biological mother did not show up to contest the adoption, nor did she respond to any attempt to reunite her family. Mrs. T. believes that Jessica may have been physically abused by her biological mother, but there is no evidence that Jessica was sexually abused. Another family that lives approximately 3 hours away from Mrs. T.'s home adopted Jessica's younger sister. Mrs. T. reported that she takes Jessica to visit her sister as frequently as possible, which is usually two to four times per year.

Jessica exhibited anger and behavioral problems for the first year that she lived with Mrs. T. By age 7, her behavior had calmed considerably, and she behaved in a generally compliant manner for several years. Mrs. T. described her home as "loving," and she said that spends her free time "doting on her daughter," including spending many volunteer hours at Jessica's school. Despite a "tight financial situation," Mrs. T. owns her own home, and the family owns two dogs and three cats. Mrs. T. described herself as being a fairly consistent and somewhat strict disciplinarian. She uses the removal or addition of privileges and treats to motivate her daughter to do her homework and to complete daily chores. Mrs. T. admitted that she yells at her daughter when she herself becomes overwhelmed. In the past year, Jessica has been talking back to her and refusing to do requested tasks. In addition, Jessica has told Mrs. T. that she feels "cheated" because she does not have a father. Her sister was adopted into a two-parent family—a fact that Jessica has brought up to Mrs. T. on many occasions. Mrs. T. reported that on one occasion she saw a scratch on Jessica's arm, and that Jessica admitted that she had made the mark herself with an opened safety pin when she felt "bored" and "upset."

Mrs. T. reported that Jessica, a seventh-grade student, has also been having difficulty at school. Her grades, usually B's and C's, have dropped in the past semester. She has received D's in physical education and in English, and her usual B in math has been lowered to a C–. Her teachers report that Jessica is frequently late for classes, and that she occasionally has cut one or more classes during the day. In general, her teachers report that she is very quiet and nonparticipatory in her classes.

Jessica admitted that she did not like school at times, and that she sometimes got into screaming fights with her mother. She described her mother as "bossy, but very nice." She said that her mother likes to sew dresses for her and was teaching her to sew. She stated that she was glad that she was adopted, but that she missed her sister a lot. She also stated that she felt sad a lot, but that she "hated" to talk about her feelings. She admitted that she did scratch her arm, and said that she did things to hurt herself "just a little" when she felt overwhelmed or upset. She denied any suicidal ideation in the past or at the current time.

At age 9, the school psychologist assessed Jessica because her teacher thought Jessica was depressed and not giving her best effort in school, even though she was earning adequate grades. The school psychologist reported that Jessica had "good self-esteem and good relationships with others." At that evaluation, Jessica was administered the WISC-IV, the WJ III ACH, and the Bender Visual–Motor Gestalt Test. Jessica earned WISC-IV index scores that were in the average range (Verbal Comprehension Index = 97, Perceptual Reasoning Index = 94, Working Memory Index = 95, and Processing Speed Index = 92). Her scaled scores were all within the average range. Scores on the WJ III ACH were basically consistent with her IQs: Broad Reading = 98 (45th percentile), Broad Mathematics = 112 (80th percentile), and Broad Written Language = 94 (34th percentile). On the Bender–Gestalt, Jessica earned a standard score of 83. She had difficulty with integration and a distortion of shape, mainly the angles. The school psychologist concluded that Jessica's achievement, as reflected in her WJ III scores and grades in school, was commensurate with her intellectual abilities.

Behavioral Observations

Jessica was carefully groomed and dressed for both of her testing sessions. She appeared slightly younger than her chronological age of 12. She is a slim and attractive girl, with straight, shoulder-length blonde hair and a shy smile. She was very quiet during the testing and did not talk unless spoken to. She tended to personalize some of the test questions. For example, during a Reading Comprehension task on the KTEA-II, she was asked how a woman lost her son. Jessica did not remember the correct answer, but stated, "She had to give her child up—like an orphan for adoption."

On many tasks, Jessica appeared to be unsure of answers. For example, on a task of written expression, she asked that all instructions be repeated two times. She erased many of her answers, then wrote, and sometimes erased them again before writing down her answer a third time. However, there were many tasks, such as one where she was asked to answer riddle-like questions, where she concentrated very hard and appeared very motivated and calm. On a task that involved using reasoning ability to complete patterns, she appeared calm, but changed her answers a few times. She was also persistent. On a task where she was asked to copy a picture with triangle-shaped pieces, she attempted all items offered, even if the task was clearly too hard. On a game-like task where she was asked to get a dog named Rover to his bone in the fewest moves possible, she answered a difficult item correctly after the allotted time had elapsed. On a task of verbal knowledge, she was willing to guess at an answer, even if she was clearly unsure whether the answer was correct. This kind of willingness to proceed when uncertain characterized her response style on virtually all tasks administered to her. On a sequential memory test, she whispered to herself during the time period when she had to remember what she had seen.

Test Results and Interpretation

Assessment of Cognitive Abilities

Jessica was administered the KABC-II, a comprehensive test of general cognitive abilities, to determine her overall level of functioning, as well as her profile of cognitive and processing abilities. The KABC-II permits the examiner to select the theoretical model that best fits assessment needs. The CHC model includes tests of acquired knowledge (crystallized ability), whereas the Luria model excludes such measures. Jessica was administered the CHC model of the KABC-II, the model of choice for children from mainstream backgrounds who have learning problems in school.

She earned a KABC-II FCI of 103, ranking her general cognitive ability at the 58th percentile and classifying it in the average range. The chances are 90% that her "true" FCI is within the 99–107 range. However, Jessica's performance on the individual scales that constitute the FCI was highly variable. Thus the FCI global score is not a very meaningful representation of her overall abilities, in light of the high degree of inconsistency among her KABC-II index scores. On the five KABC-II index scales, Jessica's standard scores ranged from a high of 120 (91st percentile, above average) on the Learning/Glr Index to a low of 88 on the Simultaneous/Gv Index (25th percentile, average range). An examination of her performance on these individual scales sheds more light on her unique abilities.

Jessica has personal relative strengths in her ability to learn new information, to store that information in long-term memory, and to retrieve it fluently and efficiently. These notable findings were apparent from her high standard score of 120 on the Learning/Glr scale because it is a personal strength as well as a normative strength (she performed better than 91% of other 12-year-olds). Her strong skills were exemplified on a subtest that required her to learn a new symbolic language efficiently. On this task, the examiner systematically taught her the words that corresponded to an array of abstract symbols. Importantly, she was also able to retain the new information over time, as she scored at a similarly high level on two supplementary delayed-recall tasks (standard score = 118, 88th percentile, above average) that measured her retention of newly learned material over a 20- to 25-minute interval. Her learning and long-term retrieval strengths are assets suggesting that she has the ability to perform at a higher level in her schoolwork than she is currently achieving. That conclusion is also supported by Jessica's relative strength in her planning (decision-making) abilities and her fluid reasoning abilities. She has a strong ability to be adaptable and flexible when drawing inferences and understanding implications to solve novel (not school-related) problems.

For example, Jessica was able to easily "fill in" the missing pictures in a story so that the complete sequence of pictures told a meaningful story. Jessica's relative personal strength in planning and reasoning was evident from her KABC-II Planning/Gf Index (111, 77th percentile, average range).

In contrast to Jessica's areas of cognitive strength, she has relative significant weaknesses in her ability to process information visually, and in her short-term memory abilities (when stimuli are presented in sequential fashion). She surpassed only 25% of other 12-year-olds in her visual processing skills—that is, in her ability to perceive, manipulate, and think with visual patterns and stimuli, and to mentally rotate objects in space (KABC-II Simultaneous/Gv standard score = 90). For example, she had difficulty assembling triangular blocks to match a picture of an abstract design; even when she was able to construct some of the more difficult designs correctly, she received no credit because she did not solve them within the time limit. Similarly, Jessica's relative weakness in visual processing was consistent with the difficulties she had on the Bender–Gestalt design-copying test at age 9 (standard score of 83; 13th percentile).

Denoting an additional personal relative weakness in her ability to take in information, hold it in immediate awareness briefly, and then use that information within a few seconds (before it is forgotten), Jessica performed better than only 34% of her age-mates on tasks of short-term memory (Sequential/Gsm Index = 94, average range). She had difficulty, for example, pointing in the correct order to pictures of common objects that were named by the examiner; as noted, she whispered to herself as an aid to recall the stimuli, but this compensatory technique could not be used for the more difficult items that incorporated an interference task (Jessica had to name colors rapidly before pointing to the sequence of pictures, so whispering was not possible), and she failed virtually all of the hard items.

Jessica's two areas of relative weakness (visual processing and short-term memory) are nonetheless within the average range compared to other 12-year-olds, and are not causes for special concern. However, one test result should be followed up with additional testing: She had unusual difficulty on a supplementary KABC-II subtest that requires *both* visual processing and short-term memory—a task that required Jessica to imitate a sequence of hand movements performed by the examiner. On that subtest, she only got the first series of three movements correct and missed all subsequent items, despite good concentration and effort. Her performance at the 1st percentile was well below the average for children her age, and also well below her scaled scores on the other 15 KABC-II subtests that were administered to her (all classifying her ability as average or above average).

In addition to her areas of cognitive strength and weakness, Jessica has average crystallized ability, which reflects her breadth and depth of specific knowledge acquired within a culture, as well as her ability to apply this knowledge effectively. Her KABC-II Knowledge/Gc Index of 100 (50th percentile) is also a measure of verbal ability, and this score is consistent with the average-level WISC-IV Verbal Comprehension Index of 97 that she earned at age 9. Similarly, her WISC-IV Perceptual Reasoning Index of 94, which is primarily a measure of visual processing, resembles her score of 88 on the KABC-II Simultaneous/Gv Index. Her WISC-IV Working Memory Index of 95 was also consistent with her KABC-II Sequential/Gsm Index score of 94. Unlike the WISC-IV, the KABC-II does not explicitly measure processing speed. It is notable that Jessica's best abilities on the KABC-II (learning abilities) are not measured in any depth on the WISC-IV.

Assessment of Achievement

To assess her current level of academic achievement, Jessica was individually administered a standardized test (the KTEA-II), and her academic abilities were compared to those of other children her age. On the KTEA-II Comprehensive Form, Jessica scored in the average range on all composite areas of achievement, ranging from a standard score of 104 (61st percentile) on the Math Composite to a standard score of 90 (25th percentile) on the Reading Composite. Her Reading Composite is a relative weakness for her, with her lowest performance on the test of Reading Comprehension (19th percentile), consistent with Mrs. T.'s specific concerns about Jessica's academic achievement. Neither Jessica's Oral Language Composite of 99 (47th percentile) nor her Written Language Composite of 102 (55th percentile) can be meaningfully interpreted because of notable variability in her scores on the subtests within each of these composites. Within the domain of Oral Language, Jessica performed significantly better in her ability to express her ideas in words (Oral Expression = 79th percentile) than in her ability to understand

what is said to her (Listening Comprehension = 21st percentile). Regarding Written Language, Jessica's performance in spelling words spoken by the examiner (Spelling = 82nd percentile) was significantly higher than her performance in expressing her ideas in writing (Written Expression = 27th percentile).

Both the Reading Comprehension and Listening Comprehension subtests measure understanding of passages via different methods of presentation (printed vs. oral). Her performance was comparable on both subtests (standard scores of 87–88), indicating that she performed at the lower end of the average range in her ability to take in information, whether by reading or listening. The KTEA-II error analysis (presented at the end of this report) showed that Jessica displayed weakness on *both* the Reading Comprehension and Listening Comprehension subtests on those items measuring *literal* comprehension—questions that require a response containing explicitly stated information from a story. In contrast, on both comprehension subtests, she performed at an average level on items requiring *inferential* comprehension—questions that require a student to use reasoning to respond correctly (e.g., to deduce the central thought of a passage, make an inference about the content of the passage, or recognize the tone and mood of the passage). The results of the error analysis are consistent with the KABC-II cognitive findings: Jessica has a strength in fluid reasoning and a weakness in short-term memory. Her difficulty with literal items relates directly to her relative weakness in short-term memory, whereas her ability to respond better to inferential items suggests that she is able to apply an area of strength (fluid reasoning) to enhance her performance on tasks that are more difficult for her (i.e., understanding what she reads and hears).

In contrast to the variability on some achievement composites, Jessica performed consistently on the Math Computation and Math Concepts and Applications subtests (58th and 68th percentiles, respectively). In addition, Jessica's scores on all KTEA-II subtests (range = 87–114) are all in the average to above-average range; they are also entirely consistent with her cognitive abilities as measured by the WISC-IV when she was 9 years old, and by the KABC-II during the present evaluation. She displayed wide variability in both the ability and achievement domains, but when her performance is viewed as a whole, she is achieving at the level that would be expected from her cognitive abilities.

Her present KTEA-II achievement scores are also commensurate with her WJ III ACH scores at age 9 (range of 94–112 on composites). Therefore, even her achievement on measures of Reading Comprehension, Listening Comprehension, and Written Expression (standard scores of 87–91) is not a cause for concern. However, the notable cognitive strengths that she displayed on measures of learning ability and fluid reasoning should be relied on to help her improve her academic achievement in her areas of relative weakness; in any case, she has too much ability to be earning grades such as her recent D in English or C– in math. Specific kinds of errors that Jessica made during the administration of the KTEA-II are listed in the error analysis at the end of this report. The categories listed as weaknesses suggest specific content areas to be targeted.

Diagnostic Impressions

Axis I: 300.4 (dysthymic disorder)
Axis II: None
Axis III: None
Axis IV: Adoption issues resurfacing at adolescence
Axis V: Global Assessment of Functioning (GAF) = 75

Summary

Jessica, a 12-year-old in the seventh grade, was referred for evaluation by her mother, Mrs. T., who has concerns about Jessica's reading comprehension, oppositional behavior, anger, irritability, and possible depression. During the evaluation, Jessica was quiet, persistent, and attentive. Although often unsure of her answers, she tried to answer virtually all items presented to her. She displayed considerable variability in her cognitive profile, which rendered Jessica's overall score on the KABC-II's FCI (103; 58th percentile, average range) as merely the midpoint of a set of diverse scores (see Table 11.5). She demonstrated cognitive strengths in the following areas: her learning ability and long-term retrieval, and her planning ability and fluid reasoning. She showed relative weaknesses in visual processing and short-term memory. However, these areas of relative weakness were in the average range of ability, and are not areas of particular concern. On the KTEA-II (see Table 11.6), she performed in the average range on all achievement composites (ranging from 90 on Reading to 104 on Mathematics). However, she

TABLE 11.5. Jessica's Scores on the KABC-II (CHC Model Interpretation)

Scale	Index (mean = 100, SD = 15)	Percentile rank
Learning/Glr	120	91st
Sequential/Gsm	94	34th
Simultaneous/Gv	88	25th
Planning/Gf	111	77th
Knowledge/Gc	100	50th
Fluid–Crystallized Index (FCI)	**103**	**58th**

displayed relative weaknesses on tests of Reading Comprehension, Listening Comprehension, and Written Expression. Her cognitive abilities and achievement are commensurate with each other, and her relative weaknesses in academic and cognitive domains are not of special concern because they are all in the average range. Nonetheless, she can improve her achievement if she is shown how to use her cognitive strengths to facilitate school learning.

TABLE 11.6. Jessica's Scores on the KTEA-II, Comprehensive Form, Form A

Scale	Standard score	Percentile rank
Reading Composite	90	25th
Letter and Word Recognition	94	34th
Reading Comprehension	87	19th
(Nonsense Word Decoding)	(93)	(32nd)
Mathematics Composite	104	61st
Mathematics Concepts and Applications	107	68th
Mathematics Computation	103	58th
Oral Language Composite	99	47th
Listening Comprehension	88	21st
Oral Expression	112	79th
Written Language Composite	102	55th
Written Expression	91	27th
Spelling	114	82nd

Note. Nonsense Word Decoding appears in parentheses because it is a supplementary subtest that does not contribute to the reading composite.

Recommendations

1. Jessica will benefit from understanding her cognitive strengths and weaknesses, and learning how to use these strengths to help her to be more successful in school. A particularly pertinent and practical source is *Helping Children Learn: Intervention Handouts for Use in School and at Home* (Naglieri & Pickering, 2010).

2. Jessica would benefit from utilizing coping mechanisms in order to help her overcome her cognitive weaknesses. Many examples of coping mechanisms could be recommended. She could write notes while listening to a lecture or when reading a textbook, making sure to capture key words and phrases that she may be called upon to remember verbatim. Whenever information is presented in a sequential fashion, Jessica would benefit from making notes in order to restructure the material into a more holistic or Gestalt-oriented presentation, so that the material is more easily accessible to her learning style. She could benefit from a tutor or learning specialist in order to help her to learn how certain kinds of note-taking skills and figure drawing can help her to overcome deficits in sequential processing and in literal reading and listening comprehension. Finally, working with a tutor or learning specialist could help Jessica to improve her writing skills. This area is extremely important, as her areas of strength in learning ability, planning ability, and problem solving will be put to better use if Jessica is able to put her knowledge in writing.

3. Jessica would benefit from further testing that would focus more on her current intrapsychic issues. Instruments such as the Rorschach, the Minnesota Multiphasic Personality Inventory for Adolescents (MMPI-A), the Thematic Apperception Test (TAT), and self-report questionnaires would yield important information regarding her interpersonal issues, as well as further diagnostic input.

4. Jessica would benefit from individual therapy at this time. As she is reluctant to talk openly at first, the therapist would benefit from the results of the personality tests mentioned above. The therapist could focus on adoption issues, adolescent issues, and skill building in the areas of modulating emotions in an appropriate manner, communication, and exploring the causes of her anger. In addition, it is important that Jessica's self-injurious behavior be examined and stopped from progressing into potential suicide attempts.

5. Mrs. T. would benefit from counseling to help support her as a single parent during this difficult time. In addition, a counselor could help her with anger management and parenting skills for the adolescent.

6. Family therapy may be indicated, if Jessica's individual therapist is in agreement.

7. It is recommended that Jessica be referred to a child psychiatrist in order to evaluate a possible need for medication.

KTEA-II Error Analysis

Jessica's responses on several KTEA-II subtests were further examined to identify possible specific strengths and weaknesses. First, her errors on each subtest were totaled according to skill categories. Then the number of errors Jessica made in each skill category was compared to the average number of errors made by the standardization sample students, similar in age, who attempted the same items. As a result, Jessica's performance in each skill category could be rated as strong, average, or weak. *Illustrative* diagnostic information obtained from Jessica's error analysis is summarized below.

Letter and Word Recognition

The following skill category was identified as a strength for Jessica:

- *Prefixes and word beginnings.* Common prefixes such as *in-, un-, pre-*; Greek and Latin morphemes used as word beginnings, such as *micro-, hyper-, penta-*. Examples: *progressive, hemisphere.*

The following skill category was identified as a weakness for Jessica:

- *Consonant blends.* Common blends that occur in the initial, medial, and final positions of words, such as *bl, st, nd, sw*. Examples: *blast, mist, send, swipe.*

Reading Comprehension

The following skill category was identified as a weakness for Jessica:

- *Literal comprehension items.* Questions that require a response containing explicitly stated information from a story. Examples: "Who is the story about? What is the animal doing? Where are the kids going?"

Nonsense Word Decoding

The following skill categories were identified as weaknesses for Jessica:

- *Vowel diphthongs.* The vowel sound in a diphthong is made by gliding or changing continuously from one vowel sound to another in the same syllable. Examples: *doubt, how, oil.*
- *Consonant–le conditional rule.* The final *e* of the consonant–*le* pattern corresponds to a schwa sound directly preceding an /l/ sound. Examples: *bumble, apple, couple, trouble.*

Math Concepts and Applications

The following skill category was identified as a strength for Jessica:

- *Geometry, shape, and space.* Problems involving geometric formulas, shapes, or computing the space contained within them. Example: "Determine the length of the diameter of a circle, given the radius."

Listening Comprehension

The following skill category was identified as a weakness for Jessica:

- *Literal comprehension items.* Questions that require a response containing explicitly stated information from a story. Examples: "Who is the story about? What is the person doing? What happened at the end of the story?"

REFERENCES

Bain, S. K., & Gray, R. (2008). Test reviews: Kaufman, A. S., & Kaufman, N. L. (2004). Kaufman Assessment Battery for Children, Second Edition. Circle Pines, MN: AGS. *Journal of Psychoeducational Assessment, 26,* 92–101.

Carroll, J. B. (1943). The factorial representation of mental ability and academic achievement. *Educational and Psychological Measurement, 3,* 307–332.

Carroll, J. B. (1993). *Human cognitive abilities: A survey of factor analytic studies.* New York: Cambridge University Press.

Carrow-Woolfolk, E. (1996). *Oral and written language scales.* Circle Pines, MN: American Guidance Service.

Cattell, R. B. (1941). The measurement of adult intelligence. *Psychological Bulletin, 40,* 153–193.

Dale, B. A. (2009). *Profile analysis of the Kaufman Assessment Battery for Children, Second Edition with African American and Caucasian preschool children.* Unpublished doctoral dissertation, Ball State University.

Flanagan, D. P., McGrew, K. S., & Ortiz, S. (2000). *The Wechsler intelligence scales and Gf-Gc theory: A contemporary approach to interpretation.* Boston: Allyn & Bacon.

Flanagan, D. P., & Ortiz, S. O. (2001). *Essentials of cross-battery assessment.* New York: Wiley.

Flanagan, D. P., Ortiz, S. O., & Alfonso, V. C. (2007). *Essentials of cross-battery assessment* (2nd ed.). Hoboken, NJ: Wiley.

Fletcher-Janzen, E. (2003, August). Neuropsychologically-based interpretations of the KABC-II. In M. H. Daniel (Chair), *KABC-II: Theory, content, and interpretation.* Symposium presented at the annual meeting of the American Psychological Association, Toronto.

Gomez, M. T. (2008). *The performance evaluation of low achieving Mexican American students on the Kaufman Assessment Battery for Children II (KABC-II): The role of English language proficiency.* Unpublished doctoral dissertation, Capella University.

Horn, J. L. (1968). Organization of abilities and the development of intelligence. *Psychological Review, 75,* 242–259.

Horn, J. L. (1985). Remodeling old models of intelligence. In B. B. Wolman (Ed.), *Handbook of intelligence: Theories, measurements, and applications* (pp. 267–300). New York: Wiley.

Horn, J. L. (1989). Cognitive diversity: A framework of learning. In P. L. Ackerman, R. J. Sternberg, & R. Glaser (Eds.), *Learning and individual differences* (pp. 61–116). New York: Freeman.

Horn, J. L., & Hofer, S. M. (1992). Major abilities and development in the adult period. In R. J. Sternberg & C. A. Berg (Eds.), *Intellectual development* (pp. 44–99). New York: Cambridge University Press.

Horn, J. L., & Noll, J. (1997). Human cognitive capabilities: Gf-Gc theory. In D. P. Flanagan, J. L. Genshaft, & P. L. Harrison (Eds.), *Contemporary intellectual assessment: Theories, tests, and issues* (pp. 53–91). New York: Guilford Press.

Hunt, M. S. (2008). A joint confirmatory factor analysis of the Kaufman Assessment Battery for Children, Second Edition, and the Woodcock–Johnson Tests of Cognitive Abilities, Third Edition, with preschool children (Doctoral dissertation, Ball State University, 2008). *Dissertation Abstracts International, 68*(11), 4605A.

Kaufman, A. S., Johnson, C. K., & Liu, X. (2008). A CHC theory-based analysis of age differences on cognitive abilities and academic skills at ages 22 to 90 years. *Journal of Psychoeducational Assessment, 26,* 350–381.

Kaufman, A. S., Kaufman, J. C., Liu, X., & Johnson, C. K. (2009). How do educational attainment and gender relate to Gf, Gc, and academic skills at ages 22 to 90 years? *Archives of Clinical Neuropsychology, 24,* 153–163.

Kaufman, A. S., & Kaufman, N. L. (1983). *K-ABC interpretive manual.* Circle Pines, MN: American Guidance Service.

Kaufman, A. S., & Kaufman, N. L. (1993). *Kaufman Adolescent and Adult Intelligence Test (KAIT).* Circle Pines, MN: American Guidance Service.

Kaufman, A. S., & Kaufman, N. L. (2004a). *Manual for the Kaufman Assessment Battery for Children—Second Edition (KABC-II),* Circle Pines, MN: American Guidance Service.

Kaufman, A. S., & Kaufman, N. L. (2004b). *Manual for the Kaufman Brief Intelligence Test—Second Edition (KBIT-2).* Circle Pines, MN: American Guidance Service.

Kaufman, A. S., & Kaufman, N. L. (2004c). *Manual for the Kaufman Test of Educational Achievement—Second Edition (KTEA-II), Comprehensive Form.* Circle Pines, MN: American Guidance Service.

Kaufman, A. S., & Kaufman, N. L. (2005). *Manual for the Kaufman Test of Educational Achievement—Second Edition (KTEA-II), Brief Form.* Circle Pines, MN: American Guidance Service.

Kaufman, A. S., Lichtenberger, E. O., Fletcher-Janzen, E., & Kaufman, N. L. (2005). *Essentials of KABC-II assessment.* New York: Wiley.

Kaufman, J. C. (2003, August). Gender and ethnic differences on the KABC-II. In M. H. Daniel (Chair), *The KABC-II: Theory, content, and administration.* Symposium presented at the annual meeting of the American Psychological Association, Toronto.

Kaufman, S. B., Liu, X., McGrew, K., & Kaufman, A. S. (2010, August). *What is the relation between Cognitive g and Academic Achievement g?* Paper presented at the annual meeting of the American Psychological Association, San Diego, CA.

Keith, T. Z. (1985). Questioning the K-ABC: What does it measure? *School Psychology Review, 14,* 9–20.

Lichtenberger, E. O., & Breaux, K. C. (2010). *Essentials of WIAT-III and KTEA-II assessment.* Hoboken, NJ: Wiley.

Lichtenberger, E. O., & Smith, D. R. (2005). *Essentials of WIAT-II and KTEA-II assessment.* Hoboken, NJ: Wiley.

Luria, A. R. (1966). *Human brain and psychological processes.* New York: Harper & Row.

Luria, A. R. (1970). The functional organization of the brain. *Scientific American, 222,* 66–78.

Luria, A. R. (1973). *The working brain: An introduction to neuropsychology.* Harmondsworth, UK: Penguin.

Malda, M., van de Vijver, F. J. R., Srinivasan, K., Transler, C., & Sukumar, P. (2010). Traveling with cognitive tests: Testing the validity of a KABC-II adaptation in India. *Assessment, 17,* 107–115.

Markwardt, F. C., Jr. (1998) *Peabody Individual Achievement Test, Revised* (Normative Update). Circle Pines, MN: American Guidance Service.

McLean, J. E. (1995). *Improving education through action research: A guide for administrators and teachers.* Thousand Oaks, CA: Corwin Press.

Morgan, K. E., Rothlisberg, B. A., McIntosh, D. E., & Hunt, M. S. (2009). Confirmatory factor analysis of the KABC-II in preschool children. *Psychology in the Schools, 46,* 515–525.

Naglieri, J. A., & Das, J. P. (1997). *Das–Naglieri Cognitive Assessment System (CAS).* Itasca, IL: Riverside.

Naglieri, J. A., & Pickering, E. B. (2010). *Helping children learn: Intervention handouts for use in school and at home* (2nd ed.). Baltimore: Brookes.

Prifitera, A., Weiss, L. G., & Saklofske, D. H. (1998). The WISC-III in context. In A. Prifitera & D. H. Saklofske (Eds.), *WISC-III clinical use and interpretation* (pp. 1–38). San Diego, CA: Academic Press.

Prifitera, A., Weiss, L. G., Saklofske, D. H., & Rolfhus, E. (2005). The WISC-IV in the clinical assessment context. In A. Prifitera, D. H. Saklofske, & L. G. Weiss (Eds.), *WISC-IV clinical use and interpretation* (pp. 3–32). San Diego, CA: Academic Press.

Psychological Corporation. (2001). *Wechsler Individual Achievement Test—Second Edition.* San Antonio, TX: Author.

Reitan, R. M. (1988). Integration of neuropsychological theory, assessment, and application. *Clinical Neuropsychologist, 2,* 331–349.

Reynolds, M. R., & Keith, T. Z. (2007). Spearman's law of diminishing returns in hierarchical models of intelligence for children and adolescents. *Intelligence, 35,* 267–281.

Reynolds, M. R., Keith, T. Z., Fine, J. G., Fisher, M. E., & Low, J. (2007). Confirmatory factor structure of the Kaufman Assessment Battery for Children—Second Edition: Consistency with Cattell–Horn–Carroll theory. *School Psychology Quarterly, 22,* 511–539.

Reynolds, M. R., Ridley, K. P., & Patel, P. G. (2008). Sex differences in latent general and broad cognitive abilities for children and youth: Evidence from higher-order MG-MACS and MIMIC Models. *Intelligence, 26,* 236–260.

Spearman, C. (1904). "General intelligence," objectively determined and measured. *American Journal of Psychology, 15,* 201–293.

Vannetzel, L. (2010). Le KABC-II. *Approche Neuropsychologique des Apprentissages Chez l'Enfant, 107–108,* 231–234.

Wechsler, D. (1991). *Wechsler Intelligence Scale for Children—Third Edition.* New York: Psychological Corporation.

Wechsler, D. (2002). *Wechsler Preschool and Primary Scale of Intelligence—Third Edition.* San Antonio, TX: Psychological Corporation.

Wechsler, D. (2003). *Wechsler Intelligence Scale for Children—Fourth Edition.* San Antonio, TX: Psychological Corporation.

Wechsler, D. (2008). *Wechsler Adult Intelligence Scale—Fourth Edition.* San Antonio, TX: Pearson.

Woodcock, R. W., McGrew, K. S., & Mather, N. (2001). *Woodcock–Johnson III.* Itasca, IL: Riverside.

CHAPTER 12

The Woodcock–Johnson III Normative Update
Tests of Cognitive Abilities and Tests of Achievement

Fredrick A. Schrank
Barbara J. Wendling

The Woodcock–Johnson III Normative Update (WJ III NU) (Woodcock, McGrew, Schrank, & Mather, 2001, 2007) is the current version of the Woodcock–Johnson III (WJ III) (Woodcock, McGrew, & Mather, 2001, 2007a). The WJ III NU includes a recalculation of normative data for the tests that are contained in, and clusters that are derived from, the WJ III Tests of Cognitive Abilities (WJ III COG; Woodcock, McGrew, & Mather, 2001, 2007c) and the WJ III Tests of Achievement (WJ III ACH; Woodcock, McGrew, & Mather, 2001, 2007b). Some of the tests are appropriate for individuals as young as 24 months; all of the tests can be used with individuals from 5 to 95 years of age.

The cognitive part of the WJ III (the acronyms WJ III and WJ III NU are used interchangeably throughout this chapter) includes 31 tests for measuring general intellectual ability, broad and narrow cognitive abilities, and related aspects of cognitive functioning. The WJ III COG includes 20 tests. Two easels house the Standard Battery (tests 1–10) and the Extended Battery (tests 11–20). The WJ III Diagnostic Supplement to the Tests of Cognitive Abilities (DS; Woodcock, McGrew, Mather, & Schrank, 2003, 2007) includes an additional 11 cognitive tests. Each of the 31 cognitive tests measures one or more narrow, or specific, abilities as

informed by the independent research efforts of Horn (1965, 1988, 1989, 1991), Horn and Stankov (1982), Cattell (1941, 1943, 1950), and Carroll (1987, 1990, 1993, 2003; see also the Appendix to this volume). Each of the tests can also be thought of as measuring a narrow aspect of a broad cognitive ability, or domain of intellectual functioning. Table 12.1 identifies the broad and narrow cognitive abilities measured by each test in the WJ III COG; it also includes brief test descriptions. The WJ III COG tests are organized into clusters for interpretive purposes; these clusters are outlined in Table 12.2.

The WJ III ACH includes 22 tests for measuring five academic domains: reading, written language, mathematics, oral language, and academic knowledge. There are two parallel, full-version forms (Form A and Form B) of the WJ III ACH; each form includes two easels. There is a third form of nine of the most commonly used reading, writing, and mathematics tests: the WJ III ACH Form C/Brief Battery (Woodcock, Schrank, Mather, & McGrew, 2007). Table 12.3 identifies the abilities measured by each test in the WJ III ACH; it also includes brief test descriptions. The WJ III ACH tests are organized into clusters for interpretive purposes; these clusters are outlined in Table 12.4.

TABLE 12.1. WJ III COG and DS Tests, CHC Broad and Narrow Abilities Measured, and Brief Test Descriptions

Test name	CHC broad/narrow abilities measured[a]	Brief test description
Test 1: Verbal Comprehension	Comprehension–knowledge (Gc) *Lexical knowledge* (VL) *Language development* (LD)	Measures aspects of language development in English, such as knowledge of vocabulary or the ability to reason using lexical (word) knowledge.
Test 2: Visual–Auditory Learning	Long-term retrieval (Glr) *Associative memory* (MA)	Measures the ability to learn, store, and retrieve a series of rebuses (pictographic representations of words).
Test 3: Spatial Relations	Visual–spatial thinking (Gv) *Visualization* (VZ) *Spatial relations* (SR)	Measures the ability to identify the two or three pieces that form a complete target shape.
Test 4: Sound Blending	Auditory processing (Ga) *Phonetic coding* (PC)	Measures skill in synthesizing language sounds (phonemes) through the process of listening to a series of syllables or phonemes and then blending the sounds into a word.
Test 5: Concept Formation	Fluid reasoning (Gf) *Induction* (I)	Measures categorical reasoning ability and flexibility in thinking.
Test 6: Visual Matching	Processing speed (Gs) *Perceptual speed* (P)	Measures speed in making visual symbol discriminations.
Test 7: Numbers Reversed	Short-term memory (Gsm) *Working memory capacity* (WM)	Measures the capacity to hold a span of numbers in immediate awareness (memory) while performing a mental operation on it (reversing the sequence).
Test 8: Incomplete Words	Auditory processing (Ga) *Phonetic coding* (PC)	Measures auditory analysis and auditory closure, aspects of phonemic awareness, and phonetic coding.
Test 9: Auditory Working Memory	Short-term memory (Gsm) *Working memory capacity* (WM)	Measures the capacity to hold information in immediate awareness, divide the information into two groups, and provide two new ordered sequences.
Test 10: Visual–Auditory Learning—Delayed	Long-term retrieval (Glr) *Associative memory* (MA)	Measures ease of relearning a previously learned task.
Test 11: General Information	Comprehension–knowledge (Gc) *Verbal information* (V)	Measures general verbal knowledge.
Test 12: Retrieval Fluency	Long-term retrieval (Glr) *Ideational fluency* (FI)	Measures fluency of retrieval from stored knowledge.
Test 13: Picture Recognition	Visual–spatial thinking (Gv) *Visual memory* (MV)	Measures visual memory of objects or pictures.
Test 14: Auditory Attention	Auditory processing (Ga) *Speech sound discrimination* (US) *Resistance to auditory stimulus distortion* (UR)	Measures the ability to overcome the effects of auditory distortion in discrimination of speech sounds.
Test 15: Analysis–Synthesis	Fluid reasoning (Gf) *General sequential reasoning* (RG)	Measures the ability to reason and draw conclusions from given conditions (or deductive reasoning).
Test 16: Decision Speed	Processing speed (Gs) *Semantic processing speed* (R4)	Measures the ability to make correct conceptual decisions quickly.

(cont.)

TABLE 12.1. *(cont.)*

Test name	CHC broad/narrow abilities measured[a]	Brief test description
Test 17: Memory for Words	Short-term memory (Gsm) *Memory span* (MS)	Measures short-term auditory memory span.
Test 18: Rapid Picture Naming	Processing speed (Gs) *Naming facility* (NA)	Measures speed of direct recall of names from acquired knowledge.
Test 19: Planning	Visual–spatial thinking (Gv)/fluid reasoning (Gf) *Spatial scanning* (SS) *General sequential reasoning* (RG)	Measures use of forethought to determine, select, or apply solutions to a series of problems presented as visual puzzles.
Test 20: Pair Cancellation	Processing speed (Gs) *Attention and concentration* (AC)	Measures the ability to control interferences, sustain attention, and stay on task in a vigilant manner by locating and marking a repeated pattern as quickly as possible.
Test 21: Memory for Names	Long-term retrieval (Glr) *Associative memory* (MA)	Measures ability to learn associations between unfamiliar auditory and visual stimuli.
Test 22: Visual Closure	Visual–spatial thinking (Gv) *Closure speed* (CS)	Measures the ability to identify a picture of an object from a partial drawing or representation.
Test 23: Sound Patterns—Voice	Auditory processing (Ga) *Sound discrimination* (U3)	Measures speech sound discrimination (whether pairs of complex voice-like sound patterns, differing in pitch, rhythm, or sound content, are the same or different).
Test 24: Number Series	Fluid reasoning (Gf) *Quantitative reasoning* (RQ)	Measures the ability to reason with concepts that depend upon mathematical relationships by completing sequences of numbers.
Test 25: Number Matrices	Fluid reasoning (Gf) *Quantitative reasoning* (RQ)	Measures quantitative reasoning ability by completing two-dimensional displays of numbers.
Test 26: Cross Out	Processing speed (Gs) *Perceptual speed* (P)	Measures the ability to scan and compare visual information quickly.
Test 27: Memory for Sentences	Short-term memory (Gsm) *Auditory memory span* (MS) *Listening ability* (LS)	Measures the ability to remember and repeat single words, phrases, and sentences.
Test 28: Block Rotation	Visual–spatial thinking (Gv) *Visualization* (Vz) *Spatial relations* (SR)	Measures the ability to view a three-dimensional pattern of blocks and then identify the two sets of blocks that match the pattern, even though their spatial orientation is rotated.
Test 29: Sound Patterns—Music	Auditory processing (Ga) *Sound discrimination* (U3)	Measures the ability to indicate whether pairs of musical patterns are the same or different.
Test 30: Memory for Names—Delayed	Long-term retrieval (Glr) *Associative memory* (MA)	Measures the ability to recall associations that were learned earlier.
Test 31: Bilingual Verbal Comprehension— English/Spanish	Comprehension–knowledge (Gc) *Lexical knowledge* (VL) *Language development* (LD)	Measures aspects of language development in Spanish, such as knowledge of vocabulary or the ability to reason using lexical (word) knowledge.

[a]Full names of narrow abilities are given in italics.

TABLE 12.2. WJ III COG and DS Clusters and Brief Cluster Descriptions

Cluster	Brief cluster description
General Intellectual Ability (GIA)	A measure of psychometric *g*. Selected and different mixes of narrow cognitive abilities constitute the GIA—Standard, GIA—Extended, GIA—Early Development, and GIA—Bilingual scales.
Broad Cognitive Ability— Low Verbal	A special-purpose, broad measure of cognitive ability that has relatively low overall receptive and expressive verbal requirements.
Brief Intellectual Ability	A brief measure of intelligence consisting of three tests measuring acquired knowledge, reasoning, and cognitive efficiency.
Verbal Ability	Higher-order language-based acquired knowledge and the ability to communicate that knowledge.
Thinking Ability	A sampling of four different thinking processes (long-term retrieval, visual–spatial thinking, auditory processing, and fluid reasoning).
Cognitive Efficiency	A sampling of two different automatic cognitive processes—processing speed and short-term memory.
Comprehension– Knowledge (Gc)	The breadth and depth of a person's acquired knowledge, the ability to communicate this knowledge (especially verbally), and the ability to reason using previously learned experiences or procedures.
Long-Term Retrieval (Glr)	The ability to store information and fluently retrieve it later.
Visual–Spatial Thinking (Gv)	The ability to perceive, analyze, synthesize, and think with visual patterns, including the ability to store and recall visual representations.
Auditory Processing (Ga)	The ability to analyze, synthesize, and discriminate auditory stimuli, including the ability to process and discriminate speech sounds that may be presented under distorted conditions.
Fluid Reasoning (Gf)	The ability to reason, form concepts, and solve problems using unfamiliar information or novel procedures.
Processing Speed (Gs)	The ability to perform automatic cognitive tasks, an aspect of cognitive efficiency.
Short-Term Memory (Gsm)	The ability to apprehend and hold information in immediate awareness and then use it within a few seconds.
Phonemic Awareness (PC)	The ability to attend to the sound structure of language through analyzing and synthesizing speech sounds (phonetic coding).
Working Memory (WM)	Capacity to hold information in immediate awareness while performing a mental operation on the information.
Numerical Reasoning (RQ)	The ability to reason with mathematical concepts involving the relationships and properties of numbers.
Associative Memory (MA)	The ability to store and retrieve associations.
Visualization (Vz)	The ability to envision objects or patterns in space by perceiving how they would appear if presented in an altered form.
Sound Discrimination (U3)	The ability to distinguish between pairs of voice-like or musical patterns.
Auditory Memory Span (MS)	The ability to listen to a presentation of sequentially ordered information and then recall the sequence immediately.
Perceptual Speed (P)	The ability to rapidly scan and compare visual symbols.
Broad Attention	A global measure of the cognitive components of attention.
Cognitive Fluency	A measure of cognitive automaticity, or the speed with which an individual performs simple to complex cognitive tasks.
Executive Processes	Measures selected aspects of central executive functions, such as response inhibition, cognitive flexibility, and planning.
Delayed Recall	Measures the ability to recall and relearn previously presented information.
Knowledge	Measures general information and curricular knowledge.

TABLE 12.3. WJ III ACH Tests, Related Curricular Areas and CHC Narrow Abilities Measured, and Brief Test Descriptions

Test name	Curricular area/CHC narrow abilities measured[a]	Brief test description
Test 1: Letter–Word Identification	Reading *Reading decoding*	Measures oral word reading (identifying and reading isolated letters and words).
Test 2: Reading Fluency	Reading *Reading speed* *Semantic processing speed*	Measures quick comprehension of simple sentences.
Test 3: Story Recall	Oral expression *Meaningful memory* *Listening ability*	Measures the ability to listen to passages and retell story elements.
Test 4: Understanding Directions	Listening comprehension *Verbal working memory* *Listening ability*	Measures the ability to listen to a series of instructions and point to objects in order.
Test 5: Calculation	Mathematics *Math achievement*	Measures calculation of simple to complex facts and equations.
Test 6: Math Fluency	Mathematics *Math achievement* *Numerical facility*	Measures rapid calculation of single-digit addition, subtraction, and multiplication facts.
Test 7: Spelling	Spelling *Spelling ability*	Measures spelling of real words presented orally.
Test 8: Writing Fluency	Writing *Writing ability* *Writing speed*	Measures the ability to write simple, short sentences incorporating three stimulus words.
Test 9: Passage Comprehension	Reading *Reading comprehension* *Cloze ability*	Measures reading comprehension by having examinee read a short passage and supply a key missing word.
Test 10: Applied Problems	Mathematics *Quantitative reasoning* *Math achievement* *Math knowledge*	Measures problem solving that requires analyzing and solving practical math problems (story problems).
Test 11: Writing Samples	Writing *Writing ability*	Measures expressive writing by having examinee write sentences in response to a series of demands.
Test 12: Story Recall–Delayed	General *Meaningful memory*	Measures recall of elements of stories presented earlier (30 minutes to 8 days earlier).
Test 13: Word Attack	Reading *Reading decoding* *Phonetic coding*	Measures the ability to pronounce phonically regular pseudowords.
Test 14: Picture Vocabulary	Oral expression *Language development* *Lexical knowledge*	Measures word knowledge by having examinee name pictured objects (object identification and naming).
Test 15: Oral Comprehension	Listening comprehension *Listening ability*	Measures listening ability by having examinee provide a missing final word to an oral passage.

(cont.)

TABLE 12.3. *(cont.)*

Test name	Curricular area/CHC Narrow abilities measured[a]	Brief test description
Test 16: Editing	Writing skills *English usage*	Measures the ability to identify and correcting errors in short written passages.
Test 17: Reading Vocabulary	Reading *Lexical knowledge* *Reading comprehension*	Measures reading vocabulary by having examinee provide synonyms and antonyms and complete analogies.
Test 18: Quantitative Concepts	Mathematics *Math knowledge* *Quantitative reasoning*	Measures aspects of math knowledge and quantitative reasoning.
Test 19: Academic Knowledge	General *General information* *Science information* *Cultural information* *Geography achievement*	Samples the breadth of knowledge in the sciences, history, geography, government, economics, arts, music, and literature.
Test 20: Spelling of Sounds	Spelling *Spelling ability* *Phonetic coding*	Measures encoding by having examinee write nonsense words presented orally.
Test 21: Sound Awareness	Reading *Phonetic coding* *Working memory*	Measures phonological awareness through rhyming, deletion, substitution, and reversal tasks.
Test 22: Punctuation and Capitalization	Writing *English usage*	Measures writing skills that require use of punctuation and capitalization marks.

[a]Names of narrow abilities are given in italics.

The WJ III NU is a comprehensive assessment system that can be used for a wide variety of assessment needs. Following a broad overview of administration and scoring principles and psychometric properties of the WJ III NU, this chapter focuses on how the WJ III can be used to generate evidence-based interventions for instructional planning. (Instructional interventions are also linked to WJ III test performance in the Woodcock Interpretation and Instructional Interventions Program [WIIIP; Schrank, Wendling, & Woodcock, 2008].)

ADMINISTRATION AND SCORING

Administration and scoring of the WJ III tests require knowledge of the exact standardized procedures and an understanding of the importance of adhering to these procedures. Each examiner's manual provides guidelines for this purpose. In addition, the test books contain an abbreviated set of instructions for administering and scoring items on each test; these are found on the introductory page of each test (the first printed page after the tab page). Additional instructions may appear on the test pages, such as in boxes with special instructions.

Administration of certain tests in the WJ III requires the examiner to use a subject response booklet and an audio recording. Directions for using the subject response booklet are provided in the test book. The audio recording is used to ensure standardized presentation of certain auditory, short-term memory, and oral language tasks. The audio equipment must have a good speaker, be in good working order, and produce a faithful, clear reproduction of the test items. Using headphones is recommended, as they were used in the standardization. Examiners can wear a monaural earphone or wear only one headphone over one ear to monitor the audio recording while the subject is also listening through his or her headphones.

TABLE 12.4. WJ III ACH Clusters and Brief Cluster Descriptions

Cluster	Brief cluster description
Brief Reading	Measures letter and word identification skills and reading comprehension.
Broad Reading	Measures reading decoding via letter and word identification skills, reading speed, and passage comprehension.
Basic Reading Skills	Measures decoding skills, using both real and phonically regular nonsense words.
Reading Comprehension	Measures comprehension at both the single-word and connected-discourse levels.
Oral Language—Standard	Measures receptive and expressive oral language skills.
Oral Language—Extended	Measures receptive and expressive oral language skills.
Listening Comprehension	Measure receptive oral language abilities.
Oral Expression	Measure expressive oral language abilities.
Brief Math	Measures math calculation skills and math reasoning.
Broad Math	Measures calculation, fluency with calculation facts, and mathematics reasoning.
Math Calculation Skills	Measures basic math skills, including computation and automaticity of math calculation facts.
Math Reasoning	Measures math knowledge and problem-solving skills.
Brief Writing	Measures spelling and written expression.
Broad Written Language	Measures written language achievement, including spelling of single-word responses, fluency of production, and quality of expression.
Basic Writing Skills	Measures encoding and editing skills.
Written Expression	Measures written expression skills, including rapid sentence formulation and quality of ideation.
Academic Knowledge	Provides a broad sample of an individual's range of scientific knowledge, social studies knowledge, and cultural knowledge.
Phoneme/Grapheme Knowledge	Measures proficiency with both phonic (sound) generalizations and common orthographic patterns (frequently occurring letter combinations).
Academic Skills	Provides an aggregate measure of reading decoding, math calculation, and spelling of single-word responses.
Academic Fluency	Provides an overall index of academic fluency in reading, math, and writing.
Academic Applications	Measures the application of academic skills to academic problems.
Brief Achievement	Measures preacademic or academic skills development, including letter and word identification skills, math reasoning, and spelling.
Total Achievement	Provides a broad measure of overall performance across reading, math, and writing achievement domains.

Examiners need to learn how to establish a basal and a ceiling for many of the tests. Basal and ceiling criteria are included in the test book for each test requiring them. If a subject fails to meet the basal criterion for any test, the examiner is directed to test backward, until the subject has met the basal criterion or until item 1 has been administered. For some tests, subjects begin with item 1 and test until they reach their ceiling level; these tests do not require a basal. Other tests are arranged with items in groups, sets, or blocks, or are timed tests; specific criteria for starting and stopping these tests are outlined in the corresponding manual, test book, and test record.

Individual test items are scored during test administration. Many tests use a 1 (correct) or 0 (incorrect) scoring rule for determining raw scores. Examiners need to learn how to score items and calculate the raw score for each test. Generally, raw scores are determined by adding the number of correctly completed items to the number of test items below the basal. Scores for sample or practice items should not be included when examiners are calculating raw scores. The correct and incorrect keys in the test books are intended to be guides to demonstrate how certain responses are scored and not all possible responses are included in the keys. Completion of the scoring procedure requires using the WJ III NU Compuscore and Profiles Program (Compuscore; Schrank & Woodcock, 2008), a computer software program that is included with each WJ III kit. Alternatively, examiners may use the WIIIP (Schrank et al., 2008) for scoring as well as for generating interpretive information and interventions.

Examiners are encouraged to use the selective testing tables (Figure 12.1 and Figure 12.2) to determine which tests to administer. Testing time will vary, depending on the number of tests that are administered (in general, about 5–10 minutes per test). Very young subjects or individuals with unique learning patterns may require more time. The tests may be administered in any order deemed appropriate, and testing may be discontinued after completion of any test.

PSYCHOMETRIC PROPERTIES

Median reliability coefficients (r_{11}) and the standard errors of measurement (SEM) are reported for the WJ III COG and DS tests in Table 12.5

and for the WJ III ACH tests in Table 12.6. The SEM values are given in standard score (SS) units. The reliabilities for all but the speeded tests and tests with multiple-point scoring systems were calculated with the split-half procedure (odd and even items) and corrected for length with the Spearman–Brown correction formula. The reliabilities for the speeded tests and tests with multiple-point scored items were calculated via Rasch analysis procedures. Most reliabilities reported in Tables 12.5 and 12.6 are .80 or higher. Table 12.7 reports median reliabilities and standard errors of measurement for the WJ III COG and DS clusters; medians for the WJ III ACH clusters are reported in Table 12.8. Most cluster reliabilities are .90 or higher.

Validity is inextricably tied to theory. John Horn and John Carroll served as expert consultants in the development of the WJ III. A synthesis of their research provided guidance for the blueprint of constructs to be measured. Identification of the broad abilities in the WJ III is historically and primarily linked to the Gf-Gc research of Cattell (1941, 1943, 1950), Horn (1965, 1988, 1989, 1991) and their associates (Horn & Masunaga, 2000; Horn & Noll, 1997; Horn & Stankov, 1982). The specification of the narrow abilities and general intellectual ability (g) construct was heavily influenced by Carroll's (1993) research.

The WJ III is supported by several sources of validity evidence as documented in the WJ III NU technical manual (McGrew, Schrank, & Woodcock, 2007), the WJ III technical manual (McGrew & Woodcock, 2001), and the DS manual (Schrank, Mather, McGrew, & Woodcock, 2003). Much of this evidence is reviewed and discussed by Floyd, Shaver, and McGrew (2003) and by Keith and Reynolds (2010). A review of the WJ III technical manual suggests that the validity of the tests is supported by reviews of content experts, psychologists, and teachers who reviewed items and made suggestions for item revision. The technical manual also presents a series of divergent growth curves to support the construct of unique abilities. A number of confirmatory factor analyses presented in the technical manual provide evidence that the structural model upon which the WJ III is based is not implausible. In addition, Taub and McGrew (2004) showed that the first- and second-order factor structure of the WJ III is invariant across the 6- to 90-year age range.

	Tests of Cognitive Abilities	General Intellectual Ability-Std	General Intellectual Ability-Ext	General Intellectual Ability-EDev	General Intellectual Ability-Bil	Broad Cognitive Ability-Low Verbal	Brief Intellectual Ability	Verbal Ability-Std	Verbal Ability-Ext	Thinking Ability-Std	Thinking Ability-Ext	Cognitive Efficiency-Std	Cognitive Efficiency-Ext	Comprehension-Knowledge (Gc)	Long-Term Retrieval (Glr)	Visual-Spatial Thinking (Gv)	Visual-Spatial Thinking 3 (Gv3)	Auditory Processing (Ga)	Fluid Reasoning (Gf)	Fluid Reasoning 3 (Gf3)	Processing Speed (Gs)	Short-Term Memory (Gsm)	Phonemic Awareness (PC)	Phonemic Awareness 3	Working Memory (WM)	Numerical Reasoning (RQ)	Associative Memory (MA)	Associative Memory-Delayed	Visualization (Vz)	Sound Discrimination (U3)	Auditory Memory Span (MS)	Perceptual Speed (P)	Broad Attention	Cognitive Fluency	Executive Processes	Delayed Recall	Knowledge
		Intellectual Ability								Cognitive Performance Model Clusters				Broad CHC Clusters												Narrow CHC Clusters									Clinical Clusters		
Standard Battery	Test 1: Verbal Comprehension	■	■	■	■		■	■	■					■																							
	Test 2: Visual–Auditory Learning	■	■							■	■				■												■										
	Test 3: Spatial Relations	■	■		■	■				■	■					■	■												■								
	Test 4: Sound Blending	■	■							■	■							■					■	■[4]													
	Test 5: Concept Formation	■	■		■	■	■			■	■								■	■															■		
	Test 6: Visual Matching	■	■	■	■	■	■					■	■								■											■					
	Test 7: Numbers Reversed	■	■		■	■						■	■									■			■								■				
	Test 8: Incomplete Words			■																			■	■[4]													
	Test 9: Auditory Working Memory																								■								■				
	Test 10: Visual–Auditory Learning—Delayed																											■								■[2]	
Extended Battery	Test 11: General Information		■						■					■																							■[3]
	Test 12: Retrieval Fluency		■								■				■																			■			
	Test 13: Picture Recognition		■								■					■	■																				
	Test 14: Auditory Attention		■								■							■															■				
	Test 15: Analysis–Synthesis		■								■								■	■																	
	Test 16: Decision Speed		■										■								■													■			
	Test 17: Memory for Words		■										■									■									■						
	Test 18: Rapid Picture Naming																																	■			
	Test 19: Planning																																		■		
	Test 20: Pair Cancellation																																■		■		
Diagnostic Supplement	Test 21: Memory for Names			■	■	■																					■										
	Test 22: Visual Closure			■													■																				
	Test 23: Sound Patterns—Voice				■	■																								■							
	Test 24: Number Series																									■											
	Test 25: Number Matrices																			■						■											
	Test 26: Cross Out																															■					
	Test 27: Memory for Sentences			■																											■						
	Test 28: Block Rotation																												■								
	Test 29: Sound Patterns—Music																													■							
	Test 30: Memory for Names—Delayed																											■									
	Test 31: Bilingual Verbal Comprehension—English/Spanish				*[1]									*[1]																							

[1]Test 31, Bilingual Verbal Comprehension, is not required for calculation of this cluster. If administered, items answered correctly on test 31 are added to the raw score for test 1, Verbal Comprehension.
[2] Also includes test 12, Story Recall—Delayed, from the WJ III Tests of Achievement.
[3] Also includes test 19, Academic Knowledge, from the WJ III Tests of Achievement.
[4] Also includes test 21, Sound Awareness, from the WJ III Tests of Achievement.

FIGURE 12.1. WJ III COG selective testing table (includes the DS).

Tests of Achievement*

Cluster categories: Reading | Oral Language | Math | Written Language | Other Clusters

Cluster columns:
Brief Reading, Broad Reading, Basic Reading Skills, Reading Comprehension, Oral Language—Standard, Oral Language—Extended, Listening Comprehension, Oral Expression, Brief Math, Broad Math, Math Calculation Skills, Math Reasoning, Brief Writing, Broad Written Language, Basic Writing Skills, Written Expression, Academic Knowledge, Phoneme/Grapheme Knowledge, Academic Skills, Academic Fluency, Academic Applications, Brief Achievement, Total Achievement

Standard Battery

- Test 1: Letter–Word Identification
- Test 2: Reading Fluency
- Test 3: Story Recall
- Test 4: Understanding Directions
- Test 5: Calculation
- Test 6: Math Fluency
- Test 7: Spelling
- Test 8: Writing Fluency
- Test 9: Passage Comprehension
- Test 10: Applied Problems
- Test 11: Writing Samples
- Test 12: Story Recall—Delayed

Extended Battery

- Test 13: Word Attack
- Test 14: Picture Vocabulary
- Test 15: Oral Comprehension
- Test 16: Editing
- Test 17: Reading Vocabulary
- Test 18: Quantitative Concepts
- Test 19: Academic Knowledge
- Test 20: Spelling of Sounds
- Test 21: Sound Awareness
- Test 22: Punctuation and Capitalization

*Test numbers refer to both Forms A and B; Form C test numbers are different.

FIGURE 12.2. WJ III ACH selective testing table.

TABLE 12.5. WJ III COG and DS Median Test Reliability Statistics

Test	Median r_{11}	Median *SEM* (SS)
Standard Battery		
Test 1: Verbal Comprehension	.92	4.24
Test 2: Visual–Auditory Learning	.86	5.61
Test 3: Spatial Relations	.81	6.54
Test 4: Sound Blending	.89	4.97
Test 5: Concept Formation	.94	3.67
Test 6: Visual Matching	.88	5.24
Test 7: Numbers Reversed	.87	5.41
Test 8: Incomplete Words	.81	6.54
Test 9: Auditory Working Memory	.87	5.41
Test 10: Visual–Auditory Learning—Delayed	.94	3.67
Extended Battery		
Test 11: General Information	.89	4.97
Test 12: Retrieval Fluency	.85	5.81
Test 13: Picture Recognition	.76	7.35
Test 14: Auditory Attention	.88	5.20
Test 15: Analysis–Synthesis	.90	4.74
Test 16: Decision Speed	.88	5.16
Test 17: Memory for Words	.80	6.71
Test 18: Rapid Picture Naming	.97	2.51
Test 19: Planning	.74	7.65
Test 20: Pair Cancellation	.96	2.92
Diagnostic Supplement		
Test 21: Memory for Names	.88	5.20
Test 22: Visual Closure	.82	6.36
Test 23: Sound Patterns—Voice	.94	3.67
Test 24: Number Series	.89	4.97
Test 25: Number Matrices	.91	4.50
Test 26: Cross Out	.72	7.94
Test 27: Memory for Sentences	.89	4.97
Test 28: Block Rotation	.82	6.36
Test 29: Sound Patterns—Music	.90	4.86
Test 30: Memory for Names—Delayed	.90	4.74
Test 31: Bilingual Verbal Comprehension—English/Spanish	.92	4.24

INTERPRETATION

The primary contribution of CHC theory has been the development of a scientifically based grammar, or professional nomenclature, for describing the existence of differentiated cognitive abilities (Keith & Reynolds, 2010; Schneider & McGrew, Chapter 4, this volume; Newton & McGrew, 2010). CHC theory—like any scientific theory—is not static, but continues to evolve as

the result of an ongoing, bidirectional interchange between psychometric and neuroscientific sources of validation. The WJ III NU technical manual (McGrew et al., 2007) introduced and described a number of inferred cognitive processes involved in performance on the WJ III tests; the inferences were derived from a number of experimental studies and related models of cognitive processing from cognitive and neuroscience research. Because the tasks used in the WJ III tests are similar (and in

TABLE 12.6. WJ III ACH Median Test Reliability Statistics

Test	Median r_{11}	Median SEM (SS)
Standard Battery		
Test 1: Letter–Word Identification	.94	3.67
Test 2: Reading Fluency	.95	3.27
Test 3: Story Recall	.87	5.41
Test 4: Understanding Directions	.83	6.18
Test 5: Calculation	.86	5.61
Test 6: Math Fluency	.98	2.36
Test 7: Spelling	.90	4.74
Test 8: Writing Fluency	.83	6.24
Test 9: Passage Comprehension	.88	5.20
Test 10: Applied Problems	.93	3.97
Test 11: Writing Samples	.75	7.52
Test 12: Story Recall—Delayed	.81	6.62
Extended Battery		
Test 13: Word Attack	.87	5.41
Test 14: Picture Vocabulary	.81	6.54
Test 15: Oral Comprehension	.85	5.81
Test 16: Editing	.90	4.74
Test 17: Reading Vocabulary	.90	4.86
Test 18: Quantitative Concepts	.91	4.50
Test 19: Academic Knowledge	.90	4.74
Test 20: Spelling of Sounds	.76	7.35
Test 21: Sound Awareness	.81	6.54
Test 22: Punctuation and Capitalization	.79	6.87

some cases identical) to tasks used in both classic and contemporary neuroscience research, the similarities between tasks provided a basis for making the inferences about the cognitive processes that are required for performance on the WJ III tests. This form of construct-and-process validation has recently been updated and expanded (Schrank, Miller, Wendling, & Woodcock, 2010) to suggest links between evidence-based instructional interventions and WJ III test scores based on cognitive processing descriptions obtained from related neuroscientific research.

As suggested by Fiorello, Hale, Snyder, Forrest, and Teodori (2008), information about processing strengths and weaknesses has potential for aligning identified limitations in cognitive capacities to targeted instructional interventions. The thesis has a broad practical implication: Educational interventions or accommodations that address cognitive processing limitations may be a key to improved performance in academic areas where learning difficulties are manifested. Similarly,

McKenna, Jurgensen, and Thurman (2008) have suggested that "to the extent that we can understand the role and functions of cognitive processes in classrooms and other applied settings, it should logically follow that instruction and consequently learning will improve" (p. 4).

Although organized in terms of broad abilities, the remainder of this chapter focuses on interpretation at the test and narrow-ability level. The alignment of cognitive processes to the WJ III and CHC theory is best accomplished at this lowest level of abstraction. In CHC theory, the narrow abilities correspond as closely as practicable to operational definitions of human cognitive capacities. In the WJ III, each test is a standardized scientific experiment that explains to the subject "what to do" and provides guidelines to the evaluator about "what to observe" to measure its effects. As a consequence, the CHC narrow abilities and descriptions of the cognitive processes required for performance on each WJ III test provide the theoretical and conceptual bases for the links be-

TABLE 12.7. WJ III COG and DS Median Cluster Reliability Statistics

Cluster	Median r_{11}	Median SEM (SS)
Standard Battery		
General Intellectual Ability—Std	.97	2.60
Brief Intellectual Ability	.96	3.00
Verbal Ability—Std	.92	4.24
Thinking Ability—Std	.95	3.35
Cognitive Efficiency—Std	.91	4.50
Phonemic Awareness (PC)	.90	4.74
Working Memory (WM)	.91	4.50
Extended Battery		
General Intellectual Ability—Ext	.98	2.12
Verbal Ability—Ext	.95	3.35
Thinking Ability—Ext	.96	3.00
Cognitive Efficiency—Ext	.92	4.24
Comprehension–Knowledge (Gc)	.95	3.35
Long-Term Retrieval (Glr)	.88	5.20
Visual–Spatial Thinking (Gv)	.81	6.54
Auditory Processing (Ga)	.91	4.50
Fluid Reasoning (Gf)	.95	3.35
Processing Speed (Gs)	.92	4.24
Short-Term Memory (Gsm)	.88	5.20
Broad Attention	.94	3.67
Cognitive Fluency	.96	3.00
Executive Processes	.96	3.00
Delayed Recall	.92	4.37
Knowledge	.94	3.67
Phonemic Awareness 3 (PC)	.90	4.74
Diagnostic Supplement		
General Intellectual Ability—Bilingual	.97	2.60
General Intellectual Ability—Early Development	.95	3.35
Broad Cognitive Ability—Low Verbal	.96	3.00
Thinking Ability—Low Verbal	.95	3.35
Visual–Spatial Thinking 3 (Gv3)	.85	5.81
Fluid Reasoning 3 (Gf3)	.96	3.00
Associative Memory (MA)	.92	4.24
Associative Memory—Delayed (MA)	.94	3.67
Visualization (Vz)	.83	6.18
Sound Discrimination (US)	.96	3.00
Auditory Memory Span (MS)	.88	5.20
Perceptual Speed (P)	.88	5.20
Numerical Reasoning (RQ)	.94	3.82
Preacademic Knowledge and Skills—Ext	.96	3.00

TABLE 12.8. WJ III ACH Median Cluster Reliability Statistics

Cluster	Median r_{11}	Median SEM (SS)
Standard Battery		
Total Achievement	.98	2.12
Oral Language—Std	.87	5.41
Broad Reading	.96	3.00
Broad Math	.95	3.35
Broad Written Language	.92	4.24
Academic Skills	.96	3.00
Academic Fluency	.96	3.00
Academic Applications	.94	3.67
Extended Battery		
Oral Language—Ext	.92	4.24
Oral Expression	.85	5.81
Listening Comprehension	.89	4.97
Basic Reading Skills	.95	3.35
Reading Comprehension	.92	4.24
Math Calculation Skills	.91	4.50
Math Reasoning	.95	3.35
Basic Writing Skills	.94	3.67
Written Expression	.85	5.90
Phoneme/Grapheme Knowledge	.90	4.74
Brief Battery		
Brief Achievement	.97	2.60
Brief Reading	.95	3.35
Brief Math	.94	3.67
Brief Writing	.90	4.62

tween the tests and a number of evidence-based instructional interventions. The importance of this relationship is echoed in the suggestion made by Wong, Harris, Graham, and Butler (2003): "An implication, borne out in research, is that student performance should improve when teachers structure instruction and academic work to cue effective processing" (p. 392).

EDUCATIONAL INTERVENTIONS RELATED TO THE WJ III COG AND DS TESTS

Although it is becoming generally accepted that an identified weakness in a particular cognitive ability may be useful for describing why a student is struggling in one academic area but not another (McGrew & Wendling, 2010), the relationship among the identified weakness, the cognitive processes required for academic performance in the affected domain, and instructional interventions is not as widely understood. As the focus of professional practice shifts from determining service eligibility to assessing basic psychological processes that inform appropriate instruction, a need exists for providing a link between cognitive assessment results and evidence-based educational interventions. This section describes an integration of the CHC theory with selected classic and contemporary cognitive neuroscience research that results in differential implications for planning appropriate interventions and/or selection of accommodations. References to research evidence for each suggested intervention are provided for further information. Table 12.9 provides an organizational schema that relates WJ III COG and DS test performance to suggested evidence-based interventions or accommodations that are conceptually related to the narrow abilities and cognitive processes identified.

Comprehension–Knowledge (Gc)

Comprehension–knowledge (Gc) is a CHC broad ability that is also sometimes referred to as *acculturation knowledge*, *crystallized intelligence*, or *verbal ability*. It is typically viewed as a store of acquired knowledge. Two of the WJ III COG tests that compose the Gc cluster are Verbal Comprehension and General Information.

The Verbal Comprehension test includes four subtests (Picture Vocabulary, Synonyms, Antonyms, and Verbal Analogies) and measures the CHC narrow abilities of lexical knowledge (i.e., vocabulary knowledge) and language development (i.e., general development of spoken language skills that do not require reading ability). Both narrow abilities (lexical knowledge and language development) are measured in the Picture Vocabulary subtest. In this task, objects are identified via access to object constructs (Martin, 2009; Murphy, 2002) in semantic memory (Tulving, 1972, 1983, 2000). The Synonyms and Antonyms subtests measure lexical knowledge via the priming process, an aspect of nondeclarative knowledge or memory (Manns & Squire, 2002). In this task, an auditory form of a stimulus word is connected to a concept via semantic access, which then activates or primes its meaning in the lexicon and consequently activates closely associated words (Caplan, 1992; Gazzaniga, Irvy, & Mangun, 1998). The Ver-

TABLE 12.9. WJ III COG and DS Tests, CHC Broad/Narrow Abilities Measured, Cognitive Processes, and Related Educational Interventions

Test	CHD broad/narrow abilities measured[a]	Cognitive processes	Related educational interventions
Test 1: Verbal Comprehension	Comprehension–knowledge (Gcf) *Lexical knowledge* *Language development*	Object recognition and reidentification; semantic activation, via priming, for semantic access and matching; verbal analogical reasoning	Creating a vocabulary-rich learning environment, particularly reading aloud to a young child and discussing new words; text talks; directed vocabulary thinking activities; explicit teaching of specific words; semantic feature analysis; semantic maps; use of computer technology to develop word knowledge; association of key words to prior knowledge; reading for a variety of purposes; independent word-learning strategies
Test 2: Visual–Auditory Learning	Long-term retrieval (Glr) *Associative memory*	Paired-associative encoding via directed spotlight attention; storage and retrieval	Active, successful learning experiences; rehearsal; overlearning; organizational strategies; mnemonics; illustrating or visualizing content
Test 3: Spatial Relations	Visual–spatial thinking (Gv) *Visualization* *Spatial relations*	Visual feature detection; manipulation of visual images in space; matching	Multisensory teaching techniques; private speech
Test 4: Sound Blending	Auditory processing (Ga) *Phonetic coding*	Synthesis of acoustic, phonological elements in immediate awareness; matching the sequence of elements to stored lexical entries; lexical activation and access	Early exposure to language sounds; promoting phonological awareness; direct instruction in sound blending; practice with blending sounds into words
Test 5: Concept Formation	Fluid reasoning (Gf) *Induction*	Rule-based categorization; rule switching; induction/inference	Categorizing with real objects; developing skills in drawing conclusions; hands-on problem-solving tasks; making meaningful associations; concrete examples of grouping objects; development of patterning skills
Test 6: Visual Matching	Processing speed (Gs) *Perceptual speed*	Speeded visual perception and matching	Emphasizing speediness; building cognitive speed via repetition, speed drills; use of technology
Test 7: Numbers Reversed	Short-term memory (Gsm) *Working memory capacity*	Span of apprehension and recoding in working memory	Chunking strategies; rehearsal
Test 8: Incomplete Words	Auditory processing (Ga) *Phonetic coding*	Analysis of a sequence of acoustic, phonological elements in immediate awareness; activation of a stored representation of the word from an incomplete set of phonological features	Promoting phonological awareness; reading aloud; games that focus on sounds and words

(cont.)

TABLE 12.9. *(cont.)*

Test	CHD broad/narrow abilities measured[a]	Cognitive processes	Related educational interventions
Test 9: Auditory Working Memory	Short-term memory (Gsm) *Working memory capacity*	Recoding of acoustic, verbalizable stimuli held in immediate awareness	Rehearsal; mnemonics; active learning
Test 10: Visual–Auditory Learning—Delayed	Long-term retrieval (Glr) *Associative memory*	Retrieval and reidentification; associative encoding (for relearning)	Active, successful learning experiences; rehearsal; overlearning; organizational strategies; mnemonics; illustrating or visualizing content
Test 11: General Information	Comprehension–knowledge (Gc) *General (verbal) information*	Semantic activation and access to mental representations of core properties of objects	Building and activating background knowledge; connecting instruction to prior knowledge; demonstration; use of visuals
Test 12: Retrieval Fluency	Long-term retrieval (Glr) *Ideational fluency* *Naming facility*	Recognition, fluent retrieval, and oral production of examples of a semantic category	Oral elaboration
Test 13: Picture Recognition	Visual–spatial thinking (Gv) *Visual memory*	Formation of iconic memories and matching of visual stimuli to stored representations	Activities designed to discriminate/match visual features and recall visual information
Test 14: Auditory Attention	Auditory processing (Ga) *Speech-sound discrimination Resistance to auditory-stimulus distortion*	Selective auditory attention	Reduction of distracting noise; modifications to listening environment
Test 15: Analysis–Synthesis	Fluid reasoning (Gf) *General sequential reasoning Quantitative reasoning*	Algorithmic reasoning; deduction	Deductive reasoning with concrete objects; hands-on problem-solving tasks; metacognitive strategies
Test 16: Decision Speed	Processing speed (Gs) *Semantic processing speed*	Object recognition and speeded symbolic/semantic comparisons	Emphasizing speediness; building cognitive speed via repetition
Test 17: Memory for Words	Short-term memory (Gsm) *Auditory memory span*	Formation of echoic memories and verbalizable span of echoic store	Rehearsal
Test 18: Rapid Picture Naming	Processing speed (Gs) *Naming facility*	Speed/fluency of retrieval and oral production of recognized objects	Increasing fluency through self-competition
Test 19: Planning	Visual–spatial thinking (Gv) and fluid reasoning (Gf) *Spatial scanning General sequential reasoning*	Means–end analysis	Use of puzzles, pegboards, dot-to-dot drawings; multisensory teaching techniques; private speech
Test 20: Pair Cancellation	Processing speed (Gs) *Attention and concentration*	Controlled, focal attention; vigilance	Speed drills; repetition

(cont.)

TABLE 12.9. *(cont.)*

Test	CHD broad/narrow abilities measured[a]	Cognitive processes	Related educational interventions
Test 21: Memory for Names	Long-term retrieval (Glr) *Associative memory*	Associative encoding via directed spotlight attention, storage, and retrieval	Active, successful learning experiences; rehearsal; overlearning; organizational strategies; mnemonics; illustrating or visualizing content
Test 22: Visual Closure	Visual–spatial thinking (Gv) *Closure speed*	Object identification from a limited set of component geons	Unknown
Test 23: Sound Patterns—Voice	Auditory processing (Ga) *Sound discrimination*	Prelexical, perceptual analysis of auditory waveform patterns	Auditory training; enhancements/modifications to listening environment
Test 24: Number Series	Fluid reasoning (Gf) *Mathematics knowledge* *Quantitative reasoning*	Representation and manipulation of points on a mental number line; identifying and applying an underlying rule/principle to complete a numerical sequence	Developing number sense; counting by increments; manipulatives
Test 25: Number Matrices	Fluid reasoning (Gf) *Quantitative reasoning*	Access to verbal–visual numerical codes; transcoding verbal and/or visual representations of numerical information into analogical representations; determining the relationship between/among numbers on the first part of the structure and mapping (projecting) the structure to complete the analogy	Seriation; patterns; explicit instruction in number reasoning skills
Test 26: Cross Out	Processing speed (Gs) *Perceptual speed*	Speeded visual matching	Emphasizing speediness; building cognitive speed via repetition
Test 27: Memory for Sentences	Short-term memory (Gsm) *Auditory memory span* *Listening ability*	Formation of echoic memories aided by a semantic, meaning-based code	Rehearsal
Test 28: Block Rotation	Visual–spatial thinking (Gv) *Visualization* *Spatial relations*	Visual matching with visual–spatial manipulation	Use of puzzles, pegboards, dot-to-dot drawings; multisensory teaching techniques; private speech
Test 29: Sound Patterns—Music	Auditory processing (Ga) *Sound discrimination* *Musical discrimination and judgment*	Prelexical, perceptual analysis of auditory waveform patterns	Auditory training; enhancements/modifications to listening environment
Test 30: Memory for Names—Delayed	Long-term retrieval (Glr) *Associative memory*	Reidentification	Interventions/accommodations to help recall previously learned information
Test 31: Bilingual Verbal Comprehension—English/Spanish	Comprehension–knowledge (Gc) *Lexical knowledge* *Language development*	Object reidentification; semantic activation, access, and matching; verbal analogical reasoning	See Test 1: Verbal Comprehension

[a]Names of narrow abilities are given in italics.

bal Analogies tasks require inductive reasoning to project (or map) the structure for the first part of each analogy onto the second—and incomplete—part of the analogy (Gentner & Markman, 1997).

In contrast, the General Information test measures the CHC narrow ability of general (verbal) information. Martin's (1998) work suggests that the type of knowledge accessed by this task is based on mental representations of one or more core properties of the objects that are stored via the visual processing system.

There are many interventions for low proficiency in Gc. Learners of any age will benefit from connecting new learning to prior knowledge and/or building background knowledge if necessary (Moje et al., 2004). For young children, suggested interventions that foster the development of knowledge and language abilities include creating a language- and experience-rich environment (Gunn, Simmons, & Kame'enui, 1995; Hart & Risley, 2003); frequent exposure to and practice with words (Gunn et al., 1995; Hart & Risley, 2003); reading aloud to the children (Adams, 1990); and text talks (Beck & McKeown, 2001).

For older children and adolescents, interventions include increased time spent reading (Cunningham & Stanovich, 1991; Herman, Anderson, Pearson, & Nagy, 1987); reading for different purposes (Anderson, 1996; National Reading Panel, 2000; Stahl, 1999); intentional, explicit word instruction (Beck, McKeown, & Kucan, 2002; Graves, Juel, & Graves, 2004; National Reading Panel, 2000); direct instruction in morphology (Anglin, 1993; Baumann, Edwards, Boland, Olejnik, & Kame'enui, 2003; Baumann, Kame'enui, & Ash, 2003; Blachowicz & Fisher, 2000; Carlisle, 2004; Graves, 2000; National Reading Panel, 2000); development of word consciousness (Anderson & Nagy, 1992; Graves & Watts-Taffe, 2002; Nagy & Scott, 2000); and use of related computer programs (Davidson, Elcock, & Noyes, 1996). Additional vocabulary-building interventions for older children and adults include semantic feature analysis (Anders & Bos, 1986; Pittelman, Heimlich, Berglund, & French, 1991) and semantic maps (Johnson & Pearson, 1984; Sinatra, Berg, & Dunn, 1985). Both of these methods provide a visual representation of the information to be studied.

Long-Term Retrieval (Glr)

Long-term retrieval (Glr) is the CHC broad ability that involves the cognitive processes of acquiring,

storing, and retrieving information. Glr reflects the efficiency with which information is initially stored and later retrieved. Two tests that compose the Glr cluster are Visual–Auditory Learning and Retrieval Fluency. Visual–Auditory Learning measures associative memory or paired-associate learning, and Retrieval Fluency measures ideational fluency and naming facility. In Visual–Auditory Learning, the initial task requires associating a visual rebus symbol with a verbal label. The controlled-learning format of this test uses directed spotlight attention (Gazzaniga et al., 1998)—the mental, attention-focusing process that prepares the examinee to encode the stimulus (Brefczynski & DeYoe, 1999; Klingberg, 2009; Sengpiel & Hubener, 1999). The retrieval phase requires the examinee to match a rebus presentation with its stored representation; this process is called *identification*. The directed-spotlight attention mechanism provides a cue to the intervention known as *active learning* (Marzano, Pinkering, & Pollock, 2001). Active learning is required for the creation of meaning-based codes that are subsequently used to relate new information or task requirements to previously acquired knowledge.

The Retrieval Fluency test requires fluent retrieval and oral production of examples of a semantic category. This task does not include the encoding and storage processes, but rather measures the rate or automaticity of retrieval. Oral elaboration (Wolf, Bowers, & Biddle, 2000; Wolfe, 2001) may be an effective intervention to improve fluency of retrieval.

Included in Table 12.9 are three additional Glr tests: Memory for Names, Visual–Auditory Learning—Delayed, and Memory for Names—Delayed. Other interventions related to limitations in encoding, storing, and retrieving information include active learning (Marzano et al., 2001); rehearsal, overlearning, and elaboration (Squire & Schacter, 2002); mnemonics (Wolfe, 2001); visual representation (Greenleaf & Wells-Papanek, 2005); and organizational strategies.

Visual–Spatial Thinking (Gv)

Visual–spatial thinking (Gv) involves visual perception (the process of extracting features from visual stimuli) and includes the processes involved in generating, storing, retrieving, and transforming visual images. Spatial Relations and Picture Recognition are two of the tests that create the Gv cluster. Spatial Relations measures the ability to use visualization (the skill to apprehend spatial forms or shapes, often by rotating or manipulating them in the imagination of the "mind's eye"). Picture Recognition is a visual memory task.

Individuals with limited proficiency in one or more of the visual–spatial thinking abilities may benefit from interventions designed to develop skills in discriminating visual features, mentally manipulating visual images, matching, and recalling visual information (Greenleaf & Wells-Papanek, 2005). Others, particularly those with very limited proficiency, may benefit from multisensory teaching techniques that make use of multiple sensory pathways to introduce and practice the information to be learned (Williams, Richman, & Yarbrough, 1992). For example, tactile/kinesthetic activities may enhance learning by incorporating multiple senses into the instructional process. For students in grades 3 and above, cognitive-behavioral interventions such as using private speech to initiate, direct, or maintain a behavior (Meichenbaum, 1977) may be applied to visual–spatial tasks.

Table 12.9 identifies and outlines the cognitive processing requirements and related educational interventions for the other WJ III COG and DS Gv tests—Planning, Visual Closure, and Block Rotation.

Auditory Processing (Ga)

Auditory processing (Ga) is a broad CHC ability that involves auditory perception (the process of extracting features from auditory stimuli) and includes a wide range of abilities that are needed to discriminate, analyze, synthesize, comprehend, and manipulate sounds. Two of the tests that compose the Ga cluster are Sound Blending and Auditory Attention. Sound Blending involves acoustic–phonetic processing, which is the ability to analyze acoustic waveforms, match the blended sequence to stored lexical entries, and identify the blended phonemes as a complete word (Caplan, 1992). Auditory Attention requires selective auditory attention, speech-sound discrimination, and resistance to auditory-stimulus distortion.

For young children, possible interventions for auditory processing limitations include early exposure to sounds, music, rhythms, and language (Glazer, 1989; Strickland, 1991); reading aloud to the children (Adams, 1990; Anderson, Hiebert, Scott, & Wilkinson, 1985); providing opportunities that encourage exploration and manipulation

of sounds, words, and language (Adams, 1990); and daily practice with language (Bridge, Winograd, & Haley, 1983).

For school-age children and some adolescents with limited phonemic awareness, interventions include explicit, systematic instruction in phonics (National Reading Panel, 2000); use of decodable texts for daily practice (Meyer & Felton, 1999); and books on tape to increase exposure to the sounds of language (Carbo, 1989). In addition, it may be beneficial to structure the students' learning environment to reduce distracting noise and increase their ability to selectively attend to relevant auditory stimuli (Bellis, 2003). Accommodations could include maintaining a low noise level in the classroom or seating a student close to the primary channels of auditory information (Zentall, 1983).

Table 12.9 identifies and outlines the cognitive processing requirements and any related educational interventions/accommodations for the other WJ III COG and DS Ga tests: Incomplete Words, Sound Patterns—Voice, and Sound Patterns—Music.

Fluid Reasoning (Gf)

Fluid reasoning (Gf) is a complex, hierarchical cognitive function that can rely on many other cognitive processes, depending on the nature and requirements of the task (Gray, Chabris, & Braver, 2003; Kosslyn & Smith, 2000). Reasoning ability is considered to be a scaffold for the development of many other cognitive abilities, particularly those in the acquired knowledge domain (Blair, 2006; Cattell, 1987; McArdle, 2001).

Concept Formation, a measure of induction, or inference, and Analysis–Synthesis, a measure of general sequential, or deductive, reasoning are two tests that compose the Gf cluster. The Concept Formation task requires rule application and frequent switching from one rule to another. Analysis–Synthesis requires drawing correct conclusions from stated conditions or premises, often from a series of sequential steps. Because of its use of specific solution keys that, if followed correctly, furnish the correct answer to each test item, Analysis–Synthesis can also be described as a measure of algorithmic reasoning. In CHC theory, algorithmic reasoning is an aspect of quantitative reasoning.

Interventions that are designed to develop skills in categorization and drawing conclusions, that involve connecting new concepts to prior knowledge, that use teacher demonstrations and guided practice, and that provide feedback on performance may positively influence the development of reasoning abilities (Klauer, Willmes, & Phye, 2002). Repeated opportunities to sort and classify objects are important in developing reasoning skills (Quinn, 2004). Particularly for young children, hands-on problem-solving tasks provide opportunities to be actively engaged in learning. These tasks need to be demonstrated by a teacher using a think-aloud procedure to model the steps involved in solving the problem. In addition, there are a wide variety of games designed to help develop patterning skills (Willis, 2008), such as finding similarities and differences, sorting, matching, and categorizing.

For older children and adults, interventions include cooperative learning groups and reciprocal teaching (Palincsar & Brown, 1984), graphic organizers (Marzano et al., 2001), and metacognitive strategies (Manning & Payne, 1996; Pressley, 1990). Cooperative learning groups and reciprocal teaching are effective ways to actively engage an individual in learning and to develop reasoning skills. Use of graphic organizers, such as Venn diagrams or concept maps, can help organize the information conceptually, linking new information to known information. Teaching metacognitive strategies and then providing opportunities to practice the strategies are important in developing higher-level reasoning skills. An individual is taught to think about the task, set goals, use self-talk, monitor progress, and then reward him- or herself when the task is accomplished. These metacognitive strategies help the individual to be aware of, monitor, and control his or her learning. Some specific strategies that might be incorporated include teaching the individual to compare new concepts to previously learned concepts or to use analogies, metaphors, or similes when approaching a task (Greenleaf, 2005).

Two additional Gf tests are included in the WJ III COG and DS. The Number Series test measures the ability to identify and apply an analogue or rule to complete a numerical sequence. The mental representations (or "number sense") that constitute this ability form the basis for the ability to learn symbols for numbers and perform simple calculations (Dehaene, 1997, 2000). Number Matrices requires a foundation in mathematics knowledge (i.e., access to the category-specific verbal and visual codes, such as knowledge of the number line); however, the verbal and/or visual codes are transcoded into analogical representations between sets of numbers. The solution to each item is obtained by mapping the relationship implied from the first part of the item onto the latter part of the item, thereby completing the matrix. Related interventions involve explicit instruction in seriation and number reasoning skills (High/Scope Educational Research Foundation, 2003; Kroesbergen & Van Luit, 2003).

Processing Speed (Gs)

Efficiency of cognitive processing is based partly on the speed of mental activity. For many years, cognitive speediness, or mental quickness, has been considered an important aspect of intelligence (Nettelbeck, 1994; Vernon, 1983). "In the face of limited processing resources, the speed of processing is critical because it determines in part how rapidly limited resources can be reallocated to other cognitive tasks" (Kail, 1991, p. 152). Two of the tests that compose the Gs cluster are Visual Matching and Decision Speed. Visual Matching is a perceptual speed measure, and Decision Speed measures speed of semantic processing (i.e., the speed of mental manipulation of stimulus content). Perceptual speed involves making comparisons based on rapid visual searches. Speed of semantic processing requires making symbolic comparisons of concepts. In contrast to decision making based on physical comparisons, the semantic or acquired knowledge (rather than perceptual information) needed for the Decision Speed test influences the decision-making process. Rapid Picture Naming and Pair Cancellation are also measures of processing speed.

There is some evidence that perceptual speed, as measured in Visual Matching or Cross Out (another Gs test), is related to the orthographic processing required for reading (McGrew, 1993; McGrew, Flanagan, Keith, & Vanderwood, 1997). Perhaps the rapid processing of visual symbols resembles the perceptual demands of reading. Research has confirmed the link between perceptual speed and reading.

Cognitive speediness can be positively influenced by repetitive practice, speed drills, and use of computer games that require an individual to make decisions quickly (Klingberg, 2009; Mahncke, Bronstone, & Merzenich, 2006; Tallal et al., 1996). More importantly, however, limitations in cognitive speediness, particularly perceptual speed, have implications for the provision of educational accommodations (Geary & Brown, 1991;

Hayes, Hynd, & Wisenbaker, 1986; Kail, 1990, 1991, 2003; Kail, Hall, & Caskey, 1999; Ofiesh, 2000; Shaywitz, 2003; Wolff, Michel, Ovrut, & Drake, 1990). Accommodations that compensate for limitations in processing or perceptual speed include providing extended time; reducing the quantity of work required (breaking large assignments into two or more component assignments); eliminating or limiting copying activities; and increasing wait times after questions are asked, as well as after responses are given (Ofiesh, 2000; Shaywitz, 2003).

Short-Term Memory (Gsm) and Working Memory Capacity

In CHC theory, short-term memory (Gsm) is the ability to apprehend and maintain awareness of elements of information in the immediate situation (the last minute or so); the term refers to a limited-capacity system that includes measures of auditory memory span and working memory capacity. Numbers Reversed, a measure of working memory capacity, and Memory for Words, a measure of memory span, are the two tests in the WJ III COG Gsm cluster. Numbers Reversed requires the ability to temporarily store and orally recode presented information, a measure of working memory capacity (Schrank et al., 2010). In this test, the individual is required to repeat a series of digits backward. Memory for Words measures the span of verbal (auditory) store by requiring the individual to repeat a series of unrelated words. Gathercole and Alloway (2008) characterize this type of task as short-term memory, but not working memory capacity because it involves storage but minimal processing. Memory for Sentences (another Gsm test) also measures the span of verbal memory, but in this test, memory is aided by context (i.e., semantic, meaning-based code).

Chunking strategies may be helpful in making more efficient use of available short-term memory capacity by recoding the information (Hardiman, 2003). Chunking strategies enable a person to group related items into units, making the information more manageable for understanding, storage, and recall. Importantly, however, accommodations may be needed to compensate for limitations in short-term memory or working memory capacity. These may include keeping oral directions short and simple, asking the student to paraphrase directions to ensure understanding, and providing visual cues for directions or steps to be followed (Gathercole & Alloway, 2008).

EDUCATIONAL INTERVENTIONS RELATED TO THE WJ III ACH TESTS

The 22 WJ III ACH tests sample the major aspects of oral language and academic achievement. In terms of CHC theory, the reading and writing tasks provide measures of a broad reading–writing construct (Grw). Newton and McGrew (2010) have defined Grw as "the breadth and depth of a person's acquired store of declarative and procedure reading and writing skills and knowledge" (p. 628). The WJ III ACH mathematics tests provide measures of a broad quantitative knowledge construct (Gq), or "the breadth and depth of a person's acquired store of declarative and procedural quantitative or numerical knowledge" (Newton & McGrew, 2010, p. 628). Oral language and knowledge tasks are also included in the WJ III ACH, providing additional measures of comprehension–knowledge (Gc). However, the WJ III ACH tests are cognitively complex tasks requiring the application of one or more narrow abilities and dynamic cognitive processes (McGrew et al., 2007). Table 12.10 is an outline of the narrow abilities defined by CHC theory and descriptions of the cognitive processes required for performance in each of the WJ III ACH tests. As in the WJ III COG and DS, the identified narrow abilities and inferred cognitive processes are used to provide a link between WJ III ACH test scores and evidence-based interventions.

Reading–Writing (Grw)

Reading–writing (Grw) is a broad cognitive ability that is based on the use of one or more shared cognitive processes (Woodcock, 1998). For example, both reading and writing involve mapping written forms of language onto phonological representations. In the normal sequence of language development, learning to read and write is mediated by phonological knowledge. For example, almost all children learn to use spoken language before written language, and research suggests that they map written language onto oral language (Caplan, 1992). Although learning to read and write is initially facilitated by phonological subword transformation processes, these processes may be discarded when the target skill has become more efficient and automatized (Baron & Strawson, 1976; Coltheart, 1978; Gough & Cosky, 1977). Consequently, Humphreys and Evett (1985) identified two routes to reading—a phonologically mediated process and a whole-word recognition process. Writing

TABLE 12.10. WJ III ACH Tests, Curricular Areas/CHC Narrow Abilities Measured, Cognitive Processes, and Related Educational Interventions

Test	Curricular area/CHC narrow abilities measured[a]	Cognitive processes	Related educational interventions
Test 1: Letter–Word Identification	Reading *Reading decoding*	Feature detection and analysis (for letters) and recognition of visual word forms and/or phonological access to pronunciations associated with visual word forms (i.e., words may or may not be familiar)	Explicit, systematic, synthetic phonics instruction; word recognition strategies (word walls, flow lists, word banks, flash cards); teaching high-frequency words; spelling-based decoding strategies; Fernald method
Test 2: Reading Fluency	Reading *Reading speed* *Semantic processing speed*	Speeded (automatic) semantic decision making requiring reading ability and generic knowledge	Repeated reading; passage previewing; assisted reading; practicing words in isolation
Test 3: Story Recall	Oral expression *Meaningful memory* *Listening ability*	Construction of propositional representations and recoding	Opportunities to hear and practice language; direct instruction in semantics, syntax, and pragmatics; role playing, games; compensatory skills
Test 4: Understanding Directions	Listening comprehension *Verbal working memory* *Listening ability*	Construction of a mental structure in immediate awareness and modification of the mental structure via mapping	Opportunities to practice listening and following directions; echo activities; auditory skill tapes; modifying the listening environment
Test 5: Calculation	Mathematics *Math achievement*	Access to and application of knowledge of numbers and calculation procedures; verbal associations between numbers represented as strings of words	Use of manipulatives; sequential direct instruction; development of number sense; cover–copy–compare method; demonstration with verbalization; cumulative review; lattice method of multiplication; mnemonic strategies; peer-assisted tutoring; concrete–representational–abstract teaching techniques; computer-assisted instruction
Test 6: Math Fluency	Mathematics *Math achievement* *Numerical facility*	Speeded (automatic) access to and application of digit–symbol arithmetic procedures (verbal associations between numbers represented as strings of words)	Development of number sense; math facts charts; explicit timings; computer-assisted instruction
Test 7: Spelling	Spelling *Spelling ability*	Access to and application of knowledge of orthography of word forms by mapping whole-word phonology onto whole-word orthography, by translating phonological segments into graphemic units, or by activating spellings of words from the semantic lexicon	Use of multisensory techniques; explicit, systematic phonics instruction; direct instruction in spelling rules; providing frequent practice; teaching common irregular words; encouraging independent reading to increase exposure to words in print; Write–Say method; Add-a-Word spelling program; group contingencies
Test 8: Writing Fluency	Writing *Writing ability* *Writing speed*	Speeded (automatic) formation of constituent sentence structures requiring fluent access to semantic and syntactic knowledge	Word, phrase, and sentence fluency-building activities; frequent practice

(cont.)

TABLE 12.10. *(cont.)*

Test	Curricular area/CHC narrow abilities measured[a]	Cognitive processes	Related educational interventions synthetic
Test 9: Passage Comprehension	Reading *Reading comprehension* *Cloze ability*	Construction of propositional representations; integration of syntactic and semantic properties of printed words and sentences into a representation of the whole passage; inferential bridging	Vocabulary enrichment; activating prior knowledge; use of graphic organizers; self-monitoring strategies; memory and imagery strategies
Test 10: Applied Problems	Mathematics *Quantitative reasoning* *Math achievement* *Math knowledge*	Construction of mental mathematics models via language comprehension, application of math knowledge, calculation skills, and/ or quantitative reasoning; formation of insight	Number talk; oral counting with sensory integration; use of pictures, graphs, and diagrams; direct instruction; strategy instruction
Test 11: Writing Samples	Writing *Writing ability*	Retrieval of word meanings via semantic access; application of psycholinguistic rules of case grammar and syntax; planning and construction of bridging inferences in immediate awareness (auditory and/or visual buffer)	Creating a literate, motivating, risk-free classroom environment; daily practice in writing; direct instruction in an expressive writing program; explicit instruction in the three key phases of the writing process; writing strategy instruction; use of dictation
Test 12: Story Recall—Delayed	General *Meaningful memory*	Reconstructive memory after a time delay; content accuracy; preservation of discourse structure	Active learning; rehearsal; overlearning; mnemonics; elaboration; visual representation
Test 13: Word Attack	Reading *Reading decoding* *Phonetic coding*	Grapheme-to-phoneme translation and accessing pronunciations of visual word forms not contained in the mental lexicon	Explicit, systematic, synthetic phonics instruction; explicit and systematic teaching of alphabetic principle; integration of phonological, orthographic, and morphological awareness
Test 14: Picture Vocabulary	Oral expression *Language development* *Lexical knowledge*	Object recognition; lexical access and retrieval	Creating a language- and experience-rich environment; frequent exposure to and practice with words; reading aloud to a child; text talks; semantic feature analysis; semantic maps; increased time spent reading; reading for different purposes; intentional, explicit word instruction; development of word consciousness; use of computerized programs
Test 15: Oral Comprehension	Listening comprehension *Listening ability*	Construction of propositional representations through syntactic and semantic integration of orally presented passages in real time; inferential bridging	Early exposure to language, particularly reading aloud to a child; direct instruction in vocabulary; directed vocabulary-building activities; outline of key points in lectures or oral instruction
Test 16: Editing	Writing skills *English usage*	Access and application of lexical and syntactic information about details of word forms and writing conventions	Strategies for proofreading; explicit instruction in the proofreading phase of the editing process; peer editing; use of technology

(cont.)

TABLE 12.10. *(cont.)*

Test	Curricular area/CHC narrow abilities measured[a]	Cognitive processes	Related educational interventions synthetic
Test 17: Reading Vocabulary	Reading *Lexical knowledge* *Reading comprehension*	Recognition of visual word forms; lexical activation and semantic access; semantic matching and verbal analogical reasoning	Semantic feature analysis; semantic maps; text talks; directed vocabulary-building activities; increased time spent reading; reading for different purposes; intentional explicit word instruction; independent word-learning strategies; development of word consciousness
Test 18: Quantitative Concepts	Mathematics *Math knowledge* *Quantitative reasoning*	Symbol recognition; access to and retrieval of category-specific representations; manipulation of points on a mental number line	Use of manipulatives; direct instruction in math concepts, symbols, and vocabulary; development of number sense; use of number line
Test 19: Academic Knowledge	General *General information* *Science information* *Cultural information* *Geography achievement*	Implicit, declarative category-specific memory	Creating a language- and experience-rich environment; frequent exposure to and practice with words used in science, social studies, and the humanities; reading aloud to a young child; text talks, particularly those that are academically related; semantic feature analysis; semantic maps; increased time spent reading; reading in the content area; intentional, explicit word instruction; direct instruction in morphology; development of word consciousness; use of computerized programs
Test 20: Spelling of Sounds	Spelling *Spelling ability* *Phonetic coding*	Translating spoken elements of nonwords into graphemic units; phonologically mediated mapping of orthography	Explicit, systematic instruction in phonics, orthography, and morphology; use of multisensory techniques; teaching common irregular words; providing frequent practice; encouraging independent reading; teaching use of a spell-checker
Test 21: Sound Awareness	Reading *Phonetic coding* *Working memory*	Access, retrieval, and application of the rules of English phonology	Early exposure to sounds, music, rhythms, and language; reading aloud to a child; providing opportunities that encourage exploration and manipulation of sounds, words, and language; instruction in rhyming, segmentation, and sound blending; manipulation and deletion of phonemes; daily practice
Test 22: Punctuation and Capitalization	Writing *English usage*	Access to and application of lexical information and details of word forms	Punctuation review exercises; self-directed attention to each punctuation mark

[a]Names of narrow abilities are given in italics.

tasks typically involve some of the same cognitive processes. "The visual word form system holds the permanent orthographic description of the word, its meaning is located in semantic memory, and a rule-governed procedure exists for mapping phonological information onto graphemic segments" (Caplan, p. 203).

The Letter–Word Identification test measures the CHC narrow ability of reading decoding. Letters are identified through feature analysis or feature detection (Gibson, 1965; McClelland & Rumelhart, 1981). Well-learned letters and words are accessed from the mental lexicon by means of automatic retrieval (Ashcraft, 2002). Caplan (1992) stated, "There is good evidence that visual word forms are largely activated on the basis of their constituent letters, that is, a reader identifies the letters in a word and then matches a representation of the word in memory against these letters" (p. 167). However, Coltheart (1978) pointed out that the nature of the task involved in Letter–Word Identification involves not only accessing words from the mental lexicon, but also the cognitive processes for activating and outputting representations of the sound patterns of the words, based on a phonological lexicon. As Caplan (1992) summarized, "It thus appears that most skilled oral reading and word recognition consists of identifying letters from a visual stimulus, using those letters to activate visual word forms stored in memory, and then accessing the pronunciation associated with the visual word form" (p. 167). Some interventions to increase the number of words contained in the mental lexicon include use of an explicit, systematic, synthetic phonics program (National Reading Panel, 2000; Stanovich, 1994; Torgesen, 1997); word recognition strategies (Adams, 1990; Moats, 1999; Pressley, 2006); teaching high-frequency words (Ehri, 1998); and spelling-based decoding strategies (Adams, 1990; Moats, 2005; Uhry & Shepherd, 1993).

The Word Attack test measures reading decoding and the narrow ability of phonetic coding, an aspect of phonemic competence (Ashcraft, 2002) that requires grapheme-to-phoneme translation of pseudowords not contained in the mental lexicon (Gazzaniga et al., 1998). Research suggests that the ability to translate nonwords such as *nat* or *ib* into sounds indicates the presence of a unique process for recognizing printed forms: assembling the pronunciation of a letter string by applying knowledge of typical correspondences between spelling units and sounds (Caplan, 1992). Use of an explicit, systematic, synthetic phonics program has proven to produce the largest gains among readers with poor decoding skills (National Reading Panel, 2000; Snow, Burns, & Griffin, 1998). These programs begin instruction at the phoneme level and then introduce graphemes. Students are explicitly taught the relationships between sounds (phonemes) and letters (graphemes), and then are taught how to blend the sounds to make words.

The Reading Vocabulary test measures the narrow abilities of verbal (printed) language comprehension and lexical, or vocabulary, knowledge. These abilities are described as functions of the mental lexicon (Ashcraft, 2002), particularly those that involve semantic memory (Quillian, 1968). Comprehension is achieved when the visual form of the word is connected to a concept by means of the semantic access and activation processes (Caplan, 1992). However, evidence suggests that this task may also be phonologically mediated. Van Orden and colleagues (Van Orden, 1987; Van Orden, Johnston, & Hale, 1988) demonstrated that the meanings of visually presented words can be activated via their sounds.

Many vocabulary words are learned indirectly through the development of oral language abilities or through reading. Incidental word learning through reading depends on the amount of time a student spends reading. Reading for different purposes and at different levels of difficulty exposes the student to new words that would never be encountered in oral language alone and helps create connections between words. Vocabulary can also be developed through explicit interventions. Intentional, explicit teaching of specific words and word-learning strategies will improve vocabulary as well as comprehension of text including those words (Graves, 2000). Other explicit interventions to increase reading vocabulary include semantic feature analysis (Anders & Bos, 1986; Pittelman et al., 1991); semantic maps (Johnson & Pearson, 1984; Sinatra et al., 1985); text talks (Beck & McKeown, 2001); increased time spent reading (Anderson, Wilson, & Fielding, 1988; Cunningham & Stanovich, 1991; Mastropieri, Leinart, & Scruggs, 1999); reading for specific purposes (Anderson, 1996; National Reading Panel, 2000; Stahl, 1999); intentional, explicit word instruction (teaching synonyms, antonyms, multiple-meaning words) (Beck et al., 2002; Graves et al., 2004; National Reading Panel, 2000); independent word-learning strategies (identification and use of context clues, use of dictionary and other reference tools, direct instruction in morphology) (Anglin, 1993; Baumann, Edwards, et al., 2003; Baumann, Kame'enui, et al., 2003; Blachowicz & Fisher, 2000; Carlisle, 2004; Graves, 2000; National Reading Panel, 2000); development of word consciousness (Anderson & Nagy, 1992; Graves & Watts-Taffe, 2002; Nagy & Scott, 2000); and use of computerized vocabulary development programs (Davidson et al., 1996).

Reading Fluency is a speeded semantic decision task that requires reading ability. This test measures the CHC narrow ability of reading speed. However, this test also requires a store of general information to be able to confirm the accuracy of a statement that is read; this helps form a decision as to whether the statement is true (Ashcraft, 2002). Fluency-building interventions include repeated reading (Begeny & Martens, 2006; O'Shea, Sindelar, & O'Shea, 1985; Rashotte & Torgesen, 1985; Samuels, 1985), passage previewing, assisted reading (Shany & Biemiller, 1995), and practicing words in isolation (Levy, Abello, & Lysynchuk, 1997). These interventions may be beneficial for use with students individually or as part of a small-group instructional program.

Passage Comprehension is a complex, conceptually driven, online comprehension task (Ashcraft, 2002; Gernsbacher, 1990) that measures the narrow ability of reading comprehension as it occurs. As the subject reads, the meaning of the passage is derived through construction of propositional representations based on concepts from stored knowledge. This aspect of the process requires the narrow ability of verbal (printed) language comprehension. Meaning is placed in immediate awareness as the passage is read. As more elements are added to the passage, they are also added to the structure held in immediate awareness via the process of mapping, a central feature of cognition (Ashcraft, 2002; Zhou & Black, 2000). The task is solved through inference (Klin, 1995)—the process by which the reader determines the referents of words and ideas, draws connections between concepts (bridging) (Clark, 1977), and derives a conclusion from the passage.

Various interventions to increase reading comprehension include activating the reader's prior knowledge (National Reading Panel, 2000; Ogle, 1986); use of graphic organizers (Berkowitz, 1986; Gardill & Jitendra, 1999; Marzano et al., 2001); self-monitoring strategies (Babbs, 1984; Brown & Palincsar, 1985; Klingner & Vaughn, 1998; National Reading Panel, 2000); and memory and imagery strategies (Gambrell & Jawitz, 1993; Mas-

tropieri & Scruggs, 1988; Peters & Levin, 1986). One strategy requires the student to summarize the central idea of a passage as a *keyword* and then to make a mental picture of that keyword (Levin, Levin, Glasman, & Nordwall, 1992). The student also uses mental imagery to connect related ideas to the keyword.

Cognitive strategy instruction has been demonstrated to increase reading comprehension (Gersten, Fuchs, Williams, & Baker, 2001). Such strategies encourage active, self-regulated, and intentional reading (Trabasso & Bouchard, 2002). One example of a reading comprehension intervention is Multipass, a metacognitive approach that a student can learn to use to better comprehend textbook content (Schumaker, Deshler, Alley, Warner, & Denton, 1982). A reading comprehension intervention that combines strategy instruction and cooperative learning is reciprocal teaching (Palinscar & Brown, 1984), a cooperative group learning strategy that helps develop critical thinking skills through reading. Such skills include setting a purpose for reading, reading for meaning, and self-monitoring of understanding.

The Writing Samples test measures the CHC narrow ability of writing ability. This test measures the ability to convey propositional meaning at the discourse level of language (Caplan, 1992). It requires retrieval of word meanings and syntactic information (i.e., knowledge of how words are combined into sentences) in the mental lexicon (Gazzaniga et al., 1998). Generation of acceptable sentences involves ideational fluency and the application of the psycholinguistic rules of grammar, particularly phrase structure. In several items, the subject must make bridging inferences in working memory to integrate the initial and final sentences into a well-formed passage. These items require planning, or tailoring the target sentence to the lexical and semantic information that is conveyed in the other portions of the sample (Ferreira, 1996).

Interventions for limited proficiency on Writing Samples include creating a literate, motivating, risk-free classroom environment (Gunn et al., 1995; Morrow, 1989); daily practice in writing (Graves, 1983; Sulzby, 1992); direct instruction in an expressive writing program (De La Paz, 1999; Englert, Raphael, Anderson, Anthony, & Stevens, 1991; Walker, Shippen, Alberto, Houchins, & Cihak, 2005); explicit instruction in the three key phases of the writing process (Gersten, Baker, & Edwards, 1999); writing strategy instruction (Chalk, Hagan-Burke, & Burke, 2005; De La Paz

& Graham, 1997a, 1997b; Graham & Harris, 1989, 2003); and use of dictation (De La Paz & Graham, 1997a).

Caplan (1992) suggests that "smooth written production of sentences depends on the temporary storage of words in a buffer that maintains information while the response is organized and executed" (p. 174). This suggests an influence of working memory on writing performance. "If the words, having been accessed, have to be held in a buffer store for a few seconds, as is likely to be the case in writing, then acoustic, as opposed to visual, coding will, according to the evidence from studies in short-term memory, be the more durable" (Hotopf, 1983, p. 166). Caplan suggested that written language production is an extremely complex task whose subprocesses function dynamically and are probably monitored by a centralized mechanism that helps preserve the structure of legitimate words (possibly working memory).

Spelling measures knowledge of the details of word forms contained in the mental lexicon (Gazzaniga et al., 1998). It often involves mapping phonology to orthographic representations of words "either by mapping whole-word phonology into whole-word orthography (if the word is contained in the lexicon), or by translating phonemic segments into graphemic units" (Caplan, 1992, p. 214). Evidence for this form of mapping was provided by Hotopf (1980, 1983), who analyzed dictation-type spelling errors and determined that a significant proportion of the errors were related to the underlying sound of the target words. Evidence also exists for a visual buffer that maintains the graphemic code in immediate awareness during spelling (Caramazza, Miceli, Villa, & Romani, 1987). Written production takes place by generating the spatial form of each letter in the correct order (Ellis, 1982). However, the orthography of entire words can also be activated entirely from their meaning (Caplan, 1992).

Some interventions for spelling include use of multisensory techniques (Carreker, 2005); use of explicit, systematic phonics instruction (Ehri, 1998; National Reading Panel, 2000); direct instruction (Edwards, 2003; Graham, 1983; Gordon, Vaughn, & Schumm, 1993); providing frequent practice (Berninger et al., 1998; Moats, 1995); teaching common irregular words (Moats, 2005); encouraging independent reading (Anderson et al., 1985; Taylor, Frye, & Maruyama, 1990); the Write–Say method (Kearney & Drabman, 2001); the Add-a-Word spelling program (McLaughlin, Reiter, Mabee, & Byram, 1991; Schermerhorn &

McLaughlin, 1997); and use of group contingencies (Popkin & Skinner, 2003; Shapiro & Goldberg, 1986; Truchlicka, McLaughlin, & Swain, 1998).

The Writing Fluency test measures the narrow abilities of writing ability and writing speed. This task requires speeded formulation of constituent structures, or fluency of combining words into phrases (Gazzaniga et al., 1998). Automaticity of writing performance is likely to be aided by mapping from semantics directly to orthography (Caplan, 1992) rather than by mapping phonology to orthography. Possible interventions related to limited performance on Writing Fluency include explicit instruction in the mechanics of writing (Graham, Berninger, Abbott, Abbott, & Whitaker, 1997); word, phrase, and sentence fluency-building activities (Hillocks, 1987); frequent practice (Graves, 1991; Gudschinsky, 1973; Moats, 1999); and use of technology (MacArthur, Graham, & Schwarz, 1993).

The Editing test requires knowledge of the details of word forms and knowledge of writing conventions (English usage); these are functions of the mental lexicon (Ashcraft, 2002). Possible interventions for low performance on Editing include strategies for proofreading (Lanham, 1992); explicit instruction in the proofreading phase of the editing process (Hillocks & Smith, 1991); peer editing (Stoddard & MacArthur, 1993); and use of editing technology (MacArthur, Ferretti, Okolo, & Cavalier, 2001). The Punctuation and Capitalization test also requires accessing and applying lexical information and details of word forms. An example of an intervention for low performance on Punctuation and Capitalization is to have the student circle every punctuation mark in a passage. This forces him or her to look at each punctuation mark and evaluate whether or not it is correct (Lane & Lange, 1993).

Two auditory processing tests measure reading- and writing-related abilities. Sound Awareness measures phonemic competence, or retrieval and application of the rules of permissible English words or sound combinations (Ashcraft, 2002). In CHC theory, this narrow ability is called phonetic coding. In addition, the requirement to manipulate phonemes during portions of the Sound Awareness test appears to place demands on working memory. For young children, possible interventions include early exposure to sounds, music, rhythms, and language (Glazer, 1989; Strickland, 1991); reading aloud to the children (Adams, 1990; Anderson et al., 1985); providing opportunities that encourage exploration and manipulation of sounds, words, and language (Adams, 1990); and daily practice with language (Bridge et al., 1983). For school-age children and some adolescents, interventions typically include explicit, systematic instruction in phonics (National Reading Panel, 2000); use of decodable texts for daily practice (Meyer & Felton, 1999); and listening to books on tape (Carbo, 1989).

Spelling of Sounds measures phonetic coding and spelling ability (or knowledge of the sound patterns of word forms), which are functions of the mental lexicon (Gazzaniga et al., 1998). This task specifically targets phonologically mediated spelling (Caplan, 1992) because the correct orthographic segment(s) is based directly on the spoken elements that constitute the stimulus. Related interventions include explicit, systematic instruction in phonics (Ehri, 1991; National Reading Panel, 2000), orthography (Moats, 2005; Templeton & Bear, 1992), and morphology (Carlisle & Stone, 2005); teaching a student how to analyze the syllables within words (graphosyllabic instruction) (Bhattacharya & Ehri, 2004); use of multisensory techniques (Carreker, 2005; Fernald, 1943); teaching common irregular words (Moats, 2005); providing frequent practice (Bridge et al., 1983); use of a spell-checker as an accommodation (MacArthur, Graham, Haynes, & De La Paz, 1996); and encouraging independent reading (Anderson et al., 1985; Taylor et al., 1990).

Mathematics (Gq)

The primary narrow CHC abilities that pertain to all of the WJ III mathematics tests are mathematics knowledge and mathematics achievement. The Calculation test requires access to and application of mathematical calculation knowledge. Math Fluency requires the rapid application of basic addition, subtraction, and multiplication procedures, which together constitute numerical facility. Simple addition and subtraction rules involve numbers coded as quantities on the number line; multiplication and division rules are based on a set of associations between numbers represented as strings of words (e.g., multiplication tables) (Dehaene, 1997, 2000).

Some possible interventions for low performance on the Calculation test and skill development in this area include sequential direct instruction (Kroesbergen & Van Luit, 2003; Maccini & Gagnon, 2000); developing number sense (Ginsburg, 1997; Griffin, 1998); use of ma-

nipulatives (Butler, Miller, Crehan, Babbitt, & Pierce, 2003; Cass, Cates, Smith & Jackson, 2003; Siegler, 1988); cover–copy–compare (Hayden & McLaughlin, 2004; Lee & Tingstrom, 1994; Skinner, Turco, Beatty, & Rasavage, 1989); demonstration with verbalization (Rivera & Deutsch Smith, 1988); mnemonic strategies (Greene, 1999; Maccini & Hughes, 2000); peer-assisted tutoring (Calhoon & Fuchs, 2003; Greenwood & Terry, 1993); concrete–representational–abstract teaching techniques (Morin & Miller, 1998); and computer-assisted instruction (Howell, Sidorenko, & Jurica, 1987).

Limited fluency with basic facts may interfere with the development of higher-level math skills and hinder later achievement. Therefore, it is important to assess this area and, when performance is limited, to provide appropriate interventions. Related interventions for low performance on Math Fluency include developing number sense (Berch, 1998; Bruer, 1997; Case, 1998; Griffin, 1998); math fact charts (Pellegrino & Goldman, 1987); explicit timings (Rathvon, 2008; Van Houten & Thompson, 1976); and computer-assisted instruction (Cummings & Elkins, 1999; Hasselbring, Goin, & Bransford, 1988).

Exact calculation and reasoning with numbers have been demonstrated to involve two different types of processes (Dehaene, Molko, Cohen, & Wilson, 2004). Besides mathematics knowledge, Applied Problems and Quantitative Concepts also require quantitative reasoning. For example, some of the more difficult items on the Number Series subtest in Quantitative Concepts require a mental manipulation of points on the number line. Applied Problems requires the construction of mental models (Johnson-Laird, Byrne, & Schaeken, 1992) to solve problems through the application of insight or quantitative reasoning. Solutions to these problems require access to complex cognitive processes and the calculation abilities that depend on them (Ashcraft, 1995). Because many Applied Problems items involve language comprehension (i.e., either listening ability or reading comprehension), the tasks are typically performed mentally by using working memory processes. Interventions related to low performance on Applied Problems and Quantitative Concepts include direct instruction (Kroesbergen & Van Luit, 2003; Maccini & Gagnon, 2000; Swanson, 2001; Tarver, 1992); use of data tables (Sellke, Behr, & Voelker, 1991); and strategy instruction (Hutchinson, 1993; Lenz, Ellis, & Scanlon, 1996; Montague, 1992; Montague & Candace, 1986).

Oral Language and Knowledge

Oral language tasks involve the integration of complex cognitive processes such as semantic memory and reasoning (Caplan, 1992). Story Recall requires comprehending and remembering the principal components of a story by constructing propositional representations (Anderson, 1976, 1985; Kintsch, 1974) and by recoding (Miller, 1956). *Recoding* is the cognitive process that is involved when we attempt to rephrase expressions in our own words. These cognitive processes provide support to the specification of the CHC narrow abilities of language development, listening ability, and meaningful memory. Examples of interventions related to limited performance on Story Recall include opportunities to hear and practice language (Hart & Risley, 1995, 2003; Moats, 2001); direct instruction in semantics, syntax, and pragmatics; role-playing games; and compensatory skills.

Story Recall—Delayed requires reconstructive memory (Ashcraft, 2002) and content accuracy; it stresses memory for the meaningful, semantic content of the material. Caplan (1992) described this process as the preservation of discourse structure. Because the storage and recall of meaningful information is an important aspect of academic competence, active learning (Marzano et al., 2001), rehearsal (Squire & Schacter, 2002), elaboration (Wolfe, 2001), mnemonics (Wolfe, 2001), and visual representations (Greenleaf & Wells-Papanek, 2005) may all be useful interventions.

Understanding Directions requires listening and mapping a series of sequential directions onto the mental structure under construction and maintaining the sequence in immediate awareness until a new directive changes the sequence (Gernsbacher, 1990, 1991, 1997); this is a function of verbal working memory. Interventions related to limited proficiency on Understanding Directions include opportunities to practice listening and following directions (Galda & Cullinan, 1991; Leung & Pikulski, 1990); echo activities (Clay, 1991); and modifying the listening environment (Hardiman, 2003).

Carroll (1993) defined listening ability primarily as listening comprehension. The Oral Comprehension test is a complex, discourse-level, online listening comprehension task that requires integration of orally presented syntactic and semantic information (Brown & Hagoort, 1999; Caplan, 1992; Gernsbacher, 1990). The task requires (1) retrieval of basic word meanings from the mental lexicon (semantic memory) to yield abstract representations; (2) assignment of words to various case roles required by the relation expressed in the sentence; and (3) formation of a propositional structure based on mapping structures within a sentence, as well as across sentences in connected discourse. Unlike the Passage Comprehension task, the Oral Comprehension Task aids the listener in dividing the discourse into meaningful segments by prosodic information. Complex cognitive processing is required to determine the right sense or meaning of the target word in the context of the discourse (Gazzaniga et al., 1998). Early interventions to help develop this skill include exposure to language (Hart & Risley, 1995; Moats, 2001), particularly reading aloud to a child (Adams, 1990; Anderson et al., 1985). Direct instruction in vocabulary (Beck & McKeown, 2001) and use of directed vocabulary thinking activities (Graves, 2000) also help develop listening comprehension skills. School-age children who have difficulties following the teacher's oral discourse in the classroom may benefit from an outline of key points (Wallach & Butler, 1994) on the board or overhead projector before the beginning of each instructional unit. Use of a directed vocabulary thinking activity (Graves, 2000) can help students learn how to use context to infer meaning of words that are not known.

Picture Vocabulary requires the cognitive processes of object recognition, lexical access, and lexical retrieval. This test is a nonreading, lexical-level language development task. Object recognition depends on an analysis of the shape and form of a visual stimulus, although nonshape cues such as color can contribute to recognition (Marr, 1982). Lexical access results when visual representations stimulate, or prime, object constructs (Martin, 2009; Murphy, 2002) that spread to semantic attributes of words. Retrieval results when the name of the object is located in the store of lexical knowledge (Gazzaniga et al., 1998) or semantic memory (Tulving, 1972, 1983, 2000).

For young children, suggested oral language interventions include creating a language- and experience-rich environment (Gunn et al., 1995; Hart & Risley, 2003); frequent exposure and practice with words (Gunn et al, 1995; Hart & Risley, 2003); reading aloud (Adams, 1990); and text talks (Beck & McKeown, 2001). For older children and adolescents, possible interventions include text talks (Beck & McKeown, 2001); increased time spent reading (Cunningham & Stanovich, 1991; Herman et al., 1987); reading for different purposes (Anderson, 1996; National Reading Panel, 2000;

Stahl, 1999); intentional, explicit word instruction (teaching synonyms, antonyms, multiple-meaning words) (Beck et al., 2002; Graves et al., 2004; National Reading Panel, 2000); direct instruction in morphology (Anglin, 1993; Baumann, Edwards, et al., 2003; Baumann, Kame'enui, et al., 2003; Blachowicz & Fisher, 2000; Carlisle, 2004; Graves, 2000; National Reading Panel, 2000); development of word consciousness (Anderson & Nagy, 1992; Graves & Watts-Taffe, 2002; Nagy & Scott, 2000); and use of computerized programs (Davidson et al., 1996). Two other examples include semantic feature analysis (Anders & Bos, 1986; Pittelman et al., 1991) and semantic maps (Johnson & Pearson, 1984; Sinatra et al., 1985).

SUMMARY

The 31 tests included in the WJ III NU COG and DS, and the 22 tests included in the WJ III NU ACH, provide measures of broad and narrow cognitive abilities as defined by CHC theory. Although the WJ III NU clusters represent broad classes of abilities that are valid and useful for many interpretive purposes, this chapter has focused primarily on test-level interpretation, homing in at the narrow-ability level of CHC theory. The narrow abilities identified by CHC theory and descriptions of the cognitive processing required for performance combine to form a theoretical and conceptual basis for suggested links between the WJ III NU tests and evidence-based educational interventions. This linkage may represent a significant advancement in assessment practice because targeted instructional interventions and/or accommodations that address appropriately identified cognitive limitations may be foundational to improved performance in areas where learning difficulties are manifested. As the focus shifts from assessment for program placement to assessment for program planning, the WJ III NU and WIIIP represent a comprehensive evaluation system that can be useful for linking test performance to educational interventions or accommodations.

REFERENCES

Adams, M. J. (1990). *Beginning to read: Thinking and learning about print.* Cambridge, MA: MIT Press

Anders, P., & Bos, C. (1986). Semantic feature analysis: An interactive strategy for vocabulary development and text comprehension. *Journal of Reading, 9,* 610–616.

Anderson, J. R. (1976). *Language, memory, and thought.* Hillsdale, NJ: Erlbaum.

Anderson, J. R. (1985). *Cognitive psychology and its implications* (2nd ed.). New York: Freeman.

Anderson, R. C. (1996). Research foundations to support wide reading. In V. Greaney (Ed.), *Promoting reading in developing countries* (pp. 55–77). Newark, DE: International Reading Association.

Anderson, R. C., Hiebert, E. H., Scott, J. A., & Wilkinson, I. A. G. (1985). *Becoming a nation of readers: The report of the commission on reading.* Champaign, IL: Center for the Study of Reading, National Institute of Education, National Academy of Education.

Anderson, R. C., & Nagy, W. E. (1992). The vocabulary conundrum. *American Educator, 16*(4), 14–18, 44–47.

Anderson, R. C., Wilson, P. T., & Fielding, L. G. (1988). Growth in reading and how children spend their time outside of school. *Reading Research Quarterly, 23,* 285–303.

Anglin, J. M. (1993). Vocabulary development: A morphological analysis. *Monographs of the Society for Research in Child Development, 58*(10, Serial No. 238), 1–66.

Ashcraft, M. H. (1995). Cognitive psychology and simple arithmetic: A review and summary of new directions. *Mathematical Cognition, 1*(1), 3–34.

Ashcraft, M. H. (2002). *Cognition* (3rd ed.). Upper Saddle River, NJ: Prentice Hall.

Babbs, P. J. (1984). Monitoring cards help improve comprehension. *The Reading Teacher, 38*(2), 200–204.

Baron, R. W., & Strawson, C. (1976). Use of orthographic and word-specific knowledge in reading words aloud. *Journal of Experimental Psychology: Human Perception and Performance, 2,* 386—393.

Baumann, J. F., Edwards, E. C., Boland, E. M., Olejnik, S., & Kame'enui, E. J. (2003). Vocabulary tricks: Effects of instruction in morphology and context on fifth-grade students' ability to derive and infer word meanings. *American Educational Research Journal, 40,* 447–494.

Baumann, J. F., Kame'enui, E. J., & Ash, G. E. (2003). Research on vocabulary instruction: Voltaire redux. In J. Flood, D. Lapp, J. R. Squire, & J. M. Jensen (Eds.), *Handbook of research on teaching the English language arts* (2nd ed., pp. 752–785). Mahwah, NJ: Erlbaum.

Beck, I. L., & McKeown, M. G. (2001). Text talk: Capturing the benefits of read-aloud experiences for young children. *The Reading Teacher, 55,* 10–20.

Beck, I. L., McKeown, M. G., & Kucan, L. (2002).

Bringing words to life: Robust vocabulary instruction. New York: Guilford Press.

Begeny, J. C., & Martens, B. K. (2006). Assisting low-performing readers with group-based reading fluency instruction. *School Psychology Review, 35*(1), 91–107.

Bellis, T. J. (2003). *Assessment and management of central auditory processing disorders in the educational setting from science to practice.* Clifton Park, NY: Thomson.

Berch, D. B. (Ed.). (1998, April). *Mathematical cognition: From numerical thinking to mathematics education.* Conference presented by the National Institute of Child Health and Human Development, Bethesda, MD.

Berkowitz, S. J. (1986). Effects of instruction in text organization on sixth-grade students' memory for expository reading. *Reading Research Quarterly, 21,* 161–178.

Berninger, V., Vaughn, K., Abbott, R., Brooks, A., Abbott, S., Rogan, L., et al. (1998). Early intervention for spelling problems: Teaching functional spelling units of varying size with a multiple-connections framework. *Journal of Educational Psychology, 90,* 587–605.

Bhattacharya, A., & Ehri, L. (2004). Grapho-syllabic analysis helps adolescent struggling readers read and spell words. *Journal of Learning Disabilities, 37,* 331–348.

Blachowicz, C., & Fisher, P. (2000). Vocabulary instruction. In M. L. Kamil, P. Mosenthal, P. D. Pearson, & R. Barr (Eds.), *Handbook of reading research* (Vol. 3, pp. 503–523). Mahwah, NJ: Erlbaum.

Blair, C. (2006). How similar are fluid cognition and general intelligence?: A developmental neuroscience perspective on fluid cognition as an aspect of human cognitive ability. *Behavior and Brain Sciences, 29*(2), 109–125; discussion, 125–160.

Brefczynski, J. A., & DeYoe, E. A. (1999). A physiological correlate of the 'spotlight' of visual attention. *Nature Neuroscience, 2,* 370–374.

Bridge, C. A., Winograd, P. N., & Haley, D. (1983). Using predictable materials vs. preprimers to teach beginning sight words. *The Reading Teacher, 36*(9), 884–891.

Brown, A. L., & Palincsar, A. S. (1985). *Reciprocal teaching of comprehension strategies: A natural history of one program to enhance learning* (Tech. Rep. No. 334). Champaign: University of Illinois at Urbana–Champaign, Center for the Study of Reading.

Brown, C., & Hagoort, P. (1999). *Neurocognition of language.* Oxford: Oxford University Press.

Bruer, J. T. (1997). Education and the brain: A bridge too far. *Educational Researcher, 26*(8), 4–16.

Butler, F. M., Miller, S. P., Crehan, K., Babbitt, B., &

Pierce, T. (2003). Fraction instruction for students with mathematics disabilities: Comparing two teaching sequences. *Learning Disabilities Research and Practice, 18*(2), 99–111.

Calhoon, M. B., & Fuchs, L. S. (2003). The effects of peer-assisted learning strategies and curriculum-based measurement on the mathematics performance of secondary students with disabilities. *Remedial and Special Education, 24,* 235–245.

Caplan, D. (1992). *Language: Structure, processing, and disorders.* Cambridge, MA: MIT Press.

Caramazza, A., Miceli, G., Villa, G., & Romani, C. (1987). The role of the grapheme buffer in spelling: Evidence from a case of acquired dysgraphia. *Cognition, 26,* 59–85.

Carbo, M. (1989). *How to record books for maximum reading gains.* Roslyn Heights, NY: National Reading Styles Institute.

Carlisle, J. F. (2004). Morphological processes influencing literacy learning. In C. A. Stone, E. R. Silliman, B. J. Ehren, & K. Apel (Eds.), *Handbook of language and literacy: Development and disorders* (pp. 318–339). New York: Guilford Press.

Carlisle, J. F., & Stone, C. A. (2005). Exploring the role of morphemes in word reading. *Reading Research Quarterly, 40*(4), 428–449.

Carreker, S. (2005). Teaching spelling. In J. Birsh (Ed.), *Multisensory teaching of basic language skills* (2nd ed., pp. 257–295). Baltimore: Brookes.

Carroll, J. B. (1987). New perspectives in the analysis of abilities. In R. R. Ronning, J. A. Glover, J. C. Conoley, & J. C. Witt (Eds.), *The influence of cognitive psychology on testing* (pp. 267–284). Hillsdale, NJ: Erlbaum.

Carroll, J. B. (1990). Estimating item and ability parameters in homogeneous tests with the person characteristic function. *Applied Psychological Measurement, 14*(2), 109–125.

Carroll, J. B. (1993). *Human cognitive abilities: A survey of factor-analytic studies.* New York: Cambridge University Press.

Carroll, J. B. (2003). The higher stratum structure of cognitive abilities: Current evidence supports g and about ten broad factors. In H. Nyborg (Ed.), *The scientific study of general intelligence: Tribute to Arthur R. Jensen* (pp. 5–22). New York: Pergamon Press.

Case, R. (1998, April). *A psychological model of number sense and its development.* Paper presented at the annual meeting of the American Educational Research Association, San Diego, CA.

Cass, M., Cates, D., Smith, M., & Jackson, C. (2003). Effects of manipulative instruction on solving area and perimeter problems by students with learning disabilities. *Learning Disabilities Research and Practice, 18*(2), 112–120.

Cattell, R. B. (1941). Some theoretical issues in adult intelligence testing. *Psychological Bulletin, 38,* 592.

Cattell, R. B. (1943). The measurement of adult intelligence. *Psychological Bulletin, 40,* 153–193.

Cattell, R. B. (1950). *Personality: A systematic theoretical and factorial study.* New York: McGraw-Hill.

Cattell, R. B. (1987). *Advances in psychology: Vol. 35. Intelligence: Its structure, growth and action.* Amsterdam: Elsevier.

Chalk, J. C., Hagan-Burke, S., & Burke, M. D. (2005). The effects of self-regulated strategy development on the writing process for high school students with learning disabilities. *Learning Disability Quarterly, 28,* 75–87.

Clark, H. H. (1977). Bridging. In P. N. Johnson-Laird & P. C. Wason (Eds.), *Thinking: Readings in cognitive science* (pp. 411–420). Cambridge, UK: Cambridge University Press.

Clay, M. M. (1991). *Becoming literate: The construction of inner control.* Portsmouth, NH: Heinemann.

Coltheart, M. (1978). Lexical access in simple reading tasks. In B. Underwood (Ed.), *Strategies of information processing* (pp. 151–215). London: Academic Press.

Cummings, J. J., & Elkins, J. (1999). Lack of automaticity in the basic addition facts as a characteristic of arithmetic learning problems and instructional needs. *Mathematical Cognition, 5*(2), 149–180.

Cunningham, A. E., & Stanovich, K. E. (1991). Tracking the unique effects of print. *Journal of Educational Psychology, 83*(2), 264–274.

Davidson, J., Elcock, J., & Noyes, P. (1996). A preliminary study of the effect of computer-assisted practice on reading attainment. *Journal of Research in Reading, 19*(2), 102–110.

Dehaene, S. (1997). *The number sense.* New York: Oxford University Press.

Dehaene, S. (2000). Cerebral bases of number processing and calculation. In M. S. Gazzaniga (Ed.), *The new cognitive neurosciences* (2nd ed., pp. 987–998). Cambridge, MA: MIT Press.

Dehaene, S., Molko, N., Cohen, L., & Wilson, A. J. (2004). Arithmetic and the brain. *Current Opinion in Neurobiology, 14*(2), 218–224.

De La Paz, S. (1999). Self-regulated strategy instruction in regular education settings: Improving outcomes for students with and without learning disabilities. *Learning Disabilities Research and Practice, 14*(2), 92–106.

De La Paz, S., & Graham, S. (1997a). Effects of dictation and advanced planning instruction on the composing of students with writing and learning problems. *Journal of Educational Psychology, 89,* 203–222.

De La Paz, S., & Graham, S. (1997b). Strategy instruction in planning: Effects on the writing performance and behavior of students with learning disabilities. *Exceptional Children, 63,* 167–181.

Edwards, L. (2003). Writing instruction in kindergarten: Examining an emerging area of research for children with writing and reading difficulties. *Journal of Learning Disabilities, 36*(2), 136–148.

Ehri, L. C. (1991). Development of the ability to read words. In R. Barr, M. Kamil, P. Mosenthal, & P. D. Pearson (Eds.), *Handbook of reading research* (Vol. 2, pp. 383–417). New York: Longman.

Ehri, L. C. (1998). Learning to read and learning to spell are one and the same, almost. In C. Perfetti, L. Rieben, & M. Fayol (Eds.), *Learning to spell: Research, theory and practice across languages* (pp. 237–269). Mahwah, NJ: Erlbaum.

Ellis, A. W. (1982). Spelling and writing (and reading and speaking). In A. W. Ellis (Ed.), *Normality and pathology in cognitive function* (pp. 113–146). London: Academic Press.

Englert, C. S., Raphael, T. E., Anderson, L. M., Anthony, H. M., & Stevens, D. D. (1991). Making writing strategies and self-talk visible: Cognitive strategy instruction in regular and special education classrooms. *American Educational Research Journal, 28,* 337–372.

Fernald, G. (1943). *Remedial techniques in basic school subjects.* New York: McGraw-Hill.

Ferreira, V. S. (1996). Is it better to give than to donate?: Syntactic flexibility in language production. *Journal of Memory and Language, 35,* 724–755.

Fiorello, C. A., Hale, J. B., Snyder, L. E., Forrest, E., & Teodori, A. (2008). Validating individual differences through examination of converging psychometric and neuropsychological models of cognitive functioning. In S. K. Thurman & C. A. Fiorello (Eds.), *Applied cognitive research in K–3 classrooms* (pp. 151–186). New York: Routledge.

Floyd, R. G., Shaver, R. B., & McGrew, K. S. (2003). Interpretation of the Woodcock–Johnson III Tests of Cognitive Abilities: Acting on evidence. In F. A. Schrank & D. P. Flanagan (Eds.), *WJ III clinical use and interpretation: Scientist-practitioner perspectives* (pp. 1–46). San Diego, CA: Academic Press.

Galda, L., & Cullinan, B. E. (1991). Literature for literacy: What research says about the benefits of using trade books in the classroom. In J. Flood, J. M. Jensen, D. Lapp, & J. R. Squire (Eds.), *Handbook of research on teaching the English language arts* (pp. 529–535). New York: Macmillan.

Gambrell, L. B., & Jawitz, P. B. (1993). Mental imagery, text illustrations, and children's story comprehension and recall. *Reading Research Quarterly, 23,* 265–273.

Gardill, M. C., & Jitendra, A. K. (1999). Advanced story

map instruction: Effects on the reading comprehension of students with learning disabilities. *Journal of Special Education, 28,* 2–17.

Gathercole, S. E., & Alloway, T. P. (2008). Working memory and classroom learning. In S. K. Thurman & C. A. Fiorello (Eds.), *Applied cognitive research in K–3 classrooms* (pp. 17–40). New York: Routledge.

Gazzaniga, M. S., Irvy, R. B., & Mangun, G. R. (1998). *Cognitive neuroscience: The biology of the mind.* New York: Norton.

Geary, D. C., & Brown, S. C. (1991). Cognitive addition: Strategy choice and speed-of-processing differences in gifted, normal, and mathematically disabled children. *Developmental Psychology, 27,* 398–406.

Gentner, D., & Markman, A. B. (1997). Structure mapping in analogy and similarity. *American Psychologist, 52*(1), 45–46.

Gernsbacher, M. A. (1990). *Language comprehension as structure building.* Hillsdale, NJ: Erlbaum.

Gernsbacher, M. A. (1991). Cognitive processes and mechanisms in language comprehension: The structure building framework. In G. H. Bower (Ed.), *The psychology of learning and motivation* (Vol. 27, pp. 217–263). New York: Academic Press.

Gernsbacher, M. A. (1997). Two decades of structure building. *Discourse Processes, 23,* 265–304.

Gersten, R., Baker, S., & Edwards, L. (1999, December). *Teaching expressive writing to students with learning disabilities.* Arlington, VA: ERIC Clearinghouse on Disabilities and Gifted Education. (ERIC/OSEP Digest E590/EDO-99-16)

Gersten, R., Fuchs, L. S., Williams, J. P., & Baker, S. (2001). Teaching reading comprehension strategies to students with learning disabilities: A review of the research. *Review of Educational Research, 71,* 279–320.

Gibson, E. J. (1965). Learning to read. *Science, 148,* 1066–1072.

Ginsburg, H. P. (1997). Mathematics learning disabilities: A view from developmental psychology. *Journal of Learning Disabilities, 30,* 20–33.

Glazer, S. M. (1989). Oral language and literacy. In D. S. Strickland & L. M. Morrow (Eds.), *Emerging literacy: Young children learn to read and write* (pp. 16–26). Newark, DE: International Reading Association.

Gordon, J., Vaughn, S., & Schumm, S. (1993). Spelling interventions: A review of literature and implications for instruction for students with learning disabilities. *Learning Disabilities and Research, 8,* 175–181.

Gough, P. B., & Cosky, M. J. (1977). One second of reading again. In N. J. Castellan, D. B. Pisoni, & G. R. Potts (Eds.), *Cognitive theory* (pp. 271–288). Hillsdale, NJ: Erlbaum.

Graham, S. (1983). Effective spelling instruction. *Elementary School Journal, 83,* 560–567.

Graham, S., Berninger, V., Abbott, R., Abbott, S., & Whitaker, D. (1997). The role of mechanics in composing of elementary school students: A new methodological approach. *Journal of Educational Psychology, 89,* 170–182.

Graham, S., & Harris, K. R. (1989). Improving learning disabled students' skills at composing essays: Self-instructional strategy training. *Exceptional Children, 56,* 201–214.

Graham, S., & Harris, K. R. (2003). Students with learning disabilities and the process of writing: A meta-analysis of SRSD studies. In H. L. Swanson, K. R. Harris, & S. Graham (Eds.), *Handbook of learning disabilities* (pp. 323–344). New York: Guilford Press.

Graves, D. H. (1983). *Writing: Teachers and children at work.* Exeter, NH: Heinemann.

Graves, D. H. (1991). *Build a literate classroom.* Portsmouth, NH: Heinemann.

Graves, M. F. (2000). A vocabulary program to complement and bolster a middle-grade comprehension program. In B. M. Taylor, M. F. Graves, & P. van den Broek (Eds.), *Reading for meaning: Fostering comprehension in the middle grades* (pp. 116–135). New York: Teachers College Press/Newark, DE: International Reading Association.

Graves, M. F., Juel, C., & Graves, B. B. (2004). *Teaching reading in the 21st century* (3rd ed.). Boston: Allyn & Bacon.

Graves, M. F., & Watts-Taffe, S. (2002). The role of word consciousness in a research-based vocabulary program. In A. Farstrup & S. J. Samuels (Eds.), *What research has to say about reading instruction* (pp. 140–165). Newark, DE: International Reading Association.

Gray, J. R., Chabris, C. F., & Braver, T. S. (2003). Neural mechanisms of general fluid intelligence. *Nature Neuroscience, 6,* 316–322.

Greene, G. (1999). Mnemonic multiplication fact instruction for students with learning disabilities. *Learning Disabilities Research and Practice, 14,* 141–148.

Greenleaf, R. K. (2005). *Brain based teaching.* Newfield, ME: Greenleaf & Papanek.

Greenleaf, R. K., & Wells-Papanek, D. (2005). *Memory, recall, the brain and learning.* Newfield, ME: Greenleaf & Papanek.

Greenwood, C. R., & Terry, B. (1993). Achievement, placement, and services: Middle school benefits of classwide peer tutoring used at the elementary school. *School Psychology Review, 22,* 497–516.

Griffin, S. A. (1998). *Fostering the development of whole number sense.* Paper presented at the annual meeting of the American Educational Research Association, San Diego, CA.

Gudschinsky, S. C. (1973). *Manual of literacy for preliterate peoples*. Ukarumpa, Papua New Guinea: Summer Institute of Linguistics.

Gunn, B. K., Simmons, D. C., & Kame'enui, E. J. (1995). *Emergent literacy: A synthesis of the research*. Eugene, OR: National Center to Improve the Tools of Educators.

Hardiman, M. M. (2003). *Connecting brain research with effective teaching*. Lanham, MD: Rowman & Littlefield.

Hart, B., & Risley, T. R. (1995). *Meaningful differences in the everyday experience of young American children*. Baltimore: Brookes.

Hart, B., & Risley, T. R. (2003). The early catastrophe: The 30 million word gap by age 3. *American Educator, 27*(1), 4–9.

Hasselbring, T. S., Goin, L., & Bransford, J. D. (1988). Developing math automaticity in learning handicapped children: The role of computerized drill and practice. *Focus on Exceptional Children, 20*, 1–7.

Hayden, J., & McLaughlin, T. F. (2004). The effects of cover, copy, and compare and flash card drill on correct rate of math facts for a middle school student with learning disabilities. *Journal of Precision Teaching and Celeration, 20*, 17–21.

Hayes, F. B., Hynd, G. W., & Wisenbaker, J. (1986). Learning disabled and normal college students' performance on reaction time and speeded classification tasks. *Journal of Educational Psychology, 78*(1), 39–43.

Herman, P. A., Anderson, R. C., Pearson, P. D., & Nagy, W. E. (1987). Incidental acquisition of word meanings from expositions with varied text features. *Reading Research Quarterly, 22*, 263–284.

High/Scope Educational Research Foundation. (2003). *Classification, seriation, and number*. Ypsilanti, MI: High/Scope Press.

Hillocks, G., Jr. (1987). Synthesis of research on teaching writing. *Educational Leadership, 44*(8), 71–82.

Hillocks, G., Jr., & Smith, M. W. (1991). Grammar and usage. In J. Flood, J. M. Jensen, D. Lapp, & J. R. Squire (Eds.), *Handbook of research on teaching the English language arts* (pp. 591–603). New York: Macmillan.

Horn, J. L. (1965). *Fluid and crystallized intelligence*. Unpublished doctoral dissertation, University of Illinois, Urbana–Champaign.

Horn, J. L. (1988). Thinking about human abilities. In J. R. Nesselroade & R. B. Cattell (Eds.), *Handbook of multivariate psychology* (2nd ed., pp. 645–865). New York: Academic Press.

Horn, J. L. (1989). Models for intelligence. In R. Linn (Ed.), *Intelligence: Measurement, theory and public policy* (pp. 29–73). Urbana: University of Illinois Press.

Horn, J. L. (1991). Measurement of intellectual capabilities: A review of theory. In K. S. McGrew, J. K. Werder, & R. W. Woodcock, *WJ-R technical manual* (pp. 197–232). Itasca, IL: Riverside.

Horn, J. L., & Masunaga, H. (2000). New directions for research into aging and intelligence: The development of expertise. In T. J. Perfect & E. A. Maylor (Eds.), *Models of cognitive aging* (pp. 125–159). Oxford: Oxford University Press.

Horn, J. L., & Noll, J. (1997). Human cognitive capabilities: Gf-Gc theory. In D. P. Flanagan, J. L. Genshaft, & P. L. Harrison (Eds.), *Contemporary intellectual assessment: Theories, tests, and issues* (pp. 53–91). New York: Guilford Press.

Horn, J. L., & Stankov, L. (1982). Auditory and visual factors of intelligence. *Intelligence, 6*, 165–185.

Hotopf, W. H. N. (1980). Slips of the pen. In U. Frith (Ed.), *Cognitive processes in spelling* (pp. 287–309). London: Academic Press.

Hotopf, W. H. N. (1983). Lexical slips of the pen and the tongue: What they tell us about language production. In B. Butterworth (Ed.), *Language production* (Vol. 2, pp. 147–199). London: Academic Press.

Howell, R., Sidorenko, E., & Jurica, J. (1987). The effects of computer on the acquisition of multiplication facts by a student with learning disabilities. *Journal of Learning Disabilities, 20*, 336–341.

Humphreys, G. W., & Evett, L. J. (1985). Are there independent lexical and nonlexical routes in word processing?: An evaluation of the dual-route theory of reading. *Behavioral and Brain Sciences, 8*, 689–740.

Hutchinson, N. L. (1993). Effects of cognitive strategy instruction on algebra problem solving of adolescents with learning disabilities. *Learning Disability Quarterly, 16*, 34–63.

Johnson, D. D., & Pearson, P. D. (1984). *Teaching reading vocabulary* (2nd ed.). New York: Holt, Rinehart & Winston.

Johnson-Laird, P. N., Byrne, R. M. J., & Schaeken, W. (1992). Propositional reasoning by model. *Psychological Review, 99*, 418–439.

Kail, R. (1990). More evidence for a common, central constraint on speed of processing. In J. Enns (Ed.), *Advances in psychology: Vol. 69. Development of attention: Research and theory* (pp. 159–173). Amsterdam: Elsevier.

Kail, R. (1991). Development of processing speed in childhood and adolescence. In H. W. Reese (Ed.), *Advances in child development and behavior* (Vol. 23, pp. 151–185). San Diego, CA: Academic Press.

Kail, R. (2003). Information processing and memory. In M. Bornstein, L. Davidson, C. L. M. Keyes, & K. A. Moore (Eds.), *Well-being: Positive development across the life course* (pp. 269–279). Mahwah, NJ: Erlbaum.

Kail, R., Hall, L. K., & Caskey, B. J. (1999). Processing speed, exposure to print, and naming speed. *Applied Psycholinguistics, 20*, 303–314.

Kearney, C. A., & Drabman, R. S. (2001). The Write–Say method for improving spelling accuracy in children with learning disabilities. *Journal of Learning Disabilities, 26*, 52–56.

Keith, T. Z., & Reynolds, M. R. (2010). Cattell–Horn–Carroll abilities and cognitive tests: What we've learned from 20 years of research. *Psychology in the Schools, 47*(7), 635–650.

Kintsch, W. (1974). *The representation of meaning in memory.* Hillsdale, NJ: Erlbaum.

Klauer, K. J., Willmes, K., & Phye, G. D. (2002). Inducing inductive reasoning: Does it transfer to fluid intelligence? *Contemporary Educational Psychology, 27*(1), 1–25.

Klin, C. M. (1995). Causal inferences in reading: From immediate activation to long-term memory. *Journal of Experimental Psychology: Learning, Memory, and Cognition, 21*, 1483–1494.

Klingberg, T. (2009). *The overflowing brain: Information overload and the limits of working memory* (N. Betteridge, Trans.). New York: Oxford University Press.

Klingner, J. K., & Vaughn, S. (1998, July–August). Using collaborative strategic reading. *Teaching Exceptional Children, 30*(6), 32–37.

Kosslyn, S. M., & Smith, E. E. (2000). Introduction to higher cognitive functions. In M. S. Gazzaniga (Ed.), *The new cognitive neurosciences* (2nd ed., pp. 961–962). Cambridge, MA: MIT Press.

Kroesbergen, E. H., & Van Luit, J. E. H. (2003). Mathematics interventions for children with special educational needs. *Remedial and Special Education, 24*(2), 97–114.

Lane, J., & Lange, E. (1993). *Writing clearly: An editing guide.* Boston: Heinle & Heinle.

Lanham, R. (1992). *Revising prose* (3rd ed.). New York: Macmillan.

Lee, M. J., & Tingstrom, D. H. (1994). A group math intervention: The modification of cover, copy, and compare for group application. *Psychology in the Schools, 31*, 133–145.

Lenz, B. K., Ellis, E. S., & Scanlon, D. (1996). *Teaching learning strategies to adolescents and adults with learning disabilities.* Austin, TX: PRO-ED.

Leung, C., & Pikulski, J. J. (1990). Incidental word learning of kindergarten and first grade children through repeated read aloud events. In J. Zutell & S. McCormick (Eds.), *Literacy, theory and research: Analyses from multiple paradigms* (pp. 491–498). Chicago: National Reading Conference.

Levin, J. R., Levin, M. E., Glasman, L. D., & Nordwall, M. B. (1992). Mnemonic vocabulary instruction: Additional effectiveness evidence. *Contemporary Educational Psychology, 17*, 156–174.

Levy, B. A., Abello, B., & Lysynchuk, L. (1997). Transfer from word training to reading in context: Gains in reading fluency and comprehension. *Learning Disabilities Quarterly, 20*, 174–188.

MacArthur, C. A., Ferretti, R. P., Okolo, C. M., & Cavalier, A. R. (2001). Technology applications for students with literacy problems: A critical review. *Elementary School Journal, 101*, 273–378.

MacArthur, C. A., Graham, S., Haynes, J. A., & De La Paz, S. (1996). Spelling checkers and students with learning disabilities: Performance comparisons and impact on spelling. *Journal of Special Education, 30*, 35–57.

MacArthur, C. A., Graham, S., & Schwarz, S. (1993). Integrating strategy instruction and word processing into a process approach to writing instruction. *School Psychology Review, 22*, 671–681.

Maccini, P., & Gagnon, J. C. (2000). Best practices for teaching mathematics to secondary students with special needs. *Focus on Exceptional Children, 32*, 1–32.

Maccini, P., & Hughes, C. A. (2000). Effects of a problem-solving strategy on the introductory algebra performance of secondary students with learning disabilities. *Learning Disabilities Research and Practice, 15*, 10–21.

Mahncke, H. W., Bronstone, A., & Merzenich, M. M. (2006). Brain plasticity and functional losses in the aged: Scientific bases for a novel intervention. In A. R. Møller (Ed.), *Progress in brain research: Vol. 157. Reprogramming the brain* (pp. 81–109). Amsterdam: Elsevier.

Manning, B., & Payne, B. (1996). *Self-talk for teachers and students: Metacognitive strategies for personal and classroom use.* Boston: Allyn & Bacon.

Manns, J. R., & Squire, L. R. (2002). The medial temporal lobe and memory for facts and events. In A. D. Baddeley, M. D. Kopelman, & B. A. Wilson (Eds.), *Handbook of memory disorders* (2nd ed., pp. 81–99). New York: Wiley.

Marr, D. (1982). *Vision: A computational investigation into the human representation and processing of visual information.* San Francisco: Freeman.

Martin, A. (1998). The organization of semantic knowledge and the origin of words in the brain. In N. Jablonski & L. Aiello (Eds.), *The origins and diversifications of language* (pp. 69–98). San Francisco: California Academy of Sciences.

Martin, A. (2009). Circuits in mind: The neural foundations for object concepts. In M. S. Gazzaniga (Ed.), *The cognitive neurosciences* (4th ed., pp. 1031–1045). Cambridge, MA: MIT Press.

Marzano, R. J., Pinkering, D. J., & Pollock, J. E. (2001). *Classroom instruction that works*. Alexandria, VA: Association for Supervision and Curriculum Development.

Mastropieri, M. A., Leinart, A., & Scruggs, T. E. (1999). Strategies to increase reading fluency. *Intervention in School and Clinic, 34*, 278–283.

Mastropieri, M. A., & Scruggs, T. E. (1998). Enhancing school success with mnemonic strategies. *Intervention in School and Clinic, 33*, 201–208.

McArdle, J. J. (2001). Growth curve analysis. In N. J. Smelser & P. B. Baltes (Eds.), *International encyclopedia of social and behavioral sciences*. New York: Pergamon Press.

McClelland, J. L., & Rumelhart, D. E. (1981). An interactive activation model of context effects in letter perception: Part 1. An account of basic findings. *Psychological Review, 88*, 375–407.

McGrew, K. S. (1993). The relationship between the Woodcock–Johnson Psycho-Educational Assessment Battery—Revised Gf–Gc cognitive clusters and reading achievement across the life span. *Journal of Psychoeducational Assessment Monograph Series: WJ–R Monograph*, pp. 39–53.

McGrew, K. S., Flanagan, D. P., Keith, T. Z., & Vanderwood, M. (1997). Beyond g: The impact of Gf–Gc specific cognitive abilities research on the future use and interpretation of intelligence tests in the schools. *School Psychology Review, 26*(2), 189–210.

McGrew, K. S., Schrank, F. A., & Woodcock, R. W. (2007). *Technical manual: Woodcock–Johnson III Normative Update*. Rolling Meadows, IL: Riverside.

McGrew, K. S., & Wendling, B. J. (2010). Cattell–Horn–Carroll cognitive–achievement relations: What we have learned from the past 20 years of research. *Psychology in the Schools, 47*(7), 651–675.

McGrew, K. S., & Woodcock, R. W. (2001). *Woodcock–Johnson III technical manual*. Rolling Meadows, IL: Riverside.

McKenna, M. C., Jurgensen, E. K., & Thurman, S. K. (2008). Cognition in the early elementary classroom. In S. K. Thurman & C. A. Fiorello (Eds.), *Applied cognitive research in K–3 classrooms* (pp. 3–14). New York: Routledge.

McLaughlin, T. F., Reiter, S. M., Mabee, W. S., & Byram, B. J. (1991). An analysis and replication of the Add-A-Word Spelling Program with mildly handicapped middle school students. *Journal of Behavior Education, 1*, 413–426.

Meichenbaum, D. H. (1977). *Cognitive-behavior modification: An integrative approach*. New York: Plenum Press.

Meyer, M. S., & Felton, R. H. (1999). Repeated reading to enhance fluency: Old approaches and new directions. *Annals of Dyslexia, 49*, 283–306.

Miller, G. A. (1956). The magical number seven, plus or minus two: Some limits on our capacity for processing information. *Psychological Review, 63*, 81–87.

Moats, L. C. (1995). *Spelling: Development, disability, and instruction*. Timonium, MD: York Press.

Moats, L. C. (1999). *Teaching reading is rocket science*. Washington, DC: American Federation of Teachers.

Moats, L. C. (2001). Overcoming the language gap. *American Educator, 25*(5), 8–9.

Moats, L. C. (2005, Winter). How spelling supports reading. *American Educator*, pp. 12–43.

Moje, E. B., Ciechanowski, K. M., Kramer, K., Ellis, L., Carrillo, R., & Collazo, T. (2004). Working toward third space in content area literacy: An examination of everyday funds of knowledge and discourse. *Reading Research Quarterly, 39*(1), 38–69.

Montague, M. (1992). The effects of cognitive and metacognitive strategy instruction on the mathematical problem solving of middle school students with learning disabilities. *Journal of Learning Disabilities, 25*, 230–248.

Montague, M., & Candace, S. B. (1986). The effect of cognitive strategy instruction on verbal math problem solving performance of learning disabled adolescents. *Journal of Learning Disabilities, 19*, 26–33.

Morin, V. A., & Miller, S. P. (1998). Teaching multiplication to middle school students with mental retardation. *Education and Treatment of Children, 21*, 22–36.

Morrow, L. M. (1989). Designing the classroom to promote literacy development. In D. S. Strickland & L. M. Morrow (Eds.), *Emerging literacy: Young children learn to read and write* (pp. 96–159). Newark, DE: International Reading Association.

Murphy, G. L. (2002). *The big book of concepts*. Cambridge, MA: MIT Press.

Nagy, W. E., & Scott, J. A. (2000). Vocabulary processes. In M. L. Kamil, P. Mosenthal, P. D. Pearson, & R. Barr (Eds.), *Handbook of reading research* (Vol. 3, pp. 269–284). Mahwah, NJ: Erlbaum.

National Reading Panel. (2000). *Teaching children to read: An evidence-based assessment of the scientific research literature on reading and its implications for reading instruction* (NIH Publication No. 00–4754). Washington, DC: National Institute of Child Health and Human Development.

Nettelbeck, T. (1994). Speediness. In R. J. Sternberg (Ed.), *Encyclopedia of human intelligence* (pp. 1014–1019). New York: Macmillan.

Newton, J. H., & McGrew, K. S. (2010). Introduction to the special issue: Current research in Cattell–Horn–Carroll based assessment. *Psychology in the Schools, 47*(7), 621–634.

O'Shea, L. J., Sindelar, P. T., & O'Shea, D. J. (1985).

The effects of repeated readings and attentional cues on the reading fluency and comprehension of learning disabled readers. *Learning Disabilities Research, 2,* 103–109.

Ofiesh, N. S. (2000). Using processing speed tests to predict the benefit of extended test time for university students with learning disabilities. *Journal of Postsecondary Education and Disability, 14*(1), 39–56.

Ogle, D. M. (1986). K-W-L: A teaching model that develops active reading of expository text. *The Reading Teacher, 39*(6), 564–570.

Palincsar, A. S., & Brown, A. L. (1984). Reciprocal teaching of comprehension-fostering and comprehension-monitoring activities. *Cognition and Instruction, 1*(2), 117–175.

Pellegrino. J. W., & Goldman, S. R. (1987). Information processing and elementary mathematics. *Journal of Learning Disabilities, 20,* 23–32, 57.

Peters, E. E., & Levin, J. R. (1986). Effects of a mnemonic imagery on good and poor readers' prose recall. *Reading Research Quarterly, 21,* 179–192.

Pittelman, S. D., Heimlich, J. E., Berglund, R. L., & French, M. P. (1991). *Semantic feature analysis: Classroom applications.* Newark, DE: International Reading Association.

Popkin, J., & Skinner, C. H. (2003). Enhancing academic performance in a classroom serving students with serious emotional disturbance: Interdependent group contingencies with randomly selected components. *School Psychology Review, 32,* 282–295.

Pressley, M. (1990). *Cognitive strategy instruction that really improves children's academic performance.* College Park: College of Education, University of Maryland.

Pressley, M. (2006). *Reading instruction that works: The case for balanced teaching* (3rd ed.). New York: Guilford Press.

Quillian, M. R. (1968). Semantic memory. In M. Minsky (Ed.), *Semantic information processing* (pp. 216–270). Cambridge, MA: MIT Press.

Quinn, P. C. (2004). Development of subordinate-level categorization in 3- to 7-month-old infants. *Child Development, 75*(3), 886–899.

Rashotte, C. A., & Torgesen, J. K. (1985). Repeated reading and reading fluency in learning disabled children. *Reading Research Quarterly, 20,* 180–188.

Rathvon, N. (2008). *Effective school interventions* (2nd ed.). New York: Guilford Press.

Rivera, D., & Deutsch Smith, D. (1988). Using a demonstration strategy to teach midschool students with learning disabilities how to compute long division. *Journal of Learning Disabilities, 21,* 77–81.

Samuels, S. J. (1985). Automaticity and repeated reading. In J. Osborn, P. T. Wilson, & R. C. Anderson (Eds.), *Reading education: Foundations of a literate America* (pp. 215–230). Lexington, MA: Lexington Books.

Schermerhorn, P. K., & McLaughlin, T. F. (1997). Effects of the Add-A-Word Spelling Program on test accuracy, grades, and retention of spelling words with fifth and sixth grade regular education students. *Child and Family Behavior Therapy, 19,* 23–36.

Schrank, F. A., Mather, N., McGrew, K. S., & Woodcock, R. W. (2003). *Manual: Woodcock–Johnson III Diagnostic Supplement to the Tests of Cognitive Abilities.* Rolling Meadows, IL: Riverside.

Schrank, F. A., Miller, D. C., Wendling, B. J., & Woodcock, R. W. (2010). *Essentials of WJ III cognitive abilities assessment* (2nd ed.). Hoboken, NJ: Wiley.

Schrank, F. A., Wendling, B. J., & Woodcock, R. W. (2008). *Woodcock Interpretation and Instructional Interventions Program* [Computer software]. Rolling Meadows, IL: Riverside.

Schrank, F. A., & Woodcock, R. W. (2008). *WJ III Compuscore and Profiles Program* (Version 3.1) [Computer software]. Rolling Meadows, IL: Riverside.

Schumaker, J. B., Deshler, D. D., Alley, G. R., Warner, M. M., & Denton, P. H. (1982). Multipass: A learning strategy for improving reading comprehension. *Learning Disability Quarterly, 5,* 295–304.

Sellke, D. H., Behr, M. J., & Voelker, A. M. (1991). Using data tables to represent and solve multiplicative story problems. *Journal for Research in Mathematics Education, 22,* 30–38.

Sengpiel, F., & Hubener, M. (1999). Visual attention: Spotlight on the primary visual cortex. *Current Biology, 9*(9), 318–321.

Shany, M. T., & Biemiller, A. (1995). Assisted reading practice: Effects on performance for poor readers in grades 3 and 4. *Reading Research Quarterly, 30,* 382–395.

Shapiro, E. S., & Goldberg, R. (1986). A comparison of group contingencies for increasing spelling performance among sixth grade students. *School Psychology Review, 15,* 546–557.

Shaywitz, S. (2003). *Overcoming dyslexia: A new and complete science-based program for overcoming reading problems at any level.* New York: Knopf.

Siegler, R. (1988). Individual differences in strategy choices: Good students, not-so-good students, and perfectionists. *Child Development, 59,* 833–851.

Sinatra, R. C., Berg, D., & Dunn, R. (1985). Semantic mapping improves reading comprehension of learning disabled students. *Teaching Exceptional Children, 17*(4), 310–314.

Skinner, C. H., Turco, T. L., Beatty, K. L., & Rasavage, C. (1989). Cover, copy, and compare: A method for increasing multiplication performance. *School Psychology Review, 18,* 412–420.

Snow, C. E., Burns, M. S., & Griffin, P. (1998). *Preventing reading difficulties in young children*. Washington, DC: National Academy Press.

Squire, L. R., & Schacter, D. L. (2002). *Neuropsychology of memory* (3rd ed.). New York: Guilford Press.

Stahl, S. A. (1999). *Vocabulary development*. Cambridge, MA: Brookline Books.

Stanovich, K. E. (1994). Romance and reality. *The Reading Teacher, 4,* 280–290.

Stoddard, B., & MacArthur, C. A. (1993). A peer editor strategy: Guiding learning-disabled students in response and revision. *Research in the Teaching of English, 27,* 76–103.

Strickland, D. S. (1991). Emerging literacy: How young children learn to read. In B. Persky & L. H. Golubchick (Eds.), *Early childhood education* (2nd ed., pp. 337–344). Lanham, MD: University Press of America.

Sulzby, E. (1992). Research directions: Transitions from emergent to conventional writing. *Language Arts, 69,* 290–297.

Swanson, H. L. (2001). Searching for the best model for instructing students with learning disabilities. *Focus on Exceptional Children, 34,* 1–15.

Tallal, P., Miller, S. L., Bedi, G., Byma, G., Wang, X., Nagarajan, S. S., et al. (1996). Language comprehension in language-learning impaired children improved with acoustically modified speech. *Science, 5,* 81–84.

Tarver, S. G. (1992). Direct instruction. In W. Stainback & S. Stainback (Eds.), *Controversial issues confronting special education: Divergent perspectives* (2nd ed., pp. 143–165). Boston: Allyn & Bacon.

Taub, G. E., & McGrew, K. S. (2004). A confirmatory factor analysis of CHC theory and cross-age invariance of the Woodcock–Johnson Tests of Cognitive Abilities III. *School Psychology Quarterly, 19*(1), 72–87.

Taylor, B. M., Frye, B. J., & Maruyama, G. M. (1990). Time spent reading and reading growth. *American Educational Research Journal, 27*(2), 351–362.

Templeton, S., & Bear, D. (Eds.). (1992). *Development of orthographic knowledge and the foundations of literacy*. Hillsdale, NJ: Erlbaum.

Tomeson, M., & Aarnoutse, C. (1998). Effects of an instructional programme for deriving word meanings. *Educational Studies, 24,* 107–128.

Torgesen, J. K. (1997). The prevention and remediation of reading disabilities: Evaluating what we know from research. *Journal of Academic Language Therapy, 1,* 11–47.

Trabasso, T., & Bouchard, E. (2002). Teaching readers how to comprehend text strategically. In C. C. Block & M. Pressley (Eds.), *Comprehension instruction: Research-based best practices* (pp. 176–200). New York: Guilford Press.

Truchlicka, M., McLaughlin, T. F., & Swain, J. C. (1998). Effects of token reinforcement and response cost on the accuracy of spelling performance with middle-school special education students with behavior disorders. *Behavioral Interventions, 13,* 1–10.

Tulving, E. (1972). Episodic and semantic memory. In E. Tulving & W. Donaldson (Eds.), *Organization of memory* (pp. 381–403). Oxford: Oxford University Press.

Tulving, E. (1983). *Elements of episodic memory*. Oxford: Oxford University Press.

Tulving, E. (2000). Introduction to memory. In M. S. Gazzaniga (Ed.), *The new cognitive neurosciences* (2nd ed., pp. 727–732). Cambridge, MA: MIT Press.

Uhry, J. K., & Shepherd, M. J. (1993). Segmentation and spelling instruction as part of a first-grade reading program: Effects on several measures of reading. *Reading Research Quarterly, 28,* 219–233.

Van Houten, R., & Thompson, C. (1976). The effects of explicit timing on math performance. *Journal of Applied Behavior Analysis, 9,* 227–230.

Van Orden, G. C. (1987). A ROWS is a ROSE: Spelling, sound, and reading. *Memory and Cognition, 15*(3), 181–198.

Van Orden, G. C., Johnston, J. C., & Hale, B. L. (1988). Word identification in reading proceeds from spelling to sound to meaning. *Journal of Experimental Psychology: Learning, Memory, and Cognition, 14*(3), 371–386.

Vernon, P. A. (1983). Speed of information processing and general intelligence. *Intelligence, 7*(1), 53–70.

Walker, B., Shippen, M. E., Alberto, P., Houchins, D. E., & Cihak, D. F. (2005). Using the Expressive Writing program to improve the writing skills of high school students with learning disabilities. *Learning Disabilities Research and Practice, 20,* 175–183.

Wallach, G. P., & Butler, K. G. (1994). Creating communication, literacy, and academic success. In G. P. Wallach & K. G. Butler (Eds.), *Language learning disabilities in school-age children and adolescents: Some principles and applications* (pp. 2–26). Boston: Allyn & Bacon.

Williams, J. K., Richman, L. C., & Yarbrough, D. B. (1992). Comparison of visual–spatial performance strategy training in children with Turner syndrome and learning disabilities. *Journal of Learning Disabilities, 25*(10), 658–664.

Willis, J. (2008). *Teaching the brain to read*. Alexandria, VA: Association for Supervision and Curriculum Development.

Wolf, M., Bowers, P. G., & Biddle, K. (2000). Naming-speed processes, timing, and reading: A conceptual review. *Journal of Learning Disabilities, 33,* 387–407.

Wolfe, P. (2001). *Brain matters*. Alexandria, VA: Association for Supervision and Curriculum Development.

Wolff, P. H., Michel, G. F., Ovrut, M., & Drake, C. (1990). Rate and timing precision of motor coordination in developmental dyslexia. *Developmental Psychology, 26*, 349–359.

Wong, B. Y. L., Harris, K. R., Graham, S., & Butler, D. L. (2003). Cognitive strategy instruction research in learning disabilities. In H. L. Swanson, K. R. Harris, & S. Graham (Eds.), *Handbook of learning disabilities* (pp. 383–402). New York: Guilford Press.

Woodcock, R. W. (1998). Extending Gf-Gc theory into practice. In J. J. McArdle & R. W. Woodcock (Eds.), *Human cognitive abilities in theory and practice* (pp. 137–156). Mahwah, NJ: Erlbaum.

Woodcock, R. W., McGrew, K. S., & Mather, N. (2001, 2007a). *Woodcock–Johnson III*. Rolling Meadows, IL: Riverside.

Woodcock, R. W., McGrew, K. S., & Mather, N. (2001, 2007b). *Woodcock–Johnson III Tests of Achievement*. Rolling Meadows, IL: Riverside.

Woodcock, R. W., McGrew, K. S., & Mather, N. (2001, 2007c). *Woodcock–Johnson III Tests of Cognitive Abilities*. Rolling Meadows, IL: Riverside.

Woodcock, R. W., McGrew, K. S., Mather, N., & Schrank, F. A. (2003, 2007). *Woodcock–Johnson III Diagnostic Supplement to the Tests of Cognitive Abilities*. Rolling Meadows, IL: Riverside.

Woodcock, R. W., McGrew, K. S., Schrank, F. A., & Mather, N. (2001, 2007). *Woodcock–Johnson III Normative Update*. Rolling Meadows, IL: Riverside.

Woodcock, R. W., Schrank, F. A., Mather, N., & McGrew, K. S. (2007). *Woodcock–Johnson III Tests of Achievement Form C/Brief Battery*. Rolling Meadows, IL: Riverside.

Zentall, S. S. (1983). Learning environments: A review of physical and temporal factors. *Exceptional Education Quarterly, 4*(2), 90–115.

Zhou, R., & Black, I. B. (2000). Development of neural maps: Molecular mechanisms. In M. S. Gazzaniga (Ed.), *The new cognitive neurosciences* (2nd ed., pp. 213–221). Cambridge, MA: MIT Press.

CHAPTER 13

The Differential Ability Scales—Second Edition

Colin D. Elliott

Psychometric assessment is one of the finer achievements of the discipline of psychology in the last 100 years. The second edition of the Differential Ability Scales (DAS-II; Elliott, 2007a) follows this tradition, and is a development of the first edition of the instrument (DAS; Elliott, 1990a). This widely used battery of tests was developed and standardized in the United States for the assessment of the cognitive abilities of children between the ages of 2 years, 6 months and 17 years, 11 months (2:6–17:11). It has a longer history than its publication date suggests, however, as it is based on a predecessor, the British Ability Scales (BAS; Elliott, 1983a, 1983b). In its turn, the BAS incorporated new features from the DAS in its second edition (BAS II; Elliott, 1996).

As its name suggests, the DAS-II was developed with a primary focus on diverse, specific abilities rather than on general "intelligence."

STRUCTURE OF THE DAS-II

The DAS-II consists of 20 individually administered subtests divided into two overlapping batteries. The Early Years battery is normed for children ages 2:6–8:11. The School-Age battery is normed for children ages 5:0–17:11. Thus the Early Years and School-Age batteries were co-normed on children ages 5:0–8:11. The overlap provides us with important advantages in terms of out-of-level testing because examiners

assessing bright younger children or less able older ones are enabled to select a battery containing subtests that are appropriate for the children's ability and level of cognitive development.

Six core subtests in each battery contribute to a composite score—General Conceptual Ability (GCA), focused on reasoning and conceptual abilities; a Special Nonverbal Composite (SNC); and three lower-level composite scores called *cluster scores*. All the core subtests are highly g-saturated.

In addition to the core subtests, up to 10 diagnostic subtests are available for children taking the Early Years battery, and up to 8 are available for those taking the School-Age battery. These diagnostic subtests yield three additional cluster scores and also measure other specific abilities that do not contribute to the composites.

Note that the youngest children (ages 2:6–3:5) take a more limited range of subtests. This age range is called the Early Years (Lower Level), and the 3:6–8:11 range is called the Early Years (Upper Level). The overall structure is summarized in Table 13.1.

CLINICAL AND THEORETICAL UNDERPINNINGS

Users of cognitive ability tests typically compare an individual's performance and responses with those of a representative population sample of the

TABLE 13.1. Number of DAS-II Subtests and Composites in Each Battery

Battery	Number of subtests	General composite	Cluster scores
Early Years (Lower Level), ages 2:6–3:5	4 core 3 diagnostic	1. GCA 2. SNC	
Early Years (Upper Level), ages 3:6–8:11	6 core 10 diagnostic	1. GCA 2. SNC	*Core clusters* 1. Verbal 2. Nonverbal Reasoning 3. Spatial *Diagnostic clusters* 4. School Readiness 5. Working Memory 6. Processing Speed
School-Age, ages 5:0–17:11	6 core 8 diagnostic	1. GCA 2. SNC	*Core Clusters* 1. Verbal 2. Nonverbal Reasoning 3. Spatial Ability *Diagnostic clusters* 4. Working Memory 5. Processing Speed

Note. GCA, General Conceptual Ability; SNC, Special Nonverbal Composite.

same age as the person being tested. Paradoxically, however, while test scores are nearly always compared with the norm, the children, students, or adults whom we assess are often extremely atypical. The bread-and-butter work of a psychologist or psychological examiner involves individuals who are having difficulties or are failing to learn under normal conditions, or whose behavior gives cause for concern.

Because the individuals who are typically referred to psychologists manifestly have a huge range of individual special needs, the *clinical* priorities in the development of the DAS-II and its predecessors have been as follows:

1. Many children referred for psychological assessment have a history of problems with attending to adult instruction (i.e., a significant number of them will be distractible). For such children, test materials need to be varied and engaging, using different formats and types of tasks. A uniform approach to the administration of all subtests (e.g., using easels) has always been deliberately avoided in the DAS-II and its predecessors, in the interest of engaging children with variety.

2. Because many low-functioning children are likely to be assessed, there need to be plenty of test items that afford an opportunity for teaching and demonstrating what is required in each task. This is to ensure as far as possible that the children who

are being assessed understand what they are supposed to be doing. Young children, and children with developmental disabilities and learning disabilities (LDs), often have difficulty in "warming up" to a task and initially understanding the task requirements. For this reason, most of the DAS-II subtests have demonstration and teaching procedures built into the administration. Such teaching items enable an examiner to tell a child that he or she is correct (if this is the case), and if the item has been failed, to give and explain the correct response or solution.

3. Again, because many low-functioning children are likely to be assessed with the DAS-II, its subtests have been designed to have low floors. A floor effect in test norms is shown when a group of individuals in an age group all get raw scores of 0 or 1 point on the test. Such individuals find even the easiest items in the test to be too difficult, and thus the test cannot discriminate among them. This results in the normative scores' being *inflated* for those who obtain such low raw scores. For example, if, say 10% of children in an age group obtain a raw score of 0 on a test, standard scores cannot reasonably go below 80. So a child who is actually at the 1st percentile in relation to his or her age group does not get a standard score that reflects this (i.e., a score of about 65), but instead gets a score of about 80. Later tables will show that the DAS-II subtests and composites have low floors.

4. Because many children have had considerable experience of failing tasks set them by adults, the tests should minimize children's experience of failure to the greatest possible extent, and should maximize their enjoyment in success. The *item set* approach to test administration, which is used throughout the DAS-II, meets this objective. This approach is unique to the DAS-II and all its predecessors.

5. At a practical level, the item set approach has two major additional advantages. First, it keeps the testing session moving briskly, with subtests ending and new ones starting more quickly than if traditional administration methods were employed. This has a positive impact on children's motivation and willingness to remain in the test situation. The second advantage is for the examiner: The battery is relatively quick to administer. The Early Years battery has a median administration time for the core subtests of 31 minutes or less, while the core subtests of the School-Age battery have a median administration time of less than 40 minutes.

6. The normative overlap between the Early Years and School-Age batteries, described earlier, is 1 year wider than it was in the first edition, and is designed to enable examiners to assess children whose developmental level is atypical for their age. Thus the Early Years battery may be given to children up to the age of 8:11, yielding composite scores with identical interpretation to those in the School-Age battery, if it is determined by the examiner that the Early Years materials are developmentally more appropriate for a child.

7. Out-of-level testing procedures and an extended GCA (taking the lowest GCA score down to 25) are provided for children with LDs and developmental disabilities. Again, therefore, a school-age child may be assessed with the Early Years materials if these are considered by the examiner to be more developmentally appropriate. These procedures are described in detail elsewhere (Dumont, Willis, & Elliott, 2009).

8. Finally, because professionals assessing children with LDs and developmental disabilities need information at a finer level of detail than an IQ score, the DAS-II and its predecessors were designed to reflect modern knowledge on the nature and structure of cognitive abilities. A pattern of *strengths and weaknesses* (PSW) approach to assessing LDs has been broadly accepted by many professionals and by the U.S. government (Individuals with Disabilities Education Improvement Act of 2004 [IDEA 2004]; Daniel, Breaux, & Frey, 2010; Hale & Fiorello, 2004). Because the DAS-II incorporates such an approach, examiners using it may obtain measures of seven broad abilities and a range of narrow abilities that reflect current theory on the structure of human cognitive abilities. This is discussed further below.

The major *technical* priority in the development of both the original DAS and the DAS-II has been to produce a battery in which subtests and cluster scores are individually interpretable. For this, they need to have substantial reliability and need to be distinctive measures of different cognitive functions. The high specificity of the DAS-II subtests and clusters (see later discussion in this chapter), which supports such interpretations of specific abilities, is a distinguishing feature of the battery.

What of the *theoretical* model? When the many theories of the structure of abilities were reviewed at the time of the DAS's initial development in the early 1980s, it was apparent that no single theory was entirely persuasive, and certainly no single theory had universal acceptance among theoreticians or practitioners. Because of this, the original DAS (and the original BAS on which it was based) were not developed solely to reflect a single model of cognitive abilities, but reflected an eclectic number of theoretical perspectives. They were designed to address processes that often underlie children's difficulties in learning, as well as what we then knew about the neurological structures underlying these abilities.

During the years since the original DAS was published, a growing consensus has developed among factor theorists of human abilities. This centers on what became widely referred to as Gf-Gc theory, after the initial theory development by Cattell (1971) and Horn (Cattell & Horn, 1978; Horn & Blankson, Chapter 3, this volume; Horn & Noll, 1997). The basic theory—that variance among multiple measures of cognitive ability can be accounted for by numerous first-order, narrow abilities and 8–10 broad, second-order factors— was also demonstrated by Carroll (1993, 2003; see also Carroll, Appendix, this volume), who showed that there are considerable similarities in the factor structures of cognitive test batteries. The contributions to this volume by Carroll and by Horn and Blankson make explicit the disagreement between Carroll and Horn about the reality of the general factor, g; Carroll supported the construct, whereas Horn considered it to be a statistical artifact. Other than this disagreement, the similarities in the factors described by these two authors are considerable and impressive.

Because of the convergence between Carroll's and Horn's theoretical positions on the hierarchical structure of human abilities, Gf-Gc theory has more recently been referred to as Cattell–Horn–Carroll (CHC) theory (McGrew, 2005; see Schneider & McGrew, Chapter 4, this volume). It also appears to be a unifying theory about which most workers in the area of the structure of human abilities broadly agree (Schneider & McGrew, Chapter 4, this volume). As a result of the development of CHC theory, and before development of the DAS-II began, McGrew (1997), McGrew and Flanagan (1998), Flanagan, McGrew, and Ortiz (2000), Alfonso, Flanagan, and Radwan (2005), and Elliott (2005) were making links between CHC theory and findings on the factor structure of the DAS. And interestingly, at about the same time as the DAS-II was published, Sanders, McIntosh, Dunham, Rothlisberg, and Finch (2007) reported a joint factor analysis of the DAS and the Woodcock–Johnson III Tests of Cognitive Abilities (WJ III COG; Woodcock, McGrew, & Mather, 2001b). Sanders et al. concluded that a three-stratum model provided the best fit to the data, with the DAS subtests measuring six of seven CHC broad ability factors.

Because of these theoretical developments, it was decided that the new DAS-II would be linked to CHC theory. Accordingly, all subtests are classified as measures of both narrow and broad CHC abilities. With one exception, all cluster scores have CHC broad ability classifications. The exception is the School Readiness cluster in the DAS-II Early Years battery, which is formed from a combination of three subtests measuring different CHC factors. It appears likely that in the early years at school, most teachers teach visual matching, early number concepts, and phonological awareness—skills that are defined by three of the DAS-II subtests. These three subtests "hang together" and form a factor that has a pragmatic rather than a theoretical basis, and that may prove useful for examiners who assess children in the early school years.

CHC theory continues to be a work in progress concerning (1) the number of factors representing independent abilities in the model; (2) the precise nature of each factor (see, e.g., the Chapter 4 discussion by Schneider and McGrew on whether Rapid Naming tests measure the broad ability of Gs or Glr); and (3) whether and to what extent subtests from different test batteries that purport to measure a given factor actually do so (see Keith & Reynolds, Chapter 32, this volume).

ORGANIZATION AND FORMAT

Test Structure and Content

The subtests in the DAS-II Early Years (Upper Level) and School-Age cognitive batteries are listed in Tables 13.2 and 13.3. In each table, the subtests are grouped according to whether they are designated *core* subtests or *diagnostic* subtests. Each subtest has a brief description of the nature of its task, including its CHC broad ability classification. The core subtests are relatively strongly g-related and therefore measure complex processing and conceptual ability.

New Subtests and Clusters in the DAS-II

All subtests that were in the original DAS are included in the DAS-II. In addition, the DAS-II has four new subtests. Recall of Sequential Order and Recall of Digits—Backward form a new diagnostic Working Memory cluster. A new Rapid Naming subtest combines with Speed of Information Processing to form a new diagnostic Processing Speed cluster. And Phonological Processing has been introduced to reflect the research done on this ability in relation to reading disability since the DAS was first published.

Moreover, the Matrices subtest has been extended downward to age 3:6 with a new set of colored pictorial items suitable for young children, thereby enabling the DAS-II Nonverbal Reasoning cluster (a measure of Gf) to extend down to age 3:6.

To a reader familiar with the first edition of the DAS, it may appear that the Block Building subtest has been dropped from the DAS-II. In fact, Block Building has been merged into the Pattern Construction subtest, enabling that subtest now to extend down to age 2:6. Technically, it was found during development that the goodness of fit to the Rasch model of the Block Building items was excellent when they and the Pattern Construction items were both included in the analysis, and they could therefore be considered to measure the same latent dimension.

The School-Age core subtests are identical to those in the original DAS. Five of the Early Years core subtests are identical, the exception being that Early Number Concepts is now designated a diagnostic subtest; its place as a core subtest has

TABLE 13.2. Subtests of the DAS-II Early Years (Upper Level) Battery (Ages 3:6–8:11), Showing Abilities Measured (and Relation of Measures to Broad CHC Ability Factors) and Their Contribution to Composites

Subtest	Description	CHC broad ability	Contribution to composite
Core subtests			
Verbal Comprehension	Using various materials, child gives a motor response to verbal commands	Gc	Verbal, GCA
Naming Vocabulary	Child sees pictures of objects and names them	Gc	Verbal, GCA
Picture Similarities	Child selects a picture or figure closest to a target picture or figure	Gf	Nonverbal Reasoning, GCA, SNC
Matrices	Child selects a picture or figure that completes a 2×2 or 3×3 matrix	Gf	Nonverbal Reasoning, GCA, SNC
Pattern Construction	Child replicates designs, using blocks or foam squares	Gv	Spatial, GCA, SNC
Copying	Child copies figure by drawing it on paper	Gv	Spatial, GCA, SNC
Diagnostic subtests			
Recall of Objects— Immediate	Examiner presents 20 objects on card; child recalls as many as possible; three trials	Glr	
Recall of Objects— Delayed	Child recalls as many objects as possible 10–30 minutes after third exposure	Glr	
Early Number Concepts	Child responds to questions requiring prenumerical and numerical concepts	Gc/Gf[a]	School Readiness
Matching Letter-Like Forms	Child matches a target figure to one of six alternatives	Gv	School Readiness
Recognition of Pictures	Child identifies previously seen pictures embedded in a larger display	Gv	School Readiness
Phonological Processing	Child rhymes, blends, deletes, and identifies sounds in words	Ga	
Recall of Digits— Forward	Child repeats spoken single-digit sequences	Gsm	
Recall of Digits— Backward	Child repeats spoken single-digit sequences in reverse order	Gsm	Working Memory
Recall of Sequential Order	Child reorganizes and repeats spoken lists of body parts and objects in correct order	Gsm	Working Memory
Speed of Information Processing	Child quickly selects the largest number of squares or the highest number in a row	Gs	Processing Speed
Rapid Naming	Child quickly names colors, objects, or colors and objects in a visual display	Gs	Processing Speed

Note. GCA, General Conceptual Ability; SNC, Special Nonverbal Composite; Gv, visual–spatial processing; Gc, crystallized intelligence or verbal ability; Gf, fluid reasoning; Gsm, auditory short-term memory; Glr, long-term storage and retrieval; Ga, auditory processing; Gs, processing speed.

[a]Note that in the DAS-II handbook (Elliott, 2007c, pp. 60–61), Early Number Concepts is characterized as measuring a mixture of Gc and Gf. However, Keith et al. (2010) have argued that Early Number Concepts is best conceived as a measure of fluid reasoning and not crystallized intelligence for ages 5 through 8. It appears that the influence of Gf on this subtest becomes stronger with increasing age.

now been taken by the downward extension of Matrices. Some of the diagnostic subtests have a lower *g* saturation and measure such less cognitively complex functions as short-term memory and speed of information processing. However, the Working Memory subtests, the Phonological Processing subtest, and the Early Number Concepts subtests have substantial *g* loadings. Subtests have

normative scores in a *T*-score metric (mean = 50, standard deviation [*SD*] = 10).

Tables 13.2 and 13.3 also show the composites that can be derived from each of the core and the diagnostic subtests. Two types of composites are provided, all in a standard score metric (mean = 100, *SD* = 15). First are lower-order cluster scores. From age 3:6 onward, the core subtests yield three

TABLE 13.3. Subtests of the DAS-II School-Age Battery (Ages 5:0–7:11), Showing Abilities Measured (and Relation of Measures to Broad CHC Ability Factors) and Their Contribution to Composites

Subtest	Description	CHC broad ability	Contribution to composite
Core subtests			
Word Definitions	Child tells the meaning of words given by the examiner	Gc	Verbal, GCA
Verbal Similarities	Child describes how three objects or concepts are similar	Gc	Verbal, GCA
Matrices	Child selects a picture or figure that completes a 2 × 2 or 3 × 3 matrix	Gf	Nonverbal Reasoning, GCA, SNC
Sequential and Quantitative Reasoning	Child completes a sequence of pictures, figures, or numbers	Gf	Nonverbal Reasoning, GCA, SNC
Pattern Construction	Child replicates designs, using blocks or foam squares	Gv	Spatial, GCA, SNC
Recall of Designs	Child draws figure after viewing it for 5 seconds	Gv	Spatial, GCA, SNC
Diagnostic subtests			
Recall of Objects—Immediate	Examiner presents 20 objects on card; child recalls as many as possible; three trials	Glr	
Recall of Objects—Delayed	Child recalls as many objects as possible 10–30 minutes after third exposure	Glr	
Recognition of Pictures	Child identifies previously seen pictures embedded in a larger display	Gv	
Phonological Processing	Child rhymes, blends, deletes, and identifies sounds in words	Ga	
Recall of Digits—Forward	Child repeats spoken single-digit sequences	Gsm	
Recall of Digits—Backward	Child repeats spoken single-digit sequences in reverse order	Gsm	Working Memory
Recall of Sequential Order	Child reorganizes and repeats spoken lists of body parts and objects in correct order	Gsm	Working Memory
Speed of Information Processing	Child quickly selects the largest number of squares or the highest number in a row	Gs	Processing Speed
Rapid Naming	Child quickly names colors, objects, or colors and objects in a visual display	Gs	Processing Speed

Note. GCA, General Conceptual Ability; SNC, Special Nonverbal Composite; Gv, visual–spatial processing; Gc, crystallized intelligence or verbal ability; Gf, fluid reasoning; Gsm, auditory short-term memory; Glr, long-term storage and retrieval; Ga, auditory processing; Gs, processing speed.

of these across the board in both Early Years and the School-Age batteries (Verbal, Nonverbal Reasoning, and Spatial). Three clusters are also derived from the diagnostic subtests (School Readiness, Working Memory, and Processing Speed). For the youngest children at the Lower Level of the Early Years battery (ages 2:6–3:5), there are just two cluster scores, Verbal and Nonverbal.

Both batteries provide two higher-order composites. For most children, the most general composite will be the GCA score. For children for whom it is judged that the verbal component of that score is inappropriate, the SNC score is provided. For the Early Years (Lower Level), this is identical to the lower-order Nonverbal cluster, formed from two subtests. For the Early Years (Upper Level) and School-Age batteries, this is formed from the four subtests in the Nonverbal Reasoning and Spatial clusters.

One major change from the first edition of the DAS is that achievement tests are no longer part of the DAS-II battery. Instead, scores from the Wechsler Individual Achievement Test—Second Edition (WIAT-II; Psychological Corporation, 2001) have been linked to the DAS-II. In addition, correlational data have been provided between the DAS-II and the Kaufman Test of Educational Achievement—Second Edition (KTEA-II; Kaufman & Kaufman, 2004), and between the DAS-II and the WJ III Tests of Achievement (WJ III ACH; Woodcock, McGrew, & Mather, 2001a). Discrepancies between ability (as measured by the DAS-II GCA or SNC) and WIAT-II achievement may be evaluated by taking either (1) the simple difference between the achievement score and the composite, or (2) the difference between predicted and observed achievement, with predicted achievement being based on the GCA or SNC score. The DAS-II norms manual (Elliott, 2007d) provides information on the statistical significance of discrepancies (i.e., their reliability), and also their frequency of occurrence (or unusualness) in the standardization sample. Dumont and colleagues (2009) provide similar tables concerning the comparison of the DAS-II with the KTEA-II and the WJ III ACH.

Subtests as Specific Ability Measures

The chief aim in designing the content of the DAS-II was to produce subtests that are individually interpretable and can stand technically as separate, specific measures of various abilities. Once a specification was made of the desired tasks and dimensions to be measured, each subtest was designed to be unidimensional and homogeneous in content and distinct from other subtests, thus aiding the interpretation of children's performance. If a subtest score is to be interpreted as a measure of a specific, identifiable ability, the items within that subtest must be of similar content and must require the examinee to perform similar operations. For example, in each item of the Naming Vocabulary subtest, a child is asked to name an object in a picture. All items are therefore homogeneous. Naming Vocabulary is distinct from Verbal Comprehension, another verbal subtest, because the former requires a verbal response and the latter does not.

Ideally, each subtest should be a clearly interpretable measure of a CHC narrow ability factor, and the clusters to which the subtests contribute should also be clearly interpretable measures of CHC broad ability factors. Subtests or clusters should not sit astride two factors, as it were, so that the interpretation of a child's performance becomes unclear (see "Factor Structure," below).

In addition to having homogeneous content that focuses on a distinct ability, each subtest should also be reliable. Because the DAS-II emphasizes the identification of cognitive strengths and weaknesses, subtests must have a sufficient amount of reliable specificity to be separately interpretable (see "Accuracy, Reliability, and Specificity," below).

Verbal Content

Although it was considered important to include measures of verbal ability in the DAS-II cognitive battery, too many verbal tasks would present problems for examiners wishing to assess children from multicultural or culturally disadvantaged backgrounds. Because of these considerations, measures of general knowledge, colloquialisms, or words with a specific meaning in the United States were eliminated as far as possible.

Because verbal abilities are a major component of cognition, it is certainly necessary to have some subtests that are purely verbally presented, particularly at the School-Age level. However, getting the balance right in a test battery is important, too. In development of the DAS-II content, only two core subtests were included with entirely verbal presentation and response (both at the School-Age level), plus the two verbally administered Recall of

Digits subtests. Other than those subtests, the aim was to have subtests with varied tasks and materials. The "Test Materials" section below shows the range and variety of DAS-II stimulus materials.

Timed or Speeded Items

The DAS-II contains a diagnostic cluster called Processing Speed, contributed to by the Speed of Information Processing and Rapid Naming subtests, which are both timed. Apart from these two subtests, the DAS-II content minimizes the use of timed or speeded items. Of the other subtests, only one—Pattern Construction—gives extra points for correct completion of the designs within specified time limits. Of course, this feature of the subtest, which is appropriate for most individuals, is inappropriate for some children. Speed of response to the Pattern Construction items may not produce a valid measure for a child with a physical disability such as cerebral palsy, or one with an attentional problem, or one who takes an extremely deliberate approach to a task. For such children, an alternative procedure is provided, in which the score is based solely on accuracy within very liberal time limits. Confirmatory factor analyses (CFAs) reported in the DAS handbook demonstrated the factorial equivalence of the standard and alternative versions of Pattern Construction, which are unchanged in the DAS-II.

Test Materials

The DAS-II test kit includes three informational volumes: an administration and scoring manual (Elliott, 2007b), an introductory and technical handbook (Elliott, 2007c), and a manual of norms (Elliott, 2007d). Separate record forms are provided for the Early Years and School-Age batteries. The kit contains four stimulus books, as well as a variety of consumable booklets and manipulable materials. Materials vary for each subtest. The materials were specifically designed to be colorful, varied and engaging for children and students of all developmental levels, while being also easy to administer.

In the Early Years battery, only one subtest, Recall of Digits, is purely verbally presented, with no additional stimulus materials. In the School-Age battery, four subtests are purely verbally presented, with no additional stimulus materials. These are Word Definitions and Verbal Similarities, which constitute the Verbal cluster, and Recall of

Digits—Forward and Recall of Digits—Backward, which measure aspects of verbal memory.

Translations

The DAS-II handbook (Elliott, 2007c, pp. 210–218) contains guidelines for the assessment of children with communication difficulties due to such causes as cultural differences, lack of proficiency in spoken English, and hearing impairments. To assist in assessing such children, the DAS-II has been published with two translations: Spanish and American Sign Language (ASL).

The manual contains an appendix in which are given the Spanish-language instructions needed to administer the subtests that do not require a verbal response from the child. The translated instructions are for the following Early Years core subtests: Copying, Matrices, Pattern Construction, and Picture Similarities. These subtests enable the Nonverbal Reasoning and Spatial cluster scores to be estimated, together with the SNC as a measure of *g*. For the School-Age battery, translated instructions are provided for Matrices, Pattern Construction, Recall of Designs, and Sequential and Quantitative Reasoning. Once again, these enable Nonverbal Reasoning, Spatial, and SNC scores to be obtained. Translations are also provided for the following diagnostic subtests: Matching Letter-Like Forms, Recognition of Pictures, and Speed of Information Processing.

The DAS-II kit includes a CD-ROM of signed administration directions in ASL for nine subtests. These include the same core subtests for the Early Years and the School-Age batteries as in the Spanish translation, thereby enabling Nonverbal Reasoning and Spatial cluster scores to be estimated, together with the SNC. In addition, three diagnostic subtests have been translated into ASL: Matching Letter-Like Forms, Recognition of Pictures, and Speed of Information Processing.

PSYCHOMETRIC PROPERTIES

The DAS-II standardization sample, the norming procedures, and data on the reliability and validity of the battery are by now well known, and are described elsewhere (Elliott, 2007c). The DAS-II followed essentially the same procedures in sampling, and in obtaining a substantial bias oversample, that were employed in the standardization of the DAS (Elliott, 1990b, 1997).

TABLE 13.4. Subtest Floors for the DAS-II Early Years (Lower Level) Battery: *T* Scores, *z* Scores, and Percentiles Produced by a Raw Score of 1 on Each Subtest for Children Ages 2:6–2:9

Clusters and subtests	*T* score	*z* score	Percentile
Verbal cluster			
Verbal Comprehension	24	–2.6	0.5
Naming Vocabulary	24	–2.6	0.5
Nonverbal cluster			
Picture Similarities	30	–2.0	2
Pattern Construction	27	–2.3	1

Subtest Floors

As explained earlier, because many low-functioning children are likely to be assessed with the DAS-II, its subtests have been designed to have low floors.

Table 13.4 shows the *T* scores, *z* scores (showing the number of standard deviations below the mean), and percentiles for a raw score of 1 on each of the four core subtests at ages 2:6–2:9, which is the lowest age group for the Early Years (Lower Level). If a child of this age happened to obtain raw scores of 1 on every subtest, this would yield standard scores of 56 and 64 on the Verbal and Nonverbal clusters, respectively, and a GCA score of 58. These three scores are at or below the 1st percentile. Clearly, because of the development of abilities in childhood, the floors of the subtests are lower than those in the table for children between the ages of 2:10 and 3:5, with lower values in the table, and with lower cluster and GCA scores.

Similarly, Table 13.5 shows the floors for children at ages 3:6–3:9—the lowest age group for the Early Years (Upper Level). These are for the six core subtests, which yield three cluster scores. Note that the two subtests that start at age 3:6 have the highest *T* scores for a raw score of 1. If a very low-functioning child were unable to understand these subtests, it is still possible to give the subtests from the Early Years (Lower Level) battery to obtain estimates of Verbal and Nonverbal ability, together with the GCA. If a child age 3:6 obtained raw scores of 1 on all six subtests, this would yield cluster standard scores of 39 (Verbal), 61 (Nonverbal Reasoning), and 60 (Spatial), with a GCA score of 47. All these scores would indicate that the child's ability in each area was below the 1st percentile.

Finally, Table 13.6 shows the floors of the DAS-II Early Years and School-Age batteries for children ages 7:0–7:5. At this age, the School-Age battery

TABLE 13.5. Subtest Floors for the DAS-II Early Years (Upper Level) Battery: *T* Scores, *z* Scores, and Percentiles Produced by a Raw Score of 1 on Each Subtest for Children Ages 3:6–3:9

Clusters and subtests	*T* score	*z* score	Percentile
Verbal cluster			
Verbal Comprehension	14	–3.6	<0.1
Naming Vocabulary	15	–3.5	<0.1
Nonverbal Reasoning cluster			
Picture Similarities	21	–2.9	0.2
Matrices	31	–1.9	3
Spatial cluster			
Copying	32	–1.8	4
Pattern Construction	18	–3.2	<0.1

would normally be given. On this battery, three of the six core subtests and three diagnostic subtests have *T* scores above the lowest possible level of 10. The *z* scores and percentile columns show that if a child obtained a raw score of 1 on any of these six subtests, he or she would be estimated to be at or below the 1st percentile for his or her age. The subtest *T* scores in Table 13.6 yield cluster standard scores as follows: Verbal, 44; Nonverbal Reasoning, 46; Spatial, 38; School Readiness, 37; Working Memory, 59; Processing Speed, 42; and GCA,

40. However, as discussed earlier, the normative overlap between the Early Years and School-Age batteries means that relatively low-functioning School-Age children ages 7:0–8:0 may be given the core subtests of the Early Years battery, which clearly has the lowest possible floors for children of that age—*T* scores of 10, four standard deviations below the mean for all subtests, which would yield a GCA score of 30.

The three age groups referred to in Tables 13.4, 13.5, and 13.6 are the lowest ages of children who

TABLE 13.6. Subtest Floors for the DAS-II Early Years and School-Age Batteries: *T* Scores, *z* Scores, and Percentiles Produced by a Raw Score of 1 on Each Subtest for Children Ages 7:0–7:5

Clusters and subtests	*T* score	*z* score	Percentile
School-Age battery			
Verbal cluster			
Word Definitions	23	−2.7	0.4
Verbal Similarities	10	−4.0	<0.1
Nonverbal Reasoning cluster			
Matrices	10	−4.0	<0.1
Seq. and Quant. Reasoning	25	−2.5	1
Spatial cluster			
Recall of Designs	16	−3.4	<0.1
Pattern Construction	10	−4.0	<0.1
Early Years (Upper Level) battery			
Verbal cluster			
Verbal Comprehension	10	−4.0	<0.1
Naming Vocabulary	10	−4.0	<0.1
Nonverbal Reasoning cluster			
Picture Similarities	10	−4.0	<0.1
Matrices	10	−4.0	<0.1
Spatial cluster			
Copying	10	−4.0	<0.1
Pattern Construction	10	−4.0	<0.1
Diagnostic clusters			
School Readiness			
Early Number Concepts	14	−3.6	<0.1
Matching Letter-Like Forms	10	−4.0	<0.1
Phonological Processing	10	−4.0	<0.1
Working Memory			
Recall of Sequential Order	24	−2.6	0.5
Recall of Digits—Backward	24	−2.6	0.5
Processing Speed			
Speed of Information Processing	27	−2.3	1
Rapid Naming	10	−4.0	<0.1

would normally be given the Early Years (Lower Level), the Early Years (Upper Level), and the School-Age batteries. Low-functioning children in these young age groups would be most likely to have the greatest difficulty with the easiest items, and would show the greatest floor effects. Children in older age groups would show lesser effects the older they became. The tables show that floor effects are minimal, and that one of the goals of test development—to provide subtests with low floors—has been met.

Accuracy and Reliability

The DAS-II uses what is termed an *item set* approach to test administration. This is a form of tailored testing that makes the assessment time-efficient while maintaining a high level of accuracy. This approach, and the procedures used in the DAS-II to achieve accuracy and reliability, are described in the DAS-II handbook (Elliott, 2007c) and in the first edition of this volume (Elliott, 1997).

Two diagnostic subtests (Recall of Objects—Immediate and Recognition of Pictures) have adequate mean internal-reliability coefficients of .79 at the Early Years level. All other Early Years subtests have internal reliabilities of .80 and above, nine of them being between .80 and .89, and five of them being .90 and over. At the School-Age level, Recognition of Pictures once again has an adequate but lower mean internal-reliability coefficient (.74) than other subtests. All other subtests have mean coefficients of .80 and above, nine of them being between .80 and .89, and six over .90.

The mean internal reliabilities of DAS-II cluster scores range from .89 to .95 for both the Early Years and School-Age levels. The mean internal reliabilities of the GCA and SNC are .95 (Early Years) and .96 (School-Age).

Without exception, the reliability coefficients improved for the DAS-II subtests retained from the first edition of the DAS; identical methods of estimation were used. Extensive further information on the reliability of the DAS-II is provided in the DAS-II handbook (Elliott, 2007c, pp. 121–140).

Specificity

The variance of test scores can be partitioned into a number of components. As described earlier, the *proportion of error variance* may be estimated and is defined as the value of 1 minus the reliability of a test. The *proportion of reliable variance* (i.e., the reliability of the test) may itself be partitioned into two components: *reliable common variance*, which is shared or overlapping with other tests in the battery, and *reliable specific variance*, which is not shared and does not overlap with other tests.

The proportion of common variance (often termed *communality*) may be estimated by the squared multiple correlation between a subtest and all others in the battery (Kaufman, 1979; Silverstein, 1976). The proportion of specific reliable variance is usually termed the *specificity* of a test and is estimated by subtracting the communality from the reliability coefficient of the test.

McGrew and Murphy (1995) consider test specificity to be high when it is (1) .25 or more (indicating that it accounts for 25% or more of the total variance of the test), and (2) greater than the proportion of error variance. Analyses of the specificity of the DAS-II (reported in detail in Elliott, 2007c, pp. 141–142) have shown every subtest to be of high specificity. For both the Early Years and the School-Age batteries, about 42% of subtest score variance is reliable specific variance. The range of subtest specificity is .31–.65 in the Early Years battery, and .31–.66 in the School-Age battery.

With one exception, the cluster scores in both batteries also show very high specificity, ranging from .37 to .57 (mean .47) for the Early Years battery and from .34 to .66 (mean .46) for the School-Age battery. The exception is the School Readiness cluster, which has a moderate specificity of .23 (falling just under the .25 criterion for high specificity). All subtest and cluster specificities substantially exceed the proportion of error variance.

Such values of specificity are very consistent with those previously found in the DAS and the BAS-II. These findings support the view that the original development goal of a battery with reliable, specific, individually interpretable subtests has been achieved. The results support the use of the DAS-II for the analysis of cognitive processing strengths and weaknesses.

Validity

The DAS-II handbook contains extensive information on the validity of the instrument. This can be broadly categorized into correlational studies, including CFAs of the structure of the battery, and studies on defined clinical samples of children with varying special needs. This section of the present chapter gives a brief description of studies on the factor structure of the DAS-II, and some data on the variety of significant strengths and weaknesses in cognitive abilities shown by children who are poor readers.

Factor Structure

The first edition of the DAS yielded only two cluster scores (Verbal and Nonverbal) at what was called the Upper Preschool level (now called the Upper Early Years battery). The downward extension of Matrices in the DAS-II was expected to produce three core cluster scores in the Early Years battery that would be equivalent to those in the School-Age battery—namely, Verbal (Gc), Nonverbal Reasoning (Gf), and Spatial (Gv).

The two new measures of working memory included in the DAS-II were also expected to form a cluster, and in addition it was thought that the new Rapid Naming subtest might cluster with Speed of Information Processing rather than with Phonological Processing when the final data were analyzed, as did similar subtests in the WJ III (McGrew & Woodcock, 2001). Thus it was anticipated that there would be two additional diagnostic clusters in the DAS-II—Working Memory and Processing Speed, measuring the CHC factors of Gsm and Gs, respectively.

Finally, the inclusion of the Phonological Processing subtest was expected to provide a measure of *auditory processing*—the CHC broad ability of Ga. This subtest would thereby fill a gap in the coverage of CHC broad ability factors that McGrew (1997, p. 160) noted in the original DAS. More importantly, it would also meet a clinical need for such a test that is relevant to reading acquisition and the assessment of reading disability.

Confirmatory Factor Analyses

Although the background of the DAS-II has remained eclectic, it was clear at the time of development that CHC theory had become the most dominant and widely accepted theory of the structure of human abilities. Accordingly, the DAS-II handbook (Elliott, 2007c) discusses the relation of the subtests and clusters to CHC theory in some detail. The major emphasis in conducting factor analyses was in using CFAs to test the correspondence of DAS-II subtests and clusters to the CHC model.

The DAS-II handbook contains details of the CFAs that were conducted to test the factor structure of the battery (Elliott, 2007c, pp. 153–162). The three clusters formed by the core subtests were confirmed as robust factors throughout the age range from 3:6 through 17:11. I have thus continued to call these clusters Verbal, Nonverbal Reasoning, and Spatial—names given them in the first edition of the DAS. In CHC terms, they measure the broad abilities of Gc (crystallized intelligence/knowledge), Gf (fluid reasoning), and Gv (visual–spatial ability), respectively.

Among the diagnostic subtests, a Working Memory factor was confirmed, formed by the subtests Recall of Digits—Forward, Recall of Digits—Backward, and Recall of Sequential Order. In CHC terms, this factor measures the broad ability of Gsm (short-term memory). This is clearly a *verbal* short-term memory factor because visual short-term memory tasks are always found under the Gv factor. Moreover, because working memory tasks are cognitively more complex than simple digit recall, we found that the working memory subtests consistently had higher loadings on the factor than Recall of Digits—Forward. In order to avoid any ambiguity in interpretation (because Recall of Digits—Forward is *not* a measure of working memory), only the two working memory subtests form the Working Memory cluster in the DAS-II.

The CFAs also confirmed the Processing Speed factor, formed by the Speed of Information Processing and Rapid Naming subtests.

As an example of the analyses that were conducted, Figure 13.1 shows the factor structure of the DAS-II School-Age battery for children ages 6:0–12:11. This is the operating age range of the Phonological Processing subtest, and is the age range in which all seven CHC broad factors are found and confirmed. Figure 13.1 represents the final model (the full CHC model), which fits the standardization data significantly better than any alternative model of one, two, three, or five factors (Elliott, 2007c, p. 156).

The robustness of the structure across age levels was confirmed in an independent study by Keith, Low, Reynolds, Patel, and Ridley (2010), using both DAS-II batteries (Early Years and School-Age) across the 4- to 17-year age range. Two of these authors commented that this detailed study demonstrated remarkable consistency of the DAS-II with CHC theory (Keith & Reynolds, 2010, p. 638). The chief difference between this study and those reported in the DAS-II handbook is that Keith et al. dropped the Phonological Processing subtest from the analysis because it is the only representative of the CHC Ga factor in the battery.

Just as the Keith and colleagues (2010) study looked at the consistency and invariance of factor structure across a wide age range, so CFA was used

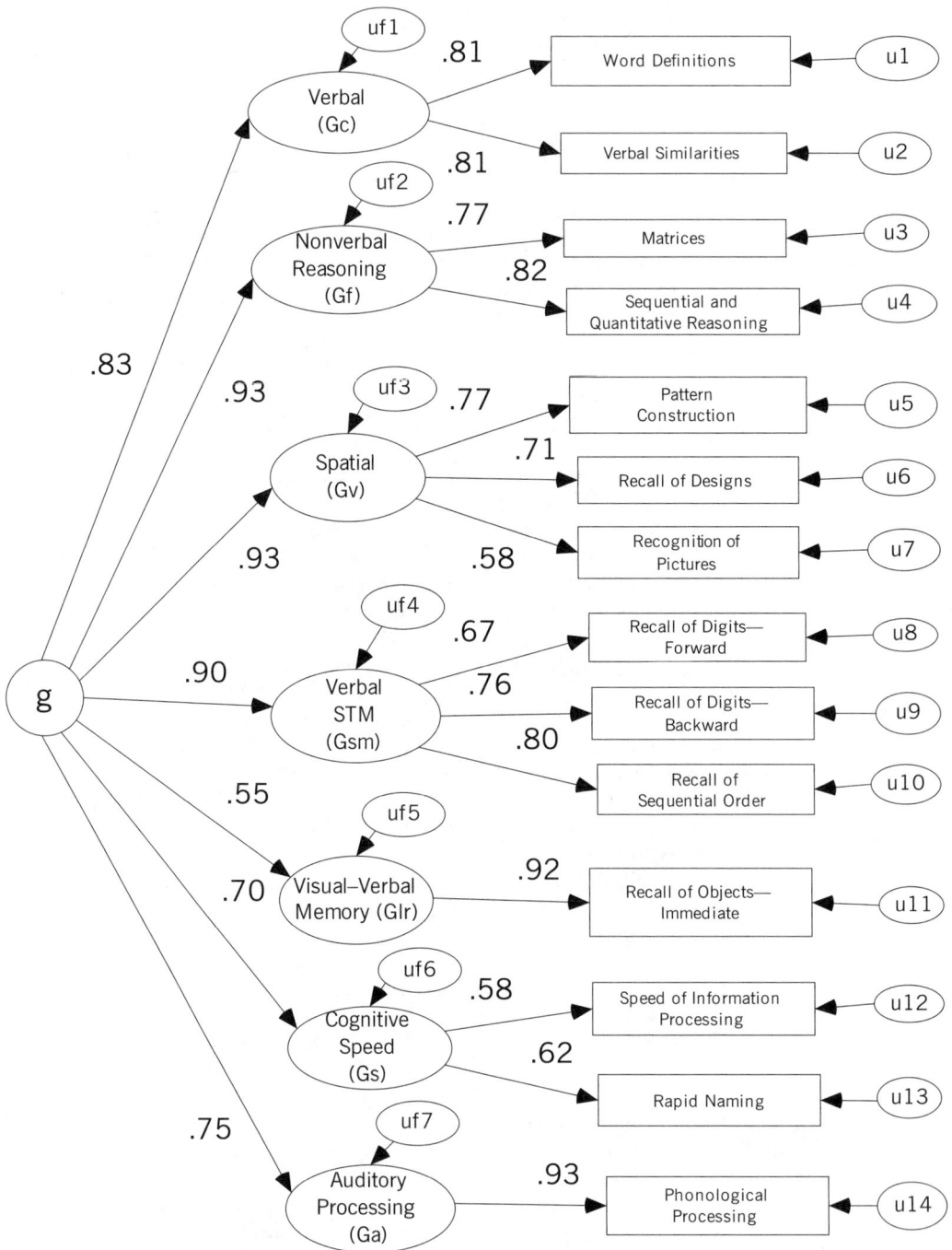

FIGURE 13.1. Factor structure of DAS-II School-Age battery for children ages 6:0–12:11, showing seven CHC broad ability factors.

to investigate construct bias in the instrument. A CFA study on the original DAS (Keith, Quirk, Schartzer, & Elliott, 1999) used the standardization sample and the bias oversample to test for construct bias. A hierarchical, multisample CFA was used to examine the constructs measured by the DAS in black, Hispanic, and white children. Results showed that the DAS measured the same constructs across all three ethnic groups across all age levels of the battery. The authors concluded that the DAS showed no construct bias, and that users of the battery could have confidence that the battery measures the same abilities for black, Hispanic, or white children and youth.

INTERPRETATION

Recommendations for Interpreting General, Broad, and Specific Cognitive Abilities

Chapters 4 and 5 in the DAS-II handbook (Elliott, 2007c) give detailed suggestions about cognitive processes underlying scores on the various DAS-II subtests and composites. The interpretive guidelines are largely (but not solely) based on the interpretation of subtests and clusters in terms of CHC broad and narrow abilities.

The DAS-II handbook also gives a systematic procedure for test interpretation. The procedure is partly based on the identification of scores that are significantly high or low at the .05 probability level. This is greatly facilitated by the design of the summary page of the record form, which shows the size of differences that are significant at $p < .05$ between achievement tests, composites, and subtest scores.

Other comparisons are made possible by tables in the DAS-II handbook. In particular, the handbook provides tables enabling discrepancies between observed and predicted achievement to be evaluated, as well as tables showing the frequency or unusualness of discrepancies. Because the development of interpretable subtests was a primary goal of the DAS-II, the handbook contains extensive interpretive guidelines for subtest scores.

Studies Conducted with Samples of Students with LDs

Research on DAS-II Score Profiles

DAS-II score profiles of 12 special populations have been reported in the handbook (Elliott, 2007b). Children were selected for each special group

sample according to specified inclusion and exclusion criteria. These studies provided the means and standard deviations of standard scores of each group on each cluster and subtest. Although such studies are of some interest—particularly when relatively homogeneous groups are being studied, such as children who are gifted and talented, or those with mild to moderate intellectual disabilities—such studies can be misleading when applied to heterogeneous groups such as those with LDs, where there are likely to be a wide range of causal influences for the disorders, resulting in a wide range of score profiles.

This is illustrated in Table 13.7, which shows that students who were poor readers and those with an LD in math had a wide range of cognitive profiles on the DAS-II. First, a sample of 293 poor readers was drawn from the DAS-II standardization sample, together with extra individuals who were tested at the time of standardization. Some of these children were surplus to the sampling requirements of the project; others belonged to the special groups referred to above and also had an LD in literacy. All 293 poor readers showed a significant discrepancy between their obtained Word Reading scores on the WIAT-II and their predicted Word Reading scores based upon their GCA scores. The second sample of 43 children consisted of the special group of children who had been identified as having an LD in math.

Score profiles on the five DAS-II cluster scores were defined as follows:

- *Low Spatial, High Verbal*: The Verbal cluster score was significantly higher ($p < .05$) than the Spatial cluster. Also, the Nonverbal Reasoning score was intermediate, being lower than Verbal, and at or above the level of the Spatial score. This pattern might possibly suggest a nonverbal LD.
- *Low Verbal, High Spatial*: The Verbal cluster score was significantly lower than the Spatial cluster. Again, the Nonverbal Reasoning score was intermediate, being lower than Spatial, and at or above the level of the Verbal score. This has been a typically reported pattern for poor readers (e.g., British Psychological Society, 1999; Snow, Burns, & Griffin, 1998).
- *High Nonverbal Reasoning*: The Nonverbal Reasoning cluster score was higher than both the Verbal and Spatial scores, and significantly higher than at least one of them. This pattern might signify good ability to process complex auditory–visual information.

TABLE 13.7. Percentage of Students with Significantly High or Low Scores on DAS-II Clusters: Comparison of Poor Readers (*n* = 293), Those with LDs in Math (*n* = 43), and the Standardization Sample for Ages 6:0–17:11 (*N* = 2,600)

Type of profile	Poor readers (with significant discrepancy)	LDs in math	DAS-II standardization sample
No significant differences between clusters	14.3	14.0	11.5
Low Spatial, high Verbal	10.2	16.3	13.3
Low Verbal, high Spatial	17.1	7.0	13.3
High Nonverbal Reasoning	17.1	16.3	18.5
Low Nonverbal Reasoning	19.8	27.9	18.8
High Processing Speed	28.0	20.9	25.3
Low Processing Speed	22.2	34.9	25.0
High Working Memory	16.7	16.3	22.1
Low Working Memory	25.9	27.9	24.2

Note. The term *poor readers* refers to children with standard scores below 85 on WIAT-II Word Reading. The term *discrepancy* refers to the presence or absence of a statistically significant difference (*p* < .05) between obtained and predicted WIAT-II Word Reading scores (the prediction was based on the GCA score).

- *Low Nonverbal Reasoning*: The Nonverbal Reasoning cluster score was lower than both the Verbal and Spatial scores, and significantly lower than at least one of them. This core cluster profile might suggest difficulty in processing complex auditory–visual information. Elliott (2005) analyzed the scores obtained from various samples of children who had been identified as having an LD in reading, and reported that approximately one-third of them had this low Nonverbal Reasoning profile.
- *High Processing Speed*: The Processing Speed cluster score was significantly higher than the GCA score.
- *Low Processing Speed*: The Processing Speed cluster was significantly lower than the GCA score.
- *High Working Memory*: The Working Memory cluster score was significantly higher than the GCA score.
- *Low Working Memory*: The Working Memory cluster score was significantly lower than the GCA score.

Table 13.7 shows the percentage of children in each sample who showed each profile. The table also shows the frequency of each profile in the total DAS-II standardization sample for ages 6:0 through 17:11. What we can conclude from an initial inspection of these profile frequencies is that

there was no common profile for poor readers or for children with an LD in math. Some children in each sample clearly had profiles that were the exact opposites of those shown by other children in the same sample.

Table 13.7 indicates that over 85% of children in the population would be expected to have one or more significantly high or significantly low cluster scores. There are also interesting differences in profile frequencies between the two samples of poor achievers.

It should be noted that the poor readers were in general *not* children who had been formally identified as having an LD in reading. About 20% had the low Nonverbal Reasoning profile previously reported to have been found in about one-third of previous samples who had an LD in reading. However, over a quarter of the sample with an LD in math had such a profile. Also, about one-third of the children in this sample also had significantly low Processing Speed scores, while very few (7%) had high Spatial ability. Both samples had a higher percentage of children with significantly low Working Memory than those with high Working Memory.

It appears that there are a number of contrasting subgroups within each group of children with reading or math difficulties. If one subgroup has significantly low mean scores on a DAS-II cluster, and the other subgroup has significantly high ones on the same cluster, the resulting mean for the total group would be attenuated, tending toward some midvalue. Correlations between this cluster and other variables would also be attenuated. Despite such likely problems, correlational studies have been conducted on samples of children with achievement problems in reading and math.

Correlational Studies

The interpretation of intelligence tests has been and remains one of the most controversial and divisive issues in cognitive assessment. Some authors (e.g., Canizez & Watkins, 1998; Glutting, McDermott, Konold, Snelbaker, & Watkins, 1998; Glutting, Watkins, Konold, & McDermott, 2006; Kahana, Youngstrom, & Glutting, 2002; Kotz, Watkins, & McDermott, 2008) dispute the validity and utility of patterns of performance, and affirm that there is little value in interpreting cognitive scores beyond a global ability estimate such as IQ or GCA.

Forty years of work on the development of the DAS-II and its predecessors run counter to this suggestion. Statistically significant intraindividual differences between subtest and cluster scores are, by definition, reliable; they indicate the presence of strengths and weaknesses in processing information that are not artifacts of measurement error. The DAS and the DAS-II standardization data indicate that a large proportion of children show such differences (see Table 13.7). The *raison d'être* of the DAS-II is that significant intraindividual differences between cluster and subtest scores should lead us to consider whether and how they illuminate processing strengths and weaknesses that may be related to the problem for which the child has been referred for assessment.

The evidence in favor of this approach is strong. CFAs conducted on the DAS-II standardization data, reviewed above, show that a model with multiple factors fits the data highly significantly better than a single-factor *g* model. The analyses demonstrate that the general factor *g* is not sufficient to explain the relationships between the subtests and clusters. Similarly, Vanderwood, McGrew, Flanagan, and Keith (2001) showed that specific cognitive abilities provide a better-fitting model for predicting reading achievement than does general cognitive ability.

Additional evidence on these issues has been provided by two studies, summarized below, which used the DAS-II (Elliott, Hale, Fiorello, Dorvil, & Moldovan, 2010; Hale et al., 2008). Interested readers can also see references in these articles to methodological criticisms of the Glutting, Watkins, and McDermott group's use of multicollinear data sets.

Prediction of WIAT-II Math Scores

Hale and colleagues (2008) used regression commonality analysis to examine the unique and shared variance components among DAS-II CHC factors in the prediction of WIAT-II Numerical Operations and Math Reasoning skills for the DAS-II normative sample and for a sample of children with a math LD. Because of the likely attenuation of correlations, it is possible (even probable) that this would reduce the number of variables found to have significant interrelationships. However, it was considered to be important to demonstrate, even from correlational data derived from heterogeneous samples, that the broad and narrow abilities represented in the DAS-II clusters and subtests would explain significantly more variance in math achievement than the GCA alone.

Results showed that the DAS-II predictors accounted for more achievement variance in typical children than in children with a math LD. The reason for this is very likely to be a restriction of range in the Math scores of the latter group. For typical children, DAS-II predictors accounted for 46% of variance in Numerical Operations and 58% of variance in Math Reasoning. On the other hand, the DAS-II predictors accounted for 33% of variance in Numerical Operations and 50% of variance in Math Reasoning for the children with a math LD. There was substantial loss of predictive validity when the GCA was used instead of cluster or subtest scores—13% loss for the typical group on both math tests, and 56% loss on Numerical Operations and 20% loss on Math Reasoning for the group with a math LD.

Prediction of WIAT-II Reading Scores

We (Elliott et al., 2010) used both commonality analysis and structural equation modeling (SEM) to investigate the effect of broad CHC abilities measured by the DAS-II, together with the effect of the general factor (*g*) on reading achievement measured by the WIAT-II.

The SEM analyses indicated that for typical children drawn from the standardization sample, four CHC-related measures were significant direct predictors of Reading Decoding (a combination of WIAT-II Word Reading and Pseudoword Decoding). These predictors were the Verbal (Gc), Nonverbal Reasoning (Gf), and Working Memory (Gsm) clusters, together with the Phonological Processing (Ga) subtest.

A similar analysis was conducted for a sample of 230 poor readers drawn from the standardization sample; children who were tested for standardization but who were surplus to requirements; and children with reading disorder, reading and written expression disorder, mathematics disorder, attention-deficit/hyperactivity disorder (ADHD), or ADHD with LD—samples gathered for studies of special populations at the time of standardization, and referred to above. For this sample, Phonological Processing was again found to be a significant predictor, together with the Spatial Ability (Gv) and Processing Speed (Gs) clusters, and the Recall of Objects—Immediate subtest (Glr).

Although Phonological Processing had a significant large effect on Reading Decoding for both samples, no other effects were significant for both samples. Each sample had three significant but different CHC factors that produced significant effects on Reading Decoding. When both analyses were considered together, the results showed that *every* CHC broad ability factor was a significant predictor in one or the other analysis. In both analyses, the effect of the general factor (*g*) was indirect. In other words, its effect was mediated through the three first-order factors measuring it (Verbal, Nonverbal Reasoning, and Spatial). The results demonstrated that children with reading problems have different cognitive predictor–reading achievement relationships than adequate readers.

The commonality analyses examined DAS-II predictors of WIAT-II Word Reading and Reading Comprehension scores. Once again, as might be expected, different commonalities were found for the typical sample and a sample of children with a specific learning disability in reading. Across all analyses, Verbal Ability (Gc), Nonverbal Reasoning Ability (Gf), Spatial Ability (Gv), Working Memory (Gsm), and Phonological Processing (Ga) showed important and significant effects, and explained significant amounts of variance over and above that explained by estimates of *g*.

The data from the studies on both math and reading suggested that practitioners should not emphasize global GCA, but should instead interpret cluster and subtest scores and their interrelationships in developing hypotheses about an individual's processing strengths and weaknesses.

BRIEF CASE STUDY

John (age 7:11), a white male in grade 2, was referred for assessment when his student assistance team reported their concern that he had not responded to the reading interventions provided as part of his regular instructional program. He struggled to name high-frequency words, and needed additional targeted instructional recommendations.[1]

John's achievement scores on the WIAT-II and his cognitive ability scores on the DAS-II are shown in Table 13.8. Examination of his WIAT-II scores shows that he has a specific difficulty with Word Reading. His higher score on Pseudoword Decoding suggests that he finds decoding regular words easier than irregular words. Such irregular words make demands on visual memory; they are often called *sight words* because they have to be remembered as a whole rather than being solvable phonetically. The initial hypothesis is that John may have visual information-processing difficulties.

On the DAS-II, the core clusters show a significant difference between Nonverbal Reasoning and both of the other clusters. Any hypothesis concerning poor processing of purely visual information is disconfirmed by John's Spatial cluster score, which is average, and at the same level as his Verbal cluster score. The subtests within each cluster have consistent scores, so the cluster scores may be interpreted without further qualification. Because of John's significantly low Nonverbal Reasoning score, it makes little sense to report his GCA score, which has little or nothing to offer in terms of describing John's cognitive processing.

The DAS-II Nonverbal Reasoning tasks are called *nonverbal* because they are presented visually. However, to solve the problems effectively, the individual needs to use internal language to encode the components of the visual stimulus, and to generate hypotheses, to test them, and to identify the correct solution. These tasks are therefore characterized in the DAS-II handbook (Elliott, 2007b) as requiring integrated analysis and complex transformation of *both* visual and verbal information. Problems in this type of processing may be at the root of John's problems in learning to read.

The diagnostic clusters of Working Memory and Processing Speed offer further information. John's Working Memory score is not significantly lower than his GCA score. However, this con-

TABLE 13.8. WIAT-II and DAS-II Subtest and Cluster Scores for John (Age 7:11)

Subtest or cluster	Score[a]
WIAT-II	
Reading	69
Word Reading	58
Pseudoword Decoding	86
Reading Comprehension	72
Written Language	83
Spelling	79
Written Expression	90
Mathematics	100
DAS-II core clusters (School-Age battery)[b]	
Verbal	102
Nonverbal Reasoning[c]	89
Spatial	102
{GCA	97}
DAS-II diagnostic clusters and subtests	
Working Memory	93
Recall of Sequential Order	$T = 40$
Recall of Digits—Backward	$T = 52$
Processing Speed	89
Speed of Information Processing	$T = 51$
Rapid Naming	$T = 38$
Additional DAS-II diagnostic subtests	
Recall of Objects— Immediate	$T = 40$
Recall of Objects—Delayed	$T = 41$
Recall of Digits—Forward	$T = 53$
Recognition of Pictures	$T = 54$
Phonological Processing	$T = 51$

[a]Standard scores except where indicated.
[b]There are no significant differences between subtests within each cluster.
[c]The Nonverbal Reasoning cluster is significantly lower than *both* the Verbal and Spatial clusters.

clusion is qualified by a significant difference between the two component subtest scores. Recall of Digits—Backward is a purely verbal subtest, and John's score on this is average for his age. On the other hand, his score on Recall of Sequential Order is 12 *T*-score points below his Recall of Digits—Backward score. This difference is highly significant ($p < .01$). Recall of Sequential Order is verbally presented, but requires the examinee to visualize the position of various parts of the body.

Based on the results from the Nonverbal Reasoning cluster, and supported by the results from the Working Memory subtests, it appears that John's processing difficulties do not appear to be shown when he is working with purely auditory–verbal or purely visual–spatial information. Our revised hypothesis is that he seems to have particular difficulties in processing auditory–visual information.

Such a view is confirmed by his scores on the Processing Speed cluster. Once again, his overall cluster score of 89 is not significantly lower than his GCA score. However, his score on the Rapid Naming subtest is 13 *T*-score points lower than his score on Speed of Information Processing, a statistically significant difference ($p < .05$). Rapid Naming presents colors and pictures that have to be named quickly, and this is another example of a subtest that requires auditory–visual processing.

The diagnostic subtest Recall of Objects is another visual–verbal task that yields separate scores for Immediate recall and Delayed recall. The subtest presents a visual array of pictures, which are then removed from view. The student is asked to recall them verbally. John's scores on Recall of Objects are below average, and significantly below the average level of the core subtests ($p < .05$). The other diagnostic subtests, on which John achieved average scores for his age, required either purely verbal or purely visual processing.

As a result of these analyses, there is now strong support for the hypothesis that John's cognitive processing difficulties center on problems with auditory–visual materials. His reading scores support this hypothesis. Reading requires a high level of visual–verbal integration in order to convert visual printed codes into sounds and words. For fluent reading, and for recognition of common words or letter strings, an individual needs information in the auditory–verbal and visual processing systems to be effectively integrated. Similarly, to perform well on the DAS-II Nonverbal Reasoning tasks (or indeed any good measures of fluid reasoning), and on the Recall of Sequential Order, Rapid Naming, and Recall of Objects subtests, one needs good integration of the visual and verbal processing systems. These tasks, like the task of reading, present visual information—but to solve the problems effectively, the use of internal language to label and to mediate the solution of the problems is generally essential. In the case of an individual who has excellent verbal and spatial abilities, if the two brain processing systems specialized for those abilities do not "talk" to each other effectively, this may have an adverse effect on performance both in reasoning and in reading acquisition.

The question now arises about appropriate intervention methods for students who have a consistent pattern of difficulties with tasks requiring auditory–visual integration. For many years, teachers of children with dyslexia have actively advocated multisensory teaching methods, despite research evidence that appeared to discredit auditory–visual integration as a cause of poor reading acquisition (e.g., Bryant, 1968). Teachers appear to have long held the view that children with dyslexia have difficulty integrating visual and verbal information. Thus it has been recommended that multisensory teaching methods should be used as much as possible in teaching John basic literacy skills. Useful references to multisensory teaching approaches are given by Thomson and Watkins (1998), Augur and Briggs (1992), Walker and Brooks (1993), Birsh (1999), and Walker (2000).

CONCLUSIONS

This chapter has outlined various ways in which the DAS-II has been designed to be appealing and accessible to children of all abilities across a very wide age range, from 2:6 to 17:11. Its good floors, and its procedures to help the least able examinees understand what is required in each task, makes the battery highly appropriate for use with clinically referred populations. It has also been designed for speed and efficiency in administration. Its cluster and subtest scores have essential qualities of reliability and interpretability. Its consistency and clarity in measuring the constructs of CHC theory make it an ideal instrument for cross-battery assessment (Flanagan, Ortiz, & Alfonso, 2007). When the DAS was first published in 1990, it was at first virtually unknown and seemed so different in its procedures that professionals probably feared it was difficult to learn. Now in its second edition, it is widely used, and is accepted as an instrument that enjoyably engages children and helps to identify their processing strengths and weaknesses with efficiency and precision.

NOTE

1. This case was kindly provided by Dr. Gloria Maccow, The Psychological Corporation, Pearson Assessments.

REFERENCES

Alfonso, V. C., Flanagan, D. P., & Radwan, S. (2005). The impact of the Cattell–Horn–Carroll theory on test development and interpretation of cognitive and academic abilities. In D. P. Flanagan & P. L. Harrison (Eds.), *Contemporary intellectual assessment: Theories. tests, and issues* (2nd ed., pp. 185–202). New York: Guilford Press.

Augur, J., & Briggs, S. (Eds.). (1992). *The Hickey multisensory language course* (2nd ed.). London: Whurr.

Birsh, J. R. (1999). *Multisensory teaching of basic language skills*. Baltimore: Brookes.

British Psychological Society. (1999). *Dyslexia, literacy and psychological assessment* (Report by a working party of the Division of Educational and Child Psychology). Leicester, UK: Author.

Bryant, P. E. (1968). Comments on the design of developmental studies of cross-modal matching and cross-modal transfer. *Cortex, 4,* 127–137.

Canivez, G. L., & Watkins, M. W. (1998). Long-term stability of the Wechsler Intelligence Scale for Children—Third Edition. *Psychological Assessment, 10,* 285–291.

Carroll, J. B. (1993). *Human cognitive abilities: A survey of factor-analytic studies*. New York: Cambridge University Press.

Carroll, J. B. (2003). The higher-stratum structure of cognitive abilities: Current evidence supports g and about ten broad factors. In H. Nyborg (Ed.), *The scientific study of general intelligence: Tribute to Arthur R. Jensen* (pp. 5–22). Amsterdam: Pergamon Press.

Cattell, R. B. (1971). *Abilities: Their structure, growth, and action*. Boston: Houghton Mifflin.

Cattell, R. B., & Horn, J. L. (1978). A check on the theory of fluid and crystallized intelligence with description of new subtest designs. *Journal of Educational Measurement, 15,* 139–164.

Daniel, M. H., Breaux, K., & Frey, F. (2010, March). *Patterns of strengths and weaknesses (PSW) models for identifying SLD*. Paper presented at the annual meeting of the National Association of School Psychologists, Chicago. Retrieved from *www.nasponline. org/conventions/handouts2010/unstated/NASP%20 2010%20PSW%20handout%202.doc*.

Dumont, R. P., Willis, J. O., & Elliott, C. D. (2009). *Essentials of DAS-II assessment*. Hoboken, NJ: Wiley.

Elliott, C. D. (1983a). *The British Ability Scales: Manual 1. Introductory handbook*. Windsor, UK: NFER-Nelson.

Elliott, C. D. (1983b). *The British Ability Scales: Manual 2. Technical handbook*. Windsor, UK: NFER-Nelson.

Elliott, C. D. (1990a). *Differential Ability Scales*. San Antonio, TX: Psychological Corporation.

Elliott, C. D. (1990b). *Differential Ability Scales: Introductory and technical handbook*. San Antonio, TX: Psychological Corporation.

Elliott, C. D. (1996). *British Ability Scales—Second Edition*. Windsor, UK: NFER-Nelson.

Elliott, C. D. (1997). The Differential Ability Scales. In D. P. Flanagan, J. L. Genshaft, & P. L. Harrison (Eds.), *Contemporary intellectual assessment: Theories. tests, and issues* (pp. 183–208). New York: Guilford Press.

Elliott, C.D. (2005). The Differential Ability Scales. In D. P. Flanagan & P. L. Harrison (Eds.), *Contemporary intellectual assessment: Theories, tests, and issues* (2nd ed., pp. 402–424). New York: Guilford Press.

Elliott, C.D. (2007a). *Differential Ability Scales—Second Edition*. San Antonio, TX: Harcourt Assessment.

Elliott, C. D. (2007b). *Differential Ability Scales—Second Edition: Administration and scoring manual*. San Antonio, TX: Harcourt Assessment.

Elliott, C. D. (2007c). *Differential Ability Scales—Second Edition: Introductory and technical handbook*. San Antonio, TX: Harcourt Assessment.

Elliott, C. D. (2007d). *Differential Ability Scales—Second Edition: Normative data tables manual*. San Antonio, TX: Harcourt Assessment.

Elliott, C. D., Hale, J. B., Fiorello, C. A., Dorvil, C., & Moldovan, J. (2010). Differential Ability Scales–II prediction of reading performance: Global scores are not enough. *Psychology in the Schools, 47*, 698–720.

Flanagan, D. P., McGrew, K. S., & Ortiz, S. O. (2000). *The Wechsler intelligence scales and Gf-Gc theory: A contemporary approach to interpretation*. Boston. Allyn & Bacon.

Flanagan, D. P., Ortiz, S. O., & Alfonso, V. C. (2007). *Essentials of cross-battery assessment* (2nd ed.). Hoboken, NJ: Wiley.

Glutting, J. J., McDermott, P. A., Konold, T. R., Snelbaker, A. J., & Watkins, M. W. (1998). More ups and downs of subtest analysis: Criterion validity of the DAS with an unselected cohort. *School Psychology Review, 27*, 599–612.

Glutting, J. J., Watkins, M. W., Konold, T. R., & McDermott, P. A. (2006). Distinctions without a difference: The utility of observed versus latent factors from the WISC-IV in estimating reading and math achievement on the WIAT-II. *Journal of Special Education, 40*, 103–114.

Hale, J. B., & Fiorello, C. A. (2004). *School neuropsychology: A practitioner's handbook*. New York: Guilford Press.

Hale, J. B., Fiorello, C. A., Dumont, R., Willis, J. O., Rackley, C., & Elliott, C. D. (2008). Differential Ability Scales—Second Edition (neuro)psychological predictors of math performance for typical children and children with math disabilities. *Psychology in the Schools, 45*, 838–858.

Horn, J. L., & Noll, J. (1997). Human cognitive capabilities: Gf-Gc theory. In D. P. Flanagan, J. L. Genshaft, & P. L. Harrison (Eds.), *Contemporary intellectual assessment: Theories. tests, and issues* (pp. 53–91). New York: Guilford Press.

Individuals with Disabilities Education Improvement Act of 2004 (IDEA 2004), Pub. L. 108-446, 118 Stat. 2647 (2004).

Kahana, S. Y., Youngstrom, E. A., & Glutting, J. J. (2002). Factor and subtest discrepancies on the Differential Ability Scales: Examining prevalence and validity in predicting academic achievement. *Assessment, 9*, 82–93.

Kaufman, A. S. (1979). *Intelligent testing with the WISC-R*. New York: Wiley.

Kaufman, A. S., & Kaufman, N. L. (2004). *Kaufman Test of Educational Achievement—Second Edition*. Circle Pines, MN: American Guidance Service.

Keith, T. Z., Low, J. A., Reynolds, M. R., Patel, P. G., & Ridley, K. P. (2010). Higher-order factor structure of the Differential Ability Scales–II: Consistency across ages 4 to 17. *Psychology in the Schools, 47*, 676–697.

Keith, T. Z., Quirk, K. J., Schartzer, C., & Elliott, C. D. (1999). Construct bias in the Differential Ability Scales?: Confirmatory and hierarchical factor structure across three ethnic groups. *Journal of Psychoeducational Assessment, 17*, 249–268.

Keith, T. Z., & Reynolds, M. R. (2010). Cattell–Horn–Carroll abilities and cognitive tests: What we've learned from 30 years of research. *Psychology in the Schools, 47*, 635–650.

Kotz, K. M., Watkins, M. W., & McDermott, P. A. (2008). Validity of the General Conceptual Ability score from the Differential Ability Scales as a function of significant and rare interfactor variability. *School Psychology Review, 37*, 261–278.

McGrew, K. S. (1997). Analysis of the major intelligence batteries according to a proposed comprehensive Gf-Gc framework. In D. P. Flanagan, J. L. Genshaft, & P. L. Harrison (Eds.), *Contemporary intellectual assessment: Theories, tests, and issues* (pp. 151–179). New York: Guilford Press.

McGrew, K. S. (2005). The Cattell–Horn–Carroll theory of cognitive abilities. In D. P. Flanagan & P. L. Harrison (Eds.), *Contemporary intellectual assessment: Theories, tests, and issues* (2nd ed., pp. 136–181). New York: Guilford Press.

McGrew, K. S., & Flanagan, D. P. (1998). *The intelligence test desk reference (IDTR): Gf-Gc cross-battery assessment*. Boston: Allyn & Bacon.

McGrew, K. S., & Murphy, S. (1995). Uniqueness and general factor characteristics of the Woodcock–

Johnson Tests of Cognitive Ability—Revised. *Journal of School Psychology, 33,* 235–245.

McGrew, K. S., & Woodcock, R. W. (2001). *Woodcock–Johnson III: Technical manual.* Itasca, IL: Riverside.

Psychological Corporation. (2001). *Wechsler Individual Achievement Test—Second Edition.* San Antonio, TX: Author.

Sanders, S., McIntosh, D. E., Dunham, M., Rothlisberg, B. A., & Finch, H. (2007). Joint confirmatory factor analysis of the Differential Ability Scales and the Woodcock–Johnson Tests of Cognitive Abilities—Third Edition. *Psychology in the Schools, 44,* 119–138.

Silverstein, A. B. (1976). Variance components in the subtests of the WISC-R. *Psychological Reports, 39,* 1109–1110.

Snow, C. E., Burns, M. S., & Griffin, P. (Eds.). (1998). *Preventing reading difficulties in young children.* Washington, DC: National Academy Press.

Thomson, M. E., & Watkins, E. J. (1998). *Dyslexia: A teaching handbook* (2nd ed.). London: Whurr.

Vanderwood, M. L., McGrew, K. S., Flanagan, D. P., & Keith, T. Z. (2001). The contribution of general and specific cognitive abilities to reading achievement. *Learning and Individual Differences, 13,* 159–188.

Walker, J. (2000). Teaching basic reading and spelling. In J. Townend & M. Turner (Eds.), *Dyslexia in practice: A guide for teachers* (pp. 93–129). New York: Kluwer Academic/Plenum.

Walker, J., & Brooks, L. (1993). *Dyslexia Institute literacy programme.* London: James & James.

Woodcock, R. W., McGrew, K. S., & Mather, N. (2001a). *Woodcock–Johnson III Tests of Achievement.* Itasca, IL: Riverside.

Woodcock, R. W., McGrew, K. S., & Mather, N. (2001b). *Woodcock–Johnson III Tests of Cognitive Abilities.* Itasca, IL: Riverside.

CHAPTER 14

The Universal Nonverbal Intelligence Test
A Multidimensional Nonverbal Alternative for Cognitive Assessment

R. Steve McCallum
Bruce A. Bracken

The Universal Nonverbal Intelligence Test (UNIT; Bracken & McCallum, 1998) is a language-free test of cognitive ability that requires no receptive or expressive language from the examiner or the examinee for administration. The need for nonverbal assessment in the United States is growing. For example, there are a large number of students with hearing impairments or other language-related limitations throughout the nation. According to 2000 figures from the National Institutes of Health (2010a), 28,600,000 Americans are deaf or have other significant hearing impairments. In 2003, about 7,500,000 Americans were reported to have speech impairments limiting their ability to communicate effectively (National Institutes of Health, 2010b). Other students have neurological and psychiatric conditions that inhibit effective verbal communications (e.g., autism spectrum disorders, traumatic brain injury, and selective mutism).

Moreover, minority populations are growing rapidly within the United States. According to the U.S. Bureau of the Census (2000), 46,951,595 people spoke a language other than English as their primary language, and almost 2,000,000 had no English-speaking ability. According to estimates from the most recent census (2010), nearly 1 of 3.6 (of the nation's 308,000,000 people at that time) was a member of a minority group—either Afri-

can American, Hispanic, Asian American, or Native American. Taken together, minority children constitute an ever-increasing percentage of public school children, particularly in many large cities. For example, minorities constitute an overwhelming percentage of the school population in Miami (approximately 84%), Chicago (89%), and Houston (88%). In addition, the population with limited English proficiency (LEP) is the fastest-growing in the nation. There are over 200 languages spoken in the greater Chicago area (Pasko, 1994), 140 in California (Unz, 1997), and 61 in Knoxville, Tennessee (S. Forrester, personal communication, March 12, 2002). In fact, in the nation's largest two school districts, students with LEP make up almost half of all students at the kindergarten level. There continue to be discrepancies in the levels of referral and placement of minority children in special education (e.g., although African Americans make up 16% of the population, they constitute 21% of the enrollment in special education). These statistics prompted the framers of the 1997 reauthorization of IDEA to state that "greater efforts are needed to prevent the intensification of problems connected with mislabeling . . . minority children with disabilities" (p. 4). In most U.S. school systems, intelligence tests are used as part of the referral-to-placement process. Because existing tests cannot be translated to accommodate all of the languages spoken, nonverbal assessment of these at-risk children's intelligence seems like the best and most viable solution. And consistent with this recommendation, IDEA 1997 admonished educators to select and administer technically sound tests that will *not* result in discriminatory practices based on racial or cultural bias. The UNIT is a viable option when examinees' characteristics preclude use of a traditional language-loaded test to assess their general cognitive abilities.

As will be apparent from the following brief review, a number of assessment experts have explored the psychometric properties of the UNIT; others have written reviews of the instrument. In general, the literature base is overwhelmingly positive, and the test has been well received. In fact, in preparation for updating this chapter, not only did we find articles addressing the utility and psychometrics of the test; we found articles that reported using the UNIT as an accepted operationalization of general intellectual ability among students with limited language abilities and other at-risk as well as not-at-risk populations (e.g., Brinton, Spackman, Fujiki, & Ricks, 2007; Fujiki, Spackman, Brinton, & Illig, 2008; Hughes & Zhang, 2007; Lienemann, Graham, Leader-Janssen, & Reid, 2006; Noland, 2009; Liew, McTigue, Barrois, & Hughes, 2009; Pendarvis & Wood, 2009). Apparently many practitioners are finding the UNIT useful.

THEORY AND STRUCTURE OF THE UNIT

The UNIT contains six subtests designed to assess functioning according to a *two-tier model of intelligence* (memory and reasoning), which incorporates *two organizational strategies* (symbolic and nonsymbolic organization). Within each of the two fundamental organizational strategies, the two cognitive abilities of memory and reasoning are assessed in a hierarchical arrangement (see Bracken & McCallum, 1998). The three memory

subtests include Object Memory, Spatial Memory, and Symbolic Memory. Similarly, three subtests were developed to assess reasoning; these subtests are Cube Design, Mazes, and Analogic Reasoning. Five of the subtests require minor motoric manipulation, and the remaining subtest (Analogic Reasoning) requires only a pointing response. With two exceptions (Cube Design and Mazes), the subtests that require motoric manipulation can be adapted to allow for a pointing response only, if necessary.

Symbolic organization strategies require the use of concrete and abstract symbols to conceptualize the environment; these symbols are typically language-related (e.g., words), although the symbols may take on any form (e.g., numbers, statistical equations, rebus characters, flags). Symbols are eventually internalized and come to label, mediate, connote, and (over time) make meaningful our experiences. *Nonsymbolic* strategies require the ability to perceive and make meaningful judgments about the physical relationships within our environment; this ability is symbol-free, or relatively so, and is closer to fluid-like intellectual abilities.

Within each of the two fundamental organizational categories included in the UNIT (nonsymbolic and symbolic), problem solution requires one of two types of abilities—memory or *reasoning*. That is, some of the items require primarily symbolic organization and rely heavily on memory (e.g., those included on the Symbolic Memory subtest). Other items require considerable symbolic organization and reasoning skills, but less memory (e.g., those included on the Analogic Reasoning subtest). Some items seem to require nonsymbolic organization strategies and memory primarily (e.g., those on the Spatial Memory subtest). Finally, others may require nonsymbolic organization and reasoning, but *little* memory (Cube Design). Consequently, the UNIT assesses four basic cognitive abilities operationalized by the six subtests (see Figure 14.1).

	Memory	Reasoning
Symbolic	Symbolic Memory Object Memory	Analogic Reasoning
Nonsymbolic	Spatial Memory	Cube Design Mazes

FIGURE 14.1. Conceptual model of the UNIT.

The rationale for using the four strategies operationalized by the UNIT to assess intelligence is supported in the literature. For example, Wechsler (1939) emphasized the importance of distinguishing between highly symbolic (verbal) and nonsymbolic perceptual (performance) means of expressing intelligence. Jensen (1980) provided rationale for a two-tiered hierarchical conceptualization of intelligence, consisting of the two subconstructs of memory (level I) and reasoning (level II). However, in contrast to many of the low-*g*-loaded level I memory tasks designed to require reproduction or recall of simple content, the UNIT memory tasks were developed to require more complex memory functioning.

The theoretical organization of the UNIT is consistent with that of several instruments that adopt the Gf-Gc model of fluid and crystallized abilities (more recently known as the *Cattell–Horn–Carroll* [CHC] model), as described by Cattell (1963), Horn (1968), Carroll (1993), and others (e.g., Woodcock, 1990; Woodcock, McGrew, & Mather, 2001). (See also Horn & Blankson, Chapter 3; Schneider & McGrew, Chapter 4; and Carroll, Appendix, this volume.) UNIT subtests tap components of strata I and II within this model, including fluid reasoning, general sequential reasoning, visual processing, visual memory, spatial scanning, spatial relations, and induction.

Intelligence consists primarily of a pervasive and fundamental ability, *g*, which provides a base for the development of somewhat unique specialized skills. Although there are many means of determining intelligence, it makes little sense to conceptualize intelligence as being either verbal or nonverbal. Rather, there are verbal and nonverbal means available to assess intelligence. Consequently, the UNIT should be considered a nonverbal measure of intelligence, not a measure of nonverbal intelligence, and was designed to be a strong measure of *g*.

The UNIT is currently being revised, and as part of that undertaking, the UNIT-2 is being modified to embody a more comprehensive theoretical model than the original test. With two new quantitative subtests, the UNIT-2 will continue to emphasize general intelligence, while representing more dimensions of the Gf-Gc model (i.e., adding quantitative reasoning). Like the original instrument, the UNIT-2 will be administered in a 100% nonverbal manner.

DESCRIPTION OF SUBTESTS

UNIT Subtests

Based on the 2×2 model, several scores can be calculated for the UNIT total test, including a Full Scale IQ (FSIQ), Memory Quotient, Reasoning Quotient, Symbolic Quotient, and Nonsymbolic Quotient. Finally, individual subtest scores can be derived for each of the six subtests for further analysis of examinees' performance. The existing UNIT subtests are described below; the first three subtests are designed to assess memory, the second three reasoning. A description of subtests, batteries, and quotients to be included in the UNIT-2 is provided in the next subsection.

1. *Symbolic Memory.* The examinee recalls and recreates sequences of visually presented universal symbols (e.g., green boy, black woman).
2. *Spatial Memory.* The examinee must remember and recreate the placement of black and/or green chips on a 3×3 or 4×4 cell grid.
3. *Object Memory.* The examinee is shown a visual array of common objects (e.g., shoe, telephone, and tree) for 5 seconds, after which he or she identifies the pictured objects from a larger array of pictured objects. This subtest is to be discontinued on the UNIT-2.
4. *Cube Design.* The examinee completes a three-dimensional block design task, using between one and nine green and white blocks.
5. *Analogic Reasoning.* The examinee completes a matrix analogies task using common objects (e.g., hand/glove, foot/__ ?) and novel geometric figures.
6. *Mazes.* The examinee completes a maze task by tracing a path through each maze from the center starting point to an exit. Mazes, like Object Memory, will not be included on the UNIT-2.

UNIT-2 Subtests

In addition to the four original UNIT subtests that will be represented on the UNIT-2 (i.e., Symbolic Memory, Object Memory, Cube Design, and Analogic Reasoning), two new subtests will be a part of the revised test. Two subtests of a quantitative reasoning nature will be added (i.e., Nonsymbolic Quantity and Numerical Series). A description of these new additions follows.

1. *Nonsymbolic Quantity.* An array of white and/ or black domino-like objects of various numerical values creates an incomplete numerical sequence, equation, analogy, or mathematical problem. The examinee points to one of four numerical options below the stimulus figures that best fits the incomplete array.
2. *Numerical Series.* An array of numbers or mathematical symbols creates an incomplete quantitative series that is either perceptual or conceptual in nature. The examinee completes the items by pointing to one of four numerical response options below the stimulus array.

With the addition of the two new subtests and the four continuing UNIT subtests, the UNIT-2 will be a new battery comprising six subtests. All six subtests in combination will form the UNIT-2 Extended Battery; two Standard batteries will be produced by combining different collections of subtests. The current UNIT Standard Battery will be represented in the UNIT-2 (i.e., the four UNIT subtests to be carried over to the UNIT-2), as well as a Standard Battery that combines the new facets of intelligence represented by the new subtests (i.e., quantitative reasoning) with the existing memory and reasoning components. This latter battery will be formed by selecting a symbolic–nonsymbolic balance of the most psychometrically sound subtests from each of the intellectual facets. Finally, the UNIT-2, like the UNIT, will include a selection of two-subtest Abbreviated Batteries, including the two most psychometrically sound, strongest measures of *g*, as well as combinations of two subtests from each of the facets (e.g., a Memory Abbreviated Battery, a Reasoning Abbreviated Battery).

ADMINISTRATION AND SCORING

Administration of UNIT Subtests

Administration of all six UNIT subtests requires approximately 45–50 minutes. Current UNIT norms allow for two- and four-subtest short-form batteries, in addition to the full six-subtest battery. The shorter batteries require approximately one-third to two-thirds less time. UNIT-2 batteries, comparable to the UNIT in size and options, will allow for a similarly brief administration as the original test (see below).

Although administration of the UNIT subtests is 100% nonverbal, the examiner may communicate with the examinee (if they have a common language) to establish rapport, discuss extratest issues, and the like, as well as to reduce the awkwardness that may otherwise occur with a nonverbal interaction. The examiner must present the UNIT stimuli nonverbally, using eight nonverbal gestures that were used during standardization and are presented in the manual (as well as on a training video available from the publisher). To aid in teaching task demands, the examiner is instructed to make liberal use of demonstration items, sample items, and so-called "checkpoint" items; checkpoint items allow feedback, but are scored.

For the Symbolic Memory subtest, stimulus plates are presented on an easel. The easel contains plates showing pictures of one or more of the following universal human figures, in a particular order: a green baby, a black baby, a green girl, a black girl, a green boy, a black boy, a green woman, a black woman, a green man, a black man. The examinee is presented with the stimulus plate and then is instructed through gestures to replicate the order shown on the stimulus plate. The examinee uses 1½" × 1½" response cards, each containing one of the universal human figures, to reproduce the array depicted on the stimulus plate. The task has no time limits other than a 5-second exposure time. Each correct item is assigned 1-point credit, and color, gender, and size are critical variables for scoring.

For the Spatial Memory subtest, the examiner briefly presents a series of grids on stimulus plates located on an administration easel. The grids show one or more green or black polka dots placed within cells (on the grid). The less difficult items use a 3 × 3 grid; the more difficult items require a 4 × 4 grid. The stimulus plate is shown for 5 seconds and then is removed from view. The examinee places response chips on a blank grid that is placed on the table top in front of him or her. Spatial Memory has no time limits, except for the 5-second exposure. Each correct response is assigned 1-point credit.

The Object Memory subtest requires presentation of pictures of common objects arranged on stimulus plates located on an administration easel. The easel is laid flat on the table, and the examinee is shown a plate containing pictures of one or more objects for 5 seconds; then the examinee is shown a second plate containing pictures from the first plate *and* pictures of distracter objects. The examinee identifies pictures on the second plate that were shown on the first plate; to create a semipermanent response, the examinee places black chips on the pictures selected. This memory task is not timed, other than the 5-second exposure. Each correct object identified on the response place is assigned 1-point credit. Again, Object Memory will not be continued on the UNIT-2.

The Cube Design subtest requires the examinee to use up to nine cubes to replicate three-dimensional designs shown on a stimulus plate. Each cube has six facets: two white sides, two green sides, and two sides that contain diagonals (triangles), one green and one white. These cubes can be arranged to replicate the three-dimensional figures depicted on the stimulus plates. This task is timed, but the time limits are liberal, to emphasize assessment of ability rather than speed. Except for the very early items, which are scored either correct or incorrect and yield a maximum of 1 point per item, examinees may earn up to 3 points (per item). Each facet of the three-dimensional construction is judged to be either correct or incorrect. Each correct facet is assigned 1-point credit.

The Analogic Reasoning subtest requires the examinee to solve analogies presented in a matrix format. The examinee is directed to indicate which one of several options best completes a two-cell or a four-cell analogy. Task solution requires the examinee to determine the relationships between objects. For example, in a four-cell matrix, the first cell may depict a fish and the second water; the third cell may show a bird, and the fourth cell is blank. The examinee selects from several options the picture that best completes the matrix. In this case, a picture of the sky is a correct response. This reasoning subtest is not timed. Each correct response is assigned 1-point credit.

The Mazes subtest requires the examinee to complete a maze using a #2 lead pencil, minus the eraser. The examinee is presented with a maze showing a mouse in the center and one or more pieces of cheese on the outside of the maze. The cheese depicts one or more possible exits from the maze. The task is to determine the correct path from the center to the (correct) piece of cheese. The examinee is stopped after the first error. The task is timed, though the time limits are quite liberal. Each decision point is scored, and correct decisions are assigned 1-point credit. Again, Mazes will not be continued on the UNIT-2.

Administration of UNIT-2 Subtests

In addition to the four UNIT subtests that will be carried over to the UNIT-2 (i.e., Symbolic Memory, Spatial Memory, Analogic Reasoning, Cube Design), two new subtests will be part of the UNIT-2, as noted earlier. Administration of the new subtests is described below.

The Nonsymbolic Quantity subtest employs an easel format and requires the examinee to solve quantitative problems represented in a nonsymbolic manner (e.g., using domino-like objects). The examinee is shown an array of stimulus dominos that collectively create a sequence, series, equation, or mathematical problem with a missing component. The examinee points to one of four response options that completes the sequence, series, or equation, or provides the dimension that contributes to solving the problem.

The Number Series subtest uses an easel format and requires the examinee to solve quantitative problems represented numerically. The examinee is shown an array of numbers that collectively create a sequence, series, equation, or mathematical problem with a missing component. The examinee points to one of four response options that completes the sequence, series, or equation, or provides the number that contributes to solving the problem.

Materials and Scoring

In addition to the manipulatives (e.g., blocks, response chips, response grids,) general materials required to administer the UNIT include a stopwatch, a #2 lead pencil, two test booklets (one for the Mazes subtest and one for recording the student's performance on the remaining five subtests), and relevant demographic information. Except for Mazes and Object Memory (optional subtests, to be administered as part of the Extended Battery only), the stimulus plates for all subtests are contained in one stand-up easel. Object Memory stimuli are presented on a small separate easel, if needed. The larger easel containing the four Standard Battery subtests contains subtest stimuli printed on front and back for efficiency and economy; colored tabs are provided to inform the examiner as to the direction of administration (e.g., tabs with subtest names in green alert the examiner that the book is oriented in the correct direction for those subtests).

Scoring is user-friendly and straightforward. Correct responses are printed on the test booklet to facilitate ease of scoring. Raw scores for each item are summed to provide a subtest total raw score. Raw scores are easily transformed to standard scores with either the tables provided in the

UNIT manual (Bracken & McCallum, 1998) or the UNIT Compuscore software (Bracken & McCallum, 2001). The Abbreviated Battery is used for screening purposes (Symbolic Memory and Cube Design); the Standard Battery for most purposes that include placement decisions (the Abbreviated Battery subtests, plus Spatial Memory, Matrix Analogies); and the Extended Battery for diagnostic purposes (the Standard Battery subtests, plus Object Memory and Mazes).

PSYCHOMETRIC PROPERTIES

Norming Procedures, Standardization Characteristics, and Technical Data

The standardization data for the UNIT were obtained from a representative sample of 2,100 children and adolescents ranging in age from 5 years, 0 months to 17 years, 11 months. These children and adolescents were carefully selected to represent the U.S. population in terms of age, sex, race, parent educational attainment, community size, geographic region, and ethnicity (see sample-to-population match data in the UNIT manual). Importantly, children and adolescents from special education categories were included to the extent that these individuals were present in the school population.

Readers are urged to consult the UNIT manual for results of numerous special studies conducted to assess the UNIT's technical adequacy, including reliability, validity, and fairness data for a variety of populations. We summarize some of the most important data from the manual below, followed by summaries of results of independent studies conducted after the manual was published.

Data from the UNIT Manual

Data from the manual provide evidence of strong reliability; the average composite scale internal-consistency coefficients range from .86 to .96 for the typical and clinical/exceptional samples across all batteries. The FSIQ internal-consistency coefficients range from .91 to .93. Test–retest stability coefficients (corrected for restriction in range) range from .79 to .84 for IQs for a sample of 197 participants. Average test–retest mean score gains due to practice effects (over approximately 3 weeks) are 7.2 for the Abbreviated Battery, 5.0 for the Standard Battery, and 4.8 for the Extended Battery. Validity data are supportive of the model

as well. For example, expected raw score age progressions for Cube Design are 13, 19, 26, and 33 for the groups ages 5–7, 8–10, 11–13, and 14–17 years, respectively.

Exploratory and confirmatory factor-analytic data have provided evidence to support the UNIT model. Using the standardization data, an exploratory analysis yielded a large first eigenvalue, 2.33; other values were below 1.0. These findings suggest the presence of a strong first factor, commensurate with the interpretation of the FSIQ as a good overall index of global intellectual ability, or g. The factor structure also supports the two-factor memory and reasoning model, particularly for the Standard Battery. When the Extended Battery subtests were factor-analyzed, all subtests loaded appropriately, although the Mazes subtest yielded a borderline low loading on the reasoning factor. Confirmatory factor-analytic procedures were equally supportive, showing strong fit statistics for a two-factor memory and reasoning model.

Strong concurrent data are also reported in the manual. For example, data from a sample of 61 children with learning disabilities yielded correlation coefficients (corrected for restriction in range) between the FSIQs from the three UNIT batteries and the Wechsler Intelligence Scale for Children—Third Edition (WISC-III; Wechsler, 1991) FSIQ from .78 to .84, and from .84 to .88 for a sample of 59 children with intellectual disabilities. Strong coefficients were obtained, showing the relationship between UNIT and other instruments for various populations (e.g., Native Americans). Coefficients between the UNIT IQs and scores from the Bateria-R (Woodcock & Muñoz-Sandoval, 1996) are more variable. Corrected coefficients between the three UNIT FSIQs and the Bateria-R Broad Cognitive Ability score (Standard Battery) ranged from .30 to .67 for 27 Spanish-speaking bilingual education students. Additional concurrent validity data are available from the manual (e.g., correlations with Raven's [1960] Progressive Matrices).

In general, predictive validity coefficients obtained between the UNIT and various achievement tests are relatively strong, and comparable to those between language-loaded tests and achievement measures. An interesting finding from the studies reported in the UNIT manual is that the magnitude of the coefficients between the UNIT global Symbolic Quotient and measures of language-based achievement (e.g., reading subtests) is often higher than the magnitude of coefficients between the UNIT Nonsymbolic Quotient and these language-loaded achievement measures. In fact, this pattern is found in 21 out of 36 comparisons (58%). This pattern would be predicted from the nature of the symbolic–nonsymbolic distinction, and provides some additional evidence for the predictive and construct validity of the test model.

Independent Studies Addressing UNIT Utility

Since the publication of the UNIT manual, results from several studies have become available showing relevant technical data. For example, Hooper and Bell (2006) have explored the relationship between the Leiter International Performance Scale—Revised (Leiter-R; Roid & Miller, 1997) and the UNIT for 100 elementary and middle school students. Correlation coefficients obtained from the comparison of the Leiter-R FSIQ and Fluid Reasoning scale and all UNIT global scales (Memory, Reasoning, Symbolic, and Nonsymbolic Quotients) are statistically significant ($p < .01$) and range from .33 for the UNIT Memory Quotient versus Leiter-R Fluid Reasoning comparison to .72 for the UNIT FSIQ versus Leiter-R FSIQ comparison. Importantly, global scale means for the two tests are similar generally, although the UNIT FSIQ is approximately 5 points higher than the Leiter-R FSIQ. The other mean global scores are more similar in magnitude across the two tests; the UNIT means range from 101.54 to 103.67, and the Leiter-R Fluid Reasoning score is 99.07.

Hooper (2002) also reported correlation coefficients ranging from .49 to .72 between the four UNIT global scores and end-of-the-year scores from the Total Reading, Total Math, and Total Language scores of the Comprehensive Test of Basic Skills (CTBS/McGraw-Hill, 1996) for 100 elementary and middle school children. Using stepwise multiple-regression analyses, Hooper found that the UNIT FSIQ predicted all three academic areas from the CTBS better than the Leiter-R FSIQ; the UNIT FSIQ entered the multiple-regression equation first, accounting for 39–55% of the variance in the three criterion scores, and the Leiter-R contributed an additional 1–2% for each.

Farrell and Phelps (2000) have compared scores from the Leiter-R and the UNIT for 43 elementary and middle school children with severe language disorders. Correlation coefficients between the UNIT quotients and Leiter-R Fluid Reasoning scale scores range from .65 to .67; the coefficients between UNIT quotients and Leiter-R Visualization Reasoning scale scores range from .73 to .80.

For this sample, Leiter-R mean scores are 65.07 and 66.33 for the Fluid Reasoning and Visualization Reasoning scales, respectively. UNIT global scale scores range from 66.71 (FSIQ) to 70 (Symbolic Quotient). Farrell and Phelps conclude that both tests show promise for providing fair and valid assessment of cognitive functioning for children with severe language impairments, and that both should be considered superior to conventional language-loaded tests (e.g., the Kaufman Assessment Battery for Children and WISC-III) for use with this population.

In an empirical study addressing this assertion for Mexican American elementary school students with LEP, Borghese and Gronau (2005) explored the convergent and discriminant validity of the UNIT by comparing it to the WISC-III. The authors concluded that the pattern of correlations between the UNIT and the WISC-III provided support for both the convergent and discriminant validity of the UNIT for this population. The UNIT mean FSIQ was significantly higher than the mean WISC-III FSIQ. As predicted, the UNIT Nonsymbolic Quotient correlated more strongly with the WISC-III Performance IQ than did the Symbolic Quotient, and the UNIT Symbolic Quotient correlated more strongly with the WISC-III Verbal IQ than with the Performance IQ. The corrected correlations ranged from .43 to .90 between the two scales, with most greater than .60. Borghese (2009) reported further evidence of convergent and discriminant validity in a subsequent study using this same population, but with data from the Stanford Achievement Test: Edition 10 reading and math scores. In general, then, these authors concluded that their data supported the validity of the UNIT for Mexican Americans with LEP.

Scardapane, Egan, Torres-Gallegos, Levine, and Owens (2002) have investigated the relationship among the UNIT, the Wide Range Intelligence Test (WRIT; Glutting, Adams, & Sheslow, 2000), and the Gifted and Talented Evaluation Scales (GATES; Gilliam, Carpenter, & Christensen, 1996) for English-speaking children and English-language learners. The correlation coefficient obtained between the WRIT Visual scale and the UNIT FSIQ of .59 can be compared to the coefficient between the UNIT FSIQ and the WRIT Verbal scale of .11. Contrary to Scardapane and colleagues' predictions, the coefficients showing the relationship between the GATES scores and the WRIT Verbal scale are not higher than the coefficients showing relationships between the UNIT

FSIQ and the four GATES scores. The coefficients between the UNIT FSIQ and the GATES scales of Intellectual Ability, Academic Skills, Creativity, Leadership, and Artistic Talent range from .50 to .57 ($p < .05$); the coefficients between the WRIT Verbal scale and these GATES scores range from .004 to .10 ($p > .05$). Scardapane and colleagues have concluded that their data support the use of the UNIT as a nonverbal measure of intelligence.

Fairness

The burden of ensuring fairness in testing is particularly salient for authors of nonverbal tests, in part because of an increasingly diverse society and the need to ensure sensitive and equally valid assessment for a wide variety of populations. The UNIT manual includes an entire chapter entitled "Fairness," and describes extensive efforts to ensure that the test is appropriate for use for all children in the United States (i.e., that construct-irrelevant variance is minimized for all relevant populations). (Also see McCallum, 1999, for additional descriptions of efforts to ensure fairness for the UNIT.)

The test model was formulated, and the test was developed, on the basis of five core fairness concepts: (1) A language-free test is less susceptible to bias than a language-loaded test; (2) a multidimensional measure of cognition is fairer than a unidimensional one; (3) a test that minimizes the influence of acquired knowledge (i.e., crystallized ability) is fairer than one that does not; (4) a test that minimizes speeded performance is fairer than one with greater emphasis on speed; and (5) a test that relies on a variety of response modes is more motivating and thereby fairer than one relying on a unidimensional response mode. Several other steps were taken to ensure fairness. For example, in the initial item development phase, items were submitted to a panel of "bias experts"—individuals sensitive to inclusion of items that might be offensive to or more difficult for individuals within certain populations (e.g., Native Americans, Hispanics). Items identified by these individuals, and those identified via statistical item bias analyses, were removed.

A number of statistical procedures were undertaken to help ensure fairness, including calculation of separate reliabilities, factor structure statistics, mean-difference analyses, and so forth. for subpopulations. Reliabilities for FSIQs for females, males, African Americans, and Hispanic Americans were all greater than .91 (uncorrected) and

.94 (corrected) for the Abbreviated Battery, and greater than .95 for the Standard and Extended Battery. Separate confirmatory factor analyses for these subpopulations have provided evidence for "a single general intelligence factor as well as the primary and secondary scales," as well as "evidence supporting the construct validity of the UNIT across sex, race, and ethnic groups" (Bracken & McCallum, 1998, p. 182).

Mean IQ difference analyses using matched groups from the UNIT standardization data have also provided evidence of fairness, as reported in the manual. The mean scores of males and females matched on age, parental educational level, and ethnicity were very similar, with effect sizes ranging from 0.02 to 0.03 across all three batteries. Mean differences, estimated via effect sizes, ranged from 0.22 to 0.43 for FSIQs across all batteries for Native Americans matched on age, sex, and parent educational levels; the largest mean difference, 6.50, was obtained from the Standard Battery. Mean differences of FSIQs, reflected via effect sizes, ranged from 0.10 to 0.14 for matched Hispanic Americans across all batteries; the largest difference, 2.13, occurred on the Standard Battery. Effect sizes for matched African Americans ranged from 0.51 to 0.65; a mean FSIQ difference of 8.63 between African Americans and European Americans was obtained using the Standard Battery. A mean FSIQ Standard Battery difference of 6.20 was found between examinees with deafness/hearing impairments and a matched nonimpaired sample; a Standard Battery FSIQ mean difference of 5.33 was found between Ecuadorian and matched non-Ecuadorian examinees. Evidence that prediction is not a function of gender and racial membership was provided by using the regression slope as a measure of the strength of the relationships between UNIT scores and achievement on the Woodcock–Johnson Psycho-Educational Battery—Revised Achievement Battery subtests in a regression equation; race and sex did not contribute significantly to the prediction ($p > .05$).

Additional data generated after the UNIT was developed also have relevance for UNIT fairness. For example, in a study using UNIT standardization data but applying a matching strategy more refined than the one reported in the manual, Upson (2003) found a further reduction of mean difference scores between Hispanic Americans and European Americans (i.e., white non-Hispanics). Matching on all relevant variables reported in the manual *and* community size *and* the educational level of both parents, rather than just one, reduced the mean between matched Hispanic Americans and European Americans considerably for the Standard Battery FSIQ, from 2.13 to 0.47. Although further refinement reduced the differences between African Americans and European Americans slightly, the reductions were not as pronounced. The Standard Battery FSIQ difference of 8.51 for 168 matched African Americans and European Americans was only slightly smaller than the 8.63 reported in the manual.

Burton (2002) investigated the utility of the UNIT for a clinical population—children with autism. She found a significantly lower mean FSIQ for a sample of 31 children diagnosed as having either autism, Asperger syndrome, or pervasive developmental disorder not otherwise specified (M = 81.85) vs. a matched control sample from the UNIT standardization sample (M = 103.89). The UNIT Nonsymbolic Quotient mean score was larger than the Symbolic Quotient, as might be predicted from the limited verbal skills of children with these diagnoses.

The UNIT has been used successfully to help identify promising students from low-socioeconomic status (low-SES) homes as well. Bracken, VanTassel-Baska, Brown, and Feng (2007) investigated the relative power of the UNIT, the Cognitive Abilities Test (CogAT; Lohman & Hagen, 2001), and a number of other school system measures for identification of gifted/promising students as part of a federally funded grant project (Project Athena). By including nonverbal measures in the assessment process, including the UNIT and the CogAT, the Project Athena assessment model identified nearly twice as many Title 1 students as gifted than the school districts' identification procedures did. Of particular note, 21% of those students with IQs of 120 and above were African American when identified by the UNIT, versus 8.8% and 9.8% identified by the CogAT Nonverbal and Verbal scales, respectively.

Although the preponderance of data from the literature is strongly supportive of the use of the UNIT for children with language limitations, those who do not have English as a first language, and those from low-SES environments, not all the studies are totally positive. Jimenez (2001) reported that five of the six UNIT subtests "failed to show acceptable internal consistency" and did not reach "the recommended coefficient of .90" (p. 5424B) for test–retest stability for 60 Puerto Rican children. The UNIT correlation coefficients with the Bateria-R Reading cluster were "moderate to low" for these children. Finally, they scored almost one-half of a standard deviation lower than a matched control group of non-Hispanic children. Jimenez concluded that although the UNIT may be a fair instrument to measure cognitive abilities of Puerto Rican children, it may not be optimal when used in isolation, and should be part of a multifaceted assessment process.

Similarly, Pendley, Myers, and Brown (2004) reported FSIQ stability coefficients for 29 children with attention-deficit/hyperactivity disorder (ADHD) to be .75, compared to .81 from a group taken from the standardization sample reported in the manual. None of the mean differences for the composite scores were significantly different from time 1 to time 2 for this sample. (Mean interval between the two administrations was 31.1 days.) As predicted in the UNIT manual, the examinees with ADHD performed better on UNIT Reasoning than Memory subtests, but a second prediction—that examinees would score higher on planning tasks than on successive processing subtests—was not supported. When an ipsative interpretation scheme was used, most examinees' identified strengths and weaknesses reverted back to the their average range on second testing. Pendley and colleagues noted limitations of using a test–retest methodology to assess the value of ipsative interpretive strategy (e.g., problems related to regression to the mean, variable practice effects, the distractibility of this particular sample). We agree with their assessment and are reminded of Kaufman's (1994, p. 31) admonition that "you get one shot" using an ipsative strategy.

Other studies have focused on more molecular analyses. For example, Maller (2000) conducted a sophisticated item analysis, using the Mantel–Haenszel (MH) procedure and item response theory (IRT), to detect differential item functioning (DIF) for 104 children and adolescents with deafness/hearing impairments. Using a group of children from the UNIT standardization sample matched on age, gender, and ethnicity to these 104 youngsters, Maller concluded that no items in the UNIT exhibited DIF when either the MH procedure or IRT was used; that is, the probability of a correct response on the UNIT items does not seem to be affected by hearing status. Consequently, she notes that the UNIT seems appropriate for this population, and there may be no need to develop special norms for children with deafness/hearing impairments. Maller and French (2004) also investigated the factor invariance across a group with deafness and the standardization group; they investigated both the primary model (memory and reasoning) and secondary model (symbolic and nonsymbolic reasoning) and reported, "The general forms of both models were invariant across group, thus supporting both theoretical models" (p. 647). However, in a follow-up molecular analysis exploring invariance of pattern coefficients, they reported one pattern coefficient to be invariant across the two samples for the primary model (for the Analogic Reasoning subtest) and three invariant patterns for the secondary model. Maller and French concluded that the primary model is to be preferred for the deaf population and note that "use of the UNIT is preferred over other published tests" (p. 657), but they caution that Analogic Reasoning scores may be lower than expected for deaf examinees and that deaf students may have difficulty with short-term memory.

Additional evidence supporting the use of the UNIT for deaf and hard-of-hearing examinees is provided by Krivitski, McIntosh, Rothlisberg, and Finch (2004). They compared children with deafness to a matched sample of hearing children from the UNIT standardization sample; the children were matched on age, race/ethnicity, SES, and gender. Results of a profile analysis showed that the children with deafness displayed similar patterns of UNIT subtest performance. Krivitski and colleagues conclude that the data support use of the UNIT for children with deafness, and add, "Evidence from this deaf sample implies that children with hearing problems are not at a disadvantage compared to their hearing counterparts when completing the measures" (p. 348). Similarly, Noland (2009) found no difference in the mean FSIQs of 21 Spanish-dominant and 18 English-dominant (for spoken language) participants.

Athanasiou (2000) has compared five nonverbal assessment instruments for psychometric integrity and fairness, including the UNIT. She concluded that all have unique strengths and weaknesses. Although Athanasiou noted that the UNIT fails to meet Bracken's (1987) criterion for test–retest stability (.90) at all ages, her assessment of the UNIT is mostly favorable. For example, she commented that the UNIT's reliance on only nonverbal directions is likely to reduce the potential for cultural bias in administration; the use of checkpoint items allows for periodic assessment of understanding during the administration; presentation of psychometric properties of subpopulations enhances the confidence users can have that the test is appropriate for a variety of examinees; and the floors, ceilings, and item gradients for the UNIT Standard

and Extended Batteries exceed minimum recommendations. But perhaps the most important observation Athanasiou offered regarding the UNIT addresses the extent to which the manual provides evidence of test fairness. She noted that all five of the tests she reviewed are generally impressive in terms of their technical adequacy, but "as a whole they present much less statistical evidence of test fairness. The UNIT appears to be an unqualified exception to this statement," and the UNIT is the only test "to provide evidence of consistent factor structure across subgroups" (p. 227).

Fives and Flanagan (2002), in an extensive review of the UNIT, noted that the test is well constructed, theoretically driven, psychometrically sound, and highly useful, and that its use will permit more effective assessment of some traditionally difficult to assess populations. They concluded their review by presenting a case study illustrating use of the UNIT for a 12-year-old Hispanic female. The examinee's UNIT IQ scores were higher than those obtained from more language-loaded tests, even those typically considered to assess nonverbal performance and fluid abilities; Fives and Flanagan remarked, "Had this particular youngster not been given the UNIT, an error might have been made and she might not have been classified learning disabled and received appropriate services" (p. 445).

Additional reviews by Bandalos (2001), Kamphaus (2001), and Sattler (2008) are generally positive, particularly regarding basic technical properties (e.g., reliability, floors, ceilings). Bandalos concluded a review reported in the Buros Institute's Mental Measurements Yearbook by noting that the UNIT provides a "much needed means of obtaining reliable and valid assessments of intelligence for children with a wide array of disabilities who cannot be tested accurately with existing instruments. It is a carefully developed instrument with excellent reliability and impressive evidence of validity for use as supplement to or substitute for more traditional measures such as the WISC-III" (p. 1298). All these reviewers note the need for certain types of validity studies, particularly ones investigating the construct validity of symbolic and nonsymbolic processing and the UNIT's ability to predict grades and/or classroom achievement.

Readers are encouraged to consult Braden and Athanasiou (2005) for a detailed review of the most commonly used nonverbal instruments, including the UNIT; traditional (and some innovative) criteria for reliability, validity, and test fairness are applied to these instruments. According to these criteria, the UNIT fares well compared to other nonverbal measures. In a more recent review, McCallum (in press) applies the Braden and Athanasiou criteria to an updated list of nonverbal tests; in addition, McCallum discusses the need for examiners to consider linguistic demand and cultural loading when choosing a nonverbal instrument, and uses the model created by Flanagan, Ortiz, and Alfonso (2007) to depict the extent to which nonverbal measures possess these characteristics.

INTERPRETING THE UNIT

Multidimensional test interpretation is complicated, partly because it requires that examiners engage in a number of steps, consult numerous tables, consider a variety of cognitive models, consider carefully the limitations of the instruments they use, and (finally and most importantly) make the test results relevant for real-world application. In addition to traditional normative interpretation, there are at least three other interpretive models available: *traditional ipsative strategies, subtest profile base rate analyses,* and *cross-battery assessment* (CBA). Traditional ipsative interpretation is controversial, but is still used by practitioners who want to get more from the instruments they use than the good predictive capabilities of an FSIQ. The goal of ipsative interpretation is to uncover relationships between cognitive strengths and weaknesses and these important academic and work-related skills. Consequently, we first describe traditional ipsative strategies, followed by brief descriptions of subtest base rate profile analyses and CBA. Citations are provided for more specific guidelines for all three methods.

Ipsative Interpretation

Because the UNIT is multidimensional, interpretation requires multiple steps. General steps for interpretation are discussed below, followed by a discussion of three specific interpretive procedures. The following guidelines are based on the psychometric strengths expressed in the UNIT manual, and detailed guidelines are provided there and on the Compuscore scoring and interpretation software (Bracken & McCallum, 2001), available from the publisher. Because of space limitations, the guidelines are presented in brief form here.

1. First, the UNIT composite or global scores should be interpreted within a normative context. The most global score, the FSIQ, should be interpreted according to its relative standing in the population, using standard scores, percentile ranks, age equivalents, and so on as indications of performance. For multidimensional tests like the UNIT, it is useful to provide some statement regarding the representativeness of the score; that is, does the FSIQ represent the examinee's overall intellectual functioning well, as operationalized by the test? Then the examiner should consider the next level of global scores, the scale scores (i.e., Reasoning Quotient, Memory Quotient, Symbolic Quotient, or Nonsymbolic Quotient). Are these scores comparable, or do they deviate significantly from one another? If these scores show considerable variability, the most global score may not represent the examinee's overall intellectual functioning very well. Considerable scatter in global and subtest scores reveals a profile with peaks and valleys, and corresponding cognitive strengths and weaknesses. These weaknesses should be determined by examining the magnitude of differences, using statistical significance and frequency-of-occurrence data.

2. The band of error of the UNIT FSIQ should be communicated next. Typically, the most reliable single score from *any* multidimensional test is the total or composite score. This global score should be considered within a band of confidence framed by one or more standard errors of measurement, determined by the level of significance desired.

3. Step 3 provides elaboration of step 1 and a transition to the more specific interpretative procedures described below. In step 3, all UNIT standard scores should be compared *systematically.* As stated above in step 1, if UNIT scale (global) scores are highly variable (i.e., if there are statistically significant differences among them), the composite score cannot be considered representative of the examinee's overall intellectual functioning. On the other hand, if there is little variability (i.e., nonsignificant amounts of variability), the composite score may be considered a reasonable estimate of the examinee's overall functioning.

Further description of the examinee's performance should be given at this point. For example, the examiner may provide additional information about the nature of the UNIT, and the abilities presumed to be measured by the instrument; in addition, the examiner may indicate that the examinee's abilities in particular areas as measured by the test (e.g., short-term memory, reasoning) are uniformly developed (or not, as the case may be). The examinee's overall level of ability should be described, and inferences about the examinee's prognosis for achievement can be made. If qualitative (e.g., intrasubtest scatter) and quantitative (i.e., variable scores) data show variability in the examinee's performance, further analyses should be performed to determine unique intrachild (ipsative) strengths and weaknesses.

More specific interpretation is possible with three other procedures (after McCallum & Whitaker, 2000), depending on the nature of the score variability. These three interpretive procedures are (1) the *pooled procedure*, (2) the *independent-factors procedure*, and (3) the *rational–intuitive procedure*. The pooled procedure is the first of the three techniques discussed. It requires computing the mean of all six UNIT subtests and individually comparing each subtest score to that mean to identify so-called "outliers" (i.e., scores that differ significantly from the overall subtest mean). The independent-factors procedure is so named because it relies on interpretation based on the (independent-factor) factor-analytic structure of the UNIT. More specifically, it is based on the factor structure obtained by maximizing the independence of the factors constituting the test. For the UNIT, the best factor-analytic solution from currently available data shows a good two-factor model (i.e., the best factor solution appears to reveal a three-subtest memory factor and a three-subtest reasoning factor). Thus the examiner should first look for the pattern of consistently higher memory (over reasoning) subtests, or the reverse, assuming little within-factor variance. The rational–intuitive procedure is so named because it relies on the interpretation of a multidimensional test based on the theoretical model that underpins the development of a test, or on other theoretical models of which the examiner is aware. In this case, users of the UNIT may find that some children will perform well on all the symbolic subtests relative to the nonsymbolic subtests, or vice versa. Examiners should keep in mind that other cognitive models can be applied to ipsative interpretation.

Interpretation of the UNIT-2 will follow the same format as the UNIT, except that there will be additional intellectual factors represented in the revised instrument. All three interpretive procedures cited above will accord with the revised test.

Base Rate Interpretation

A model of interpretation using subtest profile base rate analysis as a beginning point to interpret WISC-III performance was developed by Glutting, McDermott, and Konold (1997). They described procedures that allow an examiner to determine the extent to which an examinee's profile of subtest scores is rare in the population. First, they applied sophisticated statistical techniques to calculate common profiles in the WISC-III standardization data, and then made those profiles available to test users. Next, they provided examiners with a set of relatively straightforward calculations allowing them to determine the likelihood that a particular profile matches one or more of these common profiles. Glutting and colleagues argued that unusual profiles are more likely to have clinical significance than those that occur often in the population.

Following the logic described by Glutting and colleagues (1997), Wilhoit and McCallum (2002) have provided the information examiners need to apply the base rate method to analysis of UNIT scores. Although the base rate analysis is not particularly complicated to use, deriving the data necessary to obtain common or typical profiles is. Wilhoit and McCallum describe the lengthy cluster analysis procedures used to provide those profiles from the UNIT standardization data. Via cluster analyses, six common profiles were identified for the Standard Battery (i.e., delayed, low average, average, above average with high Memory and Symbolic Quotients, above average with high Reasoning and Nonsymbolic Quotients, and superior) and seven for the Extended Battery (i.e., delayed, low average with higher Memory and Symbolic than Reasoning and Nonsymbolic Quotients, low average with higher Reasoning and Nonsymbolic than Memory and Symbolic Quotients, average with higher Memory and Symbolic than Reasoning and Nonsymbolic Quotients, average, high average, and superior). Specific demographics are associated with each of these profiles (e.g., percentage of females, males, African Americans, European Americans, family educational levels). Because these profiles are considered typical, profiles of examinees that "fit" one of them may not be diagnostic, according to the logic from Glutting and colleagues. Examiners can determine the fit by following a few easy steps. First, each of the examinee's subtest scores is subtracted from the like subtest scores provided from the profiles in the relevant table with the closest FSIQ. These scores are squared and summed to produce a score that can be compared to a critical value (i.e., 272 for the Standard Battery and 307 for the Extended Battery). This procedure is repeated for the three profiles with FSIQs closest to the examinee's obtained FSIQ. If the obtained score from any one of these comparisons is equal to or larger than the critical value, the obtained profile is considered rare in the population, and thus potentially diagnostic. To obtain the FSIQs and subtest scores for the common profiles for both Standard and Extended Batteries, see Tables 2, 3, 5, and 6 in the Wilhoit and McCallum (2002) article in the journal *School Psychology Review*.

Cross-Battery Assessment

McGrew and Flanagan (1998) first described the rationale and procedures required to use the CBA process (for a comprehensive explanation of CBA—or XBA, as it is now referred to—see Flanagan, Alfonso, & Ortiz, Chapter 19, this volume). One important assumption of CBA is that subtests can be selected from different batteries and used to assess particular cognitive constructs, thereby increasing assessment precision and efficiency. This technique is particularly useful when there is no need to administer and interpret a particular test in its entirety (e.g., the referral question does not require that an FSIQ be obtained from a specific cognitive test). To aid in the application of CBA, McGrew and Flanagan have provided a cognitive nomenclature based on the work of several researchers, particularly Cattell (1963), Horn (1968, 1994), and Carroll (1993). This nomenclature—referred to in recent years as the CHC system or model, as noted earlier—is embedded in a three-tier hierarchical model. Stratum III represents g, the general cognitive energy presumed to underlie performance across all tasks individuals undertake. Stratum II represents relatively broad abilities that can be operationalized fairly well as factors from a factor analysis (e.g., short-term memory, long-term memory, fluid ability, acquired knowledge, visual processing, auditory processing, processing speed). Stratum I represents abilities at a more specific level, and can be assessed relatively purely by many existing subtests; two or more of these subtests can be used to operationalize stratum II abilities. Using this system, McGrew and Flanagan characterized subtests from most existing batteries as measures of stratum I and stratum II abilities, provided several caveats about the use of these operationalizations, and even provided models of worksheets to aid examiners in using CBA.

Wilhoit and McCallum (2003) have recently extended the McGrew and Flanagan (1998) model to assessment of cognitive constructs via only nonverbal tests, including the UNIT. Application of CBA is somewhat detailed, requiring the use of worksheets containing the names of tests and subtests, and the broad stratum II and stratum III abilities those subtests measure. Using the worksheets, an examiner can determine strengths and weaknesses according to operationalization of the CHC model by subtests from various nonverbal measures. Assessment of stratum II abilities is the primary focus. Typically, each subtest from nonverbal tests assesses a narrow stratum I ability, and two or more can be used to provide a good assessment of stratum II. The six stratum II abilities assessed by nonverbal tests include fluid intelligence (Gf), crystallized intelligence (Gc), visual processing (Gv), short-term memory (Gsm), long-term memory (Glr), and processing speed (Gs). The other ability typically included in CBA, auditory processing (Ga), is not assessed by nonverbal tests and is not included on the worksheets. The worksheets allow an examiner to calculate the mean performance by averaging scores from all subtests. Each stratum II ability score (determined by averaging two or more stratum I measures within that stratum II ability) can be compared to the overall stratum II average in an ipsative fashion. Assuming that all subtests use a mean of 100 and a standard deviation of 15 (or have been converted accordingly), each average stratum II ability score that is more than 15 points from the overall mean is considered a strength or a weakness, depending on the direction of the difference. Wilhoit and McCallum provide the worksheets for this application of the UNIT (and other nonverbal tests), modified from the procedure originally described by Flanagan and McGrew (1997). Importantly, the stratum II abilities have been linked to several important real-world products (e.g., processing speed and short-term memory underpin the ability to learn to decode words quickly, according to Mather & Jaffe, 2002). Consequently, using CBA can aid in diagnosing academic and other problems.

The UNIT-2 will contribute to a more comprehensive assessment of intelligence than the original UNIT does. The two newly added subtests expand the UNIT's representation of the Gf-Gc model, by adding a quantitative factor. Thus the UNIT-2 will address more of the dimensions included in the Gf-Gc model, but will do so in a completely nonverbal manner, which will allow practitioners a sound substitute for existing verbally loaded Gf-Gc assessment procedures.

ADDITIONAL CLINICAL APPLICATIONS

Administration of the UNIT to non-English-speaking populations is easy and does not require the traditional language demands of conventional intelligence tests or costly translations. Although no gestures are completely universal, we chose some gestures for the UNIT (e.g., affirmative head nods and pointing) because they seem to be ubiquitous modes of communication across most cultures. Also, an effort was made to employ universal item content (i.e., objects found in all industrialized cultures). Thus use of the UNIT with children who come into the United States from other countries is facilitated. In addition, the format is appropriate for children with deafness/hearing impairments and for those who have other types of language deficits (e.g., selective mutism, severe dyslexia, speech articulation difficulties). Additional clinical applications of the UNIT and other nonverbal tests are described in a book on nonverbal assessment (McCallum, Bracken, & Wasserman, 2001). For example, this book provides information describing how members of various populations compare on the UNIT scores; technical data such as reliability coefficients for those examinees who earn scores close to typical "cutoff points" of 70 and 130; a case study illustrating use of the test for a child with language delays; and a UNIT interpretive worksheet showing step-by-step interpretation guidelines. Another book by McCallum (2003) provides a discussion of procedures/techniques to help examiners choose the most technically appropriate and the fairest tests for assessing a range of nonverbal abilities, including nonverbally functional behaviors, academic skills, personality, cognition, and neurological functioning. This book provides chapters focusing on the nonverbal assessment of all these abilities, plus chapters describing best practices in eliminating bias in item selection for nonverbal tests; contextual and within-child influences on nonverbal performance (including pharmacological agents); and (briefly) the history and current sociological context for nonverbal assessment.

Finally, there are two book chapters now available that describe application of the UNIT in a multibattery assessment. The first focuses on a child diagnosed as having a pervasive developmental disorder (see McCallum, 2011), and the second on a child with second-language-learning problems (Bell, 2011).

INNOVATIONS IN THE MEASUREMENT OF COGNITIVE ABILITIES

Several features set the UNIT apart from all or most existing nonverbal scales.

1. The UNIT is administered solely through the use of examiner demonstrations and gestures. The liberal use of sample, demonstration, and (unique) checkpoint items ensures that the examinee understands the nature of each task prior to attempting the subtest for credit.

2. The test comprises a variety of subtests that will provide the opportunity for both motoric and motor-reduced (i.e., pointing) responses. Administration of UNIT subtests can be modified so that only a pointing response is required on four of the six subtests. The use of motoric and motor-reduced subtests facilitates administration by optimizing motivation and rapport. For example, a very shy child may be encouraged initially to point only; later, as rapport is gained, other, more motorically involved responses may be possible. Also, use of the motor-reduced subtests may be indicated for children with limited motor skills.

3. Subtests contain items that are as culturally fair as possible. We have included line drawings and objects that are recognizable to most individuals from all cultures.

4. The test is model-based. That is, we have included subtests designed to assess reasoning—a higher-order mental processing activity—as well as complex memory. Also, we have included symbolically loaded subtests as well as less symbolically laden ones. Interpretation of the UNIT is facilitated because of these theoretical underpinnings.

5. Samples of non-English-speaking individuals have been included for UNIT validation studies, collected by Riverside during the UNIT norming. Children from other cultures and children residing in the United States who had LEP and/or special education diagnoses were included in the norming and validation of the UNIT.

6. Administration time can be controlled by the examiner, depending on the number of subtests administered. The UNIT includes three administra-

tion formats: a two-subtest version, a four-subtest (standard) version, and a six-subtest (extended) version.

7. Reliability estimates were calculated for two critical cutoff points (i.e., for those with FSIQs around 70 and those with FSIQs around 130).

8. There is an unprecedented array of support resources for a nonverbal test, including a training video, a university training manual, and a computerized scoring and interpretation software program.

BRIEF CASE STUDY

Name: Sean Steven Sanders
Age: 7 years, 7 months
Date of birth: 12/07/93
Grade: Entering 1
School: Hillside Elementary
Date(s) of assessment: 07/07/01; 07/22/01; 08/06/01
Examiner: Sherry Mee Bell, PhD, NCSP

Reason for Referral and Background Information

Sean was referred to determine his current functioning and to obtain information useful in planning his educational program. He lives with both parents and an older sister. Parents report a healthy pregnancy and delivery. Birth weight was within normal limits, although developmental milestones were somewhat delayed. Sean walked independently at age 1 year, 4 months (1:4) and talked at 3:0; speech and language development was significantly delayed. Sean was toilet-trained for urination at 3:0 and for bowels between 4:0 and 5:0. He had his tonsils and adenoids removed at 4:6. Chronic middle-ear infections reportedly stopped after the tonsillectomy.

Due to apparent delays in speech and language skills, Sean was evaluated at the University Hearing and Speech Center at age 4:6. Sean exhibited a communication disorder characterized by delayed receptive and expressive language skills. He exhibited difficulty naming and identifying objects and following directions; in addition, he exhibited echolalia. Spontaneous speech was characterized by strings of unintelligible reduplicative utterances, interspersed with some intelligible words.

Testing in October 2000 yielded a standard score of 59 on the Peabody Picture Vocabulary Test—Third Edition (PPVT-III; population mean = 100). In addition, he achieved a raw score of 23 (population mean = 39) on the Templin–Darley Articulation Test. Hearing was evaluated and reported to be normal. Sean has been receiving special education services through the local school system and was identified as eligible for special education services (because of developmental delays) in April 1999.

Relevant Test Behaviors

Sean is short for his chronological age, and is slender, with dark hair and large brown eyes. He presented as somewhat shy, but he separated from his parents upon request. Sean seemed to put forth good effort during assessment and responded well to praise and encouragement, although he had difficulty following oral directions at times. At times he whispered his answers, especially when he seemed unsure of himself. Results are considered to represent a valid estimate of his current functioning level.

Assessment Test Results

On the UNIT, Sean achieved a Memory Quotient of 100, Reasoning Quotient of 98, Symbolic Quotient of 95, and Nonsymbolic Quotient of 104. His FSIQ was 98. The range of scores from 92 to 104 is believed to capture Sean's true score with 90% confidence. The Quotient and FSIQ scores of the UNIT have a mean of 100 and a standard deviation of 15, similar to many other intelligence tests. The subtests of the UNIT have a mean of 10 and a standard deviation of 3. Sean scored as follows on the subtests: Symbolic Memory, 10; Analogic Reasoning, 8; Cube Design, 11; Object Memory, 9; Spatial Memory, 11; and Mazes, 10.

Sean displayed relatively little variability on these nonverbal cognitive tasks. He performed somewhat more strongly (a little more than half a standard deviation) on nonsymbolic versus symbolic tasks. There was no difference in his performance on reasoning versus memory tasks. The slight relative strength in nonsymbolic versus symbolic abilities is consistent with Sean's deficits in language because language requires symbolic thinking/problem solving. Results of the UNIT indicate average cognitive abilities overall.

Further assessment of cognitive abilities was accomplished by administration of selected subtests from the Stanford–Binet Intelligence Scale: Fourth Edition. These subtests have a mean of 50 and a standard deviation of 8. On the Stanford–Binet, Sean achieved a standard score of 36 on the Vocabulary subtest. This score is in the borderline range of intellectual functioning. In contrast, Sean achieved a standard score of 58 on the Pattern Analysis subtest. This score is in the high average range of intellectual functioning. The Vocabulary subtest measures expressive vocabulary, whereas the Pattern Analysis subtest measures nonverbal, visual–spatial reasoning. Sean's performance on the Pattern Analysis subtest is consistent with his performance on Cube Design from the UNIT, indicating well-developed nonverbal, visual–spatial abilities. His performance on the Vocabulary subtest is consistent with previous assessments indicating significant delays or deficits in language skills.

Sean was also administered the screener portion of the Wechsler Individual Achievement Test (WIAT). Standard scores were calculated based on grade norms because Sean will be entering first grade this month. The WIAT subtests have a mean of 100 and a standard deviation of 15. Sean scored as follows on the WIAT subtests: Basic Reading, 104 (61st percentile, grade equivalent of K:7); Mathematics Reasoning, 89 (23rd percentile, grade equivalent of K:3); Spelling, 94 (34th percentile, grade equivalent of K:9).

Some caution should be used in interpreting these scores because the WIAT has a limited floor for children Sean's age. Sean performed in the average range on tasks measuring beginning reading and spelling skills. Performance was slightly weaker on tasks measuring mathematics reasoning. However, this relative weakness is most likely to be explained by Sean's difficulty with language. The WIAT Mathematics Reasoning subtest uses questions involving language rather than math calculation only.

Sean was administered the PPVT-III, Form L. Results yielded a standard score of 77, which is at the 6th percentile, and an age equivalent of 5:6. Results indicate that Sean's receptive language skills continue to be somewhat delayed, approximately 2 years below his chronological age.

Parents responded to the Vineland Adaptive Behavior Scales. Results yielded an overall Adaptive Behavior Composite standard score of 53 and age equivalent of 4:5. Domain standard scores were as follows: Communication, 60; Daily Living, 46; and Socialization, 71. The following age equivalents were calculated for the domains: Communication, 4:6; Daily Living, 3:5; and Socialization, 4:6. In addition, though no standard score could be calculated for the Motor Skills domain, an age equivalent was calculated: 3:5.

Mrs. Sanders responded to the Behavior Assessment System for Children (BASC). Validity scales were acceptable. Results yielded an overall Behavioral Symptoms Index in the average range, with scores on the Externalizing Problems, Internalizing Problems, and Adaptive Skills composites all in the average range. In addition, results on the following subscales were in the average range: Hyperactivity, Aggression, Conduct Problems, Anxiety, Depression, Atypicality, Withdrawal, Attention Problems, Adaptability, Social Skills, and Leadership. The only elevated BASC score was Somatization, which was probably elevated because Sean requires medication on a routine basis for asthma and allergies. Scores do *not* indicate atypical social development/functioning.

Summary and Recommendations

Assessment results tentatively suggest a *Diagnostic and Statistical Manual of Mental Disorders*, fourth edition, text revision (DSM-IV-TR) diagnosis of mixed receptive–expressive language disorder (Axis I, 315.32). Sean is also being referred for a neurological evaluation to assist in determining the exact nature of his developmental delay. Participation in a regular classroom with special educational support is recommended. Sean continues to be eligible for rather intensive speech and language services. In addition, he is likely to need support from the school resource teacher, either in an inclusion format or in a pull-out format. Modifications and adaptations in assignments will be needed. A multisensory approach to instruction should be most beneficial for Sean. Grading modifications may be needed, and teachers are encouraged to conduct error analysis (with Sean) to determine which kinds of tasks give him more difficulty. In the classroom, Sean may benefit from being paired with a "study buddy" who can prompt Sean on how to complete tasks and assignments. Sean's progress should be monitored routinely. A thorough reevaluation of academic progress using informal assessment strategies is recommended in 1 year.

REFERENCES

Athanasiou, M, S, (2000). Current nonverbal assessment instruments: A comparison of psychometric integrity and test fairness. *Journal of Psychoeducational Assessment, 18,* 211–299.

Bandalos, D. L. (2001). Review of the Universal Nonverbal Intelligence Test. In B. S. Plake & J. C. Impara (Eds.), *Fourteenth mental measurements yearbook* (pp. 1296–1298). Lincoln, NE: Buros Institute.

Bell, S. M. (2011). Use of nonverbal cognitive assessment to distinguish learning disabilities from second language learning difficulties. In N. Mather & L.E. Jaffe (Eds.), *Comprehensive evaluations* (pp. 553–561). Hoboken, NJ: Wiley.

Borghese, P. (2009). An analysis of predictive, convergent, and discriminant validity of the Universal Nonverbal Intelligence Test with limited English proficient Mexican-American elementary students. *Dissertation Abstracts International, 70*(3), 1962B–1970B.

Borghese, P., & Gronau, R. C. (2005). Convergent and discriminant validity of the Universal Nonverbal Intelligence Test with limited English proficient Mexican-American elementary students. *Journal of Psychoeducational Assessment, 23*, 128–139.

Bracken, B. A. (1987). Limitations of preschool instruments and standards for minimal levels of technical adequacy. *Journal of Psychoeducational Assessment, 5*, 313–326.

Bracken, B. A., & McCallum, R. S. (1998). *The Universal Nonverbal Intelligence Test.* Itasca, IL: Riverside.

Bracken, B. A., & McCallum, R. S. (2001). *UNIT Compuscore.* Itasca, IL: Riverside.

Bracken, B. A., VanTassel-Baska, J., Brown, E. F., & Feng, A. (2007). Project Athena: A table of two studies. In J. VanTassel-Baska & T. Stambaugh (Eds.), *Overlooked gems: A national perspective on low-income promising learners* (pp. 63 67). Washington, DC: National Association of Gifted Children.

Braden, J. P., & Athanasiou, M. S. (2005). A comparative review of nonverbal measures of intelligence. In D. P. Flanagan & P. L. Harrison (Eds.), *Contemporary intellectual assessment: Theories, tests, and issues* (pp. 557–577). New York: Guilford Press.

Brinton, B., Spackman, M. P., Fujiki, M., & Ricks, J. (2007). What should Chris say?: The ability of children with specific language impairment to recognize the need to dissemble emotions in social situations. *Journal of Speech, Language, and Hearing Research, 50*, 798–811.

Burton, B. (2002). *Assessment of cognitive abilities in children with a pervasive developmental disorder using the Universal Nonverbal Intelligence Test.* Unpublished doctoral dissertation, University of Tennessee, Knoxville.

Carroll, J. B. (1993). *Human cognitive abilities: A survey of factor-analytic studies.* New York: Cambridge University Press.

Cattell, R. B. (1963). Theory for fluid and crystallized intelligence: A critical experiment. *Journal of Educational Psychology, 54*, 1–22.

CTBS/McGraw-Hill. (1996). *Comprehensive Test of Basic Skills.* Monterey, CA: Author.

Farrell, M. M., & Phelps, L. (2000). A comparison of the Leiter-R and the Universal Nonverbal Intelligence Test (UNIT) with children classified as language impaired. *Journal of Psychoeducational Assessment, 18*, 268–274.

Fives, C. J., & Flanagan, R. (2002). A review of the Universal Nonverbal Intelligence Test (UNIT): An advance for evaluating youngsters with diverse needs. *School Psychology International, 23*, 425–448.

Flanagan, D. P., & McGrew, K. S. (1997). A cross-battery approach to assessing and interpreting cognitive abilities: Narrowing the gap between practice and cognitive science. In D. P. Flanagan, J. L. Genshaft, & P. L. Harrison (Eds.), *Contemporary intellectual assessment: Theories, tests, and issues* (pp. 314–325). New York: Guilford Press.

Flanagan, D. P., Ortiz, S. O., & Alfonso, V. C. (2007). *Essentials of cross-battery assessment* (2nd ed.). Hoboken, NJ: Wiley.

Fujiki, M., Spackman, M. P., Brinton, B., & Illig, T. (2008). Ability of children with language impairment to understand emotion conveyed by prosody in a narrative passage. *Internation Journal of Language and Communication Disorders, 43*(3), 330–345.

Gilliam, J. E., Carpenter, B. O., & Christensen, J. R. (1996). *Gifted and Talented Evaluation Scales: A norm referenced procedure for identifying gifted and talented students.* Austin, TX: PRO-ED.

Glutting, J., Adams, W., & Sheslow, D. (2000). *Wide Range Intelligence Test manual.* Wilmington, DE: Wide Range.

Glutting, J., McDermott, P. A., & Konold, T. R. (1997). Ontology, structure, and diagnostic benefits of a normative subtest taxonomy from the WISC-III standardization sample. In D. P. Flanagan, J. L. Genshaft, & P. L. Harrison (Eds.), *Contemporary intellectual assessment: Theories, tests, and issues* (pp. 349–372). New York: Guilford Press.

Hooper, V. S. (2002). *Concurrent and predictive validity of the Universal Nonverbal Intelligence Test and the Leiter International Performance Scale—Revised.* Unpublished doctoral dissertation, University of Tennessee, Knoxville.

Hooper, V. S., & Bell, S. M. (2006). Concurrent validity of the Universal Nonverbal Intelligence Test and the Leiter International Performance Scale revised. *Psychology in the Schools, 43*(2), 143–148.

Horn, J. L. (1968). Organization of abilities and the development of intelligence. *Psychological Review, 75*, 242–259.

Horn, J. L. (1994). Theory of fluid and crystallized intelligence. In R. J. Sternberg (Ed.), *Encyclopedia of human intelligence* (pp. 443–451). New York: Macmillan.

Hughes, J. N., & Zhang, D. (2007). Effects of the structure of classmates' perceptions of peer's academic abilities on children's perceived cognitive competence, peer acceptance, and engagement. *Contemporary Educational Psychology, 32,* 400–419.

Individuals with Disabilities Education Act Amendments of 1997, Pub. L. No. 105–17, 20 U.S.C. 33 (1997).

Jensen, A. R. (1980). *Bias in mental testing.* New York: Free Press.

Jimenez, S. (2001). An analysis of the reliability and validity of the Universal Nonverbal Intelligence Test (UNIT) with Puerto Rican children (Doctoral dissertation, Texas A&M University, 2001). *Dissertation Abstracts International, 62,* 5424B.

Kamphaus, R. W. (2001). *Clinical assessment of child and adolescent intelligence* (2nd ed.). Boston: Allyn & Bacon.

Kaufman, A. S. (1994). *Intelligent testing with the WISC-III.* New York: Wiley.

Krivitski, E. C., McIntosh, D. E., Rothlisberg, B., & Finch, H. (2004). Profile analysis of deaf children using the Universal Nonverbal Intelligence Test. *Journal of Psychoeducational Assessment, 22,* 338–350.

Liew, J., McTigue, E. M., Barrois, L., & Hughes, J. N. (2008). Adaptive and effortful control and academic self-efficacy beliefs on achievement: A longitudinal study of 1st through 3rd graders. *Early Childhood Research Quarterly, 23,* 515–526.

Lienemann, T. O., Graham, S., Leader-Janssen, B., & Reid, R. (2006). Improving the writing performance of struggling writers in second grade. *Journal of Special Education, 40,* 66–78.

Lohman, D. F., & Hagen, E. P. (2001). *Cognitive Abilities Test (CogAT), Form 6.* Itasca, IL: Riverside.

Maller, S. J. (2000). Item invariance in four subtests of the Universal Nonverbal Intelligence Test (UNIT) across groups of deaf and hearing children. *Journal of Psychoeducational Assessment, 18,* 240–254.

Maller, S. J., & French, B. F. (2004). Universal Nonverbal Intelligence Test factor invariance across deaf and standardization samples. *Educational and Psychological Measurement, 64,* 647–660.

Mather, N., & Jaffe, L. E. (2002). *Woodcock–Johnson III: Reports, recommendations, and strategies.* New York: Wiley.

McCallum, R. S. (1999). A "baker's dozen" criteria for evaluating fairness in nonverbal testing. *The School Psychologist, 53,* 40–43.

McCallum, R. S. (Ed.). (2003). *Handbook of nonverbal assessment.* New York: Kluwer Academic/Plenum.

McCallum, R. S. (2011). Assessing a child with a nonspecific pervasive development disorder: Can a nonverbal cognitive measure help? In N. Mather & L.E. Jaffe (Eds.), *Comprehensive evaluations* (pp. 553–561). Hoboken, NJ: Wiley.

McCallum, R. S. (in press). Assessing intelligence nonverbal. In K. F. Geisinger (Ed.), *APA Handbook of testing and assessment.* Washington, DC: American Psychological Association.

McCallum, R. S., Bracken, B. A., & Wasserman, J. (2001). *Essentials of nonverbal assessment.* New York: Wiley.

McCallum, R. S., & Whitaker, D. A. (2000). Using the Stanford–Binet: FE to assess preschool children. In B. A. Bracken (Ed.), *The psychoeducational assessment of preschool children* (3rd ed.). Boston: Allyn & Bacon.

McGrew, K. S., & Flanagan, D. P. (1998). *The intelligence test desk reference (ITDR): Gf-Gc cross-battery assessment.* Boston: Allyn & Bacon.

National Institutes of Health. (2010a). Hearing disorders and deafness. Bethesda, MD: National Library of Medicine. Retrieved from *www.nlm.nih.gov/medlineplus/hearingdisordersanddeafness.html.*

National Institutes of Health (2010b). Speech and communication disorders. Bethesda, MD: National Library of Medicine. Retrieved from *www.nlm.nih.gov/medlineplus/speechandcommunicationdisorders.html.*

Noland, R. M. (2009). When no bilingual examiner is available: Exploring the use of ancillary examiners as a viable testing solution. *Journal of Psychoeducational Assessment, 27,* 29–45.

Pasko, J. R. (1994). Chicago—don't miss it. *Communique, 23,* 2.

Pendarvis, E., & Wood, E. W. (2009). Eligibility of historically underrepresented students referred for gifted education in a rural school district: A case study. *Journal for the Education of the Gifted, 32*(4), 495–514.

Pendley, J. D., Myers, C. L., & Brown, R. D. (2004). The Universal Nonverbal Intelligence Test with children with attention-deficit hyperactivity disorder. *Journal of Psychoeducational Assessment, 22,* 124–135.

Raven, J. C. (1960). *Guide to standard progressive matrices.* London: Lewis.

Roid, G. H., & Miller, L. J. (1997). *Leiter International Performance Scale—Revised.* Wood Dale, IL: Stoelting.

Sattler, J. M. (2001). *Assessment of children: Cognitive applications* (4th ed.). San Diego, CA: Jerome M. Sattler.

Sattler, J. M. (2008). *Assessment of children: Cognitive foundations* (5th ed.). San Diego, CA: Author.

Scardapane, J. R., Egan, A., Torres-Gallegos, M., Levine, N., & Owens, S. (2002, March). *Relationships among WRIT, UNIT, and GATES scores and language proficiency.* Paper presented at the meeting of the Council for Exceptional Children, New York.

Unz, R. (1997). Perspective on education: Bilingual is a damaging myth, a system that ensures failure is kept alive by the flow of federal dollars. A 1998 initiative would bring change. *Los Angeles Times*, Section M, p. 5.

Upson, L. M. (2003). *Effects of an increasingly precise socioeconomic match on mean score differences in nonverbal intelligence test scores.* Unpublished doctoral dissertation, University of Tennessee, Knoxville.

U.S. Bureau of the Census. (2000). Language use. Washington, DC: Author. Retrieved from *www.census.gov/population.www.socdemo/lang_use.html*.

U.S. Bureau of the Census. (2010). 2010 census data. Washington, DC: Author. Retrieved from *http://2010.census.gov/2010census/data*.

Wechsler, D. (1939). *The measurement of adult intelligence.* Baltimore: Williams & Wilkins.

Wechsler, D. (1991). *Wechsler Intelligence Scale for Children—Third Edition.* San Antonio, TX: Psychological Corporation.

Wilhoit, B. E., & McCallum, R. S. (2002). Profile analysis of the Universal Nonverbal Intelligence Test standardized sample. *School Psychology Review, 31*, 263–281.

Wilhoit, B. E., & McCallum, R. S. (2003). Cross-battery analysis of the UNIT. In R. S. McCallum (Ed.), *Handbook of nonverbal assessment* (pp. 63–83). New York: Kluwer Academic/Plenum.

Woodcock, R. W. (1990). Theoretical foundations of the WJ-R measures of cognitive ability. *Journal of Psychoeducational Assessment, 8*, 231–258.

Woodcock, R. W., McGrew, K. S., & Mather, N. (2001). *Woodcock–Johnson III Tests of Cognitive Abilities.* Itasca, IL: Riverside.

Woodcock, R. W., & Muñoz-Sandoval, A. F. (1996). *Bateria Woodcock–Muñoz Pruebas de habilidad cognoscitiva—Revisada.* Itasca, IL: Riverside.

CHAPTER 15

The Cognitive Assessment System
From Theory to Practice

Jack A. Naglieri
Tulio M. Otero

THEORY AND STRUCTURE

Theory

The Cognitive Assessment System (CAS; Naglieri & Das, 1997a) is built on the Planning, Attention, Simultaneous, and Successive (PASS) theory (see Naglieri, Das, & Goldstein, Chapter 7, this volume). This theory describes four basic psychological processing abilities, following largely from the neuropsychological work of A. R. Luria (1966a, 1966b, 1973, 1980, 1982). Luria (1973) viewed the brain as a functional mosaic, which means that various parts interact in different combinations to apply varying combinations of cognitive processing abilities. Thus he contended that no area of the brain functions without input from other areas. Integration of processing abilities is a key principle of brain functioning within the Lurian framework. Cognition and behavior therefore result from an interaction of complex brain activity across various areas. Naglieri and Das (1997a) used Luria's work as a base to redefine intelligence from a multiability perspective. The PASS theory has strong empirical support, produced both before the publication of the CAS (see Das, Kirby, & Jarman, 1979; Das, Naglieri, & Kirby, 1994) and since the CAS was published (see Naglieri, 1999a; Naglieri & Conway, 2009; Naglieri & Otero, 2011).

The four CAS scales are designed to measure ability as defined by the PASS theory. PASS theory itself is based on a fusion of cognitive and neuropsychological constructs, such as various aspects of executive functioning (planning); selective, sustained, and shifting attention (attention); visual–spatial tasks (simultaneous), and serial features of language and memory (successive) (Naglieri & Das, 2005; Naglieri & Otero, 2011). These cognitive and neuropsychological functions are composed of flexible and interactive subcomponents that are mediated by equally flexible, interactive neural networks. The four PASS abilities measured by the CAS are considered the basic building blocks of human intellectual functioning (Naglieri, 1999a) and, as such, provide a viable underpinning for the measurement of ability (see Chapter 7 for a more complete discussion of the theory). During development of both the CAS and the forthcoming CAS-2 (Naglieri, Das, & Goldstein, 2012), the primary goal has been to apply these cognitive and neuropsychological constructs to the measurement of ability. Each of the four PASS scales included in the CAS is more fully described below.

The Planning scale of the CAS is intended to measure cognitive control; use of strategies, knowledge, and skills; intentionality; and self-regulation. In essence, the scale measures a child's ability to determine how to solve a problem, execute that solution, monitor its effectiveness, and modify as needed to achieve the goal. Planning ability includes impulse control, as well as generation, evaluation, and execution of a plan. Planning is essential to all activities that require solving a problem. The Planning scale measures how well a child can solve problems of varying complexity that may involve control of attention, simultaneous, and successive processes, as well as acquisition of knowledge and skills.

Planning is measured with tests that require the child to develop a plan of action, evaluate the value of the method, execute the plan, monitor its effectiveness, revise the plan as necessary to meet the demands of the task, and control the impulse to act without careful consideration, all of which are important components of executive functioning. Planning subtests included in the CAS are similar to other assessments used to measure these components, such as the Trail Making subtest of the Delis–Kaplan Executive Functioning System (Delis, Kaplan, & Kramer, 2001), the Inhibition subtest of the NEPSY-II (Korkman, Kirk, & Kemp, 2007), and the Porteus Mazes (Porteus, 1965).

The Attention scale of the CAS is intended to measure a child's ability to demonstrate focused, selective cognition over time, with resistance to distraction. In other words, attention occurs when the child must demonstrate focused, selective, sustained, and effortful activity. *Focused* attention involves concentration directed toward a particular activity, and *selective* attention is important for the inhibition of responses to distracting stimuli. *Sustained* attention refers to the variation of performance over time, which can be influenced by the varying amounts of effort required to solve the test. An effective measure of attention thus presents children with competing demands on their attention and requires sustained focus. The Attention scale subtests included in the CAS are similar to those used to measure attentional aspects of executive function, such as color–word interference tests (Delis et al., 2001), and the Ruff 2&7 selective attention test (Ruff & Allen, 1996).

The components of attention are subserved by subcortical and frontal brain regions in an interactive manner. Executive attention includes maintaining behavior goals and using these goals as a basis for choosing what aspects of the environment or tasks to attend to and which action to select. Paying attention is the first step in the learning process. Attention is a very complicated process with many parts to it. Understanding the parts may help children know what they need to do in school to pay attention and learn more easily.

The Simultaneous scale of the CAS is designed to measure a child's ability to integrate interrelated but separate stimuli into groups or into a whole,

an essential aspect of simultaneous processing ability. Simultaneous processing tests have strong visual–spatial aspects for this reason, but this ability is also used to solve tasks with verbal content (e.g., reading comprehension), as long as the cognitive demands of the task include integration of information into a coherent whole. Simultaneous processing underlies the use and comprehension of grammatical statements because they demand comprehension of word relationships, prepositions, and inflections, so that the person can obtain meaning based on the whole idea. Other aspects of verbal reasoning tasks, such as those in which an examinee is given two to four clues and asked to deduce the object or concept being described, also require simultaneous processing.

The ability to recognize patterns as interrelated elements is made possible by several posterior brain regions, and for this reason many visual–spatial tasks involve simultaneous processing ability. For example, Block Design on the Wechsler Intelligence Scale for Children—Fourth Edition (WISC-IV; Wechsler, 2003), progressive matrices, and object assembly subtests involve simultaneous processing (Naglieri, Kamphaus, & Kaufman, 1983) and are also often described as nonverbal (Naglieri, 2008). Children who have difficulty integrating visual information are likely to have poor simultaneous processing and may be given a diagnosis of nonverbal learning disabilities. These children have been found to do more poorly on such measures as visual–motor integration and visual–perceptual skill tests than normally developing children do (Wilkinson & Semrud-Clikeman, 2008).

Simultaneous processing, then, is measured with tasks that require integration of parts into a single whole and understanding of logical and grammatical relationships. The abilities measured by this scale on the CAS are similar to those measured by nonverbal scales of intelligence tests, such as the Wechsler Nonverbal Scale of Ability (WNV; Wechsler & Naglieri, 2006), the Naglieri Nonverbal Ability Test—Individual Form (Naglieri, 2003), the Perceptual Reasoning Index of the WISC-IV (Wechsler, 2003), the Simultaneous scale of the Kaufman Assessment Battery for Children—Second Edition (KABC-II; Kaufman & Kaufman, 2004), and the Nonverbal Reasoning and Spatial scales of the Differential Ability Scales—Second Edition (DAS-II; Elliott, 2007)

The Successive scale of the CAS is intended to evaluate how well a child can work with stimuli in a specific serial order, where each element is only related to those that precede it and these stimuli are not interrelated. Successive processing ability involves both the perception of stimuli in sequence and the formation of sounds and movements in order. For example, successive processing is involved in the decoding of unfamiliar words, production of syntactic aspects of language, and speech articulation. For this reason, successive processing is involved with activities such as phonological skills (Das et al., 1994) and the syntax of language. This process is measured with tests that demand use, repetition, or comprehension of information based on order. Following a sequence such as the order of operations in a math problem is another example of successive processing.

The ability measured by the Successive scale on the CAS is similar to that measured by the Sequential scale of the KABC-II (Kaufman & Kaufman, 2004) and by tests that require recall of serial information, such as Digit Span Forward on the WISC-IV (Wechsler, 2003). Sequential processing may also be required on some visual–spatial tasks, such as the Spatial Span subtest of the WNV (Wechsler & Naglieri, 2006).

It is clear from this description of the PASS scales that CAS is not based on the same conceptualization used to build traditional IQ tests, such as those developed by Wechsler and Binet. The result is that instead of having subtests organized by content (verbal or nonverbal) or modality (visual or auditory), the CAS has subtests that are organized according to the underlying demands of the subtests. If a subtest demands that a child develop and use efficient solutions for solving the questions, then planning ability is required. When the test requires focused cognitive activity and resistance to distraction, then attention is measured. When the child has to appreciate the way in which information is organized into a coherent whole, simultaneous ability is used. When the child has to work with and understand information based on the order in which that information is structured, successive ability is required. Thus the CAS measures the basic psychological processing abilities that underlie human function, making this a unique type of ability test.

Structure

The CAS (Naglieri & Das, 1997a) is an individually administered measure of ability designed for children and adolescents ages 5 through 17 years. The 12 regularly administered subtests are orga-

nized into the four PASS scales described above. The PASS scale scores and a total score called the Full Scale (FS) are expressed as standard scores (mean of 100, standard deviation [SD] of 15). There are two forms of the test: the Basic Battery (8 subtests, 2 per PASS scale), and the Standard Battery (all 12 subtests). The scales and subtests are briefly described below.

- *Full Scale.* The FS score is an overall measure of cognitive processing based on the combination of either 8 or 12 subtests from the four PASS scales.
- *PASS scales.* The PASS scale scores are computed on the basis of the sum of subtest scaled scores included in each respective scale. These scales represent a child's cognitive processing in specific areas and are used to examine cognitive strengths and/or weaknesses.
- *Subtests.* Each of the 12 subtests measures the specific PASS process corresponding to the scale on which it is found. The subtests are not considered to represent their own sets of specific abilities, but rather are measures of one of the four types of processes. They vary in content (some are verbal, some involve memory, etc.), but each is an effective measure of a specific PASS process. A fuller description of the subtests follows.

DESCRIPTION OF SUBTESTS

Subtests for the CAS were developed specifically to operationalize the PASS theory over a period of about 25 years (summarized in three sources: Das et al., 1979, 1994; Naglieri & Das, 1997c). Each subtest's correspondence to the theoretical framework of the PASS theory, and the relationships between that subtest and others, formed the basis of selection and modification during construction. Development of the subtests was accomplished by following a carefully prescribed sequence of item generation, experimental research, test revision, and reexamination until the instructions, items, and other dimensions were refined over a series of pilot tests, research studies, national tryouts, and national standardization. This allowed for the identification of subtests that provide an efficient way to measure each of the processes (Das et al., 1994; Naglieri & Das, 1997c). Descriptions of the experimental tasks that became the CAS subtests, and efforts to evaluate their practical utility and validity, are contained in more than 100 published papers and several books (see Naglieri & Das, 1997c, for references). Each subtest is more completely described below.

The Planning Subtests

All of the CAS Planning subtests require the child to create and apply some plan, verify that the approach achieves the original goal, and modify the plan as needed. These subtests contain tasks that are relatively easy to perform, but require the individual to make a decision (or decisions) about how to solve the novel tasks.

- *Matching Numbers* consists of four pages, each consisting of eight rows of numbers with six numbers per row. Children are instructed to underline the two numbers in each row that are the same. Numbers increase in length across the four pages from one digit to seven digits, with four rows for each digit length. Each item (defined as a page of eight rows) has a time limit. The subtest score is based on the combination of time and number correct for each page.
- *Planned Codes* contains two pages, each with a distinct set of codes and arrangement of rows and columns. A legend at the top of each page shows how letters correspond to simple codes (e.g., A, B, C, and D correspond to OX, XX, OO, and XO, respectively). Each page contains seven rows and eight columns of letters without codes. Children fill in the appropriate codes in empty boxes beneath each letter. On the first page, all the A's appear in the first column, all the B's in the second column, all the C's in the third column, and so on. On the second page, letters are configured in a diagonal pattern. Children are permitted to complete each page in whatever fashion they desire. The subtest score is based on the combination of time and number correct for each page.
- *Planned Connections* contains eight items. The first six items require children to connect numbers appearing in a quasi-random order on a page in sequential order. The last two items require children to connect both numbers and letters in sequential order alternating between numbers and letters (e.g., 1-A-2-B-3-C). The items are constructed so that children never complete the sequence by crossing one line over the other. The score is based on the total amount of time in seconds used to complete the items.

The Attention Subtests

The Attention subtests require the focus of cognitive activity, detection of a particular stimulus, and inhibition of responses to irrelevant competing stimuli. These subtests always involve examination of the features of the stimulus, as well as a decision to respond to one feature and not to other competing features in a complex environment.

- *Expressive Attention* consists of two different sets of items, depending on the age of the child. Children 5 though 7 years of age are asked to identify whether each animal depicted in the item is big or small. In the first item, the animals are the same size (approximately 1 inch high and 1 inch wide). In the second item, the animals are sized appropriately (big animals are approximately 1 inch high and 1 inch wide, and small animals are about ½ inch by ½ inch). In the third item, where selective attention is being measured, the realistic sizes of the animals usually differ from the relative sizes they appear to be in the item. In each instance, the child responds based upon the size of these animals in real life, ignoring their relative size on the page. For children 8 years of age and older, the stimuli are color words. On the first item children are asked to read 40 words (BLUE, YELLOW, GREEN, and RED) from the stimulus page. In the next item children are asked to name the colors of a series of rectangles (printed in blue, yellow, green, and red). In the final item the words BLUE, YELLOW, GREEN, and RED are printed in ink of a different color from the colors the words name. The child is instructed to name the color the word is printed in, rather than to read the word. The last item administered at each age is used as the measure of selective attention. The raw score on this subtest is the ratio of the accuracy (total number correct) and time on the final item.
- *Number Detection* consists of a page of specially formatted numbers. Children are asked to underline specific numbers when they are printed in an outlined typeface. There are 18 rows of 10 numbers with 45 targets (25% targets) in each of the first two pages (treated as one item each), and 15 rows of 12 numbers in the third and fourth pages (items), with a total of 45 targets (25% targets) in each item. Children must complete each page by working from left to right and top to bottom, and may not go back to check the page upon completion. The raw score for Number Detection is the ratio of the accuracy (total number correct minus

the number of false detections) and the total time for each item, summed across the items.

• *Receptive Attention* is a two-page paper-and-pencil subtest written in two versions, depending on the age of the child. The version for children ages 5 through 7 is contained on four pages of pictures arranged in pairs. In the first condition (item 1), a child is asked to underline pairs of drawings that are identical in appearance. In the second condition (item 2), the child is required to underline the pairs of pictures that are the same from a lexical perspective (i.e., they have the same name). Children ages 8 years and above are also presented with two conditions (items 1 and 2). One page contains 200 pairs of letters with 50 targets (25% targets), and the second page also has 200 pairs of letters with 50 targets (25% targets). Although the targets are different on these two pages, the distractors are the same. In the first condition, a child underlines pairs of letters that are identical in appearance (e.g., AA, not Aa). In the second condition, the child circles all the pairs of letters that have the same name (e.g., Aa, not Ba). At all ages, the child must complete the subtest by working from left to right and top to bottom. The child may not go back to check the page upon completion. The raw score is the ratio of the accuracy (total number correct minus the number of false detections) and the total time for each item, summed across the items.

The Simultaneous Subtests

The Simultaneous subtests require that the examinee comprehend the organization of information as a group. This may involve either questions of a visual–spatial type or verbal statements that describe how objects are arranged in space. The Simultaneous subtests always involve examination of the interrelationships among parts.

• *Nonverbal Matrices* is a 33-item progressive matrix test; it utilizes shapes and geometric elements that are interrelated through spatial or logical organization. Children are required to comprehend the relationships among the parts of the item and respond by choosing the best of six options. Items are scored as correct or incorrect (1, 0). The raw score is the total number of items answered correctly.

• *Verbal–Spatial Relations* is composed of 27 items that require the comprehension of logical and grammatical descriptions of spatial relation-

ships. Children are shown items that depict six drawings and a printed question at the bottom of each page. The items involve both objects and shapes that are arranged in a specific spatial configuration. The examiner reads the question aloud, and the child is required to select the option that matches the verbal description. The raw score is the total number of items correctly answered.

• *Figure Memory* is a 27-item subtest where a child is shown a page that contains a two- or three-dimensional geometric figure for 5 seconds. The figure is then removed and the child is presented with a response page that contains the original design embedded in a larger, more complex geometric pattern. Children are required to identify the original design that is embedded within the larger figure by tracing over the appropriate lines with a red pencil. For a response to be scored correct, all lines of the design have to be indicated without any additions or omissions. Items are scored as either correct or incorrect (1, 0).

The Successive Subtests

The Successive subtests require that the examinee recall and/or understand the sequence of information. This may involve either simple repetition of words in the order provided by the examiner, or repetition and comprehension of verbal statements. The Successive subtests always evaluate a child's ability to work with information arranged in a specific linear sequence.

• *Word Series* consists of 27 items, each of which uses from two to nine single-syllable, high-frequency words. The child is asked to repeat the words in the same order as stated by the examiner. Each series is read at the rate of one word per second. Each item is scored as either correct or incorrect (1, 0). The child must reproduce the entire word series in the order presented to receive credit for the item. The raw score is the total number of items repeated correctly.

• *Sentence Repetition* consists of 20 sentences composed of color words (e.g., "The blue is yellowing") that are read to the child. The child is required to repeat each sentence verbatim. Each item is scored as either correct or incorrect (1, 0).

• *Speech Rate* is an eight-item, timed subtest used at ages 5–7 years. In each item, children are required to repeat a three-word series of high-imagery, single- or double-syllable words in order, 10 times in a row. The examiner begins timing when the child says the first word in the series and stops timing when the child finishes repeating the last word in the 10th repetition. The total time taken to repeat the eight items 10 times each is the total raw score.

- *Sentence Questions* is a 21-item subtest that is used in place of Speech Rate for children ages 8–17 years. The subtest uses the same type of sentences as those in Sentence Repetition. Children are read a sentence and then asked a question about it (e.g., "The blue is yellowing," "Who is yellowing?"). Each item is scored as either correct or incorrect (1, 0), based upon rules defined on the record form. The raw score is the total number of questions answered correctly.

ADMINISTRATION AND SCORING

Administration

The directions for administration are provided in the CAS administration and scoring manual (Naglieri & Das, 1997c). These instructions include both verbal statements and nonverbal actions to be used by the examiner. The combination of oral and nonverbal communication is designed to ensure that all children understand each task.

The CAS subtests are carefully sequenced to ensure the integrity of the subtests and to reduce the influence of extraneous variables on a child's performance. The Planning tests are administered first because the child is given flexibility to solve the subtest in any manner. Attention subtests must be completed in the prescribed order (i.e., left to right, top to bottom), so they are given later in the test.

All Planning subtests include strategy assessment, which is conducted during and after the administration of each Planning subtest. Observed strategies are those seen by the examiner through careful observation of the child completing the items. Reported strategies are obtained following completion of an item. The examiner obtains this information by saying, "Tell me how you did these," or "How did you find what you were looking for?" or some similar statement. The child can communicate the strategies by either verbal or nonverbal (gesturing) means. Strategies are recorded in the "Observed" and "Reported" sections of the Strategy Assessment Checklist included in the record form.

Several methods have been used to ensure that a child understands what is being requested. These include sample and demonstration items, as well as opportunities for the examiner to clarify the requirements of the task. If, however, the child does not understand the demands of the subtest or appears in any way confused or uncertain, the examiner is instructed to "provide a brief explanation if necessary" (Naglieri & Das, 1997c, p. 8). This instruction gives the examiner the freedom to explain what the child must do in whatever terms are considered necessary to ensure that the child understands the task. This type of instruction can be given in any form—including gestures, as well as the use of a language other than English. However, it is important to remember that these alternative instructions are meant to ensure that the child understands what to do; they are not intended to teach the child how to do the test.

Scoring

The CAS is scored via a standard method of subtest raw scores to subtest scaled scores to composite (PASS scale and CAS FS) standard scores. The CAS subtest raw scores are calculated in various ways: the total number correct (Nonverbal Matrices, Verbal–Spatial Relations, Figure Memory, Word Series, Sentence Repetition, and Sentence Questions); time in seconds (Planned Connections and Speech Rate); and ratio scores that combine time and number correct (Matching Numbers, Planned Codes, and Expressive Attention) or time, number correct, and number of false detections (Number Detection and Receptive Attention). *False detections* are defined as the number of times a child underlines a stimulus that is not a target.

The CAS subtest scaled scores are obtained by using the appropriate table for the child's chronological age in years, months, and days. The PASS and FS standard scores are obtained from the sum of the subtests on either the Standard (12-subtest) or Basic (8-subtest) Battery. Conversions from raw to standard scores are made easier by use of the CAS Rapid Score (Naglieri, 2002). This program computes the ratio scores (where applicable), sums the raw scores for each subtest, sums the subtest scores, calculates all subtest scaled scores, and calculate PASS as well as FS standard scores. In addition, the CAS Rapid Score computes all the values needed to make comparisons among CAS scores and to compare CAS and achievement test scores.

The CAS Rapid Score is a record-form-based program designed on the premise that computer scoring, interpretation, and report generation should be managed in a clear and easily understood environment. When the program is opened, the first page that appears is one that looks very much like the first page of the CAS record form. Data entry requires the examiner to enter actual item data. For example, when time scores and number correct are entered for each Matching Numbers page, the program computes the ratio score, and then the sum of the ratio scores is calculated automatically. Alternatively, subtest raw scores can be entered directly on the front of the record form.

Once the subtest raw scores are entered, the subtest scaled scores and PASS Scale standard scores are computed, and analysis of the differences among the scores is completed. A text description of the results is also provided, as are handouts for teachers and parents that describe the four PASS scales. The program performs all the interpretive tasks described by Naglieri (1999a), and it also provides some of the intervention handouts included in the book *Helping Children Learn: Intervention Handouts for Use in School and at Home* (2nd ed.; Naglieri & Pickering, 2010).

PSYCHOMETRIC PROPERTIES

Standardization

The CAS was standardized on a sample of 2,200 children ages 5–17 years. A stratified random sampling plan was used, resulting in a sample that closely matched the U.S. population. The CAS sample was stratified on the following variables: age (5 years, 0 months through 17 years, 11 months); gender (female, male); race (black, white, Asian, Native American, other); Hispanic origin (Hispanic, non-Hispanic); region (Midwest, Northeast, South, West); community setting (urban/suburban, rural); classroom placement (full-time regular classroom, part-time special education resource, full-time self-contained special education); educational classification (learning disability, speech–language impairment, social-emotional disability, intellectual disability, giftedness, and non-special-education); and parental educational attainment (less than high school degree, high school graduate or equivalent, some college or technical school, 4 or more years of college).

Reliability

The CAS subtests and scales have high reliability and meet or exceed minimum values suggested by

Bracken (1987). The FS reliability coefficients for the Standard Battery range from a low of .95 to a high of .97, and the average reliabilities for the Standard Battery PASS scales are .88 (Planning and Attention scales) and .93 (Simultaneous and Successive scales). The Basic Battery reliabilities are as follows: FS, .87; Planning, .85; Simultaneous, .90; Attention, .84; and Successive, .90.

Validity

The CAS is distinguished among all measures of ability by its association with the specific PASS theory of intelligence, which in turn is based on Luria's neuropsychological framework of three functional units. The foundational research was described by Das (1972), Das, Kirby, and Jarman (1975, 1979), and Das and colleagues (1994). The considerable research base that followed is described in detail by Naglieri and Das (1997b), Naglieri (1999a, 1999b), Naglieri and Conway (2009), Naglieri and Otero (2011), and Naglieri and Goldstein (2011). Interested readers should review these sources for a more complete examination of the validity of the PASS theory as measured by the CAS.

Relationships to Achievement

The CAS can be used to understand current academic performance, to predict future performance, and to design or select appropriate interventions based upon the child's cognitive characteristics. For these reasons, the relationship between CAS and achievement test scores is one of the most important aspects of validity (Brody, 1992; Cohen, Swerdlik, & Smith, 1992). In order to better appreciate the relationship between the PASS scales of the CAS and achievement, two important facts need to be considered. First, how strongly do traditional IQ tests correlate with achievement? According to Brody (1992) and Naglieri and Bornstein (2003), the relationship between ability and intelligence has been found to be about .55–.60. Second, it is important to recognize that traditional IQ tests and achievement tests have similar content. For example, verbal IQ tests and achievement tests both contain measures of vocabulary, general information, and arithmetic. This similarity in content serves to inflate the correlations between these two types of tests (for more details, see Naglieri & Bornstein, 2003; Naglieri & Rojahn, 2004). Given that the CAS (like the KABC-II) does not include achievement-like test items, the study of the relationship between ability as measured using basic psychological processes and achievement can be more efficiently accomplished. The research on the relationship between the CAS and achievement has suggested that the PASS processes are strongly related to academic scores.

Naglieri and Rojahn (2004) studied the relationship between the PASS processing scores of the CAS and the Woodcock–Johnson Psycho-Educational Battery—Revised (WJ-R) Tests of Achievement (Woodcock & Johnson, 1989), using a nationally representative sample of 1,559 students ages 5–17 years. The correlation of the CAS FS with the WJ-R Tests of Achievement was .71 for the Standard Battery (all 12 subtests) and .70 for the Basic Battery (8 subtests). Naglieri and Rojahn (2004) also found that using the four PASS scales in a multiple-regression analysis to predict achievement test scores yielded higher values than using the CAS FS did. These findings suggested that the four PASS scales correlate more strongly with achievement than the FS score does. In addition, the predictive power of the combination of the four PASS scales was weakened when any one of the PASS scales was excluded in the prediction equation (Naglieri & Rojahn, 2004). This suggests that each of the PASS scales has additive value in predicting achievement, and further supports the validity of the interrelated nature of these neuropsychologically derived cognitive processes as described by Luria.

Naglieri, Goldstein, DeLauder, and Schwebach (2006) further studied the relationship between PASS and achievement for children ages 6–16 years who were referred for learning and emotional problems. They compared the WISC-III (Wechsler, 1991) and the CAS to the Woodcock–Johnson III (WJ III) Test of Achievement (Woodcock, McGrew, & Mather, 2001). The correlation of the WJ III achievement scores with the WISC-III Full Scale IQ (FSIQ) scores was .63, but the correlation with achievement was .83 for the CAS FS. The results indicate that when the same children took the two tests and those scores were correlated with the same achievement scores, both showed a strong relationship between ability and achievement, but the CAS FS score correlations were significantly higher (Naglieri et al., 2006).

In summary, these findings provide strong evidence for the construct validity of the CAS. What is especially important is that the measures of the PASS processes do not include achievement-like subtests (e.g., vocabulary and arithmetic). This is especially important for children who come from disadvantaged environments, as well as those who have had a history of academic failure. A discussion of the CAS's fairness is presented next.

Fairness

As the characteristics of the U.S population continues to become more diverse, the need for fair assessment of children from culturally and linguistically diverse backgrounds has become progressively more important. Suzuki and Valencia (1997) have suggested that processing tests such as the CAS hold a particular advantage over ability tests that have verbal questions (e.g., vocabulary) and quantitative (e.g., arithmetic word problems) content for linguistically diverse students. Verbal and quantitative content can create an unfair disadvantage for many children, such as those living in non-English-speaking homes and impoverished environments. Reducing the amount of knowledge needed to answer the questions on intelligence tests correctly is a useful way to ensure appropriate and fair assessment of diverse populations (Naglieri, 2008). The CAS scores earned by children from culturally and linguistically diverse backgrounds have been studied in a series of research reports.

Naglieri, Rojahn, Matto, and Aquilino (2005) compared CAS scores for samples composed of 298 black and 1,691 white children. In order to control statistically for demographic variables, regression analyses were used. The results showed an estimated CAS FS mean score difference of 4.8, which is smaller than those found with traditional tests of ability. Importantly, the correlations between the CAS scores and scores on the WJ-R Tests of Achievement were very similar for blacks (.70) and whites (.64) (Naglieri et al., 2005).

Naglieri, Rojahn, and Matto (2007) examined CAS scores for 244 Hispanic and 1,956 non-Hispanic children. They found that the two groups differed by 6.1 points when the samples were unmatched samples, 5.1 with samples matched on basic demographic variables, and 4.8 points when demographic differences were statistically controlled. We (Naglieri, Otero, DeLauder, & Matto, 2007) compared the English and Spanish versions of the CAS for bilingual Hispanic children. The children in this study earned very similar CAS FS scores (84.6 and 87.6 on the English and Spanish versions, respectively), and deficits in Successive processing were found (78.0 and 83.1 on the English and Spanish versions, respectively). The FS scores for the English and Spanish versions of the CAS correlated .96. Importantly, 90% of children who had a PASS weakness on one version of the CAS also had the same PASS weakness on the other version of the CAS. A second study of the English and Spanish versions of the CAS yielded very similar findings. We (Otero, Gonzales, & Naglieri, in press) examined the performance of referred Hispanic English-language learners (N = 40) on the English and Spanish versions of the CAS and found no significant differences in the FS scores or in any of the PASS scales. Students earned their lowest scores in Successive processing, regardless of the language in which the test was administered. These findings suggest that the CAS may be a useful measure for Hispanic children with underdeveloped English-language proficiency.

Naglieri and Taddei (see D'Amico, Cardaci, Di Nuovo, & Naglieri, in press) examined English and Italian versions of the CAS for Italian (N = 809) and U.S. (N = 1,174) samples matched by age and gender. Small differences between the two samples were found on the PASS and FS standard scores when the U.S. norms were used. The differences between the samples for the PASS scores were trivial except for the Attention scale (d = 0.26), where the Italian sample had slightly higher scores. The FS standard scores (using the U.S. norms) for the Italian (100.9) and U.S. (100.5) samples were nearly identical. Negligible differences were found for 9 of the 13 subtests; three showed small d ratios (two in favor of the Italian sample); and one showed a large ratio (in favor of the U.S. sample).

The findings for the English–Spanish and English–Italian studies suggest that the PASS theory as measured by CAS yields similar mean scores for samples that differ on cultural and linguistic characteristics. In sum, the research on race and ethnic differences strongly demonstrates the utility of PASS theory as a way to fairly assess diverse populations.

Factor Analysis

The factor structure of the CAS, and by implication the PASS theory, has been a topic of some discussion. In the CAS interpretive handbook, Naglieri and Das (1997c) reported information about the factor structure of the CAS, using both exploratory and confirmatory factor-analytic methods. They provided evidence that the PASS four-factor solution was the best solution, based on the convergence of both types of factor-analytic results, clinical utility of the four separate scores,

evidence of strategy use, and theoretical interpretation of the subtests. Keith and Kranzler (1999) challenged this position and argued that there was insufficient support for the PASS structure. Naglieri (1999b) responded with evidence in defense of the structure of the test and the validity of the theory. The issue has since been examined with an alternative to the methods used both by Naglieri and Das and by Keith and Kranzler. This factor technique is considered more objective than the statistical approaches previously used (Blaha, 2003).

Blaha (2003) conducted an examination of the CAS subtest assignment, using an exploratory hierarchical factor-analytic method described by Blaha and Wallbrown (1996). This method is less subjective and follows the data more closely, allowing for the most probable factor-analytic model (Carroll, 1993). Blaha found a general factor that he equated to the CAS FS and interpreted as a general intelligence factor. This represents the overlap among the diverse PASS scales. After removal of the variance caused by the general factor, two factors emerged. The first consisted of the Simultaneous and Successive subtests, and the second included the Planning and Attention subtests. At the third level, four primary factors were found that consisted of each of the four PASS scales. Blaha (2003) concluded that the results "provide support for maintaining the Full Scale as well as Planning, Attention, Simultaneous, and Successive standard scores of the CAS" (p. 1).

It is important to recognize that the technique of factor analysis is far from objective. In fact, Carroll (1994) wrote that "analyzing factor-analytic data is in many respects an art rather than a science" (p. 49). Even his important work, based on factor analysis, illustrates the problem with the method. For example, Carroll noted that not all the analyses included in his 1993 book were conducted with the same methodologies. He noted that

> in the course of the project, over more than 5 years, various refinements in techniques were discovered or devised, but it was not deemed feasible to go back and apply these refinements uniformly to all datasets that had already been analyzed at a given stage of the work. . . . Perhaps partly for this reason, but mostly because of characteristics inherent in the data, the reanalyses resulted in many indeterminacies and questions that the data left unresolved. (Carroll, 1993, p. 113)

Variety in the exact methods, assumptions, and decisions made by investigators can lead to different results. Factor-analytic methods are therefore far from decisive, and factor analysis should not be given inordinate weight as a method for establishing or discrediting the validity of any instrument. At best, it provides one piece of evidence that must be part of a balanced examination of validity. Other types of validity evidence—such as relationships to achievement, issues of fair assessment, diagnostic utility, and relevance to instructional interventions—should also be considered. We have already discussed the first two of these; we now examine the others.

Diagnostic Utility

There are several reasons to examine profiles of ability test scale variability: to discern variations in characteristics that help understand the cognitive profiles of specific groups of exceptional children; to determine whether specific profiles can be used as aids in diagnosis; and to make decisions about interventions that are consistent with a child's cognitive strengths and weaknesses. The profiles of PASS scores on the CAS that have been suggested for special populations of children are amply discussed in Chapter 7 of this book. In summary, the research conducted thus far on the CAS suggests that groups of children with specific reading decoding failure have obtained low Successive scores (Naglieri, 1999a; Naglieri, Otero, DeLauder, & Matto, 2007; Naglieri et al., 2010); groups of children diagnosed with attention-deficit/hyperactivity disorder (ADHD) have earned low scores in Planning (Dehn, 2000; Naglieri, Goldstein, Iseman, & Schwebach, 2003; Naglieri, Salter, & Edwards, 2004; Paolitto, 1999); and that groups with autism spectrum disorders have scored specifically low in Attention (Goldstein & Naglieri, 2009).

In this section of the chapter, we contextualize the findings on reading disorders and ADHD in relation to other tests of ability and processing. In order to do so, we obtained data from various test manuals and related sources. The data presented here were obtained from the test manuals for the KABC-II (Kaufman & Kaufman, 2004), the fifth edition of the Stanford–Binet (SB5; Roid, 2003), and the WISC-IV (Wechsler, 2003), or from book chapters on the CAS (Naglieri & Conway, 2009) and the WJ III (Wendling, Mather, & Schrank, 2009). These data need to be examined with an understanding of their limitations. For example, different samples were used; none of these children was administered more than one of these tests; the methods of diagnosis may have been dif-

ferent; and the demographic composition of the groups was not matched. The goal here, however, is to present an initial examination of these data as the best approximation of our current state of knowledge about this topic. Much more research is needed to fully and more completely understand the extent to which these various tests are sensitive to the cognitive impairments associated with reading disabilities and attention deficits.

Reading Disorders

The comparisons of profiles for scales included in these various tests of ability for individuals with reading disorders are shown in Figure 15.1. The mean scores by scale and ability test suggests that some of the scales detect specific weaknesses in cognitive characteristics of individuals with reading disorders more readily than other scales do. Two tests showed overall low scores and the least variability across the scales it yields. The SB5 (mean FSIQ = 84) and KABC-II (mean Mental Processing Index [MPI] = 83) showed relatively little intratest variability, with a range of scale means of 3.8 standard scores for both tests. The WISC-IV (mean FSIQ = 89), WJ III (mean General Intellectual Ability [GIA] = 92), and CAS (mean FS = 88) showed larger ranges of scale means (7.4, 10.0, and 10.3, respectively). The sample of individuals with reading disorders earned their lowest scores on the WJ III Long-Term Retrieval scale (mean = 90), the WISC-IV Working Memory Index (mean = 87), and the CAS Successive scale (mean = 83). These children earned other scores that clustered around 90 on the WISC-IV and the WJ III. Interestingly, the WISC-IV Working Memory Index standard score was below the average range, as was the CAS Successive scale. These findings suggest that the CAS showed the most internal variability, and that the group earned the lowest score on the CAS Successive scale than on any of the other tests.

The CAS profile, and to a lesser extent the WISC-IV profile, for this sample of students with reading disabilities suggested that this group had a specific cognitive weakness in successive ability. That is, there was considerable variability within the scales, *and* the lowest score was in successive processing and was considerably below the normal range. This means that as a group, these individuals had difficulty working with stimuli arranged in a specific serial order, such as sequences of sounds that make words, sequences of letters to spell words, and sequences of groups of sounds and let-

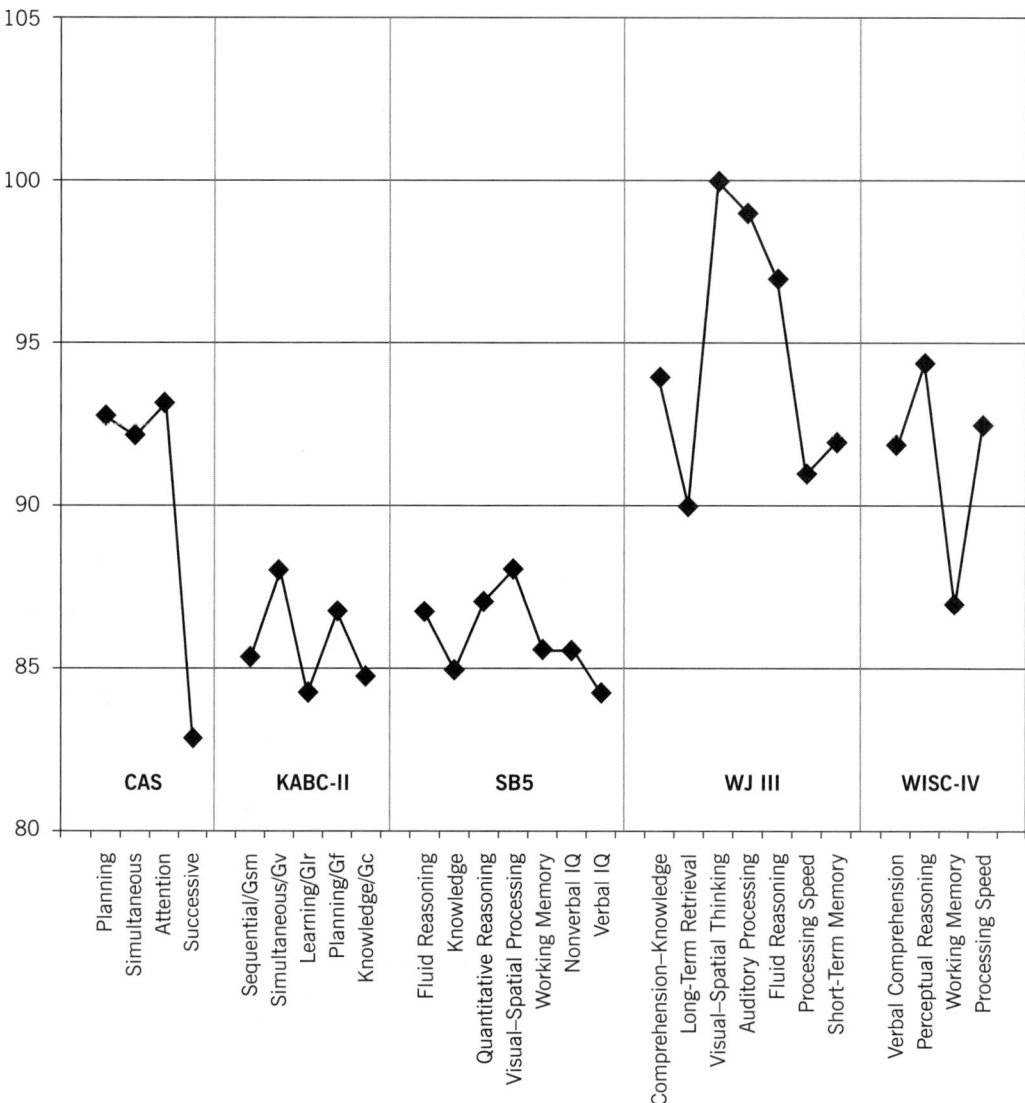

FIGURE 15.1. Graphic representation of mean scores for individuals with reading disorders across several ability tests.

ters needed to make words (see Naglieri & Gold-stein, 2011). The two scales reflecting this specific weakness were the CAS Successive scale and the WISC-IV Working Memory Index. That is, in both tests the group of children with reading dis-abilities earned relatively low scores on a scale taht requires sequencing of information. This is logical, given that both of these scales have subtests that require the repetition of sequential information (e.g., words in CAS Word Series or numbers in WISC-IV Digit Span). Surprisingly, the KABC-II

scales did not show much variability, but the Se-quential scale was lower than the Simultaneous scale.

Attention-Deficit/Hyperactivity Disorder

The mean scores across these various ability tests for individuals with ADHD are provided in Fig-ure 15.2. These results suggest that scores for most of the tests were within the 90–100 range. The WISC-IV, SB5, and KABC-II showed relatively little intratest variability (range means were 6.7, 5.7, and 3.4 standard score points, respectively). The WJ III showed more variability (range of 9), with the lowest score in Long-Term Retrieval (90) and the highest in Visual–Spatial Thinking (100). The Long-Term Retrieval score measures "a person's facility in storing and recalling associations" (Wendling et al., 2009, p. 192); the test requires a child to associate simple shapes and drawings with words and then to use those shapes to make a statement. The CAS showed the most vari-

ability (range of 11.3) of the various tests, with the lowest score on the Planning scale (85) and highest on the Successive scale (97). This finding indicates that the sample with ADHD had considerable difficulty with use of strategies for solving problems, self-monitoring, and self-regulation. The CAS is the only test providing a measure of a neuropsychologically derived ability (planning) that is critical when a person has to demonstrate self-monitoring and impulse control, as well as the generation, evaluation, and execution of strategies.

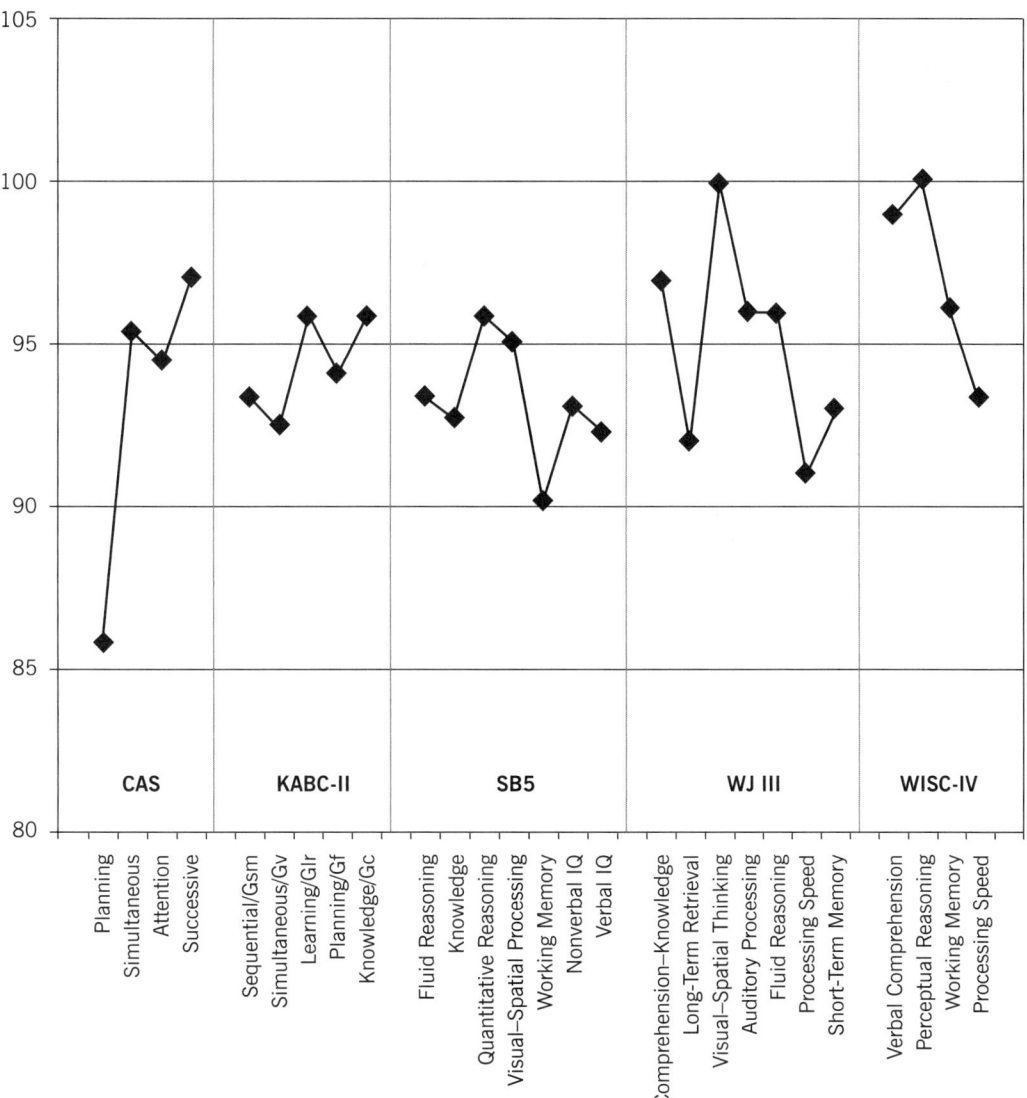

FIGURE 15.2. Graphic representation of mean scores for individuals with ADHD across several ability tests.

This is consistent with Barkley's (1997, 2006) conceptualization of individuals with ADHD, that is, they have difficulty with planning and anticipation, organization, development and use of organizational strategies, and self-regulation, which, according to Goldberg (2009), is associated with the prefrontal areas of the brain and can be assessed using the CAS (Goldstein & Naglieri, 2006).

The findings for children with ADHD suggest that these various tests of ability yield different information about the cognitive characteristics of this diagnostic group. Like the findings for individuals with reading disorders, the results provide some evidence that individuals with ADHD have a specific cognitive disorder detected by the CAS (Naglieri & Das, 1997a). These findings not only augment our understanding of the diagnostic group, but have considerable relevance to eligibility determination (see Naglieri, 2011) and have been shown to provide valuable implications for intervention (see Naglieri, 2011; Naglieri & Pickering, 2010).

Instructional Implications

There are three main sources of information for linking PASS theory to academic instruction and intervention: (1) Planning Strategy Instruction, now known as the Planning Facilitation Method (Naglieri & Pickering (2010); (2) the PASS Reading Enhancement Program (PREP; Das, 1999); and (3) Naglieri and Pickering's (2010) book of instructional handouts for teachers and parents. The first two methods are based on empirical studies, while the book contains empirically supported approaches to academic interventions that are related to PASS theory.

Planning Strategy Instruction/ Planning Facilitation Method

The connection between planning and intervention has been well illustrated by research that has examined the relationship between strategy instruction and CAS Planning scores. The studies have involved both math and reading achievement scores. These intervention studies focused on the concept that children can be encouraged to be more planful when they complete academic tasks and that the facilitation of plans has a positive impact on academic performance. The initial concept for Planning Strategy Instruction was based on the work of Cormier, Carlson, and Das (1990) and Kar, Dash, Das, and Carlson (1992).

These authors taught children to discover the value of strategy use without being specifically instructed to do so. The children were encouraged to examine the demands of the task in a strategic and organized manner. The research demonstrated that students differentially benefited from the technique that facilitated planning. Children who performed poorly on measures of planning demonstrated significantly greater gains than those with higher planning scores. These initial results indicated that PASS scores could help predict response to instruction.

The Planning Strategy Instruction/Planning Facilitation Method was shown to improve children's performance in math calculation by Naglieri and Gottling (1995, 1997). All children in these studies attended a special school for those with learning disabilities. In the investigations, students completed mathematics worksheets in sessions over about a 2-month period. The method designed to teach planning indirectly was applied in individual tutoring sessions (Naglieri & Gottling, 1995) or in the classroom by the teacher (Naglieri & Gottling, 1997) about two to three times per week in 30-minute blocks. Students were encouraged to recognize the need to plan and use strategies when completing mathematic problems during the intervention periods. The teachers provided probes that facilitated discussion and encouraged the children to consider various ways to be more successful. More details about the method are provided by Naglieri and Gottling (1995, 1997) and by Naglieri and Pickering (2010).

The relationship between the Planning Strategy Instruction/Planning Facilitation Method and the PASS profiles for children with learning disabilities and mild mental impairments was studied by Naglieri and Johnson (2000). The purpose of this study was to determine whether children with cognitive weaknesses in each of the four PASS processes, and children with no cognitive weaknesses, would show different rates of improvement in math when given the same instructional method in a group format. The findings from this study showed that children with a cognitive weakness in planning improved considerably over baseline rates, while those with no cognitive weakness improved only marginally. Similarly, children with cognitive weaknesses in simultaneous, successive, and attention processes showed substantially lower rates of improvement. The importance of this study was that the five groups of children responded very differently to the same intervention. Thus the PASS scores were predictive of the children's response to this math intervention (Naglieri & Johnson, 2000).

Another study examining the effects of this instructional method was reported by Haddad and colleagues (2003). This study assessed whether an instruction designed to facilitate planning would have differential benefit on reading comprehension, and whether improvement would be related to the PASS scores of each child. The researchers used a sample of general education children sorted into three groups, based on their PASS scale profiles from the CAS. Even though the groups did not differ by CAS FS scores or pretest reading comprehension scores, children with low Planning scores benefited substantially (effect size of 1.52) from the instruction designed to facilitate planning. In contrast, children with no PASS weakness or low Successive scores did not benefit as much (effect sizes of 0.52 and 0.06, respectively). These results further support previous research suggesting that the PASS profiles are relevant to instruction.

Iseman and Naglieri (2011) examined the Planning Strategy Instruction/Planning Facilitation Method for children with learning disabilities and ADHD. Students in the experimental group engaged in this instructional approach to encourage effective strategies in mathematics. A comparison group received additional math instruction by the regular teacher. Following the intervention, an analysis examined students with and students without low Planning scores on the CAS. Students with low Planning scores in the experimental group improved considerably on math worksheets. In contrast, students with low Planning scores in the comparison group did not improve. In addition, students with ADHD and low Planning scores in the experimental group improved considerably on the worksheets, whereas students with ADHD but without a cognitive weakness in planning in the comparison group did not improve. Thus individuals with a cognitive weakness on the Planning scale, with and without ADHD, benefited more from this instructional method than from normal instruction (Iseman & Naglieri, 2011).

The results of these the Planning Strategy Instruction/Planning Facilitation Method studies using academic tasks suggest that changing the way aptitude is conceptualized (i.e., in terms of PASS theory rather than traditional IQ) and measured (i.e., with the CAS) provided a way to predict response to intervention. Past efforts to show a relationship between IQ scores and instruction suffered from inadequate conceptualizations of abilities (e.g., verbal or nonverbal) based on the general intelligence approach, which is very different from the basic psychological processing view represented by the PASS theory and measured by the CAS. The studies summarized here are particularly different from previous intervention research that found students with low general ability to improve little, and those with high general ability to improve more, with instruction (see Fuchs & Young, 2006). In contrast, children with a weakness in one of the PASS processes (planning) benefited more from planning-based instruction than did children who had no weakness or a weakness in a different PASS process. The results of these studies strongly suggest that CAS Planning scores can predict which children will respond to academic instruction and which will not when the intervention is designed to improve strategy use.

PASS Reading Enhancement Program

Based on the PASS theory of cognitive functioning (Das et al., 1994), the PREP was developed as a cognitive remedial program and is supported by a line of research beginning with Brailsford, Snart, and Das (1984), D. Kaufman and Kaufman (1979), and Krywaniuk and Das (1976). These researchers demonstrated that students could be trained to use successive and simultaneous processes more efficiently, which resulted in an improvement in their performance on those processes, and "some transfer to specific reading tasks also occurred" (Ashman & Conway, 1997, p. 169). The PREP aims to improve the information-processing strategies (specifically, simultaneous and successive processing) that underlie reading, while at the same time avoiding the direct teaching of word-reading skills such as phoneme segmentation or blending. The tasks in the program teach children to focus their attention on the sequential nature of many academic tasks, including reading. This helps the children better utilize successive processing, which is a very important cognitive process needed in reading decoding.

Empirical support for the PREP has been established by studies examining its effectiveness for children with reading decoding problems. Carlson and Das (1997) and Das, Mishra, and Pool (1995) studied children with reading disabilities who were divided into PREP and control groups. A total of 15 PREP sessions were given to small groups of four children. Word attack and word identification tests were administered pre- and posttreatment. In both studies, the PREP groups outperformed the control groups. Similarly, Boden and Kirby (1995) studied children with learning disabilities who were randomly assigned to a PREP training group or a control group that received regular instruction. Again, the results showed significant differences between the two groups in reading decoding of real and pseudowords. Similarly, Das, Parrila, and Papadopoulos (2000) found that children who received the PREP improved significantly more in pseudoword reading than did a control group. Parrila, Das, Kendrick, Papadopoulos, and Kirby (1999) reported a significant improvement of reading (word identification and word attack) for their PREP group, and the gain in reading was greater than it was for a control group that received meaning-based instruction. Specific relevance to the children's CAS profiles was also demonstrated by the fact that those children with higher Successive scores at the beginning of the program benefited the most from the PREP instruction, but those with the most improvement in the meaning-based program were characterized by higher Planning scores (Parrila et al., 1999).

All of these experimental studies of the PREP "suggest that process training can assist in specific aspects of beginning reading" (Ashman & Conway, 1997, p. 171). Taken together, these studies support the PREP's effectiveness in remediating deficient reading skills during the elementary school years. In addition, they illustrate the connection between the PASS theory and intervention.

Naglieri and Pickering's Intervention Handouts

The Naglieri and Pickering (2010) book includes approximately 100 empirically supported, PASS-theory-based instructional handouts in both English and Spanish for teachers and parents. The book begins with an explanation of the PASS theory designed for teachers and parents, and continues with case studies illustrating how the theory can be used to understand and teach children with learning problems. The second part of the book contains handouts that describe the four PASS abilities; academic interventions in reading, spelling, writing, and math; and test-taking and memory interventions. Handouts for the students are also included, to help them learn about their own abilities.

Neuropsychological Research

An increasing amount of neuropsychological research supports the validity of the PASS theory as

measured by the CAS. According to Luria (1973), a person who suffers traumatic brain injury (TBI) is likely also to experience impairments in such processes as organization and planning. One of the main reasons why an assessment tool such as the CAS would be particularly useful for the population with TBI is that typical intelligence tests only yield results that reflect general intelligence. "Although results from intelligence measures reflect general ability, they do not provide systematic measurement of, for example, the attentional and planning impairments that interfere with the academic performance of children with TBI" (Savage & Wolcott, 1994, cited in Gutentag, Naglieri, & Yeates, 1998, p. 265). Gutentag and colleagues (1998) studied children with TBI and found deficits in their performance on the CAS, compared to that of a matched control group drawn from the CAS normative population. Neurocognitive deficits were most pronounced on the Attention and Planning scales, and less severe in the Simultaneous and Successive scales.

The CAS has been increasingly used in other clinical neuropsychology studies. In Spain, Perez-Alvarez, Timoneda-Gallart, and Baus-Rosell (2006) used the CAS in a study assessing the effects of topiramate (a pharmacological treatment for epilepsy) on cognitive processes and behavior. The 35 patients, ages 5–15, were assessed with the CAS at baseline and at 6 and 12 months. The parents were given behavior rating scales at each point as well. At all three time points, patients had lower Successive scores. However, at 12 months Planning scores had increased significantly, and there was a concomitant improvement on behavior as measured by rating scales.

McCrea (2007) studied three patients with unilateral focalized stroke lesions on the CAS subtests at 1 month and 6 months postinfarct, so that each patient functioned as his or her own baseline. Patient 1, with a left temporal pole lesion, had a severe syntactic comprehension deficit on the Sentence Questions subtest. Patient 2 had a rare right anterior cerebral artery aneurysm culminating in an orbitofrontal syndrome and impairments on Expressive Attention and Word Series, as well as a praxis-based figure–ground reversal phenomenon on Figure Memory. Patient 3 suffered a right frontoparietal lesion with resulting representational difficulties, as well as elements of motor neglect and impairments on Matching Numbers, Number Detection, and Receptive Attention. The patients' lesions were all entirely consistent with the nature of their cognitive neuropsychological symptoms, suggesting that the CAS subtests are unique and also sensitive and specific to focalized cortical lesions.

INTERPRETATION

Before we discuss interpretation of profiles on the CAS, it is important to emphasize two points. First, although profile analysis of intelligence test results has traditionally been conducted with *subtests*, profile analysis of the CAS is conducted at the theoretical *PASS scale* level. Second, a specific method called the discrepancy–consistency model (Naglieri, 1999a, 2011) is used to determine whether PASS scores differ significantly and whether these differences have diagnostic utility. This method requires two important findings. First, at least one of the four PASS scores must be significantly below the child's mean PASS score; second, that score must be substantially below normal (e.g., at least a standard score of 90). A finding such as this provides evidence of a disorder in one or more of the basic psychological processes, as specified in the definition of a specific learning disability (SLD) in the Individuals with Disabilities Education Improvement Act of 2004 (IDEA 2004) (Naglieri, 2011).

A summary of CAS interpretation methods is provided in this section, but a complete discussion can be found in Naglieri (1999a, 2011). These interpretive steps should be applied within the context of all available information about a child, so that a comprehensive assessment (diagnosis and treatment planning) of the child is achieved. All the values needed to conduct interpretation of CAS are provided by the CAS Rapid Score (Naglieri, 2002).

Interpretation of CAS scores begins with an analysis of the test scores, followed by integration of those scores with other data obtained from a comprehensive evaluation (see Figure 15.3). The first step, therefore, is the examination of the child's levels of performance on the four separate PASS scores, interpreted according to the PASS theory (see Naglieri, 1999a; Naglieri & Otero, 2011). It is important to note that the CAS FS score is intended to be an overall estimate of processing based on the combination of the four PASS scales. This score will be a good overall description of a child's cognitive processing when the four PASS scale scores are similar. However, when there is significant variability among the PASS scale standard scores, the FS score should be deemphasized

because it is not necessarily representative of the parts of which it is comprised.

The second step in the preliminary analysis of the CAS is examination of differences in the four PASS scale scores. This will determine whether cognitive strengths or weaknesses are found. Variation in PASS scores is accomplished by examining the statistical significance of the score profile, using an intraindividual or ipsative method to determine when the variation in PASS scores is meaningful. When the variation is not significant, any differences are assumed to reflect measurement error. Meaningful, or reliable, variation can be (1) interpreted within the context of the theory, (2) related to strategy use, (3) evaluated in relation to achievement tests, and (4) used for treatment planning.

When a child's score on one of the PASS subtests is significantly above his or her mean score, then a cognitive processing strength is found. When a PASS subtest score is significantly lower than the child's mean score, then a weakness is detected. In other words, strengths and weaknesses are determined in relation to the child's own average level of performance. The steps needed to determine whether a child's PASS profile is significant are provided in Figure 15.3. Note that the values needed for significance for the Standard and Basic Batteries are provided by Naglieri (1999a) and Naglieri and Das (1997b), and by the CAS Rapid Score interpretive software (Naglieri, 2002). The flow chart provides a graphic representation of the decision-making steps for analyzing the PASS scores and using the results for instructional and/ or eligibility determination.

Using PASS Variability for Eligibility Determination

It is important to note that using PASS variability for diagnosis or eligibility determination should be done when the weakness is well below the child's mean *and* is also below the average range. When a child has significant PASS variability (with a weakness) *and* the lowest score is below average (<90), then the child is more likely to have significantly lower achievement scores and more likely to be in need of special education (Naglieri, 2000). Using this method ensures that the deficit in basic psychological processing is found in relation to peers, not just in relation to the child him- or herself. That is, the PASS weakness provides evidence of a disorder in one of the four PASS basic psychological processes—evidence that, when paired

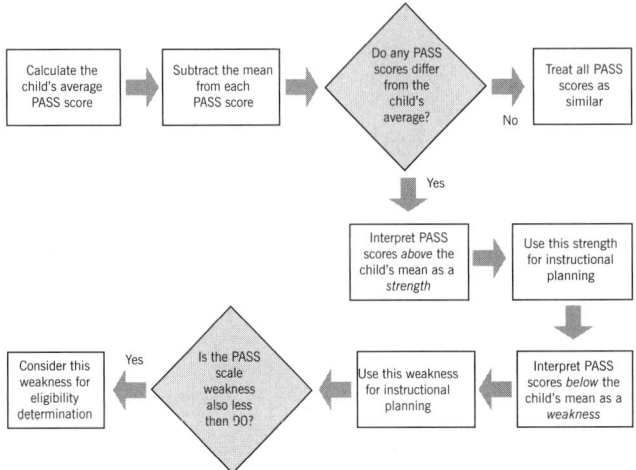

FIGURE 15.3. Steps for analysis of PASS scale standard scores on the CAS. Copyright 2011 by Jack A. Naglieri. Reprinted by permission.

with a deficit in achievement, can form the basis of eligibility determination according to IDEA 2004 (see Naglieri, 2011). When a child has (1) significant variability among the four PASS cognitive processing scores, (2) a significant discrepancy between good ability scores and achievement scores, and (3) consistency between a low PASS score and low academic skills, then the child fits the discrepancy–consistency model for SLD eligibility as proposed by Naglieri (1999a, 2011). That is, this model (shown in Figure 15.4, which is very similar to the discrepancy–consistency model for diagnosis depicted in Figure 7.2 in Chapter 7) sug-

gests that a child has a specific cognitive and specific academic weakness, and may therefore meet criteria for having an SLD.

Merging PASS with Other Concepts

Comprehensive examination of academic learning problems often involves integration of information from many different sources (home, school, teacher reports, classroom observations, etc.) and often time across different tests. Table 15.1 is provided as a way to help practitioners relate the subtest scores obtained from the CAS to other commonly used concepts, so that similarities or differences can be uncovered. For example, if a child's poor performance in the classroom appears to be related to working with tasks that require memory, it would be reasonable to ask whether the child's scores on the CAS subtests that involve memory (as well as PASS processing abilities) are low. Similarly, if another professional has suggested that the child does poorly in auditory tasks, analysis of the CAS subtests along this dimension can be conducted. Table 15.2 is intended for comparing CAS and WISC-IV scores. That is, with this table, WISC-IV index scores can be related to particular CAS subtest scores. This more clinical approach to test interpretation can be used to help develop hypotheses about the child's performance that will require additional support. Understanding how CAS scores relate to other concepts can often help a practitioner better understand the extent to which a PASS cognitive weakness may be seen in a child's performance on other test scores.

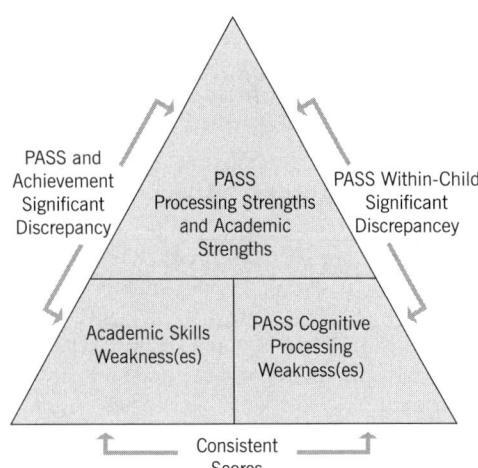

FIGURE 15.4. Discrepancy–consistency model for SLD eligibility determination. Copyright 2011 by Jack A. Naglieri. Reprinted by permission.

TABLE 15.1. Similarity of PASS Subtest Scores from the CAS to Commonly Used Concepts

PASS scale/subtest	Executive function	Working memory	Verbal content	Nonverbal content	Working with numbers	Auditory tasks	Visual–spatial tasks	Tasks involving speed
Planning								
Planned Codes	×			×				
Matching Numbers	×			×	×			
Planned Connections	×	×			×		×	
Attention								
Expressive Attention	×		×					Items 1–2 only
Receptive Attention	×							
Number Detection	×				×			
Simultaneous								
Nonverbal Matrices				×			×	
Verbal–Spatial Relations			×					
Figure Memory		×		×			×	
Successive								
Word Series		×				×		
Sentence Repetition		×	×			×		
Sentence Questions		×	×			×		
Speech Rate								×

TABLE 15.2. Similarity of PASS Subtest Scores from the CAS to the WISC-IV Index Scales

PASs scale/subtest	Verbal Comprehension	Perceptual Reasoning	Working Memory	Processing Speed
Planning				
Planned Codes				
Matching Numbers			×	
Planned Connections			×	
Attention				
Expressive Attention				Items 1–2 only
Receptive Attention				
Number Detection				
Simultaneous				
Nonverbal Matrices		×		
Verbal–Spatial Relations	×	×		
Figure Memory			×	
Successive				
Word Series			×	
Sentence Repetition			×	
Sentence Questions	×			
Speech Rate				×

CASE STUDY

The following case illustrates how the PASS constructs can be used to identify a cognitive processing weakness and aid in SLD eligibility determination. It also shows how a weakness in PASS ability can be related to academic failure and how these two findings can be used for instructional planning. The approach is intentionally limited to CAS, WISC-IV, and achievement test results for the purposes of efficiency and brevity. In actuality, a comprehensive assessment would include more than is presented in this illustration.

Adolfo is a fourth grader of Hispanic origin with a history of learning difficulties who has been receiving several types of support in reading. He is an English-language learner who can converse in both English and Spanish, and whose parents only speak Spanish. Adolfo speaks Spanish at home and mostly English at school. The results of Adolfo's yearly language proficiency testing indicate that he is still developing cognitive–academic English-language skills. His teacher describes him as a hard worker and as someone who likes to try new things; he often volunteers for different classroom chores and activities. He enjoys being in school and is happy and inquisitive. His teacher also notes that he often has trouble remembering information like directions and math facts, and is especially struggling with sounding out words and spelling. The most recent districtwide testing indicated that Adolfo's overall reading skills are below grade level. His reading comprehension is typically better than his decoding and reading fluency. His math reasoning skills, assessed with word problems, are also poor. Adolfo is also described as often having difficulty following what is said in a conversation and keeping up with classroom lectures, and he usually does not understand lengthy instructions. Difficulties on math tasks, particularly word problems, are reported as stemming from his problem with keeping all elements of the word problem in memory in order before he can decide how to go about solving the problem. Socially, however, he is described as outgoing, as well liked, and as having many friends both in and out of school. He plays on a soccer team as a goalie. His coach has placed him in this position because of his difficulty in following specific directions when he played other positions on the field.

Adolfo's teacher has attempted to assist him in reading and math by giving tasks that are shorter in length, lower in difficulty level, and fewer in number. He also receives small-group instruction

for 15–20 minutes a day from a classroom aide. Adolfo has told the school psychologist that he enjoys the extra attention, but gets frustrated when he sees others getting all their work done while he sees himself as just starting. He typically has to take work home to complete and often is unable to complete it entirely. He has an older brother who helps him with his work, but not consistently. Both his parents have very limited educational experience, work many hours, and are not home to provide further support. Adolfo has been showing signs of becoming anxious about his performance in school. He has begun to have somatic complaints, and looks for approval while working on reading and math tasks. Although he does not refuse to engage in schoolwork, he has been noticed to procrastinate about starting a task, to be more vigilant about the time of day for lunch and recess periods, and to be more distractible than usual.

Aldolfo was administered the CAS (in both English and Spanish by a bilingual psychologist), the WISC-IV, and achievement tests over the course of several weeks as efforts to assist him were made. He was friendly and cooperative, and he put forth his best effort during the evaluation. Adolfo was well oriented and displayed a good range of emotion, but his attention and concentration were variable, depending on the complexity of questions or task demands. Of note was the need to repeat instructions and check for understanding across several subtests. Adolfo had difficulty understanding multicomponent questions and keeping information in sequential order. For example, he had difficulty keeping details of information in order; in such situations, he showed a clear increase in anxiety, limited attention, and a tendency to avoid or withdraw from the situation. This was especially noticeable on math calculation tasks when he was required to listen to a problem, recognize the procedure to be followed, and then perform the calculations. Because many of the problems included extraneous information, Adolfo needed to decide not only the appropriate order of operations to use, but also what information to include in the calculation.

The results of the ability measures (provided in Table 15.3) help clarify the nature of Adolfo's cognitive ability weakness, how that weakness is related to academic problems, and how that weakness is demonstrated across measures of intelligence. Each of the three tests was examined by first computing Adolfo's mean standard score for each test. The differences between scales were compared to values needed for significance reported by Naglieri

(1999a) for the CAS and by Naglieri and Paolitto (2005) for the WISC-IV. The values needed for significance are included in Table 15.3.

The results for the CAS administered in both English and Spanish strongly show that Adolfo has a cognitive weakness in successive ability. He earned CAS Successive scores of 72 (English) and 77 (Spanish) that were significantly below his PASS mean and substantially below the average range. Clearly, he has considerable problems working with nonacademic as well as academic tasks that demand sequencing of information. Interestingly, Adolfo also earned a low score on the WISC-IV Working Memory Index (79), which also demands, in part, sequencing of information.

Closer examination of Adolfo's scores on the WISC-IV Digit Span subtest revealed some important results. According to the WISC-IV technical manual, the Working Memory subtests Digit Span Forward and Backward require different degrees of working memory. The manual states that Digit Span Backward requires greater working memory than Digit Span Forward. Importantly, Schofield and Ashman (1986) found that Digit Span Forward was strongly related to successive processing ability and that Digit Span Backward to be equally related to successive and planning abilities (from PASS theory). Comparison of these two scores can therefore yield important clinical information about how to interpret a child's performance. In this case, Adolfo earned a score on Digit Span Forward (raw score = 3) that was significantly lower than his Digit Span Backward score (raw score = 8). In other words, Adolfo did better on the task requiring more working memory (Digit Span Backward) than on the less complex task (Digit Span Forward). Recall of digits forward, like recall of words in sequence (Word Recall from CAS), can be interpreted as measuring successive processing ability. Therefore, Adolfo's low Working Memory Index score could be better viewed as being influenced by successive processing ability. Said another way, his well-documented cognitive weakness in successive ability (i.e., on the CAS Successive scale) also influenced his performance on the WISC-IV Working Memory Index.

Figure 15.5 shows Adolfo's standardized academic achievement test results in both English and Spanish (which are consistent with the reports from the classroom teacher), and contrasts these with his CAS and WISC-IV scores. Adolfo's results in both English and Spanish reveal low scores in basic reading, spelling, and math reasoning skills. Taken together, the results demonstrate consistency in relation to his cognitive processing skills. That is, his reading and spelling scores are consistent with his low Successive processing scale score and these were substantially below his cogni-

TABLE 15.3. Intelligence Test Results for Adolfo

Test	Score	Difference from mean	Difference needed	Strength or weakness
WISC-IV				
Verbal Comprehension	86	−4.8	8.6	
Perceptual Reasoning	99	8.3	9.1	
Working Memory	79	−11.8	9.3	W
Processing Speed	99	8.3	10.7	
CAS (English)				
Planning	101	12.5	10.8	S
Simultaneous	97	8.5	9.6	
Attention	84	−4.5	11.1	
Successive	72	−16.5	9.5	W
CAS (Spanish)				
Planning	101	10.2	10.8	
Simultaneous	101	10.2	9.6	S
Attention	84	−6.6	11.1	
Successive	77	−13.8	9.5	W

Note. Values for significance of each scale's difference from the child's mean ($p = .05$) for the CAS are from Naglieri (1999a) and WISC-IV from Naglieri and Paolitto (2005).

tive and academic strengths. These data indicate that his scores form the three components of the Discrepancy/Consistency model shown in Figure 15.5.

Several interventions from *Helping Children to Learn: Intervention Handouts for Use in School and at Home* (Naglieri & Pickering, 2010) were suggested, based on Adolfo's cognitive processing strengths and weaknesses. His teacher was very receptive and willing to try anything in order to help Adolfo in attaining academic success. Using the handouts about successive processing to teach Adolfo about this processing ability was the first step. This allowed him to feel a sense of self-efficacy and to feel successful in spite of his cognitive weakness.

Adolfo's poor successive processing was then addressed with several other handouts, such as Teaching Students about Successive Processing (p. 62), More Strategies for Math Word Problems (p. 120), Seven-Step Strategy for Math Word Problems (p. 177), and Improving Reading Skills Online (p. 92). The math handouts taught Adolfo that developing systematic strategies while mentally keeping information in order would aid him in the successful completion of word problems. Finally, Adolfo learned that he could work on improving his reading decoding and sequencing skills by playing online games that are engaging, require multiple cognitive processes, and make reading fun (see also Naglieri & Pickering, 2010, pp. 96–97).

Teaching Adolfo's parents to understand what successive processing is was also deemed impor-

tant. They were given the Spanish versions of the handouts Successive Processing Explained (p. 132) and Seven-Step Strategy for Math Word Problems (p. 154). These handouts helped Adolfo's parents to recognize that information is often organized in a sequence, and that maintaining such information in order is the key to understanding and learning.

CONCLUSIONS

This chapter is based on the assumption that a cognitive approach to conceptualizing and measuring basic psychological processing abilities offers today's school and clinical psychologists a theoretically and empirically sound solution for efficient diagnosis and treatment of learning problems. Advances in cognitive psychology and neuropsychology have provided the opportunity for change, and the PASS theory, as represented by the CAS, reflects this modern view of abilities. The research summarized in this chapter demonstrates that the CAS offers a strong alternative to traditional tests, as evidenced by four major findings. First, children with disabilities (particularly reading disabilities and ADHD) have PASS profiles that are distinctive and relevant to diagnosis. Second, the CAS is an excellent predictor of achievement, despite the fact that it does not contain verbal and achievement-based tests like those found in traditional IQ tests. Third, the CAS yields the smallest differences between white and black as well as between Hispanic and non-Hispanic children, and across cultures, among the various tests of ability that are available. And, fourth, the PASS theory provides information that is relevant to intervention and instructional planning. The advantages offered by the CAS are timely, appropriate to the demands placed on practitioners today, and important to help children maximize academic success.

REFERENCES

Ashman, A. F., & Conway, R. N. F. (1997). *An introduction to cognitive education: Theory and applications.* London: Routledge.

Barkley, R. A. (1997). *ADHD and the nature of self-control.* New York: Guilford Press.

Barkley, R. A. (2006). *Attention-deficit hyperactivity disorder: A handbook for diagnosis and treatment* (2nd ed.). New York: Guilford Press.

Blaha, J. (2003). *What does the CAS really measure?: An*

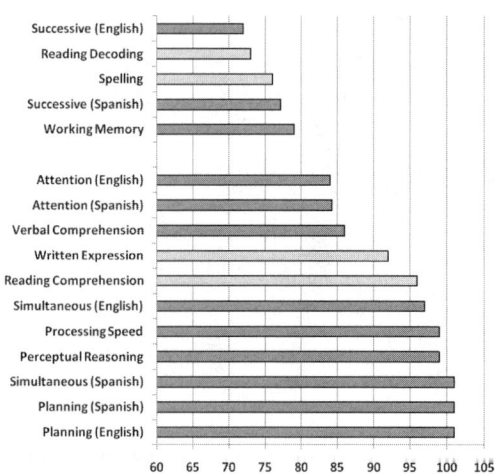

FIGURE 15.5. Adolfo's intelligence and achievement test scores.

exploratory hierarchical factor analysis of the Cognitive Assessment System. Paper presented at the annual convention of the National Association of School Psychologists, Chicago.

Blaha, J., & Wallbrown, F. H. (1996). Hierarchical factor structure of the Wechsler Intelligence Scale for Children—III. *Psychological Assessment, 8,* 214–218.

Boden, C., & Kirby, J. R. (1995). Successive processing, phonological coding and the remediation of reading. *Journal of Cognitive Education, 4,* 19–31.

Bracken, B. A. (1987). Limitations of preschool instruments and standards for minimal levels of technical adequacy. *Journal of Psychoeducational Assessment, 5,* 313–326.

Brailsford, A., Snart, F., & Das, J. P. (1984). Strategy training and reading comprehension. *Journal of Learning Disabilities, 17,* 287–290.

Brody, N. (1992). *Intelligence.* San Diego, CA: Academic Press.

Carlson, J., & Das, J. P. (1997). A process approach to remediating word decoding deficiencies in Chapter 1 children. *Learning Disability Quarterly, 20,* 93–102.

Carroll, J. B. (1993). *Human cognitive abilities: A survey of factor-analytic studies.* New York: Cambridge University Press.

Carroll, J. B. (1994). Cognitive abilities: Constructing a theory from data. In D. K. Detterman (Ed.), *Current topics in human intelligence: Vol. 4. Theories of intelligence* (pp. 43–63). Norwood, NJ: Ablex.

Cohen, R. J., Swerdlik, M. E., & Smith, D. K. (1992). *Psychological testing and assessment.* Mountain View, CA: Mayfield.

Cormier, P., Carlson, J. S., & Das, J. P. (1990). Planning ability and cognitive performance: The compensatory effects of a dynamic assessment approach. *Learning and Individual Differences, 2,* 437–449.

D'Amico, A., Cardaci, M., Di Nuovo, S., & Naglieri, J. A. (in press). Differences in achievement not intelligence in the north and south of Italy: Comments on Lynn (2010). *Learning and Individual Differences.*

Das, J. P. (1972). Patterns of cognitive ability in nonretarded and retarded children. *American Journal of Mental Deficiency, 77,* 6–12.

Das, J. P. (1999). *PASS Reading Enhancement Program.* Deal, NJ: Sarka Educational Resources.

Das, J. P., Kirby, J. R., & Jarman, R. F. (1979). *Simultaneous and successive cognitive processes.* New York: Academic Press.

Das, J. P., Mishra, R. K., & Pool, J. E. (1995). An experiment on cognitive remediation or word-reading difficulty. *Journal of Learning Disabilities, 28,* 66–79.

Das, J. P., Naglieri, J. A., & Kirby, J. R. (1994). *Assessment of cognitive processes.* Needham Heights, MA: Allyn & Bacon.

Das, J. P., Parrila, R., & Papadopoulos, R. (2000). Cognitive education and reading disability. In A. Kozulin & Y. Rand (Eds.), *Experiences of mediated learning* (pp. 274–291). Amsterdam: Pergamon Press.

Dehn, M. (2000). *Cognitive assessment system performance of children with ADHD.* Poster presented at the annual convention of the National Association of School Psychologists, New Orleans, LA.

Delis, D. C., Kaplan, E., & Kramer, J. H. (2001). *Delis–Kaplan Executive Function System (D-KEFS).* San Antonio, TX: Pearson.

Elliott, C. D. (2007). *Differential Ability Scales—Second Edition.* San Antonio, TX: Harcourt Assessment.

Fuchs, D., & Young, C. L. (2006). On the irrelevance of intelligence in predicting responsiveness to reading instruction. *Exceptional Children, 73,* 8–30.

Goldberg, E. (2009). *The new executive brain: Frontal lobes in a complex world.* New York: Oxford University Press.

Goldstein, S., & Naglieri, J. A. (2006). The role of intellectual processes in the DSM-V diagnosis of ADHD. *Journal of Attention Disorders, 10,* 3–8.

Goldstein, S., & Naglieri, J. A. (2009). *Autism Spectrum Rating Scale.* Toronto: Multi-Health Systems.

Gutentag, S., Naglieri, J. A., & Yeates, K. O. (1998). Performance of children with traumatic brain injury on the Cognitive Assessment System. *Assessment, 5,* 263–272.

Haddad, F. A., Garcia, Y. E., Naglieri, J. A., Grimditch, M., McAndrews, A., & Eubanks, J. (2003). Planning facilitation and reading comprehension: Instructional relevance of the PASS theory. *Journal of Psychoeducational Assessment, 21,* 282–289.

Iseman, J., & Naglieri, J. A. (2011). A cognitive strategy instruction to improve math calculation for children with ADHD: A randomized controlled study. *Journal of Learning Disabilities, 44*(2), 184–195.

Kar, B. C., Dash, U. N., Das, J. P., & Carlson, J. S. (1992). Two experiments on the dynamic assessment of planning. *Learning and Individual Differences, 5,* 13–29.

Kaufman, A. S., & Kaufman, N. L. (2004). *Kaufman Assessment Battery for Children—Second Edition.* Circle Pines, MN: American Guidance Service.

Kaufman, D., & Kaufman, P. (1979). Strategy training and remedial techniques. *Journal of Learning Disabilities, 12,* 63–66.

Keith, T. Z., & Kranzler, J. H. (1999). Independent confirmatory factor analysis of the Cognitive Assessment System (CAS): What does the CAS measure? *School Psychology Review, 28,* 117–144.

Korkman, M., Kirk, U., & Kemp, S. (2007). *NEPSY—Second Edition (NEPSY-II).* San Antonio, TX: Harcourt Assessment.

Krywaniuk, L. W., & Das, J. P. (1976). Cognitive strategies in native children: Analysis and intervention. *Alberta Journal of Educational Research, 22,* 271–280.

Luria, A. R. (1966a). *Higher cortical functions in man.* New York: Basic Books.

Luria, A. R. (1966b). *Human brain and psychological processes.* New York: Harper & Row.

Luria, A. R. (1973). *The working brain: An introduction to neuropsychology.* New York: Basic Books.

Luria, A. R. (1980). *Higher cortical functions in man* (2nd ed.). New York: Basic Books.

Luria, A. R. (1982). *Language and cognition.* New York: Wiley.

McCrea, S. M. (2007). Measurement of recovery after traumatic brain injury: A cognitive-neuropsychological comparison of the WAIS-R with the Cognitive Assessment System (CAS) in a single case of atypical language lateralization. *Applied Neuropsychology, 14,* 296–304.

Naglieri, J. A. (1999a). *Essentials of CAS assessment.* New York: Wiley.

Naglieri, J. A. (1999b). How valid is the PASS theory and CAS? *School Psychology Review, 28,* 145–162.

Naglieri, J. A. (2000). Can profile analysis of ability test scores work?: An illustration using the PASS theory and CAS with an unselected cohort. *School Psychology Quarterly, 15*(4), 419–433.

Naglieri, J. A. (2002). *CAS Rapid Score.* Austin, TX: PRO-ED.

Naglieri, J. A. (2003). *Naglieri Nonverbal Ability Test—Individual Form.* San Antonio, TX: Psychological Corporation.

Naglieri, J. A. (2008). Traditional IQ: 100 years of misconception and its relationship to minority representation in gifted programs. In J. VanTassel-Baska (Ed.), *Alternative assessments with gifted and talented students* (pp. 67–88). Waco, TX: Prufrock Press.

Naglieri, J. A. (2011). The discrepancy/consistency approach to SLD identification using the PASS theory. In D. P. Flanagan & V. C. Alfonso (Eds.), *Essentials of specific learning disability identification* (pp. 145–172). Hoboken, NJ: Wiley.

Naglieri, J. A., & Bornstein, B. T. (2003). Intelligence and achievement: Just how correlated are they? *Journal of Psychoeducational Assessment, 21,* 244–260.

Naglieri, J. A., & Conway, C. (2009). The Cognitive Assessment System. In J. A. Naglieri & S. Goldstein (Eds.), *A practitioner's guide to assessing of intelligence and achievement* (pp. 3–10). Hoboken, NJ: Wiley.

Naglieri, J. A., & Das, J. P. (1997a). *Cognitive Assessment System.* Itasca, IL: Riverside.

Naglieri, J. A., & Das, J. P. (1997b). *Cognitive Assessment System: Administration and scoring manual.* Itasca, IL: Riverside.

Naglieri, J. A., & Das, J. P. (1997c). *Cognitive Assessment System: Interpretive handbook.* Itasca, IL: Riverside.

Naglieri, J. A., Das, J. P., & Goldstein, S. (2012). *Cognitive Assessment System—Second Edition.* Austin, TX: PRO-ED.

Naglieri, J. A., & Goldstein, S. (2011). Assessment of cognitive and neuropsychological processes. In S. Goldstein & J. A. Naglieri (Eds.), *Understanding and managing learning disabilities and ADHD in late adolescence and adulthood* (2nd ed.). New York: Wiley.

Naglieri, J. A., Goldstein, S., DeLauder, B., & Schwebach, A. (2006). WISC-III and CAS: Which correlates higher with achievement for a clinical sample? *School Psychology Quarterly, 21,* 62–76.

Naglieri, J. A., Goldstein, S., Iseman, J. S., & Schwebach, A. (2003). Performance of children with attention deficit hyperactivity disorder and anxiety/depression on the WISC-III and Cognitive Assessment System (CAS). *Journal of Psychoeducational Assessment, 21,* 32–42.

Naglieri, J. A., & Gottling, S. H. (1995). A cognitive education approach to math instruction for the learning disabled: An individual study. *Psychological Reports, 76,* 1343–1354.

Naglieri, J. A., & Gottling, S. H. (1997). Mathematics instruction and PASS cognitive processes: An intervention study. *Journal of Learning Disabilities, 30,* 513–520.

Naglieri, J. A., & Johnson, D. (2000). Effectiveness of a cognitive strategy intervention to improve math calculation based on the PASS theory. *Journal of Learning Disabilities, 33,* 591–597.

Naglieri, J. A., Kamphaus, R. W., & Kaufman, A. S. (1983). The Luria–Das simultaneous–successive model applied to the WISC-R. *Journal of Psychoeducational Assessment, 1,* 25–34.

Naglieri, J. A., & Otero, T. (2011). Cognitive Assessment System: Redefining intelligence from a neuropsychological perspective. In A. Davis (Ed.), *Handbook of pediatric neuropsychology* (pp. 320–333). New York: Springer.

Naglieri, J. A., Otero, T., DeLauder, B., & Matto, H. (2007). Bilingual Hispanic children's performance on the English and Spanish versions of the Cognitive Assessment System. *School Psychology Quarterly, 22,* 432–448.

Naglieri, J. A., & Paolitto, A. W. (2005). Ipsative comparisons of WISC-IV Index scores. *Applied Neuropsychology, 12,* 208–211.

Naglieri, J. A., & Pickering, E. (2010). *Helping children learn: Intervention handouts for use in school and at home* (2nd ed.). Baltimore: Brookes.

Naglieri, J. A., & Rojahn, J. (2004). Validity of the PASS theory and CAS: Correlations with achievement. *Journal of Educational Psychology, 96,* 174–181.

Naglieri, J. A., Rojahn, J., & Matto, H. (2007). Hispanic and non-Hispanic children's performance on PASS cognitive processes and achievement. *Intelligence, 35,* 568–579.

Naglieri, J. A., Rojahn, J., Matto, H., & Aquilino, S. A. (2005). Black–white differences in intelligence: A study of the PASS theory and Cognitive Assessment System. *Journal of Psychoeducational Assessment, 23,* 146–160.

Naglieri, J. A., Salter, C. J., & Edwards, G. (2004). Assessment of ADHD and reading abilities using the PASS theory and Cognitive Assessment System. *Journal of Psychoeducational Assessment, 22,* 93–105.

Otero, T. M., Gonzales, L., & Naglieri, J. A. (in press). The neurocognitive assessment of Hispanic English language learners with reading failure. *Archives of Clinical Neuropsychology.*

Paolitto, A. W. (1999). Clinical validation of the Cognitive Assessment System with children with ADHD. *ADHD Report, 7,* 1–5.

Parrila, R. K., Das, J. P., Kendrick, M., Papadopoulos, T., & Kirby, J. (1999). Efficacy of a cognitive reading remediation program for at-risk children in grade 1. *Developmental Disabilities Bulletin, 27,* 1–31.

Perez-Alvarez, F., Timoneda-Gallart, C., & Baus-Rosell, J. (2006). Topiramate and epilepsy in the light of Das–Naglieri Cognitive Assessment System. *Revisto de Neurología, 42,* 3–9.

Porteus, S. D. (1965). *Porteus Maze Test: Fifty years' application.* New York: Psychological Corporation.

Roid, G. H. (2003). *Stanford–Binet Intelligence Scales, Fifth Edition.* Itasca, IL: Riverside.

Ruff, R. M., & Allen, C. C. (1996). *Ruff 2 & 7 Selective Attention Test professional manual.* Odessa, FL: Psychological Assessment Resources.

Savage, R. C., & Wolcott, G. F. (Eds.). (1994). *Educational dimensions of acquired brain injury.* Austin, TX: PRO-ED.

Schofield, N. J., & Ashman, A. F. (1986). The relationship between digit span and cognitive processing across ability groups. *Intelligence, 10,* 59–73.

Suzuki, L. A., & Valencia, R. R. (1997). Race-ethnicity and measured intelligence. *American Psychologist, 52,* 1103–1114.

Wechsler, D. (1991). *Wechsler Intelligence Scale for Children—Third Edition.* San Antonio, TX: Psychological Corporation.

Wechsler, D. (2003). *Wechsler Intelligence Scale for Children—Fourth Edition.* San Antonio, TX: Psychological Corporation.

Wechsler, D., & Naglieri, J. A. (2006). *Wechsler Nonverbal Scale of Ability.* San Antonio, TX: Harcourt Assessment.

Wendling, B. J., Mather, N., & Schrank, F. A. (2009). Woodcock–Johnson III Tests of Cognitive Abilities. In J. A. Naglieri & S. Goldstein (Eds.), *A practitioner's guide to assessment of intelligence and achievement* (pp. 191–232). New York: Wiley.

Wilkinson, A., & Semrud-Clikeman, M. (2008, February). *Motor speed in children and adolescents with nonverbal learning disabilities.* Paper presented at the annual meeting of the International Neuropsychological Society, Kona, Hawaii.

Woodcock, R. W., & Johnson, M. B. (1989). *Woodcock–Johnson Psycho-Educational Battery—Revised Tests of Achievement: Standard and supplemental batteries.* Chicago: Riverside.

Woodcock, R. W., McGrew, K. S., & Mather, N. (2001). *Woodcock–Johnson III Tests of Cognitive Abilities.* Itasca, IL: Riverside.

CHAPTER 16

The Reynolds Intellectual Assessment Scales and the Reynolds Intellectual Screening Test

Ceil R. Reynolds
Randy W. Kamphaus
Tara C. Raines

This chapter provides the reader with an extensive introduction to the Reynolds Intellectual Assessment Scales (RIAS; Reynolds & Kamphaus, 2003), an increasingly popular measure of intelligence for children and adults. A brief overview of the subtests is provided, followed by a review of the theory and structure of the RIAS, framed primarily around its goals for development. A more extensive description is then provided of the subtests and their administration and scoring. Psychometric characteristics of the RIAS are next presented, along with guidelines for interpretation and clinical applications. The chapter closes with a case study using the RIAS as the featured measure of intelligence.

The RIAS is an individually administered test of intelligence appropriate for ages 3 years through 94 years, with a co-normed, supplemental measure of memory. The RIAS includes a two-subtest Verbal Intelligence Index (VIX) and a two-subtest Nonverbal Intelligence Index (NIX). The scaled sums of T scores for the four subtests are combined to form the Composite Intelligence Index (CIX), which is a summary estimate of global intelligence. Administration of the four intelligence scale subtests by a trained, experienced examiner requires approximately 20–25 minutes. A Composite Memory Index (CMX) is derived from the two supplementary memory subtests, which require approximately 10–15 minutes of additional testing time. The CIX and the CMX represent combinations of verbal and nonverbal subtests. Table 16.1 provides an overview of the indexes and subtests of the RIAS.

The Reynolds Intellectual Screening Test (RIST; Kamphaus & Reynolds, 2003) is a two-subtest screening version of the RIAS that covers the same age range. The RIST is designed to allow users to make the decision regarding the need for a full RIAS evaluation in about 10 minutes or less (see Reynolds & Kamphaus, 2003, for complete RIST administration, scoring, and interpretation procedures).

THEORY AND STRUCTURE

The RIAS was designed to meld practical and theoretical aspects of the assessment of intelligence. Although the models of Carroll (1993) and Cattell and Horn (Horn & Cattell, 1966; Kamphaus, 2001) were the primary theoretical guides, the RIAS also followed closely the division of intelligence into verbal and nonverbal domains, due to the practical benefits of assessing verbal and nonverbal intelligence. Memory was included as a

TABLE 16.1. RIAS Composite Scores and Subtests

Composite Intelligence Index (CIX)

Subtests of the Verbal Intelligence Index (VIX)

Guess What. Examinees are given a set of two or three clues, and are asked to deduce the object or concept being described. This subtest measures verbal reasoning in combination with vocabulary, language development, and overall fund of available information.

Verbal Reasoning. Examinees listen to a propositional statement that essentially forms a verbal analogy, and are asked to respond with one or two words that complete the idea or proposition. This subtest measures verbal-analytical reasoning ability, but with fewer vocabulary and general knowledge demands than Guess What.

Subtests of the Nonverbal Intelligence Index (NIX)

Odd-Item Out. Examinees are presented with a picture card containing five to seven pictures or drawings, and are asked to designate which one does not belong or go with the others. This subtest measures nonverbal reasoning skills, but also requires the use of spatial ability, visual imagery, and other nonverbal skills on various items. It is a form of reverse nonverbal analogy.

What's Missing. A redesign of a classic task present on various ability measures. Examinees are shown a picture with some key element or logically consistent component missing, and are asked to identify the missing essential element. This subtest assesses nonverbal reasoning: The examinee must conceptualize the picture, analyze its Gestalt, and deduce what essential element is missing.

Composite Memory Index (CMX)

Subtests

Verbal Memory. In this verbal memory subtest, depending upon the examinee's age, a series of sentences or brief stories are read aloud by the examiner and then recalled by the examinee. This task assesses the ability to encode, store briefly, and recall verbal material in a meaningful context where associations are clear and evident.

Nonverbal Memory. This visual memory subtest contains a series of items in which a stimulus picture is presented for 5 seconds, following which an array of pictures is presented. The examinee must identify the target picture from the new array of six pictures. It assesses the ability to encode, store, and recognize pictorial stimuli that are both concrete and abstract or without meaningful referents.

Note. From Reynolds and Kamphaus (2003). Copyright 2003 by Psychological Assessment Resources, Inc. Adapted by permission.

separate scale on the RIAS, due to the growing importance of working memory in models of intelligence and the practical aspects of memory to everyday diagnostic questions faced by the practitioner (see, e.g., Bigler & Clement, 1997; Goldstein & Reynolds, 2011; Reynolds & Bigler, 1994; Reynolds & Fletcher-Janzen, 1997). To clarify the theoretical underpinnings of the RIAS as well as its practical aspects and structure, a review of the goals for development of the test provides a strong heuristic.

Development Goals

We (Reynolds & Kamphaus, 2003) described a set of eight primary goals for development of the RIAS. The eight core development goals were derived from our experiences over the years in teaching intelligence testing, use of many different intelligence tests in clinical practice, and the current literature surrounding theoretical models of intelligence and research on intelligence test interpretation (for more extensive review and discussion, see Reynolds & Kamphaus, 2003, especially Chs. 1 and 6).

1. Provide a reliable and valid measurement of *g* and its two primary components, verbal and nonverbal intelligence, with close correspondence to crystallized and fluid intelligence.
2. Provide a practical measurement device in terms of efficacies of time, direct costs, and information needed from a measure of intelligence.
3. Allow continuity of measurement across all developmental levels from ages 3 years through 94 years for both clinical and research purposes.
4. Substantially reduce or eliminate dependence on motor coordination and visual–motor speed in the measurement of intelligence.
5. Eliminate dependence on reading in the measurement of intelligence.
6. Provide for accurate prediction of basic academic achievement, at levels at least comparable to those of intelligence tests twice the length of the RIAS.
7. Apply familiar, common concepts that are clear and easy to interpret, coupled with simple administration and scoring.
8. Eliminate items that show differential item functioning (DIF) associated with gender or ethnicity.

In addition to tasks targeting *g* and its two primary components, the RIAS was designed to assess basic memory functions in the verbal and nonverbal domains. Brief assessments of the integrity of memory have appeared on intelligence tests since Binet first asked children to recall a single picture and repeat a sentence of 15 words (Binet & Simon, 1905). Traditionally, scores on these tasks have been included as a component of IQ; the RIAS assesses memory function in a separate scale. The RIAS includes assessment of memory function because it is crucial to the diagnostic process for numerous disorders of childhood (Goldstein & Reynolds, 2011; Reynolds & Fletcher-Janzen, 1997) and adulthood, particularly later adulthood (Bigler & Clement, 1997). The RIAS CMX does not provide a comprehensive memory assessment, but it does cover the two areas of memory that are historically assessed by intelligence tests and are considered by many to be the two most important memory functions to assess (e.g., Bigler & Clement, 1997; Reynolds & Bigler, 1994): memory for meaningful verbal material and visual memory. Memory assessment co-norming presents the best possible scenario for contrasting test scores (Reynolds, 1984–1985), allowing the clinician to compare general intelligence directly with key memory functions.

Theory

The RIAS is a measure of intelligence that focuses on the measurement of *g*, or general intelligence (the CIX), and the two major components of general intelligence: verbal intelligence (the VIX) and nonverbal intelligence (the NIX). As with any measure of intelligence, many other basic but subsidiary cognitive processes, such as auditory and visual perception, logical reasoning, language processing, spatial skills, visual imagery, attention, and the like, play a role in performance on the RIAS. These skills are the building blocks of the primary intellectual functions assessed by the RIAS. The RIAS CMX is offered as a basic overall measure of short-term memory skills, with the Verbal Memory subtest measuring recall in the verbal associative domain, and the Nonverbal Memory subtest measuring ability to recall pictorial stimuli in both concrete (i.e., meaningful) dimensions and abstract dimensions (where concrete referents are not provided or easily derived).

The RIAS was designed to measure four important aspects of intelligence: *general intelligence* (of which the major component is *fluid* or *reasoning abilities*); *verbal intelligence* (sometimes referred to as *crystallized abilities*, a closely related though not identical concept); *nonverbal intelligence* (referred to in some theories as *visualization* or *spatial abilities*, and closely allied with fluid intelligence); and *memory* (subtests measuring this ability have been labeled variously as assessing *working memory*, *short-term memory*, or *learning*). These four constructs are measured by combinations of the six RIAS subtests (see Table 16.1).

The RIAS subtests were selected and designed to measure intelligence constructs that have a substantial history of scientific support. In addition, Carroll's (1993) seminal and often-cited three-stratum theory of intelligence informed the creation of the RIAS by demonstrating that many of the latent traits tapped by intelligence tests were test-battery-independent. He clearly demonstrated, for example, that numerous tests measured the same crystallized, visual-perceptual, and memory abilities. However, Kamphaus (2001) concluded that these same test batteries did not measure fluid abilities to a great extent.

The RIAS focuses on the assessment of stratum III and stratum II abilities from Carroll's (1993) three-stratum theory (see also Carroll, Appendix, this volume). Stratum III is composed of one construct only, *g*. Psychometric *g* accounts for the major portion of variance assessed by intelligence test batteries. More important, however, is the consistent finding that the correlations of intelligence tests with important outcomes, such as academic achievement and occupational attainment, are related to the amount of *g* measured by the test battery. In other words, so-called "g-saturated" tests are better predictors of important outcomes than are tests with low *g* saturation. One theory posits that *g* is actually a measure of working memory capacity (Kyllonen, 1996), whereas another theory posits that it is a measure of reasoning ability (Gustafson, 1999). Regardless of the theory that will eventually be supported, the utility of psychometric *g* remains, much in the same way that the usefulness of certain pharmaceutical drugs will continue before their mechanisms of action are fully understood. For these reasons, the RIAS places great emphasis on the assessment of psychometric *g* and on the assessment of its theorized main components (i.e., verbal and nonverbal reasoning and working memory).

The second stratum in Carroll's (1993) hierarchy consists of traits that are assessed by combinations of subtests, or stratum I measures. There are, however, several stratum II traits to choose from.

These second-stratum traits include fluid intelligence, crystallized intelligence, general memory and learning, broad visual perception, broad auditory perception, broad retrieval ability, broad cognitive speed, and processing speed (i.e., reaction time or decision speed). Of importance, however, is the suggestion (from the findings of hundreds of investigations) that these abilities are ordered by their assessment of *g* (Kamphaus, 2001). Specifically, subtests that tap fluid abilities are excellent measures of *g*, whereas tests of psychomotor speed are the weakest. If one accepts the aforementioned finding that *g* saturation is related to predictive validity, then the first few stratum II factors become the best candidates for inclusion in an intelligence test battery like the RIAS, especially one that seeks to be a time-efficient test. This logic informed subtest selection as well as item writing throughout the RIAS developmental process. Any test of *g* must measure so-called "higher-order" cognitive abilities—those associated with fluid abilities, such as general sequential reasoning, induction, deduction, syllogisms, series tasks, matrix reasoning, analogies, quantitative reasoning, and so on (Carroll, 1993). Kamphaus (2001) has advocated the following definition of *reasoning*: "that which follows as a reasonable inference or natural consequence; deducible or defensible on the grounds of consistency; reasonably believed or done" (*New Shorter Oxford English Dictionary*, 1993). This definition emphasizes a central cognitive requirement to draw inferences from knowledge. This characteristic of general intelligence is measured best by two RIAS subtests, Verbal Reasoning and Odd-Item Out, although all of the subtests have substantial *g* saturation (see Reynolds & Kamphaus, 2003, especially Ch. 6).

First-order factors of crystallized ability typically have one central characteristic: They involve language abilities (Vernon, 1950). These language abilities range from vocabulary knowledge to spelling to reading comprehension. On the other hand, it is not possible to dismiss this type of intelligence as a general academic achievement factor (see Reynolds & Kamphaus, 2003, for a discussion of this point). Kamphaus (2001) has proposed that the *verbal* factor be defined as "oral and written communication skills that follow the system of rules associated with a language" (p. 45), including comprehension skills.

Nonverbal tests have come to be recognized as measures of important spatial and visual-perceptual abilities—abilities that may need to be assessed for a variety of clients, including those with brain injuries. In the 1963 landmark Educational Testing Service Kit of Factor-Referenced Cognitive Tests, *spatial ability* was defined as "the ability to manipulate or transform the image of spatial patterns into other visual arrangements" (cited in Carroll, 1993, p. 316). The RIAS What's Missing and Odd-Item Out subtests follow in this long tradition of tasks designed to measure visual–spatial abilities. Digit recall, sentence recall, geometric design recall, bead recall, and similar measures loaded consistently on a *general memory and learning* stratum II factor identified by Carroll (1993) in his numerous analyses. The RIAS Verbal Memory and Nonverbal Memory subtests are of this same variety, although they are more complex than simple confrontational memory tasks such as pure digit recall. Carroll's findings suggest that the RIAS Verbal Memory and Nonverbal Memory subtests should be good measures of the memory construct that has been identified previously in so many investigations of a diverse array of tests. Memory is typically considered a complex trait with many permutations, including visual, verbal, long term, and short term. Carroll's analysis of hundreds of datasets supports the organization of the RIAS, in that he found ample evidence of a general memory trait that may be subdivided further for particular clinical purposes.

Description of Subtests

Subtests with a familiar look and feel, and with essentially long histories in the field of intellectual assessment, were chosen for inclusion on the RIAS. There are a total of four intelligence subtests and two memory subtests. The intelligence subtests were also chosen because of their complex nature: Each assesses many intellectual functions and requires their integration for successful performance (see also a later section of this chapter, "Evidence Based on Response Processes"). The memory subtests were chosen not only for complexity, but also due to their representation of the primary content domains of memory.

- *Guess What.* This subtest measures vocabulary knowledge in combination with reasoning skills that are predicated on language development and fund of information. For each item, the examinee listens to a question containing clues presented orally by the examiner, and then gives a verbal response (one or two words) consistent with the clues. The questions pertain to physical objects, abstract concepts, and well-known places and historical figures from a variety of cultures, geographic locations, and disciplines.

- *Verbal Reasoning.* The second verbal subtest measures analytical reasoning abilities. More difficult items also require advanced vocabulary knowledge. For each item, the examinee is asked to listen to an incomplete sentence presented orally by the examiner, and then to give a verbal response, typically one or two words, that completes the sentence (most commonly completing a complex analogy). Completion of the sentences requires the examinee to evaluate the various conceptual relationships that exist between the physical objects or abstract ideas contained in the sentences.

- *Odd-Item Out.* This subtest measures general reasoning skills emphasizing nonverbal ability. For each item, the examinee is presented with a picture card containing from five to seven figures or drawings. One of the figures or drawings on the picture card has a distinguishing characteristic, making it different from the others. For each item, the examinee is given two chances to identify the figure or drawing that is different from the others. Two points are awarded for a correct response given on the first attempt. One point is awarded for a correct response given on the second attempt (i.e., if the first response was incorrect).

- *What's Missing.* This subtest measures nonverbal reasoning skills through the presentation of pictures in which some important component of the pictured object is missing. Examinees must understand or conceptualize the pictured object, assess its Gestalt, and distinguish essential from nonessential components. For each item the examinee is shown a picture card, asked to examine the picture, and then asked to indicate (in words or by pointing) what is missing from the picture. Naming the missing part correctly is not required, so long as the examinee can indicate the missing component correctly. For each item, the examinee is given two chances to identify what is missing from the picture.

- *Verbal Memory.* This subtest measures the ability to encode, briefly store, and recall verbal material in a meaningful context. Young children (ages 3–4 years) are asked to listen to sentences of progressively greater length read aloud by the examiner, and then asked to repeat each sentence word for word immediately after it is read aloud. Older children and adults listen to two stories read aloud by the examiner, and then repeat each story back to the examiner immediately after it is read

aloud. The sentences and stories were written to provide developmentally appropriate content and material of interest to the targeted age group. Specific stories are designated for various age groups.

- *Nonverbal Memory.* This subtest measures the ability to encode, briefly store, and recall visually presented material, whether the stimuli represent concrete objects or abstract concepts. For each item, the examinee is presented with a target picture for 5 seconds, and then with a picture card containing the target picture and an array of similar pictures. The examinee is asked to identify the target picture among the array of pictures presented on the picture card. For each item, the examinee is given two chances to identify the target picture. The pictures are primarily abstract at the upper age levels, and pictures of common objects at the lower age levels. The use of naming and related language strategies is not helpful, however, due to the design of the distracters.

ADMINISTRATION AND SCORING

The RIAS was specifically designed to be easy to administer and objective to score. For all subtests except Verbal Memory, there are clear, objective lists of correct responses for each test item, and seldom are any judgment calls required. Studies of the interscorer reliability of these five subtests produced interscorer reliability coefficients of 1.00 by trained examiners (Reynolds & Kamphaus, 2003). On Verbal Memory, some judgment is required when examinees do not give verbatim responses; however, the scoring criteria provide clear examples and guidelines for such circumstances, making the Verbal Memory subtest only slightly more difficult to score. The interscorer reliability study of this subtest produced a coefficient of .95.

The time required to administer the entire RIAS (including both the intelligence and the memory subtests) averages 30–35 minutes once an examiner has practiced giving the RIAS and has become fluent in its administration. The RIST averages about 10–12 minutes. As with most tests, the first few administrations are likely to take longer. The four intelligence subtests alone (i.e., Guess What, Odd-Item Out, Verbal Reasoning, and What's Missing) can be administered to most examinees in about 20–25 minutes. The two memory subtests can typically be administered in about 10 minutes. However, significant time variations can occur as a function of special circumstances (e.g., very low-functioning individuals will probably take much less time to complete the battery, and very bright individuals may take longer). Basal and ceiling rules along with age-designated starting points were employed to control the administration time, and each was derived empirically from the responses of the standardization sample. Also, to facilitate ease and efficiency of administration, the RIAS and RIST record forms contain all of the necessary instructions and examiner guides necessary to administer the tests.

PSYCHOMETRIC PROPERTIES

Due to the length restrictions in a single book chapter, a discussion of the developmental process of the tests simply cannot be provided. However, the RIAS underwent years of development, including tryout and review of the items on multiple occasions by school psychologists, clinical psychologists, neuropsychologists, and others. Items were written to conform to clear specifications consistent with the goals for development of the test as given previously in this chapter. Items were reviewed by panels of expert psychologists for content and construct consistency, and by expert minority psychologists to ascertain the cultural saliency of the items and any potential problems of ambiguity or offensiveness. The developmental process speaks directly to the psychometric characteristics of the tests, and is described in far more detail in Reynolds and Kamphaus (2003). It should be considered carefully in any full evaluation of the instrument.

Standardization

The RIAS was normed on a sample of 2,438 participants residing in 41 states between the years of 1999 and 2002. U.S. Bureau of the Census characteristics of the U.S. population projected initially to the year 2000, and then updated through 2001, were used to select a population-proportionate sample. Age, gender, ethnicity, educational level (parental educational level was used for ages 3 years through 16 years, and the participants' actual educational level was used at all other ages), and region of residence were used as stratification variables. The resulting norms for the RIAS and the RIST were calculated on a weighted sampling that provided a virtually perfect match to the census data. The overall sample was a close match to the population statistics in every regard (see Reynolds & Kamphaus, 2003, especially Tables 4.2–4.5).

Norm Derivation and Scaling

All standard scores for the RIAS were derived via a method known as *continuous norming*. Continuous norming is a regression-based methodology used to mitigate the effects of any sampling irregularities across age groupings and to stabilize parameter estimation. An important feature of continuous norming is that it uses information from all age groups, rather than relying solely on the estimates of central tendency, dispersion, and the shape of the distributions of a single age grouping for producing the norms at each chosen age interval in the normative tables for a particular test. As such, the continuous-norming procedure maximizes the accuracy of the derived normative scores and has become widespread in its application to the derivation of test norms over the last 20 years (see, e.g., Reynolds, 2003; Roid, 2003; Zachary & Gorsuch, 1985). Calculation of normative scores via continuous norming essentially involves calculating these things, sequentially: the lines or curves of best fit for the progression of means and standard deviations across age groupings of the norming variables (using polynomial regression); the mean, standard deviation, skewness, and kurtosis of the distribution of scores for each normative age group; and percentiles and scaled scores based on the estimates obtained from the prior steps.

For the RIAS and the RIST, census-weighted means and standard deviations of the subtest raw scores for the 52 age groups in the normative sample were analyzed separately to determine the best-fitting polynomial regression equations. Mean subgroup age and its powers up to the sixth power were used as predictors. Visual inspection of the polynomial curves derived from the group standard deviations, and those previously derived from the individuals' raw scores, showed considerable congruence. Means and standard deviations were then calculated for each normative age group, using the polynomial regression equations derived above. The method of continuous norming assumes that the best estimate of distribution shape is derived from the composite skewness and kurtosis aggregated across groupings of the normative variables (Angoff & Robertson, 1987). Composite estimates of skewness and kurtosis were thus calculated from the averages of these respective values in the 52 age groups. Percentiles and normalized standardized scores corresponding to raw scores were calculated for every normative age group, using the respective mean and standard deviation values obtained in step 2. *T* scores were derived to have a mean of 50 and a standard deviation of 10 for each of the RIAS subtests. These scores were then combined into the various composite and index scores described previously (see Table 16.1) and scaled via a similar procedure to a mean of 100 and standard deviation of 15.

T scores were chosen for the RIAS subtests over the more traditional scaled scores (mean = 10) popularized by Wechsler (e.g., Wechsler, 1949), due to the higher reliability coefficients obtained for the RIAS subtest scores. With high degrees of reliability of test scores, the use of scales that make finer discriminations among individuals is possible, producing a more desirable range of possible scores. For the convenience of researchers and examiners who wish to use other types of scores for comparative, research, or other purposes, the RIAS manual (Reynolds & Kamphaus, 2003, App. B) provides several other common types of scores for the RIAS and RIST indexes, including percentiles, *T* scores, *z* scores, normal curve equivalents, and stanines, along with a detailed explanation of each score type.

Score Reliability

Since the RIAS is a power test (i.e., items are presented in order of difficulty, from least to most difficult, and individuals' scores depend entirely on how many items they respond to correctly), the internal-consistency reliability of the items on the RIAS subtests was investigated by using Cronbach's coefficient alpha. Alpha reliability coefficients for the RIAS subtest scores and the Nunnally reliability estimates for the index scores are presented in Tables 16.2 and 16.3, respectively, for 16 age groups from the total standardization sample. The reliability estimates are rounded to two decimal places and represent the lower limits of the internal-consistency reliability of the RIAS scores.

According to the tables, 100% of the alpha coefficients for the RIAS subtest scores reach .84 or higher for every age group. As the data in Table 16.2 show, the median alpha reliability estimate for each RIAS subtest across age equals or exceeds .90. This point is important because many measurement experts recommend that reliability estimates above .80 are necessary and those above .90 are highly desirable for tests used to make decisions about individuals. All RIAS subtests meet these

TABLE 16.2. Reliability Coefficients of the RIAS Subtests by Age Group

Age (years)	Subtest					
	Guess What (GWH)	Verbal Reasoning (VRZ)	Odd-Item Out (OIO)	What's Missing (WHM)	Verbal Memory (VRM)	Nonverbal Memory (NVM)
3	.89	.84	.93	.84	.93	.93
4	.92	.87	.91	.89	.94	.93
5	.95	.86	.90	.85	.95	.94
6	.93	.86	.94	.92	.89	.96
7	.93	.89	.95	.94	.93	.96
8	.92	.88	.94	.92	.90	.95
9	.92	.90	.95	.93	.92	.96
10	.91	.88	.94	.93	.92	.96
11–12	.89	.90	.94	.93	.90	.95
13–14	.90	.92	.94	.93	.91	.96
15–16	.91	.92	.95	.92	.93	.95
17–19	.92	.92	.94	.90	.94	.90
20–34	.92	.94	.95	.93	.94	.95
35–54	.95	.94	.95	.93	.94	.96
55–74	.91	.93	.95	.91	.93	.95
75–94	.94	.93	.95	.92	.94	.96
Median	.92	.90	.94	.92	.93	.95

Note. From Reynolds and Kamphaus (2003). Copyright 2003 by Psychological Assessment Resources, Inc. Reprinted by permission.

TABLE 16.3. Reliability Estimates of the RIAS Indexes by Age Group

Age (years)	Index			
	VIX	NIX	CIX	CMX
3	.91	.92	.94	.94
4	.94	.93	.95	.95
5	.94	.92	.96	.95
6	.94	.94	.96	.94
7	.94	.95	.97	.95
8	.94	.94	.96	.93
9	.94	.95	.97	.95
10	.93	.95	.95	.95
11–12	.94	.95	.96	.93
13–14	.95	.95	.97	.95
15–16	.95	.95	.97	.95
17–19	.95	.94	.96	.93
20–34	.96	.96	.97	.96
35–54	.97	.96	.98	.97
55–74	.95	.95	.97	.95
75–94	.96	.96	.98	.97
Median	.94	.95	.96	.95

Note. VIX, Verbal Intelligence Index; NIX, Nonverbal Intelligence Index; CIX, Composite Intelligence Index; CMX, Composite Memory Index. From Reynolds and Kamphaus (2003). Copyright 2003 by Psychological Assessment Resources, Inc. Reprinted by permission.

recommended levels. As shown in Table 16.3, the reliability estimates for all RIAS indexes have median values across age that equal or exceed .94. These reliability estimates are viewed as excellent and often exceed the reliability values presented for the composite indexes or IQs of tests two or three times the length of the RIAS.

One cannot always assume that because a test is reliable for a general population, it will be equally reliable for every subgroup within that population. Therefore, test developers should demonstrate whenever possible that their test scores are indeed reliable for subgroups, especially those subgroups that because of gender, ethnic, or linguistic differences, might experience test bias (Reynolds, 2000). As noted in the *Standards for Educational and Psychological Testing* (American Educational Research Association [AERA], American Psychological Association [APA], & National Council on Measurement in Education [NCME], 1999) these values may also provide information relevant to the consequences of test use. When calculated separately for male and female examinees, the reliability coefficients are high and relatively uniform (see

Table 5.4 of Reynolds & Kamphaus, 2003, for the full table of values), with no significant differences in test score reliability at any age level as a function of gender. For male and female examinees, the RIAS subtests and the indexes are highly comparable across groups. Reliability estimates were also calculated separately for European American and African American ethnic/racial group members (see Reynolds & Kamphaus, 2003).

The stability of RIAS scores over time was investigated via the test–retest method with 86 individuals ages 3 years through 82 years. The intervals between the two test administrations ranged from 9 to 39 days, with a median test–retest interval of 16 days. The correlations for the two testings, along with mean scores and standard deviations, are reported in detail in the RIAS manual (Reynolds & Kamphaus, 2003) in Tables 5.7–5.11 for the total test–retest sample and for four age groups: 3–4 years, 5–8 years, 9–12 years, and 13–82 years. The obtained coefficients are of sufficient magnitude to allow confidence in the stability of RIAS test scores over time. In fact, the values are quite good for all of the subtests, but especially for the index scores. The uncorrected coefficients are all higher than .70, and 6 of the 10 values are in the .80s. The corrected values are even more impressive, with all but 2 values ranging from .83 to .91. When viewed across age groups, the values are generally consistent with the values obtained for the total test–retest sample.

Validity of RIAS Test Scores as Measures of Intelligence

The *Standards* volume (AERA et al., 1999, pp. 11–17) suggests a five-category scheme for organizing sources of evidence to evaluate proposed interpretations of test scores, although clearly recognizing that other organizational systems may be appropriate. The RIAS manual (Reynolds & Kamphaus, 2003) provides a thorough analysis of the currently available validity evidence associated with the RIAS/RIST scores as measures of intelligence organized according to the recommendations just noted.

Evidence Based on Test Content

Evidence with respect to the content validity of the RIAS subtests may be gleaned from the item review and item selection processes. As the *Standards* volume (AERA et al., 1999) notes, expert judgments may be used to assess agreement with test specifications and constructs in evaluating validity based on test content. During the first item tryout, a panel of minority psychologists, all with experience in assessment, reviewed all RIAS items for appropriateness as measures of their respective constructs and for applicability across various U.S. cultures. Another panel of five psychologists with doctoral degrees in school psychology, clinical psychology, clinical neuropsychology, and measurement also reviewed all items in the item pool for appropriateness. Items questioned or found faulty were either eliminated outright or modified. The RIAS items in the published version thus passed a series of judgments by expert reviewers. Final items were then chosen on the basis of traditional item statistics derived from true-score theory. Analyses of item characteristics across age, gender, and ethnicity were also undertaken to ensure appropriateness of content across various nominal groupings.

Evidence Based on Response Processes

Evidence based on the response processes of the tasks is concerned with the fit between the nature of the performance or actions in which the examinee is actually engaged and the constructs being assessed. For heavily g-loaded and memory tasks on the RIAS, the best evidence related to the response process is gleaned from an examination of these tasks themselves, as well as from their correlates (see the later section on relations to external variables).

The four RIAS intelligence subtests are designed to measure general intelligence in the verbal and nonverbal domains. As such, the tasks are complex and require the integration of multiple cognitive skills, thereby avoiding contamination by irrelevant, noncognitive response processes.

Because of their relationship to crystallized intelligence, the two verbal subtests invoke vocabulary and language comprehension. However, clearly academic or purely acquired skills such as reading are avoided. The response process requires integration of language and some general knowledge to deduce relationships; only minimal expressive language is required. One- or two-word responses are acceptable for virtually all items. The response process also is not contaminated by nonintellectual processes, such as motor acuity, speed, and coordination. Rather, problem solving through the processes of deductive and inductive reasoning is emphasized.

Likewise, the two nonverbal tasks avoid contamination by extraneous variables such as motor

acuity, speed, and coordination. Examinees have the response options of pointing or giving a one- or two-word verbal indication of the correct answer. As with any nonverbal task, some examinees may attempt to use verbal encoding to solve these tasks, and some will do so successfully. However, the tasks themselves are largely spatial and are known to be more affected by right- than by left-hemisphere impairment (e.g., Joseph, 1996; Reynolds & French, 2003)—a finding that supports the lack of verbal domination in strategies for solving such problems.

Response processes of the two RIAS memory subtests also avoid contamination from reading and various aspects of motor skills. Although good language skills undoubtedly facilitate verbal memory, they are not the dominant skills involved. The RIAS memory tasks are very straightforward, with response processes that coincide with their content domain—verbal in the Verbal Memory subtest and nonverbal in the Nonverbal Memory subtest. Even so, in the latter case, examinees who have severe motor problems may give a verbal indication of the answer they have selected.

Evidence Based on Internal Structure

The RIAS provides an index score (CIX) that purports to be a measure of g. The RIAS additionally provides indexes that focus on verbal ability (VIX), a construct closely related to crystallized intelligence, and nonverbal ability (NIX), a construct closely related to fluid intelligence. A separate memory index (CMX) is also provided. The CIX, which is derived from the four intelligence subtests of the RIAS, presupposes a common underlying construct that reflects overall intelligence. The other index scores likewise presuppose some meaningful, identifiable dimension underlying their construction. The extent to which a composite score can be evaluated internally is directly related to the dimensionality of the scores that make up the composite. Therefore, evidence based on the internal structure of the RIAS is provided from two sources: item coherence (or internal consistency), and factor analyses of the intercorrelations of the subtests. The internal-consistency evidence has been reviewed in the section on the reliability of test scores derived from the RIAS. Factor analysis is another method of examining the internal structure of a scale that lends itself to assessing the validity of recommended score interpretations.

Factor analysis is a common method of examining the patterns of relationships among a set of variables. It is a commonly recommended analytical approach to evaluating the presence and structure of any latent constructs among a set of variables, such as subtest scores on a test battery (see Cronbach, 1990; Kamphaus, 2001). Two methods of factor analysis have been applied to the intercorrelation matrix of the RIAS subtests—first with only the four intelligence subtests examined, and then with all six subtests examined under both techniques of analysis. Exploratory analyses were undertaken first and were followed by a set of confirmatory analyses to assess the relative goodness of fit of the chosen exploratory results to mathematically optimal models. For the exploratory factor analyses, the method of *principal factors* was chosen. In such analyses, the first unrotated factor to be extracted is commonly interpreted as g. The correlations of each subtest with this factor (i.e., the factor loadings) are indicators of the degree to which each subtest measures general intelligence as opposed to more specific components of ability.

For purposes of factor analyses of the RIAS subtests' intercorrelations, the sample was divided into five age groups (rather than 1-year interval groups) to enhance the stability and the generalizability of the factor analyses of the RIAS scores. These age groupings reflect common developmental stages. The five age groupings were early childhood, ages 3 years through 5 years; childhood, ages 6 years through 11 years; adolescence,

ages 12 years through 18 years; adulthood, ages 19 years through 54 years; and senior adulthood, ages 55 years through 94 years. A Pearson correlation between each possible pair of RIAS subtest scores within each age level was determined, and factor analyses were performed.

When the two-factor and three-factor solutions were subsequently obtained, the two-factor varimax solution made the most psychological and psychometric sense for both the set of four intelligence subtests and for all six RIAS subtests. In the four-subtest three-factor solution, no variables consistently defined the third factor across the four age groupings. In the six-subtest three-factor solutions, singlet factors (i.e., factors with a single salient loading) appeared, commonly representing a memory subtest; What's Missing tended to behave in an unstable manner as well. Summaries of the two-factor varimax solutions are presented for the four-subtest and six-subtest analyses in Table 16.4. In each case, the first, unrotated factor is a representation of g as measured by the RIAS.

The g factor of the RIAS is quite strong. Only the intelligence subtests have loadings that reach into the .70s and .80s. All four intelligence subtests are good measures of g; however, of the four, the verbal subtests are the strongest. Odd-Item Out and What's Missing follow, the latter being the weakest measure of g among the four intelligence subtests. The strength of the first unrotated factor

TABLE 16.4. Two-Factor Solutions for the Four-Subtest and Six-Subtest Analyses of the RIAS

Subtest	g^a 3–5 years	6–11 years	12–18 years	19–54 years	55–94 years	Factor 1 3–5 years	6–11 years	12–18 years	19–54 years	55–94 years	Factor 2 3–5 years	6–11 years	12–18 years	19–54 years	55–94 years
RIAS intelligence subtest loadings from a principal-factors solution by age group															
Guess What	.71	.77	.88	.87	.82	.66	.73	.78	.74	.65	.34	.32	.44	.48	.50
Verbal Reasoning	.78	.81	.85	.84	.85	.69	.74	.78	.73	.80	.40	.37	.39	.45	.38
Odd-Item Out	.70	.60	.60	.73	.74	.36	.32	.30	.42	.50	.63	.57	.58	.62	.55
What's Missing	.60	.49	.63	.66	.69	.30	.21	.32	.36	.33	.58	.53	.60	.60	.67
RIAS intelligence and memory subtest loadings from a principal-factors solution by age group															
Guess What	.70	.77	.84	.82	.82	.66	.74	.77	.77	.68	.29	.33	.38	.35	.47
Verbal Reasoning	.79	.79	.86	.83	.83	.78	.70	.83	.78	.76	.29	.39	.34	.36	.40
Odd-Item Out	.67	.63	.58	.71	.74	.41	.26	.23	.44	.48	.57	.67	.64	.58	.57
What's Missing	.59	.44	.57	.64	.68	.37	.21	.38	.46	.32	.47	.44	.43	.45	.66
Verbal Memory	.54	.48	.41	.58	.60	.51	.48	.40	.49	.56	.22	.18	.15	.31	.28
Nonverbal Memory	.49	.48	.57	.66	.61	.16	.23	.26	.28	.31	.59	.47	.59	.71	.56

Note. From Reynolds and Kamphaus (2003). Copyright 2003 by Psychological Assessment Resources, Inc. Adapted by permission.
g^a, or general intelligence factor, reported as the subtests' loadings on the first unrotated principal factor. Loadings for both factor 1 and factor 2 are those following varimax rotation.

is, however, indisputable; it indicates that first and foremost, the RIAS intelligence subtests are measures of g, and that the strongest interpretive support is given in these analyses to the CIX. At the same time, the varimax rotation of the two-factor solution clearly delineates two components of the construct of g among the RIAS intelligence subtests. For every age group, the verbal and nonverbal subtests clearly break into two distinct factors that coincide with their respective indexes, VIX and NIX. The six-subtest solution also breaks along content dimensions, with Verbal Memory joining the two verbal intelligence subtests on the first rotated factor, and Nonverbal Memory joining the two nonverbal intelligence subtests on the second rotated factor. However, in view of the analysis of the content and response processes as well as other evidence presented throughout the RIAS manual (Reynolds & Kamphaus, 2003), it remains sensible to separate the Verbal Memory and Nonverbal Memory subtests into a separate memory index (i.e., CMX). This decision is further supported by the outcomes of a recent analysis of the RIAS factor structure demonstrating the alignment of the subtests with their factors and the separation of the CMX from the others (Dombrowski, Watkins, & Brogan, 2009). Memory is clearly a component of intelligence. The two memory tasks that were chosen for the RIAS are relatively complex, and both are strong predictors of broader composites of verbal and nonverbal memory (Reynolds & Bigler, 1994)—characteristics that are at once an asset and a liability. Although these two memory tasks are good measures of overall or general memory skill, they tend to correlate more highly with intelligence test scores than do very simple, confrontational measures of working memory, such as digit repetition. Given the purpose of providing a highly reliable assessment of overall memory skill, such a compromise is warranted.

The stability of the two-factor solution across other relevant nominal groupings and the potential for cultural bias in the internal structure of the RIAS were also assessed. For this purpose, the factor analyses were also calculated separately for males and females and for European Americans and African Americans, according to recommendations and procedures outlined in detail by Reynolds (2000). Tables 6.3–6.6 in Reynolds and Kamphaus (2003) present these results for each comparison. The similarity of the factor-analytic results across gender and across ethnicity was also assessed. Two indexes of factorial similarity were calculated for the visually matched rotated factors

and for the first unrotated factor—the coefficient of congruence (r_c) and Cattell's (1978) salient variable similarity index—as recommended in several sources (e.g., Reynolds, 2000). In all cases, the factor structure of the RIAS was found to be highly consistent across gender and ethnicity.

Subsequent to the exploratory factor analyses, several confirmatory factor analyses were conducted to examine the fit of exploratory analyses to a more purely mathematical model (see Reynolds & Kamphaus, 2003, for table values and a thorough discussion). Based on the theoretical views of the structure of the RIAS discussed earlier in this chapter, three theoretical models were tested. The models were defined as follows: (1) The RIAS is a measure of general intellectual abilities; (2) the RIAS is a measure of verbal and nonverbal abilities; and (3) the RIAS is a measure of verbal, nonverbal, and memory abilities.

The resulting chi-square (χ^2), residuals, root mean square error of approximation (RMSEA), and other model-fitting statistics were then compared; the LISREL-VI program (Joreskog & Sorbom, 1987) was used to test the relative fit of the three models. Model 1, general intelligence, clearly fit better when only the four intelligence subtests were included ($\chi^2 = 8.17$ to 20.57 and RMSEA ranging from .10 to .14, depending on the age range studied) than when six subtests were included. Although these models suggested, much in the same way as the exploratory factor analyses showed, that the RIAS is dominated by a large first factor, the RMSEAs were still high enough to suggest that models 2 and 3 should be explored.

Model 2 was a very good fit to the data, particularly when four subtests were included in the model versus six subtests. For the model that included four subtests, the chi-square values were between .22 and 1.49. Similarly, the RMSEAs were less than .01 for the first four age groups (i.e., 3 years to 54 years) and .04 for ages 55 years and older—values suggesting that two factors explained virtually all of the variance between the four subtests. These findings indicated that the fit of a three-factor model was not likely to be as good.

In fact, model 3 with six subtests included ($\chi^2 = 14.14$ to 37.48, and RMSEA ranging from .01 to .09) did not fit nearly as well as model 2. There were some indications that the six-subtest two-factor model was also plausible for the population 19 years and older. Although the four-subtest two-factor model is recommended, these results suggest that use of all six subtests for assessing verbal and nonverbal intelligence may be defensible for adults as well. In cases where memory problems are part of the referral question for adults, the use of six subtests may be beneficial; however, integrating the memory subtests into the VIX and NIX is not recommended. With clinical populations, we continue to prefer the division of the RIAS subtests into the VIX, NIX, and CMX, even though placing the memory subtests into the VIX and NIX may have a reasonable mathematical foundation in the confirmatory factor analyses.

In summary, the results of the confirmatory factor analyses suggest that the CIX, VIX, and NIX possess evidence of factorial validity. The CMX, in particular, requires further research with a variety of clinical and nonclinical samples. Although factor-analytic results are often open to alternate interpretations, it is our opinion, based on the findings just described as well as the conceptual distinctions we have drawn previously, that it is best not to use all six subtests to measure general intelligence.

Evidence Based on Relations with Other (External) Variables

Another important area in the validation process is the evaluation of the relationship of scores on the instrument of interest to variables that are external to the test itself. This evaluation may include, for example, relationships with other tests that measure similar or dissimilar constructs, diagnostic categorizations, and relationships with developmental constructs such as age. The *Standards* volume (AERA et al., 1999) emphasizes that a wide range of variables are of potential interest, and that different relationships will have different degrees of importance to examiners who work in different settings or are using the test for different purposes. As with other areas of evidence, test users ultimately have the responsibility of evaluating the evidence and determining its saliency and adequacy for their own intended use of the instrument. Several different external variables were chosen for investigation with the RIAS, including developmental variables (i.e., age), demographic variables, relations with other tests, and clinical status.

Developmental Trends

As a developmental construct, intellectual ability grows rapidly in the early years, begins to plateau in the teens but shows some continued growth (particularly in verbal domains), and eventually declines in the older years. This decline generally begins sooner and is more dramatic for nonverbal, or fluid, intelligence (Kaufman, McLean, Kaufman-Packer, & Reynolds, 1991; Kaufman, Reynolds, & McLean, 1989; Reynolds, Chastain, Kaufman, & McLean, 1987). If raw scores on the tasks of the RIAS reflect such a developmental process or attribute, then relationships with age should be evident. The relationship between age (a variable external to the RIAS) and performance on the RIAS was investigated in two ways.

First, the correlation between age and raw score for each subtest was calculated for the primary developmental stage, ages 3 years through 18 years. The correlations for all groups were uniformly large, typically exceeding .80 and demonstrating that raw scores on the RIAS increase with age and in a relatively constant manner across subtests (see Reynolds & Kamphaus, 2003). To examine the issue in more detail, lifespan developmental curves were generated for each subtest from ages 3 years through 94 years. These curves are presented in the RIAS manual (Reynolds & Kamphaus, 2003) and show a consistent pattern of score increases and declines (with aging) across all groups.

Correlations with the Wechsler Scales

Edwards and Paulin (2007) found that the RIAS indexes all correlated highly with the Wechsler Intelligence Scale for Children—Fourth Edition (WISC-IV; Wechsler, 2003) Full Scale IQ (FSIQ), with correlations ranging from a low of .60 (NIX–FSIQ) to a high of .78 (VIX–FSIQ). The pattern of correlations was much as predicted; namely, the highest correlations were between those aspects of the tests most closely associated with *g* (from their respective factor analyses).

In another study, a group of 31 adults were administered the RIAS and the Wechsler Adult Intelligence Scale—Third Edition (WAIS-III; Wechsler, 1997) in a counterbalanced design. All but two of the correlations exceeded .70; the VIX–PIQ correlation was the lowest at .61. All of the RIAS indexes correlated at or above .70 with the WAIS-III FSIQ. Furthermore, there were no significant differences among any of the correlations. This finding is most likely a function of the *g* saturation of both the RIAS and WAIS-III. These findings were corroborated by a recent comparison of the RIAS and the WAIS-III, where the scales on the two measures were found to have the following correlations: CIX–FSIQ, .94; VIX–VIQ, .89; NIX–PIQ, .88 (Umphress & Taylor, 2008). Functionally, both the RIAS and WAIS-III appear to measure the same intelligence constructs.

Correlations with the Woodcock–Johnson III Tests of Cognitive Abilities

Krach, Loe, Jones, and Farrally (2009) found that the RIAS indexes also correlated highly with the Woodcock–Johnson III Tests of Cognitive Abilities (WJ III COG; Woodcock, McGrew, & Mather, 2001). Correlations ranged from a low of .54 (Gf–NIX) to a high of .88 (Gc–CIX). The WJ III COG relies on the use of abstract geometric structures and colors for the Gf scale, in contrast to the use of many concrete items as seen on the subtests used to derive the NIX.

Correlations with Measures of Academic Achievement

One of the major reasons for the development of the early, individually administered intelligence tests was to predict academic achievement levels. Intelligence tests have done well as predictors of school learning, with typical correlations in the mid-.50s and .60s (for summaries, see Kamphaus, 2001; Sattler, 2001). To evaluate the relationship between the RIAS and academic achievement, 78 children and adolescents were administered the RIAS and the Wechsler Individual Achievement Test (WIAT; Wechsler, 1992).

School learning is fundamentally a language-related task, and this fact is clearly evident in these data. Although all of the RIAS indexes correlated well with all of the WIAT composite scores, the highest correlations were consistently between the VIX and CIX and the WIAT composites. These correlations were predominantly in the .60s and .70s, indicating that the RIAS has strong predictive value for educational achievement.

Evidence Based on the Consequences of Testing

The final area of the validation process is the most controversial of all the aspects of this process, as presented in the *Standards* volume (AERA et al., 1999). It is most applicable to tests designed for selection and may deal with issues of bias or loss of opportunity. How these applications should be evaluated for clinical diagnostic tests is largely unclear. However, accurate diagnosis might be one anticipated consequence of testing and should be

the key to evaluating the "consequential" validity of a clinical instrument. The evidence reviewed in the preceding sections demonstrates the ability of the RIAS to provide an accurate estimate of intellectual ability and certain memory skills, and to do so accurately across such nominal groupings as gender and ethnicity. Cultural biases in the format and content of tests, when apparent, have also been found to produce undue consequences of testing. Evidence pointing toward a lack of cultural bias in the RIAS is extensive for male and female examinees, as well as for European Americans, African Americans, and Hispanic Americans. This evidence has been provided previously in this chapter and in Chapter 4 of the RIAS manual (Reynolds & Kamphaus, 2003), where results of item bias studies are reported. The studies of potential cultural bias in the RIAS items were extensive in both objective and subjective formats and resulted in the removal of many items and modification of others, as described in detail in the manual. Evidence based on consequences is thus supportive, but work remains to be done in this arena, particularly with as yet unstudied ethnic groups.

In evaluating evidence for test score interpretations, examiners must always consider their purposes for using objective tests. Evidence clearly supports the use of the constructs represented on the RIAS. The potential consequences of knowing how an individual's performance compares to that of others are many and complex, and are not always anticipated. The RIAS was designed to eliminate or minimize any cultural biases in the assessment of intelligence and memory for individuals reared and educated in the United States (who are fluent in the English language). The data available to date indicate that the RIAS precludes undue consequences toward diverse individuals who fit the target population. Examiners must nevertheless act wisely, consider the need for objective testing of intelligence and memory, and work to minimize or eliminate unsupported interpretations of scores on such tests.

CRITIQUES OF THE RIAS

Much as other standardized instruments have been, the RIAS has been the focus of some criticisms (Beaujean, McGlaughlin, & Margulies, 2009; Nelson, Canivez, Lindstrom, & Hatt, 2007). Most of these have centered on the methods utilized to determine the validity of the VIX, NIX, CIX, and CMX scales. Limitations of the research conducted that has challenged the validity of the RIAS include the use of both small sample sizes and specific populations. Thus it is difficult to determine whether the findings of these critiques are generalizable. Researchers, however, have urged continuing investigation of the validity of RIAS score inferences because of the test's promising features (Beaujean et al., 2009; Edwards & Paulin, 2007; Nelson et al., 2007).

APPLICATIONS OF THE RIAS

As a measure of intelligence, the RIAS is appropriate for a wide array of purposes and should be useful when assessment of an examinee's intellectual level is needed. The RIAS will be useful with preschool and school-age children for purposes of educational placement, as well as for diagnosis of various forms of childhood psychopathology (especially developmental disorders) where intellectual functioning is an issue. Diagnosis of specific disorders—such as intellectual disabilities, learning disabilities, the various dementias, and the effects of central nervous system (CNS) injury or compromise—most often calls for the use of an intelligence test as a component of patient evaluation, and the RIAS is appropriate for such applications. Clinicians who perform general clinical and neuropsychological evaluations will find the RIAS very useful when a measure of intelligence is needed. Practitioners will also find the RIAS useful in disability determinations under various state and federal programs, such as the Social Security Administration's disability program and Section 504 regulations. The RIAS was already being used consistently in such disability exams almost immediately following its publication (M. Shapiro, personal communication, April 2003).

Although the RIAS is rapid to administer, relative to the majority of other comprehensive measures of intelligence, it is not an abbreviated measure or a short form of intellectual assessment. The RIAS is regarded as an instrument that "substantially lessens the time to assess intelligence without compromising statistical integrity" (Elliot, 2004, p. 328). The RIAS is a comprehensive measure of verbal and nonverbal intelligence and of general intelligence, providing the same level of useful information often gleaned from much longer intelligence tests. When the memory subtests are also administered, the RIAS can provide even more useful information than typical intelligence tests currently used.

The major clinical uses of intelligence tests are generally classification (most commonly, diagnostic) and selection. The RIAS has broad applicability in each of these areas. Some of the more common uses in these areas are discussed here.

Learning Disabilities

For the evaluation of a learning disability, assessment of intelligence is a common activity. However, when a child or adult is evaluated for the possible presence of a learning disability, both verbal and nonverbal intelligence should be assessed. Individuals with learning disabilities may have spuriously deflated IQ estimates in one or the other domain, due to the learning disabilities themselves. Lower verbal ability is the more common type of learning disability in the school population and among adjudicated delinquents (Kaufman, 1994). However, the concept of nonverbal learning disabilities is gaining momentum. For individuals with such disabilities, verbal ability will often exceed nonverbal ability. The assessment of functioning in both areas is important, and the RIAS provides a reliable assessment of these domains, as well as a composite intelligence index.

Intellectual Disabilities

Most definitions—including those of the American Association on Intellectual and Developmental Disabilities (2009) and the *Diagnostic and Statistical Manual of Mental Disorders*, fourth edition, text revision (DSM-IV-TR; American Psychiatric Association, 2000)—require the administration of an individually administered test of intelligence for diagnosis of an intellectual disability. The RIAS is applicable to this diagnosis, for which the evaluation of verbal and nonverbal intelligence as well as adaptive functioning is necessary. Intellectual disabilities are pervasive problems and not limited to serious problems in only the verbal or nonverbal domain. The range of scores available on the RIAS will also make it useful in distinguishing levels of severity of intellectual disabilities. Lower levels of functioning, such as profound intellectual disability, are difficult to assess accurately on nearly all tests of intelligence; this is likewise true of the RIAS. Although normed on children as young as 3 years of age, the RIAS also has limited discriminative ability below mild levels of intellectual disability in the 3-year-old age group.

Intellectual Giftedness

Many definitions of giftedness include reference to superior levels of performance on measures of intelligence. Here again, measures of both the verbal and nonverbal domains are useful, due to the influences of schooling and educational opportunity on verbal intelligence. The range of index scores available on the RIAS is adequate at all ages for identifying persons with significantly above-average levels of overall intellectual functioning, as well as in the verbal and nonverbal domains.

Physical/Orthopedic Impairment

The RIAS will be particularly useful in the evaluation of intellectual functioning among individuals with any significant degree of physical or motor impairment. The RIAS has no real demands for speed or accuracy of fine motor movements. If necessary, the pointing responses by the examinee on the RIAS nonverbal tasks can all be replaced with simple verbal responses, designating the location of the chosen response. It is, however, very important for an examiner to have knowledge of the physical impairments of any examinee and to make any necessary modifications in the testing environment, doing so in a manner consistent with appropriate professional standards (e.g., the *Standards for Educational and Psychological Testing*; AERA et al., 1999).

Neuropsychological and Memory Impairment

The information gleaned from evaluating memory functions can provide valuable clinical information above and beyond what is traditionally obtained with IQ measures. Memory is generally recognized as a focal or discreet subset of cognitive functions, and as such is often quite vulnerable to CNS trauma and various other CNS events. Disturbances of memory and attention are the two most frequent complaints of children and adults following traumatic brain injury at all levels of severity, as well as other forms of CNS compromise (e.g., viral meningitis, AIDS dementia complex, and other systemic insults). Therefore, it is not unusual for memory functioning to be affected, even when there is little or no impact on general intellectual ability. The memory measures on the RIAS offer clinicians

valuable assessment tools with which to evaluate recent or more immediate memory functioning in both the auditory (i.e., verbal memory) and visual (i.e., nonverbal memory) modalities.

Emotional Disturbance

Individuals with various forms of emotional and/ or psychotic disturbance (e.g., depression, schizophrenia) may exhibit cognitive impairments to varying degrees. Often clinicians do not assess the intelligence of such individuals because of the time required to do so. The RIAS offers clinicians a more efficient means of gathering information on the psychometric intelligence of individuals with emotional problems.

Job Performance

In personnel settings, IQ tests are sometimes used to predict success in job training programs; in other instances, lower limits are set on IQ levels for specific jobs. The RIAS and the RIST are strong predictors of academic performance, and the tasks involved and constructs assessed on these instruments match up well with known predictors of job performance in the form of other IQ tests. When intelligence level is a question in such situations, the RIAS and the RIST are appropriate choices.

CASE STUDY (ABBREVIATED)

Carl Last, age 6, was referred to the clinic by his parents, Jamie and Harold Last, for a psychoeducational evaluation. Carl's parents are concerned about his behavioral, emotional, and academic functioning. Six months prior to the current evaluation, Carl was diagnosed with attention and anxiety disorders. The Lasts are interested in verifying these diagnoses and hope to find out whether Carl is experiencing learning problems. Mr. and Mrs. Last are interested in receiving a better understanding of his difficulties, so that they can help him be successful in school and at home.

Parent Interview

Carl's past medical history includes colic, occasional constipation, and complaints of itchy skin. Currently, Carl is in good physical health and wears glasses for corrective vision while reading. Mr. Last reported that results of Carl's previous hearing screenings have been within normal limits, but that his hearing has not been checked recently. Family history is significant for a variety of health problems.

According to Mr. Last, Carl has always been a hyperactive child. He reported that Carl "learned to hop before he could walk" and frequently bounces when he is excited. Furthermore, he noted that Carl has not taken naps since the age of 2 and is overly active, such as rocking back and forth and fidgeting with things in his hands. Mr. Last also noted that Carl often waves his fingers back and forth, especially when he is frustrated or doing an undesirable activity. Mr. Last indicated that Carl's rocking and finger waving could be due to anxiety related to school, as he often engages in these behaviors when doing school activities. Mrs. Last indicated that in addition to hyperactivity, Carl is easily distracted and pays too much attention to minute details. She described Carl as making many careless mistakes and answering questions impulsively.

In addition, Mr. Last reported that Carl displays atypical and compulsive behaviors. Carl has specific places for all of his belongings; he is disturbed when things are misplaced and must immediately return them to their desired place. Moreover, Mrs. Last indicated that Carl is "anal" at times about organization and neatness, and insists on placing his belongings (such as his trophies) in a perfect line. She noted that Carl engages in cleaning rituals one or two times a month. Mrs. Last described the cleaning as repetitive, with Carl frequently moving objects as if they are "just not quite right." Mr. Last also indicated that Carl says phrases repetitively, such as muttering a phrase he has heard to himself over and over.

In addition to difficulties with hand washing, cleaning, and repetitive speech patterns, Mr. Last noted that Carl has unusual feelings and spells where he stares blankly. Specifically, Carl often claims, "Here comes that feeling. I don't like that feeling." At this point, Carl closes his eyes and is still for a couple of seconds until the feeling passes. He describes the experience as feeling "all shivery in my body and my brain." These experiences have occurred since Carl was 2 or 3 years old; they currently fluctuate from happening a couple of times a week to a couple of times a day. Mr. Last also reported that a couple of times a month, Carl appears to lose touch with reality and stares blankly for a few minutes. When he comes out of the stares, he does not rejoin the conversation in a normal matter; instead, he frequently asks about details from the past.

The Lasts reported that during kindergarten and first grade, Carl has experienced difficulties with inattention and concentration—specifically, problems with following directions and staying focused. The Lasts indicated that due to these problems, Carl has had difficulty with reading comprehension and formerly received tutoring services after school. They are currently not concerned about his reading performance. Carl is currently receiving B's and C's.

Behavioral Observations

Carl appeared for the evaluation well groomed and appropriately dressed on both days of testing. Consistent with the reports from his parents, Carl was hyperactive. He frequently rocked back and forth repetitively in his seat and moved about the testing room on occasion. He fidgeted with his hands during most of the 2-day evaluation, often rolling a pencil back and forth on his legs. At times, Carl seemed focused on the breaks that he was allowed during testing; he frequently asked to take a break. He engaged in age-appropriate social interaction and was generally well behaved throughout the sessions. He seemed comfortable with the examiners, and rapport was easily established. Carl required frequent redirection to the task at hand, but upon redirection he could maintain focus. He answered questions impulsively and was talkative throughout the evaluation.

Overall, Carl presented himself as well behaved and cooperative during testing. He seemed engaged in most testing procedures and appeared to put forth his best effort. Results of the evaluation are viewed as valid estimates of Carl's intellectual abilities, academic achievement, and social-emotional adjustment.

Teacher Interview

Carl's teacher, Mrs. Taylor, provided information regarding his overall functioning in the school setting. She noted that Carl is having learning problems, specifically with reading and reading comprehension. During the teacher interview, Mrs. Taylor noted that Carl has made adequate progress throughout the school year, but still seems to be having difficulties with reading. She indicated that Carl was hyperactive in the beginning of the year, but appears to have calmed down somewhat. However, she noted that he often does not seem relaxed and appears to feel "uncomfortable in his own body." Mrs. Taylor indicated that Carl's attention is variable, depending on the nature of the task; however, she noted that he often fails to give close attention to his assignments, such as failing to go back and check his work. Mrs. Taylor noted that Carl is well liked by his peers and does not have any behavior problems.

Intelligence Testing

The RIAS and the Wechsler Abbreviated Scale of Intelligence (WASI) were given to evaluate Carl's intelligence. As Table 16.5 indicates, Carl earned a low average to average RIAS VIX score of 89 (23rd percentile) and an average NIX score of 105 (63rd percentile). Taken together, the VIX and NIX scores yielded a CIX score of 95 (37th percentile), which falls in the average range. There was significant scatter within RIAS subtests, with scores ranging from high average to below average (see Table 16.6). For example, Carl had difficulty on a verbal subtest requiring him to complete verbal analogies, earning a below-average score. There is a significant discrepancy between Carl's verbal and performance intellectual ability scores, suggesting that his nonverbal reasoning skills as measured by the RIAS are more highly developed. Carl earned an average CMX score of 107, indicating that he has an average ability to learn and remember material.

Due to the considerable scatter on the subtests of the RIAS, Carl was administered the WASI as a second measure of cognitive ability. This instrument is an abbreviated version of the WISC-III. Carl earned a Verbal composite score of 98 (45th percentile), which falls in the average range. His score of 78 (7th percentile, significantly below-average range) on the Performance component was

TABLE 16.5. Carl's Composite Scores on the RIAS

Composites	Standard score	Confidence interval	Percentile
VIX	89	84–95	23rd
NIX	105	99–110	63rd
CIX	95	90–109	37th
CMX	107	101–112	68th

Note. The RIAS yields standard scores with a mean of 100 and a standard deviation of 15. Standard scores between 85 and 115, which include 68% of the general population, are considered to be within the average range.

TABLE 16.6. Carl's Subtest Scores on the RIAS

Subtest	Age-adjusted *T* score
Guess What	49
Odd-Item Out	57
Verbal Reasoning	33
What's Missing	47
Verbal Memory	48
Nonverbal Memory	59

significantly different from his Verbal IQ. Again, Carl's performance was variable and produced significant subtest scatter. Carl's Performance IQ was negatively affected by the timed nature of the Block Design task. Qualitatively, it was noticed that Carl was not interested by the blocks and was inattentive and off task during this subtest. He earned a significantly below-average score on this subtest, which affected his overall Performance IQ. Verbal and Performance IQ scores combined to yield an overall Full Scale IQ of 86, which is considered to be low average when compared to that of his same-age peers.

Overall, Carl appears to be functioning in the average to low average range of intelligence and conceptual reasoning skills. His performance seems to be adversely affected by difficulties with attention and off-task behaviors. During administration of both the RIAS and the WASI, Carl answered questions impulsively, failing to listen to detailed directions for the tasks. His scores on both verbal and performance tasks were variable, depending on the nature of each task. In general, however, Carl should be able to make age-appropriate progress in learning and remembering new information, given his cognitive abilities.

Parent and Teacher Rating Scales

Carl's mother and father both completed the Behavior Assessment System for Children—Parent Rating Scales (BASC-PRS), and Mr. Last completed the Conners Parent Rating Scale—Revised: Long Version (CPRS-R:L). On the BASC-PRS, they rated Carl as having attention problems in the at-risk range. Specifically, they indicated that Carl is easily distracted and sometimes has difficulties with listening to directions, completing work on time, listening attentively, and forgetfulness. In order to help clarify the results of the BASC-PRS, Carl's father also completed the CPRS-R:L. Although ratings were within the average range, Mr. Last endorsed items indicative of inattention and cognitive problems, such as failing to give close attention to details and making careless mistakes. This is consistent with information obtained during the parent interview.

Mrs. Taylor, Carl's first-grade teacher, completed the Behavior Assessment System for Children—Teacher Rating Scales (BASC-TRS) to evaluate his attentional skills. Mrs. Taylor did not rate him as having any clinically significant problems with attention on the BASC-TRS. However, she noted that Carl is easily distracted from classwork and often has trouble concentrating. Furthermore, during her interview, she noted (as indicated earlier) that Carl often does not pay close attention to his assignments, failing to check over his work for any potential errors. It should be noted that both the parents and the teacher completed their rating scales after Carl had been on medication for a substantial amount of time. Therefore, it is possible that ratings of attention, which were below the clinically significant level, were influenced by the positive effects noticed since Carl has been taking atomoxetine hydrochloride (Strattera). Carl's parents and teacher indicated that they have noticed an increased ability to sustain attention and concentrate since he began taking Strattera. From the conversations with the teacher and parents, as well as the rating scales, however, it seems that Carl is still having difficulty with inattention. These difficulties are interfering with his ability to perform in the classroom and at home.

Achievement Testing

Broad reading, basic reading skills, and reading comprehension were assessed by the Woodcock–Johnson III Tests of Achievement (WJ III ACH). Carl's overall reading achievement was commensurate with his overall intellectual functioning as measured by the RIAS and the WASI. Carl demonstrated average letter–word identification skills, average passage comprehension skills, and low average skills on a subtest measuring reading fluency or speed. These scores combined to form a WJ III Broad Reading Composite of 89 (24th percentile), which is in the average to low average range. Carl's decoding skills were assessed through a portion of the WJ III ACH. He was asked to pronounce nonwords to further measure phonic and structural analysis skills in the Word Attack subtest. This subtest assessed Carl's ability to match sound blends to letter combinations. Carl was asked to read such nonwords as *zoop* and *rox*. He earned a standard score of 102 (55th percentile), a score in the average range of functioning. These scores suggest that Carl's overall reading achievement falls within age-appropriate limits.

Carl's basic writing skills, such as spelling, sentence construction, and writing fluency, were also assessed by the WJ III ACH. The Spelling subtest measured Carl's ability to write orally presented words correctly. Carl earned an average to low average standard score of 88. The Writing Fluency subtest measured his skill in formulating and writing short, simple sentences quickly. He earned a standard score of 91, which is in the average range. Carl was also asked to produce writing samples consisting of a sentence describing a given picture or using specific words. On this Writing Samples subtest, Carl earned an 84, in the low average range. He did not appear to be paying attention to the task or directions. When asked to write sentences, he frequently wrote fragments or single words. Overall, Carl demonstrated average to low average writing abilities. His lack of attention to the directions of the task had an adverse impact on his writing scores.

Carl's mathematical skills, such as calculation, applied problems, and math fluency, were likewise assessed with the WJ III ACH. Carl earned a significantly below-average score on the Calculation subtest (72, 3rd percentile); a below-average score on the Math Fluency subtest (77, 6th percentile); and a low-average score on the Applied Problems subtest (84, 15th percentile). When these subtests were examined, it was noticed that Carl failed to give close attention to detail, specifically regarding the addition or subtraction signs. For example, on the Math Fluency portion, which required him to do simple addition and subtraction quickly, Carl added all of the numbers. He was given oral instructions to pay attention to the signs, but Carl did not take notice of the changing signs.

Overall, achievement testing indicates that Carl's academic achievement is in the average to low average range and is consistent with his general cognitive ability. Carl demonstrated age-appropriate reading, writing, and mathematics skills. However, he failed to pay close attention to details and listen attentively to directions. Again, Carl's inattention seems to be having a negative impact on his academic performance.

Behavioral, Social, and Emotional Functioning

In order to better understand Carl's functioning across behavioral, social, and emotional domains, several measures of social and emotional functioning were given. As noted earlier, Mr. and Mrs. Last completed the BASC-PRS, and Mr. Last completed the CPRS-R:L. Also as noted earlier, Carl's teacher, Mrs. Taylor, was interviewed and completed the BASC-TRS to provide information regarding Carl's social, emotional, and behavioral functioning at school. Finally, Carl himself was interviewed and completed two self-report measures—the Revised Children's Manifest Anxiety Scale (RCMAS) and the Children's Depression Inventory (CDI)—to discern his thoughts and feelings regarding numerous issues. The results of these latter two measures suggested that Carl generally perceives himself as a well-adjusted child. He reported that he is happy with himself, his family, and his friends. He further indicated that he enjoys school and likes his teacher. He does not indicate any significant problems with depression or anxiety. However, during the child interview, Carl noted that he is sometimes afraid of nightmares, blood, and skulls.

Mr. and Mrs. Last indicated that Carl demonstrates problems with hyperactivity, attention, perfectionism, and atypicality. Mrs. Taylor, Carl's first-grade teacher, also endorsed items indicative of difficulties with hyperactivity, attention, and atypicality. In the area of hyperactivity, Mr. Last indicated that Carl often talks excessively, is overly active, fidgets with his hands, and has difficulty playing in leisure activities quietly. Furthermore, the Lasts noted that Carl often interrupts others when they are speaking and occasionally blurts out answers to questions before the questions have been completed. Mrs. Taylor rated Carl as being overly active and often tapping his foot or pencil. She further indicated that at times he hurries through assignments, is unable to wait his turn, and acts without thinking. These symptoms of hyperactivity and impulsivity are consistent with information obtained during the parent interview and with observations of Carl during testing.

Carl's parents and teacher all also noted that Carl is displaying atypical behaviors. For example, they indicated that Carl will repeat one activity or thought over and over, and that he stares blankly at times. Furthermore, they noted that Carl often rocks back and forth and waves his fingers repeatedly when he seems excited. During time spent

at the clinic, Carl indeed frequently rocked back and forth in his seat during testing. The Lasts also indicated that Carl complains about being unable to block out unwanted thoughts and feelings. For example, Carl often claims that he gets "shivery" feelings that he does not like and that he cannot block out. Moreover, the Lasts described Carl as having an acute sense of hearing and as often hearing sounds that they do not hear. They also described Carl as "particular" and endorsed items suggesting that he displays perfectionistic behaviors. Specifically, Mr. Last noted that everything has to be just right, that he gets upset if someone rearranges his things, and that things must be done the same way every time. This information is consistent with that obtained during the parent interview, when Mr. Last described obsessive–compulsive behaviors. In addition, the Lasts described Carl as repetitively cleaning and lining up his belongings, and they indicated past difficulties with hand washing. During time spent at the clinic, Carl was observed going to the bathroom to wash his hands after playing with bubbles that made his hands "smell like throw-up." Furthermore, Mrs. Taylor indicated that Carl went to the bathroom more frequently than his classmates, approximately six times a day. The teacher also noted that Carl's desk is very organized, but that she did not see this neatness or his trips to the bathroom as interfering with his schoolwork. Similarly, the Lasts noted that Carl's compulsive behaviors are not having a significant impact on his functioning at home. Overall, Carl appears to be experiencing problems with hyperactivity and inattention, and is displaying some atypical behaviors.

Summary

The results of this evaluation reveal that Carl's developed intelligence is in the average to low average range. This suggests that Carl will be able to benefit from instruction, although difficulties with attention, impulsivity, and off-task behaviors are affecting his daily school performance. Carl is demonstrating average perceptual and visual–motor skills commensurate with cognitive functioning. Carl is functioning in the average to significantly below-average range on tests of attention and executive functioning measuring his ability to plan, organize, and regulate his mental activity. Specifically, Carl appears to have difficulty paying attention to speech sounds and using attention to hold and process information. Carl's difficulties with attention and executive functioning are likely to impede his academic progress.

Overall, Carl is achieving academically at a level that is expected for his cognitive abilities. Specifically, his reading, writing, and mathematics achievement skills are in the average to low average range. Consistent with his cognitive profile, his test performance was adversely affected by his difficulties with attention. He often failed to pay close attention to details, such as mathematical signs, and did not attend to the specific directions of the task. In all, Carl is achieving in the average to low average range, which is commensurate with his cognitive abilities. Therefore, Carl does not meet diagnostic criteria for a specific learning disability in any area.

Behaviorally, Carl appears to be experiencing significant problems with inattention, hyperactivity, and impulsivity. Parent and teacher reports indicate that Carl fails to give close attention to details in schoolwork and is easily distracted. Furthermore, they noted that he fails to finish schoolwork and chores, dislikes tasks that require sustained mental effort, and is often forgetful. This pattern of inattention was likewise observed during testing in the clinic.

Mr. and Mrs. Last and Mrs. Taylor also reported that Carl is hyperactive and impulsive. Specifically, he often talks excessively, is overly active, fidgets with his hands, and has difficulty playing in leisure activities quietly. In addition, he often interrupts others when they are speaking and occasionally blurts out answers to questions before the questions have been completed. During his evaluation at the clinic, Carl was overactive, frequently rocking back and forth in his seat, and answered questions impulsively. The Lasts and Mrs. Taylor indicated that Carl's ability to concentrate and attend has improved since he began taking Strattera. However, this pattern of behavior is still consistent with a DSM-IV-TR diagnosis of attention-deficit/hyperactivity disorder, combined type (314.01).

According to the Lasts and Mrs. Taylor, Carl displays a pattern of atypical behaviors. Mr. Last described Carl as often staring blankly and not making sense when he comes out of his stares. The Lasts noted that Carl often complains of unwanted "shivery" feelings and is extremely sensitive to sounds, hearing things that others do not hear. Furthermore, he often does not seem to listen when he is spoken to and has occasional days where he does not act like his usual self. On one occasion, Mr. Last noted that Carl seemed completely sedated and lethargic all day, and at times talked in nonsensical, incomplete thoughts. Moreover, Carl has a history of engaging in obsessive–compulsive, repetitive behaviors. Carl engaged in repetitive hand-washing and lining-up behaviors as a toddler. He currently has occasional days, a couple of times a month, where he engages in repetitive cleaning rituals. Specifically, he must line up his toys and trophies in his room over and over as if they are not exactly right. Carl also engages in repetitive body rocking and often waves his fingers back and forth. Mr. Last indicated that these behaviors are worse when Carl is frustrated or when he is doing undesirable activities. He further indicated that these behaviors could be related to anxiety about school. In addition, Carl uses repetitive speech patterns, such as muttering a specific phrase over and over. Hand washing was noticed during the clinic evaluation, and the Lasts indicated that there are occasions when he feels that he must wash his hands due to smells. These behaviors are indicative of compulsions; however, it is unclear at this time whether Carl feels driven to perform these actions to reduce anxiety or distress. In addition, Carl's parents and teachers do not report that these behaviors significantly interfere in his daily life, and it is unclear at this time whether these behaviors cause Carl marked distress. Furthermore, Carl's compulsions are not time-consuming, lasting less than 1 hour a day.

DSM-IV-TR Diagnosis

314.01   Attention-deficit/hyperactivity disorder, combined type
300.3 Obsessive–compulsive disorder (rule out)

REFERENCES

American Association on Intellectual and Developmental Disabilities. (2009). *Intellectual disability: Definition, classification, and systems of supports* (11th ed.). Washington, DC: Author.

American Educational Research Association (AERA), American Psychological Association (APA), and National Council on Measurement in Education (NCME). (1999). *Standards for educational and psychological testing.* Washington, DC: AERA.

American Psychiatric Association. (2000). *Diagnostic and statistical manual of mental disorders* (4th ed., text rev.). Washington, DC: Author.

Angoff, W. H., & Robertson, G. R. (1987). A procedure for standardizing individually administered tests, normed by age or grade level. *Applied Psychological Measurement, 11*, 33–46.

Beaujean, A., McGlaughlin, S. M., & Margulies, A. S. (2009). Factorial validity of the Reynolds Intellectual Assessment Scales for referred students. *Psychology in the Schools, 46*(10), 932–950.

Bigler, E. D., & Clement, P. F. (1997). *Diagnostic clinical neuropsychology* (3rd ed.). Austin: University of Texas Press.

Binet, A., & Simon, T. (1905). New methods for the diagnosis of the intellectual level of subnormals. *L'Année Psychologique, 11*, 191–244.

Carroll, J. B. (1993). *Human cognitive abilities: A survey of factor-analytic studies.* New York: Cambridge University Press.

Cattell, R. B. (1978). Matched determiners vs. factor invariance: A reply to Korth. *Multivariate Behavioral Research, 13*(4), 431–448.

Cronbach, L. J. (1990). *Essentials of psychological testing* (5th ed.). New York: Harper & Row.

Dombrowski, S. C., Watkins, M. W., & Brogan, M. J. (2009). An exploratory investigation of the factor structure of the Reynolds Intellectual Assessment Scales (RIAS). *Journal of Psychoeducational Assessment, 27*(6), 494–507.

Edwards, O. W., & Paulin, R. V. (2007). Referred students' performance on the Reynolds Intellectual Assessment Scales and the Wechsler Intelligence Scale for Children Fourth Edition. *Journal of Psychoeducational Assessment, 25*, 334–340.

Elliot, R. W. (2004). Test review: Reynolds Intellectual Assessment Scales. *Archives of Clinical Neuropsychology, 19*, 325–328.

Goldstein, S., & Reynolds, C. R. (Eds.). (2011). *Handbook of neurodevelopmental and genetic disorders in children* (2nd ed.). New York: Guilford Press.

Gustafsson, J. E. (1999). Measuring and understanding g: Experimental and correlational approaches. In P. L. Ackerman, P. C. Kyllonen, & R. D. Roberts (Eds.), *Learning and individual differences: Process, trait, and content determinants* (pp. 275–291). Washington, DC: American Psychological Association.

Horn, J. L., & Cattell, R. B. (1966). Refinement and test of the theory of fluid and crystallized general intelligences. *Journal of Educational Psychology, 57*(5), 253–270.

Joreskog, K. G., & Sorbom, D. (1987). *LISREL 6.13: User's reference guide.* Chicago: Scientific Software.

Joseph, R. (1996). *Neuropsychiatry, neuropsychology, and clinical neuroscience: Emotion, evolution, cognition,* language, memory, brain damage, and abnormal behavior (2nd ed.). Baltimore: Williams & Wilkins.

Kamphaus, R. W. (2001). *Clinical assessment of child and adolescent intelligence* (2nd ed.). Boston: Allyn & Bacon.

Kamphaus, R. W., & Reynolds, C. R. (2003). *Reynolds Intellectual Screening Test.* Lutz, FL: Psychological Assessment Resources.

Kaufman, A. S. (1994). *Intelligent testing with the WISC-III.* New York: Wiley.

Kaufman, A. S., McLean, J. E., Kaufman-Packer, J., & Reynolds, C. R. (1991). Is the pattern of intellectual growth and decline across the adult lifespan different for men or women? *Journal of Clinical Psychology, 47*(6), 801–812.

Kaufman, A. S., Reynolds, C. R., & McLean, J. E. (1989). Age and WAIS-R intelligence in a national sample of adults in the 20 to 74 year range: A cross-sectional analysis with education level controlled. *Intelligence, 13*(3), 235–253.

Krach, S., Loe, S. A., Jones, W., & Farrally, A. (2009). Convergent validity of the Reynolds Intellectual Assessment Scales (RIAS) using the Woodcock–Johnson Tests of Cognitive Ability, Third Edition (WJ-III) with university students. *Journal of Psychoeducational Assessment, 27*(5), 355–365.

Kyllonen, P. C. (1996). Is working memory capacity Spearman's *g*? In I. Dennis & P. Tapsfield (Eds.), *Human abilities: Their nature and measurement* (pp. 49–75). Mahwah, NJ: Erlbaum.

New shorter Oxford English dictionary. (1993). Portsmouth, NH: Oxford University Press.

Nelson, J. M., Canivez, G. L., Lindstrom, W., & Hatt, C. V. (2007). Higher-order exploratory factor analysis of the Reynolds Intellectual Assessment Scales with a referred sample. *Journal of School Psychology, 45*, 439–456.

Reynolds, C. R. (1984–1985). Critical measurement issues in learning disabilities. *Journal of Special Education, 18*, 451–476.

Reynolds, C. R. (2000). Methods for detecting and evaluating cultural bias in neuropsychological tests. In E. Fletcher-Janzen, T. Strickland, & C. R. Reynolds (Eds.), *Handbook of cross-cultural neuropsychology* (pp. 249–286). New York: Plenum Press.

Reynolds, C. R. (2003, August). *Twenty years of continuous norming: An author's perspective.* Paper presented at the annual meeting of the American Psychological Association, Toronto.

Reynolds, C. R., & Bigler, E. D. (1994). *Test of Memory and Learning.* Austin, TX: PRO-ED.

Reynolds, C. R., Chastain, R. L., Kaufman, A. S., &

McLean, J. E. (1987). Demographic influences on adult intelligence at ages 16 to 74 years. *Journal of School Psychology, 25*(4), 323–342.

Reynolds, C. R., & Fletcher-Janzen, E. (Eds.). (1997). *Handbook of clinical child neuropsychology* (2nd ed.). New York: Plenum Press.

Reynolds, C. R., & French, C. L. (2003). The neuropsychological basis of intelligence. In A. M. Horton & L. C. Hartlage (Eds.), *Handbook of forensic psychology* (pp. 35–92). New York: Springer.

Reynolds, C. R., & Kamphaus, R. W. (2003). *Reynolds Intellectual Assessment Scales.* Lutz, FL: Psychological Assessment Resources.

Roid, G. H. (2003). *Stanford–Binet Intelligence Scales, Fifth Edition.* Itasca, IL: Riverside.

Sattler, J. M. (2001). *Assessment of children: Cognitive applications* (4th ed.). San Diego, CA: Author.

Umphress, T., & Taylor, S. (2008). A comparison of low IQ scores from the Reynolds Intellectual Assessment Scales and the Wechsler Adult Intelligence Scale—Third Edition. *Intellectual and Developmental Disabilities, 46*(3), 229–233.

Vernon, P. E. (1950). *The structure of human abilities.* New York: Wiley.

Wechsler, D. (1949). *Wechsler Intelligence Scale for Children.* New York: Psychological Corporation.

Wechsler, D. (1992). *Wechsler Individual Achievement Test.* San Antonio, TX: Psychological Corporation.

Wechsler, D. (1997). *Wechsler Adult Intelligence Scale—Third Edition.* San Antonio, TX: Psychological Corporation.

Wechsler, D. (2003). *Wechsler Intelligence Scale for Children—Fourth Edition.* San Antonio, TX: Psychological Corporation.

Woodcock, R. W., McGrew, K. S., & Mather, N. (2001). *Woodcock–Johnson III.* Itasca, IL: Riverside.

Zachary, R., & Gorsuch, R. (1985). Continuous norming: Implications for the WAIS-R. *Journal of Clinical Psychology, 41,* 86–94.

CHAPTER 17

The NEPSY-II

Robb N. Matthews
Cynthia A. Riccio
John L. Davis

STRUCTURE

Case conceptualization often requires that the scope of an evaluation go beyond traditional measures of general characteristics (e.g., intellectual functioning) and include targeted assessment of specific traits or skills (e.g., divided attention, ideational fluency). In such cases, practitioners must choose assessment techniques that effectively target the various aspects of traits or skills under consideration, in order to gather relevant information and to develop ecologically valid recommendations related to the examinees' needs (Rhodes, D'Amato, & Rothlisberg, 2009). The NEPSY-II (Korkman, Kirk, & Kemp, 2007) is an integrated battery of subtests designed to complement other measures and techniques typically used in assessing the needs of children ages 3–16 years (Kemp & Korkman, 2010). Because of its structure, the NEPSY-II provides one of the few avenues for targeted assessment of specific cognitive skills in younger populations (Brooks, Sherman, & Strauss, 2010; Titley & D'Amato, 2008). Based on the general neuropsychological principles put forth by Luria (1980) and operationalized through a flexible multidomain design, the NEPSY-II allows examination of the subcomponents of complex cognitive processes. The structure and development of the NEPSY-II have been informed by current literature surrounding child development, child psychology, and pediatric neuropsychology (Korkman et al., 2007). As such, this battery provides a method for merging quantitative measures and qualitative observations of performance into a fuller description of an examinee's functioning.

The NEPSY-II is intended to assist clinicians of varying proficiency levels with understanding the complex and often multilayered aspects of cognitive processing. The flexible structure allows the clinicians to address the specific issues raised in referral questions, to identify basic and interactive cognitive subcomponents of functional skills, and to extrapolate their impact on current and future functioning (Kemp & Korkman, 2010; Luria, 1980). The NEPSY-II structure reflects six theoretically derived domains of cognitive processing thought to be key areas contributing to a child's success in meeting the expectations of diverse environments (Brooks, Sherman, & Strauss, 2010; Hooper, 2010). The particular set of subtests administered can be based either on a predetermined battery as specified in the manual, or on a clinician's conceptualization of a referral question and its related primary functional components (e.g., attention) or secondary subcomponents (e.g., memory); however, it never encompasses all 36 subtests. Suggested referral batteries listed in the scoring assistant and assessment planner are combinations of subtests the authors believe may be useful for particular "classes" of difficulties and those components most likely to be affected (Korkman et al., 2007). In some populations, a short-battery or a fixed-battery approach can be an efficient way to answer referral questions. The flexible design of the NEPSY-II allows the clinician to use other information and the presenting problem to select which domains or combinations of subtests will be most useful for a specific referral. Although the NEPSY-II is not designed to assess for specific diagnoses (e.g., learning disorders), its flexible structure may contribute to a diagnostic conclusion based on identified patterns (i.e., diagnostic clusters) of cognitive processing consistent with a particular condition (Kemp & Korkman, 2010; Titley & D'Amato, 2008). Most importantly, the structure of the NEPSY-II allows for more in-depth examination of specific cognitive processing areas that may be helpful in selection of well-designed intervention programs (Titley & D'Amato, 2008).

THEORETICAL UNDERPINNINGS

The NEPSY-II, like the original NEPSY (Korkman, Kirk, & Kemp, 1998) and the original NEPS in Finnish, are based on Luria's (1980) model of functional systems and an integrated theory of brain function. The initial 36 tasks and 30 performance areas were intended to correspond to components of complex cognitive functions (Korkman, 1999) that were drawn from Luria's model of functional systems. A *functional system* is made up of multiple brain regions and their interconnections; the regions and interconnections working together form the substrate for a complex psychological function or process (e.g., attention, language). The integration of the individual components (i.e., brain structures and connections) is what allows for complex thought and processes (Luria, 1980). From a clinical perspective, the nature of the individual's impaired performance is determined by the specific location of damage or developmental difference within the affected functional system(s), as well as the effects of this damage or difference to the rest of the functional systems (Bauer, 2000; Pramuka & McCue, 2000).

Luria believed that the fundamental purpose of a neuropsychological assessment was to better describe the function of the neuropsychological symptoms (i.e., the presenting problems that result in referral for assessment). In effect, the assessment is designed to present various opportunities, thus identifying those contexts in which an individual's deficits become significant (Bauer, 2000). In this regard, Luria's approach is considered to be client- and problem-centered, with examination of performance across and within the various functional systems. As part of this process, there is a need to examine performance or function at simple, complex, and integrated levels, as well as with varying input and output demands. The interpretation is to some extent qualitative; it is not based on the number of problems solved or on a total score, but rather on which problems were and were not solved. The emphasis on complex patterns of functioning (i.e., strengths or weaknesses) is a key component of the Luria model. It is the examination of the pattern of strengths and weaknesses, believed to represent intact or disrupted systems, on which the interpretation is based (Bauer, 2000).

As noted above, specific combinations of the NEPSY-II subtests are intended to represent the various functional systems in an effort to better understand and quantify which brain functions are intact and which are impaired. Five of the six content domains of the NEPSY-II were also in the original NEPSY and correspond to specific functional systems identified by Luria. With the NEPSY-II, the sixth domain of social perception, representing some aspects of social-emotional functioning, was created to address concerns specific to the autism spectrum. Thus the six domains are consistent with the cognitive domains; moreover, these domains have associated correlates in everyday functioning (Pramuka & McCue, 2000). At the same time, with the NEPSY-II there has been some movement away from the original theoretical model, in that the domain scores have been eliminated. The domain scores have been replaced with subtest-level scores—primary, process, and contrast scores—as well as behavioral observations. At the same time, however, subtests continue to be organized by domain in order to facilitate subtest selection (Korkman et al., 2007). For the NEPSY-II, the domains of interest are Attention and Executive Functioning, Language, Memory and Learning, Visuospatial Processing, Sensorimotor, and Social Perception.

It is important to note that these six domains are theoretically based, rather than statistically based (Korkman et al., 2007); this is one reason why it was determined that the domain scores were not appropriate. In effect, the authors recognized that no single subtest only measures one of the functional domains, and that because of the differing components measured by each subtest, the correlations within and across domains vary considerably. With subtests measuring some overlapping skills, one strength of the theoretical rather than statistical design is the ability to assess deficits underlying impaired performance both within and across functional domains (Korkman et al., 2007). Consistent with developmental considerations, differing subtests or formats are deemed appropriate for differing age levels within each domain. Given that specific functional systems have been implicated for differing neurodevelopmental disorders, there is also flexibility in the combinations of subtests that can be administered based on the presenting problem. Although domain scores are no longer calculated, the provision of contrast scores (an indication of whether differences between subtest scores are meaningful) allows for examination of patterns (i.e., the syndrome analysis).

ORGANIZATION AND FORMAT

Within the six domains, the NEPSY–II includes 32 individually administered and autonomous subtests, with an additional four delayed-recall subtests. These wide-ranging subtests are designed to assess neuropsychological functioning across the six domains, as presented in Table 17.1. Each subtest is theoretically derived to assess specific skill strengths and weaknesses. Input, output, and processing demands vary across subtests and within domains; the combination of subtest scores and differences in performance is what is important. The manual provides suggested batteries to assist in planning assessments for specific referral questions. These eight tailored batteries are based on information obtained in special group studies for deficits in reading, math, attention, social/interpersonal skills, behavioral management, school readiness, and perceptual–motor delays. These suggested batteries are empirically based, and designed to align with profiles of children known to possess deficits in the aforementioned areas. The format of the NEPSY-II is designed to offer flexible administration of subtests to explore specific facets of neurological functioning in children. In terms of demands placed on the examinee, the subtests range from oral responding to individual paper-and-pencil work. The NEPSY-II is very well designed in terms of providing test material that promotes engagement across the range of ages it is intended to assess. Due to the wide range of potential subtests, users should carefully consider

each child's profile and assessment needs prior to administration. Examiners should also pay special attention to the age range of examinees appropriate for each subtest, as the NEPSY-II varies considerably in format in this area. This variation is a strength of the NEPSY-II; because it offers a wide range of tests that are appropriate across different ages and developmental levels, it affords examiners complete coverage of the intended construct. However, this variation has the potential to create confusion or misadministration of subtests. The NEPSY-II offers 17 subtests for ages 3–4, 22 subtests and two delayed tasks for ages 5–6, 23 subtests and two delayed tasks for ages 7–12, and 24 subtests and three delayed tasks for ages 13–16. For specific information on the age range for each subtest, see Table 17.1.

SCORING

Most subtests of the NEPSY-II provide multiple score options that allow for a variety of applications, including general performance, error rates, or measures of subcomponent skills necessary for task completion. Scores in the NEPSY-II include (but are not limited to) primary scores, process scores, combined scaled scores, and contrast scaled scores. Primary scores describe the overall ability assessed by each subtest. Process scores are intended to provide additional insight into the child's ability or error rates for the subtest. The combined scaled scores were developed to assist the clinician with understanding the unique contributions of specific subcomponents of a process and with determining whether they fall within expected limits. Combined scaled scores are similar to index scores on many other popular instruments, but interpretation is achieved by considering both the domain being measured and the subcomponents being combined in the score (Korkman et al., 2007). Several subtests of the NEPSY-II provide multiple primary scores; therefore, the contrast scaled scores allow comparison of scores within subtests. Contrast scaled scores were designed to hold the impact of one characteristic constant while performance on another is considered. These scores indicate the degree to which examinees' performance is within expectations, given their performance on a related subcomponent or skill (Kemp & Korkman, 2010). This aspect of scoring provides clinicians with additional information to discriminate between higher-level and lower-level skill deficits within a single subtest.

TABLE 17.1. NEPSY-II Subtests and Descriptions

Domain	Subtest	Descriptions
Attention and Executive Functioning	Animal Sorting	Assesses the ability to group pictures based on self-initiated sorting criteria.
	Auditory Attention	Assesses selective auditory attention and the ability to sustain attention.
	Response Set	Assesses the ability to shift and maintain attention.
	Clocks	Assesses the ability to organize, execute, and recreate the expression of time on an analog clock.
	Design Fluency	Assesses the child's ability to generate unique designs presented in structured or random arrays.
	Inhibition	Assesses the ability to inhibit automatic responses in favor of novel responses and the ability to switch between response types.
	Statue	Assesses motor persistence and inhibition.
Language	Body Part Naming and Identification	Assesses expressive and receptive language for identifying body parts with self-prompts and with picture prompts.
	Comprehension of Instructions	Assesses the ability to follow oral instruction with increasing complexity.
	Oromotor Sequences	Assesses oral–motor coordination.
	Phonological Processing	Assesses the child's understanding of phonological processing through repeating or recreating words with substitute words or phonemes.
	Repetition of Nonsense Words	Assesses phonological decoding skills.
	Speeded Naming	Assesses the child's ability to rapidly name common material when presented visually.
	Word Generation	Assesses the child's ability to rapidly generate verbal responses.
Memory and Learning	List Memory	Assesses verbal learning and memory, rate of learning, and the role of interference in recall for words.
	List Memory Delayed	Assesses long-term memory for words.
	Memory for Designs	Assesses spatial memory for novel visual material.
	Memory for Designs Delayed	Assesses long-term visual–spatial memory.
	Memory for Faces	Assesses discrimination and recognition of facial features.
	Memory for Faces Delayed	Assesses long-term memory for faces.
	Memory for Names	Assesses the child's memory for names, with three trials to rehearse.
	Memory for Names Delayed	Assesses long-term memory for names.
	Narrative Memory	Assesses memory for verbally presented material with free-recall and cued conditions.
	Sentence Repetition	Assesses rote memory for sentences that increase in complexity and length.
	Word List Interference	Assesses working memory and recall for verbally presented material.

(cont.)

TABLE 17.1. *(cont.)*

Domain	Subtest	Descriptions
Sensorimotor	Fingertip Tapping	Assesses the child's finger dexterity and motor speed.
	Imitating Hand Positions	Assesses the ability to imitate hand/finger positions.
	Manual Motor Sequences	Assesses the ability to imitate hand movement sequences.
	Visuomotor Precision	Assesses motor speed and accuracy.
Social Perception	Affect Recognition	Assesses the child's ability to recognize affect from a picture cue.
	Theory of Mind	Assesses ability to understand and properly attribute mental states.
Visuospatial Processing	Arrows	Assesses the ability to identify and infer line directionality.
	Block Construction	Assesses the ability to construct three-dimensional models from a two-dimensional picture prompt.
	Design Copying	Assesses the ability to reproduce images from a two-dimensional picture prompt.
	Geometric Puzzles	Assesses mental rotation and visual–spatial skills.
	Picture Puzzles	Assesses visual discrimination and visual–spatial skills.
	Route Finding	Assesses visual planning and directionality.

Additional scores available from the NEPSY-II include percentile ranks, cumulative percentages, and behavioral observations. Korkman and colleagues (2007) used percentile ranks in place of standard scores on some subtests, due to the level of skewness present in the distribution. In other words, subtests yielding only percentile ranks tend to assess those skills generally seen early in the typical developmental process and were therefore generally at an advanced level in the standardization sample (Kemp & Korkman, 2010). NEPSY-II percentile ranks are presented in ranges, so that scores falling in the 26th–50th or 51st–75th percentile should be interpreted as falling in the expected range of performance. Cumulative percentages represent the base rates or probability of occurrence of a particular performance, characteristic, or profile (Sattler, 2008) and should be interpreted with regard to the "rareness" of a particular outcome; this is discussed further in the section on interpretation.

In keeping with the Lurian tradition, the NEPSY-II also allows for structured qualitative observations of an examinee's performance. Some of the coded observations are simply descriptive of performance, while others are formalized observation measures. The set of behavioral observations coded on the NEPSY-II protocol are based on the clinical experience of the test authors and the behavior of typically developing children in the normative sample (Korkman et al., 2007). For example, cumulative percentages permit clinicians to compare instances of "out-of-seat behavior" with those for the normative group by age. Reviewing behavioral observations can give a reference point from which to develop hypotheses about an examinee's performance (Kemp & Korkman, 2010). Those behaviors tallied and summed in the protocol are converted to cumulative percentages (or base rates) and are included in an appendix in the test manual.

PSYCHOMETRIC PROPERTIES

Item Generation

With the revision of the NEPSY-II, several modifications were made to the original NEPSY, including the addition of several subtests and the omission of others. The manual appropriately describes the theoretical basis that necessitated these modifications, as well as the development of new subtests and additional items to existing subtests. The examination of items was conducted in multiple phases. This allowed the test authors to examine the psychometric impact of the changes in items and subtests. Specific item evaluation procedures or item evaluation outputs are not available in the manual.

Ceiling and Floors

One component of item generation involves assurance of appropriate floors and ceilings of each subtest. This is important in order to ensure assessment sensitivity across a broad range of abilities in children (Korkman et al., 2007). To this goal, the NEPSY-II provides additional items to ensure appropriate floors and ceilings in every subtest. For younger ages and lower levels of ability, additional subtests have been specifically included (e.g., Body Part Naming and Identification for 3- to 4-year-olds). Each six primary domains offer developmentally appropriate items for children between 3 and 16 years old.

Standardization

The NEPSY-II normative data were collected from 2005 to 2006. The normative data for the NEPSY-II were derived from a sample that closely matched the U.S. census data of children ages 3–16. An analysis of data gathered in the October 2003 census provided the basis for stratification across the variables of age, race/ethnicity, geographic region, and parent education level. Twelve hundred examinees were assessed for the normative sample, with 100 children from each of the 12 age groups ranging from 3 through 16. Ages 3–12 were divided by 6-month intervals, with 50 cases collected from children in the first 6 months of each year of age and 50 cases collected from children in the last 6 months of that same year. For each age group in the normative sample, examinees were further separated by the race/ethnicity category. Each child in the normative sample was categorized as belonging to one of the following groups: white (i.e., European American), African American, Hispanic, or other.

The groups were also stratified by gender to include 50% males and 50% females. Children were also stratified by four major geographic regions of the United States: Northeast, Midwest, South, and West. Children were further selected for the normative group to represent the proportions of children living in each region. Finally, the sample was stratified by parental educational level; the children were grouped according to the parents' reported educational attainment. For children in two-parent homes, the average of the parents' educational level was used (Korkman et al., 2007).

In the renorming of the NEPSY-II, several new subtests were added (Animal Sorting, Clocks, Inhibition, Memory for Designs, Word List Interference, Affect Recognition, Theory of Mind, Geometric Puzzles, and Picture Puzzles). For many of the subtests in the NEPSY-II, items were carried over from the original NEPSY and renormed. For several subtests in the NEPSY-II (Design Fluency, Repetition of Nonsense Words, List Memory, List Memory Delayed, and Imitating Hand Positions), the normative data from the original NEPSY continue to be used, with no renorming conducted. The rationale provided was that these subtests were not expected to be subject to the Flynn effect (Flynn, 1984, 1987) or changes in the population demographics; however, no empirical examination is offered to support this decision.

Reliability

Data are available in the manual for interrater reliability in scoring protocols, test–retest stability, decision consistency of classification, and internal consistency. Each of these reliability coefficients are listed for both the primary and process scores for subtests that were evaluated (Korkman et al., 2007). Interrater reliability in scoring the NEPSY-II protocol was assessed through percent agreement. Agreement rates ranged from 93% to 99%, with *Word Generation* at the lowest level (93%) and *Memory for Names* at the highest level (99%).

Test–retest stability was calculated on both the primary and process scores. A diverse group of 165 children (52% male, 48% female) took the NEPSY-II on two occasions. The sample was then divided into six age groups: 3–4 years, 5–6 years, 7–8 years, 9–10 years, 11–12 years, and 13–16 years. Test–retest intervals ranged from 12 to 51 days, with a mean of 21 days between administrations. Several indices for evaluating test–retest stability are provided. Test–retest scores showed generally adequate stability across time for all age groups in subtests assessed. Despite a very thorough treatment of subtest stability, the manual does not provide stability data for two of the subtests in the Sensorimotor domain (Manual Motor Sequences and Fingertip Tapping). Stability estimates for several subtests (Design Fluency, Repetition of Nonsense Words, List Memory, List Memory Delayed, and Imitating Hand Positions) are based on data collected for the NEPSY, as these were not renormed (Korkman et al., 2007).

A decision consistency index was also used to document reliability for several subtests. This alternative to standard test–retest reliability estimates was used because of skewed score distribution or restricted variance within particular subtests that may artificially lower reliability estimates. For these subtests, raw scores were converted to percentile ranks, combined scaled scores, or contrast scaled scores. Decision consistency shows the agreement between converted raw scores by two separate administrators. The test authors set two classification ranges as the criteria for judging decision consistency. For percentile ranks, the authors categorized scores as either above or below the 10th percentile. Combined or contrast scores were categorized as above or below a scaled score of 6. To achieve reliability with this index, a child would be assessed by two separate administrators, and the raw score would be converted to a percentile rank, combined score, or contrast score (where appropriate). If the resulting converted score was in the 6th percentile on the first administration and the 9th on the second, the subtest was said to be reliable. Decision consistency between raters was moderate to high on each subtest across all age groups. For three subtests (Oromotor Sequences, Manual Motor Sequences, and Route Finding), the analysis of decision consistency from the NEPSY is reported; notably, these subtests have the lowest decision consistency (Korkman et al., 2007).

In addition to stability coefficients and decision consistency procedures, split-half (Spearman–Brown) and alpha methods were used to calculate internal consistency when appropriate. The manual reports reliability coefficients for primary and process scores across individual age groups, and provides an average across the six age bands noted earlier (3–4, 5–6, 7–8, 9–10, 11–12, and 13–16). The reliability data indicated adequate to high internal consistency for a majority of subtests (r_{12} range = .21–.91). The highest internal-consistency scores were found on Comprehension of Instructions, Design Copying, and Fingertip Tapping. The lowest internal-consistency scores were found on the Inhibition and Memory for Designs subtests (Korkman et al., 2007).

Validity

Due to the wide array of specific skill areas examined on the NEPSY-II, evidence of concurrent validity is provided through a series of correlation studies on separate instruments designed to measure cognitive ability, academic achievement, neuropsychological functioning, and behavior. For example, concurrent validity of intellectual functioning was assessed with the Wechsler Intelligence Scale for Children—Fourth Edition (WISC-IV; Wechsler, 2003), the Differential Ability Scales—Second Edition (DAS-II; Elliott, 2007), and the Wechsler Nonverbal Scale of Ability (WNV; Wechsler & Naglieri, 2006). Correlations between these instruments suggested that the NEPSY-II scores correlate well with cognitive performance in both verbal and nonverbal applications. Correlations with the Verbal Comprehension Index of the WISC-IV ranged from a low on the *Auditory Attention* subtest (–.02) to a high on the *Narrative Memory* subtest (.58). Concurrent validity in academic domains was assessed with the Wechsler Individual Achievement Test—Second Edition (WIAT-II; Psychological Corporation, 2001). Results yielded a low to moderate link between the NEPSY-II Attention and Executive Functioning domain and the WIAT-II tests of Mathematics Reasoning (r = .09–.43), Oral Expression (r = .03–.52), and Written Language (r = .08–.47). Within the NEPSY-II Memory and Learning domain, the Sentence Repetition subtest strongly correlated with the WIAT-II tests of Reading Comprehension (r = .87) and Pseudoword Decoding (r = .87). The Narrative Memory subtest of the NEPSY-II varied in correlation (r = .04–.61) with the Children's Memory Scale (CMS; Cohen, 1997). Moderate correlations were shown between subtest scores of the CMS and the Auditory Attention subtest (r = .03–.42). The variability reflects the range of constructs the NEPSY-II is designed to assess. It would not be expected that all NEPSY-II subtests would correlate with any specific measure; however, the presence of high to moderate correlations for each of the constructs mentioned above provides reasonable evidence of validity.

Additional concurrent and construct validity coefficients were derived from a variety of other measures. Results of the NEPSY-II ranged in correlation (r = –.45–.65) to the content of various measures, including the Delis–Kaplan Executive Function System (D-KEFS; Delis, Kaplan, & Kramer, 2001); the Bracken Basic Concept Scale—Third Edition: Receptive (BBCS-3:R; Bracken, 2006a); the Bracken Basic Concept Scale—Expressive (BBCS:E; Bracken, 2006b); the Devereux Scales of Mental Disorders (DSMD; Naglieri, LeBuffe,

& Pfeiffer, 1994); the Children's Communication Checklist—Second Edition (CCC–2; Bishop, 2006); the Brown Attention-Deficit Disorder Scales for Children and Adolescents (Brown ADD Scales; Brown, 2001); and the Adaptive Behavior Assessment System—Second Edition (ABAS-II; Harrison & Oakland, 2003). The highest levels of association were found between the Memory for Designs Delayed subtest of the NEPSY-II and the School Readiness (.61) and Receptive Total (.64) composites of the BBCS-3:R. In addition, the Inhibition—Switching subtest of the NEPSY-II correlated highly (.59) with the Color Word Interference subtest of the D-KEFS. In contrast, correlation coefficients were moderate but negative for the Affect Recognition subtest of the NEPSY-II in relation to the Conduct scale (–.45) and Externalizing composite (–.40) of the DSMD. The Inhibition—Switching combined scaled score also had a moderate negative correlation (–.41) with the Focus cluster of the ABAS-II.

The authors also conducted several studies of "special groups" to test criterion validity, or the scale's clinical utility in yielding information that supports a diagnosis or disability classification. Children with the following diagnoses/educational classifications were included: attention-deficit/hyperactivity disorder (ADHD), reading disorder, language disorder, mathematics disorder, mild intellectual disability, autistic disorder, Asperger syndrome, traumatic brain injury, deafness/hearing impairment, and emotional disturbance. Small-group studies compared each of the score indices for each of the subtests between a group of children with a specific condition and a control group. The control group was matched with the normative sample on demographic categories. By examining differences in mean scale scores between children identified with a particular condition and the matched controls, the test authors identified specific subtests where children within an identified diagnosis/classification group diverged from the norm. These studies helped to form the empirical basis for recommended subtests for each condition. The NEPSY-II does not provide a diagnostic recommendation for any particular condition; rather, the test authors recommend using the information from suggested batteries as a method to conceptualize deficits commonly associated with a particular condition. The authors emphasize that the NEPSY-II should not be used as the sole source to diagnose or classify for educational purposes (Korkman et al., 2007).

INTERPRETATION

General Principles

Consistent with common assessment practice, levels of test performance are typically described and categorized statistically, to allow comparison between an individual's performance and levels of performance in the general population (Sattler, 2008). At the same time, the importance of understanding that mild deficits (e.g., low average functioning) may significantly interfere with daily functioning cannot be understated in interpreting performance on measures such as the NEPSY-II (Riccio, Sullivan, & Cohen, 2010; Yeates, Ris, Taylor, & Pennington, 2010). Furthermore, the probability that any given technique or instrument samples (and that scores are therefore affected by) more than one closely related skill set or domain is quite high. Paramount to skilled interpretation of performance is an understanding of the component processes being sampled, their interrelation, and how these processes may be manifest across circumstances or domains. Therefore, familiarity with current cognitive theories as well as with ongoing research is essential to the adequate interpretation and integration of results of the NEPSY-II.

Differentiating specific narrow characteristics or comorbid conditions can be difficult, and may result in several plausible conclusions about an examinee's performance or the relationship between the examinee's skills. Consequently, hypotheses or conclusions regarding particular performances or the interaction of characteristics may also vary between clinicians. As the number of subtests administered, observations recorded, or comparisons made between scores increases, it is also important to remember that the likelihood that spurious results will arise also increases (Crocker & Algina, 2006). To offset the impact of spurious results, consistency among the findings across measures or techniques is the most stable method (i.e., the most resistant to erroneous conclusions) of conceptualizing results in a coherent and practical manner that is useful for describing an examinee's needs, drawing diagnostic conclusions, and developing effective recommendations (Korkman et al., 2007; Riccio et al., 2010; Sattler, 2008; Yeates et al., 2010).

Moreover, the NEPSY-II allows a clinician to make a developmental comparison of the subcomponents of a given characteristic by examining underlying individual processes, although it was not designed to examine all potential characteristics or interactions of characteristics within or across cognitive domains (Kemp & Korkman, 2010; Korkman et al., 2007). Considering the developmental differences between a beginning reader's skills and an established reader's skills elucidates these principles. The beginning reader is deliberate in applying sound–symbol association, directed attention, and working memory, whereas the established reader probably uses only sight recognition of overlearned material (Kemp & Korkman, 2010). Thus the chain of skills used by both these readers may have been similar in the beginning, but has shifted with maturation, so that the readers now differ in their application and level of automaticity of reading skills. Considering only the outcome of a reading measure would be insufficient evidence on which to base a conclusion or develop recommendations. Targeted examination of skills allows a clinician to clarify the nature of an examinee's primary and secondary difficulties (according to Luria's model), and subsequently allows for improved recommendations and intervention development. The ability to differentiate the root cause (primary) of a deficit, such as poor phonological processing, from its impact (secondary), such as slow processing speed, effectively becomes a function of the clinician's knowledge and expertise in the areas under consideration. Thus, although clinicians of varying levels of training and experience can administer and score the NEPSY-II with proficiency (Brooks, Sherman, & Strauss, 2010), both choosing the appropriate subtests and interpreting performance across subtests or domains require a higher degree of expertise in neuropsychological constructs, developmental theory, and the professional literature (Titley & D'Amato, 2008).

Results

With these basic principles in mind, the next consideration for interpretation is at the level of the scores generated. The successful interpretation of NEPSY-II results begins with looking for patterns of scores at the subtest level, then moving to combined scaled scores, percentile ranks, and finally behavioral observation base rates (Kemp & Korkman, 2010). Although each of these scores is standardized along the same metric (mean of 10, standard deviation of 3), and therefore could result in the same descriptions of range (e.g., low average, average, high average), interpretation of the scores varies considerably (Korkman et al., 2007). In keeping with conventional assessment results,

scaled scores compare an individual's performance to that of same-age peers (Sattler, 2008). These scores can be used to compare the examinee's skills to the population, identify patterns of strengths and weaknesses, and/or identify a pattern of performance consistent that may suggest potential intervention strategies. The conventional method of score analysis may be the final level of analysis for evaluators with little training in neuropsychology, or the beginning of analysis for evaluators with a greater depth of training (Kemp & Korkman, 2010). Beyond the scale scores, techniques such as consideration of error types (i.e., error analyses) or examination of differences in performance across subtests or domains (i.e., profile analyses) may help to clarify an examinee's needs. This higher level of analysis is supported by examining the overall profile of an examinee as it is related to the identified difficulties; the combined and contrast scaled scores are useful in this regard.

The combined scaled scores allow the clinician to consider not only the outcome of performance, but the chain of events leading to that outcome (Korkman et al., 2007). The contrast scaled scores then allow the clinician to understand the examinee's range of functioning and more clearly identify potential contributing factors. Caution is warranted in the interpretation of contrast scores, however, as they only represent *differences* in level of functioning. Thus a performance on one subtest in the superior range (e.g., Memory for Faces) versus a performance on another subtest in the average range (e.g., Memory for Faces Delayed) can result in a similar contrast scaled score to that produced with performance differences of average versus below average. Although the contrast scaled score values will be similar, the implications for functioning in these two scenarios are significantly different.

Another consideration involves the cumulative percentage scores or the base rates, as these provide important information in the interpretation process. Although the observed difference between scores can be statistically significant, the base rate indicates how meaningful that difference is. For a difference to be considered rare (i.e., clinically meaningful), Sattler (2008) has suggested a base rate of no more than 15%, while Kemp and Korkman (2010) have supported using a more stringent rate of 10%. Finally, in addition to interpretation of the various scores provided, the behavioral observations need to be considered to lend additional qualitative insights into an examinee's functioning.

Integration

NEPSY-II results should be considered only in light of other standardized measures, as well as historical, observational, and functional information (Titley & D'Amato, 2008). Integrating NEPSY-II results with other psychometric and functional data into a comprehensive discussion of an examinee's strengths and weaknesses can be a difficult task, especially for less experienced clinicians (Hooper, 2010). Selecting a battery of tests/techniques designed to address the referral issue(s) efficiently and effectively is the first step in this process. Appropriate selection allows for comparison across subtests, within and across domains, and with other measures (e.g., intellectual) to identify the patterns of performance. Poor performance in a single area or on a single measure, without corroborating evidence, is insufficient for identifying a developmental deviation or a diagnostic conclusion; typical children show developmental differences over time, without significant impact on their daily life (Meltzer, 2007). Significant findings across measures of similar or related characteristics (e.g., subtests and coded observations) give informational consistency and internal support to hypotheses and conclusions (Kemp & Korkman, 2010). Selection of measures and methods should ensure coverage of all functional domains, with specific subtests of the NEPSY-II providing supplemental coverage.

One approach to integration would follow the model of cross-battery assessment (Flanagan, Ortiz, & Alfonso, 2007), which aligns various subtests across measures based on broad and narrow abilities. The NEPSY-II was co-normed with the WISC-IV; this should facilitate its use in cross-battery assessment. Although the NEPSY is included in software available for such assessment, the NEPSY-II subtests are not included as yet. For clinicians deriving their own combinations of subtests for narrow and broad abilities, the information provided in Table 17.1 can be helpful in placing the NEPSY-II subtests into this type of integrative model. Alternatively, the cognitive hypothesis-testing model (e.g., Flanagan, Fiorello, & Ortiz, 2010; Flanagan, Ortiz, Alfonso, & Mascolo, 2006)—which identifies normative deficits, considers plausible contributing or causal factors (e.g., lack of motivation vs. a cognitive deficit), and links current results to ecological deficits identified in the referral question—is another model that can be used.

Regardless of the model employed, the general idea is that of moving from the simple to the complex, with emphasis on consistencies, to facilitate the identification of patterns of performance and the integration of performance on the NEPSY-II with other information gathered during the evaluation process. To facilitate the integrative process, the clinician will need to be familiar with research on the chosen instruments or techniques (i.e., what is being measured) and how the instruments relate to each other (Hooper, 2010).

Some examples from research on the NEPSY or NEPSY-II reinforce the idea that assessment of higher-level cognitive processes is far more complex than simply administering one or more subtests and generating a score in a particular range. In their review of bilingual children's performance on NEPSY subtests, Garratt and Kelly (2008) found significant performance differences from monolingual children. Bilingual children demonstrated lower visual attention, naming speed, and verbal comprehension; however, their performance on the Imitating Hand Positions and Design Copying subtests was superior to that of their monolingual peers. In addition, Dixon and Kelly (2001) found potential cultural influences on the NEPSY, as British children were noted to demonstrate better phonological processing, visual attention, and verbal comprehension skills than their American counterparts. These differences may be in part due to differences in educational strategies in different cultures, to the use of theoretically versus empirically derived domains, due to homogeneity in the norming samples, or to the interaction of these or other unidentified issues. Regardless of the causes of these differences, these findings underscore the need to consider results of the NEPSY-II in the broader context of all other information.

Gifford, Mahaney, and Gorman (2008) found that children with ADHD performed significantly better than children with an autism spectrum disorder (ASD) on NEPSY-II tests of motor speed and dexterity, whereas children with an ASD outperformed children with ADHD on tests of visual–spatial analysis and attention to detail. Gifford and colleagues (2008) commented that these findings diverged from their expectations, as no significant differences between these groups were noted on NEPSY-II tests of attention and concentration or of executive skills. In a second study, Gifford, Mahaney, and Gorman (2009) found that children with ADHD performed better on visual memory tasks than children with an ASD and children with seizure disorders, while the children with an ASD performed better than children with seizure disorders on tests of phonological processing. Among children with an ASD, differences were also found for subgroups on the spectrum; the meaning of these differences is the subject of theoretical discussion and additional research.

Finally, Brooks, Sherman, and Iverson's (2010) research supports the notion that typically developing children's performance can fall well below expectations on a given day or subtest. When the seven subtests for 3- to 4-year-olds were considered together, 71.5% of the sample had one or more scores below the 25th percentile, and 40% of the sample had two or more scores below the 10th percentile. The number of low scorers in this group was mediated by parental education level, with lower levels of parental educational attainment being associated with increased rates of NEPSY-II scale scores falling below the expected range. Stamina also appears to play a role in typically developing children's NEPSY-II performance. When a 1-hour battery consisting of eight subtests was used, 70.3% of participants ages 5–6 had one or more scale scores below the 25th percentile, and 37.2% of participants had two or more scale scores below the 10th percentile. When a 2-hour battery consisting of 12 scale scores was used, 82.6% of these participants had one or more scores below the 25th percentile, and 49.3% had two or more scores below the 10th percentile. Once again, the base rates of children with low scores decreased as a function of their parents' educational attainment. The authors found similar relationships between parental education and the lowered score base rate in the 7- to 16-year-old group as well.

BEYOND TRADITIONAL INTELLECTUAL ASSESSMENT

Traditional intellectual assessment is concerned with quantifying general ability (g), and is most often used in determining intellectual disability or as one component of identifying learning disability. The NEPSY-II is not a measure of intelligence, but a supplemental measure to increase the extent to which the assessment process examines all functional systems. The majority of intellectual assessment instruments do not effectively measure the full range of cognitive abilities (Flanagan et al., 2007); thus the use of a traditional intelligence test with the NEPSY-II provides the means for obtaining a comprehensive assessment of domains of function (Pramuka & McCue, 2000). It provides additional information on the narrow abilities that may otherwise be ignored and are important for development of appropriate interventions.

The NEPSY-II, in combination with a general measure of ability, is consistent with a focus on the need to integrate cognitive and behavioral data. It thus increases clinicians' ability to deal with the multidimensionality of individuals (Riccio & Reynolds, in press) and to translate this understanding into educationally relevant information (Goldstein & Naglieri, 2008). As noted earlier, the NEPSY-II permits systematic variation of the inputs, outputs, and levels of complexity, to maximize the likelihood of dissociating the potential underlying problem that is presenting as impaired performance. It is not solely a deficit-based approach; it is consistent with Luria's assertion that neuropsychological assessment is a valuable approach for determining not only deficits, but individual strengths or intact cognitive functions, as they relate to everyday functioning. Focusing on strengths lends itself to compensatory models that focus not on the underlying impairment, but on ways to compensate for the impairment to improve everyday living (Glisky & Glisky, 2002). Compensation approaches identify methods to bypass deficit skills through the use of intact functions or alternative methods of reaching the same goal (Anderson, 2002).

A more unified picture of the individual should increase the predictive value of the assessment as it relates to achievement as well as realistic life planning (Silver et al., 2006; Teeter & Semrud-Clikeman, 1997). By not only emphasizing how well a student does or doesn't do, but gaining an understanding of the types of problems (i.e., inputs, outputs) that are most difficult for the individual, a clinician can identify interventions that focus on circumventing the problems (i.e., accommodations, modifications). The more comprehensive picture typically associated with neuropsychological assessment examines individual performance across a range of functional domains, including linguistic, perceptual, sensory–motor, attention, memory, learning, executive control/planning, speed of processing, and emotional functioning (Riccio & Reynolds, in press; Silver et al., 2006).

Following in the traditions of Luria, neuropsychological assessment such as that provided by the NEPSY-II looks beyond the failure to attain a specific skill to the underlying brain–behavior relation that contributes to this difficulty. This is seen as important, in that this same problem within the functional system may indicate increased likelihood of failure in attaining other academic, functional, social, or behavioral skills (Riccio & Reynolds, 1998, in press). At the same time, Kemp and Korkman (2010) have warned against drawing conclusions about specific brain function based on NEPSY-II results: A child's brain is still developing, and the long-term effects of a congenital or acquired injury on brain development will differ, depending on a number of factors that may vary over the lifespan.

Neuropsychological assessment (e.g., with the NEPSY-II) may be appropriate to establish initial functioning, as well as to track progress; it may serve to clarify intervention needs and result in referrals to other specialists (Berkelhammer, 2008). Intervention planning goes beyond the labeling or eligibility/placement process to include the identification of specific management or rehabilitation techniques, medical management approaches, outcome-related goals, and modifications that need to be addressed (Silver et al., 2006). Changes in functioning on the various subtests of the NEPSY-II, due to their developmental sensitivity, may be more apparent than on the traditional full-scale score of an intelligence test. The flexibility of being able to select specific subtests, rather than having to administer the full battery, also renders the NEPSY-II more suitable for follow-up evaluation.

CONCLUSIONS

The NEPSY-II is one of the few flexible, child-friendly batteries of tests available for the assessment of higher-level cognitive functions (Brooks, Sherman, & Strauss, 2010; Davis & Matthews, 2010). It is best used to supplement rather than to replace traditional standardized intelligence tests, in order to obtain a more comprehensive picture of multilayered abilities. It should be kept in mind that theoretical as well as statistical and psychometric bases need to be considered in using the NEPSY-II. Developmental and cultural contexts must also be considered. Without considering expected developmental or cultural differences, a clinician could easily draw erroneous conclusions and develop baseless recommendations. Similarly, convergent validity (i.e., consistency across subtests and measures) is important in decreasing the likelihood of potentially spurious results.

Although some may rightly argue against various statistical properties of this battery or the norming choices made by the authors (Titley & D'Amato, 2008), the NEPSY-II ultimately demonstrates excellent clinical utility through an integrated battery of subtests and a variety of scores

allowing for in-depth assessment of an examinee's skill set (Hooper, 2010). The NEPSY-II represents continuing strides forward in the integration of qualitative and quantitative information in the comprehensive evaluation of children. Building on the foundation of the NEPSY, the NEPSY-II continues to enhance the breadth and depth of available assessment instruments for children and adolescents. However, several areas in need of additional consideration remain.

Defining the NEPSY-II domains via factor analysis would lend significant power to the battery's predictive validity. The problem with such a task is the lack of agreement in the literature regarding the definitions or methods of assessment for particular skills. For instance, although executive functions are frequently discussed in the literature, and are generally agreed to be of great importance, a widely accepted formal definition of these skills has not been established (Jurado & Rosselli, 2007; Kenworthy, Black, Harrison, Rosa, & Wallace, 2009). Furthermore, common differences in the definition of executive skills leads to differences in the validity of particular evaluation methods, as well as the ecological validity of resulting recommendations.

Developing suggested batteries and assessment practices based on research defining expected performance could also enhance the predictive and diagnostic power of the NEPSY-II. Although social perception is a concern in a variety of conditions, how would a child with a given condition perform on the NEPSY-II? Could the degree of impairment related to a given condition be ascertained on the basis of NEPSY-II performance? What impact would the level of chronicity have on a performance profile? Broadening the stratification to factors beyond those typically employed (e.g., race, socioeconomic status) could also lend insight into NEPSY-II performance. As discussed above, different cultural or familial experiences can significantly affect a performance profile. Along this line, the applicability of the NEPSY-II would probably be broadened if it were considered in relation to instruments developed for assessing English-language learners for instance. Moreover, how do the methods of assessment used in NEPSY-II subtests (e.g., Theory of Mind) influence expected performance? How should methods of assessment be expected to vary by language or cultural background? Finally, how do NEPSY-II results translate into ecologically valid recommendations? Would a particular pattern of performance suggest one recommendation or strategy over another? These types of questions (and surely others) require ongoing research related to underlying neuropsychological characteristics of the individuals being evaluated, as well as how the NEPSY-II measures those characteristics and how those measurements translate into improved recommendations.

REFERENCES

Anderson, P. (2002). Assessment and development of executive function (EF) during childhood. *Child Neuropsychology*, 8, 71–82.

Bauer, R. M. (2000). The flexible battery approach to neuropsychological assessment. In R. D. Vanderploeg (Ed.), *Clinician's guide to neuropsychological assessment* (2nd ed., pp. 419–448). Mahwah, NJ: Erlbaum

Berkelhammer, L. D. (2008). Pediatric neuropsychological evaluation. In M. Hersen & A. M. Gross (Eds.), *Handbook of clinical psychology* (pp. 497–519). Hoboken, NJ: Wiley.

Bishop, D. V. M. (2006). *Children's Communication Checklist—Second Edition* (U.S. ed.). San Antonio, TX: Harcourt Assessment.

Bracken, B. A. (2006a). *Bracken Basic Concept Scale: Expressive*. San Antonio, TX: Harcourt Assessment.

Bracken, B. A. (2006b). *Bracken Basic Concept Scale—Third edition: Receptive*. San Antonio, TX: Harcourt Assessment.

Brooks, B. L., Sherman, E. M. S., & Iverson, G. L. (2010). Healthy children get low scores too: Prevalence of low scores on the NEPSY-II in preschoolers, children, and adolescents. *Archives of Clinical Neuropsychology*, 25, 182–190.

Brooks, B. L., Sherman, E. M. S., & Strauss, E. (2010). NEPSY-II: A developmental neuropsychological assessment, second edition. *Child Neuropsychology*, 16, 80–101.

Brown, T. E. (2001). *Brown Attention-Deficit Disorder Scales for Children and Adolescents*. San Antonio, TX: Psychological Corporation.

Cohen, M. J. (1997). *Children's memory scale*. San Antonio, TX: Psychological Corporation.

Crocker, L., & Algina, J. (2006). *Introduction to classical and modern test theory*. Mason, OH: Wadsworth.

Davis, J. L., & Matthews, R. N. (2010). Test review: NEPSY—Second Edition (NEPSY-II). *Journal of Psychoeducational Assessment*, 28(2), 175–182.

Delis, D. C., Kaplan, E., & Kramer, J. H. (2001). *Delis–Kaplan Executive Function System*. San Antonio, TX: Psychological Corporation.

Dixon, L. A., & Kelly, T. P. (2001). A comparison of the performance of preschool children from England and the USA on the NEPSY: Developmental neuropsychological assessment. *Clinical Neuropsychological Assessment*, 2, 43–60.

Elliott, C. D. (2007). *Differential Ability Scales—Second Edition*. San Antonio, TX: Harcourt Assessment.

Flanagan, D. P., Fiorello, C. A., & Ortiz, S. O. (2010). Enhancing practice through application of Cattell–Horn–Carroll theory and research: A "third" method approach to specific learning disabilities identification. *Psychology in the Schools*, 47, 739–760.

Flanagan, D. P., Ortiz, S. O., & Alfonso, V. C. (2007). *Essentials of cross-battery assessment* (2nd ed.). Hoboken, NJ: Wiley.

Flanagan, D. P., Ortiz, S. O., Alfonso, V. C., & Mascolo, J. T. (2006). *The achievement test desk reference: A guide to learning disability identification* (2nd ed.). Hoboken, NJ: Wiley.

Flynn, J. R. (1984). The mean IQ of Americans: Massive gains 1932 to 1978. *Psychological Bulletin*, 95, 29–51.

Flynn, J. R. (1987). Massive IQ gains in 14 nations: What IQ tests really measure. *Psychological Bulletin*, 101, 171–191.

Garratt, L. C., & Kelly, T. P. (2008). To what extent does bilingualism affect children's performance on the NEPSY? *Child Neuropsychology*, 14, 71–81.

Gifford, K. A., Mahaney, T. R., & Gorman, P. W. (2008, October). *Differentiating between seizure disorder, ADHD, and PDD in children using the NEPSY-II*. Poster presented at the annual conference of the National Academy of Neuropsychology, New York.

Gifford, K. A., Mahaney, T. R., & Gorman, P. W. (2009, November). *Using the NEPSY-II to assess ADHD, seizure disorder, and autism spectrum disorders in children*. Poster presented at the annual conference of the National Academy of Neuropsychology, New Orleans, LA.

Glisky, E. L., & Glisky, M. L. (2002). Learning and memory impairments. In P. J. Eslinger (Ed.), *Neuropsychological interventions: Clinical research and practice* (pp. 137–162). New York: Guilford Press.

Goldstein, S., & Naglieri, J. A. (2008). The school neuropsychology of ADHD: Theory, assessment, and intervention. *Psychology in the Schools*, 45, 859–874.

Harrison, P. L., & Oakland, T. (2003). *Adaptive Behavior Assessment System—Second Edition*. San Antonio, TX: Psychological Corporation.

Hooper, S. R. (2010). Strengths and weaknesses of the NEPSY-II. In S. L. Kemp, & M. Korkman, *Essentials of NEPSY-II assessment* (pp. 227–247). Hoboken, NJ: Wiley.

Jurado, M. B., & Rosselli, M. (2007). The elusive nature of executive functions: A review of our current understanding. *Neuropsychological Review*, 17, 213–233.

Kemp, S. L., & Korkman, M. (2010). *Essentials of NEPSY-II assessment*. Hoboken, NJ: Wiley.

Kenworthy, L., Black, D. O., Harrison, B., Rosa, A. D., & Wallace, G. L. (2009). Are executive control functions related to autism symptoms in high-functioning children? *Child Neuropsychology, 15,* 425–440.

Korkman, M. (1999). Applying Luria's diagnostic principles in the neuropsychological assessment of children. *Neuropsychology Review, 9,* 89–105.

Korkman, M., Kirk, U., & Kemp, S. (1998). *NEPSY.* San Antonio, TX: Psychological Corporation.

Korkman, M., Kirk, U., & Kemp, S. (2007). *NEPSY— Second Edition (NEPSY-II).* San Antonio, TX: Harcourt Assessment.

Luria, A. R. (1980). *Higher cortical functions in man* (2nd ed.). New York: Basic Books.

Meltzer, L. (2007). *Executive function in education: From theory to practice.* New York: Guilford Press.

Naglieri, J., LeBuffe, P., & Pfeiffer, S. I. (1994). *Devereux Scales of Mental Disorders (DSMD).* San Antonio, TX: Psychological Corporation.

Pramuka, M., & McCue, M. (2000). Assessment to rehabilitation: Communicating across the gulf. In R. D. Vanderploeg (Ed.), *Clinician's guide to neuropsychological assessment* (2nd ed., pp. 337–356). Mahwah, NJ: Erlbaum.

Psychological Corporation. (2001). *Wechsler Individual Achievement Test—Second Edition.* San Antonio, TX: Author.

Rhodes, R. L., D'Amato, R. C., & Rothlisberg, B. A. (2009). Utilizing a neuropsychological paradigm for understanding common educational and psychological tests. In C. R. Reynolds & E. Fletcher-Janzen (Eds.), *Handbook of clinical child neuropsychology* (pp. 321–348). New York: Springer.

Riccio, C. A., & Reynolds, C. R. (1998). Neuropsychological assessment of children. In A. S. Bellack & M. Hersen (Series Eds.) & C. R. Reynolds (Ed.), *Comprehensive clinical psychology* (Vol. 4, pp. 267–301). New York: Pergamon Press.

Riccio, C. A., & Reynolds, C. R. (in press). Principles of neuropsychological assessment in children and adolescents. In D. Saklofske & V. L. Schwean (Eds.), *Oxford handbook of psychological assessment of children and adolescents.* New York: Oxford University Press.

Riccio, C. A., Sullivan, J. R., & Cohen, M. J. (2010). *Neuropsychological assessment and intervention for childhood and adolescent disorders.* Hoboken, NJ: Wiley.

Sattler, J. M. (2008). *Assessment of children: Cognitive foundations* (5th ed.). San Diego, CA: Author.

Silver, C. H., Blackburn, L. B., Arffa, S., Barth, J. T., Bush, S. S., Koffler, S. P., et al. (2006). The importance of neuropsychological assessment for the evaluation of childhood learning disorders: NAN Policy and Planning Committee. *Archives of Clinical Neuropsychology, 21,* 741–744.

Teeter, P. A., & Semrud-Clikeman, M. (1997). *Child neuropsychology: Assessment and interventions for neurodevelopmental disorders.* Boston: Allyn & Bacon.

Titley, J. E., & D'Amato, R. C. (2008). Understanding and using the NEPSY-II with young children, children, and adolescents. In R. C. D'Amato & L. C. Hartlage (Eds.), *Essentials of neuropsychological assessment: Treatment planning for rehabilitation* (pp. 149–172). New York: Springer.

Wechsler, D. (2003). *Wechsler Intelligence Scale for Children—Fourth Edition.* San Antonio, TX: Psychological Corporation.

Wechsler, D., & Naglieri, J. A. (2006). *Wechsler Nonverbal Scale of Ability.* San Antonio, TX: Harcourt Assessment.

Yeates, K. O., Ris, M. D., Taylor, H. G., & Pennington, B. F. (2010). *Pediatric neuropsychology: Research, theory, and practice* (2nd ed.). New York: Guilford Press.

CHAPTER 18

The Wechsler Nonverbal Scale of Ability
Assessment of Diverse Populations

Jack A. Naglieri
Tulio M. Otero

MEASUREMENT OF GENERAL ABILITY

The concept of *general ability*, as measured by traditional IQ tests such as the Wechsler scales, has had a long and successful history in psychology and education—so much so that the tests have been used to define intelligence. There is strong support for a view of the Wechsler scales as good measures of general ability, using verbal and nonverbal (i.e., visual–spatial) test questions. The visual–spatial tests (e.g., Block Design and Object Assembly) are often described as measures of "nonverbal ability," and the verbal tests (e.g., Vocabulary and Similarities) are often described as measures of "verbal ability," even though Wechsler did not have any intention to measure verbal and nonverbal abilities. In fact, Wechsler did not view verbal and nonverbal tests as measures of two types of intelligence, despite the fact that for years his tests yielded Verbal and nonverbal (Performance) IQ scores. Wechsler stated that "the subtests are different measures of intelligence, not measures of different kinds of intelligence" (1958, p. 64), and he "viewed verbal and performance tests as equally valid measures of intelligence" (Wechsler & Naglieri, 2006, p. 1). Furthermore, Bracken and Naglieri (2003) and Naglieri (2003a, 2003b, 2008a, 2008b) have clarified that the term *nonverbal* refers to the *content* of the test, not a type of ability, and that the goal is to measure general ability.

Wechsler believed that nonverbal tests help to "minimize the over-diagnosing of feeble-mindness that was, he believed, caused by intelligence tests that were verbal in content . . . and he viewed verbal and performance tests as equally valid measures of intelligence and criticized the labeling of performance [nonverbal] tests as measures of special abilities" (Boake, 2002, p. 396). Those individuals who have not had the chance to acquire verbal skills in the language used to give an IQ test do poorly on verbal tests of general ability because of a limited opportunity to learn (or a developmental or acquired neurological condition). As a result, the test score will not be a good reflection of their general ability to learn after having had ample instruction. The problem is complicated by the fact that the content of traditional IQ test questions is often very similar to that of questions found in tests of achievement.

Traditional IQ tests often include tests of word knowledge that are used to measure intelligence—for example, tests that ask the examinee to define vocabulary words or determine how two words are alike. A good example of the similarity of test questions across ability and achievement tests can be found in the Woodcock–Johnson

III Tests of Cognitive Abilities (WJ III COG; Woodcock, McGrew, & Mather, 2001a) and the Woodcock–Johnson III Tests of Achievement (WJ III ACH; Woodcock, McGrew, & Mather, 2001b). For example, the WJ III COG contains a Verbal Comprehension subtest item similar to "Tell me another word for *small*," and the W JIII ACH contains a Reading Vocabulary question similar to: "Tell me another word for *little*." Also included in the WJ III ACH Reading Vocabulary subtest is something like "Tell me another word for [examiner points to the word *big*]," and in the WJ III COG Verbal Comprehension test, the examiner asks something like "Tell me another word for *tiny*." Additionally, the WJ III COG Verbal Comprehension test contains 23 picture vocabulary items, and the WJ III ACH Reading Vocabulary test includes 44 picture vocabulary questions. This overlap in content artificially increases the correlation between these tests of ability and achievement (thereby distorting the validity of the tests) and raises important questions about the utility of measuring ability with questions that are clearly achievement-laden. More importantly, however, these test questions pose particular problems for those individuals with limited English-language and academic skills.

It is particularly important to recognize the role of knowledge and skills when ability tests are given to diverse populations. One way to assess ability without the confounding variables of language and knowledge is to use a nonverbal test of ability. A nonverbal test of general ability provides a way to assess individuals from diverse linguistic groups, especially those who have limited language skills, as well as children with language impairments. In addition, children who cannot tolerate a lengthy test battery—such as those with autism, those who are significantly inattentive and/or hyperactive, or those who fatigue easily due to traumatic brain injury—are more easily evaluated with nonverbal tests, especially brief ones. Importantly, therefore, nonverbal tests give practitioners a way to evaluate individuals who on other intelligence tests would fare poorly due to poor language, academic, and/or other skills.

Nonverbal tests can be particularly important when Hispanic children are assessed, as these children are more likely to have varying histories of educational opportunity and vary with respect to academic English language proficiency. In order to equitably evaluate the ability levels of Hispanics (the largest minority group in the United States

(Ramirez & de la Cruz, 2002), tests that do not measure intelligence on the basis of verbal skills are absolutely necessary.

MEASUREMENT OF GENERAL ABILITY WITH NONVERBAL TESTS

The greatest advantage of a nonverbal test of general ability is that it measures intelligence without using test questions that are unduly reliant on verbal skills. The test questions evaluate *general* ability *nonverbally*—not *nonverbal ability*—via subtests with strong spatial requirements (e.g., blocks to make a design or progressive matrices). The specific administration format and subtests may vary, but the basic concept remains the same. For example, Bracken and McCallum (1998) suggest that an entire ability test must be administered nonverbally and that pantomimed instructions must be used. Others suggest that test directions for administration may be spoken, but that the content of the test questions should not require knowledge of a specific language (Naglieri, 1997). Another method is to use pictorial directions, as found in the Naglieri Nonverbal Ability Test— Second Edition (NNAT-2; Naglieri, 2008a) and the Wechsler Nonverbal Scale of Ability (WNV; Wechsler & Naglieri, 2006). Nonverbal tests of general ability also differ in the diversity of their subtests. For example, some nonverbal tests consist of one type of item such as the progressive matrix (e.g., the NNAT-2), given in either a group or an individual format (e.g., the Naglieri Nonverbal Ability Test—Individual Form [NNAT-I]; Naglieri, 2003b). Another method is to use several different types of nonverbal subtests, as found in the WNV (as well as the Universal Nonverbal Intelligence Test [UNIT]; Bracken & McCallum, 1998). Despite their differences in administration methods and subtest content, these nonverbal tests of general ability provide a way to assess a wide variety of individuals fairly, regardless of their educational or linguistic backgrounds and/ or disabilities. The goal of fair and equitable assessment is as critical today as it was when the concepts of verbal and nonverbal assessment were initiated in the early 1900s.

Assessment of ability for populations of individuals who vary in educational and linguistic skills has been and continues to be one of the most important problems facing psychology and education. The initial conceptualization was clearly stated by

Yoakum and Yerkes (1920) when they wrote that nonverbal (Army Beta) tests were used to assess soldiers during World War I because a person could fail verbal (Army Alpha) tests because of limited skills in English. To avoid "injustice by reason of relative unfamiliarity with English" (Yoakum & Yerkes, 1920, p. 19), these persons were tested with nonverbal (Army Beta) tests to ensure accurate measurement of their general ability. Rather than attempting to measure verbal and nonverbal intelligences, the Army Alpha and Beta tests were used to measure general ability. Today, there are several different types of nonverbal tests of general ability (for a review, see Naglieri & Goldstein, 2009). In the remainder of this chapter, we describe an individually administered measure of general ability, WNV (Wechsler & Naglieri, 2006).

STRUCTURE AND ADMINISTRATION OF THE WNV

The WNV consists of six subtests that are organized into two forms (one for ages 4–7 years and the other for ages 8–21 years) and two versions (a two-subtest and a four-subtest version), as shown in Figure 18.1. The subtests measure general ability with tasks that vary in specific requirements. Some of the subtests have a strong visual–spatial requirement; others demand recall of spatial information or recall of the sequence of information; and still others involve paper-and-pencil skills. The multidimensionality of these tasks distinguishes the WNV from tests such as the NNAT-2 (Naglieri, 2008a), which exclusively uses progressive matrices.

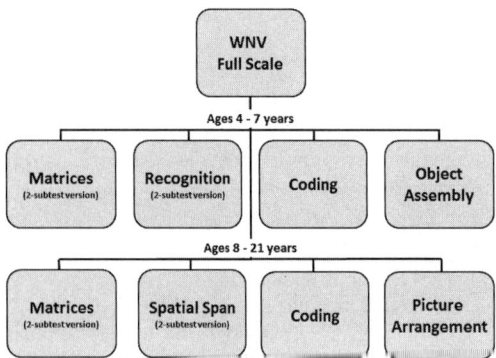

FIGURE 18.1. Organization of WNV two- and four-subtest versions by age.

Subtests

Most of the WNV subtests have appeared in previous editions of the Wechsler scales and have an established record of reliability and validity for the nonverbal measurement of general ability. The origins and descriptions of the WNV subtests are provided in Table 18.1. Adaptation of the subtests was necessary to accommodate the new pictorial-directions format, identify items that were most appropriate for the specific ages, and provide directions in several languages. WNV subtest norms (mean of 50 and standard deviation [SD] of 10) and Full Scale score norms (mean of 100 and SD of 15) are based on standardization samples collected in the United States and Canada. The subtests are briefly described below.

- *Matrices.* The Matrices subtest requires the examinee to discover how different geometric shapes are spatially or logically interrelated. The multiple-choice items are constructed of geometric figures such as squares, circles, and triangles, in some combination of the colors black, white, yellow, blue, and green. Matrices is always administered (i.e., it is given to examinees in both age bands and is included in both the four- and two-subtest batteries).

- *Coding.* The Coding subtest requires the examinee to copy symbols (e.g., two vertical lines, a dash) that are paired with simple geometric shapes or numbers according to a key provided at the top of the page. Form A is used in the four-subtest battery for ages 4 years, 0 months to 7 years, 11 months (4:0–7:11), and Form B is used in the four-subtest battery for ages 8:0–21:11.

- *Object Assembly.* The Object Assembly subtest consists of items that require the examinee to complete pieces of a puzzle to form a recognizable object, such as a ball or a car. Object Assembly is included in the four-subtest battery of the WNV for examinees ages 4:0–7:11.

- *Recognition.* The Recognition subtest was created for use in the WNV and is included in both the four- and two-subtest batteries for examinees ages 4:0–7:11. It requires the examinee to examine a stimulus (e.g., a square with a small circle in the center) for 3 seconds and then to choose which option is identical to the stimulus that was just seen. The figures are colored black, white, yellow, blue, and/or green to maintain interest and minimize the likelihood that impaired color vision will influence the scores.

TABLE 18.1. Origins and Description of WNV Subtests

Subtest	Origin and description
Matrices	This subtest was adapted from the Naglieri Nonverbal Ability Test—Individual Form (NNAT-I; Naglieri, 2003b). The examinee chooses an option that solves a progressive matrix.
Coding	This subtest was adapted from the Wechsler Intelligence Scale for Children—Fourth Edition (WISC-IV; Wechsler, 2003). The examinee copies symbols that are paired with simple geometric shapes or numbers using a key that appears at the top of the page.
Object Assembly	This subtest was adapted from the Wechsler Preschool and Primary Scale of Intelligence—Third Edition (WPPSI-III; Wechsler, 2002) and the Wechsler Intelligence Scale for Children—Third Edition (WISC-III; Wechsler, 1991). The child assembles puzzle pieces that make an object (e.g., a car).
Recognition	This is a new match-to-stimulus subtest. The child looks at a page with a design containing geometric patterns for 3 seconds. Then the child chooses which of several options matches the previously viewed stimulus.
Spatial Span	This subtest was adapted from the Wechsler Memory Scale—Third Edition (WMS-III; Wechsler, 1997a). The examinee repeats the examiner's touching of a series of blocks, either in the same order as the examiner or in the reverse order.
Picture Arrangement	This subtest is adapted from the Wechsler Adult Intelligence Scale—Third Edition (WAIS-III; Wechsler, 1997b) and a research version of the Wechsler Intelligence Scale for Children—Fourth Edition—Integrated (WISC-IV Integrated; Wechsler et al., 2004). The examinee puts picture cards in the correct order to tell a logical story within a specified time limit.

• *Spatial Span.* The Spatial Span subtest requires the examinee to touch a group of blocks arranged in an irregular pattern on an 8½-inch by 11-inch board in the same and reverse order demonstrated by the examiner. Spatial Span is included in both the four- and two-subtest batteries for ages 8:0–21:11.

• *Picture Arrangement.* The Picture Arrangement subtest involves cartoon-like illustrations, which must be put into a sequence that is logical and makes sense. Picture Arrangement is included in the four-subtest battery for examinees ages 8:0–21:11.

Administration

Administration of the WNV starts with short standardized introductions that tell examinees (1) to look at the pictorial directions to understand what to do, and (2) to ask the examiner questions if necessary. These introductions can be provided in English, French, Spanish, Chinese, German, or Dutch.

1. The first step in administration includes standardized directions that are always given as instructed and should never be changed. These directions include gestures that correspond to the pictorial directions. Pictorial directions are used at step 1 to provide a standardized method of communicating the demands of each task. These pictorial directions (see Figure 18.2) show a scene like the one the examinee is currently in. The pictures show an examinee being presented with the question, then thinking about the item, and finally choosing the correct solution. These instructions include actions by the examiner that must be carefully followed to ensure that the examinee understands the correspondence between the materials and the task. Gestures are used to direct the examinee's attention to specific portions of the pictorial directions and to the stimulus materials, and sometimes to demonstrate the task itself. Sometimes simple statements are also included to convey the importance of both time and accuracy to the examinee.

2. Additional directions are used *as needed* after the standard directions are provided. These instructions must also be followed exactly and are only given when an examinee is unclear about what he or she is being asked to do. These directions include simple sentences and gestures for further communicating the requirements of the task. The verbal instructions provide another way

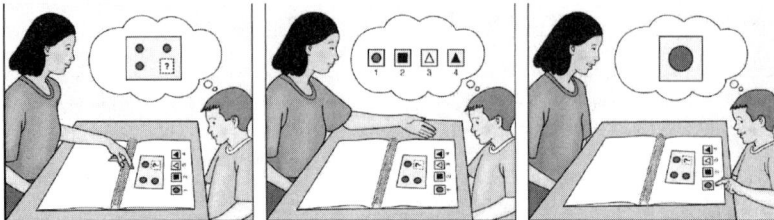

FIGURE 18.2. WNV Matrices pictorial directions. From Wechsler and Naglieri (2006). Copyright 2006 by Harcourt Assessment. Reprinted by permission of Pearson.

to ensure that the examinee understands the demands of the tasks; again, they can be given in English, Spanish, German, French, Chinese, or Dutch. These instructions are only used when two conditions are both met: first, if the WNV is being administered to an examinee who speaks one of the languages and, second, if the examiner or a professional interpreter speaks the same language.

3. Should additional assistance be necessary, special instructions to provide help are given, but these directions are only used after the previous two steps have been taken. This is the only step of administration that gives an examiner flexibility to communicate the demands of the task in any form. In general, examiners are given the opportunity to communicate in whatever manner they think will best clarify the demands of the subtest, based on their judgment of an examinee's needs. This may include providing further explanation or demonstration of the task, restating or revising the verbal directions, or using additional words (in a combination of languages, including sign language) to describe the requirements of the task. At no time, however, should an examiner teach an examinee how to solve the items. Instead, the goal is to provide additional help to ensure that the examinee understands the demands of the task. The amount of help provided and the determination about when to stop should both be based on professional judgment.

Using an Interpreter

When an interpreter is used to facilitate communication prior to and during administration, it is important for the interpreter to understand what is and what is not permitted. The person should translate a general explanation of the testing situation for the examinee, and especially the introductory paragraph at the beginning of Chapter 3 in the WNV Administration and Scoring Manual, before administration begins. The interpreter must also recognize the boundaries of his or her role in administration. For example, although it is appropriate for the interpreter to translate the examiner's responses to an examinee's response to a sample item, it is not acceptable for the interpreter to make additional statements unless instructed to do so. Importantly, at no time should the interpreter communicate any information that could influence the examinee's scores. See Brunnert, Naglieri, and Hardy-Braz (2009) for more information about working with translators, especially in testing examinees who are deaf or hard of hearing.

Subtest Administration Tips

Administration of the WNV subtests is designed to be simple and easy. The WNV Administration and Scoring Manual includes a section prior to actual administration directions for each subtest that describes the subtest; the materials needed; start, stop, and reverse rules; scoring; and issues unique to each subtest. The manual also provides considerable discussion of the physical materials; uses and applications for the two versions of the WNV; and general testing, administration, and scoring issues. Below, we highlight some of the most important points about individual subtest administration.

- *Matrices.* Matrices is a straightforward subtest to administer, but examiners should always be aware of possible responses that may suggest concern. For example, some students who are particularly impulsive may select the option that is mostly but not completely correct because the options were written with varying degrees of accuracy. If an examinee is not looking at the options closely, one of the almost-correct answers may be selected.

Similarly, if an examinee takes a long time to respond, the examiner may (after about 30 seconds) prompt a response.

• *Coding.* The examiner should ensure that the examinee works from left to right and from top to bottom without skipping any items or rows, by providing the appropriate instruction when needed. The examinee is allowed to correct mistakes by crossing out the incorrect symbol and writing the new response next to it, so the pencil without an eraser needs to be used for the Coding subtest. The examiner also briefly instructs the examinee to work as quickly as possible. For this reason, examinees should not be allowed to spend too much time making corrections.

• *Object Assembly.* The examiner should set up the puzzle pieces on the same side of the stimulus book as the examinee's dominant hand, and should then remove the stimulus book before administering the sample item. The examiner should also ensure that the examinee works as quickly as possible. If the examinee is still completing a puzzle when the time limit expires, the examiner should place his or her hand over the puzzle to stop the examinee's progress, and record the examinee's answer. If the examinee seems upset at that point, the examiner should allow the examinee to finish, but should not consider any additional work for scoring purposes. It is also important to remember to begin timing after the last word of the instruction is provided. Assembling the pieces for the examinee requires a specific method fully articulated in the WNV Administration and Scoring Manual. Essentially, the method requires that the puzzle pieces are put before the child in a specific format *face down*. Once all the pieces are before the child, then they are turned over in the order indicated by the number on the back of each piece.

• *Recognition.* The examiner must be sure to expose each stimulus page for exactly 3 seconds. To do so, the examiner should expose the page when the stopwatch strikes an exact second, and then be prepared to turn the page exactly when the 3 seconds have elapsed. Examinees should not be allowed to turn the pages, and it may be necessary to tell them to look at the stimulus page.

• *Spatial Span.* It is important to arrange the Spatial Span board so that an examinee can easily reach all cubes on the board and so that only the examiner can see the numbers on the back of each blue block. Also, the Spatial Span board should always be set on the same side of the stimulus book as the examinee's dominant hand. The blocks must be tapped at a rate of one per second, and the examiner should raise the hand approximately 1 foot above the Spatial Span board between each tap. If the examinee does not respond after the examiner taps a sequence, the examiner can say, "It's your turn." The examiner should always administer both Spatial Span Forward and Spatial Span Backward, regardless of the examinee's performance on Spatial Span Forward, and should always administer both trials of an item, regardless of the examinee's performance on the first trial.

• *Picture Arrangement.* The examiner should always place the Picture Arrangement cards on the same side of the stimulus book as the examinee's dominant hand, and should then remove the stimulus book with pictorial directions before administering the sample item. Having the cards in the box in the order in which they are to be exposed to the examinee is the best way to deliver the items. When the examinee completes the item, the examiner should record the sequence and then re-sequence the cards in the presentation order for the next administration. If the examinee is working too slowly, it is permissible to inform the examinee realizes that he or she should work as quickly as possible. If the examinee orders the cards from right to left instead of left to right, the examiner should ask, "Where does it start?" If the examinee is still working when the time limit expires, the examiner should place his or her hand over the story to stop the examinee's progress, and record the examinee's answer. If the examinee seems upset at being stopped while completing the story, the examiner should allow the examinee to finish. No credit can be given for any work completed after the time has expired, however.

SCORING

Scoring the WNV is straightforward and easily completed. Five of the six subtests (i.e., Matrices, Coding, Recognition, Spatial Span, and Picture Arrangement) are scored by summing the number of points earned during administration. The sixth subtest (i.e., Object Assembly) has time bonuses for some items that may be part of the raw score. The raw scores are converted to T scores. The sum of T scores is converted to a Full Scale score. Percentile ranks and confidence intervals are included in the conversion table. The WNV Scoring Assistant is a computer scoring program that obtains all derived scores based on the U.S. as well as the Canadian samples. The report-writing feature of the software provides reports that are appropriate for clinicians as well as parents. The parent report is available in English, French, and Spanish. The software also provides links between the WNV and the Wechsler Individual Achievement Test—Second Edition (Wechsler, 2001) for all the comparisons of ability to achievement.

PSYCHOMETRIC PROPERTIES

Standardization

The WNV was standardized in the United States and Canada. The U.S. sample consisted of 1,323 children and adolescents stratified across five demographic variables: age (4:0–21:11), sex, race/ethnicity (described as black, white, Hispanic, Asian, and other), education level (8 years or less of school, 9–11 years of school, 12 years of school [high school degree or equivalent], 13–15 years of school [some college or associate's degree], and 16 or more years of school [college or graduate degree]), and geographic region (Northeast, North Central, South, and West). Educational level was determined by parental education for examinees ages 4:0–17:11 and by the examinees' own education for ages 18:0–21:11. Approximately 4% of the U.S. normative sample consisted of individuals with limited English skills.

The Canadian sample consisted of 875 examinees stratified across five demographic variables: age (4:0–21:11), sex, race/ethnicity (described as Caucasian, Asian, First Nations, and other), education level (less than a high school diploma; high school diploma or equivalent; college/vocational diploma or some university, but no degree obtained; and a university degree), and geographic region (West, Central, and East). In addition, the Canadian sample consisted of 70% English speakers, 18% French speakers, and 12% speakers of other languages. See the WNV manual (Wechsler & Naglieri, 2006) for more details.

Reliability

WNV coefficients are provided by subtest and Full Scale scores by age and over all ages for the U.S. and Canadian normative samples, and for all the special groups in the WNV Technical and Interpretive Manual. The reliability coefficients for the U.S. normative sample were .91 for both the two-subtest and four-subtest versions' Full Scale scores

across ages, and ranged from .74 to .91 for the subtests. The reliability estimates for the Canadian normative sample ranged from .73 to .90 for the subtests, .90 for the Full Scale score (four-subtest version), .91 for the Full Scale score (two-subtest version). The reliability estimates for the studies of examinees with various classifications (gifted, mild and moderate of intellectual disabilities, reading and written expression disorders, language disorders, English-language learners, deaf, and hard of hearing are provided in the manual. Other information, such as the standard error of measurements (SEM), confidence intervals, and test–retest stability estimates for both the U.S. and the Canadian normative samples, is also provided in the WNV technical and Interpretive Manual (as well as the Administration and Scoring Manual).

Validity

English as a Second Language

As the United States continues to become more diverse, the number of individuals whose primary language is not English has also increased substantially. The largest of these groups is the Hispanic population, as noted earlier (Ramirez & de la Cruz, 2002). This population of Hispanics is dominated by individuals of Mexican origin (66.9%), who reside in the Western (44.2%) and Southern (34.8%) regions of the country. Hispanics ages 25 and older are less likely to have a high school diploma than white non-Hispanics (57.0% and 88.7%, respectively). These facts make clear the need for psychological tests that are appropriate for examinees from working-class homes with parents who have limited academic and English-language skills. Nonverbal tests of general ability such as the WNV are particularly useful for assessment of minority children because they yield smaller race and ethnic differences (which can be attributed to the difference in content) while retaining good correlations with achievement. In particular, they can help identify minority children for gifted programs, as noted below (Bracken & McCallum, 1998; Naglieri & Ford, 2003; Naglieri & Ronning, 2000a, 2000b).

Wechsler and Naglieri (2006) provide studies of the utility of the WNV for a sample of individuals speaking English as a second language (ESL), in comparison to a matched group from the WNV standardization sample. The ESL sample included 55 examinees ages 8–21 years whose native language was not English, who spoke a language other than English at home, and whose parents had resided in the United States less than 6 years. There were 27 Hispanics and 28 examinees whose primary language was Cantonese, Chinese, Korean, Russian, or Urdu. This sample earned very similar scores to their matched counterparts from the normative sample, with negligible effect sizes for the Full Scale scores from both WNV test batteries, as shown in Table 18.2. Additional information about this sample is available in the WNV Technical and Interpretive Manual.

Giftedness

The fact that minority children are underrepresented in classes for the gifted has been and continues an important educational problem (Ford, 1998; Naglieri & Ford, 2003, 2005). Discussion of this problem have sometimes focused on the types of tests used to evaluate children who may be eligible for gifted programming. Some researchers have argued that the verbal and quantitative content of some of the ability tests used and procedures followed are inconsistent with the characteristics of culturally, ethnically, and linguistically diverse populations (Naglieri & Ford, 2005). That is, since IQ has traditionally been measured with verbal, quantitative, and nonverbal questions, students with limited English-language and math skills earn lower scores on the verbal and quantitative scales these tests include because they do not have sufficient knowledge of the language or training in math, not because of low ability (Bracken & Naglieri, 2003; Naglieri, 2008a). One way to address this issue is to include tests that measure general ability nonverbally. Naglieri and Ford (2003) demonstrated the effectiveness of using a group nonverbal measure of general ability (the NNAT; Naglieri, 1997) for increasing the identification of Hispanic and black students as gifted. Similarly,

the WNV provides an individually administered way to assess general ability nonverbally and increase the participation of minorities in gifted classes.

The WNV manual reports a study involving gifted children who were carefully matched to control subjects included in the standardization sample on the basis of age, race/ethnicity, and education level. The differences between the means were calculated by using Cohen's (1988) formula (i.e., the difference between the means of the two groups divided by the square root of the pooled variance). The study included 41 examinees, all of whom had already been identified as gifted via a standardized ability measure where they performed at 2 SD above the mean or more. The students in the gifted programs performed significantly better than their matched counterparts from the normative sample, with large effect sizes for the Full Scale score on both the two- and four-subtest batteries. See Table 18.2 for more details.

Deafness/Hearing Impairments

The issues of limited spoken language and educational attainment are also relevant to those with deafness or hearing impairments. A more complete discussion of assessing such individuals with the WNV can be found in Brunnert and colleagues (2009). In general, however, the assessment issues center on (1) content of the test and (2) communicating test requirements to the examinees. The former issue has been covered in the previous section above on evaluation of the gifted. The issue of communicating test requirements has also been discussed in the "Administration" section of this chapter. In essence, because the directions are given pictorially and can be augmented with additional statements and/or communication in sign language, the WNV offers considerable advan-

TABLE 18.2. WNV Means, *SD*s, and Effect Sizes for Diverse Populations and Matched Control Groups

	Diverse sample			Control group			
	Mean	SD	n	Mean	SD	n	Effect size
Gifted students	123.7	13.4	41	104.2	12.3	41	1.5
English-language learners	101.7	13.4	55	102.1	13.4	55	0.0
Hard-of-hearing students	96.7	15.9	48	100.5	14.2	48	0.3
Profoundly deaf students	102.5	9.0	37	100.8	14.3	37	0.1

Note. Effect size = (X1 – X2)/SQRT [(n1 * SD12 + n2 * SD22)/(n1 + n2)]

tages for appropriate evaluation of individuals who are deaf or hard of hearing, as the research studies described below illustrate.

Wechsler and Naglieri (2006) reported two studies involving individuals who were deaf or hard of hearing. The first study involved a sample of profoundly deaf examinees who were compared with a group from the standardization sample of the WNV matched on a number of important demographic variables. The deaf sample consisted of 37 examinees who "must not have been able to hear tones to interpret spoken language after the age of 18 months, must not lip read, must not be trained in the oral or auditory–verbal approach, and must not use cued speech (i.e., they must have routine discourse by some means of communicating other than spoken language). They must have had severe to profound deafness (hearing loss measured with dB, Pure Tone Average greater than or equal to 55)" (WNV Technical and Interpretive Manual, p. 65). These examinees performed very similarly to their matched counterparts from the normative sample, with negligible effect sizes (Cohen's d) for the Full Scale score for both the two- and four-subtest batteries, as shown in Table 18.2.

Wechsler and Naglieri (2006) also described a study of individuals who were hard of hearing and compared them to a demographically matched group from the standardization sample. This study included 48 examinees who "could have a unilateral or bilateral hearing loss or deafness, and the age of onset of their inability to hear could be any age and [they] could have cochlear implants" (WNV Technical and Interpretive Manual, pp. 65–66). This group also performed similarly to the matched counterparts from the normative sample, again with negligible effect sizes (Cohen's d) for both batteries, as shown in Table 18.2.

INTERPRETATION

Like all test results, the WNV scores should be interpreted within the full context of the examinee and the administration setting. Issues such as the behaviors observed during testing, relevant educational and environmental backgrounds, physical and emotional status, and reason for referral must be considered when the results are examined. In order to obtain the greatest amount of information from the WNV, some interpretive methods that should be used are the same for the four- and two-subtest batteries, whereas others are unique to each version. These are discussed next.

Interpretation of Both Versions

The WNV subtests are set at a mean of 50 and SD of 10. These scores are combined to yield the Full Scale score (see below). The WNV is the first of the Wechsler tests to express the subtest scores on the T-score metric (as opposed to a traditional scaled score with a mean of 10 and SD of 3). This format was selected because the individual subtests had a sufficient range of raw scores to allow for the use of T scores which have a greater range and precision than scaled scores. The use of T scores also provides greater precision on each subtest, allowing for higher reliability coefficients of the Full Scale score. The subtest and Full Scale T scores are based on the U.S. or Canadian standardization sample.

The WNV Full Scale is set to have a mean of 100 and SD of 15, regardless of whether the four- or two-subtest battery is used. This score provides a nonverbal estimate of general ability that has excellent reliability and validity. It is important to recognize that even though the WNV subtests have different demands—that is, some are spatial (e.g., Matrices or Object Assembly), whereas others involve sequencing (Picture Arrangement and Spatial Span), require memory (e.g., Recognition and Spatial Span), or use symbol associations (Coding)—they all measure general ability. General ability, as represented by the Full Scale standard score, provides an estimate for predicting how well a person, for example, will be able to understand spatial as well as verbal and mathematical concepts, remember visual relationships as well as quantitative or verbal facts, and work with sequences of information of all kinds (Naglieri, Brulles, & Lansdowne, 2009). The content of the questions may be visual or verbal, and require memory or recognition, but general ability (sometimes referred to as g) underlies performance on all these kinds of tasks.

WNV Interpretation—Level 1

In the first interpretive step, the Full Scale score should be reported with its associated percentile score, categorical description (average, above average, etc.), and confidence interval. The following illustrates how this information could be included in a written document:

Annie obtained a WNV Full Scale score of 91, which is ranked at the 27th percentile and falls within the average classification. This means that she performed as well as or better than 27% of examinees her age in the normative sample. There is a 90% chance that her true Full Scale score falls within the range 85–99.

The second step in interpretation of the four-subtest version of the WNV is to examine the *T* scores the examinee earned on the subtests, taking into consideration the lower reliability of these scores. Examination of the four WNV subtests should also take into consideration that even though the subtests are all nonverbal measures of general ability, they do have unique attributes, as noted above. In addition, statistical guidelines should be followed to ensure that any differences interpreted are beyond those that could be expected by chance. The values needed for significance when comparing a WNV subtest for an examinee to that examinee's mean *T* score are provided in the WNV Administration and Scoring Manual (Table B.1) and in more detail by Brunnert and colleagues (2009), and should be used in examining subtest variability. The following steps should be used to compare each of the four WNV subtest *T* scores to the examinee's mean subtest *T* score:

1. Calculate the mean of the four subtest *T* scores.
2. Calculate the difference between each subtest *T* score and the mean.
3. Subtract the mean from each of the subtest *T* scores (retain the sign).
4. Find the value needed for significance, using the examinee's age group and the desired significance level in Table 12.3 of the WNV manual.
5. If the absolute value of the difference is equal to or greater than the value in the table, the result is statistically significant.
6. If the subtest difference from the mean is lower than the mean, then the difference is a weakness; if the subtest difference from the mean is greater than the mean, then the difference is a strength.

When there is significant variability in the WNV subtests, it is also important to determine whether a weakness relative to the examinee's overall mean is also sufficiently below the average range. Determining whether a child has significant variability relative to his or her own average score is a valuable way to determine strengths and weaknesses, but Naglieri (1999) has cautioned that a relative weakness could also be significantly below the

normative mean. He recommends that any subtest score that is low relative to the child's mean score should also fall below the average range to be considered a noteworthy weakness (i.e., at least 1 *SD* below the normative mean).

WNV Interpretation—Level 2

Spatial Span Forward and Backward

The WNV Spatial Span Forward and Backward scores can be interpreted separately. This can be useful when relating these findings to those for similar tests, such as Digit Span Forward and Backward (see the WISC-IV manual; Wechsler, 2003). The sizes of the differences required for statistical significance by age and for the U.S. and Canadian standardization samples are 11 and 13 for the .10 and .05 levels for the U.S. sample, and 10 and 13 for these levels for the Canadian sample, for the combined ages 8:0–21:11. The comparisons are accomplished with Table C.1 of the WNV Administration and Scoring Manual, which provides a way to convert the raw scores to *T*-score equivalents for Spatial Span Forward and Backward. A difference of 9 *T*-score points is needed at the .15 level (13 at the .05 level) for significance. (Note that base rate data by the direction of the difference are provided in the WNV manual.)

Information about Spatial Span Forward and Backward *T* scores may provide useful information, but it should be integrated within the greater context of a comprehensive assessment. For example, if a difference between Spatial Span Forward and Backward is found, it may be expected that similar results will be found on similar tests (e.g., WISC-IV Digit Span Forward vs. Digit Span Backward). The Backward scores may also be related to the Planning Scale of the Cognitive Assessment System (CAS; see Naglieri, 1999) and may suggest that the examinee has difficulty with development and utilization of strategies for reversing the order of serial information. In addition, Digit Span and Spatial Span Forward may be considered measures of sequencing, whereas Digit Span and Spatial Span Backward may be considered measures of sustained concentration and visual–spatial working memory, respectively (Miller, 2007, 2010).

In fact, Spatial Span can be considered a non-verbal version of the WISC-IV Digit Span subtest, even though the task has a distinct spatial component. For Spatial Span Forward, the child touches a sequence of blocks randomly arranged on an 8½-by 11-inch board in the same order as demonstrated by the examiner. For Spatial Span Backward, the child repeats a sequence in the reverse order of that demonstrated by the examiner. Again, then, Spatial Span Backward can be viewed as a task that requires visual–spatial working memory. Goldberg (2009) defines working memory "as the selection of task-relevant information" (p. 94), and it is the selection process incorporated into the task that demands strategy use. Observing the child's performance on Spatial Span Forward can reveal information about how well the child initially commits sequenced visual–spatial information to memory. Spatial Span Backward allows the examiner to observe visual working memory capacity and efficiency in the selection of the sequence executed. Normative information for comparisons of Spatial Span Forward and Backward, as well as normative sample base rates found in the WNV manual, should be used to calibrate any differences found.

Coding

The WNV Coding subtest also provides the opportunity for finer clinical interpretation. For example, Koziol and Budding (2009) hypothesized that a task such as coding places demands on working memory because there are numbers and symbols, and that quick performance may be facilitated by "holding this information online in working memory in the course of performing the task" (p. 261). The associations between symbols and numbers are maintained within working memory, and a short-term plan of action is activated. If the number–symbol associations are made quickly, it is assumed that less conscious effort is required for the task. This observation is consistent with Gabrieli, Stebbins, Singh, Willingham, and Goetz's (1997) formulation that working memory capacity facilitates fast performance and the attainment of procedural learning.

A child who completes the Coding subtest accurately but very slowly is approaching the task differently from a child who completes the task quickly but with many errors (making the wrong number–symbol association, skipping), who in turn is different from a child who completes the task quickly and accurately. Useful ways to interpret this kind of performance may be in terms of attention to the instructions (e.g., whether the instruction to "do the task as fast as you can" is ignored) or of conscious effort or concentration. The child who works faster for the 120 seconds and gives more responses has approached the task

very differently from the child who works more slowly and gives fewer responses. These subjects have completed the tasks at different rates over the same time interval. From this we can hypothesize that the child who works more slowly has to put forth greater conscious control and effort, which may be related to recruitment of more brain area (Saling & Philips, 2007). The child who works more slowly has to concentrate harder, and the child who works quickly has probably expended less effort. In this way, the subtest score for Coding may be viewed as a measure of efficiency of concentration.

Matrices

The WNV Matrices subtest is similar to others that have a long history as good measures of general ability as measured by high g loadings (Jensen, 1998). Tests like Matrices can be viewed as measures of visual-perceptual reasoning. Matrices can also be considered a test of simultaneous processing, a mental activity by which a person integrates stimuli into interrelated groups or a whole (Naglieri, 1999). Simultaneous processing tests typically have strong visual–spatial aspects. The cognitive demand of the task requires the integration of information (Naglieri & Otero, 2011).

CASE STUDY

Reason for Referral

Lorena was seen in connection with a multidisciplinary evaluation to assess her educational needs. The examiner (Tulio M. Otero) was specifically requested to evaluate Lorena in the areas of cognitive and academic functioning. Lorena is a third grader who is currently in a regular education class with English-language learner (ELL) services. A review of her files indicated that she suffered a closed head injury at age 3 in a motor vehicle accident. There was brief loss of consciousness (approximately 10 minutes). At the time of this evaluation, no further medical history was available. Despite interventions that included 8 weeks of Lexia Reading and Symphony Math, Lorena has been making only limited progress in both reading and math.

Observations

Lorena is a 9-year-old Hispanic female who speaks both English and Spanish. At home, Lorena speaks only Spanish, since neither of her parents speaks English. As noted above, she is in a regular classroom setting with ELL services. Lorena preferred to converse with the examiner in English, but during the evaluation both languages needed to be used. Although both languages were used, her performance did not improve on verbal portions of the tests. She was alert, oriented, friendly, and cooperative. Her range of emotion was good, and she did not report any significant worries or concerns. Lorena reported that she had gone to bed late the night before because the family had gone to a party. She further indicated that she sometimes naps in the afternoon and then stays awake watching TV until very late in the evening. Although she put forth good effort on all tasks, it was obvious that she struggled from time to time because of fatigue. She did not have any negative reaction to failure and became quite animated when she did well on tasks.

Lorena struggled on academic achievement tests. During word-reading tasks, she read slowly. Her reading errors can be described as approximations to words based on what they looked like. For example, she read "ground" instead of *around*, "worm" for *wrong*, and "throw" for *threw*. Reading comprehension was deficient and very slow. She did not seem to benefit from the visual stimuli accompanying the passage she needed to read in order to complete the missing word. On math reasoning tasks, Lorena took a long time to initiate a response, needed prompting to use paper and pencil to assist her in deriving the answer, and often used ineffective strategies. Relatively simple items took her several minutes to work through. On calculation tasks she also did poorly initially because of either treating subtraction as addition or providing a result that did not make sense. During testing of the limits, Lorena was guided to notice her errors and the operation sign. She correctly reworked five items for which she could not receive credit. Her spelling skills seem typical of ELL students who are using sounds in Spanish to spell English words that may not follow a similar sound structure. Yet she also missed sounds or sound clusters. Examples of some of her errors were "joump" for *jump*, "forrise" for *forest*, "unfar" for *unfair*, and "meniger" for *manager*.

Tests Administered

- Reynolds Intellectual Assessment Scales (RIAS)
- Cognitive Assessment System (CAS)
- Wechsler Nonverbal Test of Ability (WNV)
- WJ III Tests of Achievement (WJ III)
- Batería III Pruebas de Aprovechamiento

Ability Results

Lorena was administered the RIAS in English with Spanish support, using select items from the Spanish version of the RIAS. The RIAS is an individually administered measure of intellectual functioning normed for individuals between the ages of 3 and 94 years. It contains several individual tests of intellectual problem solving and reasoning ability, which are combined to form a Verbal Intelligence Index (VIX) and a Nonverbal Intelligence Index (NIX). These two indexes of intellectual functioning are then combined to form an overall Composite Intelligence Index (CIX). Each of these indexes is expressed as an age-corrected standard score that is scaled to a mean of 100 and an *SD* of 15. The RIAS also contains Verbal Memory and Nonverbal Memory subtests, which are combined to form a Composite Memory Index (CMX).

Lorena earned a CIX score of 81 on the RIAS. This level of performance falls within the range of scores designated as below average and exceeds the performance of 10% of individuals Lorena's age. Lorena earned a VIX score of 79, which falls within the moderately below-average range of verbal intelligence skills and exceeds the performance of 8% of individuals Lorena's age. Lorena earned an NIX score of 88, which falls within the below-average range of nonverbal intelligence skills and exceeds the performance of 21% of individuals Lorena's age. Lorena's VIX and NIX scores are not significantly different.

Lorena also earned a CMX score of 86, which falls within the low average range of working memory skills. This exceeds the performance of 18% of individuals Lorena's age. Within the subtests making up the CMX, Lorena's performance in the Nonverbal Memory domain significantly exceeded her performance within the Verbal Memory domain. This difference is reliable and indicates that Lorena functions at a significantly higher level when asked to recall or engage in working memory tasks that are easily adapted to visual–spatial cues (*T* score = 51) and other nonverbal memory features, as opposed to tasks relying on verbal linguistic strategies (*T* score = 33). Lorena's RIAS performance is presented in Table 18.3.

The CAS was also administered to Lorena in Spanish, in order to understand her functioning from a neurocognitive perspective. The CAS is an

TABLE 18.3. Reynolds Intellectual Assessment Scales (RIAS) Results for Lorena

Subtest	T score		
Guess What	34		
Odd-Item Out	40		
Verbal Reasoning	35		
What's Missing	43		
Verbal Memory	33		
Nonverbal Memory	51		

Scale	T score	90% confidence interval	Percentile rank
Verbal Intelligence Index	79	75–86	8
Nonverbal Intelligence Index	88	83–94	21
Composite Intelligence Index	81	77–87	10
Composite Memory Index	86	81–92	18

Note. Lorena's Verbal Memory score is significantly lower than her Nonverbal Memory score.

individually administered test designed to measure intelligence as a group of cognitive processes. It is based on the PASS theory of intelligence. The basic premise of the theory is that human cognitive functioning includes Planning, Attention, Simultaneous processing, and Successive processing (PASS) abilities.

Lorena earned a CAS Full Scale score of 87, which is within the low average classification and is ranked at the 19th percentile. This means that her performance is equal to or greater than 19% of those obtained by children her age in the standardization group. There is a 90% probability that Lorena's true Full Scale score is within the range of 81–96. The CAS Full Scale score is made up of four separate scales, each measuring one of the PASS processes. There was no significant variation among the separate PASS scales of the CAS; this indicates that she performed similarly when using planning, attention, simultaneous, and successive cognitive processes. It also means that the Full Scale score is a good description of her overall performance on this test. It is noteworthy to mention that although no significant discrepancies are noted relative to her average performance across cognitive processing domains, normative weaknesses are evident in both planning and successive processes. Furthermore, Lorena did particularly poorly on a subtest requiring the simultaneous understanding and integration of verbal and spatial information (Verbal–Spatial Relations).

The Planning scale of the CAS measures cognitive control, use of strategies, knowledge and skills,

intentionality, and self-regulation. In essence, the scale measures a child's ability to determine how to solve a problem, execute that solution, monitor its effectiveness, and modify the approach as needed to achieve the goal. This includes impulse control, as well as generation, evaluation, and execution of a plan. The Planning scale measures how well a child can solve problems of varying complexity that may involve control of attention, simultaneous, and successive processes, as well as acquisition of knowledge and skill. This ability is associated with the brain area known as the prefrontal cortex. Lorena earned a CAS Planning standard score of 85, which is within the low average classification and is ranked at the 16th percentile. This means that Lorena did as well as or better than 16% of children her age in the standardization group. There is a 90% probability that Lorena's true Planning score is within the range of 79–95.

The Attention scale of the CAS measures a student's ability to demonstrate focused, selective cognition over time, with resistance to distraction. That is, attention can be described as focused, selective, sustained, and effortful activity. *Focused* attention involves concentration directed toward a particular activity, and *selective* attention is important for the inhibition of responses to distracting stimuli. *Sustained* attention refers to the variation of performance over time, which can be influenced by the varying amounts of *effort* required to solve the test. An effective measure of attention presents children with competing demands and requires sustained focus. The components of attention are subserved by subcortical and frontal brain regions in an interactive manner. *Executive attention* is defined as maintaining behavior goals and using these goals as a basis for choosing what aspects of the environment or tasks to attend to and which action to select. Paying attention is the first step in the learning process. Lorena earned a CAS Attention standard score of 100, which is within the average classification and is ranked at the 50th percentile. This means that Lorena did as well as or better than 50% of children her age in the standardization group. There is a 90% probability that Lorena's true Attention score is within the range of 92–109.

The Simultaneous scale of the CAS is designed to measure the child's ability to integrate separate but interrelated stimuli into groups or into a whole. Simultaneous processing tests have strong visual–spatial aspects for this reason, but this ability is also used to solve tasks with verbal content (e.g., reading comprehension), as long as the tasks require integration of information into a coherent whole. Simultaneous processing underlies the use and comprehension of grammatical statements because they demand comprehension of word relationships, prepositions, and inflections, so that the person can obtain meaning based on the whole idea. Select aspects of verbal reasoning tasks, such as those in which an examinee is given two to four clues and asked to deduce the object or concept being described, also require simultaneous processing. Lorena earned a CAS Simultaneous standard score of 94, which is within the average classification and is ranked at the 34th percentile. This means that Lorena did as well as or better than 34% of children her age in the standardization group. There is a 90% probability that Lorena's true Simultaneous score is within the range of 87–102.

The Successive scale of the CAS evaluates how well the child can work with stimuli in a specific serial order, where each element is only related to those that precede it and these stimuli are not interrelated. Successive processing ability involves both the perception of stimuli in sequence and the formation of sounds and movements in order. For example, successive processing is involved in the decoding of unfamiliar words, production of syntactic aspects of language, and speech articulation. This process is measured with tests that demand use, repetition, or comprehension of information based on order. Following a sequence such as the order of operations in a math problem is another example of successive processing. Lorena earned

a CAS Successive standard score of 84, which is within the low average classification and is ranked at the 14th percentile. This means that Lorena did as well as or better than 14% of children her age in the standardization group. There is a 90% probability that Lorena's true Successive score is within the range of 78–93. Lorena's overall CAS performance is presented in Table 18.4.

In order to assess Lorena's overall cognitive ability by eliminating or minimizing the impacts of limited language proficiency, she was administered the WNV. The WNV is used to assess the general cognitive ability of individuals ages 4–21 years. Lorena's WNV Full Scale score is 95; she scored higher than approximately 37 out of 100 individuals her age. Her general cognitive ability, as assessed by the WNV, is in the average range. These results suggest that her general cognitive ability is somewhat higher than that measured by other measures, which require the student to process language both receptively and expressively. This is an example of how nonverbal tests can be particularly important when Hispanic children are assessed, as these students are more likely to have varying histories of educational opportunity and levels of academic English-language proficiency. Lorena's WNV performance is presented in Table 18.5.

Academic Skills Results

Lorena was administered select subtests from the WJ III and Bateria III. These tests provide measures of Lorena's academic achievement. Relative strengths and weaknesses among her academic skills are described below.

Assessment in English

The WJ III Broad Reading cluster includes reading decoding, reading speed, and the ability to comprehend connected discourse while reading. Her standard score for this cluster is 61, which falls within the very low range (percentile rank range of <1–1; standard score range of 58–63) for her age. Lorena's overall reading ability is very limited; reading tasks above the age 7:5 level will be quite difficult for her. Lorena is likely to require intensive instructional support and targeted interventions in reading. The Letter–Word Identification subtest measured Lorena's ability to identify words. Lorena seemed unable to apply phoneme–grapheme relationships. Passage Comprehension measured Lorena's ability to understand what she had read. The items required Lorena to read a

TABLE 18.4. Cognitive Assessment System (CAS) Results for Lorena

Subtest	Scaled score
Planning	
Matching Numbers	8
Planned Codes	7
Simultaneous	
Nonverbal Matrices	11
Verbal–Spatial Relations	7
Attention	
Expressive Attention	11
Number Detection	9
Successive	
Word Series	6
Sentence Repetition	8

Scale	Scaled score	90% confidence interval	Percentile rank	Difference
Planning	85	79–95	16	5.75
Simultaneous	94	87–102	34	–3.25
Attention	100	92–109	50	–9.25
Successive	84	78–93	14	6.75
Full Scale	87	81–96	19	—

Note. Lorena's mean PASS score = 90.75. Verbal–Spatial Relations is a significant weakness within the Simultaneous scale.

short passage and identify a missing keyword that made sense in the context of the passage. Lorena appeared to read each passage very slowly and had difficulty identifying the missing word. Reading Fluency measured Lorena's ability to read simple sentences quickly. Lorena appeared to read and respond to the sentences slowly.

The WJ III Broad Math cluster includes mathematics reasoning and problem solving, number facility, and automaticity. Although her standard score in this cluster is within the very low range (58), her performance varied on different types of math tasks. Lorena's performance was very limited on tasks requiring the ability to analyze and

TABLE 18.5. Wechsler Nonverbal Scale of Ability (WNV) Results for Lorena

	Standard score	Percentile rank	90% confidence interval		
Full Scale score	95	37	89–102		

Subtest	Subtest *T* score	Difference from mean	Critical value	Variability	Base rate
Matrices	51	3	8	NS	32.8
Coding	47	–1	10	NS	47.2
Spatial Span	42	–6	8	NS	18.6
Picture Arrangement	52	4	10	NS	27.7
Within-subtests analysis					
Spatial Span Forward–Backward	39	–8	13	NS	21.6

Note. The mean WNV subtest score is 48.0.

solve applied mathematics problems (the Applied Problems subtest; standard score = 80). Her performance was limited to negligible on tasks requiring knowledge of how to perform mathematical computations, either with or without time limits (the Math Calculation Skills cluster, including the Calculation and Math Fluency subtests; standard score = 39). Intensive instructional support in math, including targeted interventions, is likely to be needed for Lorena. Calculation measured Lorena's ability to perform mathematical computations; she worked very slowly and relied on the use of strategies that appeared to be inefficient for her age level. To solve each item in Applied Problems, Lorena was required to listen to the problem, recognize the procedure to be followed, and then perform relatively simple calculations. Because many of the problems included extraneous information, Lorena needed to decide not only the appropriate mathematical operations to use, but also what information to include in the calculation. Lorena appeared to have limited understanding of age-appropriate math application tasks. Finally, Math Fluency measured Lorena's ability to solve a series of simple addition, subtraction, and multipli-

cation problems quickly (in a 3-minute time limit). Lorena appeared to take longer to work on such problems than is typical for her age peers.

In the area of Brief Writing, Lorena attained a standard score within the low range (79), suggesting underdeveloped writing skills. Her Spelling score was significantly lower than her Writing Samples score. Spelling measured Lorena's ability to write orally presented words correctly; Lorena spelled words in a laborious manner. Writing Samples measured Lorena's skill in writing responses to meet a variety of demands. She was asked to produce written sentences that were evaluated with respect to the quality of expression. Lorena was not penalized for any errors in basic writing skills, such as spelling or punctuation. Many of her sentences were inadequate to meet the task demands. Yet she managed to score within the average range on this particular subtest.

Overall, Lorena's academic skills in English are negligible (see Table 18.6 for a summary). For example, her spelling is very limited. Her sight-reading ability and math calculation skills are negligible. Lorena's overall ability to apply her academic skills is limited. Specifically, her writing ability is limited

TABLE 18.6. Woodcock–Johnson III Normative Update Tests of Achievement Results for Lorena

CLUSTER/test	AE	Easy	to	diff.	SS (90% confidence interval)	GE
ACHIEVEMENT	7:4	7:0	to	7:8	67 (65–70)	2:0
BROAD READING	7:1	6:9	to	7:5	61 (58–63)	1:7
BROAD MATH	6:11	6:4	to	7:7	58 (55–62)	1:6
MATH CALC. SKILLS	6:4	5:11	to	7:0	39 (32–45)	1:1
BRIEF WRITING	7:7	7:2	to	8:2	79 (76–82)	2:2
ACADEMIC SKILLS	6:11	6:7	to	7:3	58 (55–61)	1:6
ACADEMIC APPLICATIONS	7:6	7:1	to	8:1	72 (69–76)	2:2
Letter–Word Identification	7:2	6:11	to	7:5	67 (65–70)	1:8
Applied Problems	7:10	7:4	to	8:4	80 (76–83)	2:5
Spelling	7:2	6:10	to	7:7	72 (68–76)	1:9
Passage Comprehension	6:11	6:7	to	7:2	67 (62–71)	1:6
Math Fluency	7:1	<5:1	to	9:0	70 (66–73)	1:8
Calculation	6:3	6:1	to	6:6	38 (31–46)	1:0
Writing Samples	8:5	7:6	to	10:4	92 (87–97)	3:1
Reading Fluency	7:3	6:1	to	8:2	71 (65–76)	1:9

	SS			Variation		
Variations	Actual	Predicted	Difference	PR	SD	Significant at ±1.50 SD (SEE)
Intra-Achievement (Brief) BROAD MATH	58	79	–20	5	–1.63	Yes

Note. Norms based on ages 9–10. AE, age equivalent; SS, standard score; GE, grade equivalent.

to average. Her passage comprehension ability and quantitative reasoning are very limited.

Academic Assessment in Spanish

On the Batería III, Breve Lectura includes reading decoding and the ability to comprehend connected discourse while reading. Lorena's standard score in this area is within the very low range (66; percentile rank range of 1–2; standard score range of 64–69) when compared to others of her age. Her reading skill is negligible; reading tasks above the age 7:6 level will be quite difficult for her.

Ortografía measures Lorena's ability to write orally presented words correctly in Spanish. Her standard score is within the low range (74; percentile rank range of 3–7; standard score range of 71–78) for her age. Lorena's spelling ability is very limited; spelling above the age 7:9 level will be quite difficult for her. Lorena's Batería III performance is presented in Table 18.7.

Summary

Lorena's RIAS CIX score (81) indicates mild deficits in general intelligence relative to others of her age when ability is measured with verbal and nonverbal tests. Students earning a CIX score in the 80s frequently experience at least some difficulty acquiring information through traditional educational methods provided in the classroom setting. Although her verbal and nonverbal cognitive skills are relatively equally developed, according to statistical analysis, her verbal skills are qualitatively lower. Her score on the RIAS Nonverbal Memory scale is higher than her Verbal Memory score. Importantly, however, the WNV results (95) suggest that Lorena's general ability when language-processing requirements are mark-

edly reduced is within the average range. Lorena's English achievement test scores suggest academic skills within the low range. When compared to those of others at her age level, Lorena's standard score is low in writing, and her standard scores are very low in broad reading, broad mathematics, and math calculation skills. Lorena demonstrated a significant weakness in mathematics, particularly because she confused the operation signs and made calculation errors when borrowing and regrouping. Among the Spanish achievement test results, Lorena's standard score is very low in reading.

Possible Instructional Recommendations and Interventions

- Lorena will probably gain the most from reading instruction presented within the middle- to late-first-grade range. Increased time spent reading may increase Lorena's exposure to printed words and may result in an increase in the number of words that she can recognize orthographically.
- Translating written words into speech—orally reading words in isolation—may be helpful to Lorena in activating and outputting the sound representations of printed words.
- Repeated reading is a fluency-building intervention. Lorena should read a short passage several times until she can read the passage with ease. The instructor should select material that is at Lorena's instructional reading level; have her read through the passage aloud; record the number of errors, as well as the time it took to read the passage; and, when Lorena completes the passage, review the misread words and then have her read it again. This approach should be continued until Lorena has read the passage

TABLE 18.7. Batería III Normative Update Pruebas de Aprovechamiento Results for Lorena

CLUSTER/test	AE	Easy to diff.	SS (90% confidence interval)	GE
LECTURA (READING)	7:2	6:11 to 7:6	66 (64–69)	1:9
Ident de Letras y Palabras (Letter–Word Identification)	7:3	7:1 to 7:6	70 (68–73)	2:0
Ortografía (Spelling)	7:4	7:0 to 7:9	74 (71–78)	2:0
Comprensión de Textos (Reading Comprehension)	7:1	6:9 to 7:5	71 (68–75)	1:8

Note. See footnote to Table 18.6.

three to five times or has reached a preestablished goal for accuracy or rate.

- Lorena and her parents should be encouraged to spend time reading every day outside of school.
- In order to address Lorena's weaknesses in planning and successive abilities, reading strategies described by Naglieri and Pickering (2010) should be used. Lorena's teachers and parents can help her follow the instructions in the handouts (e.g., Summarization Strategy for Reading Comprehension, Chunking for Reading/Decoding, Word Families for Reading/Decoding).
- Math instruction presented within the middle-first-grade to early-second-grade range will be likely to produce the greatest gains for Lorena.
- Use of a concrete–representational–abstract sequence will ensure that Lorena understands a computation or math fact: first by using manipulatives, then by drawing representations (pictures or tallies) of the problem, and finally by solving the problem with actual numbers.
- Teachers and parents should consider using math techniques described by Naglieri and Pickering (2010), such as Touch Math, the Part–Whole Strategy, and the Seven-Step Strategy. These methods will help Lorena to solve math problems in a variety of settings.
- The cover–copy–compare intervention requires teacher-made worksheets that provide correctly completed problems on the left side of the paper and the unsolved problem on the right side of the paper. The teacher will instruct Lorena to study the correctly completed problem, then cover it with an index card, complete the matching problem to the right, and check her work by comparing it to the model problem.
- Writing instruction presented within the early- to middle-second-grade level is appropriate for Lorena.
- The Write–Say method may be helpful in addressing Lorena's spelling skills. This intervention will require Lorena to study a spelling list on her own on Monday and then to participate in an orally administered spelling test on Tuesday. The teacher will provide verbal feedback, and Lorena will then say and write the correct spelling of missed words, letter by letter, five times. The same procedure is to be followed Wednesday and Thursday; however, Lorena will then practice incorrectly spelled words 10 times and 15 times, respectively. Finally, the teacher will administer a summative spelling test on Friday.
- The Add-a-Word spelling program may assist Lorena in developing better spelling skills. To implement this intervention, Lorena's teacher will provide five daily spelling words. Each word must be correctly spelled 5 days in a row before an individual word is replaced with a new spelling word. If on subsequent spelling tests a previously learned word is missed, that word will be placed back onto the current spelling list until it is mastered again.
- Lorean needs to devote more time to writing. Daily writing practice at school and at home facilitates writing for different purposes and for different audiences. Making the connection between writing and real-world applications should be an important motivator in developing Lorena's writing skills.
- Because Lorena has earned a low score on the Planning scale of the CAS, she should be provided with strategies for writing. The following descriptive handouts of specific methods (Naglieri & Pickering, 2010) should be provided to the teachers and parents: Story Plans for Written Composition, Story Grammar for Writing, and Plans for Writing. These will help Lorena acquire strategies for communicating her ideas in writing. These and other handouts are available in Spanish for use by Lorena's parents.
- Lorena will probably gain the most from Spanish reading instruction presented within the late-first-grade to early-second-grade range.
- Further analysis will be undertaken, and specific recommendations will be made, by the school's multidisciplinary team.

Examined by Tulio M. Otero, PhD, NCSP, ABSNP

SUMMARY AND CONCLUSIONS

Assessment of diverse populations of children and adults with ability tests that include verbal questions is particularly problematic for those with limited language skills and/or educational opportunities. The WNV was designed to provide a nonverbal measure of general ability that would be appropriate for a wide variety of culturally and linguistically diverse populations and would be useful in a number of assessment settings, including identification of gifted minority students. The selection of subtests, the use of pictorial directions, and inclusion of supplemental oral directions in several languages provides a unique approach to measuring general ability nonverbally. This chapter has summarized some of the validity evidence provided in the test manual, which supports the utility of the WNV for fair assessment of cognitive ability in several groups (students from culturally diverse backgrounds and/or with language differences, gifted students, and students who are deaf or hard of hearing). Within the context of a comprehensive evaluation, the WNV can provide critically important information about an examinee's level of general ability.

REFERENCES

Boake, C. (2002). From the Binet–Simon to the Wechsler–Bellevue: Tracing the history of intelligence testing. *Journal of Clinical and Experimental Neuropsychology, 24*, 383–405.

Bracken, B. A., & McCallum, R. S. (1998). *Universal Nonverbal Intelligence Test*. Itasca, IL: Riverside.

Bracken, B. A., & Naglieri, J. A. (2003). Assessing diverse populations with nonverbal tests of general intelligence. In C. R. Reynolds & R. W. Kamphaus (Eds.), *Handbook of psychological and educational assessment of children* (pp. 243–273). New York: Guilford Press.

Brunnert, K., Naglieri, J. A., & Hardy-Braz, S. (2009). *Essentials of WNV assessment*. Hoboken, NJ: Wiley.

Cohen, J. (1988). *Statistical power analysis for the behavioral sciences* (2nd ed.). San Diego, CA: Academic Press.

Ford, D. Y. (1998). The underrepresentation of minority students in gifted education: Problems and promises in recruitment and retention. *Journal of Special Education, 32*, 4–14.

Gabrieli, J. D., Stebbins, G. T., Singh, J., Willingham, D. B., & Goetz, C. G. (1997). Intact mirror-tracing and impaired rotary-pursuit skill learning in patients with Huntington's disease: Evidence for dissociable memory systems in skill learning. *Neuropsychology, 11*, 272–281.

Goldberg, E. (2009). *The new executive brain: Frontal lobes in a complex world*. New York: Oxford University Press.

Jensen, A. R. (1998). *The g factor: The science of mental ability*. Westport, CT: Praeger.

Koziol, L., & Budding, D. E. (2009). *Subcortical structures and cognition: Implications for neuropsychological assessment*. New York: Springer.

Miller, D. C. (2007). *Essentials of school neuropsychology assessment*. Hoboken, NJ: Wiley.

Miller, D. C. (2010). *Best practices in school neuropsychology: Guidelines for effective practice, assessment, and evidence-based intervention*. Hoboken, NJ: Wiley.

Naglieri, J. A. (1997). *Naglieri Nonverbal Ability Test— Multilevel Form*. San Antonio, TX: Psychological Corporation.

Naglieri, J. A. (1999). *Essentials of CAS assessment*. New York: Wiley.

Naglieri, J. A. (2003a). Naglieri Nonverbal Ability Tests: NNAT and MAT-EF. In R. S. McCallum (Ed.), *Handbook of nonverbal assessment* (pp. 175–190). New York: Kluwer.

Naglieri, J. A. (2003b). *Naglieri Nonverbal Ability Test— Individual Form*. San Antonio, TX: Psychological Corporation.

Naglieri, J. A. (2008a). *Naglieri Nonverbal Ability Test— Second Edition*. San Antonio, TX: Pearson.

Naglieri, J. A. (2008b). Traditional IQ: 100 years of misconception and its relationship to minority representation in gifted programs. In J. VanTassel-Baska (Ed.), *Critical issues in equity and excellence in gifted education series alternative assessment of gifted learners* (pp. 67–88). Waco, TX: Prufrock Press.

Naglieri, J. A., Brulles, D., & Lansdowne, K. (2009). *Helping all gifted children learn: A teacher's guide to using the NNAT2*. San Antonio, TX: Pearson.

Naglieri, J. A., & Ford, D. Y. (2003). Addressing underrepresentation of gifted minority children using the Naglieri Nonverbal Ability Test (NNAT). *Gifted Child Quarterly, 47*, 155–160.

Naglieri, J. A., & Ford, D. Y. (2005). Increasing minority children's participation in gifted classes using the NNAT: A response to Lohman. *Gifted Child Quarterly, 49*, 29–36.

Naglieri, J. A., & Goldstein, S. (Eds.). (2009). *Practitioner's guide to assessing intelligence and achievement*. New York: Wiley.

Naglieri, J. A., & Otero, T. (2011). Cognitive Assessment System: Redefining intelligence from a neuropsychological perspective. In A. Davis (Ed.), *Handbook of pediatric neuropsychology* (pp. 320–333). New York: Springer.

Naglieri, J. A., & Pickering, E. (2010). *Helping children learn: Intervention handouts for use in school and at home* (2nd ed.). Baltimore: Brookes.

Naglieri, J. A., & Ronning, M. E. (2000a). Comparison of white, African-American, Hispanic, and Asian children on the Naglieri Nonverbal Ability Test. *Psychological Assessment, 12*, 328–334.

Naglieri, J. A., & Ronning, M. E. (2000b). The relationships between general ability using the NNAT and SAT Reading Achievement. *Journal of Psychoeducational Assessment, 18*, 230–239.

Ramirez, R. R., & de la Cruz, G. (2002). *The Hispanic population in the United States: March 2002* (Current Population Reports No. 20-545). Washington, DC: U.S. Bureau of the Census.

Saling, L. L., & Philips, J. G. (2007). Automatic behavior: efficient not mindless. *Brain Research Bulletin, 73,* 1–20.

Wechsler, D. (1958). *The measurement and appraisal of adult intelligence* (4th ed.). Baltimore: Williams & Wilkins.

Wechsler, D. (1991). *Wechsler Intelligence Scale for Children—Third Edition.* San Antonio, TX: Psychological Corporation.

Wechsler, D. (1997a). *Wechsler Adult Intelligence Scale—Third Edition,* San Antonio, TX: Psychological Corporation.

Wechsler, D. (1997b). *Wechsler Memory Scale—Third Edition.* San Antonio, TX: Pearson

Wechsler, D. (2001). *Wechsler Individual Achievement Test—Second Edition.* San Antonio, TX: Psychological Corporation.

Wechsler, D. (2002). *Wechsler Preschool and Primary Scale of Intelligence—Third Edition.* San Antonio, TX: Psychological Corporation.

Wechsler, D. (2003). *Wechsler Intelligence Scale for Children—Fourth Edition.* San Antonio, TX: Psychological Corporation.

Wechsler, D., Kaplan, E., Fein, D., Kramer, J., Morris, R., Delis, D. C., et al. (2004). *Wechsler Intelligence Scale for Children—Fourth Edition—Integrated.* San Antonio, TX: Harcourt Assessment.

Wechsler, D., & Naglieri, J. A. (2006). *Wechsler Nonverbal Scale of Ability.* San Antonio, TX: Harcourt Assessment.

Woodcock, R. W., McGrew, K. S., & Mather, N. (2001a). *Woodcock–Johnson III Test of Achievement.* Itasca, IL: Riverside.

Woodcock, R. W., McGrew, K. S., & Mather, N. (2001b). *Woodcock–Johnson III Test of Cognitive Abilities.* Itasca, IL: Riverside.

Yoakum, C. S., & Yerkes, R. M. (1920). *Army mental tests.* New York: Holt.

PART IV

CONTEMPORARY INTERPRETIVE APPROACHES AND THEIR RELEVANCE FOR INTERVENTION

CHAPTER 19

The Cross-Battery Assessment Approach
An Overview, Historical Perspective, and Current Directions

Dawn P. Flanagan
Vincent C. Alfonso
Samuel O. Ortiz

AN OVERVIEW OF THE XBA APPROACH

The Cattell–Horn–Carroll (CHC) cross-battery assessment approach (hereafter referred to as the XBA approach) was introduced by Flanagan and her colleagues well over a decade ago (Flanagan & McGrew, 1997; Flanagan, McGrew, & Ortiz, 2000; Flanagan & Ortiz, 2001; McGrew & Flanagan, 1998). The XBA approach provides practitioners with the means to make systematic, reliable, and theory-based interpretations of cognitive batteries, and to augment them with academic ability tests and neuropsychological instruments, to gain a more complete understanding of an individual's strengths and weaknesses (Flanagan, Ortiz, & Alfonso, 2007, 2012). Moving beyond the boundaries of a single cognitive, achievement, or neuropsychological battery by adopting the theoretically and psychometrically sound principles and procedures outlined in the XBA approach represents a significant improvement over single-battery assessment because it allows practitioners to focus on measurement of the cognitive constructs and neurodevelopmental functions that are most germane to referral concerns (e.g., Carroll, 1998; Decker, 2008; Kaufman, 2000; Wilson, 1992).

According to Carroll (Appendix, this volume), the CHC taxonomy of human cognitive abilities "appears to prescribe that individuals should be assessed with regard to the *total range* of abilities the theory specifies" (p. 889; emphasis in original). However, because Carroll recognized that "any such prescription would of course create enormous problems," he indicated that "[r]esearch is needed to spell out how the assessor can select what abilities need to be tested in particular cases" (p. 889). Flanagan and colleagues' XBA approach was developed to "spell out" how practitioners can conduct assessments that approximate the total range of cognitive and academic abilities and neuropsychological processes more adequately than what is possible with most collections of co-normed tests.

In a review of the XBA approach, Carroll (1998) stated that it "can be used to develop the most appropriate information about an individual in a given testing situation" (p. xi). In Kaufman's (2000) review of XBA, he stated that the approach is based on sound assessment principles, adds theory to psychometrics, and improves the quality of the assessment and interpretation of cognitive abilities and processes. More recently, Decker (2008) stated that the CHC XBA approach "may improve school psychology assessment practice and facilitate the integration of neuropsychological methodology in school-based assessments . . . [because it] shift[s] assessment practice from IQ composites to neurodevelopmental functions" (p. 804).

Noteworthy is the fact that assessment professionals "crossed" batteries well before Woodcock (1990) recognized the need, and before Flanagan and her colleagues introduced the XBA approach in the late 1990s based, in part, on Woodcock's suggestion. Neuropsychologists have long adopted the practice of crossing various standardized tests in an attempt to measure a broader range of brain functions than that offered by any single instrument (Lezak, 1976, 1995; Lezak, Howieson, & Loring, 2004; see Wilson, 1992, for a review). Nevertheless, several problems with crossing batteries plagued assessment-related fields for years. Many of these problems have been circumvented by Flanagan and colleagues' XBA approach (see Table 19.1 for examples). But unlike the XBA approach, the various so-called "cross-battery" techniques applied within the field of neuropsychological assessment, for example, are not typically grounded in a systematic approach that is theoretically and psychometrically sound. Thus, as Wilson (1992) cogently pointed out, the field of neuropsychological assessment was in need of an approach that would guide practitioners through the selection of measures that would result in more specific and delineated patterns of function and dysfunction—an approach that would provide more clinically useful information than one "wedded to the utilization of subscale scores and IQs" (p. 382) would. Indeed, all fields involved in the assessment of cognitive and neuropsychological functioning have some need for an approach that would aid practitioners in their attempt to "touch all of the major cognitive areas, with emphasis on those most suspect on the basis of history, observation, and ongoing test findings" (Wilson, 1992, p. 382). The XBA approach meets this need. The definition of and rationale for XBA is presented in this chapter, followed by a description of the XBA method. Figure 19.1 provides an overview of the information presented in this chapter.

DEFINITION

The XBA approach is a method of assessing cognitive and academic abilities and neuropsychological processes that is grounded mainly in CHC theory and research. It allows practitioners to measure reliably a wider range (or a more in-depth but selective range) of ability constructs than that represented by any given stand-alone assessment battery. The XBA approach is based on three foundational sources of information (Flanagan et al., 2007, 2012) that together provide the knowledge base necessary to organize theory-driven, comprehensive assessment of cognitive, academic, and neuropsychological constructs.

THE FOUNDATION OF THE XBA APPROACH

The foundation of the XBA approach is contemporary CHC theory—specifically, the broad and narrow CHC ability classifications of all subtests constituting current cognitive, achievement, and selected neuropsychological batteries.

CHC Theory

The CHC theory was selected to guide assessment and interpretation because it is based on a more thorough network of validity evidence than any other contemporary multidimensional model of intelligence within the psychometric tradition (see Carroll, 1993; Horn & Blankson, Chapter 3, this volume; McGrew, 2005; Messick, 1992; Schneider & McGrew, Chapter 4, this volume; Sternberg & Kaufman, 1998). According to Daniel (1997), the strength of the multiple-cognitive-abilities (CHC) model is that it was arrived at "by synthesizing hundreds of factor analyses conducted over decades by independent researchers using many different collections of tests. Never before has a psychometric ability model been so firmly grounded in data" (pp. 1042–1043). Because CHC theory is discussed in detail by Schneider and McGrew in Chapter 4 of this volume, it is not described in detail here.

CHC Broad (Stratum II) Classifications of Major Ability Tests

Using the results of a series of cross-battery confirmatory factor analysis (CFA) studies of the major intelligence batteries (see Keith & Reynolds, 2010, for a review) and the task analyses of many cognitive test experts, Flanagan and colleagues classified the subtests of the major cognitive, neuropsychological, and achievement batteries according to the particular CHC broad abilities they measured (e.g., Flanagan, Alfonso, Ortiz, & Dynda, 2010; Flanagan, Ortiz, Alfonso, & Mascolo, 2006; Flanagan et al., 2007, 2012; McGrew, 1997; McGrew & Flanagan, 1998; Reynolds, Keith, Flanagan, & Alfonso, 2011). To date, hundreds of CHC broad-ability classifications have been based on the results of these studies. These

TABLE 19.1. Parallel Needs in Assessment-Related Fields Addressed by the Cross-Battery Assessment (XBA) Approach

Need within assessment-related fields[a]	Need addressed by the XBA approach
School psychology, clinical psychology, and neuropsychology have lagged in the development of conceptual models of the assessment of individuals. There is a need for the development of contemporary models.	The XBA approach provides a contemporary model for measurement and interpretation of cognitive and academic abilities and neuropsychological processes.
It is likely that there is a need for events external to a field of endeavor to give impetus to new developments and real advances in that field.	Carroll and Horn's fluid–crystallized theoretical models and systematic programs of research in cognitive psychology provided the impetus for the XBA approach and led to the development of better assessment instruments and interpretive procedures.
There is a need for truly unidimensional assessment instruments for children and adults. Without them, valid interpretations of test scores are problematic at best.	Several scale and composite measures on ability batteries are mixed, containing excess reliable variance associated with a construct irrelevant to the one intended for interpretation. The XBA approach ensures that assessments include composites or clusters that are relatively pure representations of Cattell–Horn–Carroll (CHC) broad and narrow abilities, allowing for valid measurement and interpretation of multiple, relatively distinct abilities.
There is a need to utilize a conceptual framework to direct any approach to assessment. This would aid both in the selection of instruments and methods, and in the interpretation of test findings.	The XBA approach to assessment is based mainly on CHC theory as well as sound measurement and interpretive procedures. Since this approach links all the major intelligence batteries, academic achievement tests, and selected neuropsychological instruments to this theory, both selection of tests and interpretation of test findings are made within the context of an overarching conceptual framework.
It is necessary for the conceptual framework or model underlying assessment to incorporate various aspects of neuropsychological and cognitive functioning, which can be described in terms of constructs that are recognized in the neuropsychological and cognitive psychology literature.	The XBA approach incorporates various aspects of neuropsychological and cognitive ability functions, which are described in terms of constructs that are recognized in the related literature.
There is a need to adopt a conceptual framework that allows for the measurement of the full range of behavioral functions subserved by the brain. Unfortunately, in neuropsychological assessment there is no inclusive set of measures that is standardized on a single normative population.	XBA allows for the measurement of a wide range of broad and narrow cognitive abilities specified in CHC theory. Although an XBA norm group does not exist, the method of crossing batteries to obtain a broad assessment of human cognitive abilities is grounded in sound psychometric principles and procedures.
Because there are no truly unidimensional measures in psychological assessment, there is a need to select subtests from standardized instruments that appear to reflect the neurocognitive function of interest. In neuropsychological assessment, therefore, the aim is to select those measures that, on the basis of careful task analysis, appear mainly to tap a given construct.	The XBA approach is defined in part by a CHC classification system. Subtests from the major intelligence batteries, academic achievement tests, and selected neuropsychological instruments were classified as measures of broad and narrow CHC constructs. Use of these classifications allows practitioners to be reasonably confident that a given test taps a given construct.

(cont.)

TABLE 19.1. *(cont.)*

Need within assessment-related fields[a]	Need addressed by the XBA approach
It is clear that an eclectic approach is needed in the selection of measures—preferably subtests rather than the omnibus IQs, in order to gain more specificity in the delineation of patterns of function and dysfunction.	The XBA approach ensures that two or more relatively pure, but qualitatively different, indicators of each *broad* cognitive ability are represented in an assessment of broad CHC constructs. Two or more qualitatively similar indicators are necessary to make inferences about specific or *narrow* CHC constructs. The XBA approach is eclectic in its selection of measures, but attempts to represent all broad and narrow abilities and processes of interest by using a subset of measures from one battery to augment another battery.
There is a need to solve the potential problems that can arise from crossing normative groups as well as sets of measures that vary in reliability.	In the XBA approach, one can typically achieve baseline data in cognitive functioning across seven or eight CHC broad abilities and processes through the use of two well-standardized batteries that were normed within a few years of one another; this minimizes the effects of error due to norming differences. Also, since interpretation of both broad and narrow CHC abilities is made at the cluster (rather than subtest) level, issues related to low reliability are less problematic in this approach. Also, because confidence intervals are used for all broad- and narrow-ability clusters, the effects of measurement error are reduced further. Additionally, any and all evidence of weakness, deficit, or dysfunction must have ecological validity (see Flanagan et al., 2012, for details).

[a]Information obtained, in part, from Wilson (1992).

classifications of cognitive, neuropsychological, and achievement batteries assist practitioners in identifying measures that assess the various broad and narrow abilities represented in CHC theory. Classification of tests at the broad-ability level is necessary to improve upon the validity of cognitive assessment and interpretation. Specifically, broad-ability classifications ensure that the CHC constructs underlying assessments are minimally affected by *construct-irrelevant variance* (Messick, 1989, 1995). In other words, knowing what tests measure what abilities enables clinicians to organize tests into *construct-relevant* clusters—clusters that contain only measures that are relevant to the construct or ability of interest (McGrew & Flanagan, 1998).

To clarify, construct-irrelevant variance is present when an "assessment is too broad, containing excess reliable variance associated with other distinct constructs . . . that affects responses in a manner irrelevant to the interpreted constructs" (Messick, 1995, p. 742.) For example, the Wechsler Intelligence Scale for Children—Fourth Edition (WISC-IV; Wechsler, 2003) Perceptual Reasoning Index (PRI) has construct-irrelevant variance because, in addition to its two indicators of Gf

(i.e., Picture Concepts, Matrix Reasoning), it has an indicator of Gv (i.e., Block Design). Therefore, the PRI is a mixed measure of two relatively distinct, broad CHC abilities (Gf and Gv); it contains reliable variance (associated with Gv) that is irrelevant to the interpreted construct of Gf. The PRI represents a grouping together of subtests on the basis of factor analysis and face validity (e.g., grouping tests together that appear to measure the same common construct) the latter of which may result in an inappropriate aggregation of subtests that can actually decrease reliability and validity (Epstein, 1983). Through CHC-driven CFA, Keith, Fine, Reynolds, Taub, and Kranzler (2006) showed that a five-factor model that included Gf and Gv (not PRI) fit the WISC-IV standardization data equally well as the four-factor Wechsler model. As a result of their analysis, Gf and Gv composites for the WISC-IV were provided in Flanagan and Kaufman (2004, 2009) and are recommended in the XBA approach because they contain only construct-relevant variance (Flanagan et al., 2012).

Construct-irrelevant variance can also operate at the subtest (as opposed to composite) level. For example, a Verbal Analogies test (e.g., "Sun

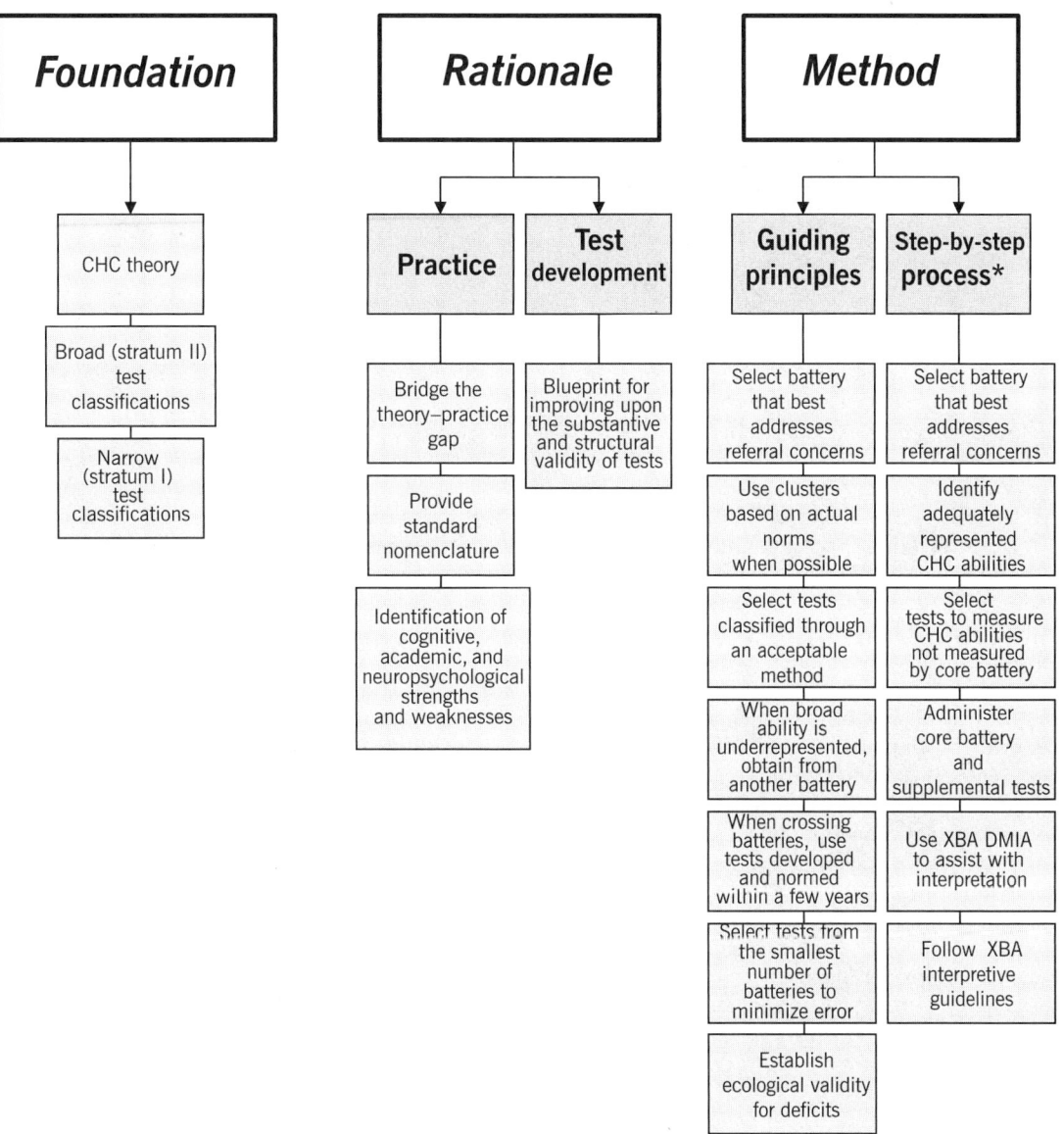

FIGURE 19.1. Overview of the CHC XBA approach. XBA DMIA is the XBA Data Management and Interpretive Assistant. This program (described in Table 19.6) automates the XBA approach. *These steps are described in *Essentials of Cross-Battery Assessment* (Flanagan et al., 2007, 2012).

is to day as moon is to _____") measures both Gc and Gf. That is, in theory-driven factor-analytic studies, Verbal Analogies tests have significant loadings on both the Gc and Gf factors (e.g., Woodcock, 1990). Therefore, this test is considered factorially complex—a condition that complicates interpretation. For example, is poor performance due to low vocabulary knowledge [Gc] or to poor reasoning ability [Gf], or both?

In short, interpretation is less complicated when composites are derived from relatively pure measures of the underlying construct. Conversely, "any test that measures more than one common factor to a substantial degree yields scores that are psychologically ambiguous and very difficult to interpret" (Guilford, 1954, p. 356; cited in Briggs & Cheek, 1986). Therefore, cross-battery assessments are typically designed using only empirically strong or moderate (but not factorially complex or mixed) measures of CHC abilities (Flanagan et al., 2007, 2012; McGrew & Flanagan, 1998).

CHC Narrow (Stratum I) Classifications of Major Ability Tests

Narrow-ability classifications were originally reported in McGrew (1997), then later reported in McGrew and Flanagan (1998) and Flanagan and colleagues (2000) after minor modifications. Flanagan and her colleagues continued to gather content validity data on cognitive ability tests and expanded their analyses to include tests of academic achievement (Flanagan, Ortiz, Alfonso, & Mascolo, 2002; Flanagan et al., 2006) and, more recently, tests of neuropsychological processes (Flanagan et al., 2010, 2012). Classifications of cognitive ability tests according to content, format, and task demand at the narrow-ability (stratum I) level were necessary to improve further upon the validity of cognitive ability assessment and interpretation. Specifically, these narrow-ability classifications were necessary to ensure that the CHC constructs underlying assessments are well represented (McGrew & Flanagan, 1998). According to Messick (1995), *construct underrepresentation* is present when an "assessment is too narrow and fails to include important dimensions or facets of the construct" (p. 742).

Interpreting the Woodcock–Johnson III Tests of Cognitive Abilities (WJ III; Woodcock, McGrew, & Mather, 2001, 2007) Concept Formation (CF) test as a measure of fluid intelligence (i.e., the broad Gf ability) is an example of construct underrepresentation. This is because CF measures *one* narrow aspect of Gf (viz., inductive reasoning). At least one other Gf measure (i.e., subtest) that is qualitatively different from inductive reasoning is necessary to include in an assessment to ensure adequate representation of the Gf construct (e.g., a measure of general sequential [or deductive] reasoning). Two or more qualitatively different indicators (i.e., measures of two or more narrow abilities subsumed by the broad ability) are needed for adequate construct representation (see Comrey, 1988; Messick, 1989, 1995). The aggregate of CF (a measure of inductive reasoning at the narrow-ability level) and the WJ III Analysis–Synthesis test (a measure of deductive reasoning at the narrow-ability level), for example, would provide an adequate estimate of the broad Gf ability because these tests are strong measures of Gf and represent qualitatively different aspects of this broad ability.

The Verbal Comprehension Index (VCI) of the Wechsler Adult Intelligence Scale—Fourth Edition (WAIS-IV; Wechsler, 2008) is an example of good construct representation. This is because the VCI includes Vocabulary (lexical knowledge), Similarities (language development/lexical knowledge), and Information (general information), which represent qualitatively different aspects of Gc.

Most intelligence batteries yield construct-relevant composites, although some of these composites underrepresent the broad ability intended to be measured. This is because construct underrepresentation can also occur when the composite consists of two or more measures of the *same* narrow (stratum I) ability. For example, the Number Recall and Word Order subtests of the Kaufman Assessment Battery for Children—Second Edition (KABC-II; Kaufman & Kaufman, 2004) were intended to be interpreted as a representation of the broad Gsm ability. However, these subtests primarily measure memory span, a narrow ability subsumed by Gsm. Thus the Gsm cluster of the KABC-II is more appropriately interpreted as memory span (a narrow ability) than as an estimate of the broad ability of short-term memory.

"A scale [or broad CHC ability cluster] will yield far more information—and, hence, be a more valid measure of a construct—if it contains more differentiated items [or tests]" (Clarke & Watson, 1995, p. 311). The XBA approach circumvents the misinterpretations that can result from underrepresented constructs by specifying the use of two or more qualitatively different indicators to represent each broad CHC ability. In order to ensure that qualitatively different aspects of broad abilities are represented in assessment, classification of cognitive and academic ability tests at the narrow-ability (stratum I) level was necessary (McGrew & Flanagan, 1998). The subtests of current cognitive batteries, special-purpose tests (including neuropsychological tests), and achievement tests have been classified at both the broad- and narrow-ability levels (see Flanagan et al., 2006, 2007, 2010; Flanagan, Alfonso, & Mascolo, 2011).

In sum, the classifications of tests at the broad- and narrow-ability levels of CHC theory guard against two ubiquitous sources of invalidity in assessment: construct-irrelevant variance and construct underrepresentation. Taken together, CHC theory and the CHC classifications of tests that underlie the XBA approach provide the necessary foundation from which to organize assessments that are theoretically driven, comprehensive, and supported by research.

RATIONALE FOR THE XBA APPROACH

The XBA approach has significant implications for practice, research, and test development (see Figure 19.1). A brief discussion of these implications follows.

Practice

The XBA approach provides "a much needed and updated bridge between current intellectual theory and research and practice" (Flanagan & McGrew, 1997, p. 322). The need for the XBA "bridge" became evident following a review of the results of several cross-battery factor analyses conducted prior to 2000. In particular, the results demonstrated that none of the intelligence batteries in use at that time contained measures that sufficiently approximated the full range of broad abilities defining the structure of intelligence specified in contemporary psychometric theory (see Table 19.2; see also Alfonso, Flanagan, & Radwan, 2005, for a comprehensive discussion of these findings). Indeed, the joint factor analyses conducted by Woodcock (1990) suggested that it might be necessary to "cross" batteries to measure a broader range of cognitive abilities than that provided by a single intelligence battery.

As may be seen in Table 19.2, most batteries fell far short of measuring all seven of the broad cognitive abilities listed. Of the major intelligence batteries in use prior to 2000, most failed to measure three or more broad CHC abilities (viz., Ga, Glr, Gf, Gs) that were (and are) considered important in understanding and predicting school achievement (Flanagan et al., 2006; McGrew & Wendling, 2010). In fact, Gf, often considered to be the *essence* of intelligence, was either not measured or not measured adequately by most of the intelligence batteries included in Table 19.2 (i.e., WISC-III, WAIS-R, WPPSI-R, K-ABC, and CAS) (Alfonso et al., 2005).

The finding that the abilities *not measured* by the intelligence batteries listed in Table 19.2 are important in understanding children's learning difficulties provided much of the impetus for developing the XBA approach (McGrew & Flanagan, 1998). In effect, the XBA approach was developed to systematically replace the dashes in Table 19.2 with tests from another battery. As such, this approach guides practitioners in the selection of tests that together provide measurement of abilities that can be considered sufficient in both breadth and depth for the purpose of addressing referral concerns.

Another contribution of the XBA approach to practice was that it facilitated communication among professionals. Most scientific disciplines have a standard nomenclature (i.e., a common set of terms and definitions) that facilitates communication and guards against misinterpretation (McGrew & Flanagan, 1998). For example, the standard nomenclature in chemistry is reflected in the periodic table of elements; in biology, it is reflected in the classification of animals according to phyla; in psychology and psychiatry, it is reflected in the *Diagnostic and Statistical Manual of Mental Disorders*; and in medicine, it is reflected in the *International Classification of Diseases*. Underlying the XBA approach is a standard nomenclature or *table of human cognitive abilities* (McGrew & Flanagan, 1998) that includes classifications of hundred of tests according to the broad and narrow CHC abilities they measure (see also Alfonso et al., 2005; Flanagan & Ortiz; 2001; Flanagan et al., 2002, 2006, 2007, 2010, 2012). The XBA classification system has had a positive impact on communication among practitioners; has improved our understanding of and guided the research on the relations between cognitive and academic abilities (Flanagan et al., 2011; McGrew & Wendling, 2010); and has resulted in improvements in the measurement of cognitive constructs, as may be seen in the design and structure of current cognitive batteries.

Finally, the XBA approach offers practitioners a psychometrically sound means to identifying population-relative (or normative) strengths and weaknesses. Because the approach focuses interpretation on cognitive ability clusters (i.e., via combinations of construct-relevant subtests) that contain either qualitatively different indicators of each CHC broad-ability construct (to represent broad-ability domains) or qualitatively similar indicators of narrow abilities (to represent narrow- or specific-ability domains), the identification of normative strengths and weaknesses via XBA is possible. Adhering closely to the guiding principles of the approach (described later) will help to ensure that the identified strengths and weaknesses may be interpreted in a theoretically and psychometrically sound manner. In sum, the XBA approach addresses the long-standing need within the entire field of assessment, from learning disabilities

TABLE 19.2. Representation of Broad CHC Abilities on Nine Intelligence Batteries Published Prior to 2000

Battery	Gf	Gc	Gv	Gsm	Glr	Ga	Gs
WISC-III	—	Vocabulary Information Similarities Comprehension	Block Design Object Assembly Picture Arrangement Picture Completion Mazes	Digit Span	—	—	Symbol Search Coding
WAIS-R	—	Vocabulary Information Similarities Comprehension	Block Design Object Assembly Picture Completion Picture Arrangement	Digit Span	—	—	Digit–Symbol
WPPSI-R	—	Vocabulary Information Similarities Comprehension	Block Design Object Assembly Picture Completion Mazes Geometric Design	Sentences	—	—	Animal Pegs
KAIT	Mystery Codes Logical Steps	Definitions Famous Faces Auditory Comprehension Double Meanings	Memory for Block Designs	—	Rebus Learning Rebus Delayed Recall Auditory Delayed Recall	—	—
K-ABC	Matrix Analogies	—	Triangles Face Recognition Gestalt Closure Magic Window Hand Movements Spatial Memory Photo Series	Number Recall Word Order	—	—	—

CAS	—	—	Figure Memory Verbal–Spatial Relations Nonverbal Matrices	Word Series Sentence Repetition Sentence Questions	—	—	Matching Numbers Receptive Attention Planned Codes Number Detection Planned Connections Expressive Attention
DAS	Matrices Picture Similarities Sequential and Quantitative Reasoning	Similarities Verbal Comprehension Word Definitions Naming Vocabulary	Pattern Construction Block Building Copying Matching Letter-Like Forms Recall of Designs Recognition of Pictures	Recall of Digits	Recall of Objects	—	Speed of Information Processing
WJ-R	Concept Formation Analysis–Synthesis	Oral Vocabulary Picture Vocabulary Listening Comprehension Verbal Analogies	Spatial Relations Picture Recognition Visual Closure	Memory for Words Memory for Sentences Numbers Reversed	Memory for Names Visual–Auditory Learning Delayed Recall: Memory for Names Delayed Recall: Visual–Auditory Learning	Incomplete Words Sound Blending Sound Patterns	Visual Matching Cross Out
SB-IV	Matrices Equation Building Number Series	Verbal Relations Comprehension Absurdities Vocabulary	Pattern Analysis Bead Memory Copying Memory for Objects Paper Folding and Cutting	Memory for Sentences Memory for Digits	—	—	—

Note. WISC-III, Wechsler Intelligence Scale for Children—Third Edition (Wechsler, 1991); WAIS-R, Wechsler Adult Intelligence Scale—Revised (Wechsler, 1981); WPPSI-R, Wechsler Preschool and Primary Scale of Intelligence—Revised (Wechsler, 1989); KAIT, Kaufman Adolescent and Adult Intelligence Test (Kaufman & Kaufman, 1993); K-ABC, Kaufman Assessment Battery for Children (Kaufman & Kaufman, 1983); CAS, Cognitive Assessment System (Naglieri & Das, 1997); DAS, Differential Ability Scales (Elliott, 1990); WJ-R, Woodcock-Johnson Psycho-Educational Battery—Revised (Woodcock & Johnson, 1989); SB-IV, Stanford–Binet Intelligence Scale: Fourth Edition (Thorndike, Hagen, & Sattler, 1986).

to neuropsychological assessment, for methods that "provide a greater range of information about the ways individuals learn—the ways individuals receive, store, integrate, and express information" (Brackett & McPherson, 1996, p. 80; see also Decker, 2008).

Test Development

Although there was substantial evidence of at least eight or nine broad cognitive CHC abilities by the late 1980s, the tests of the time did not reflect this diversity in measurement. For example, Table 19.2 shows that the WPPSI-R, K-ABC, KAIT, WAIS-R, and CAS batteries (see the footnotes to this and subsequent tables for full names of most test batteries from this point on) only measured two or three broad CHC abilities adequately. The WPPSI-R primarily measured Gv and Gc. The K-ABC primarily measured Gv and Gsm, and to a much lesser extent Gf; the KAIT primarily measured Gc and Glr, and to a much lesser extent Gf and Gv. The CAS measured Gs, Gsm, and Gv.[1] Finally, while the DAS, SB-IV, and WISC-III did not provide sufficient coverage of abilities to narrow the gap between contemporary theory and practice, their comprehensive measurement of approximately four CHC abilities was nonetheless an improvement over the previously mentioned batteries. Table 19.2 shows that only the WJ-R included measures of all broad cognitive abilities as compared to the other batteries available at that time. Nevertheless, most of the broad abilities were not measured adequately by the WJ-R (Alfonso et al., 2005; McGrew & Flanagan, 1998).

In general, Table 19.2 shows that Gf, Gsm, Glr, Ga, and Gs were not measured well by the majority of intelligence batteries published before 2000. Therefore, it was clear that most test authors did not use contemporary psychometric theories of the structure of cognitive abilities to guide the development of their intelligence batteries. As such, a substantial theory–practice gap existed; that is, theories of the structure of cognitive abilities were far in advance of the instruments used to operationalize them. In fact, prior to the mid-1980s, theory seldom played a role in intelligence test development. The numerous dashes in Table 19.2 exemplify the theory–practice gap that existed in the field of intellectual assessment at that time (Alfonso et al., 2005).

In the past decade particularly, CHC theory has had a significant impact on the revision of old and development of new intelligence batter-

ies. For example, a wider range of broad and narrow abilities is represented in current intelligence batteries than in previous editions of these tests. Table 19.3 provides several salient examples of the impact that CHC theory and the XBA classifications have had on intelligence test revision over the past two decades. This table lists the major intelligence tests that have been revised since 2000 in the order in which they were revised, beginning with those tests with the greatest number of years between revisions (i.e., K-ABC). Not included in Table 19.3 are fairly dated tests that have yet to be revised (e.g., the CAS). As is obvious from a review of Table 19.3, CHC theory and XBA classifications have had a significant impact on test development (Alfonso et al., 2005).

Of the seven intelligence batteries that were revised since 2000, the test authors of four clearly used CHC theory and XBA classifications as a blueprint for test development (i.e., the WJ III, SB5, KABC-II, and DAS-II). Only the authors of the Wechsler scales (i.e., the WPPSI-III, WISC-IV, and WAIS-IV) did not state explicitly that CHC theory was used as a guide for revision. Nevertheless, the authors of the Wechsler scales have acknowledged the research of Cattell, Horn, and Carroll in their most recent test manuals (Wechsler, 2002, 2003, 2008). Presently, as Table 19.3 suggests, nearly all intelligence batteries that are used with some regularity subscribe either explicitly or implicitly to CHC theory (Alfonso et al., 2005; Flanagan et al., 2006, 2012).

Convergence toward the incorporation of CHC theory is also seen clearly in Table 19.4. This table is similar to Table 19.2 except that it includes all intelligence battery revisions published after 2000. A comparison of Table 19.2 and Table 19.4 shows that many of the gaps in measurement of broad cognitive abilities have been filled in the revisions. Specifically, the majority of test revisions published after 2000 now measure four or five broad cognitive abilities adequately (see Table 19.4), as compared to two to three (see Table 19.2). For example, Table 19.4 shows that the WISC-IV measures Gf, Gc, Gv, Gsm, and Gs, while the KABC-II measures Gf, Gc, Gv, and Glr adequately, and to a lesser extent Gsm. The WAIS-IV measures Gc, Gv, Gsm, and Gs adequately, and to a lesser extent Gf, while the WPPSI-III measures Gf, Gc, Gv, and Gs adequately. Finally, the SB5 measures four CHC broad abilities (i.e., Gf, Gc, Gv, Gsm) (Alfonso et al., 2005).

Table 19.4 shows that the DAS-II and the WJ III include measures of all the major broad cognitive

TABLE 19.3. Impact of CHC Theory and XBA on Intelligence Test Revision

Test (year of publication) CHC and XBA impact	Revision (year of publication) CHC and XBA impact
K-ABC (1983) No obvious impact.	**KABC-II (2004)** Provides a second global score that includes fluid and crystallized abilities. Includes several new subtests measuring reasoning. Interpretation of test performance may be based on CHC theory or Luria's theory. Provides assessment of five CHC broad abilities.
SB-IV (1986) Used a three-level hierarchical model of the structure of cognitive abilities to guide construction of the test. The top level included a general reasoning factor or g; the middle level included three broad factors called Crystallized Abilities, Fluid-Analytic Abilities, and Short-Term Memory; the third level included more specific factors, including Verbal Reasoning, Quantitative Reasoning, and Abstract/Visual Reasoning.	**SB5 (2003)** CHC theory has been used to guide test development. Increases the number of broad factors from four to five. Includes a Working Memory factor, based on research indicating its importance for academic success.
WPPSI-R (1989) No obvious impact.	**WPPSI-III (2002)** Incorporates measures of Processing Speed that yield a Processing Speed Quotient, based on recent research indicating the importance of processing speed for early academic success. Enhances the measurement of fluid reasoning by adding the Matrix Reasoning and Picture Concepts subtests.
WJ-R (1989) Modern Gf-Gc theory was used as the cognitive model for test development. Included two measures of each of seven broad abilities.	**WJ III (2001)** CHC theory has been used as a "blueprint" for test development. Includes two or three qualitatively different narrow abilities for each broad ability. The combined cognitive and achievement batteries of the WJ III include nine broad abilities comprised in CHC theory.
WISC-III (1991) No obvious impact.	**WISC-IV (2003)** Eliminates Verbal and Performance IQs. Replaces the Freedom from Distractibility Index with the Working Memory Index. Replaces the Perceptual Organization Index with the Perceptual Reasoning Index. Enhances the measurement of fluid reasoning by adding the Matrix Reasoning and Picture Concepts subtests. Enhances the measurement of Processing Speed with the Cancellation subtest.
DAS (1990) No obvious impact.	**DAS-II (2007)** Five CHC broad abilities are well represented in the DAS-II. Others are represented by diagnostic subtests.
WAIS-III (1997) Enhances the measurement of fluid reasoning by adding the Matrix Reasoning subtest. Includes four index scores that measures specific abilities more purely than the traditional IQs. Includes a Working Memory Index, based on research indicating its importance for academic success.	**WAIS-IV (2008)** Eliminates Verbal and Performance IQs. Replaces the Perceptual Organization Index with the Perceptual Reasoning Index. Enhances the measurement of fluid reasoning by adding the Figure Weights and Visual Puzzles subtests. Enhances measurement of Processing Speed with the Cancellation subtest.

Note. K-ABC, Kaufman Assessment Battery for Children (Kaufman & Kaufman, 1983); KABC-II, Kaufman Assessment Battery for Children—Second Edition (Kaufman & Kaufman, 2004); SB-IV, Stanford–Binet Intelligence Scale: Fourth Edition (Thorndike, Hagen, & Sattler, 1986); SB5, Stanford–Binet Intelligence Scales, Fifth Edition (Roid, 2003); WAIS-III, Wechsler Adult Intelligence Scale—Third Edition (Wechsler, 1997); WAIS-IV, Wechsler Adult Intelligence Scale—Fourth Edition (Wechsler, 2008); WPPSI-R, Wechsler Preschool and Primary Scale of Intelligence—Revised (Wechsler, 1989); WPPSI-III, Wechsler Preschool and Primary Scale of Intelligence—Third Edition (Wechsler, 2002); WJ-R, Woodcock–Johnson Psycho-Educational Battery—Revised (Woodcock & Johnson, 1989); WJ III, Woodcock Johnson III Tests of Cognitive Abilities (Woodcock, McGrew, & Mather, 2001); WISC-III, Wechsler Intelligence Scale for Children—Third Edition (Wechsler, 1991); WISC-IV, Wechsler Intelligence Scale for Children—Fourth Edition (Wechsler, 2003); DAS, Differential Ability Scales (Elliott, 1990); DAS-II, Differential Ability Scales—Second Edition (Elliott, 2007).

TABLE 19.4. Representation of Broad and Narrow CHC Abilities on Seven Intelligence Batteries Revised after 2000

Battery	Gf	Gc	Gv	Gsm	Glr	Ga	Gs
WISC-IV	Matrix Reasoning (I, RG) Picture Concepts (I) Arithmetic (RQ, Gsm-MW)	Vocabulary (VL) Information (K0) Similarities (VL, LD, Gf-I) Comprehension (K0, LD) Word Reasoning (VL, Gf-I)	Block Design (SR, Vz) Picture Completion (CF, Gc-K0)	Digit Span (MS, MW) Letter–Number Sequencing (MW)			Symbol Search (P, R9) Coding (R9) Cancellation (P, R9)
WAIS-IV	Matrix Reasoning (I, RG) Arithmetic (RQ, Gsm-MW) Figure Weights (RQ)	Vocabulary (VL) Information (K0) Similarities (VL, LD, Gf-I) Comprehension (K0, LD)	Block Design (SR, Vz) Picture Completion (CF, Gc-K0) Visual Puzzles (SR, Vz)	Digit Span (MS, MW) Letter–Number Sequencing (MW)			Symbol Search (P, R9) Coding (R9) Cancellation (P, R9)
WPPSI-III	Matrix Reasoning (I, RG) Picture Concepts (Gc-K0, I)	Vocabulary (VL) Information (K0) Similarities (VL, LD, Gf-I) Comprehension (K0, LD) Receptive Vocabulary (VL, LD) Picture Naming (VL, K0) Word Reasoning (VL, Gf-I)	Block Design (SR, VZ) Object Assembly (CS, SR) Picture Completion (CF, Gc-K0)				Coding (R9) Symbol Search (P, R9)
KABC-II	Pattern Reasoning (I, Gv-Vz) Story Completion (I, RG, Gv-Vz, Gc-K0)	Expressive Vocabulary (VL) Verbal Knowledge (VL, K0) Riddles (VL, LD, Gf-RG)	Face Recognition (MV) Triangles (SR, Vz) Gestalt Closure (CS) Rover (SS, Gf-RG, Gq-A3) Block Counting (Vz, Gq-A3) Conceptual Thinking (Vz, Gf-I)	Number Recall (MS) Word Order (MS, MV) Hand Movements (MS, Gv-MV)	Atlantis (MA) Rebus (MA) Atlantis—Delayed (MA) Rebus—Delayed (MA)		

WJ III	Concept Formation (I) Analysis–Synthesis (RG)	Verbal Comprehension (VL, LD) General Information (K0)	Spatial Relations (SR, Vz) Picture Recognition (MV) Planning (SS, Gf-RG)	Memory for Words (MS) Numbers Reversed (MW) Auditory Working Memory (MW)	Visual–Auditory Learning (MA) Retrieval Fluency (FI, NA) Visual–Auditory Learning—Delayed (MA) Rapid Picture Naming (NA, Gs-P)	Sound Blending (PC:S) Auditory Attention (US/U3) Incomplete Words (PC:A. PC:S)	Visual Matching (P, R9) Decision Speed (RE) Pair Cancellation (P)
SB5	Nonverbal Fluid Reasoning (I, RG, Gv) Verbal Fluid Reasoning (I, RG, Gc-CM) Nonverbal Quantitative Reasoning (RQ, Gq-Km, Gq-VL) Verbal Quantitative Reasoning (RQ, Gq-A3)	Nonverbal Knowledge (K0, LS, Gf-RG) Verbal Knowledge (VL)	Nonverbal Visual–Spatial Processing (SR, CS) Verbal Visual–Spatial Processing (Vz, Gc-VL, K0)	Nonverbal Working Memory (MS, MW, Gv-MV) Verbal Working Memory (MS, MW, Gc-LD)			
DAS-II	Matrices (I) Picture Similarities (I) Sequential and Quantitative Reasoning (RQ)	Early Number Concepts (VL, Gq-KM) Naming Vocabulary (VL) Word Definitions (VL, LD) Verbal Comprehension (LS) Verbal Similarities (LD, Gf-I)	Pattern Construction (SR) Recall of Designs (MV) Recognition of Pictures (MV) Copying (Vz) Matching Letter-Like Forms (Vz)	Recall of Digits—Forward (MS) Recall of Digits—Backward (MW) Recall of Sequential Order (MW)	Rapid Naming (NA, Gs-P) Recall of Objects—Immediate (M6) Recall of Objects—Delayed (M6)	Phonological Processing (PC:S, PC:A)	Speed of Information Processing (N, R9)

Note. CHC classifications are based on primary sources, such as Carroll (1993), Flanagan, Ortiz, Alfonso, and Mascolo (2006), Horn (1991), Keith, Fine, Reynolds, Taub, and Kranzler (2006), McGrew (1997), and McGrew and Flanagan (1998). WISC-IV, Wechsler Intelligence Scale for Children—Fourth Edition (Wechsler, 2003); WAIS-IV, Wechsler Adult Intelligence Scale—Fourth Edition (Wechsler, 2008); WPPSI-III, Wechsler Preschool and Primary Scale of Intelligence—Third Edition (Wechsler, 2002); KABC-II, Kaufman Assessment Battery for Children—Second Edition (Kaufman & Kaufman, 2004); WJ III, Woodcock–Johnson III Tests of Cognitive Abilities (Woodcock, McGrew, & Mather, 2001); SB5, Stanford–Binet Intelligence Scales, Fifth Edition (Roid, 2003); DAS-II, Differential Ability Scales—Second Edition (Elliott, 2007). Gf, fluid intelligence; Gc, crystallized intelligence; Gv, visual processing; Gsm, short-term memory; Glr, long-term storage and retrieval; Ga, auditory processing; Gs, processing speed; Gq, quantitative knowledge; RQ, quantitative reasoning; I, induction; RG, general sequential reasoning; RE, speed of reasoning; VL, lexical knowledge; K0, general (verbal) knowledge; LD, language development; LS, listening ability; MV, visual memory; SR, spatial relations; Vz, visualization; SS, spatial scanning; CF, flexibility of closure; CS, closure speed; MW, working memory; MS, memory span; MA, associative memory; LI, learning abilities; FI, ideational fluency; NA, naming facility; M6, free-recall memory; PC:S, phonetic coding: synthesis; PC:A, phonetic coding: analysis; US, speech sound discrimination; U3, general sound discrimination; P, perceptual speed; R9, rate of test taking; N, number facility; KM, math knowledge; A3, math achievement.

abilities and now measures these abilities. The WJ III measures all broad abilities adequately whereas the DAS-II measures five adequately, leaving two (Ga, Gs) underrepresented. Also, a comparison of Tables 19.2 and 19.4 indicates that two broad abilities not measured by many intelligence batteries prior to 2000 are now measured by the majority of revised intelligence batteries available today—that is, Gf and Gsm. These broad abilities may be better represented on revised (and new) intelligence batteries because of the accumulating research evidence regarding their importance in overall academic success (see Flanagan & Alfonso, 2011). Finally, Table 19.4 reveals that these intelligence batteries continue to fall short in their measurement of three CHC broad abilities—specifically, Glr, Ga, and Gs. In addition, these batteries do not provide adequate measurement of most specific or narrow CHC abilities, many of which are important in predicting academic achievement. Thus, although there is greater coverage of CHC broad abilities now than there was just a few years ago, the need for the XBA approach to assessment remains, particularly to ensure better measurement and interpretation of narrow abilities (Alfonso et al., 2005; Flanagan et al., 2007, 2012).

APPLICATION OF THE XBA APPROACH

Guiding Principles

In order to ensure that XBA procedures are theoretically and psychometrically sound, it is recommended that practitioners adhere to several guiding principles (McGrew & Flanagan, 1998). These principles are listed in Figure 19.1 and are defined briefly below.

First, a practitioner should select a comprehensive intelligence battery as the core battery in assessment. It is expected that the battery of choice will be one that is deemed most responsive to referral concerns. These batteries may include (but are certainly not limited to) the Wechsler scales, WJ III, SB5, DAS-II, and KABC-II. It is important to note that the use of co-normed tests (e.g., the WJ III Tests of Cognitive Abilities and Tests of Achievement, the KABC-II and Kaufman Test of Educational Achievement—Second Edition [KTEA-II]) may allow for the widest coverage of broad and narrow CHC abilities and processes.

Second, practitioners should use subtests and clusters/composites from a single battery whenever possible to represent broad CHC abilities. In other

words, best practices involve using actual norms whenever they are available, in lieu of arithmetic averages of scaled scores from different batteries. In the past, it was necessary to convert subtest scaled scores from different batteries to a common metric and then average them (after determining that there was a nonsignificant difference between the scores) in order to build construct-relevant CHC broad-ability clusters. Because the development of current intelligence batteries has benefited greatly from CHC theory and research, this practice is seldom necessary at the broad-ability level. It continues to be necessary at the narrow-ability level and for testing hypotheses about aberrant performance within broad-ability domains (see Flanagan et al., 2007, 2012, for details).

Third, when constructing CHC broad- and narrow-ability clusters, practitioners should select tests that have been classified through an acceptable method, such as through CHC theory-driven factor analyses or expert-consensus content validity studies. All test classifications included in the works of Flanagan and colleagues have been classified through these acceptable methods (Flanagan et al., 2007, 2012). For example, when practitioners are constructing broad-ability (stratum II) ability composites or clusters, *relatively pure CHC indicators* should be included (i.e., tests that had either *strong* or *moderate* [but not mixed] loadings on their respective factors in theory-driven within- or cross-battery factor analyses). Furthermore, to ensure appropriate construct representation when practitioners are constructing broad-ability (stratum II) composites, *two or more qualitatively different* narrow-ability (stratum I) indicators should be included to represent each domain. Without empirical classifications of tests, constructs may not be adequately represented; therefore, inferences about an individual's broad (stratum II) ability cannot be made confidently. Of course, the more broadly an ability is represented (i.e., through the derivation of composites based on *multiple* qualitatively different narrow-ability indicators), the more confidence practitioners can have in drawing inferences about the broad ability underlying a composite. A minimum of two qualitatively different indicators per CHC broad ability is recommended in the XBA approach for practical reasons (viz., time-efficient assessment). Noteworthy is the fact that most intelligence tests also include only two qualitatively different indicators (subtests) to represent broad abilities, which is why constructing broad-ability clusters in the XBA approach is seldom necessary.

Fourth, when at least two qualitatively different indicators of a broad ability of interest is not available on the core battery, then a practitioner should supplement the core battery with at least two qualitatively different indicators of that broad ability from another battery. In other words, if an evaluator is interested in measuring auditory processing (Ga), and the core battery includes only one or no Ga subtests, then the evaluator should select a Ga cluster from another battery to supplement the core battery. This practice ensures that actual norms are used for interpreting broad-ability performance whenever they are available.

Fifth, when crossing batteries (e.g., augmenting a core battery with relevant CHC clusters from another battery) or when constructing CHC narrow-ability clusters using tests from different batteries (e.g., averaging scores when the narrow-ability cluster of interest is not available), practitioners should select tests that were developed and normed within a few years of one another, to minimize the effect of spurious differences between test scores that may be attributable to the "Flynn effect" (Flynn, 1984, 2010). The tests recommended by Flanagan and her colleagues in their most recent XBA book include only those that were normed within 10 years of one another (Flanagan et al., 2012).

Sixth, practitioners should select tests from the smallest possible number of batteries, to minimize the effect of spurious differences between test scores that may be attributable to differences in the characteristics of independent norm samples (McGrew, 1994). In most cases, using selected tests from a single battery to augment the constructs measured by any other major cognitive battery is sufficient to represent the breadth of broad cognitive abilities adequately, as well as to allow for at least two or three qualitatively different narrow-ability indicators of most broad abilities (Flanagan et al., 2007).

Seventh, practitioners should establish ecological validity for any and all test performances that are suggestive of normative weaknesses or deficits. The finding of a cognitive weakness or deficit is largely meaningless without evidence of how the weakness manifests in activities of daily living, including academic achievement (Flanagan et al., 2011). The validity of test findings is bolstered when clear connections are made between the cognitive dysfunction (as measured by standardized tests) and the educational impact of that dysfunction, for example, as observed in classroom performance and as may be gleaned from a student's work samples. To demonstrate, Table 19.5 includes information about (1) the major cognitive domains of functioning comprising CHC theory, (2) how deficits in these domains manifest in general as well as how they manifest in specific academic areas, and (3) interventions and recommendations that can be tailored to the unique learning needs of the individual when such weaknesses are found.

Noteworthy is the fact that when the XBA guiding principles are implemented systematically and the recommendations for development, use, and interpretation of clusters are adhered to, the potential error introduced through the crossing of norm groups is negligible (Flanagan et al., 2007). Additionally, the authors of *Essentials of Cross-Battery Assessment* included software with their book to facilitate the implementation of the XBA method and aid in the interpretation of cross-battery data (see Flanagan et al., 2007). (The XBA approach may be carried out following a straightforward set of steps, which are detailed in Flanagan and colleagues, 2007, 2012.)

HISTORICAL PERSPECTIVE AND CURRENT DIRECTIONS OF THE XBA APPROACH

The preceding discussion was designed to provide readers with an overview of the foundation, rationale, and guiding principles that underlie the XBA approach. Because a definitive discussion regarding all aspects of the approach was beyond the scope of this chapter, the reader is referred to other sources for comprehensive step-by-step XBA procedures (i.e., Flanagan et al., 2007, 2012). But beyond what the XBA approach is, and the manner in which it is implemented, an understanding of its evolution provides the perspective necessary to appreciate its impact and influence on applied domains of psychology, in particular cognitive evaluation and interpretation. To that end, we offer Table 19.6. This table provides an annotated chronology of some of the more significant past and present contributions of the XBA approach and how it has evolved in response to practice-based changes in the field. For example, Flanagan and McGrew (1997) originally developed the XBA approach based on the need within the field to narrow the theory–practice gap. That is, because the major intelligence tests of the time did not measure the breadth of abilities inherent in contemporary theory on the structure of cog-

TABLE 15.5. CHC Broad Ability Definitions, Manifestations of CHC Weaknesses, and Suggested Recommendations and Interventions

CHC broad-ability	CHC broad-ability definition	General manifestations of the CHC broad-ability weakness	Specific manifestations of the CHC broad-ability weakness in academic areas	Recommendations/interventions
Fluid Reasoning (Gf)	• Novel reasoning and problem solving • Processes are minimally dependent on learning and acculturation • Involves manipulating rules, abstracting, generalizing, and identifying logical relationships	*Difficulties with:* • Higher-level thinking • Transferring or generalizing learning • Deriving solutions for novel problems • Extending knowledge • Perceiving and applying underlying rules or process(es) to solve problems	***Reading Difficulties:*** • Inferential reading comprehension • Abstracting main idea(s) ***Math Difficulties:*** • Math reasoning (word problems) • Internalizing procedures and processes used to solve problems • Apprehending relationships between numbers ***Writing Difficulties:*** • Essay writing and generalizing concepts • Developing a theme • Comparing and contrasting ideas	• Develop student's skill in categorizing objects and drawing conclusions • Use demonstrations to externalize the reasoning process • Gradually offer guided practice (e.g., guided questions list) to promote internalization of procedures or process(es) • Targeted feedback • Cooperative learning • Reciprocal teaching • Graphic organizers to arrange information in visual format • Metacognitive strategies • Comparison of new concepts to previously learned (same vs. different) • Using analogies, similes, and metaphors when presenting tasks
Crystallized Intelligence (Gc)	• Breadth and depth and knowledge of a culture • Developed through formal education and general learning experiences • Stores of information and declarative and procedural knowledge • Ability to verbally communicate and reason with previously learned procedures	*Difficulties with:* • Vocabulary acquisition • Knowledge acquisition • Comprehending language • Fact-based/informational questions • Using prior knowledge to support learning	***Reading Difficulties:*** Decoding and comprehension ***Math Difficulties:*** • Understanding math concepts and the "vocabulary of math" ***Writing Difficulties:*** • Grammar (syntax) • Bland writing with limited descriptors • Verbose writing with repetitions • Inappropriate word usage ***Language Difficulties:*** • Understanding class lessons • Expressive language—"poverty of thought"	• Provide an environment rich in language and experiences • Frequent practice with and exposure to words • Read aloud to children • Vary reading purpose (leisure, information) • Work on vocabulary building • Teach morphology • Use text talks
Auditory Processing (Ga)	• Ability to analyze and synthesize auditory information	*Difficulties with:* • Hearing information presented orally, initially processing oral information	***Reading Difficulties:*** • Acquiring phonics skills • Decoding and comprehension • Using phonetic strategies ***Math Difficulties:***	• Phonemic awareness activities • Emphasis on sight-word reading • Teach comprehension monitoring (e.g., does the word I heard/read make sense in context?)

- Paying attention, especially in the presence of background noise
- Discerning the direction from which auditory information is coming
- Foreign language acquisition
- Acquiring receptive vocabulary

- Word problems

Writing Difficulties:
- Spelling
- Note-taking
- Poor quality of writing

- Annunciating sounds in words in an emphatic manner when teaching new words for reading or spelling
- Use work preview/text preview to clarify unknown words
- Provide guided notes during note-taking activities
- Build in time for clarification questions related to "missed" or "misheard" items during lecture
- Supplement oral instructions with written instructions
- Shortening instructions
- Preferential seating
- Localizing sound source for student
- Minimizing background noise

Long-Term Retrieval (Glr)

- Ability to store information (e.g., concepts, words, facts) and fluently retrieve it later through association

Difficulties with:
- Learning new concepts
- Retrieving or recalling information by using association
- Performing consistently across different task formats (e.g., recognition vs. recall formats)
- Speed with which information is retrieved and/or learned
- Paired learning (visual–auditory)
- Recalling specific information (words, facts)

Reading Difficulties:
- Accessing background knowledge to support new learning while reading (Associative Memory deficit)
- Slow to access phonological representations during decoding (RAN deficit)

Math Difficulties:
- Recalling procedures to use for math problems
- Memorizing and recalling math facts

Writing Difficulties:
- Accessing words to use during essay writing
- Specific writing tasks (compare and contrast; persuasive writing; conceptual)
- Note-taking

Language Difficulties:
- Expressive—circumlocutions, speech fillers, "interrupted" thought, pauses
- Receptive—making connections throughout oral presentations (e.g., class lectures)

- Repeated practice with and review of newly presented information
- Teach memory strategies (verbal rehearsal to support encoding, use of mnemonic devices)
- Use multiple modalities when teaching new concepts (pair written with verbal information)
- Limit the amount of new material to be learned; introduce new concepts gradually and with a lot of context
- Be mindful of when new concepts are presented
- Make associations between newly learned and prior explicit information
- Use lists to facilitate recall (prompts)
- Expand vocabulary to minimize impact of word-retrieval deficits
- Build in wait-time for student when fluency of retrieval is an issue
- Use text previews to "prime" knowledge
- Provide background knowledge first before asking a question to "prime" student for retrieval

(cont.)

TABLE 19.5. (cont.)

CHC broad-ability	CHC broad-ability definition	General manifestations of the CHC broad-ability weakness	Specific manifestations of the CHC broad-ability weakness in academic areas	Recommendations/interventions
Processing Speed (Gs)	• Speed of processing, particularly when required to pay focused attention to tasks that require rapid processing, but are relatively easy. Usually measured by	*Difficulties with:* • Efficient processing of information • Quickly perceiving relationships (similarities and differences between stimuli or information) • Working within time parameters • Completing simple, rote tasks quickly	***Reading Difficulties:*** • Slow reading speed • Impaired comprehension • Need to reread for understanding ***Math Difficulties:*** • Automatic computations • Computational speed is slow despite accuracy • Slow speed can result in reduced accuracy due to memory decay ***Writing Difficulties:*** • Limited output due to time factors • Labored process results in reduced motivation to produce ***Language Difficulties:*** • Cannot retrieve information quickly—slow, disrupted speech as cannot get out thoughts quickly enough • Is slow to process incoming information, puts demands on memory store, which can result in information overload and loss of meaning	• Repeated practice • Speed drills • Computer activities that require quick, simple decisions • Extended time • Reducing the quantity of work required • Increasing wait-times both after questions are asked and after responses are given
Visual Processing (Gv)	• Ability to generate, perceive, analyze, synthesize, manipulate, transform, and think with visual patterns and stimuli	*Difficulties with:* • Recognizing patterns • Reading maps, graphs, and charts • Attending to fine visual detail	***Reading Difficulties:*** • Orthographic coding (using visual features of letters to decode) • Sight-word acquisition • Using charts and graphs within a text in conjunction with reading	• Capitalize on students phonemic skills for decoding tasks • Teach orthographic strategies for decoding (e.g., word length, shape of word) • Provide oral explanation for visual

Ability	Characteristics	Academic Difficulties	Instructional Strategies/Interventions
	• Recalling visual information • Appreciation of spatial characteristics of objects (e.g., size length) • Recognition of spatial orientation of objects	• Comprehension of text involving spatial concepts (e.g., social studies text describing physical boundaries, movement of troops along a specified route) **Math Difficulties:** • Number alignment during computations • Reading and interpreting graphs, tables, and charts **Writing Difficulties:** • Spelling sight words • Spatial planning during writing tasks (e.g., no attention to margins, words that overhang a line) • Inconsistent size, spacing, position, and slant of letters	concepts • Review spatial concepts and support comprehension through use of hands-on activities and manipulatives (e.g., using models to demonstrate the moon's orbital path) • Highlight margins during writing tasks • Provide direct handwriting practice • Use graph paper to assist with number alignment
Short-Term Memory (Gsm)	• Ability to hold information in immediate awareness and use or transform it within a few seconds	*Difficulties with:* • Following oral and written instructions • Remembering information long enough to apply it • Remembering the sequence of information • Rote memorization **Reading Difficulties:** • Reading comprehension • Decoding multisyllabic words • Orally retelling or paraphrasing what one has read **Math Difficulties:** • Rote memorization of facts • Remembering mathematical procedures • Multistep problems and regrouping • Extracting information to be used in word problems **Writing Difficulties:** • Spelling multisyllabic words • Redundancy in writing (word and conceptual levels) • Note-taking	• Provide opportunities for repeated practice and review • Provide supports (e.g., lecture notes, study guides, written directions) to supplement oral instruction • Break down instructional steps for student • Provide visual support (e.g., times table) to support acquisition of basic math facts • Outline math procedures for student and provide procedural guides or flashcards for the student to use when approaching problems • Highlight important information within a word problem • Have student write all steps and show all work for math computations

TABLE 19.6. Past and Present Contributions of the XBA Approach to Psychological Evaluation

Source	Contribution
Flanagan, Genshaft, and Harrison (1997)	• First attempt at merging the Cattell–Horn Gf–Gc theory and Carroll's three-stratum theory (McGrew, 1997), which represented the foundation of Cross-Battery Assessment (XBA). • First expert consensus study regarding the narrow abilities measured by intelligence tests (McGrew, 1997), an important component of XBA. • Introduced the need for XBA and the assumptions, foundations, and operationalized set of principles that comprise it (Flanagan & McGrew, 1997).
McGrew and Flanagan (1998)	• Introduced a step-by-step approach to XBA in an attempt to improve upon the measurement of cognitive constructs. • Demonstrated how the XBA approach guarded against two ubiquitous sources of invalidity in assessment: construct irrelevant variance and construct underrepresentation. • Provided worksheets for organizing assessments according to contemporary Gf–Gc theory and for conducting XBA. • Provided a review of the research on the relations between broad and narrow Gf–Gc abilities and academic (reading and math) and occupational outcomes. • Provided a desk reference of all the major intelligence tests, which provided important information for each subtest as a means of informing interpretation of XBA data (e.g., reliability, validity, standardization sample characteristics, test floors and ceilings, item gradients, variables influencing subtest performance, g loadings, broad and narrow abilities measured by subtest). • Provided the first comprehensive set of theory-based classifications of tests in an attempt to further establish a Gf–Gc nomenclature for the field. • Highlighted the importance of joint or cross-battery confirmatory factor analytic studies for understanding the Gf–Gc broad abilities underlying intelligence tests. • Provided the first set of systematic classifications of ability tests according to degree of cultural loading and degree of linguistic demand.
Flanagan, McGrew, and Ortiz (2000)	• Introduced the "Integrated Cattell–Horn and Carroll Gf–Gc Model" as the foundation for cross-battery assessment based on analyses conducted by McGrew (e.g., McGrew, 1997). This integrated model was renamed "Cattell–Horn–Carroll (CHC) theory" shortly thereafter (see McGrew, 2005, for details). • Applied Gf–Gc theory to interpretation of the Wechsler scales. • Demonstrated that the Wechsler scales included redundancy in the assessment of certain constructs (e.g., Gc and Gv) and omitted measurement of other important constructs (e.g., Gf, Ga, and Glr). • Offered step-by-step XBA guidelines for augmenting a Wechsler scale so that a broader range of cognitive abilities could be measured as deemed relevant and necessary vis à vis referral concerns. • Provided a set of worksheets for conducting XBA with the Wechsler scales.
Flanagan and Ortiz (2001)	• Used CHC theory as the foundation for XBA. • Expanded test classifications to include a variety of special-purpose tests in addition to the major intelligence tests. • Included more comprehensive coverage of test interpretation. • Provided updated and improved XBA worksheets. • Expert consensus studies provided the basis for narrow-ability classifications of cognitive tests. • Refined classifications of ability tests according to degree of cultural loading and degree of linguistic demand.
Flanagan, Ortiz, Alfonso, and Mascolo (2002)	• Extended the XBA approach to achievement tests. • Included the largest expert consensus study of the narrow abilities underlying ability tests. • Provided an updated review of the literature on the relations between cognitive abilities and reading and math achievement. Review was expanded to include the area of written language. • Demonstrated how to use the XBA approach within the context of a CHC-based operational definition of SLD. • Provided a desk reference of achievement tests, which provided important information for each subtest (e.g., reliability, validity, standardization sample characteristics, test floors and ceilings, broad and narrow abilities measured by each subtest). • Included tables of the qualitative characteristics of individual achievement subtests from 48 batteries—information that informs test selection for XBA as well as interpretation.

(cont.)

TABLE 19.6. *(cont.)*

Source	Contribution
Flanagan and Kaufman (2004, 2009)	• Provided a CHC interpretive framework for the WISC-IV, thereby facilitating the use of this instrument in the XBA approach. • Included actual norms for seven CHC-based clinical clusters, including narrow-ability clusters that were incorporated into the XBA approach. • Automated the CHC-interpretation method for the WISC-IV (program included on CD that accompanies the book).
Flanagan and Harrison (2005)	• Detailed origins of the XBA approach and the theoretical and research foundation upon which it was based (McGrew, 1997, 2005). • Detailed the manner in which CHC theory and the XBA approach influenced test development (Alfonso, Flanagan, & Radwan, 2005). • Highlighted the XBA approach as an example of the current "wave" of intelligence test interpretation: application of theory (Kamphaus, Winsor, Rowe, & Kim, 2005)
Flanagan, Ortiz, Alfonso, and Mascolo (2006)	• Included variation in task characteristics of the subtests of over 50 achievement batteries—information that informs test selection for XBA as well as interpretation. • Updated CHC-based classifications of achievement tests. • Provided a desk reference of achievement tests, which provided important information for each subtest (e.g., reliability, validity, standardization sample characteristics, test floors and ceilings, broad and narrow abilities measured by each subtest). • Revised and refined the operational definition of SLD and demonstrated how to use the XBA approach within the context of this definition. • Introduced Academic Clinical Clusters according to the eight areas of specific learning disability listed in IDEA 2004.
Flanagan, Ortiz, and Alfonso (2007)	• Introduced automated XBA worksheets in a program called the *XBA Data Management and Interpretive Assistant (DMIA)*. • Introduced an automated *Culture–Language Interpretive Matrix (C-LIM)* program to evaluate whether test performance systematically declines as a function of increased culture and language demands for English language learners. • Introduced an automated program called the *SLD Assistant*. This program was intended to assist in determining whether an individual was of at least average overall intellectual ability despite cognitive deficits in one or more specific areas. • Uses core tests (and supplemental tests as may be necessary) from a single battery, rather than selected components of a battery, as part of the assessment because (1) current intelligence tests have better representation of the broad CHC abilities and use only two or three subtests to represent them; and (2) the broad abilities measured by current intelligence batteries are typically represented by qualitatively different indicators that are relevant only to the broad ability intended to be measured. • Greater emphasis placed on use of actual norms, rather than averages. Averages are obtained under a selected few circumstances (e.g., narrow-ability level). • Expanded coverage of CHC theory to include abilities typically measured on achievement tests (e.g., Grw, Gq, Ga), providing additional information useful in the identification of specific learning disabilities. • Addressed the "disorder in a basic psychological process" language of IDEA (2004). • Demonstrated how the XBA approach might be used to operationalize the "pattern of strengths and weaknesses" language of the Federal Regulations (2006).
Flanagan, Alfonso, Ortiz, and Dynda (2010)	• Extended CHC classifications to neuropsychological instruments, thus expanding the range of instruments that might be used in the XBA approach. • Applied neuropsychological domain classifications to cognitive tests, which was intended to expand the interpretive options for XBA data. • Application of XBA principles to neuropsychological evaluation.
This volume	• Expanded CHC theory to include 16 broad abilities and over 80 narrow abilities (Schneider & McGrew, Chapter 4) • Emphasized the relevance of the XBA approach for augmenting stand-alone batteries (e.g., McCallum & Bracken, Chapter 14)

(cont.)

TABLE 19.6. *(cont.)*

Source	Contribution
Flanagan, Ortiz, and Alfonso (2012)	• Expands coverage of CHC theory to include abilities not measured by most major intelligence and cognitive batteries (e.g., Gh-tactile abilities, Gk-kinesthetic abilities). • Incorporates and integrates all current intelligence batteries (i.e., WJ III, WPPSI-III, WISC-IV, SB5, KABC-II, DAS-II, and WAIS-IV), tests of academic achievement, and selected neuropsychological instruments. • Provides a stronger emphasis on using actual norms when available. • Includes more stringent guidelines for averaging subtest scores from the same or different batteries under specific circumstances. • Summarizes current research on the relations between cognitive abilities and processes and academic skills and places even greater emphasis on forming narrow CHC ability clusters given their importance in understanding academic outcomes. • The DMIA was revised and incorporates and integrates all features of the XBA approach and includes interpretive statements. It also includes tabs for all current intelligence batteries, major achievement tests (e.g., WJ III Tests of Achievement), and co-normed (e.g., KABC-II and KTEA-II) or linked (WISC-IV and WIAT-III) batteries. Additionally, the DMIA now uses a variety of criteria to determine whether within-battery clusters are cohesive. • Revised the SLD Assistant and renamed it the *Ability, Aptitude, and Response to Intervention Estimator (AARTIE)*. This program allows practitioners to estimate the likelihood that a student with a specific pattern of strengths and weaknesses, for example, will respond to high-quality instruction and intervention in a manner that approximates the rate and level of learning typical of average same-grade peers. • Revised and updated the C-LIM to include current cognitive tests, special-purpose tests, and selected neuropsychological instruments. The C-LIM now provides additional features for evaluating individuals based on varying levels of language proficiency, acculturative knowledge, and/or giftedness. The C-LIM also allows for an examination of cognitive performance by the influences of language or culture independently. • Classifies current cognitive batteries according to neuropsychological domains of functioning (e.g., sensorimotor, visual–spatial, speed and efficiency, executive). • Includes examples of how the XBA approach is used within the context of various state and district criteria for SLD identification. • Includes guidelines for linking findings of cognitive weaknesses or deficits to intervention.

nitive abilities, there was a need to systematically supplement these batteries with tests from other batteries to broaden an assessment of cognitive functioning and thereby address referral concerns more comprehensively and directly. Also, because research on the relations between cognitive abilities and processes demonstrated the importance of narrow (rather than broad) abilities in explaining academic skill acquisition and development, there was a need in the field to measure narrow abilities reliably and validly. Flanagan and colleagues (2006, 2007) presented the research on the narrow abilities that are most important in understanding reading, math, and writing achievement and provided a means of measuring these narrow abilities as part of the XBA approach.

The information in Table 19.6 also reflects how the XBA approach has served to engender changes in practice. For example, in the past, the lack of theoretical clarity of widely used intelligence tests (e.g., the Wechsler scales) confounded interpreta-

tion and adversely affected the examiner's ability to draw clear and useful conclusions from the data. The principles and procedures of XBA put forth by Flanagan, McGrew, and their colleagues (e.g., Flanagan, McGrew, & Ortiz, 2000) aided test authors and publishers in clarifying the theoretical underpinnings of their instruments. The XBA approach has also influenced test construction (Alfonso et al., 2005). In particular, the XBA approach was designed to reduce major sources of invalidity in assessment known as construct irrelevant variance and construct underrepresentation. Test authors and publishers have addressed these problems in the current editions of their intelligence tests and cognitive batteries. To illustrate, two composites (containing construct-irrelevant variance) on the Wechsler scales that were interpreted routinely over a period of several decades—the Verbal IQ and Performance IQ—were dropped from the current editions of the WISC and the WAIS. As another example, the WJ-R Gc cluster was underrepresented because it contained two tests that measured only lexical knowledge. The current WJ III Gc cluster provides an adequate representation of this broad ability because it contains two qualitatively different measures of Gc (i.e., the cluster was expanded to measure general information in addition to lexical knowledge).

The XBA approach continues to shape the field of applied psychology and influence cognitive evaluation. Greater integration of neuropsychological constructs, more psychometric rigor behind assessing and interpreting cognitive constructs, expanded application to the evaluation of SLD as well as evaluation of other populations (e.g., preschool), and more emphasis on the relations between the narrow CHC abilities and specific academic skills are just some examples of how the XBA approach continues to evolve. We believe that such developments will enhance both the reliability and validity of evaluations in future practice while at the same time provide information that is directly relevant to the learning and instructional needs of examinees.

SUMMARY

In this chapter we presented the XBA approach as a method that allows practitioners to augment or supplement any major ability test (e.g., cognitive, neuropsychological, academic, speech-language) to ensure measurement of a wider range of broad and narrow cognitive abilities in a manner that is consistent with contemporary theory and research and that is predicated upon sound psychometric principles. The foundational sources of information upon which the XBA approach was formulated (e.g., CHC theory and the classifications of ability tests according to this theory), coupled with straightforward step-by-step procedures, provide a way to systematically construct a theoretically driven, comprehensive, and valid assessment of a wide range of cognitive abilities and processes. When the XBA approach is applied to the Wechsler Intelligence Scales, for example, it is possible to measure important abilities that would otherwise not be assessed (e.g., Ga, Glr)—abilities that are important in understanding school learning and certain vocational and occupational outcomes (e.g., Flanagan et al., 2006; Flanagan & Kaufman, 2009).

The XBA approach allows for the measurement of the major cognitive areas specified in CHC theory with emphasis on those considered most critical on the basis of history, observation, response to intervention, and other available sources of data. The CHC classifications of a multitude of ability tests bring stronger content and construct validity evidence to the evaluation and interpretation process. As test development continues to evolve and becomes increasingly more sophisticated (psychometrically and theoretically), batteries of the future will undoubtedly possess stronger content and construct validity. (The above comparison of Tables 19.2 and 19.4 illustrated this point.) Improvements in test construction notwithstanding, it is unrealistic from an economic and practical standpoint to develop a battery that operationalizes contemporary CHC theory fully (Carroll, 1998; Flanagan et al., 2007). Therefore, it is likely that the XBA approach will remain important as the empirical support for CHC theory mounts and the need to evaluate comprehensively a greater range of abilities continues (Reynolds et al., 2011).

NOTE

1. Das and Naglieri developed the CAS from PASS theory; therefore, their test is based on an information-processing theory, rather than any specific theory within the psychometric tradition (see Naglieri & Otero, Chapter 15, this volume).

REFERENCES

Alfonso, V. C., Flanagan, D. P., & Radwan, S. (2005). The impact of the Cattell–Horn–Carroll theory on test development and interpretation of cognitive and academic abilities. In D. P. Flanagan & P. L. Harrison (Eds.), *Contemporary intellectual assessment: Theories, tests, and issues* (2nd ed., pp. 185–202). New York: Guilford Press.

Borgas, K. (1999). Intelligence theories and psychological assessment: Which theory of intelligence guides your interpretation of intelligence test profiles? *The School Psychologist, 53*, 24–25.

Brackett, J., & McPherson, A. (1996). Learning disabilities diagnosis in postsecondary students: A comparison of discrepancy-based diagnostic models. In N. Gregg, C. Hoy, & A. F. Gay (Eds.), *Adults with learning disabilities: Theoretical and practical perspectives* (pp. 68–84). New York: Guilford Press.

Briggs, S. R., & Cheek, J. M. (1986). The role of factor analysis in the development and evaluation of personality scales. *Journal of Personality, 54*(1), 106–148.

Carroll, J. B. (1993). *Human cognitive abilities: A survey*

of factor-analytic studies. Cambridge, UK: Cambridge University Press.

Carroll, J. B. (1998). Foreword. In K. S. McGrew & D. P. Flanagan, *The intelligence test desk reference: Gf-Gc cross-battery assessment* (pp. xi–xii). Boston: Allyn & Bacon.

Clarke, L. A., & Watson, D. (1995). Constructing validity: Basic issues in objective scale development. *Psychological Assessment, 7*, 309–319.

Comrey, A. L. (1988). Factor-analytic methods of scale development in personality and clinical psychology. *Journal of Consulting and Clinical Psychology, 56*, 754–761.

Daniel, M. H. (1997). Intelligence testing: Status and trends. *American Psychologist, 52*, 1038–1045.

Decker, S. L. (2008). School neuropsychology consultation in neurodevelopmental disorders. *Psychology in the Schools, 45*, 799–811.

Elliott, C. D. (1990). *Differential Ability Scales*. San Antonio, TX: Psychological Corporation.

Elliott, C. D. (2007). *Differential Ability Scales—Second Edition*. San Antonio, TX: Harcourt Assessment.

Epstein, S. (1983). Aggression and beyond: Some basic issues on the prediction of behavior. *Journal of Personality, 51*, 360–392.

Esters, E. G., Ittenbach, R. F., & Han, K. (1997). Today's IQ tests: Are they really better than their historical predecessors? *School Psychology Review, 26*, 211–223.

Flanagan, D. P., & Alfonso, V. C. (Eds.). (2011). *Essentials of specific learning disability identification* Hoboken, NJ: Wiley.

Flanagan, D. P., Alfonso, V. C., & Mascolo, J. T. (2011). A CHC-based operational definition of SLD: Integrating multiple data sources and multiple data-gathering methods. In D. P. Flanagan & V. C. Alfonso (Eds.), *Essentials of specific learning disability identification* (pp. 233–298). Hoboken, NJ: Wiley.

Flanagan, D. P., Alfonso, V. C., Ortiz, S. O., & Dynda, A. M. (2010). Integrating cognitive assessment in school neuropsychological evaluations. In D. C. Miller (Ed.), *Best practices in school neuropsychology: Guidelines for effective practice assessment, and evidence-based intervention* (pp. 101–140). Hoboken, NJ: Wiley.

Flanagan, D. P., Genshaft, J. L., & Harrison, P. L. (Eds.). (1997). *Contemporary intellectual assessment: Theories, tests and issues*. New York: Guilford Press.

Flanagan, D. P., & Harrison, P. L. (Eds.). (2005). *Contemporary intellectual assessment: Theories, tests and issues* (2nd ed.). New York: Guilford Press.

Flanagan, D. P., & Kaufman, A. S. (2004). *Essentials of WISC-IV assessment*. Hoboken, NJ: Wiley.

Flanagan, D. P., & Kaufman, A. S. (2009). *Essentials of WISC-IV assessment* (2nd ed.). Hoboken, NJ: Wiley.

Flanagan, D. P., & McGrew, K. S. (1997). A cross-battery approach to assessing and interpreting cognitive abilities: Narrowing the gap between practice and cognitive science. In D. P. Flanagan, J. L. Genshaft, & P. L. Harrison (Eds.), *Contemporary intellectual assessment: Theories, tests, and issues* (pp. 314–325). New York: Guilford Press.

Flanagan, D. P., McGrew, K. S., & Ortiz, S. O. (2000). *The Wechsler intelligence scales and Gf-Gc theory: A contemporary approach to interpretation*. Needham Heights, MA: Allyn & Bacon.

Flanagan, D. P., & Ortiz, S. O. (2001). *Essentials of cross-battery assessment*. New York: Wiley.

Flanagan, D. P., Ortiz, S. O., & Alfonso, V. C. (2007). *Essentials of cross-battery assessment* (2nd ed.). New York: Wiley.

Flanagan, D. P., Ortiz, S. O., & Alfonso, V. C. (2012). *Essentials of cross-battery assessment* (3rd ed.). Hoboken, NJ: Wiley.

Flanagan, D. P., Ortiz, S. O., Alfonso, V. C., & Mascolo, J. T. (2002). *The achievement test desk reference (ATDR): Comprehensive assessment and learning disabilities*. Boston: Allyn & Bacon.

Flanagan, D. P., Ortiz, S. O., Alfonso, V. C., & Mascolo, J. T. (2006). *The achievement test desk reference (ADTR): A guide to learning disability identification*. Boston: Allyn & Bacon.

Flynn, J. R. (1984). The mean IQ of Americans: Massive gains 1932 to 1978. *Psychological Bulletin, 95*, 29–51.

Flynn, J. R. (2010). Problems with IQ gains: The huge vocabulary gap. *Journal of Psychoeducational Assessment, 28*, 412–433.

Genshaft, J. L., & Gerner, M. (1998). CHC cross-battery assessment: Implications for school psychologists. *Communique, 26*(8), 24–27.

Guilford, J. P. (1954). *Psychometric methods* (2nd ed.). New York: McGraw-Hill.

Horn, J. L. (1991). Measurement of intellectual capabilities: A review of theory. In K. S. McGrew, J. K. Werder, & R. W. Woodcock, *Woodcock–Johnson technical manual* (pp. 197–232). Chicago: Riverside.

Kamphaus, R. W., Winsor, A. P., Rowe, E. W., & Kim, S. (2005). A history of intelligence test interpretation. In D. P. Flanagan & P. L. Harrison (Eds.), *Contemporary intellectual assessment* (2nd ed., pp. 23–38). New York: Guilford Press.

Kaufman, A. S. (2000). Foreword. In D. P. Flanagan, K. S. McGrew, & S. O. Ortiz, *The Wechsler intelligence scales and Gf-Gc theory: A contemporary approach to interpretation*. Needham Heights, MA: Allyn & Bacon.

Kaufman, A. S., & Kaufman, N. L. (1983). *Kaufman Assessment Battery for Children*. Circle Pines, MN: American Guidance Service.

Kaufman, A. S., & Kaufman, N. L. (1993). *Kaufman*

Adolescent and Adult Intelligence Test. Circle Pines, MN: American Guidance Service.

Kaufman, A. S., & Kaufman, N. L. (2004). *Kaufman Assessment Battery for Children—Second Edition*. Circle Pines, MN: American Guidance Service.

Keith, T. Z., Fine, J. G., Reynolds, M. R., Taub, G. E., & Kranzler, J. H. (2006). Hierarchical, multi-sample, confirmatory factor analysis of the Wechsler Intelligence Scale for Children-Fourth edition: What does it measure? *School Psychology Review, 35*, 108–127.

Keith, T. Z., & Reynolds, M. R. (2010). CHC and cognitive abilities: What we've learned from 20 years of research. *Psychology in the Schools, 47*, 635–650.

Lezak, M. D. (1976). *Neuropsychological assessment*. New York: Oxford University Press.

Lezak, M. D. (1995). *Neuropsychological assessment* (3rd ed.). New York: Oxford University Press.

Lezak, M. D., Howieson, D. B., & Loring, D. W. (2004). *Neuropsychological assessment* (4th ed.). New York: Oxford University Press.

McGrew, K. S. (1994). *Clinical interpretation of the Woodcock–Johnson Tests of Cognitive Ability—Revised*. Boston: Allyn & Bacon.

McGrew, K. S. (1997). Analysis of the major intelligence batteries according to a proposed comprehensive CHC framework. In D. P. Flanagan, J. L. Genshaft, & P. L. Harrison (Eds.), *Contemporary intellectual assessment: Theories, tests, and issues* (pp. 151–180). New York: Guilford Press.

McGrew, K. S. (2005). The Cattell–Horn–Carroll theory of cognitive abilities: Past, present, and future. In D. P. Flanagan & P. L. Harrison (Eds.), *Contemporary intellectual assessment: Theories, tests, and issues* (2nd ed., pp. 136–182). New York: Guilford Press.

McGrew, K. S., & Flanagan, D. P. (1998). *The intelligence test desk reference (ITDR): CHC cross-battery assessment*. Boston: Allyn & Bacon.

McGrew, K. S., & Wendling, B. J. (2010). Cattell–Horn–Carroll cognitive–achievement relations: What we have learned from the past 20 years of research. *Psychology in the Schools, 47*, 651–675.

Messick, S. (1989). Validity. In R. Linn (Ed.), *Educational measurement* (3rd ed., pp. 104–131). Washington, DC: American Council on Education.

Messick, S. (1992). Multiple intelligences or multilevel intelligence?: Selective emphasis on distinctive properties of hierarchy: On Gardner's *Frames of Mind* and Sternberg's *Beyond IQ* in the context of theory and research on the structure of human abilities. *Psychological Inquiry, 3*, 365–384.

Messick, S. (1995). Validity of psychological assessment: Validation of inferences from persons' responses and performances as scientific inquiry into score meaning. *American Psychologist, 50*, 741–749.

Naglieri, J. A., & Das, J. P. (1997). *Cognitive Assessment System*. Itasca, IL: Riverside.

Reynolds, M. R., Keith, T. Z., Flanagan, D. P., & Alfonso, V. C. (2011). *CHC taxonomy: Invariance of selection of variables and population*. Manuscript in preparation.

Roid, G. H. (2003). *Stanford–Binet Intelligence Scales, Fifth Edition*. Itasca, IL: Riverside.

Sternberg, R. J., & Kaufman, J. C. (1998). Human abilities. *Annual Review of Psychology, 49*, 479–502.

Thorndike, R. L., Hagen, E. P., & Sattler, J. M. (1986). *Stanford–Binet Intelligence Scale: Fourth Edition*. Chicago: Riverside.

Wechsler, D. (1981). *Wechsler Adult Intelligence Scale—Revised*. New York: Psychological Corporation.

Wechsler, D. (1989). *Wechsler Preschool and Primary Scale of Intelligence—Revised*. San Antonio, TX: Psychological Corporation.

Wechsler, D. (1991). *Wechsler Intelligence Scale for Children—Third Edition*. San Antonio, TX: Psychological Corporation.

Wechlser, D. (1997). *Wechsler Adult Intelligence Scale—Third Edition*. San Antonio, TX: Psychological Corporation.

Wechsler, D. (2002). *Wechsler Preschool and Primary Scale of Intelligence—Third Edition*. San Antonio, TX: Psychological Corporation.

Wechsler, D. (2003). *Wechsler Intelligence Scale for Children—Fourth Edition*. San Antonio, TX: Psychological Corporation.

Wechsler, D. (2008). *Wechsler Adult Intelligence Scale—Fourth Edition*. San Antonio, TX: Pearson.

Wilson, B. C. (1992). The neuropsychological assessment of the preschool child: A branching model. In I. Rapin & S. I. Segalowitz (Vol. Eds.), *Handbook of neuropsychology: Vol. 6. Child neuropsychology* (pp. 377–394). Amsterdam: Elsevier.

Woodcock, R. W. (1990). Theoretical foundations of the WJ-R measures of cognitive ability. *Journal of Psychoeducational Assessment, 8*, 231–258.

Woodcock, R. W., & Johnson, M. B. (1989). *Woodcock–Johnson Psycho-Educational Battery—Revised*. Chicago: Riverside.

Woodcock, R. W., McGrew, K. S., & Mather, N. (2001, 2007). *Woodcock–Johnson III Tests of Cognitive Abilities*. Itasca, IL: Riverside.

CHAPTER 20

Cognitive Hypothesis Testing
Linking Test Results to the Real World

Catherine A. Fiorello
James B. Hale
Kirby L. Wycoff

IMPORTANCE OF COMPREHENSIVE COGNITIVE ASSESSMENT

This chapter presents a model, *cognitive hypothesis testing* (CHT), which is a balanced approach to assessment and intervention (Hale & Fiorello, 2004). Cognitive assessment rests on a foundation of cognitive, neuropsychological, and neuroscientific research, and can inform our interventions with children displaying academic and behavioral difficulties. Research into the neuropsychology of specific learning disabilities (SLD) has made tremendous strides over the last 20 years (Hale, Fiorello, Miller, et al., 2008), and provides support for cognitive and neuropsychological assessment that can lead to the development of truly individualized education programs.

The CHT model described in this chapter encourages the use of Response to Intervention (RTI) as a *prevention* and *intervention* program, although not a *diagnostic* one (Hale, Wycoff, & Fiorello, 2010). We hope that a balanced practice model that includes CHT will provide the basis for a new paradigm shift—a multitiered model that combines academic and behavioral interventions for all children who need them, with comprehensive psychoeducational evaluations for those who do not respond to those interventions

(Hale, 2006). For students who do not respond to increasingly intensive intervention approaches, a comprehensive evaluation that includes assessment of cognitive processing will allow us to examine their learning and psychosocial needs, as well as to determine whether or not they have SLD (Fiorello, Hale, Snyder, Forrest, & Teodori, 2008; Fuchs & Deshler, 2007; Hale, Fiorello, Dumont, et al., 2008; Hain, Hale, & Glass-Kendorski, 2009; Miller & Hale, 2008). This model acknowledges that students may fail to respond to interventions for a variety of reasons, one of which is SLD, a set of neuropsychological disabilities requiring individualized instruction designed to meet students' unique needs (Hale, Flanagan, & Naglieri, 2008). Students who do not respond to RTI service delivery approaches are a heterogeneous group, and a comprehensive CHT evaluation of neuropsychological relationships will aid in both differential diagnosis and intervention for these children.

Diagnosis

The Education for All Handicapped Children Act (Pub. L. No. 94-142, 1975) defined SLD as a deficit in the basic psychological processes that adversely affects academic achievement, and its regulatory language required the presence of a severe discrepancy between ability and achievement. The formal definition was deemphasized, and instead the regulatory language of "severe discrepancy" was emphasized (e.g., Mercer, Jordan, Alsopp, & Mercer, 1996), as was the case in most subsequent research and practice. Unfortunately, the process deficits presumed to underlie the academic difficulties were not given the same attention as the ability–achievement discrepancy—partly because there was little consensus as to what processes were involved in learning, and partly because good measures of basic psychological processes were not available at the time (Hale & Fiorello, 2004). Much has changed since then, as there are now many well-standardized tools with excellent technical quality to assess psychological processes (Hale & Fiorello, 2004; Hale, Wycoff, & Fiorello, 2010).

As the SLD definition and implementation of the severe-discrepancy method differed among districts and states (Reschly & Hosp, 2004) and identification of processing disorders was not required, SLD became anything but "specific," and there was an enormous increase in prevalence (MacMillan, Gresham, Lopez, & Bocian, 1996; MacMillan & Speece, 1999). Students with SLD eventually accounted for about half of all special education students (Kavale, Holdnack, & Mostert, 2005). In response, there were calls for a paradigm shift (e.g., Reschly & Ysseldyke, 2002) that would focus on intervention for learning problems rather than diagnosis of them. There are unquestionably problems with the severe-discrepancy methodology; in particular, the lack of specificity and sensitivity of measures leads to overclassification (e.g., MacMillan, Siperstein, & Gresham, 1996). We do not believe that this condemns all cognitive assessment, however. Instead, we argue that we need to use our well-standardized cognitive assessment tools more wisely, within the context of a comprehensive CHT approach (Fiorello, Hale, & Snyder, 2006; Hale & Fiorello, 2004).

RTI advocates suggest that many learning problems are due to delays that can be remedied by more intensive instruction (e.g., Barnett, Daly, Jones, & Lentz, 2004). However, there are many reasons why children might not respond to intervention, only one of which is SLD (Hale, Kaufman, Naglieri, & Kavale, 2006). SLD and other neuropsychological disorders are characterized by specific deficits, not just delays (Berninger & Richards, 2002; Collins & Rourke, 2003; Fiez & Petersen, 1998; Filipek, 1999; Fine, Semrud-Clikeman, Keith, Stapleton, & Hynd, 2007; Francis, Shay-

witz, Stuebing, Shaywitz, & Fletcher, 1996; Geary, Hoard, & Hamsom, 1999; Hale & Fiorello, 2004; Naglieri & Bornstein, 2003; Nicholson & Fawcett, 2001; Pugh et al., 2000; Shaywitz, Lyon, & Shaywitz, 2006; Simos et al., 2005; Stein, 2001). These specific deficits are markers that differentiate SLD from simple delays or lack of instruction. These deficits require comprehensive evaluation, according to the law (e.g., Dixon, Eusebio, Turton, Wright, & Hale, 2011) and to a recent survey of renowned SLD experts (Hale, Alfonso, et al., 2010).

Children with SLD have specific cognitive deficits in the presence of cognitive integrities that can be ascertained during comprehensive evaluations with well-standardized cognitive and neuropsychological tests (Fiorello, Hale, & Snyder, 2006; Hale, 2006). Research by Hale and colleagues has demonstrated significant profile variability, and more predictive validity for subtests over global composites like IQ, for students with SLD, attention-deficit/hyperactivity disorder (ADHD), and traumatic brain injury (Elliott, Hale, Fiorello, Dorvil, & Moldovan, 2010; Fiorello, Hale, McGrath, Ryan, & Quinn, 2001; Fiorello et al., 2006, 2007; Hale, Fiorello, Dumont, et al., 2008; Hale, Fiorello, Kavanagh, Holdnack, & Aloe, 2007), indicating that empirically based interpretation of strengths and weaknesses is necessary for these students. Research on the diagnostic role of cognitive and neuropsychological assessment will continue to be important, especially for students who do not respond to intervention (Berninger, 2006; Hale et al., 2006; Hale, Fiorello, Dumont, et al., 2008; Kavale et al., 2005; Semrud-Clikeman, 2005; Willis & Dumont, 2006).

The Individuals with Disabilities Education Improvement Act of 2004 (IDEA 2004) no longer requires an ability–achievement discrepancy for identification of SLD, allows the use of an RTI methodology, and also allows a "third-method" approach. The final IDEA 2004 regulations (34 C.F.R. Parts 300 and 301; U.S. Department of Education, 2006) indicate that states "may permit the use of other alternative research-based procedures" (p. 46786) for identifying SLD. Although the language is nonspecific, it has typically been interpreted to refer to a "pattern of strengths and weaknesses" approach to identification (Flanagan, Fiorello, & Ortiz, 2010; Hale, Flanagan, & Naglieri, 2008) and is considered an appropriate alternative for SLD classification by several state boards of education (Zirkel & Thomas, 2010). Evaluation of cognitive and neuropsychological processing, as well as academic achievement, for patterns of strengths and weaknesses that are diagnostic of SLD is therefore consistent with the IDEA 2004 SLD definition (Fiorello et al., 2008; Hale, Fiorello, Dumont, et al., 2008; Kavale et al., 2005). This type of comprehensive evaluation is also helpful in identifying other possible disorders or difficulties that may be interfering with academic achievement because there are many reasons for nonresponse in an RTI model, not just SLD (Hale et al., 2006).

Recent work by Hale and colleagues (Hale, Betts, Morley, & Chambers, 2010; Hale & Morley, 2009) has demonstrated that not all nonresponders in an RTI model have SLD. These researchers successfully used a combined RTI–CHT approach to provide RTI services to all children, and dramatically reduced referrals for special education evaluation. Although all of the nonresponders in their multitiered RTI approach did meet IDEA 2004 criteria for a disability, the comprehensive CHT evaluation revealed that these children had many different types of disorders (e.g., ADHD, anxiety disorder) or different subtypes of SLD (e.g., orthographic SLD, working memory SLD). Not only did the CHT evaluation help identify each child's unique pattern of strengths and weaknesses and disabling condition, but it also led to targeted interventions designed to meet each child's unique needs, and ultimately to treatment efficacy.

The third-method pattern of strengths and weaknesses approach to identifying SLD is supported by a white-paper consensus of SLD experts (Hale, Alfonso, et al., 2010); representative samples of school psychology practitioners (Caterino, Sullivan, Long, & Bacal, 2008; Machek & Nelson, 2007); and several national organizations, including the National Association of School Psychologists (2007), the American Academy of School Psychology (Schrank, Miller, Caterino, & Desrochers, 2006), and the Learning Disabilities Association of America (Hale, Alfonso, et al., 2010).

Intervention Development

Evaluations for students who do not respond to intervention must be comprehensive, and we define *comprehensive* as including cognitive and neuropsychological measures in addition to other data sources. The goal of the comprehensive evaluation before tier III service delivery is not just differential diagnosis or determination of special education eligibility, but also development of targeted interventions designed to meet a child's unique needs. Most eligibility assessment procedures have

not been directly linked to intervention and have poor validity for this purpose (Bocian, Beebe, MacMillan, & Gresham, 1999). Although early special education research suggested that there were no "aptitude–treatment interactions" (Reschly & Ysseldyke, 2002), neuropsychological research has been more fruitful in linking assessment to intervention (see a summary in Hale, Fiorello, Miller, et al., 2008). In fact, a recent special issue of the *Journal of Learning Disabilities*, titled *Cognitive and Neuropsychological Assessment Data That Inform Educational Intervention* (see Fuchs, Hale, & Kearns, 2011), attests to recent advances in the area of linking these types of data to intervention. Of course, there is no easy "cookbook" approach for linking assessment results to interventions. Our CHT model calls for a complete problem-solving process: collaborative development of interventions, regular monitoring of progress/results, and recycling of the process until a successful intervention is found for each individual child.

MODELS OF COGNITIVE FUNCTIONING: CHC THEORY AND NEUROPSYCHOLOGY

Cattell–Horn–Carroll (CHC) theory, based in psychometrics and large-scale factor analyses, is the predominant model of cognitive functioning today (Newton & McGrew, 2010). The broad and narrow cognitive abilities identified in CHC theory have been linked with a variety of educational outcomes (Elliott et al., 2010; Hale, Fiorello, Dumont, et al., 2008; McGrew & Wendling, 2010). Most measures of cognitive functioning today are designed to measure a variety of constructs, rather than simply to provide a single IQ or *g* measure (Elliott et al., 2010; Fiorello et al., 2001, 2007; Flanagan, Ortiz, & Alfonso, 2007; Hale et al., 2006, 2007; Hale, Fiorello, Dumont, et al., 2008; Hale, Fiorello, Miller, et al., 2008; McGrew & Wendling, 2010), and CHC theory is often the model used for that development (Keith & Reynolds, 2010).

At the same time as CHC has been coming into prominence as a psychometric theory of cognitive functioning, neuropsychological research has burgeoned; much of it has examined learning disabilities, ADHD, and other high-prevalence disorders (e.g., D'Amato, Fletcher-Janzen, & Reynolds, 2005; Feifer & Rattan, 2009; Hale & Fiorello, 2004; Miller, 2010). The convergence of evidence that cognitive and neuropsychological processes can be reliably and validly measured and linked to outcomes is leading to a synthesis of the psychometric and neuropsychological approaches to assessment (Fiorello et al., 2008). This knowledge can be used during CHT evaluations for nonresponders in a multitiered RTI model—an approach that includes the strengths of both CHT and RTI models, or, as we (Hale, Wycoff, & Fiorello, 2010) suggest, the "best of both worlds" (p. 173).

COGNITIVE HYPOTHESIS TESTING

Overview of the Model

The CHT model is based on the idea that professionals must *intervene* to *assess* (Hale & Fiorello, 2004). A multitiered RTI model, implemented with fidelity, will ensure that the number of students referred for comprehensive evaluations will be relatively small. When professionals are completing an assessment on every child who is at risk for school failure, they do not have time to complete the kind of comprehensive assessment that we recommend. However, if most students are served through an RTI process, the number who require an assessment for diagnosis and placement eligibility should be manageable. School psychologists operating in typical public schools are often faced with an overwhelming number of students who are referred for full psychoeducational evaluations. Many of these clinicians cringe at the thought of having to do additional testing on top of what is already a very demanding caseload. However, the CHT model does not simply advocate for "more testing." The model is not intended to place more responsibility on school psychologists, but rather to help redistribute that responsibility back to general education teachers, special educators, and others who are

intervening at tiers I and II. When RTI is correctly implemented, all team members are responsible for data collection. When other team members are responsible for interventions and data collection at tiers I and II, the number of referrals for full evaluations will decrease, and school psychologists will have more time to assess the small subset of the student population with true, neurologically based learning disabilities. An RTI model that includes both standard protocol and collaborative problem-solving approaches (that also include participation from special educators across tier levels) will ultimately maximize external and internal validity in the decision-making process (Hale, Flanagan, & Naglieri, 2008). This position is advocated by a majority of leading researchers in SLD (Hale, Alfonso, et al., 2010).

The CHT model (Hale & Fiorello, 2004; see Figure 20.1) uses cognitive and neuropsychological measures to assess students who do not respond to intervention. Based on a scientist-practitioner approach, the CHT model uses the scientific method to assess children over time; this mitigates some of the difficulties with one-shot assessments, and establishes concurrent and ecological validity in the process. Any hypotheses about processing weaknesses derived from the initial cognitive battery or other data sources are tested further with more specific measures, and are evaluated to ensure their ecological and treatment validity (Hale & Fiorello, 2004). Although we do recommend empirical profile analysis (Elliott et al., 2010), CHT avoids many of the difficulties of that process by confirming or disconfirming hypotheses with further data collection, including further testing of psychological processes beyond a single cognitive test.

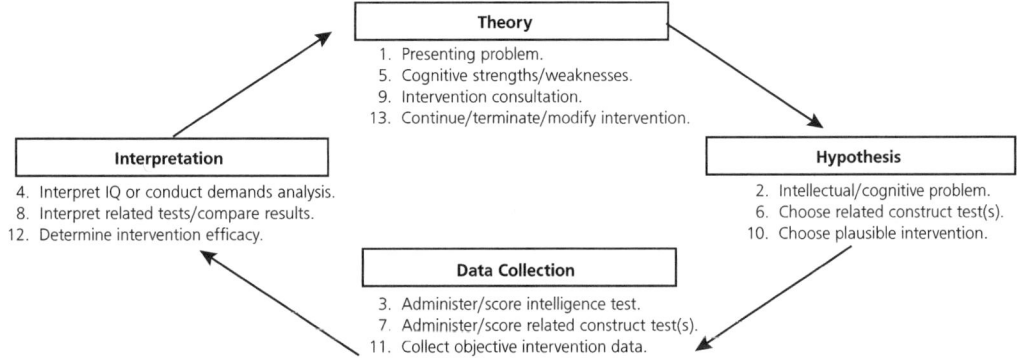

FIGURE 20.1. The cognitive hypothesis testing (CHT) model. From Hale and Fiorello (2004). Copyright 2004 by The Guilford Press. Reprinted by permission.

The beginning stages of CHT are similar to typical assessment practices. A student who has failed to respond to instruction and intervention is referred for formal evaluation. The referral question is considered together with historical records, classroom permanent products, and RTI data to develop a theory of the problem. Hypotheses are proposed to explain the academic or behavioral deficits, and if the hypothesis revolves around a question of cognitive functioning, a cognitive/intelligence test is used during the first round of data collection. The initial battery should be chosen to cover a broad range of cognitive processes, and to be a fair measure of the student's functioning based on his or her cultural and linguistic background. That measure should be scored and interpreted to identify possible processing strengths and weaknesses—using clinical references to generate initial hypotheses (such as Dehn, 2006; Flanagan et al., 2007; Hale & Fiorello, 2004; Miller, 2007; Naglieri & Goldstein, 2009; Sattler, 2008), and using *demands analysis* (see below) as needed to determine what cognitive processes are being assessed by a given measure.

Although large-group studies can provide valuable information about what particular tests measure, they are often based on the standardization samples of cognitive batteries (e.g., McGrew & Wendling, 2010) and therefore do not capture the differences in what is measured that may be found in individuals or subgroups. Students with disabilities, in particular, may use different cognitive processes to complete complex tasks from those used by the typically developing majority (e.g., Elliott et al., 2010; Hale, Fiorello, Dumont, et al., 2008; Shaywitz et al., 1998). Recent neuroimaging research confirms that most students use multiple brain areas to solve complex tasks, but that different brain areas are primarily responsible for different components of cognitive tests (Glascher et al., 2009). In addition, most complex cognitive tasks can be completed in a variety of ways, so using a "cookbook" approach by listing all potential processing possibilities is not helpful in intervention development. For example, poor Wechsler Intelligence Scale for Children—Fourth Edition (WISC-IV) Processing Speed performance may result from many different problems, including attention, visual acuity, visual scanning, visual–spatial functioning, visual memory, associative learning, somatosensory function, processing speed, psychomotor speed, fine motor coordination, and/or graphomotor skills. Further testing and comparison to ecological information should

evaluate these hypotheses to allow development of appropriate interventions.

Practically speaking, this process may unfold in the following way: The school psychologist generates hypotheses about the potential reasons for a student's poor WISC-IV Processing Speed score. Next, the school psychologist consults with the special educator who was responsible for the tier II interventions. The special educator provides work samples, classroom examples, and progress-monitoring data to suggest that the student's visual memory and visual–spatial functioning are poor, but that graphomotor skills appear intact. The school psychologist can then choose specific subtests (e.g., Wide Range Assessment of Memory and Learning, Second Edition subtests for Visual Memory; NEPSY-II Arrows, Design Copy) from different neuropsychological and cognitive measures to test the specific hypotheses about the underlying processes—visual memory, visual–spatial processing, and graphomotor skills—that may be responsible for poor Processing Speed scores on the WISC-IV. If the visual memory hypothesis is confirmed, then the school psychologist is in a better position to recommend very specific, clear recommendations and accommodations focusing on poor visual memory. On the other hand, if the school psychologist stops the process prematurely and simply reports back to the team that this child has "poor processing speed," little headway will be made with regard to providing appropriate, practical suggestions to help this child learn.

Clinical interpretation that takes into account a variety of empirical information about what tests measure, together with deep knowledge of the tests themselves and close observation of *how* a student performs the required tasks, can identify potential strengths and weaknesses. Both level (i.e., nomothetic) and pattern (i.e., idiographic) of performance are examined to determine the student's cognitive, neuropsychological, academic, and behavioral state at the time of the evaluation (Hale & Fiorello, 2004). Note that it is not assumed that the psychologist is assessing unchanging *traits* of the student, but obtaining a picture of the student's current *state* of functioning. Since cognitive states are measured, it is important to administer measures over more than one session to confirm or refute the hypotheses derived from any given session, which is why CHT is so critical for interpretation. However, at this point in a typical psychoeducational assessment, most clinicians write a report describing the purported strengths and weaknesses and make recommendations for placement and interventions. But this is only the beginning of the CHT process because any hypotheses developed need to be confirmed or disconfirmed by using additional data sources and conducting additional testing (Hale & Fiorello, 2004).

Many supplemental tests are brief neuropsychological processing measures with adequate sensitivity and more specificity, so this additional testing need not take an inordinate amount of time. The results of the additional testing are examined in light of all the data collected about the child, and a theory about a likely intervention approach is developed (Hale & Fiorello, 2004). Through a process of collaborative consultation with the teacher and/or parent, an intervention plan is devised. The intervention is implemented with regular progress monitoring, and evaluated to determine efficacy. If the intervention is not effective, the psychologist revises the plan or recycles through the process until a successful intervention is found (Hale & Fiorello, 2004). In this way, CHT combines information about cognitive and neuropsychological functioning within a collaborative problem-solving approach, and uses single-subject methodology to evaluate the effectiveness of interventions (Fiorello et al., 2006; Hale et al., 2006; Reddy & Hale, 2007).

CHT can be used to link assessment to intervention for students with difficulties in various areas, including reading (Fiorello et al., 2006), math (Hale et al., 2006), and attention (Reddy & Hale, 2007). CHT has also been recommended for use in neuropsychological settings (Fletcher-Janzen, 2005; Miller, Getz, & Leffard, 2006) as well as in schools (Elliott et al., 2010; Hale, Fiorello, Dumont, et al., 2008). Because CHT is incorporated within the context of a collaborative problem-solving approach, it is inherently self-correcting and leads to successful intervention for children with a number of disabilities (Fiorello et al., 2006; Hale, Fiorello, Miller, et al., 2008).

Demands Analysis

Interpreting an IQ score is simple, but it seldom is reflective of a child's ability, nor is it the most predictive of academic achievement (Fiorello et al., 2007; Hale, Fiorello, Miller, et al., 2008). Instead, we must acknowledge that interpretation of intelligence/cognitive subcomponent scores is necessary, and that it is not a simple or straightforward process. Various intelligence tests involve different tasks, different cognitive demands, different cultural and linguistic loading, and different administration procedures. In addition, every test measures, to a greater or lesser extent, a combination of ability and achievement; therefore, an examinee's background and exposure to similar tasks must be taken into account during interpretation. Scores are not interchangeable and should not be interpreted as a measure of a student's *trait* of intelligence, but as a measure of the student's current *state* of cognitive functioning (Hale, Wycoff, & Fiorello, 2010). The choice of a battery should be based on a priori information about the student's prior RTI data, prior experience and education, cultural and linguistic background, and any sensory or motor difficulties, in order to minimize the construct-irrelevant variance that these factors can introduce.

After administration and scoring, the profile should be examined for significant variability. If there is significant subtest or factor variability, the global IQ score should not be interpreted. But even factor scores are complex, and should not be interpreted as unitary clusters if they too show significant subtest variability within the factors. Factor scores should only be interpreted if they hold together, or are reliable, for the child being evaluated. Of course, we do not mean to imply that variability implies a disability, as the majority of people show significant variability on complex batteries like our current IQ tests (Fiorello et al., 2007; Hale, Fiorello, Dumont, et al., 2008). We simply mean that profiles should be interpreted as indicating cognitive strengths and weaknesses when there is significant variability present. In fact, it may even be necessary to examine differences *within* a subtest if it contains disparate tasks, such as Digits Forward and Digits Backward on the WISC-IV Digit Span subtest. For instance, research has shown that the difference between Digits Forward and Backward can be useful in identification of children with SLD (e.g., Hain et al., 2009) and attention problems (Hale, Hoeppner, & Fiorello, 2002), suggesting that interpretation of a Digit Span score may not accurately reflect a child's functioning.

Many school psychologists report using factor scores, profile analysis, or both to examine cognitive strengths and weaknesses in practice (Pfeiffer, Reddy, Kletzel, Schmelzer, & Boyer, 2000). However, we need a consistent methodology for interpreting the pattern of strengths and weaknesses to increase the reliability and validity of those conclusions. We derived our CHT model in such a way as to increase the reliability and validity by systematically testing our hypotheses, and evaluating ecological and treatment validity. *Demands analysis* (see Figure 20.2) systematizes the process of identifying the input, processing, and output demands of individual tasks. Rather than just basing interpretation on a score and the test maker's description of what a subtest measures, demands analysis provides a wide range of possible interpretive factors to be considered in evaluating a student's strengths and weaknesses. After testing these hypotheses with further evaluation, demands analysis allows professionals to develop an individualized education program that will truly meet a student's individual needs.

Demands analysis is a combination of the "intelligent testing" approach begun by Alan Kaufman (1979) and in widespread use in school psychology (e.g., Sattler, 2008), along with the CHC cross-battery approach advocated by McGrew, Flanagan, and colleagues (e.g., Flanagan et al., 2007; McGrew & Wendling, 2010), and a neuropsychological assessment "process approach" (e.g., Groth-Marnat, Gallagher, Hale, & Kaplan, 2000; Hebben & Milberg, 2002). This emphasis on the neuropsychological processes underlying task completion has become more widespread in school psychology since our introduction of the process in *School Neuropsychology: A Practitioner's Handbook* (Hale & Fiorello, 2004; see, e.g., D'Amato et al., 2005; Dehn, 2006; Miller, 2007, 2010).

To complete a demands analysis, a professional must first consider the *input* demands of the task.

This refers to the directions and stimulus materials—what modalities are used; the presence of pictures, manipulatives, oral directions, or written materials; how abstract or meaningful the content is; how much English-language mastery is called for; and how much cultural loading there is in the task. Next, the *processing* demands must be considered. It is important not to depend on the primary process suggested in the test manual or the loading on CHC abilities indicated by factor-analytic research, but to consider other neurological processing demands, such as executive and working memory skills. As Goldberg (2001) suggests, several brain processes are typically involved in any given task, so it is important to interpret this interrelationship among cognitive processes when examining any given test result. Also, it is important to consider the different ways that examinees can solve a given task. Some students use the visual Gestalt to solve Block Design on the Wechsler scales; others use a trial-and-error approach; still others talk their way through the problem in a linear, sequential, manner and instead focus on stimulus details.

Finally, it is important to consider the *output* demands of the task. What modalities and skills are required to complete the task—simple pointing, a complex motoric task, a complex verbal explanation? Taking copious notes on the student's actual behavior on the task, even at the level of individual items, is required for this fine-grained

Student's Name: _____ Age: _____ Grade: _____

	Test/subtest	Input	Process	Output
Strengths				
Weaknesses				

FIGURE 20.2. Demands analysis. From Hale and Fiorello (2004). Copyright 2004 by The Guilford Press. Reprinted by permission.

interpretation. A poor score on the Wechsler Information subtest may be due to memory retrieval problems or lack of general knowledge—but it may also be due to lack of knowledge in one specific area, like science. Once a professional has noted the demands of a student's strong and weak tasks, it is important to examine the notes for commonalities and contradictions. The practitioner must keep in mind that input and output difficulties are most likely due to sensory or motor difficulties or even to cultural or linguistic differences, whereas processing difficulties are characteristic of neuropsychological disorders (e.g., SLD, ADHD, or depression).

After a theory of the student's strengths and weaknesses is developed, the practitioner will then determine what measures are necessary to confirm or refute this theory during subsequent testing. Tasks that assess these specific hypotheses are more sensitive and specific for the processes in question. Then these results are compared to data from history, work samples, behavior observations, or rating forms to confirm or refute initial findings. Comparing the conclusions about input, processing, and output demands that are drawn from a child's test performance to indicators of classroom performance and behavior will help establish the accuracy of interpretation and establish ecological validity of findings. Tests that are specifically designed to cleanly assess narrow abilities (like the Woodcock–Johnson III [WJ III] Tests of Cognitive Abilities and Diagnostic Supplement) or neuropsychological instruments that yield a variety of process scores (like the WISC-IV Integrated, the NEPSY-II, and the Delis–Kaplan Executive Function System) are good places to look for tasks that can test hypotheses.

Concordance–Discordance Model

In order to identify SLD, our concordance–discordance model (C-DM; Hale & Fiorello, 2004) (see Figure 20.3) provides practitioners with an empirical approach to examining patterns of performance on cognitive and academic measures to establish that a processing deficit is the cause of the SLD, and therefore meets the IDEA 2004 statutory definition for the disorder (Hale et al., 2006). Establishing this pattern of strengths and weaknesses, and associated achievement deficit(s), appears to be the preferred method among those advocating "third-method" approaches to SLD identification (Flanagan et al., 2010; Hale, Alfonso, et al., 2010; Hale, Flanagan, & Naglieri, 2008), and is growing in popularity across states (Zirkel & Thomas, 2010). By identifying a pattern of cognitive and academic strengths and weaknesses, and evaluating whether they are statistically and clinically different from each other, practitioners can determine the presence of SLD as part of the CHT model.

A step-by-step approach for using the C-DM model can be found in Hale, Wycoff, and Fiorello (2010). The C-DM approach establishes a pattern of cognitive strength(s) together with a cognitive weakness(es) that is associated with an academic weakness. Each component should be composed of a test or cluster score that is reliable and valid for individual, high-stakes decision making. A cluster score may be provided by the test itself, like a General Ability Index score from the WISC-IV or a Nonverbal Index score from the Kaufman Assessment Battery for Children—Second Edition in the cognitive area, or practitioners may have to construct a cluster themselves, such as separat-

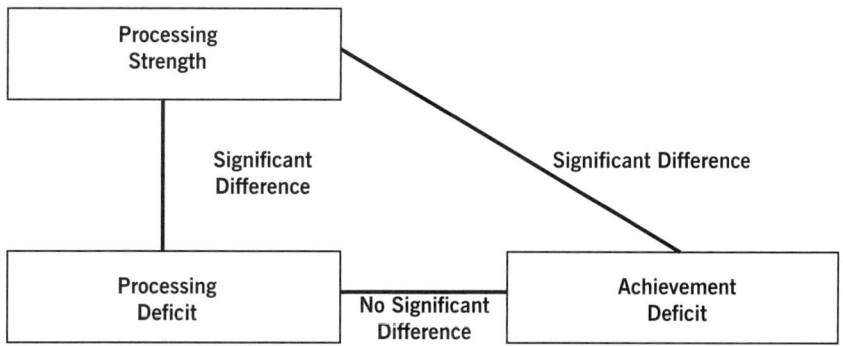

FIGURE 20.3. The concordance–discordance model of SLD identification. Based on Hale and Fiorello (2004).

ing out the fluid reasoning subtests from the visual processing subtests in the Perceptual Reasoning Index on the WISC-IV (Hale, Fiorello, Miller, et al., 2008). In most cases, if professionals do this, they will have to calculate the mean cluster score and reliability coefficient themselves, using Fischer's z' transformation (Hale, Fiorello, Miller, et al., 2008). The WJ III Tests of Cognitive Abilities Third Edition has software available that allows the calculation of cluster scores that take intercorrelations and regression to the mean into effect (Schneider, 2010).

It is important that practitioners not merely use the highest and lowest cognitive scores and lowest academic scores to calculate the C-DM differences. The cognitive strength should be one that the literature indicates is seldom related to the academic weakness (e.g., visual processing and reading comprehension), while the cognitive weakness should be empirically linked to the academic weakness (e.g., working memory and reading comprehension). Following the standard error of the difference (SED) formula (Anastasi & Urbina, 1997), $SED = SD\sqrt{2 - r_{xx} - r_{yy}}$, the practitioner then calculates the SED between the cognitive strength and the academic weakness, using the reliability of those cluster scores. This value is then multiplied by 1.96 to obtain the $p < .05$ difference score (or 2.58 for $p < .01$). If the cognitive strength score minus academic weakness score is equal to or greater than that number, there is a significant difference. Then the same SED formula is applied to the cognitive strength and the cognitive weakness to see whether there is a significant difference. Then the calculation is performed again using the cognitive weakness and the academic weakness, and these scores should not be significantly different. If the pattern of results fits the pattern shown in Figure 20.3, this is evidence for the presence of SLD. The null hypothesis is that this pattern will not be found, indicating that something other than SLD is responsible for the learning difficulties.

Establishing Ecological and Treatment Validity

We recommend direct behavior observations in natural environments (e.g., classroom) and behavior rating scales to help establish the ecological validity of assessment findings. If a student has a true neuropsychological disorder, it should manifest itself in some form across settings. Of course, behavior is interactional, so a student's behavior will vary in environments with differing demands;

however, if difficulties observed during individual testing are not present in the classroom environment, findings need to be evaluated more closely. Sattler and Hoge (2005) present a variety of methods for systematically observing student behavior in the classroom, and there are formal coding systems available as well, such as the Achenbach System of Empirically Based Assessment (ASEBA) Direct Observation Form (McConaughy & Achenbach, 2009) and the Behavior Assessment System for Children, Second Edition (BASC-2) Student Observation System (Reynolds & Kamphaus, 2004). Behavior rating scales sample behavior across settings and over a period of time, and so add important data to an evaluation. We recommend starting with a general rating scale so as to evaluate a broad range of behaviors, such as the ASEBA Teacher Report Form (Achenbach & Rescorla, 2001), the BASC-2 Teacher Rating Scale (Reynolds & Kamphaus, 2004), or the Clinical Assessment of Behavior (Bracken & Keith, 2004). If practitioners later want more detailed information about a specific class of behaviors, they can follow up with a more focused rating scale. However, it is important to note that the indirect data gained through behavior ratings are quite different from those obtained through direct assessment, so clinical judgment will be necessary to reconcile differences obtained on these measures (e.g., Hale et al., 2009).

Intervention must occur within the context of a collaborative problem-solving approach, and therefore the importance of ongoing progress monitoring to evaluate treatment efficacy cannot be overstated. Gone are the days when a school psychologist would file an evaluation report and not check back for 1 or even 3 years. Effective practitioners must be involved in treatment implementation and monitoring to ensure that what was recommended is actually implemented with fidelity and is effective; if not, consultation skills are necessary to recycle the plan as necessary until treatment efficacy is obtained (Hale & Fiorello, 2004).

Using the CHT model to link cognitive and neuropsychological assessment data to intervention on an individual level can ensure that the students served will obtain the individualized services they need. But more group and single-subject research is needed to establish the utility of the CHT approach, and to identify intervention approaches that are effective with students displaying specific patterns of SLD, especially since there are numerous SLD subtypes (e.g., Fiorello et al.,

2006; Hain et al., 2009; Hale, Fiorello, Dumont, et al., 2008). The evidence is just now emerging that cognitive and neuropsychological processes are relevant for academic and behavioral intervention, and considerable empirical work is needed to establish the validity of these relationships (e.g., Fuchs et al., 2011). Only then will the true promise of special education be realized.

REFERENCES

Achenbach, T. M., & Rescorla, L. A. (2001). *Manual for the ASEBA school-age forms and profiles*. Burlington: University of Vermont Research Center for Children, Youth, and Families.

Anastasi, A., & Urbina, S. (1997). *Psychological testing* (7th ed.). Upper Saddle River, NJ: Prentice Hall.

Barnett, D. W., Daly, E. J., Jones, K. M., & Lentz, F. E. (2004). Response to intervention: Empirically based special service decisions from single-case designs of increasing and decreasing intensity. *Journal of Special Education, 38*, 66–79.

Berninger, V., & Richards, T. L. (2002). *Brain literacy for educators and psychologists*. Boston: Academic Press.

Berninger, V. W. (2006). Research-supported ideas for implementing reauthorized IDEA with intelligent professional psychological services. *Psychology in the Schools, 43*, 781–796.

Bocian, K., Beebe, M., MacMillan, D., & Gresham, F. M. (1999). Competing paradigms in learning disabilities classification by schools and the variations in the meaning of discrepant achievement. *Learning Disabilities Research and Practice, 14*, 1–14.

Bracken, B. A., & Keith, L. K. (2004). *Examiner's manual: Clinical Assessment of Behavior*. Lutz, FL: Psychological Assessment Resources.

Caterino, L., Sullivan, A., Long, L., & Bacal, E. (2008). A survey of school psychologists' perceptions of the reauthorization of IDEA 2004. *The School Psychologist, 62*(2), 45–49.

Collins, D. W., & Rourke, B. P. (2003). Learning-disabled brains: A review of the literature. *Journal of Clinical and Experimental Neuropsychology, 25*, 1011–1034.

D'Amato, R. C., Fletcher-Janzen, E., & Reynolds, C. R. (Eds.). (2005). *Handbook of school neuropsychology*. Hoboken, NJ: Wiley.

Dehn, M. J. (2006). *Essentials of processing assessment*. Hoboken, NJ: Wiley.

Dixon, S. G., Eusebio, E. C., Turton, W. J., Wright, P. W. D., & Hale, J. B. (2011). *Forest Grove School District v. T. A.* Supreme Court case: Implications for school psychology practice. *Journal of Psychoeducational Assessment, 29*(2), 103–113.

Education for All Handicapped Children Act, Pub. L. No. 94-142, 20 U.S.C. 1401 et seq. (1975).

Elliott, C. D., Hale, J. B., Fiorello, C. A., Dorvil, C., & Moldovan, J. (2010). Differential Ability Scales—Second Edition prediction of reading performance: Global scales are not enough. *Psychology in the Schools, 47*, 698–720.

Feifer, S. G., & Rattan, G. (Eds.). (2009). *Emotional disorders: A neuropsychological, psychopharmacological, and educational perspective*. Middletown, MD: School Neuropsych Press.

Fiez, J. A., & Petersen, S. E. (1998). Neuroimaging studies of word reading. *Proceedings of the National Academy of Sciences USA, 95*, 914–921.

Filipek, P. A. (1999). Neuroimaging in the developmental disorders. The state of the science. *Journal of Child Psychology and Psychiatry, 40*, 113–128.

Fine, J. G., Semrud-Clikeman, M., Keith, T. Z., Stapleton, L. M., & Hynd, G. W. (2007). Reading and the corpus callosum: An MRI family study of volume and area. *Neuropsychology, 21*, 235–241.

Fiorello, C. A., Hale, J. B., Holdnack, J. A., Kavanagh, J. A., Terrell, J., & Long, L. (2007). Interpreting intelligence test results for children with disabilities: Is global intelligence relevant? *Applied Neuropsychology, 14*, 2–12.

Fiorello, C. A., Hale, J. B., McGrath, M., Ryan, K., & Quinn, S. (2001). IQ interpretation for children with flat and variable test profiles. *Learning and Individual Differences, 13*, 115–125.

Fiorello, C. A., Hale, J. B., & Snyder, L. E. (2006). Cognitive hypothesis testing and response to intervention for children with reading disabilities. *Psychology in the Schools, 43*, 835–854.

Fiorello, C. A., Hale, J. B., Snyder, L. E., Forrest, E., & Teodori, A. (2008). Validating individual differences through examination of converging psychometric and neuropsychological models of cognitive functioning. In S. K. Thurman & C. A. Fiorello (Eds.), *Applied cognitive research in K–3 classrooms* (pp. 151–186). New York: Routledge.

Flanagan, D. P., Fiorello, C. A., & Ortiz, S. O. (2010). Enhancing practice through application of CHC theory and research: A "third method" approach to SLD identification. *Psychology in the Schools, 47*, 739–760.

Flanagan, D. P., Ortiz, S. O., & Alfonso, V. C. (2007). *Essentials of cross-battery assessment* (2nd ed.). Hoboken, NJ: Wiley.

Fletcher-Janzen, E. (2005). The school neuropsychological examination. In R. C. D'Amato, E. Fletcher-Janzen, & C. R. Reynolds (Eds.), *Handbook of school neuropsychology* (pp. 172–212). Hoboken, NJ: Wiley.

Francis, D. J., Shaywitz, S. E., Stuebing, K. K., Shaywitz, B. A., & Fletcher, J. M. (1996). Developmental delay versus deficit models of reading disability: A longitudinal, individual growth curve analysis. *Journal of Educational Psychology, 88,* 3–17.

Fuchs, D., & Deshler, D. D. (2007). What we need to know about responsiveness to intervention (and shouldn't be afraid to ask). *Learning Disabilities Research and Practice, 22,* 129–136.

Fuchs, D., Hale, J. B., & Kearns, D. (2011). On the importance of a cognitive processing perspective: An introduction. *Journal of Learning Disabilities, 44,* 99–104.

Geary, D. C., Hoard, M. K., & Hamsom, C. O. (1999). Numerical and arithmetic cognition: Patterns of functions and deficits in children at risk for a mathematical disability. *Journal of Experimental Child Psychology, 74,* 213–239.

Glascher, J., Tranel, D., Paul, L. K., Rudrauf, D., Rorden, C., Hornaday, A., et al. (2009). Lesion mapping of cognitive abilities linked to intelligence. *Neuron, 61,* 681–691.

Goldberg, E. H. (2001). *The executive brain: Frontal lobes and the civilized mind.* New York: Oxford University Press.

Groth-Marnat, G., Gallagher, R. E., Hale, J. B., & Kaplan, E. (2000). The Wechsler intelligence scales. In G. Groth-Marnat (Ed.), *Neuropsychological assessment in clinical practice: A guide to test interpretation and integration* (pp. 129–194). New York: Wiley.

Hain, L. A., Hale, J. B., & Glass-Kendorski, J. (2009). Comorbidity of psychopathology in cognitive and academic SLD subtypes. In S. G. Feifer & G. Rattan (Eds.), *Emotional disorders: A neuropsychological, psychopharmacological, and educational perspective* (pp. 199–226). Middletown, MD: School Neuropsych Press.

Hale, J. B. (2006). Implementing IDEA with a three-tier model that includes response to intervention and cognitive assessment methods. *School Psychology Forum: Research and Practice, 1,* 16–27.

Hale, J. B., Alfonso, V., Berninger, V., Bracken, B., Christo, C., Clark, E., et al. (2010). Critical issues in response-to-intervention, comprehensive evaluation, and specific learning disabilities identification and intervention: An expert white paper consensus. *Learning Disability Quarterly, 33,* 223–236.

Hale, J. B., Betts, E. C., Morley, J., & Chambers, C. (2010, March). *SLD third method approaches for combining RTI and comprehensive evaluation.* Mini Skills Workshop presented at the annual convention of the National Association of School Psychologists, Chicago.

Hale, J. B., & Fiorello, C. A. (2004). *School neuropsychology: A practitioner's handbook.* New York: Guilford Press.

Hale, J. B., Fiorello, C. A., Dumont, R., Willis, J. O., Rackley, C., & Elliott, C. (2008). Differential Ability Scales—Second Edition (neuro)psychological predictors of math performance for typical children and children with math disabilities. *Psychology in the Schools, 45,* 838–858.

Hale, J. B., Fiorello, C. A., Kavanagh, J. A., Holdnack, J. A., & Aloe, A. M. (2007). Is the demise of IQ interpretation justified?: A response to special issue authors. *Applied Neuropsychology, 14,* 37–51.

Hale, J. B., Fiorello, C. A., Miller, J. A., Wenrich, K., Teodori, A. M., & Henzel, J. (2008). WISC-IV assessment and intervention strategies for children with specific learning disabilities. In A. Prifitera, D. H. Saklofske, & L. G. Weiss (Eds.), *WISC-IV clinical assessment and intervention* (2nd ed., pp. 109–171). Amsterdam: Elsevier.

Hale, J. B., Flanagan, D. P., & Naglieri, J. A. (2008). Alternative research-based methods for IDEA (2004) identification of children with specific learning disabilities. *Communiqué, 36*(8), 1, 14–17.

Hale, J. B., Hoeppner, J. B., & Fiorello, C. A. (2002). Analyzing Digit Span components for assessment of attention processes. *Journal of Psychoeducational Assessment, 20,* 128–143.

Hale, J. B., Kaufman, A., Naglieri, J. A., & Kavale, K. A. (2006). Implementation of IDEA: Integrating response to intervention and cognitive assessment methods. *Psychology in the Schools, 43,* 753–770.

Hale, J. B., & Morley, J. (2009, February). *Combining RTI with cognitive hypothesis testing for effective classroom instruction.* Invited workshop at the Annual Convention of the National Association of School Psychologists, Boston.

Hale, J. B., Reddy, L. A., Decker, S. L., Thompson, R., Henzel, J., Teodori, A., et al. (2009). Development and validation of an executive function and behavior rating screening battery sensitive to ADHD. *Journal of Clinical and Experimental Neuropsychology, 31,* 897–912.

Hale, J. B., Wycoff, K. L., & Fiorello, C. A. (2010). RTI and cognitive hypothesis testing for specific learning disabilities identification and intervention: The best of both worlds. In D. P. Flanagan & V. C. Alfonso (Eds.), *Essentials of specific learning disability identification* (pp. 173–202). Hoboken, NJ: Wiley.

Hebben, N., & Milberg, W. (2002). *Essentials of neuropsychological assessment.* New York: Wiley.

Kaufman, A. S. (1979). *Intelligent testing with the WISC-R.* New York: Wiley.

Kavale, K. A., Holdnack, J. A., & Mostert, M. P. (2005). Responsiveness to intervention and the identification of specific learning disability: A critique and alternative proposal. *Learning Disability Quarterly, 28,* 2–16.

Keith, T. Z., & Reynolds, M. R. (2010). Cattell–Horn–Carroll abilities and cognitive tests: What we've learned from 20 years of research. *Psychology in the Schools, 47,* 635–650.

Machek, G. R., & Nelson, J. M. (2007). How should reading disabilities be operationalized?: A survey of practicing school psychologists. *Learning Disabilities Research and Practice, 22,* 147–157.

MacMillan, D. L., Gresham, F. M., Lopez, M. F., & Bocian, K. M. (1996). Comparison of students nominated for prereferral interventions by ethnicity and gender. *Journal of Special Education, 30,* 133–151.

MacMillan, D. L., Siperstein, G., & Gresham, F. M. (1996). Mild mental retardation: A challenge to its viability as a diagnostic category. *Exceptional Children, 62,* 356–371.

MacMillan, D. L., & Speece, D. (1999). Utility of current diagnostic categories for research and practice. In R. Gallimore, L. Hernheimer, D. MacMillan, D. Speece, & S. Vaughn (Eds.), *Developmental perspectives on children with high-incidence disabilities* (pp. 111–133). Mahwah, NJ: Erlbaum.

McConaughy, S. H., & Achenbach, T. M. (2009). *Manual for the ASEBA Direct Observation Form.* Burlington: University of Vermont Research Center for Children, Youth, and Families.

McGrew, K. S., & Wendling, B. J. (2010). Cattell–Horn–Carroll cognitive–achievement relations: What we have learned from the past 20 years of research. *Psychology in the Schools, 47,* 651–675.

Mercer, C. D., Jordan, L., Alsopp, D. H., & Mercer, A. R. (1996). Learning disabilities definitions and criteria used by state education departments. *Learning Disability Quarterly, 19,* 217–232.

Miller, D. C. (2007). *Essentials of school neuropsychological assessment.* Hoboken, NJ: Wiley.

Miller, D. C. (Ed.). (2010). *Best practices in school neuropsychology: Guidelines for effective practice, assessment, and evidence-based intervention.* Hoboken, NJ: Wiley.

Miller, D. C., & Hale, J. B. (2008). The neuropsychological applications of the Wechsler Intelligence Scale for Children—Fourth Edition. In A. Prifitera, D. H. Saklofske, & L. G. Weiss (Eds.), *WISC-IV Advanced Clinical Interpretation 2e* (pp. 445–495). San Diego, CA: Academic Press.

Miller, J. A., Getz, G., & Leffard, S. A. (2006, February). *Neuropsychology and the diagnosis of learning disabilities under IDEA 2004.* Poster presented at the 34th annual meeting of the International Neuropsychological Society, Boston.

Naglieri, J. A., & Bornstein, B. T. (2003). Intelligence and achievement: Just how correlated are they? *Journal of Psychoeducational Assessment, 21,* 244–260.

Naglieri, J. A., & Goldstein, S. (Eds.). (2009). *Practitioner's guide to assessing intelligence and achievement.* Hoboken, NJ: Wiley.

National Association of School Psychologists. (2007). *Identification of students with specific learning disabilities (Position statement).* Bethesda, MD: Author.

Newton, J. H., & McGrew, K. S. (2010). Introduction to the special issue: Current research in Cattell–Horn–Carroll-based assessment. *Psychology in the Schools, 47,* 621–634.

Nicholson, R. I., & Fawcett, A. J. (2001). Dyslexia, learning, and the cerebellum. In M. Wolf (Ed.), *Dyslexia, fluency, and the brain.* (pp. 159–188). Timonium, MD: York Press.

Pfeiffer, S. L., Reddy, L. A., Kletzel, J. E., Schmelzer, E. R., & Boyer, L. M. (2000). The practitioner's view of IQ testing and profile analysis. *School Psychology Quarterly, 15,* 376–385.

Pugh, K. R., Mencl, W. E., Shaywitz, B. A., Shaywitz, S. E., Fulbright, R. K., Constable, R. T., et al. (2000). The angular gyrus in developmental dyslexia: Task-specific differences in functional connectivity within posterior regions. *Psychological Science, 11,* 51–56.

Reddy, L. A., & Hale, J. B. (2007). Inattentiveness. In A. R. Eisen (Ed.), *Clinical handbook of childhood behavior problems: Case formulation and step-by-step treatment programs* (pp. 156–211). New York: Guilford Press.

Reschly, D. J., & Hosp, J. L. (2004). State SLD policies and practices. *Learning Disability Quarterly, 27,* 197–213.

Reschly, D. J., & Ysseldyke, J. E. (2002). Paradigm shift: The past is not the future. In A. Thomas & J. Grimes (Eds.), *Best practices in school psychology* (4th ed., pp. 3–21). Bethesda, MD: National Association of School Psychologists.

Reynolds, C. R., & Kamphaus, R. (2004). *Behavior Assessment System for Children, Second Edition (BASC-2).* San Antonio, TX: Harcourt Assessment.

Sattler, J. M. (2008). *Assessment of children: Cognitive foundations* (5th ed.). La Mesa, CA: Author.

Sattler, J. M., & Hoge, R. D. (2005). *Assessment of children: Behavioral, social, and clinical foundations* (5th ed.). San Diego, CA: Jerome M. Sattler, Publisher.

Schneider, W. J. (2010). *The Compositator* (Version 1.0) [Computer software]. Available from *www.woodcock-munoz-foundation.org/press/compositator.html.*

Schrank, F. A., Miller, J. A., Caterino, L., & Desrochers, J. (2006). American Academy of School Psychology survey on the independent educational evaluation for a specific learning disability: Results and discussion. *Psychology in the Schools, 43,* 771–780.

Semrud-Clikeman, M. (2005). Neuropsychological aspects for evaluating learning disabilities. *Journal of Learning Disabilities, 38,* 563–568.

Shaywitz, B. A., Lyon, G. R., & Shaywitz, S. E. (2006). The role of functional magnetic resonance imaging in understanding reading and dyslexia. *Developmental Neuropsychology, 30,* 613–632.

Shaywitz, S. E., Shaywitz, B. A., Pugh, K. R., Fulbright, R. K., Constable, R. T., Mencl, W. E., et al. (1998). Functional disruption in the organization of the brain for reading in dyslexia. *Proceedings of the National Academy of Sciences USA, 95,* 2636–2641.

Simos, P. G., Fletcher, J. M., Sarkari, S., Billingsley, R. L., Francis, D. J., Castillo, E. M., et al. (2005). Early reading development of neurophysiological processes involved in normal reading and reading disability: A magnetic source imaging study. *Neuropsychology, 19,* 787–798.

Stein, J. F. (2001). The neurobiology of reading difficulties. In M. Wolf (Ed.), *Dyslexia, fluency, and the brain* (pp. 3–22). Timonium, MD: York Press.

U.S. Department of Education. (2006, August 14). 34 C.F.R. Parts 300 and 301: Assistance to states for the education of children with disabilities and preschool grants for children with disabilities: Final rule. *Federal Register, 71*(146), 46539–46845.

Willis, J. O., & Dumont, R. (2006). And never the twain shall meet: Can response to intervention and cognitive assessment be reconciled? *Psychology in the Schools, 43,* 901–908.

Zirkel, P., & Thomas, B. (2010). State laws and guidelines for implementing RTI. *Teaching Exceptional Children, 43*(1), 60–73.

CHAPTER 21

Processing Approaches to Interpretation of Information from Cognitive Ability Tests
A Critical Review

Randy G. Floyd
John H. Kranzler

In his famous presidential address to the American Psychological Association titled "The Two Disciplines of Scientific Psychology," Cronbach (1957) stated that "two historic streams of method, thought, and affiliation . . . run through the last century of our science. One is *experimental psychology*; the other, *correlational psychology*" (p. 671; emphases in original). The aim of research and theory in experimental psychology is to discover laws of nature that apply to all humans. Experimental psychologists test hypotheses about the functional relations between a dependent variable and carefully manipulated independent variables, often in a scientific laboratory. Nearly all experiments are within-subjects designs, sometimes with a sample size of $N = 1$, wherein the effect of stimuli upon some behavioral response for a given individual is observed. Extraneous situational variables are controlled to the greatest extent possible to minimize individual differences (i.e., error variance). Well-designed experiments lead to "rigorous tests of hypotheses and confident statements about causation" (Cronbach, 1957, p. 672).

The aim of research and theory in correlational psychology (also known as *differential psychology*), in contrast, is to classify and quantify the differences that exist between individuals on virtually every measurable biological and psycho-logical characteristic. Differential psychologists largely employ between-subjects designs, wherein the conditions of experimentation are held constant across participants, and individual differences among them are measured. The goal is to predict within-subject variability, primarily with correlational techniques, while holding treatment variability constant. Research in differential psychology leads to discoveries of the essential nature or structure of individual differences, usually in terms of a smaller number of underlying constructs (Jensen, 1998).

Given differences in the aims and methods between these two disciplines, Cronbach (1957) argued that "psychology continues to this day to be limited by the dedication of its investigators to one or the other method of inquiry rather than to scientific psychology as a whole" (p. 671). Perhaps nowhere in psychology were the differences between these two disciplines reflected more clearly than in the fields of learning and intelligence, despite the fact that individual differences in the level of performance on learning tasks are the essence of the definition of intelligence (e.g., Jensen, 1989; Snyderman & Rothman, 1987). Until only recently, research in the fields of learning and intelligence progressed with quite different basic assumptions, methodologies, and theories.

Within the past 30 years, however, advancements in experimental cognitive psychology on *information processing* have provided the unifying framework for these two disciplines. Theory and research on information processing concern the testing of hypotheses about how *information* (i.e., the stimulus inputs that must precede the acquisition of knowledge and skills) is apprehended, encoded, stored, organized, retrieved, and mentally manipulated to enable a person to perform cognitive tasks (Jensen, 1998). Differential psychologists, primarily using the techniques of mental chronometry, have examined individual differences in speed and variability of these information processes to inform theory and research on intelligence (e.g., see Jensen, 2006). Moreover, applied psychologists have used well-established findings in experimental cognitive psychology on information processing to better understand the results of cognitive ability tests. Of particular interest is the identification of processing deficits that can lead to effective interventions (e.g., Dehn, 2006). This attention to the processing of information that underlies cognitive ability test performance has been driven in part by the federal guidelines for identifying learning disabilities (Individuals with Disabilities Education Improvement Act of 2004 [IDEA 2004]), which postulate that "basic psychological processes" are the underlying causes of deficits in academic achievement seen in those with such disabilities.

The goal of this chapter is to review some of the most prominent information-processing approaches to the interpretation of cognitive ability tests. We first outline three predominant models of information processing and describe widely agreed-upon principles in experimental and differential psychology. We then discuss several general approaches designed to guide practitioners' consideration of cognitive processes during assessment. Last, we provide a critique of current practices in processing assessment and offer suggestions for clinicians and researchers.

APPROACHES TO UNDERSTANDING HUMAN COGNITION

Experimental Cognitive Psychology Approaches

In the 1970s and 1980s, there was a surge of interest by experimental psychologists in information processing as an alternative technology for understanding the measurement of human cognitive competencies. According to Sternberg (1981), "information processing is generally defined as the sequence of mental operations and their products involved in performing a cognitive task" (p. 1182). Consistent with this definition, information-processing models of cognitive functioning emerged in which a computer system was used as the analogy (Hunt, Frost, & Lunneborg, 1973; Neisser, 1967; Newell & Simon, 1972). These models provided a description of the stages through which information is transformed from sensations to mental representations, analyzed within the cognitive system, and expressed via some response. These stages of information processing were often represented in box-and-arrow models (Logan, 2000), with each stage typically representing an elementary information process (Newell & Simon, 1972).

An *elementary information process* can be considered the fundamental mental event in which information is operated on to produce a response (Carroll, 1993; Posner & McLeod, 1982). For example, these processes may include the *encoding* of external information into the cognitive system, *retrieval* of information stored in memory (e.g., names of letters), *comparison* of the new information to retrieved information , selection of a response (e.g., either "same" or "different"), and *execution* of that response (saying either "same" or "different") (see Logan, 2000). Models of information processing, such as the stage model of memory, the working memory model, and the ACT-R theory, represent some of the most widely accepted descriptions of the human information-processing system and its processes.

Stage Model of Memory

Over 40 years ago, Atkinson and Shiffrin (1968) presented a *multistore model of memory* (see Figure 21.1). Since its initial presentation, this model has stimulated a large body of research, which has led to support for its postulations as well as to modifications (Estes, 1999; Healy & McNamara, 1996; Raaijmakers, 1993; Shiffrin, 1999). Specifying both structural features and control processes, the model focuses on how information is stored in memory across three stages of processing. The structural features represent the hardware and built-in stages of the cognitive processing system; they include the *sensory register*, multiple *short-term stores*, and the *long-term store*. The sensory register represents the temporary holding space for all stimuli from the environment detected by

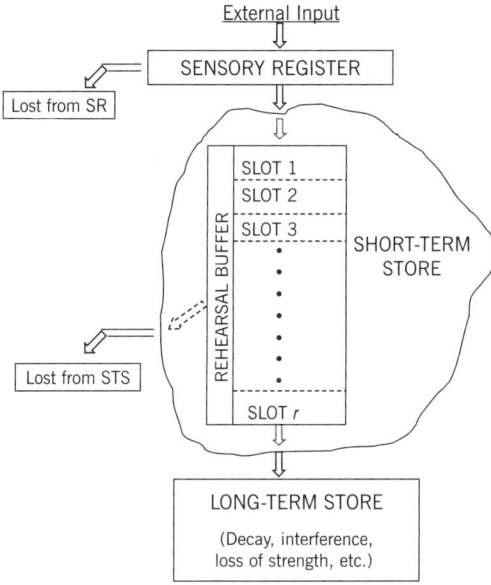

FIGURE 21.1. The multistore model of memory. From Atkinson and Shiffrin (1968, p. 113). Copyright 1968 by Academic Press. Reprinted by permission of Elsevier.

the sense organs (e.g., sounds and images). If unattended, this information is lost in milliseconds. If attended to, information from the sensory register is copied into one of the short-term memory stores.

Atkinson and Shiffrin referred to these stores as *auditory–verbal–linguistic memory*, the *visual short-term store*, and the *haptic* (touch-related) *short-term store*. Because oral communication is ubiquitous and the objects of our attention are frequently labeled or coded verbally, the auditory–verbal–linguistic memory store is perhaps the most vital to adaptive information processing. The limited-capacity stores are temporary holding areas for information in one's immediate awareness—*active* information. Such information, stored in a finite number of slots in the stores, is lost within approximately 30 seconds if it is not rehearsed (i.e., the process of cycling through information held in short-term memory) or reactivated in some way. With the use of storage strategies, information in the short-term stores is copied into the long-term memory. The long-term store is considered a relatively permanent storage area—a warehouse of memories and acquired knowledge and skills. The information in the long-term store may appear to be lost for a number of reasons: decay of the in-

formation, interference due to subsequent experiences, or weakening of the bonds between related units of information. According to this theory, processing occurs in a serial, discontinuous manner as information moves from one stage to the next. Control processes in the multistore model of memory describe acquired programs that drive the operation of the structural system. Examples of control processes include rehearsal of information in the short-term store, verbal coding of stimuli, and memory storage and retrieval strategies. According to this model, the individual coordinates control processes to accomplish cognitive goals.

Working Memory Model

Baddeley's *working memory model* (Baddeley, 1986, 1994, 1996, 2001; Baddeley & Hitch, 1974, 1994) is a modification and extension of Atkinson and Shiffrin's (1968) multistore theory of memory. Baddeley and colleagues developed the working memory model to increase the understanding of the functional or "working" operations carried out in the short-term stores. As such, working memory facilitates the manipulation and storage of information in the larger memory system, which includes sensory stores and a long-term store. According to Baddeley, working memory is composed of three subcomponents: the *central executive* and two slave systems, the *phonological loop* and the *visuo-spatial sketchpad*. These slave systems largely represent two of the short-term stores identified by Atkinson and Shiffrin.

After receiving information via the auditory sensory store, the phonological loop holds and manipulates phonological (speech-based) stimuli. The phonological loop consists of two components: the *phonological short-term store* and the *articulatory rehearsal process*. The phonological short-term store retains speech-based information for a brief time according to its phonological structure. Baddeley (1986) suggested that this information gains obligatory access to the phonological store and becomes an auditory memory trace. Consistent with the auditory–verbal–linguistic memory store of Atkinson and Shiffrin (1968), the phonological store retains the structure of the information for 2–3 seconds before the corresponding memory trace fades. The articulatory rehearsal process functions to maintain or refresh the fading information in the phonological store through subvocal articulation.

The visuo-spatial sketchpad functions to hold and to manipulate visual and spatial information.

Baddeley (1986) proposed that visual and spatial information are operated on by separate elements of this system. Visual information is thought to rely on sensory coding and spatial information on motoric processes (Wilson & Emmorey, 1997). The visuo-spatial sketchpad has a structure similar to that of the phonological loop, in which one area holds visual and spatial information, and another element facilitates rehearsal of such information.

The central executive is described as an attentional control system that coordinates information processes performed in working memory. It represents, in effect, a *homunculus*—a miniature person who manipulates the workings of the cognitive system (Baddeley, 1996). The central executive performs two functions: processing and storage capabilities, and control activities (Gathercole, 1994). The processing and storage capabilities of the central executive include maintenance rehearsal, the analysis of information, and the storage and retrieval of memories held in the long-term store. The control activities include the management of attention and behavior, as well as the regulation of information in the memory system.

Anderson's ACT-R

In contrast to models of memory, which attempt to explain the processing of information across stages of the mind, the *adaptive control of thought—rational theory* (ACT-R, pronounced "act R") is more ambitious in its breadth and explanatory power (Anderson, 1983; Anderson & Lebiere, 1998). This evolving architecture[1] forms the basis for computer modeling of the higher-level cognitive processes leading to complex human behavior (Anderson, 1976, 1983, 1990; Anderson & Lebiere, 1998). For example, ACT-R has simulated behavior on several tasks like those seen on intelligence tests, such as mathematical problem solving, spatial reasoning, sentence memory, and nonverbal reasoning (Anderson et al., 2004).

The foundation of ACT-R is based on units of procedural knowledge and units of declarative knowledge that are entered into the processing system. *Procedural knowledge* is conceptualized as knowing how to perform a behavior, and in ACT-R it comprises a repository of productions, which are if–then rules or strategies used to achieve goals. *Declarative knowledge* is conceptualized as knowing what and what to do, and in ACT-R it comprises memories and other explicit knowledge called *chunks*. As evident in the representation of ACT-R in Figure 21.2, visual information from the environment enters the cognitive system through activation of the visual module. *Modules* represent programs or storehouses of knowledge used by the cognitive system. Following the model, in-

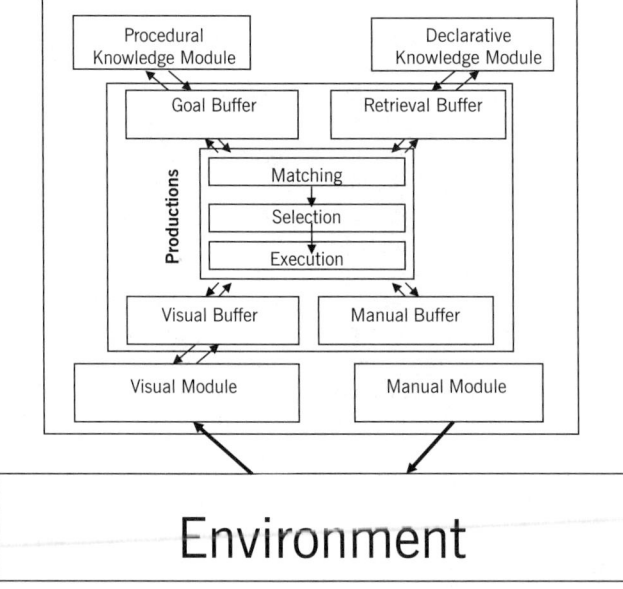

FIGURE 21.2. The adaptive control of thought—rational (ACT-R) architecture. From Anderson et al. (2004). Copyright 2004 by the American Psychological Association. Adapted by permission.

formation is then placed in a visual buffer. *Buffers in ACT-R* are similar to the sensory register and short-term stores of Atkinson and Shiffrin (1968) and the slave systems of Baddeley (1986). (Figure 21.2 emphasizes visual information processing and not phonological processing.) Once in the buffer, information may be acted upon by any number of productions from the central processing system, such as matching and selection. These productions are extracted from the procedural knowledge module and its associated buffer, and, if needed, information from the declarative knowledge module may be extracted to assist in understanding the new information and reacting to it in an adaptive manner. When the central processing system prepares a response, the execution production may be activated in the manual (or motor) buffer, and the manual module can make a response.

Summary: Basic Principles

Despite the fact that there are widely varying views within experimental cognitive psychology on models of information processing, we believe that there are basic principles that most researchers would agree upon. The most basic of these principles is the limited capacity of short-term memory. Short-term memory refers to the restriction of information from the perceptual system and of information retrieved from long-term memory stores that can be simultaneously processed. Miller (1956) originally estimated the capacity of short-term memory at about seven items or chunks of information. In addition to limited capacity, information in short-term memory rapidly decays without continuous rehearsal (Brown, 1958; Murdock, 1961; Muter, 1980; Peterson & Peterson, 1959) or is lost as a result of interference (Klatzky, 1975; Reitman, 1974). In order to compensate for limited capacity, rapid decay, and interference, one must either continually process information in short-term memory or store it in long-term memory. But the storage process itself takes time and channel capacity, so there is a tradeoff between the amount of information that can be stored and processed at one time (Baddeley, 1972; Baddeley & Hitch, 1974). Throughout the various stages of information processing, higher-order components or *metacomponents* oversee elementary processing (e.g., Sternberg, 1985). These metacomponents control, monitor, and evaluate cognitive processing. Last, memory is enhanced by the depth with which it was processed (e.g., Craik & Lockhart, 1972). Information that is processed at a deeper, more meaningful level is more likely to be remembered than information that is simply rehearsed because information processed at deeper levels creates networks of associations with other memory traces that facilitate retention and retrieval.

It is important to note that these basic principles are based on research on information processing in experimental cognitive psychology, the primary focus of which is to discover laws of nature that apply to all individuals. In other words, research in this area is concerned with how individuals process information, not with how and why they differ when processing information. In contrast, the differential psychology approaches target these differences in processing information; and intelligence tests are developed and validated with the goal of measuring individual differences on cognitive tasks.

Differential Psychology Approaches

In differential psychology, the psychometric approach to studying human cognitive abilities "has not only inspired the most research and attracted the most attention . . . but is by far the most widely used in practical settings" (Neisser et al., 1996, p. 77). Research from this perspective has shown that any time a diverse collection of cognitive ability tests (i.e., objectively scored tests on which individual differences are not due to sensory acuity or motor deftness) is administered to a large representative sample of the population, scores on those tests are almost always positively correlated (e.g., Jensen, 1998). This pattern of correlations is an empirical fact of nature that is known as the *positive manifold*. The positive manifold indicates that a common source of variance underlies individual differences on all tests and performances of cognitive ability. Spearman (1904) invented factor analysis to estimate the degree to which tests of cognitive ability correlate with this common source of variance, which he referred to as the general factor, or psychometric *g*. No test or performance involving cognitive ability measures only psychometric *g*, however. The reliable (non-error-related) variance from tests also reflects group factors and specificity. *Group factors* are common only to tests that require similar content (e.g., verbal, numerical, or spatial content) or cognitive processes (e.g., short-term memory for phonological information), whereas *specificity* refers to the variance that is unique to each test.

At the current time, the most widely accepted theory of the structure of individual differences in human cognitive abilities is Carroll's (1993) three-stratum theory. This theory is essentially a taxonomy in which cognitive abilities are classified at three levels of generality (i.e., general, broad, and narrow). Psychometric *g* occupies the apex of a pyramid-like hierarchical structure of abilities (stratum III). Stratum II consists of eight broad cognitive abilities (e.g., fluid and crystallized intelligence), comparable to those specified in the extended Gf-Gc model (e.g., Horn & Blankson, Chapter 3, this volume). Last, stratum I is composed of approximately 70 narrow abilities (e.g., inductive reasoning, memory span, etc.). Similarities between the broad abilities specified in the three-stratum theory and in the extended Gf-Gc theory have led some researchers to combine the two theories into what is referred to as *Cattell–Horn–Carroll* (CHC) theory (for reviews, see Horn & Blankson, Chapter 3; Schneider & McGrew, Chapter 4; Schrank & Wendling, Chapter 12; and Carroll, Appendix, this volume). Results of psychometric research clearly indicate that individual differences in "intelligence" are multidimensional and do not reflect one underlying source of variance.

Measurements of cognitive abilities have long been used to predict a number of socially important outcomes, such as academic attainments, occupational and social status, job performance, and income, to name a few (e.g., Gottfredson, 2002; Jensen, 1998; Neisser et al., 1996). In addition, in recent years, the interpretation of scores from cognitive abilities tests has increasingly relied upon the CHC theory for understanding the underlying constructs measured across different standardized tests (e.g., McGrew & Flanagan, 1998; Sattler, 2008; see Flanagan, Alfonso, & Ortiz, Chapter 19, this volume).

From the psychometric perspective, an *ability* is defined as a "developed skill, competence, or power to do something, especially . . . existing capacity to perform some function, whether physical, mental, or a combination of the two, without further education or training" (Colman, 2001, p. 1). According to Jensen (1998), an ability is a directly observable behavior that can be judged in terms of level of proficiency, that is stable over time, and that is consistently displayed across varying opportunities to perform the behavior (see pp. 51–52). At its most basic level, an ability may be viewed as the consistent performance of a discrete behavior in appropriate contexts (e.g., saying the word "No" in response to a question or writing the letter X when asked to do so), but under different conditions of task difficulty, individuals typically vary considerably in abilities (Carroll, 1993), and these

individual differences are the foundation of ability measurement. From the structure provided by factor analysis and accompanying factor labels, the underlying sources of these individual differences on abilities can be inferred. As an extension of this definition, *cognitive ability* is defined as "any ability that concerns some . . . class of tasks in which correct or appropriate processing of mental information is critical to successful performance" (Carroll, 1993, p. 10).

In contrast to cognitive abilities, which are defined in terms of differences across individuals, cognitive processes are inferred from the performance of individuals. Jensen (1998) stated:

> Information processes are defined as hypothetical constructs used by cognitive theorists to describe how persons apprehend, discriminate, select, and attend to certain aspects of the vast welter of stimuli that impinge on the sensorium to form internal representations that can be mentally manipulated, transformed, related to previous internal representations, stored in memory . . . and later retrieved from storage to govern the person's decision and behavior in a particular situation. (pp. 205–206)

Although individual differences on cognitive ability tests are quantified by examining variability in performance across individuals, an individual's cognitive processes can be inferred only by examining the item stimuli, the task demands, and the response requirements of these cognitive ability tests.

Summary: Cognitive Abilities and Processes

Cognitive abilities are inferred from directly observable behaviors on objectively scored tests that require information processing for successful performance. Specific cognitive processes, such as apprehension, discrimination, and selection, are hypothesized to underlie performance on these tasks. Individual differences on tests of cognitive ability are best described by a taxonomy in which cognitive abilities are classified at three levels of generality (i.e., general, broad, and narrow) as described in Carroll's (1993) three-stratum theory. There are logical, as well as empirical, links between some sequences of processes and narrow (stratum I) cognitive abilities (Carroll, 1988, 1993, 1998, and Appendix, this volume; Deary, 2001; Sternberg, 1977). With commonalities in use of stimulus materials, presumed cognitive processes, and kinds of outcomes and products, *some* narrow (stratum I) abilities may provide a means of representing sequences of cognitive processes (Carroll, 1976, 1987). Toward this end, Sternberg (1977) presented a schematic using Thurstone's (1938) *primary mental abilities* to indicate the importance of tasks and components below the level of general, broad, and narrow ability factors. Figure 21.3 is an extension of both Sternberg's and Floyd's (2005) schematic that integrates characteristics from both Carroll's three-stratum theory and CHC theory at the ability level and provides examples of hypothesized processes for tasks measuring abilities associated with reasoning (Sternberg, 1977) and reaction time (Carroll, 1993).

CONTEMPORARY INTERPRETIVE FRAMEWORKS FOR PROCESSING DURING TESTS

Both the experimental and differential psychology approaches to understanding human cognition have been applied to the practice of psychology in schools, clinics, and other settings (Milberg, Hebben, & Kaplan, 2009). This section reviews some of the interpretive frameworks that have been developed to facilitate the possible identification and interpretation of the cognitive processes reflected on cognitive ability tests.

These interpretive frameworks generally fall along two related dimensions. One dimension reflects the contrast between *quantitative* and *qualitative* interpretive approaches. Quantitative approaches draw meaning from the numbers derived from assessment. Norm-referenced standardized scores and frequency counts are examples of quantitative data that are the foundation of this interpretive approach. In contrast, qualitative approaches draw meaning from differences in the kinds of behaviors exhibited by those being tested. Written narrative descriptions of odd test behaviors, recordings of vocalizations, or patterns of errors across items are examples of qualitative data. The second dimension reflects the contrast between a group-based or *nomothetic* approach and an individual-based or *idiographic* approach (Allport, 1937). Thus comparison of the total number of items correct or total number of errors accumulated on a task with the performance of a norm group is consistent with the nomothetic approach, whereas noting the types of errors made on a subtest—regardless of the expected performance of others—is consistent with the idiographic approach.

Cognitive ability test interpretation has strong nomothetic and quantitative foundations. Scores on such tests have typically been interpreted in relation to some norm group, and individual differences in abilities are inferred from the deviation of an individual's performance from the average performance of that group. Most readers are likely to

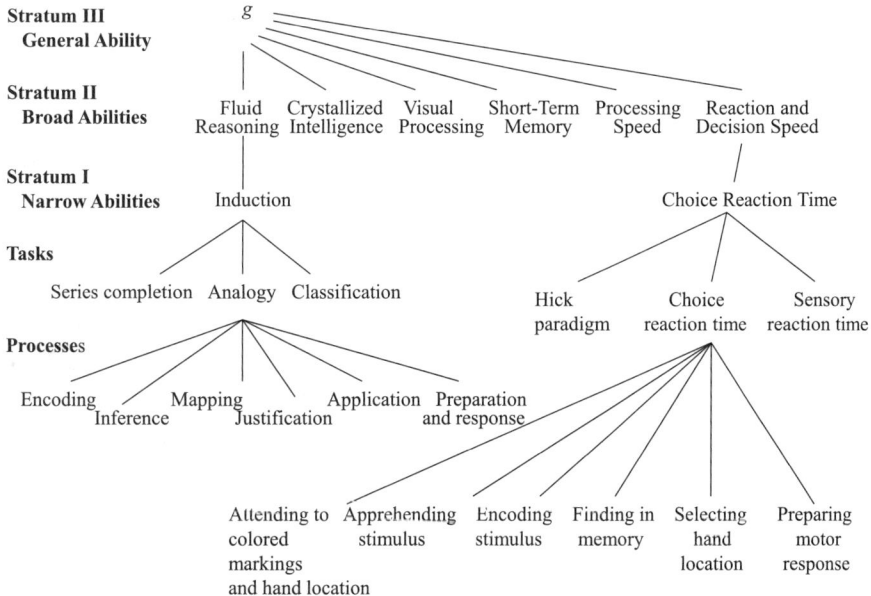

FIGURE 21.3. Possible relations among the three-stratum model described in the Cattell–Horn–Carroll theory, cognitive tasks, and processes underlying them. Based on Sternberg (1977).

be intimately familiar with this approach to interpreting age-based standardized scores and percentile ranks. In contrast, there is a strong tradition in clinical neuropsychology of applying qualitative and idiographic approaches to interpretation of cognitive ability tests and related assessment instruments (Semrud-Clikeman, Wilkinson, & Wellington, 2005). Neuropsychology is the study of brain–behavior relations, and inferences made about these relations by clinical neuropsychologists are typically drawn from behaviors during testing and variation across items and tasks. Thus clinical neuropsychology is consistent with the experimental approach described previously in its focus on understanding how and why an individual's performance differs as a function of stimulus input or output or task demands when processing information (Miller, 2007).

The neuropsychologist Luria (1966, 1973) was one of the first to propose an approach for examining the cognitive processes used by individuals during testing via analysis of errors and supplemental test requirements, called *testing of limits*. According to Luria, an examiner should develop hypotheses, based on observation of task performance, regarding the reasons for errors on that task and present the same task that produced these errors under varying conditions to test those hypotheses (Semrud-Clikeman et al., 2005). Thus, if performance improved in one of these varied task conditions, it could be inferred that an omitted or otherwise errant cognitive process led to the initial errors. Using this qualitative method, which is consistent with the experimental psychology methodologies, an examiner could construct and test varied hypotheses across tasks and draw conclusions thought to be clinically meaningful.

Luria's (1966, 1973) qualitative approach had a significant impact on neuropsychologists in their selection of comprehensive batteries of neuropsychological tests (producing quantitative indexes) and accompanying qualitative interpretation of them (Groth-Marnat, 2000), and these techniques and accompanying technology were advanced substantially in the work of Kaplan and others. Kaplan was one of the foremost advocates of the Boston Process Approach (Kaplan, 1998; Milberg et al., 2009), and she and others developed tests, modified others with supplemental instructions and requirements, and trained clinicians to "test the limits" by using special encouragement and other motivational strategies to facilitate better understanding of the patterns of errors demonstrated by examinees. In particular, the Boston Process

Approach increased emphasis on idiosyncratic behaviors during the test sessions, called *qualitative indicators*, as reflective of the correct or errant cognitive processes. For example, research reported by Kaplan (1998) revealed that adults with damage to one brain hemisphere would display characteristic errors on subtests, such as the Wechsler Block Design subtests, whereas those with damage on the other side would display other types of errors. Test authors influenced by this research have increasingly provided metrics to quantify the frequency of qualitative indicators, as well as to compare these frequencies to normative data (Miller, 2007).

Considering the quantitative–qualitative and nomothetic–idiographic dimensions to assessment, we review four frameworks for representing cognitive processes in the section that follows: (1) creating test batteries designed to produce scores representing cognitive processes; (2) applying processing models to interpretation of scores designed to measure cognitive abilities; (3) adapting existing test batteries to allow for qualitative testing of hypotheses regarding cognitive processes; and (4) identifying processes based on qualitative analysis of item-level performance.

Creating Test Batteries to Measure Cognitive Processes

During the past several decades, several test batteries have been developed to operationalize select cognitive processes via their scores. Two test batteries, whose authors have drawn on this top-down approach to test development, are discussed in this section.

Tests Based on the PASS Theory

Derived from Luria's (1966, 1973, 1980) work in neuropsychology, the planning, attention, simultaneous, successive (PASS) theory of human cognition is one of the few theories of information processing that has been used to guide test development (e.g., Das, 1992; Das & Varnhagen, 1986). As described by Naglieri, Das, and Goldstein (Chapter 7, this volume), this theory posits four interrelated cognitive processes—*planning, attention, simultaneous* processes, and *successive* processes. Planning processes are the actions of executive control involved in governing the information-processing system, such as searching the long-term store for existing strategies and problem solving. This process mirrors the productions outlined in ACT-R (Anderson & Lebiere, 1998) and other production systems (Schunn & Klahr, 1998). Attention processes include the modulation of arousal and maintenance of mental focus across time. Simultaneous processing include perceiving, encoding, transforming, or otherwise utilizing bits of information occurring concurrently or as a group, whereas successive processing refers to the same processes involving bits of information presented in serial order (one after another).

Although the PASS model began as a relatively confined description of types of information processing (Das, Kirby, & Jarman, 1979), it was later expanded into a theory of intelligence (Das, Naglieri, & Kirby, 1994; Naglieri & Das, 1997). The model maintains characteristics of an information-processing model by specifying input, processing, and output stages and knowledge stores (e.g., Das et al., 1994), but the PASS processes are conceptualized as nonhierarchical; that is, all may be performed at the memory, conceptual, and perceptual levels. For example, simultaneous processes may be expressed at the memory level by drawing an image from memory. Finally, output mechanisms can be expressed in either a simultaneous or a successive manner. For instance, writing sentences typically requires successive motor output to group letters and words in the correct order on the written page.

The only commercially published test that is currently available based solely on the PASS theory is the Cognitive Assessment System (CAS; Naglieri & Das, 1997; see Naglieri & Otero, Chapter 15, this volume). The CAS was designed to assess the PASS processes in children ages 5–17. Scores from its 12 subtests contribute to four scales representing each of the PASS processes. Research on the structure of the CAS, however, suggests that it does not measure the constructs it was designed to measure (Carroll, 1995; Keith & Kranzler, 1999; Keith, Kranzler, & Flanagan, 2001; Kranzler & Keith, 1999; Kranzler, Keith, & Flanagan, 2000; Kranzler & Weng, 1995a, 1995b). For example, Keith and colleagues (2001) conducted a series of joint confirmatory factor analyses of the CAS and the Woodcock–Johnson III (WJ III) Tests of Cognitive Abilities (Woodcock, McGrew, & Mather, 2001b). Results of their analyses indicated that the underlying constructs measured on the CAS were better explained by CHC theory than by the PASS model. Their findings indicate that although the CAS may have been derived from an information-processing theory, individual difference on the test reflect the same sources of variance as that measured by other tests. Concerns regarding the

adequacy of the PASS model as a theory of intelligence were voiced by Sternberg (1984) in his review of the Kaufman Assessment Battery for Children (K-ABC; Kaufman & Kaufman, 1983), which is based on a partial PASS model. As Sternberg stated, "I am not aware of any empirical support in the cognitive–experimental literature that should lead me to accept Luria's theory, either as a psychological theory or as a basis for an intelligence test" (p. 272).

Nonetheless, it is important to note that despite the questions surrounding the PASS theory, research indicates that the CAS (Naglieri & Das, 1997) and the revision of the K-ABC (Kaufman & Kaufman, 1983), the Kaufman Assessment Battery for Children—Second Edition (KABC-II; Kaufman & Kaufman, 2004), are excellent measures of psychometric *g* and a number of CHC factors at stratum II of the three-stratum theory (e.g., Keith et al., 2001; Reynolds, Keith, Fine, Fisher, & Low, 2007). In fact, the KABC-II allows for interpretation of scores in terms of the four postulated PASS processes *and* in terms of CHC theory. In a recent confirmatory factor analysis of the standardization sample, Reynolds and colleagues (2007) found that the underlying structure of the KABC-II was explained quite well by CHC theory. The authors of the CAS and KABC-II are to be applauded for their attempts to develop tests of intelligence derived from information-processing theories, but until further work in experimental cognitive psychology is conducted, it would appear that individual differences in the cognitive processes underlying the currently available tests based on the PASS model are similar to (if not the same as) those measured by other widely used tests of cognitive abilities.

Cognitive Ability Measurement

In order to measure a range of cognitive abilities during research studies examining personnel selection and training and the effects of stressors on cognition, Kyllonen and colleagues (Chaiken, Kyllonen, & Tirre, 2000; Kyllonen, 1995, 2002) developed the Cognitive Ability Measurement (CAM) battery. The battery includes almost 60 individual tests, and all are administered with a computer-based user interface. Tests were developed to operationalize the major elements and processes represented in early versions of the ACT architecture (ACT*; Anderson, 1983) via measurement of seven cognitive abilities: working memory capacity; rate of learning of declarative knowledge (fact acquisition); rate of learning of procedural knowledge (skill acquisition); consolidated declarative knowledge; consolidated procedural knowledge; mental processing speed; and time estimation.

The CAM battery is structured according to a detailed taxonomy that highlights aspects of the tests that may influence performance on them (and accompanying scores). They include test paradigms, domains of knowledge, input modality, and response format (Kyllonen, 1995). To ensure broad construct representation in measurement of the elements and operations of the ACT architecture, and to avoid "method variance" stemming primarily from similar test paradigms, the CAM battery draws from varying test paradigms to assess cognitive abilities. For example, in order to assess the rate of learning of declarative knowledge, test paradigms requiring free-recall learning, paired-associates learning, and implicit learning are employed. In order to avoid the measurement of abilities tied closely to the content acted upon by the information processes, tests that vary in terms of the domain of knowledge (i.e., verbal, quantitative, and spatial), but that measure the same ability and draw from the same test paradigm, are included. Following the example regarding assessing rate of learning of declarative knowledge, the tests using the free-recall learning paradigm require working with representations of words or sentences, numbers, or visual–spatial stimuli. Similarly, tests may vary systematically according to the nature in which the test items are presented (e.g., in a visual or auditory input modality). Finally, tests are selected to vary systematically in their response formats. For example, response formats include pressing a key, touching a computer screen, manipulating a mouse, and vocalizing an answer. The authors of the CAM battery sought to develop at least one test that measures each of the seven cognitive abilities and that falls into each cell of this four-dimension taxonomy. As a result, the number of possible tests designed to measure *each* cognitive ability through different methods are many. This number would logically equal (1) the number of test paradigms multiplied by (2) the number of domains of knowledge multiplied by (3) the number of input modalities multiplied by (4) the number of response formats.

The CAM battery has a well-supported architecture from which it was developed. It is also innovative because it was designed to tap into general levels of abilities by balancing out test-related influences. Unlike no other assessment battery, it allows for distinctions to be made between those

influences due to test demands, test content, input modality, and response format and those influences associated with a specific type of cognitive ability (and perhaps cognitive process). However, the CAM battery has been used primarily for research purposes and is not commercially available. Its multitude of individual tests (and an administration time of 5–12 hours; Kyllonen, 1995, 2002) would probably be too unwieldy for use by most psychologists and other professionals involved in psychoeducational assessments. Furthermore, it is unclear how users would interpret the numerous scores stemming from the CAM. Additional research examining the reliability, validity, and utility of the CAM scores is needed before it can be used across applied settings.

Applying Processing Models to Interpretation of Test Scores

Woodcock and Dean's Information-Processing Model

In a series of articles, chapters, and other publications, Woodcock, Dean, and colleagues have offered an information-processing model that outlines the organization of and interactions among cognitive abilities (as specified in the CHC theory) and external and internal influences on cognitive performance (Brinkman, Decker, & Dean, 2005; Dean, Decker, Woodcock, & Schrank, 2003; Dean & Woodcock, 1999; Mather & Woodcock, 2001; Woodcock, 1993, 1997, 1998). Consistent with classic information-processing models and architectures, a horizontal dimension of the model represents the *input–processing–output loop*. It begins with physical stimuli being registered by the senses. If attended to, this information is encoded into immediate awareness, which is represented by the CHC broad cognitive ability *short-term memory* (Gsm) in the model. It represents the short-term store described in the multistore model of memory (Atkinson & Shiffrin, 1968) and the phonological loop described in the working memory model (Baddeley, 1986, 1994, 1996, 2001; Baddeley & Hitch, 1994). Information then may be acted upon and expressed via motor or oral output, or entered again into the processing loop. A vertical dimension of the model represents complexity of information processing, ranging from reflexes at the automatic level to complex mental operations, such as reasoning at the highest levels.

The Woodcock and Dean model includes components reflecting 10 cognitive abilities from

CHC theory. As noted above, immediate awareness is represented by short-term memory (Gsm). The *processing speed* (Gs) ability is purported to represent the speed with which the individual is able to move information across stages in the cognitive system. The *thinking abilities* in the model require application of programs devoted to sensory perception, storage and retrieval of information in the long-term store, and novel problem solving. These abilities include *tactile and kinesthetic thinking* (Gtk), *visual–spatial thinking* (Gv), *auditory processing* (Ga), *long-term retrieval* (Glr), and *fluid reasoning* (Gf). The model also includes *stores of acquired knowledge*, which represents the information stored in the largely permanent long-term store. Consistent with ACT-R (Anderson & Lebiere, 1998), Woodcock and Dean have referred to the stores of acquired knowledge as storehouses of declarative and procedural knowledge (Brinkman et al., 2005; Dean et al., 2003; Dean & Woodcock, 1999; Mather & Woodcock, 2001; Woodcock, 1993, 1997, 1998). Although these stores could contain numerous specific content areas, Woodcock and Dean have focused on only three: *reading and writing* (Grw), *quantitative knowledge* (Gq), and *comprehension knowledge* (Gc). However, it is likely that the thinking abilities, which are differentiated from the stores of acquired knowledge, are the result of related procedural memory modules and the action rules contained in them (i.e., productions).

In addition to these measurable abilities operationalized by existing assessment instruments (viz., the WJ III; Woodcock et al., 2001a, 2001b), Woodcock and Dean have also included an *executive control* component in the model, which is consistent with Baddeley's central executive (Baddeley, 1986, 1994, 1996, 2001; Baddeley & Hitch, 1994). Executive control governs the choice and sequence of cognitive processes. For example, it can activate the metaknowledge filter to search the stores of acquired knowledge (i.e., the long-term store) for existing strategies or knowledge to be used during completion of a cognitive task. Finally, Woodcock and Dean have stressed the potential impact of situational and contextual factors on cognitive performance by the inclusion of *facilitators–inhibitors* in the model. Examples include distractions during testing and noncognitive person variables (e.g., sensory acuity deficits, fatigue, motivation, and behavioral styles).

Woodcock and Dean's information-processing model serves as the basis for the Gf-Gc Diagnostic Worksheet (Woodcock, 1993, 1998), the WJ III Diagnostic Worksheet (Mather & Woodcock, 2001; Schrank & Woodcock, 2002), and the Dean–Woodcock Neuropsychological Assessment System neuropsychology model. One version of this model and its accompanying worksheet focus on the interactions among cognitive abilities as measured by the WJ III Tests of Cognitive Abilities (Woodcock, McGrew, & Mather, 2001b) and the WJ III Tests of Achievement (Woodcock, McGrew, & Mather, 2001a); sensory–motor scores from the Dean–Woodcock Sensory–Motor Battery (Dean & Woodcock, 2003b); and facilitators–inhibitors from the Dean–Woodcock Structured Interview (Dean & Woodcock, 2003c) and the Dean–Woodcock Emotional Status Exam (Dean & Woodcock, 2003a).

Woodcock and Dean's information-processing model contains almost all of the components as prominent information-processing models described previously, as well as more recent components from cognitive science research. It is a very plausible organization of the interactions among processes associated with the broad cognitive ability factors specified in CHC theory and other influences on cognitive performance. It seems, however, that there are several problems with the organization of the model. As noted previously, it is unclear how thinking abilities in this model differ from procedural knowledge and related productions held in the stores of acquired knowledge. Review of prominent information-processing models also indicates that a short-term store for visual information (in Baddeley's working memory model, the visuo-spatial sketchpad; Baddeley & Hitch, 1994) is probably necessary in comprehensive information-processing models, but it is absent in Woodcock and Dean's model. A component representing this structure and related processes could be represented along with short-term memory to represent the holding areas for active information.

The operationalization of the processes via cognitive ability measures—and especially broad-ability measures—in the Woodcock and Dean model also seems problematic. For example, the inclusion of broad cognitive abilities, rather than more specific narrow abilities, leads to uncertainty about its accuracy in guiding test interpretation. For example, consistent with covariance structural analyses, the Picture Recognition test from the Woodcock–Johnson III Tests of Cognitive Abilities (Woodcock et al., 2001b) is typically grouped with another test as a measure of visual–spatial thinking in the Woodcock and Dean model. Picture Recognition requires examinees to hold images in mind and, soon afterward, identify them in an array of images presented on a page. In the nomenclature of CHC theory, this test measures visual memory (or, more generally, visual short-term memory span). Thus this test should probably be placed in an area of the model representing the visuo-spatial sketchpad, as described previously. In addition, cognitive abilities reflecting expressive and receptive language are grouped under the same factor, comprehension–knowledge, as are measures of cultural knowledge. Just because tests measuring similar processes covary to the degree that they measure a single factor, this does not mean that they should be grouped together in a fine-grained processing analysis, given that processing differences may or may not be related to the same source of individual differences (see Jensen, 1987). Without focus on the specific influences on item- and task-level performance, the interpretation of cognitive ability measures as reflecting distinct sets of processes is questionable.

Processing Assessment

In a book titled *Essentials of Processing Assessment*, Dehn (2006) has presented guidelines for test score interpretation based on recent models of cognitive abilities and neuropsychological functioning. He has argued that "we need not wait until we have a proven theory of processing before we begin to routinely assess processing and apply processing models to diagnosis and treatment. . . . There is adequate evidence in support of cognitive processing constructs and the relationships various processes have with learning" (p. 3). In his model, Dehn has described an array of processes, derived from both CHC theory and neuropsychological models, such as PASS theory, to consider. They include attention, auditory processing, executive processing, fluid reasoning, long-term retrieval, phonemic awareness, planning, processing speed, short-term memory, simultaneous processing, successive processing, visual processing, and working memory. In doing so, Dehn has equated processes with select CHC broad abilities and introduced the term *cognitive processing abilities*. In describing the connection between cognitive abilities and processes, he states:

> Cattell–Horn Carroll (CHC) theory is a contemporary theory of intelligence and human cognitive abilities, not a processing theory per se. . . . The [CHC] model is applicable to processing assessment because

most of the broad abilities identified by the theory can also be considered cognitive processes. The cognitive processing abilities include visual processing, auditory processing, short-term memory, long-term storage and retrieval, fluid intelligence, and processing speed. Crystallized intelligence, quantitative knowledge, and reading and writing ability are also broad cognitive abilities but are not considered types of processing for the purposes of this book. Decision/Reaction Time/Speed is also a type of processing but will not be included in this book's proposed assessment model because psychometric scales seldom measure it. (p. 17)

Dehn's (2006) guidelines for *processing assessment* appear to be influenced only minimally by the information-processing frameworks derived from experimental cognitive psychology research. Instead, Dehn's model seems to rely primarily on interpretation of ability measures at a broad-ability level—not unlike the CHC cross-battery approach (Flanagan, Ortiz, & Alfonso, 2007; McGrew & Flanagan, 1998), which is a quantitative, nomothetic approach to interpreting ability scores. The so-called "processing" components of his model appear to be derived from the inclusion of measures purported to measure constructs not included in cognitive ability models (e.g., CHC theory), such as those from the neuropsychological tradition (e.g., attention, executive processing, and planning). Thus it is a model not unlike those advocating for the application of clinical neuropsychological practices in the schools (e.g., Miller, 2007). In addition, the identification of "processing" elements in Dehn's model seems to stem from his classification of tests according to their targeting abilities associated with procedural knowledge (i.e., "processes") and those targeting abilities associated with declarative knowledge (i.e., "content"). Doing so is consistent with Kaplan's (1998) approach, which was based in part on Werner's (1937) developmental theory, but this dichotomy has no sound empirical support from cognitive ability research. Finally, the model seems to misapply the term *process* throughout, such as the reference to "processing abilities" and reference to global processes and individual processes, when all processes by definition are specific to a presumed cognitive operation. Although this approach to processing assessment draws on some sound research supporting the interpretation of cognitive ability measures and integrates tests from the clinical neuropsychological tradition, several of the key assumptions do not appear to be well founded.

Adapting Existing Tests to Allow for Qualitative Testing of Hypotheses

Several existing intelligence tests have been modified to isolate some of the processes that may be interfering with performance or leading to weaknesses in abilities. Drawing on the tenets of Luria's (1966, 1973) clinical method and the Boston Process Approach (Kaplan, 1998), the Wechsler Adult Intelligence Scale—Revised as a Neuropsychological Instrument (WAIS-R NI; Kaplan, Fein, Morris, & Delis, 1991); the Wechsler Intelligence Scale for Children—Third Edition as a Process Instrument (WISC-III PI; Kaplan, Fein, Kramer, Delis, & Morris, 1999); and, most recently, the Wechsler Intelligence Scale for Children—Fourth Edition Integrated (WISC-IV Integrated; Kaplan, et al., 2004) were all developed to aid clinicians in identifying cognitive processes. Thus their intent has been to facilitate a "finer analysis of problem-solving behaviors and the parsing of component factors contributing to performance [in a way that can] provide the examiner a deeper understanding of the child's level of processing as well as a basis for generating tailored, individual interventions" (Kaplan et al., 1999, p. 2). As evident from the test titles, they draw upon the subtests from the Wechsler intelligence scales, but the task paradigms of their subtests are modified slightly with the goal of isolating some processes through a systematic testing of limits.

The most recently published battery of this group is the WISC-IV Integrated (Kaplan et al., 2004). It contains 16 *process tests*, which reflect slight changes in the task requirements of subtests through adaptations to their stimulus input, to steps in responding, and to the nature of the cognitive task itself. Table 21.1 lists some of these adaptations. The battery also offers eight additional scoring criteria and provides the option of add-on administration procedures. Performance on most of these process tests yields norm-based scores that can be compared to those stemming from the original standardized administration of subtests from the Wechsler scales. At the idiographic level of interpretation, higher scores on the process tests than on the original subtests indicate that the process targeted by the adaptation must have interfered with performance on the original subtest. For example, a examiner would probably conclude that children who performed notably better on the Information subtest after being provided with multiple-choice options (see Table 21.1)

experienced memory retrieval problems that interfered with their initial performance on the subtest. Observations of performance during subtests during the WISC-IV Integrated can also yield the quantitative measures and norm-based scores representing some qualitative indicators, such as requests for item repetition, pointing responses, and (on the Block Design subtest) use of extra blocks and breaks in the final configurations. In addition, there are several checklists of behaviors during the test administration that promote the recording of information about the examinee's language skills, sensory responses, motor stereotypies, social skills, cooperativeness, attention/concentration, and confidence.

The WAIS-R NI (Kaplan et al., 1991), the WISC-III PI (Kaplan et al., 1999), and the WISC-IV Integrated (Kaplan et al., 2004) are certainly innovative in that they combine quantitative and qualitative approaches as well as normative and idiographic approaches. The detailed guidelines for their use lessen the need for intensive clinical training (e.g., in neuropsychology; Milberg et al., 2009) for standard test interpretation, and they sensitize examiners to processes that may affect cognitive performance. The wealth of quantitative information stemming from them also promotes research examining the reliability and validity evidence supporting their interpretation. However, the practical benefit of (1) engaging in the deductive process to determine reasons for poor performance, such as why a child performed poorly on the Block Design subtest or (2) knowing that a child more often engaged in idiosyncratic responses to certain test stimuli (e.g., pointing versus verbalizing) while responding than others, is unclear. Furthermore, as with all testing-of-limits approaches, it appears that practice effects (and other carryover effects) are often not considered as potential confounds affected the repeated presentation of similar tasks. Like other methods derived from the Boston Process Approach (Kaplan, 1998), these instruments have not been substantiated by research supporting their use for differential diagnosis or treatment utility (Milberg et al., 2009).

Identifying Processes Based on Qualitative Analysis of Item-Level Performance

Numerous interpretive schemes have been developed over the decades to aid practitioners in their interpretation of test scores, and some of the most

TABLE 21.1. Descriptions of the WISC-IV Subtests and Their Modifications in the WISC-IV Integrated

WISC-IV subtest	Typical task requirements	Modifications to subtest or subtest scoring
Information	Children are required to answer orally presented questions about people, places, and things from U.S. culture.	Division of items by content categories: number facts, calendar facts, geography, science, and history. Provision of response options in multiple-choice format.
Vocabulary	Children are required to define orally presented words.	Words in items presented in images. Provision of response options in multiple-choice format.
Similarities	Children are required to describe the common characteristic associated with orally presented words.	Provision of response options in multiple-choice format.
Comprehension	Children are required to answer orally presented questions regarding everyday problems or understanding of social rules and concepts.	Provision of response options in multiple-choice format.
Block Design	Children are required to construct geometric patterns from a model or visual image, using cubes, during a timed administration.	Provision of overlay on stimulus design that distinguishes individual blocks. No time bonus option. Provision of response options in multiple-choice format.
Digit Span	Children are required to repeat orally presented digits in sequence or in reversed sequence.	Visual presentation of items via numbers printed on a page. Blocks tapped rather than numbers presented. Letters presented orally rather than digits. Analysis of types of errors.
Letter–Number Sequencing	Children are required to repeat orally presented letters in alphabetical order digits in ascending order.	Word cues embedded in letter–number sequence.
Arithmetic	Children are required to solve orally presented arithmetic problems without the use of paper and pencil.	Visual supplement to oral item presentation. Provision of pencil and paper for hand calculations. Problems isolated from "word problems" and put in standard arithmetic format.
Coding	Children are required to draw symbols that are paired with a series of shapes or numbers according to a key during a timed administration.	Requirement to recall symbols when presented with numbers. Requirement to recall symbols with no prompt. Requirement to recall numbers when presented with symbols. Requirement to copy symbols.
Elithorn Mazes	Children are required to connect dots to complete mazes.	

comprehensive interpretive schemes have relied on task-analytic methods to meet this goal. This section reviews three of these interpretive schemes.

Carroll's Coding Scheme for Cognitive Tasks

After completing a comprehensive review of the research examining elementary information processes, Carroll (1976) amended an information-processing model proposed by Hunt (1971) and, from it, developed a coding scheme for cognitive tasks (see Table 21.2). Carroll specified six general elements in his coding scheme. The first element targets characteristics of the stimuli presented at the outset of a task, such as the number and nature of the stimuli used in an item. The second element focuses on the types of overt responses that must be made to respond to an item and the manner in which they are judged for accuracy. The third element targets the temporal parameters of steps in the task. For example, a time delay between presentation of the item and recall of its content would be coded. The fourth element focuses on the elementary information processes likely to be employed when performing the task. The fifth element targets speed-related influences or conditions on task performance. The final element focuses on the primary memory stores involved during task completion and their content, including short-term memory, long-term memory, and intermediate-term memory stores (i.e., working memory involving memory storage and retrieval). Content of the stores may range from simple stimuli, such as one-dimensional lines, to information focusing on word meaning.

Carroll (1976) used this scheme to deconstruct the steps involved in completing items from 48 tests found in the group-administered Kit of Reference Tests for Cognitive Factors (French, Ekstrom, & Price, 1963). He chose tests as "pure" measures of 24 factors and randomly selected two tests of each factor for coding. In order to delineate the probable "causes" of individual differences on these tests, Carroll presented a portion of the results organized according to the factors measured by the tests. These results included the descriptions of the primary memory store involved, the cognitive operations implied in task directions, and strategies that may contribute to performance. In the coding scheme, Carroll (1976) distinguished between *operations*, which are "control processes that are explicitly specified, or implied, in the task instructions and fore-exercises that must be per-

formed if the task is to be completed successfully" and *strategies*, which are "control processes that are not specified by task instructions, but may or may not be used (discovered) by a particular subject" (p. 42).

Table 21.3 presents results for four factors frequently measured by intelligence tests. For example, the factor *lexical knowledge* is measured on tasks like Vocabulary from the WISC-IV (Wechsler, 2003) and the Wechsler Adult Intelligence Scale— Fourth Edition (WAIS-IV; Wechsler, 2008). According to Carroll's (1976) coding scheme, items on tests measuring this factor tap lexical–semantic information stored in the long-term store, and the operation performed is retrieval of the meanings of the words presented. The factor *memory span* is measured by tasks such as Digits Forward from the WISC-IV and WAIS-IV Digit Span subtest. Items measuring memory span require that the information be held in short-term memory, and individual differences are thought to stem at least partially from the speed with which information to be held is encoded, refreshed, and retrieved from the stores; the nature of that information (e.g., numbers, letters, and words); and the capacity of the memory stores. Individuals may engage in strategies such as grouping information and vocal or subvocal rehearsal. *Perceptual speed* is measured by tasks like the WISC-IV and WAIS-IV Coding and Symbol Search subtests. These tasks require that the information be held in short-term memory (whether coded as visual images or coded verbally as words). The primary operation would include searching for items, and individual differences would stem primarily from speed in doing so. *Induction* is measured by tasks such as the WISC-IV and WAIS-IV Matrix Reasoning subtest. Although tasks measuring this factor are typically considered measures of novel reasoning, such tasks, according to Carroll, tap abstract or logical information stored in the long-term store—perhaps procedural knowledge. The primary operation used is the search for information to form hypotheses for solving items, and individual differences stem primarily from the depth and breadth of this information stored in memory and the speed in which the information is retrieved and hypotheses tested. A strategy may include using a systematic–deductive manner of testing hypotheses.

Carroll's (1976) coding scheme provides one method for identifying possible process-level characteristics underlying performance on test items. In our minds, of particular importance are his descriptions of the processes implied in task direc-

TABLE 21.2. Carroll's Provisional Coding Scheme for Cognitive Tasks

 I. Types of stimuli presented at outset of task
   A. Number of stimulus classes
     a. One stimulus class (a word, picture, etc.)
     b. Two stimulus classes (as in many types of multiple-choice items, paired-associates learning, etc.)
   B. Description of the stimulus class(es)
     a. Complete
     b. Degraded (with visual or auditory "noise")
   C. Interpretability
     a. Unambiguous (immediately interpretable)
     b. Ambiguous (coded several ways)
     c. Anomalous (not immediately codable)
 II. Overt responses to be made at end of task
   A. Number and type
     a. Select response from presented alternatives
     b. Produce one correct answer from operations to be performed
     c. Produce as many responses as possible (all different)
     d. Produce a specified number of responses (all different)
   B. Response mode
     a. Indicate choice of alternative (in some conventional way)
     b. Produce a single symbol (letter, numerical quantity)
     c. Write word
     d. Write phrase or sentence
     e. Write paragraph or more
     f. Make spoken response
     g. Make line or simple drawing
   C. Criterion for response acceptability
     a. Identity
     b. Similarity (or nonsimilarity) with respect to one or more features
     c. Semantic opposition
     d. Containment
     e. Correct result of serial operation
     f. Instance (subordinate of stimulus class)
     g. Superordinate
     h. Correct answer to verbal question ("fill in wh-")
     i. Comparative judgment
     j. Arbitrary association established in task
     k. Semantic and/or grammatical acceptability ("makes sense")
     l. Connectedness of lines or paths
III. Task structure
   A. Unitary (each item is completed on a single occasion)
   B. A temporal structure, such that stimuli are presented on one occasion and responses are made on another occasion (as in memory and learning tasks)
IV. Operations and strategies
   A. Number of operations and strategies for the task
   B. Type or description
     a. Identify, recognize, and interpret stimulus

     b. Educe identities or similarities between two or more stimuli
     c. Retrieve name, description, or instance from memory
     d. Store item in memory
     e. Retrieve associations, or general information, from memory
     f. Retrieve or construct hypotheses
     g. Examine different portions of memory
     h. Perform serial operations with data from memory
     i. Record intermediate result
     j. Use visual inspection strategy (examine different parts of visual stimulus)
     k. Reinterpret possibly ambiguous item
     l. Image, imagine, or otherwise form abstract representation of a stimulus
     m. Mentally rotate spatial configuration
     n. Comprehend and analyze language stimulus
     o. Judge stimulus with respect to specified characteristic
     p. Ignore irrelevant stimuli
     q. Use a special mnemonic aid (specify)
     r. Rehearse associations
     s. Develop a specific search strategy (visual)
     t. Chunk or group stimuli or data from memory
   C. Is the operation specified in the task instructions?
     a. Yes, explicitly
     b. Implied but not explicitly stated
     c. Not specified or implied in instructions
   D. How dependent is acceptable performance on this operation or strategy?
     a. Crucially dependent
     b. Helpful, but not crucial
     c. Of dubious effect (may be positive or negative)
     d. Probably a hindrance, counterproductive
 V. Temporal aspects of the operation strategy
   A. Duration (range of average duration)
     a. Irrelevant or inapplicable
     b. Very short (e.g., <200 msec)
     c. Middle range (e.g., >1 sec)
     d. Long (e.g., 1–5 sec)
     e. Longer (e.g., >5 sec)
   B. Individual differences in duration (or probability of strategy)
     a. Probably inconsequential
     b. Possibly relevant
     c. Probably wide individual differences (in likely test population)
   C. Criterion for termination of operation
     a. Irrelevant
     b. Upon arrival at recognizably correct solution (self-terminating)
     c. Not self-terminating in sense of (b) (i.e., the solution may be a guess, or subject may be satisfied with what is actually an incorrect solution)

(cont.)

TABLE 21.2. *(cont.)*

VI. Memory storage involved
  A. Term
    a. Memory store involved
    b. Sensory buffer
    c. Short-term memory (a matter of seconds)
    d. Intermediate-term memory (a matter of minutes)
    e. Long-term or permanent memory (programs/production system housed there)—contents:
      i. Visual-representational (images or other abstract representations derived from visual perceptions
      ii. Auditory-representational (analogous to visual-representational, but in the auditory mode)
      iii. Lexical–semantic information (abstract representation of words, and their semantic and grammatical features and rules in English)
      iv. Quantitative information (abstract representation of numbers, number operations, and algorithms for dealing with quantitative information)
      v. Abstract concepts and "general logic" information (representations of various concepts, principles, and rules having to do with implication, inference, causality, sequencing, attributes, patterning, etc.)
      vi. Experiential information (related to an individual's general store of information about the self and the environment, and past experiences)
  B. Contents
    a. Nonspecific
    b. Visual in nature (general, nonspecific)
      i. Points, positions of points
      ii. Lines (one-dimensional)
      iii. Lines and curves (two-dimensional)
      iv. Geometric patterns and shapes
      v. Pictorial (objects, etc.)
        1. Subcategory (e.g., tools)
      vi. Real two-dimensional items
      vii. Maps, charts, grids
      viii. Representation of three-dimensional geometric shapes
        1. Pictures of three-dimensional geometric objects or situations
        2. Faces
      ix. Real objects in three dimensions
    c. Auditory
    d. Graphemic, general
      i. Letters
      ii. Words (apart from their semantic information)
      iii. Alphabetic order information
    e. Linguistic, general (of native language)
      i. Lexical
      ii. Syntactic
      iii. Grammatical rules and features, general
      iv. Semantic (meanings of words, syntactic features, etc.)
      v. Nonverbal semantics (e.g., meanings of pictorial symbols)
    f. Numerical, mathematical, general
      i. Digit symbols with meaning
      ii. Elementary number operations and symbols
      iii. Algorithms for dealing with quantitative relations
    g. Logic, general
      i. Various abstract patterns (alternation, sequence, etc.)
      ii. Attributes in which stimuli could vary
    h. Movements, kinesthetic "concepts"
    i. "Real-world" experiences, situation, facts, information
      i. Subcategories (e.g., mechanical and electrical information)
    j. Arbitrary, new codings and associations established in the task situation
  C. Relevance of individual differences in the store
    a. Most subjects will have required store
    b. Doubtful that most subjects will have required store
    c. Wide individual differences in this memory store are likely

Note. From Carroll (1976). Copyright 1976 by Lawrence Erlbaum Associates. Adapted by permission of Taylor and Francis.

TABLE 21.3. Results for Select Latent Factors from Carroll's Coding of Cognitive Tasks

| | | Cognitive processes/operations | | | |
Factor	Principal type of memory involved	Addressing sensory buffers (attentional processes)	Addressing intermediate-term memory or long-term memory	Manipulations in executive and short-term memory	Strategies
Lexical knowledge	Long-term memory (lexical–semantic)		Retrieve word meanings (content)		
Memory span	Short-term memory (nonspecific)			Store in short-term memory (time, content) Retrieve from short-term memory (time, content)	Chunk or group stimulus items
Perceptual speed	Short-term memory (visual)	Visual search for specified items (time)		Comparison of visual stimuli	
Induction	Long-term memory (abstract logical)		Search hypotheses (content, time)		Serial operations to construct new hypotheses (probability that strategy would be used, time)

Note. Carroll's (1976) factor label for *lexical knowledge* was originally *verbal comprehension*. Based on Carroll (1987), "comparison of visual stimuli" was added to the *perceptual speed* entry. From Carroll (1976). Copyright 1976 by Lawrence Erlbaum Associates. Adapted by permission of Taylor and Francis.

tions (i.e., operations) and his specification of the primary memory store involved in item-level performance. However, the model might benefit from integration of more recent conceptualizations from cognitive psychology and cognitive science, such as *productions* (i.e., rules guiding operations or strategy use). Despite its potential, we identified only one published refereed journal article (Stankov, 1980) in which this method was applied. No other articles, chapters, or tests appear to have utilized Carroll's coding scheme to classify items from intelligence tests, and we have no evidence that this coding scheme has influenced test developers' or practitioners' interpretations of tests.

Kaufman and Lichtenberger's Shared-Abilities Analysis

Kaufman and Lichtenberger's (Kaufman, 1994; Kaufman & Lichtenberger, 1999, 2000, 2002) *shared-abilities analysis* has been most consistently applied to the subtests from the Wechsler intelligence scales. It has integrated existing factor-

analytic evidence and conceptions of intelligence and personality into a processing model to promote the classification of cognitive tasks according to the abilities they measure. In developing their methods, Kaufman and Lichtenberger drew upon a processing model that is a synthesis of (1) Silver's (1993) model explaining deficiencies and deficits displayed by children with learning disabilities, and (2) Osgood's (1957) conception of channels of communication. Following an information-processing perspective, Silver's model includes *input*, *integration*, *storage*, and *output* stages. Input refers to the manner in which information enters the cognitive system (i.e., auditory–verbal or visual–motor channels). Integration refers to the mental operations facilitating the interpretation and processing of information that has entered the cognitive system. Such operations include sequencing encoded information, inferring meaning from the encoded information, and integrating new information with information stored in memory. Storage represents the depositing of information in either the short-term store or the long-term store. Finally, output refers to the manner in which a response is expressed, typically through language or motor activity.

Similar to Silver's model, Osgood's (1957) psycholinguistic approach refers to *channels of communication* and describes information processing in terms of *reception, association,* and *expression.* Osgood's conception of channels of communication refers to the pathways in when types of meaningful information travel. These channels include auditory–verbal or visual–motor pathways. The information-processing component reception is comparable to Silver's input stage and refers to the perception and encoding of external information that is seen or heard. Association mirrors Silver's integration stage and refers to the mental manipulations used to relate the new information to existing knowledge or to transform the new information. Finally, expression is similar to Silver's output stage and refers to the manifestation of a response (viz., a vocal or motor response) stemming from information processing.

Based on their synthesis of these two models, Kaufman and Lichtenberger (2000, 2002) have asserted that any cognitive task can be classified according to five criteria.[2] The first is specification of the channel of communication: auditory–verbal or visual–motor. The second is input/reception. The third is integration/association. The fourth is storage/memory. The fifth is output/expression. As part of the classification of each cognitive task, the level of emphasis on a criterion can be identified, and ties between performance on one task and another can be made according to their shared abilities. For example, the WISC-IV and WAIS-IV Comprehension subtest, which requires the examinee to answer detailed questions about cultural phenomena, would follow the auditory–verbal channel, require adequate input/reception to understand the question, draw upon a complex interplay between integration/association and storage/memory processes to reason by using prior knowledge, and probably lead to output/expression via verbalization. In contrast, the WISC-IV and WAIS-IV Picture Completion subtest, which requires the identification of missing stimuli in pictures, would follow the visual–motor channel, require adequate reception to encode stimuli in the pictures, draw upon integration/association to compare the stimulus pictures to existing images of objects and settings, require little storage of information via storage/memory processes, and lead to output/expression via verbalization or motoric response (i.e., pointing). In order to develop hypotheses regarding cognitive performance, Kaufman and Lichtenberger (Kaufman, 1994; Kaufman & Lichtenberger, 1999, 2000, 2002) have integrated the processing framework with existing factor-analytic evidence and conceptions of intelligence (cf. Bannatyne, 1974; Guilford, 1967; Horn, 1989). Table 21.4 presents the specific abilities or components listed under each information-processing category.

Although the shared-abilities analysis and the information-processing model upon which it is based may sensitize those interpreting intelligence tests (1) to the construct-irrelevant influences related to input (e.g., visual acuity problems) and output (e.g., motor deficits) and (2) to the fine-grained processes affecting performance, they have a number of limitations.[3] First, the approach stems primarily from theoretically and logically derived analysis of subtests. We have found no reviews or critical evaluations of the information-processing component of this interpretive approach. Although such creative work is necessary to guide the initial development of interpretive frameworks, there is little or no evidence supporting its use in terms of diagnostic or eligibility accuracy or intervention development. Second, the information-processing model upon which it was based is somewhat dated and does not reflect the complexity of processing in more contemporary models. As a result, it does not include an array of processing steps (e.g., memory retrieval) and necessary model components (e.g., long-term store and control processes) like those outlined previously. It also tends to focus on general categories of processing (related to cognitive abilities) rather than specific processes. In addition, the integration of factor-analytic research in the model to represent the elementary processes seems too vague and loosely integrated to be useful.

Hale and Fiorello's Demands Analysis

In the cognitive hypothesis-testing approach to neuropsychological assessment offered by Hale and Fiorello (2004), the *demands analysis* of task-level performance is a central component. This method is consistent with (1) Luria's (1966, 1973) clinical method and the Boston Process Approach (Kaplan, 1998) in its primary focus on the qualitative aspects of performance, not on the resulting test scores; and with (2) Kaufman and Lichtenberger's shared-abilities approach (Kaufman, 1994; Kaufman & Lichtenberger, 1999, 2000, 2002) in its ultimate goal of identifying reasons for the patterns of

TABLE 21.4. Kaufman and Lichtenberger's Integrative Shared Abilities Organized by Information-Processing Categories

Input	Integration/association and storage/memory (continued)
Attention/concentration	Integrating brain function
Auditory–vocal channel	Learning ability
Complex verbal directions	Long-term memory
Distinguishing essential from nonessential detail	Memory
Encode information for processing	Nonverbal reasoning
Simple verbal directions	Planning ability
Understanding long questions	Reasoning
Understanding words	Reproduction of models
Visual–motor channel	Semantic cognition
Visual perception of abstract material	Semantic content
Visual perception of complete meaningful stimuli	Sequential
Visual perception of meaningful stimuli	Short-term memory (auditory or visual)
	Simultaneous processing
Integration/association and storage/memory	Social comprehension
Achievement	Spatial
Acquired knowledge	Spatial visualization
Cognition	Symbolic content
Common sense	Synthesis
Concept formation	Trial-and-error learning
Convergent production	Verbal concept formation
Crystallized intelligence	Verbal conceptualization
Culture-loaded knowledge	Verbal reasoning
Evaluation	Visual memory
Facility with numbers	Visual processing
Figural cognition	Visual sequencing
Figural evaluation	
Fluid intelligence	**Output**
Fund of information	Much verbal expression
General ability	Simple vocal expression
Handling abstract verbal concepts	Visual organization
Holistic (right-brain) processing	Visual–motor coordination

Note. From Kaufman and Lichtenberger (2002). Published by Allyn and Bacon, Boston, MA. Copyright 2002 by Pearson Education. Adapted by permission of Alan S. Kaufman.

errors across tasks. Thus hypotheses regarding the reasons for poor performance on cognitive tasks can be developed by considering their demand characteristics. In particular, Hale and Fiorello (2004) encourage examiners to consider the input and output demands of tasks, as well as to infer what specific "neuropsychological processes" were required by those tasks. They claim that "research is clearly demonstrating that the underlying neuropsychological processing demands are essential for understanding and helping many children with their learning and behavior problems" (p. 128). As in the shared-abilities approach, it is recommended that users identify similarities and contradictions in scores associated with the particular demands required across subtests included in the battery.

Hale and Fiorello (2004) have provided well-designed worksheets to guide the clinician's com-

pletion of the demands analysis, and the details regarding its three components are evident in them. Input demands are considered those demands associated with a subtest's stimulus materials as well as its directions, including those associated with demonstrations and teaching items. Hale and Fiorello's worksheets guide users to consider the nature of the instructions (e.g., demonstration and modeling, gestures, and oral directions); timing requirements (e.g., time limits and bonus points for speedy performance); teaching requirements (e.g., inclusion of sample items, feedback regarding performance, and querying); the stimulus modality for item presentation (e.g., visual stimuli in the form of pictures, abstract figures, and print and auditory stimuli in the form of spoken directions and directions played by audio recordings); and item content (e.g., infusion of narrow cultural or emotional content). Output demands, conversely, refer to the requirements associated with producing a response to test items. Hale and Fiorello's worksheets assist clinicians when comparing the response type (e.g., oral, fine motor, and written) and response formats (e.g., free-recall or multiple-choice).

In contrast to the inferences that can be made about input and output demands from reviewing the test requirements and an examinee's responses to them, inferences about processing demands require substantially more training (in neuropsychology) and a much higher degree of inference to identify. In Hale and Fiorello's (2004) Psychological Processes Worksheet, they present four general classes of processes and encourage users to select the processes associated with an examinee's identified learning deficits and those associated with the examinee's strengths. One set of processes is labeled "attention and executive frontal lobe processes," which include 34 processes, such as sustained attention, planning, organization, monitoring, inhibition, maintenance and change, motor overactivity and underactivity, apraxia in varying forms, aphasia in varying forms, working memory, perseveration, and problem solving. The second set of processes is labeled "concordant/convergent left-hemisphere processes"; these encompass 26 processes, such as sensory memory, phonemic awareness and manipulation, comprehension, math fact automaticity, sight word recognition, aphasia and its variants, neologism, and left–right confusion. The final set of processes is labeled "discordant/divergent right-hemisphere processes," which encompass 35 processes, such as sensory memory, visual and spatial processes, ambiguity, neglect, grapheme awareness, inference, social perception/judgment and metaphor/idiom/humor, aphasia and its variants, and neologism.

Hale and Fiorello's demands analysis presents a broad array of processes for examiners to consider, but it is supported by what we consider to be the most comprehensive set of materials for conducting such an analysis. It has strong roots in Luria's (1966, 1973) and the Boston Process Approach's (Kaplan, 1998) qualitative methods, and its frequent employment of terms from neuropsychology may well be foreign to many examiners and inconsistent with those found in the most prominent information-processing theories. It is important to note that Hale and Fiorello's demands analysis is only one component of the cognitive hypothesis-testing approach, which is nested in a self-correcting problem-solving model in which assessment results are used to generate

hypotheses that are evaluated as interventions are implemented. The reliance on the problem-solving model certainly lessens the potential negative impact of errant hypotheses generated from demands analysis. At present, primary concerns with this method are (1) that examiners using this approach must engage in complex interpretive strategies (e.g., across a multitude of different subtests) to develop high-inference hypotheses (about ability levels and brain functioning) stemming from each examinee's idiosyncratic reactions to test content; and (2) that there is an absence of research supporting the diagnostic accuracy or treatment utility of these methods.

GENERAL CONCLUSIONS AND RECOMMENDATIONS

Can the modern versions of the box-and-arrow models and a focus on information processes facilitate better understanding of the reasons for individual differences in test scores? The information we have reviewed so far has revealed that some progress has been made toward greater understanding. However, we are not convinced that interpretive strategies based on the interpretive frameworks reviewed in this chapter have progressed to a point at which we can place confidence in them during clinical decision making. We highlight some of the key points from our study of these frameworks in this section.

Measurement of Distinct Processes

How should psychologists and other professionals involved in psychoeducational assessments view cognitive processes and their measurement? We should view them as hypothetical constructs inferred from observation of test performance, which is consistent with Jensen's (1998) definition of *information processes* at the beginning of the chapter. In the case of cognitive processes, they occur inside the "black box" of the mind (see Shaw, 2004). Although we can infer the existence of processes from an individual's responses and program computers can simulate them, representing and measuring an individual's cognitive processes accurately with traditional, individually administered cognitive ability tests is an exceedingly difficult challenge.

The successful completion of any mental task requires three things: (1) elemental cognitive processes (such as stimulus encoding, short-term memory scanning, and retrieval of information from long-term memory, among others); (2) task-relevant knowledge; and (3) a program or strategy (see Jensen, 1987). Failure on any cognitive task could be related to a deficiency in any one of the three. In order to adequately measure elemental cognitive processes, therefore, one must rule out deficiencies in task-relevant knowledge and strategies. At present, this conclusion can only be drawn adequately in laboratory settings on what are called *elementary cognitive tasks* (ECTs; for a review, see Jensen, 2006). These ECTs are so simple that the only source of individual differences is response latency, or reaction time. On ECTs, the roles played by task-relevant knowledge and strategies in task performance are either eliminated or reduced to a minimum. There are also different types of ECTs that can be manipulated to measure disparate cognitive processes (see, e.g., Posner, 1980, and Vernon, 1987, for reviews). Research on the use of these techniques in applied settings, however, has not begun. Traditional cognitive ability tests, such as the WISC-IV (Wechsler, 2003) and WJ III (Woodcock et al., 2001b), are much too complex for the measurement of elemental cognitive processes (Jensen, 2006). Not only are individual differences on these tests related to underlying factors of mental ability (e.g., Carroll, 1993), but numerous processes are implicated in any score derived from such tests (including subtest scaled scores). Scores on traditional tests also reflect only the end products of mental activity and thereby confound basic processing with item content. Thus identifying deficient processes with the currently available tests will in all likelihood be problematic until the advent of batteries of ECTs that can be applied in the field.

Norm-Referenced Scores as Abilities, Not Processes

Clinicians should avoid the interpretation of norm-referenced scores from intelligence tests as indicating distinct cognitive processes. Because of the complexity of processing required for completion of any cognitive task, summary scores (stemming from responses to multiple items or multiple trials across a subtest or sets of subtests) are best seen as measures of individual differences in cognitive abilities. Because of this aggregation, norm-referenced intelligence test scores should not be viewed as measures of distinct cognitive processes. This recommendation was reinforced by Carroll (1976):

> Nearly all cognitive tasks are complex, in the sense that they involve different kinds of memories and control processes. . . . It may be impossible, in principle, to identify "pure" factors of individual differences probably not, at any rate, through the application of typical group-administered tests [and typical individually administered tests]. . . . The often-noted observation that all psychometric tests in the cognitive domain tend to be more or less positively correlated probably reflects the multifaceted nature of the tasks sampled in these tests. (p. 52)

Thus it seems prudent to conclude that during complex cognitive tasks, like those from intelligence tests, an examinee's performance is far too multifaceted to deconstruct to the process level.

There is little doubt that measures of cognitive abilities reflect information processes. For example, evidence abounds that tasks requiring attention to individual sounds measure a factor like broad auditory perception (see Carroll, 1993). However, we do not know whether this factor emerges because of a common set of information processes used during task completion because of similar task stimuli and related task paradigms, or because of some combination of these or other influences (cf. Kyllonen, 1995, 2002). Careful review of the different tasks measuring broad auditory perception indicates that many require somewhat different operations and strategies and draw on different types of knowledge for task completion. However, the task stimuli are the most similar among tasks measuring this factor. Perhaps the common processes at the input stage of information processing form a common bond across these tasks. On the other hand, the body of evidence examining tasks designed to measure processes, such as those measuring planning and attention in the PASS model, should be examined with experimental cognitive approaches to determine whether the processes they purportedly measure are in fact common across tasks varying in task stimuli, task paradigms, and task response formats. Research showing that the same sources of variance underlie individual differences on the CAS (Naglieri & Das, 1997) and on CHC-based tests (e.g., Kaufman & Kaufman, 2004; Keith et al., 2001) suggests that further research on the information processes that are involved on these measures is needed.

Subtests from commercially published cognitive ability tests may isolate groups of relatively distinct processes. These subtests are relatively simple tasks (1) focusing on processes associated closely with sensory information held in short-term stores and (2) requiring relatively few processes to complete items. One of the best examples is the Picture Recognition test from the WJ III (Woodcock et al., 2001b; see also Schrank & Wendling, Chapter 12, this volume). Each item requires examinees to study images of groups of people, animals, foods, plants, or objects for 5 seconds and then identify the images within a larger array after their removal. When considering possible processes, the examinee must sense and encode the images into the short-term store, retain that information for a brief period of time, match the mental representation of those images to those seen in the array, and respond by pointing or naming letters of the pictures in the array. (A facilitative strategy would include coding the images to be remembered according to some verbal label, in order to draw upon the phonological store in addition to the visual store.) It seems logical that this test measures individual differences in the capacity of the short-term store most closely associated with visual information, like Baddeley's (1986) visuo-spatial sketchpad. We suppose that all scores associated with such tasks that tap into small groups of processes would have relatively low *g* loadings because they involve fewer steps and components of the information-processing system. For example, as reported in Floyd, Shaver, and McGrew (2003), the WJ III Picture Recognition test has a *g* loading of only .38 (*g* loadings below .50 are considered poor; see Kaufman, 1994). Some of the least complex cognitive tasks, such as those measuring reaction time, often also demonstrate very low *g* loadings (e.g., Carroll, 1993; Jensen, 1998). Although some test users may believe that measuring a distinct group of related information processes is very useful, it is probable that in practice, the resulting scores will not possess the predictive power of more complex measures. As a result, evidence for the clinical utility of these measures of narrow sets of processes is needed.

Nonetheless, as Jensen (2006) has noted in his review of mental chronometry (i.e., the scientific study of cognitive processing speed), different ECTs held to measure different stages of processing (e.g., encoding, scanning information held in short-term memory, and long-term memory retrieval) have been used to investigate the relations between reaction time and intelligence. These ECTs have been found to correlate modestly, albeit significantly, with intelligence, typically in the range of .30–.50. The correlation between these ECTs and intelligence may in fact be somewhat higher after correction for the attenuating effects of restriction of range and measurement error. Multiple correla-

tions between intelligence and various measures of reaction time are approximately .60, which is comparable to the correlation typically observed between different intelligence tests. These results suggest that the measurement of a battery of ECTs is an avenue for the development of future tests of cognitive abilities.

Processes as Steps

We should use the term *process* in the most informed way possible: to refer to the many unseen steps in completing a task and not to the sum or outcome of those steps (as reflected in individual differences in ability). Shaw (2004) has argued that the term *process* and its derivatives are too often substituted for more meaningful terms in scientific and clinical parlance, while producing no added value. He states, "*Language processing* means language. *Reading processing* means reading. *Information processing* means thinking. *Memory processing* means memory. The word [processing] adds nothing" (p. 34; emphasis in original). Furthermore, it is apparent (e.g., Dehn, 2006) that the terms *process* and *processing* are sometimes combined with *ability*, which is inconsistent with widely held definitions of cognitive process. Perhaps replacing *process* with *step*, and *processing* with *steps* or *series of steps*, would promote clarity. If the goal is to consistently label and interpret measures of cognitive abilities that are more specific and orthogonal to the *g* factor (e.g., group factors or abilities unique to specific tests), using the emerging standard nomenclature from CHC theory (see McGrew, 2009, and Schneider & McGrew, Chapter 4, this volume)—which includes labels for classes of processes, such as *auditory processing abilities*—would be beneficial to enhance communication in research and practice.

Risk due to Variability across Individuals and High-Level Inferences

We recognize that all types of assessment results are subject to random error, but we believe that idiographic interpretation methods designed to identify cognitive processes leave clinicians at great risk for errors in interpretation. Not only are inferences often drawn from item-level performance, which has well-known problems with reliability, but there is also ample evidence to expect (1) variability in the processes individuals use across items within tasks and (2) variability in processes across individuals at different ability levels (see Lohman, 2000). Although some processes may be very simple and elicit little variability across items and individuals (e.g., subtraction with borrowing), most cognitive tasks are complex and elicit great variability within and across individuals (Corno et al., 2002). It requires a high degree of inference to interpret the performance on complex psychometric tasks in terms of underlying cognitive processes for a given individual—even when these tasks are considered at the item level. In the case of memory stores and related operations, it may be possible to isolate the capacity to retain information in the short-term store for a brief period of time before producing a response (i.e., short-term memory). However, once information reaches a "deeper level" in the information-processing system or that information is transformed in some way (e.g., Craik & Lockhart, 1972), there are few ways to distinguish between different content and operations of the varying memory structures. For example, during tasks in which previously retained information must be recalled, the breadth and depth of information stored in the long-term store would be targeted. However, other processes, such as retention or rehearsal of the item in the short-term store, information search and retrieval operations, and construction of the response before output, must all be employed. All of these processes are thought to be controlled by a central executive. In sum, the information-processing system may be far too complex—and our methods based on observation of behavior too insensitive—to permit us to draw inferences about cognitive processes with any fidelity.

Perhaps we should recognize that hypotheses about an examinee's processing will always be ones based on reasoning and high levels of inference, as personified in some of the qualitative approaches described previously. To us, many of the inferences about processes drawn from task-level performance of individuals seem as if they are intuitive and idiosyncratic to those developing them, and as if they are without a strong theoretical or empirical base. Although it is evident that practitioners consider the varied processes elicited by commonly administered cognitive ability subtests, their classifications of these subtests appear to be general and somewhat coarse, focusing on their being timed or not timed and their containing lots of language-based content (i.e., verbal content) or images and manipulatives (i.e., performance content; Frisby & Parkin, 2007). Many of the approaches we have reviewed, such as the

task-analytic approaches, require the examiner to formulate the same kind of high-level inferences that may lead to comparisons with the high-level inferences involved in protective techniques, such as human figure drawings. Inferences about attention and executive frontal lobe processes, concordant/convergent left-hemisphere processes, and so on, from cognitive ability test performance, are similar to inferences about drives, needs, and intrapsychic conflicts from projective techniques (see also Mann, 1979). Although inferences about cognitive processes are based on the science of experimental and differential psychology, whereas inferences about the unconscious mind are based on the pseudoscience of psychoanalysis, inferences about cognitive processes gleaned from cognitive ability tests appear to go beyond the currently available evidence. Such associations between cognitive ability test interpretation and projective test interpretation are worrisome, considering the evidence of heuristics, biases, and decision-making errors to which protective techniques are particularly susceptible (see Barnett, Macmann, & Lentz, 2003; Watkins, 2009). We also wonder whether the qualitative approaches and inferences drawn about cognitive processes would be able to stand up the empirical scrutiny that has gradually whittled away at the once widespread use of projective techniques in psychological practice.

A more conservative, but perhaps more useful, approach to problem solving would be to exhaust low-inference hypotheses related to directly observable behaviors displayed in the environment in which the "referral concerns" are occurring (e.g., reading comprehension problems in classroom settings) before turning to high-inference hypotheses generated in test sessions (Christ, 2008). Once testing has been initiated, however, it seems to make practical sense to examine the influences associated with *input* of information into the cognitive system and the *output* via responses when clinicians are evaluating item-level performance; these influences are observable for the most part. Labeling of these steps is modeled well by the interpretive approaches of Kaufman and Lichtenberger (Kaufman, 1994; Kaufman & Lichtenberger, 1999, 2000, 2002) and of Hale and Fiorello (2004). At a minimum, attention to the initial and the final steps (i.e., input and output) taken when examinees are completing items will likely be very beneficial in identifying influences that interfere with the measurement of the targeted cognitive abilities, such as sensory acuity problems impairing accurate input of information and motor impairments impairing response speed (see McGrew & Flanagan, 1998). Furthermore, tasks requiring the same operations but using different types of stimuli and different response options may be helpful in testing hypotheses regarding the reasons for poor performance (see Kaplan et al. 1999; Kyllonen, 1995, 2002).

Risk Due to the Absence of Evidence

From our review of the literature, it appears that the processing-based approaches to interpretation are not supported by a strong enough body of evidence to recommend their routine use for high-stakes decisions. For example, there is no direct evidence of the interrater reliability of clinicians' identification of cognitive processes based on qualitative analysis of test performance (Groth-Marnat, 2000). In addition, although carryover effects during testing of limits may confound accurate measurement, these effects appear to be frequently overlooked. Furthermore, there is no evidence that process-based interpretive approaches improve the predictive or diagnostic accuracy of assessment results, or that they provide unique information that informs intervention development. From a practical perspective, there is presently little convincing evidence that the devotion of additional time and effort to processing approaches yields dividends for clinicians or their clients. Overall, further research is needed before inferences about cognitive processes can be made with confidence. We firmly believe that researchers and clinicians alike should generate evidence to substantiate their inferences (about processes and other psychological constructs) before they are applied to practices with children and youth in schools, clinics, and hospitals.

Final Comments

Because processes are hypothetical constructs that can be inferred only from behaviors, there are inherent challenges facing processing-based approaches applied to responses from cognitive ability tests. Enhancing assessment practices to facilitate identification of the nature and causes of an individual's cognitive deficits to improve differential diagnosis and treatment is an extremely important goal. Further research on information processing, reflecting the disciplines of both experimental and correlational psychology, will undoubtedly lead to advances in both assessment and intervention.

NOTES

1. Earlier incarnations of ACT-R include ACT-E (Anderson, 1976) and ACT* (Anderson, 1983). The most recent version of ACT-R is 5.0.
2. In earlier descriptions, the integration/association and storage/memory classifications were merged, due to difficulty in differentiating these processes.
3. It is notable that this interpretive approach is no longer advocated by Kaufman or Lichtenberger in their most recent publications focusing on interpretation of the scores from intelligence tests. Thus, these authors have replaced this approach to interpretation wiht newer, theory-based approaches (A. S. Kaufman, personal communication, August 19, 2011).

REFERENCES

Allport, G. W. (1937). *Personality: A psychological interpretation.* New York: Wiley.

Anderson, J. R. (1976). *Language, memory and thought.* Hillsdale, NJ: Erlbaum.

Anderson, J. R. (1983). *The architecture of cognition.* Cambridge, MA: Harvard University Press.

Anderson, J. R. (1990). *The adaptive character of thought.* Hillsdale, NJ: Erlbaum.

Anderson, J. R., Bothell, D., Byrne, M. D., Douglas, S., Lebiere, C., & Qin, Y. (2004). An integrated theory of the mind. *Psychological Review, 111,* 1036–1060.

Anderson, J., & Lebiere, C. (1998). *The atomic components of thought.* Mahwah, NJ: Erlbaum.

Atkinson, R. C., & Shiffrin, R. M. (1968). Human memory: A proposed system and its control processes. In K. W. Spence & J. T. Spence (Eds.), *The psychology of learning and motivation* (pp. 89–195). New York: Academic Press.

Baddeley, A. D. (1972). Retrieval cues and semantic coding in short-term memory. *Psychological Bulletin, 78,* 379–385.

Baddeley, A. D. (1986). *Working memory.* New York: Oxford University Press.

Baddeley, A. D. (1994). Working memory: The interface between memory and cognition. In D. L. Schacter & E. Tulving (Eds.), *Memory systems 1994* (pp. 351–367). Cambridge, MA: MIT Press.

Baddeley, A. D. (1996). Exploring the central executive. *Quarterly Journal of Experimental Psychology, 49A,* 5–28.

Baddeley, A. D. (2001). Is working memory still working? *American Psychologist, 56,* 851–864.

Baddeley, A. D., & Hitch, G. (1974). Working memory. In G. H. Bower (Ed.), *Psychology of learning and motivation* (Vol. 8, pp. 47–89). New York: Academic Press.

Baddeley, A. D., & Hitch, G. J. (1994). Development in the concept of working memory. *Neuropsychology, 8,* 485–493.

Bannatyne, A. (1974). Diagnosis: A note on recategorization of the WISC scaled scores. *Journal of Learning Disabilities, 7,* 272–274.

Barnett, D. W., Macmann, G. M., & Lentz, F. E. (2003). Personality assessment research: Applying criteria of confidence and helpfulness. In C. R. Reynolds & R. W. Kamphaus (Eds.), *Handbook of psychological and educational assessment of children: Personality, behavior, and context* (2nd ed., pp. 3–29). New York: Guilford Press.

Brinkman, J. J., Decker, S. L., & Dean, R. S. (2005). Assessing and understanding brain function through neuropsychologically based ability tests. In R. C. D'Amato, E. Fletcher-Janzen, & C. R. Reynolds (Eds.), *Handbook of school neuropsychology* (pp. 303–326). Hoboken, NJ: Wiley.

Brown, J. A. (1958). Some tests of the decay theory of immediate memory. *Quarterly Journal of Experimental Psychology, 10,* 12–21.

Carroll, J. B. (1976). Psychometric tests as cognitive tasks: A new structure of intellect. In L. B. Resnick (Ed.), *The nature of intelligence* (pp. 27–56). Hillsdale, NJ: Erlbaum.

Carroll, J. B. (1987). Psychometric approaches to cognitive abilities and processes. In S. H. Irvine & S. E. Newstead (Eds.), *Intelligence and cognition: Contemporary frames of reference* (pp. 217–251). Boston: Martinus Nijhoff.

Carroll, J. B. (1988). Cognitive abilities, factors, and processes. *Intelligence, 12,* 101–109.

Carroll, J. B. (1993). *Human cognitive abilities: A survey of factor analytic studies.* New York: Cambridge University Press.

Carroll, J. B. (1995). [Review of Das, J. P., Naglieri, J. A., & Kirby, J. R. (1994). *Assessment of cognitive processes: The PASS theory of intelligence*]. *Journal of Psychoeducational Assessment, 13,* 397–409.

Carroll, J. B. (1998). Human cognitive abilities: A critique. In J. J. McCardle & R. W. Woodcock (Eds.), *Human cognitive abilities in theory and practice* (pp. 5–24). Mahwah, NJ: Erlbaum.

Chaiken, S. R., Kyllonen, P. C., & Tirre, W. (2000). Organization and components of psychomotor ability. *Cognitive Psychology, 40,* 198–226.

Christ, T. J. (2008). Best practices problem analysis. In A. Thomas & J. Grimes (Eds.), *Best practices in school psychology* (5th ed., Vol. 2, pp. 159–176). Bethesda, MD: National Association of School Psychologists.

Colman, A. M. (2001). *A dictionary of psychology.* New York: Oxford University Press.

Corno, L., Cronbach, L. J., Kupermintz, H., Lohman, D. F., Mandinach, E. B., Porteus, A. W., et al. (2002). *Remaking the concept of aptitude: Extending the legacy of Richard E. Snow.* Mahwah, NJ: Erlbaum.

Craik, F., & Lockhart, R. (1972). Levels of processing: A framework for memory research. *Journal of Verbal Thinking and Verbal Behavior, 11,* 671–684.

Cronbach, L. J. (1957). The two disciplines of scientific psychology. *American Psychologist, 12,* 671–684.

Das, J. P. (1992). Beyond a unidimensional scale of merit. *Intelligence, 16,* 137–150.

Das, J. P., Kirby, J. R., & Jarman, R. F. (1979). *Simultaneous and successive cognitive processes.* New York: Academic Press.

Das, J. P., Naglieri, J. A., & Kirby, J. R. (1994). *Assessment of cognitive processes: The PASS theory of intelligence.* Needham Heights, MA: Allyn & Bacon.

Das, J. P., & Varnhagen, C. K. (1986). Neuropsychological functioning and cognitive processing. *Child Neuropsychology, 1,* 117–140.

Dean, R. S., Decker, S. L., Woodcock, R. W., & Schrank, F. A. (2003). A cognitive neuropsychology assessment system. In F. A. Schrank & D. P. Flanagan (Eds.), *WJ III clinical use and interpretation* (pp. 345–376). New York: Academic Press.

Dean, R. S., & Woodcock, R. W. (1999). *The WJ-R and Bateria-R in neuropsychological assessment* (Research Report No. 3). Itasca, IL: Riverside.

Dean, R. S., & Woodcock, R. W. (2003a). *Dean–Woodcock Emotional Status Exam.* Itasca, IL: Riverside.

Dean, R. S., & Woodcock, R. W. (2003b). *Dean–Woodcock Sensory–Motor Battery.* Itasca, IL: Riverside.

Dean, R. S., & Woodcock, R. W. (2003c). *Dean–Woodcock Structured Interview.* Itasca, IL: Riverside.

Deary, I. J. (2001). Human intelligence differences: Toward a combined experimental–differential approach. *Trends in Cognitive Science, 4,* 164–170.

Dehn, M. J. (2006). *Essentials of processing assessment.* Hoboken, NJ: Wiley.

Estes, W. K. (1999). Models of human memory: A 30-year retrospective. In C. Izawa (Ed.), *On human memory: Evolution, progress, and reflections on the 30th anniversary of the Atkinson–Shiffrin model* (pp. 59–86). Mahwah, NJ: Erlbaum.

Flanagan, D. P., Ortiz, S. O., & Alfonso, V. C. (2007). *Essentials of cross-battery assessment* (2nd ed.). Hoboken, NJ: Wiley.

Floyd, R. G. (2005). Information-processing approaches to interpretation of contemporary intellectual assessment instruments. In D. P. Flanagan & P. Harrison (Eds.), *Contemporary intellectual assessment* (2nd ed., pp. 203–233). New York: Guilford Press.

Floyd, R. G., Shaver, R. B., & McGrew, K. S. (2003).

Interpretation of the Woodcock–Johnson III Tests of Cognitive Abilities: Acting on evidence. In F. A. Schrank & D. P. Flanagan (Eds.), *WJ III clinical use and interpretation* (pp. 1–46, 403–408). Boston: Academic Press.

French, J. W., Ekstrom, R. B., & Price, L. A. (1963). *Kit of reference tests for cognitive factors*. Princeton, NJ: Educational Testing Service.

Frisby, C. L., & Parkin, J. R. (2007). Identifying similarities in cognitive subtest functional requirements: An empirical approach. *Journal of School Psychology, 45*, 385–400.

Gathercole, S. E. (1994). Neuropsychology and working memory: A review. *Neuropsychology, 8*, 494–505.

Gottfredson, L. S. (2002). g: Highly general and highly practical. In R. J. Sternberg & E. L. Grigorenko (Eds.), *The general factor of intelligence: How general is it?* (pp. 331–380). Mahwah, NJ: Erlbaum.

Groth-Marnat, G. (2000). Introduction to neuropsychological assessment. In G. Groth-Marnat (Ed.), *Neuropsychological assessment in clinical practice: A guide to test interpretation and integration* (pp. 3–20). New York: Wiley.

Guilford, J. P. (1967). *The nature of human intelligence*. New York: McGraw-Hill.

Hale, J. B., & Fiorello, C. A. (2004). *School neuropsychology: A practitioner's handbook*. New York: Guilford Press.

Healy, A. F., & McNamara, D. S. (1996). Verbal learning and memory: Does the modal model still work? *Annual Review of Psychology, 47*, 143–172.

Horn, J. L. (1989). Cognitive diversity: A framework for learning. In P. T. Ackerman, R. J. Sternberg, & R. Glaser (Eds.), *Learning and individual differences* (pp. 61–116). New York: Freeman.

Hunt, E. (1971). What kind of computer is man? *Cognitive Psychology, 2*, 57–98.

Hunt, E., Frost, N., & Lunneborg, C. (1973). Individual differences in cognition: A new approach to intelligence. In G. H. Bower (Ed.), *The psychology of learning and motivation: Advances in research and theory* (pp. 87–122). New York: Academic Press.

Individuals with Disabilities Education Improvement Act of 2004 (IDEA 2004), Pub. L. No. 108-446, 118 Stat. 2647 (2004).

Jensen, A. (1987). Process differences and individual differences in some cognitive tasks. *Intelligence, 11*, 107–136.

Jensen, A. (1989). The relationship between learning and intelligence. *Learning and Individual Differences, 1*, 37–62.

Jensen, A. (1998). *The g factor: The science of mental ability*. Westport, CT: Praeger.

Jensen, A. (2006). *Clocking the mind: Mental chronometer individual differences*. Amsterdam: Elsevier.

Kaplan, E. (1998). A process approach to neuropsychological assessment. In T. Boll & B. K. Bryant (Eds.), *Clinical neuropsychology and brain function: Research, measurement, and practice* (pp. 125–167). Washington, DC: American Psychological Association.

Kaplan, E., Delis, D., Fein, D., Maerlender, A., Morris, R., & Kramer, J. (2004). *WISC-IV Integrated*. San Antonio, TX: Harcourt Assessment.

Kaplan, E., Fein, D., Kramer, J., Delis, D., & Morris, R. (1999). *WISC-III as a Process Instrument*. San Antonio, TX: Psychological Corporation.

Kaplan, E., Fein, D., Morris, R., & Delis, D. (1991). *WAIS-R as a Neuropsychological Instrument*. San Antonio, TX: Psychological Corporation.

Kaufman, A. S. (1994). *Intelligent testing with the WISC-III*. New York: Wiley.

Kaufman, A. S., & Kaufman, N. L. (1983). *Kaufman Assessment Battery for Children*. Circle Pines, MN: American Guidance Service.

Kaufman, A. S., & Kaufman, N. L. (2004). *Kaufman Assessment Battery for Children—Second Edition*. Circle Pines, MN: American Guidance Service.

Kaufman, A. S., & Lichtenberger, E. O. (1999). *Essentials of WAIS-III assessment*. New York: Wiley.

Kaufman, A. S., & Lichtenberger, E. O. (2000). *Essentials of WISC-III and WPPSI-R assessment*. New York: Wiley.

Kaufman, A. S., & Lichtenberger, E. O. (2002). *Assessing adolescent and adult intelligence* (2nd ed.). Boston: Allyn & Bacon.

Keith, T. Z., & Kranzler, J. H. (1999). The absence of structural fidelity precludes construct validity: Rejoinder to Naglieri on what the Cognitive Assessment System does and does not measure. *School Psychology Review, 28*, 303–321.

Keith, T. Z., Kranzler, J. H., & Flanagan, D. P. (2001). What does the Cognitive Assessment System (CAS) measure?: Joint confirmatory factor analysis of the CAS and the Woodcock–Johnson Tests of Cognitive Ability (3rd ed.). *School Psychology Review, 30*, 89–119.

Klatzky, R. L. (1975). *Human memory: Structures and processes*. San Francisco: Freeman.

Kranzler, J. H., & Keith, T. Z. (1999). Independent confirmatory factor analysis of the Cognitive Assessment System (CAS): What does the CAS measure? *School Psychology Review, 28*, 117–144.

Kranzler, J. H., Keith, T. Z., & Flanagan, D. P. (2000). Independent examination of the factor structure of the Cognitive Assessment System (CAS): Further evidence disputing the construct validity of the CAS. *Journal of Psychoeducational Assessment, 18*, 143–159.

Kranzler, J. H., & Weng, L. (1995a). The factor structure of the PASS cognitive tasks: A reexamination of Naglieri et al. (1991). *Journal of School Psychology, 33*, 143–157.

Kranzler, J. H., & Weng, L. (1995b). A reply to the commentary by Naglieri and Das on the factor structure of a battery of PASS cognitive tasks. *Journal of School Psychology, 33*, 169–176.

Kyllonen, P. C. (1995). CAM: A theoretical framework for cognitive abilities measurement. In D. Detterman (Ed.), *Current topics in human intelligence: Vol. 4. Theories of intelligence* (pp. 307–359). Norwood, NJ: Ablex.

Kyllonen, P. C. (2002). Item generation for repeated testing of human performance. In S. Irvine & P. C. Kyllonen (Eds.), *Generating items for cognitive tests: Theory and practice* (pp. 251–275). Hillsdale, NJ: Erlbaum.

Logan, G. (2000). Information-processing theories. In A. E. Kazdin (Ed.), *Encyclopedia of psychology* (pp. 294–297). Washington, DC: American Psychological Association.

Lohman, D. F. (2000). Complex information processing and intelligence. In R. J. Sternberg (Ed.), *Handbook of intelligence* (pp. 285–340). Cambridge, UK: Cambridge University Press.

Luria, A. R. (1966). *Human brain and psychological processes.* New York: Harper & Row.

Luria, A. R. (1973). *The working brain: An introduction to neuropsychology.* New York: Basic Books.

Luria, A. R. (1980). *Higher cortical functions in man* (2nd ed.). New York: Basic Books.

Mann, L. (1979). *On the trail of process: A historical perspective on cognitive processes and their training.* New York: Grune & Stratton.

Mather, N., & Woodcock, R. W. (2001). *Examiner's manual: Woodcock–Johnson III Tests of Cognitive Abilities.* Itasca, IL: Riverside.

McGrew, K. S. (2009). Editorial: CHC theory and the Human Cognitive Abilities project: Standing on the shoulders of the giants of psychometric intelligence research. *Intelligence, 37*, 1–10.

McGrew, K. S., & Flanagan, D. P. (1998). *The intelligence test desk reference (ITDR): Gf-Gc cross-battery assessment.* Boston: Allyn & Bacon.

Milberg, W. P., Hebben, N., & Kaplan, E. (2009). The Boston Process Approach to neuropsychological assessment. In I. Grant & K. M. Adams (Eds.), *Neuropsychological assessment of neuropsychiatric and neuromedical disorders* (3rd ed., pp. 42–65). New York: Oxford University Press.

Miller, D. C. (2007). *Essentials of school neuropsychological assessment.* Hoboken, NJ: Wiley.

Miller, G. A. (1956). The magical number seven, plus or minus two: Some limits on our capacity for processing information. *Psychological Review, 63*, 81–97.

Murdock, B. B., Jr. (1961). The retention of individual items. *Journal of Experimental Psychology, 62*, 618–625.

Muter, P. (1980). Very rapid forgetting. *Memory and Cognition, 8*, 174–179.

Naglieri, J. A., & Das, J. P. (1997). *Das–Naglieri Cognitive Assessment System.* Itasca, IL: Riverside.

Neisser, U. (1967). *Cognitive psychology.* Englewood Cliffs, NJ: Prentice-Hall.

Neisser, U., Boodoo, G., Bouchard, T. J., Boykin, A. W., Brody, N., Ceci, S. J., et al. (1996). Intelligence: Knowns and unknowns. *American Psychologist, 51*, 77–101.

Newell, A., & Simon, H. A. (1972). *Human problem solving.* Englewood Cliffs, NJ: Prentice-Hall.

Osgood, C. E. (1957). A behavioristic analysis of perception and language as cognitive phenomena. In J. S. Bruner, E. Brunswick, E. Festinger, K. F. Muenzinger, C. E. Osgood, & D. Rapaport (Eds.), *Contemporary approaches to cognition* (pp. 75–118). Cambridge, MA: Harvard University Press.

Peterson, L. R., & Peterson, M. J. (1959). Short-term retention of individual verbal items. *Journal of Experimental Psychology, 58*, 193–198.

Posner, M. I. (1980). Orienting of attention. *Quarterly Journal of Experimental Psychology, 32*, 3–25.

Posner, M. I., & McLeod, P. (1982). Information processing models: In search of elementary operations. *Annual Review of Psychology, 22*, 477–514.

Raaijmakers, J. G. W. (1993). The story of the two-store model of memory: Past criticisms, current status, and future directions. In D. E. Meyer & S. Kornblum (Eds.), *Attention and performance XIV: Synergies in experimental psychology, artificial intelligence, and cognitive neuroscience* (pp. 467–487). Cambridge, MA: MIT Press.

Reitman, J. S. (1974). Without surreptitious rehearsal: Information and short term memory decay. *Journal of Verbal Learning and Verbal Behavior, 13*, 365–377.

Reynolds, M. R., Keith, T. Z., Fine, J. G., Fisher, M. E., & Low, J. (2007). Confirmatory factor structure of the Kaufman Assessment Battery for Children—Second Edition: Consistency with Cattell–Horn–Carroll Theory. *School Psychology Quarterly, 22*, 511–539.

Sattler, J. M. (2008). *Assessment of children: Cognitive foundations* (5th ed.). San Diego, CA: Author.

Schrank, F. A., & Woodcock, R. W. (2002). *Report Writer for the WJ III Compuscore and Profiles Program* [Computer software]. Itasca, IL: Riverside.

Schunn, C. D., & Klahr, D. (1998). Production systems. In W. Bechtel & G. Graham (Eds.), *A companion to cognitive science* (pp. 542–551). Malden, MA: Blackwell.

Semrud-Clikeman, M., Wilkinson, A., & Wellington, T. M. (2005). Evaluating and using qualitative approaches to neuropsychological assessment. In R. C. D'Amato, E. Fletcher-Janzen, & C. R. Reynolds (Eds.), *Handbook of school neuropsychology* (pp. 287–302). Hoboken, NJ: Wiley.

Shaw, S. R. (2004). Disordered processing. *NASP Communiqué, 32*(5), 33–34.

Shiffrin, R. M. (1999). 30 years of memory. In C. Izawa (Ed.), *On human memory: Evolution, progress, and reflections on the 30th anniversary of the Atkinson–Shiffrin model* (pp. 17–33). Mahwah, NJ: Erlbaum.

Silver, L. B. (1993). Introduction and overview to the clinical concepts of learning disabilities. *Child and Adolescent Psychiatric Clinics of North America, 2,* 181–192.

Snyderman, M., & Rothman, S. (1987). Survey of expert opinion on intelligence and aptitude testing. *American Psychologist, 42,* 137–144.

Spearman, C. (1904). General intelligence, objectively determined and measured. *American Journal of Psychology, 15,* 201–293.

Stankov, L. (1980). Psychometric factors as cognitive tasks: A note on Carroll's new "structure of intellect." *Intelligence, 4,* 65–71.

Sternberg, R. (1977). *Intelligence, information processing, and analogical reasoning.* Hillsdale, NJ: Erlbaum.

Sternberg, R. (1981). Testing and cognitive psychology. *American Psychologist, 36,* 1181–1189.

Sternberg, R. (1984). The Kaufman Assessment Battery for Children: An information-processing analysis and critique. *Journal of Special Education, 18,* 269–279.

Sternberg, R. (1985). *Beyond IQ: A triarchic theory of human intelligence.* New York: Cambridge University Press.

Thurstone, L. L. (1938). *Primary mental abilities* (Psychometric Monographs No. 1). Chicago: University of Chicago Press.

Vernon, P. E. (Ed.). (1987). *Speed of information processing and intelligence.* Norwood, NJ: Ablex.

Watkins, M. W. (2009). Errors in diagnostic decision making and clinical judgment. In T. B. Gutkin & C. R. Reynolds (Eds.), *The handbook of school psychology* (4th ed., pp. 210–229). Hoboken, NJ: Wiley.

Wechsler, D. (2003). *Wechsler Intelligence Scale for Children—Fourth Edition.* San Antonio, TX: Psychological Corporation.

Wechsler, D. (2008). *Wechsler Adult Intelligence Scale—Fourth Edition.* San Antonio, TX: Pearson.

Werner, H. (1937). Process and achievement. *Harvard Educational Review, 7,* 353–368.

Wilson, M., & Emmorey, K. (1997). A visuo-spatial "phonological loop" in working memory: Evidence from American Sign Language. *Memory and Cognition, 25,* 313–320.

Woodcock, R. W. (1993). An information processing view of the Gf-Gc theory. *Journal of Psychoeducational Assessment Monograph Series: Woodcock–Johnson Psycho-Educational Assessment Battery—Revised* (pp. 80–102). Cordova, TN: Psychoeducational Corporation.

Woodcock, R. W. (1997). The Woodcock–Johnson Tests of Cognitive Ability—Revised. In D. P. Flanagan, J. L. Genshaft, & P. L. Harrison (Eds.), *Contemporary intellectual assessment: Theories, tests, and issues* (pp. 230–246). New York: Guilford Press.

Woodcock, R. W. (1998). Extending Gf-Gc theory into practice. In J. J. McArdle & R. W. Woodcock (Eds.), *Human cognitive abilities in theory and practice* (pp. 137–156). Mahwah, NJ: Erlbaum.

Woodcock, R. W., McGrew, K. S., & Mather, N. (2001a). *Woodcock–Johnson III Tests of Achievement.* Itasca, IL: Riverside.

Woodcock, R. W., McGrew, K. S., & Mather, N. (2001b). *Woodcock–Johnson III Tests of Cognitive Abilities.* Itasca, IL: Riverside.

CHAPTER 22

Testing with Culturally and Linguistically Diverse Populations
Moving beyond the Verbal–Performance Dichotomy into Evidence-Based Practice

Samuel O. Ortiz
Salvador Hector Ochoa
Agnieszka M. Dynda

The racial and ethnic diversity of the U.S. population continues to grow at a rapid pace. Across the nation, children from ethnic minority groups have now become the majority group in various areas (e.g., some New Jersey counties and Washington, D.C.) (Llorente & Sheingold, 2010; Smith, 2008), and the precollege-grade-level population of Hispanics currently exceeds whites in Arizona, California, and Nevada (U.S. Census Bureau, 2009). Reports from the U.S. Census Bureau (2009) also indicate that one-fourth of children presently in U.S. public school kindergarten classes are Hispanic, and that ethnic minority children will become the majority by 2023. The time when practitioners might only encounter ethnic minority children on rare occasions has long since passed. The data make it clear that diversity within the population is already high, increasing quickly, and ultimately unavoidable.

In a survey of current practices in psychological assessment of students with limited English proficiency (LEP), Ochoa, Riccio, Jimenz, Garcia de Alba, and Sines (2004) found that practitioners engaged in the assessment of diverse individuals utilized a variety of instruments. The most commonly used combination included an intelligence scale (most often a Wechsler scale administered completely in English), a test of visual–motor integration, an informal pro-

jective drawing test, and a nonverbal intelligence instrument. Interestingly, Ochoa and colleagues noted that this makeshift battery is not substantially different from the instruments employed in the evaluation of mainstream, monolingual English speakers. Indeed, even when a practitioner had professional bilingual capability, the battery remained largely the same; the only notable changes occurred in the language version or language of administration of the tests. The similarity in test usage suggests that practitioners are effectively ignoring major factors that differ markedly in the testing of students with LEP as compared to mainstream students. These factors include inadequately representative norms and inappropriate comparison groups for students with LEP, as well as linguistic and cultural confounds that manifest themselves in unequal levels of age- and grade-expected language and acculturative knowledge acquisition. Because these different levels of performance occur primarily as a function of limited experience and exposure, not actual lack of ability, they have not been well understood. It had been thought that these factors posed threats to the inherent reliability of tests in areas such as factor structure, difficulty level, or prediction, but such bias was rarely found (Figueroa, 1983; Reynolds & Ramsay, 2003; Sandoval, Frisby, Geisinger, Scheuneman, & Grenier, 1998).

The failure to identify bias as defined in terms of reliability is not surprising. First, race and ethnicity are only partially correlated with differences in cultural experiences and dual-language exposure, but are clearly not acceptable proxies. Second, cultural knowledge and language acquisition (both first and second) are developmental processes already well reflected by the inherent structure of ability tests that are expressly designed to follow a pattern of difficulty aligned with known development. And third, simply because a test is reliable does not make it valid. Thus, if differences in test performance relative to cultural and linguistic influences are to be properly understood, it appears that it will need to occur primarily through the lens of validity.

In contrast to the extensive studies on reliability, the degree to which cultural and linguistic factors pose any threat to issues of validity has been largely overlooked. Whereas it can be said that a low score on an IQ test predicts an individual's general performance in school quite well, notions regarding exactly what caused the low score become much less clear in the case of culturally and linguistically diverse children. Questions about the causal influence of latent variables (such as intelligence) that may be confounded by differences in experiential background, particularly those rooted in language and acculturative knowledge development (Ortiz, 2008; Rhodes, Ochoa, & Ortiz, 2005; Salvia & Ysseldyke, 1991; Valdés & Figueroa, 1994), are issues of validity and do not appear to be accounted for by any of the instruments or procedures reported in current use by practitioners. Even when practitioners turn to the use of native-language tests or utilize a translator/interpreter in assessment, the question of validity remains prominent and is not automatically or significantly resolved (Lopez, 1997, 2002; McCallum & Bracken, 1997).

The survey by Ochoa and colleagues (2004) highlights an important point: Practitioners are not simply choosing the "wrong" tests because in fact there is no "right" one. Rather, regardless of what tests are selected, practitioners appear to administer tests (including in the native language) and interpret them with cultural/ethnic minority students in much the same way as they do with any other individuals. In another recent survey, it was noted that 98% of school psychologists who evaluate culturally and linguistically diverse individuals stated that they consider both the "validity of test scores" and "an examinee's level of English language proficiency before selecting a test and interpreting test scores" (Sotelo-Dynega, Cuskley, Geddes, Mc-

Swiggan, & Soldano, 2011). But when asked how they actually evaluate examinees so that the relevant issues are properly considered, the vast majority simply reported differences in test selection. For example, 88% reported using nonverbal tests, 40% reported use of an interpreter to administer a test, 20% report use of a native-language test, and 2% reported "on-the-fly" translation of a test. Practitioners appear to be presuming that validity issues are addressed merely by decisions regarding test selection. In short, there are few indications that practitioners are actually examining issues of validity directly or attempting to integrate current research regarding the manner in which cultural and linguistic factors are known to influence test performance. As a consequence, there is often no defensible or scientific basis for the types of interpretations, conclusions, and diagnoses rendered based on the use of tests in such practice.

The purpose of this chapter is to describe the current issues pertaining to the use of standardized, norm-referenced tests in attempts to evaluate the abilities (intellectual, cognitive, academic, and neuropsychological) of individuals from culturally and linguistically diverse backgrounds. All issues are evaluated in light of evidence-based practice to assess the degree to which research can be used to enhance methods and procedures for evaluation and interpretation. Specific discussion topics in this chapter include (1) evaluating current standards of practice; (2) evaluating the advantages and disadvantages of current practices; and (3) integrating research into defensible practice.

EVALUATING CURRENT STANDARDS OF PRACTICE

Changing demographics will continue to place pressure on graduate training programs and their trainees to acquire the requisite multicultural competency necessary for conducting fair and equitable evaluations of individuals from culturally and linguistically diverse backgrounds (Ortiz, 2008). It is unclear at present whether sufficient faculty and supervisors exist, or sufficient resources are available, to ensure that all graduate students will gain adequate experience in formulating appropriate knowledge and skills, but it seems safe to say that supervised experience with multicultural populations is likely to be somewhat limited. When practitioners find themselves at a loss or in need of guidance on the matter, they are likely to refer to the usual sources of information. For example, the American Psychological Association (APA, 1990) publishes *Guidelines for Providers of Psychological Services to Ethnic, Linguistic, and Culturally Diverse Populations*, which emphasizes the need for psychologists to acknowledge the influences of language and culture on behavior, and to consider those factors when working with diverse groups. The guidelines also include admonitions regarding appraisal of the validity of the methods and procedures used for assessment and interpretation. But exactly what should or can be done when validity is deemed questionable, or what specific steps exist to reduce bias and maintain validity in the first place, are unfortunately absent from this set of guidelines.

The search for more definitive answers invariably leads practitioners to the *Standards for Educational and Psychological Testing* (American Educational Research Association [AERA], APA, & National Council on Measurement in Education [NCME], 1999), known simply as "the *Standards*." At first glance, the *Standards* volume seems to provide some definitive guidance for practitioners faced with evaluating the knowledge and abilities of individuals from culturally and linguistically diverse backgrounds. Chapter 1, for example, provides some discussion on validity evidence related to response processes as well as consequences of testing. These two issues are central to understanding the performance of individuals from diverse backgrounds, but are not discussed at length in this regard. Chapter 4 addresses issues of norm-referenced score interpretation and norm sample comparability, but the ensuing standards are geared more toward test developers than practitioners. Consider Standard 4.5, where it is noted that "norms, if used, should refer to clearly described populations. These populations should include individuals or groups to whom test users will ordinarily wish to compare their own examinees" (p. 55). Whereas the simplicity of the language suggests straightforward approaches for compliance (i.e., stratified random sampling), there is actually significantly greater operational complexity in meeting the standard. Test developers have dutifully included individuals of different races and ethnicities in their norm samples for quite some time. But have such attempts created "clearly described populations" as noted in Standard 4.5? The answer is no. Socially constructed categories, such as race and ethnicity, do little in achieving accurate representation along the relevant and important dimensions that actually affect test performance. Neither skin color nor an individual's ethnic heritage affects test performance directly. It is the individual's developmental background, particularly with respect to linguistic and acculturative experiences, that influences the individual's responding on standardized, norm-referenced tests. Salvia and Ysseldyke (1991) make this point clear in their statement regarding the *assumption of comparability*:

> When we test students using a standardized device and compare them to a set of norms to gain an index of their relative standing, we assume that the students we test are similar to those on whom the test was standardized; that is, we assume their acculturation is comparable, but not necessarily identical, to that of the students who made up the normative sample for the test. When a child's general background experiences differ from those of the children on whom a test was standardized, then the use of the norms of that test as an index for evaluating that child's current performance or for predicting future performances may be inappropriate. (p. 18)

Controlling for racial or ethnic differences via stratified random sampling may provide a desired measure of "face validity" for the norm sample, but in fact it only ensures that proportionate numbers of individuals from such backgrounds are included in the norm sample. It does not ensure that individuals from such backgrounds have comparable experiences, particularly as related to linguistic development and acculturative experiences. It is unfortunate that current research continues to use groups based exclusively on racial or ethnic categories (e.g., Hispanic) to examine a multitude of issues related to test performance. When constructed in such a manner, such studies lack generalizability, do not inform practice in any substantive way, and are effectively flawed in methodology. As described recently by Lohman, Korb, and Lakin (2008),

> Most studies compare the performance of students from different ethnic groups . . . rather than ELL [English-language learner] and non-ELL children within those ethnic groups. . . . A major difficulty with all of these studies is that the category Hispanic includes students from diverse cultural backgrounds with markedly different English-language skills. . . . This reinforces the need to separate the influences of ethnicity and ELL status on observed score differences. (pp. 276–278)

In a manner quite similar to differences in language skills, differences in test performance related to acquisition of cultural knowledge also preclude valid comparisons of performance. Validity can only be inferred when an examinee's background and experiences are comparable to those of the individuals who compose the norm sample.

Whenever this assumption is not met, conclusions regarding the meaning of test results become dubious at best. This notion has also been described by Salvia and Ysseldyke:

> Incorrect educational decisions may well be made. It must be pointed out that acculturation is a matter of experiential background rather than of gender, skin color, race, or ethnic background. When we say that a child's acculturation differs from that of the group used as a norm, we are saying that the *experiential background* differs, not simply that the child is of different ethnic origin, for example, from the children on whom the test was standardized. (1991, p. 18; emphasis in original)

It would seem that if they are to advance our scientific understanding, empirical investigations that make their way into academic journals in the future need to begin acknowledging this issue and incorporate subject groupings that are more representative of the true linguistic and cultural differences that play a pivotal role in how an individual performs on a test.

Perhaps a more utilitarian discussion for practitioners can be found in Chapter 7 of the *Standards*, which deals with fairness in testing and test use. In addition to the ubiquitous discussions regarding psychometric bias, the introductory section provides an important definition and analysis of *fairness* as "opportunity to learn" and the absence of "response-related sources of test bias." In Chapter 7, for the purposes of testing in educational settings, it is noted that "when test takers have not had the opportunity to learn the material tested, the policy of using their test scores . . . is viewed as unfair" (AERA et al., 1999, p. 76). Individuals who move between a home environment where the language and content emanate from the heritage culture and a school environment where the language and content emanate from the majority/mainstream culture are likely to fall into this category of having limited opportunity to learn. Parents who do not speak English at all or well, were not raised in the cultural mainstream, and were not educated in the content of the school curriculum can do little to transmit to their children the incidental knowledge or language skills that often accompany the requirements of academic and cognitive tests. When an individual comes from such circumstances, test performance will be adversely affected.

But how does this help the practitioner? The *Standards* volume acknowledges that "the definition of *opportunity to learn* is difficult in practice, especially at the level of individuals. Opportunity is a matter of degree" (AERA et al., 1999, p. 76; emphasis in original). Likewise, the volume addresses problems that arise when a test requires an ability that is not the intended construct under measurement. It is noted that "test performance may rely on some capability (e.g., English language proficiency or fine-motor coordination) that is irrelevant to the intent of the measurement but nonetheless poses impediments for some examinees" (p. 78). However, practitioners are left without guidance on either matter in terms of what can be done to account for differences along the lines of limited opportunity for learning and bias related to response processes. It is recommended only that test developers and users rely on "credible research" and information related to problems in the meaning of score differences, construct-irrelevant variance, differential item functioning, differential prediction, and outcomes. Of course, if a test developer finds such problems, they are likely to be addressed before final publication—and in some cases, such as differential prediction, there is already a large body of literature suggesting that the problem is exceedingly rare (Cummins, 1984; Figueroa, 1983, 1990b; Jensen, 1976, 1980; Reynolds, 2000; Reynolds & Kamphaus, 1990; Sandoval, 1979; Sattler, 1992; Valdés & Figueroa, 1994).

Moreover, in recognizing that the concept of degree is critical in these matters, a curious contradiction remains embedded in the *Standards*. For example, in discussing response-related sources of test bias, the volume notes that "a test of quantitative reasoning that makes inappropriately heavy demands on verbal ability would probably be biased against examinees whose first language is other than that of the test" (p. 78). Later, in Standard 7.7, it is recommended that "in testing applications where the level of linguistic or reading ability is not part of the construct of interest, the linguistic or reading demands of the test should be kept to the minimum necessary for the valid assessment of the intended construct" (p. 82). Just what constitutes an appropriate level of linguistic demand is not explained, and adopting a stance that there is even a minimal level of language that would not in some way affect performance is inconsistent with language as a developmental process. Such a stance seems to view language proficiency as a threshold ability, beyond which further development provides no benefit to test performance. The well-known correlation between level of education and IQ contradicts such a view (Brody, 1997; Gustafsson & Undheim, 1996; Neisser et al., 1996; Ormrod, 2008; Sattler, 2001). Indeed, the fact is that all tests, including nonverbal ones, require some level of communication between the examiner and examinee; thus some tests will indeed be subject to heavy linguistic demands (e.g., expressive vocabulary), and some tests will be less so (e.g., block construction). Test performance is thus likely to be affected continually and linearly, and not in an either–or manner (i.e., affected vs. not affected), as is implied by the *Standards*.

Perhaps the most important and detailed discussion in the *Standards* with respect to evaluating diverse individuals is Chapter 9, "Testing Individuals of Diverse Linguistic Backgrounds." This chapter covers a variety of relevant concerns: test translation, adaptation, and modification; issues of equivalence in test scores; language proficiency testing; testing bilingual individuals; administration and examiner variables; use of interpreters in testing; and cultural differences in individual testing. The chapter provides an excellent overview of the salient issues and emphasizes the point that language differences (between the language of the test and norm sample, and the language or languages of the examinee) may lead to significant problems in reliability and validity. This notion is captured best in Standard 9.1: "Testing practice should be designed to reduce threats to the reliability and validity of test score inferences that may arise from language differences" (p. 97). The commentary that follows, however, is noteworthy in both its extreme brevity and lack of guidance for practitioners. It begins, "Some tests are inappropriate for use with individuals whose knowledge of the language of the test is questionable" (p. 97). This statement implies that some tests are appropriate for use with individuals whose knowledge of the language of the test is questionable; perhaps it alludes to the less verbally demanding tasks often found on nonverbal instruments. For practitioners who are interested in measuring visual processing, memory, or reasoning abilities, this would be sufficient guidance. But what about evaluations where the referral concern involves reading difficulties, which create a need to measure phonological processing skills, extent of vocabulary, and facility with language (e.g., with verbal analogies)? Such abilities cannot be measured in a nonverbal way. They are verbal by definition, and language development and proficiency are integral parts of what they intend to measure. Strict application of Standard 9.1 would effectively eliminate use of substantial portions of standardized intelligence, cognitive ability, neuropsychological, and academic batteries, and virtually all language batteries, with linguistically diverse individuals.

The commentary under Standard 9.1 ends with the statement that "assessment methods together with careful professional judgment are required to determine when language differences are relevant. Test users can judge how best to address this standard in a particular testing situation" (p. 97). Beyond the use of nonverbal tests, what assessment methods are likely to comply with this standard? What factors should professionals take into account when making a decision about language differences and whether they are relevant? Would not language differences of any kind always be relevant, especially in connection with potential limited opportunity for learning?

The standards in Chapter 9 appear to alternate between specific guidance and vague suggestions, and at times they seem to be based on faulty notions regarding language development and proficiency. For example, Standard 9.2 discusses the need for collecting validity evidence for test scores that differ in meaning across linguistic subgroups. It does not define, however, what a *linguistic subgroup* is: Is it a group of individuals who use a different language (e.g., Spanish vs. Polish), or who have a different level of proficiency within the same language (e.g., beginning, intermediate, advanced)? The latter represents an extremely important variable in performance and has strong implications for the meaning of test score differences and norm sample development, yet it remains significantly underresearched. Standard 9.3 states that individuals who are "proficient" in two languages should be tested in their more proficient language. Such a recommendation suggests that doing so eliminates all problems with validity, when instead it conveniently ignores the fact that an individual who is proficient in two languages does not have a background that is similar, let alone comparable, to an individual who speaks only one language. Likewise, problems exist in being able to determine what level of language development constitutes proficiency in the first place. Just how proficient is proficient? Is it enough to be conversational or is full literacy required? Once again, the matter is reduced to an either–or proposition, when language actually represents a continuum of development. Standard 9.6 admonishes test developers to provide evidence when a test is recommended for use with linguistically diverse test takers, as well as to "provide the information necessary for appropriate test use and interpretation" (p. 99). Such recommendations generally come from publishers of nonverbal tests, who often overstate these tests' utility and validity with diverse learners (Lohman et al., 2008). Even then, information and evidence regarding appropriate test interpretation are conspicuously absent; this absence implies that the test is valid for any diverse learner, including all linguistic subgroups (whether these are defined by language or by proficiency level). As noted by Figueroa (1990b), "tests developed without accounting for language differences are limited in their validity and on how they can be interpreted" (p. 94).

In reality, very little of Chapter 9 in the *Standards* provides information that is directly applicable to psychological and educational testing practices with diverse individuals. The only exception is that test publishers are correctly instructed to consider the impact of language differences in test development (including threats to reliability, validity, and score comparability), and to provide evidence of the manner in which their tests are affected by these variables. It seems unlikely, however, that test publishers would be willing to publish this type of information, given that it might be misconstrued as evidence of poor test design, inappropriate for certain populations, or deficient in comparison to other tests that do not publish the same information. But for practitioners who are looking for specific guidance on practical standards for testing in psychological practice with culturally and linguistically diverse individuals, there remains a need to look beyond the *Standards*.

Without question, the *Standards* volume is an important and significant work. And in all fairness, by the time this chapter goes to press, an updated version of the *Standards* will be close to publication. There are some indications that in the next edition fairness will become an important and central issue cutting across all aspects of psychological and educational testing. However, given the degree to which significant changes are necessary in the understanding and accommodation of experiential differences in the assessment of culturally and linguistically diverse populations, and the degree to which they will affect nearly every aspect of test development, construction, administration, and use, it seems unlikely that the new edition will provide all the guidance evaluators currently require to engage in practice that fully mitigates all concerns regarding fairness, particularly those related to validity. Instead, practitioners will probably still need to review and evaluate empirical evidence independently and find a manner in which such evidence can be used to make critical decisions in testing and interpretation. The final section of this chapter provides a discussion along these lines, but first, a critical examination of current testing and interpretive practices is necessary.

EVALUATING CURRENT METHODS OF PRACTICE

The problems inherent in applying tests developed in the U.S. cultural milieu and normed primarily on monolingual English speakers to examinees from other cultures and who speak other languages were noted at the very advent of psychological testing (Brigham, 1923; Goddard, 1913; Yerkes, 1921), but they appear to have been either ignored or simply dismissed in the face of prevailing beliefs and arguments to the contrary (Sanchez, 1934). Despite a persistent pattern of lower performance among culturally and linguistically diverse individuals than among native English speakers, the matter of differential performance remained largely confined to notions regarding genetic differences (Jensen, 1974, 1976). Perhaps spurred by the spirit of social justice and civil rights that permeated the 1960s, researchers in the 1970s began to reexamine the issue (e.g., Oakland & Laosa, 1976)—particularly in light of the passage of the original Education for All Handicapped Children Act (1975), most recently reauthorized as the Individuals with Disabilities Education Improvement Act of 2004 (IDEA 2004). In the early forays into "nondiscriminatory assessment," the problem was broadly defined as "one dimension of the more general problem of valid assessment of any child" (Oakland, 1976, p. 1).

Despite the fact that earlier examinations of test bias had been largely focused on issues of reliability, Oakland (1976) noted that the most important aspect in testing of diverse individuals was validity. The issues described in the preceding section regarding the various recommendations outlined in the *Standards* all reinforce the importance and centrality of the concept of validity in fairness, far more so than the concept of reliability. But as also noted previously, the *Standards* volume is rather silent regarding the manner in which test results are to be examined for evidence of validity, and practitioners have historically been forced to resort to a variety of methods in attempts to address it—often without any empirical support to defend their use. Indeed, many of the methods in current use appear to be based on the mistaken idea that validity, like reliability, is a continuous variable. From a strict psychometric standpoint, a measure or scale can be considered valid or not, depending on whether there is sufficient evidence to support it one way or the other. Viewing validity as shades of gray instead of as a dichotomous concept is easily forgiven in light of the fact that practitioners are simply trying to do whatever can be done to ensure the validity of their obtained test results. Thus doing more should be better than doing less or nothing at all in accomplishing the goal. Unfortunately, more often than not, practitioners cannot actually evaluate the success of their efforts in establishing validity. That is, the extent to which factors such as LEP or differences in opportunity for learning cultural knowledge actually affect the results of testing is rarely addressed in reports, apart from the ubiquitous but hollow warnings that "results should be interpreted with extreme caution." Use of a particular method or strategy may lead practitioners to assume that validity has been "increased" or "maintained," but typical methods simply do not permit independent verification that this is in fact the case. As we discuss, such unverified assumptions (i.e., that validity has been achieved when in fact it has not) are common to all current approaches and limit their utility as avenues for achieving fairness.

In general, a review of the literature reveals four basic approaches that have been touted as viable methods for dealing with validity issues stemming from cultural and linguistic differences. Each approach is intended in some manner to address questions of fairness, so that test results emerge as valid—and each method has its own particular advantages and disadvantages, many of which do not appear to be acknowledged or recognized by those who employ them. It is especially important that the limitations of each approach be well understood by any practitioner with a desire to implement any of them in actual testing practice.

Modified or Adapted Testing

Perhaps some of the first attempts to address the various problems inherent in the evaluation of culturally and linguistically diverse individuals with standardized tests involved modifications or adaptations of the tests or testing protocols themselves. In this approach, tests are administered primarily in English but modified in some way so as to increase their fairness. Among the various adaptations that have been suggested, the most common include eliminating or not administering certain test items with presumed culturally biased content; mediating culturally based task concepts prior to administration; repeating verbal instructions to ensure full comprehension; accepting responses in either the native language or the language of the test; administering only subtests that do not rely

on oral expression; and eliminating or modifying time constraints (Figueroa, 1983, 1990a, 1990b; Sattler, 1992, 2001). Such procedures are extensions of what is often referred to as "testing the limits" and represent a clinical approach to evaluating diverse individuals. These procedures are designed to aid examinees in performing to the true extent of their actual ability by reducing aspects of the testing process that might attenuate the scores. Unfortunately, any time a test is administered with such alterations, when not specifically permitted or directed by the test's standardized administration protocol, by definition it no longer remains standardized. Unknown amounts of error are introduced into the testing situation, resulting in a loss of confidence in the test's psychometric properties, especially those that determine its validity. Despite the benevolent intent of such procedures, any results derived from their application are rendered suspect at best and effectively preclude valid and defensible interpretation.

Another common testing adaptation involves attempts to overcome the language barrier via use of a translator/interpreter. Up to 20% of practitioners working with culturally and linguistically diverse children indicate that they employ this method (Sotelo-Dynega et al., 2011). The presumption that testing will be valid as long as an individual comprehends what is being said or asked has intuitive appeal; however, it neglects the culturally based aspects of the testing process itself, as well as the fact that the test remains culturally bound. More importantly, even if we ignore the significant problems in translating tests "on the fly" with or without the aid of trained and untrained interpreters and the presence of third-party observers, tests have yet to be standardized with the use of a translator/interpreter. That is, the use of a translator/interpreter in the testing process represents another violation of standardized procedures, which again by itself undermines the reliability and validity of the results and continues to prevent interpretation.

Beyond issues related to test administration and modification, it is important to note that such procedures do nothing to address problems related to norm sample representation. Even if modification of the test or its administration protocol did not invalidate the process, could the test scores be interpreted fairly? Even if threats to validity are controlled in some areas, it does not mean that validity has been addressed in all areas. This is particularly true with respect to the adequacy of the norm sample against whom the test scores will be compared. Test developers often attempt to control for cultural or linguistic differences by including individuals from diverse racial and ethnic backgrounds. But race and ethnicity are not the same as culture or cultural differences and do not directly account for differences in experience that affect language or acculturative knowledge development, as noted by Salvia and Ysseldyke (1991) and discussed in the preceding section. Representation within a test's norm sample on the basis of racial or ethnic categories is simply not a sufficient proxy for the degree to which an individual is or is not familiar with the culture of the test. Likewise, neither race nor ethnicity provides specific information about the extent of an individual's proficiency in English. Despite demonstration of high-quality technical characteristics and the use of sophisticated sampling techniques, norm samples that are stratified on the basis of race or ethnicity, but that contain individuals who are predominantly or exclusively monolingual English speakers, are unlikely to meet the necessary standards for adequate representation of genuinely "bilingual" and "bicultural" individuals. For the most part, test developers and researchers have not addressed or recognized this issue, but this may not be the case much longer. Until norm samples for tests are built upon stratification variables that matter to culturally and linguistically diverse individuals, the results simply cannot be construed as valid, even when tests are carefully modified, adapted, or translated.

Because altering the standardized requirements of the testing process in any manner effectively precludes the assignment of meaning to the collected data, modifications or adaptations in testing are of limited utility. Even if such adaptations could be seen as valid, the significant problems with norm sample adequacy would still preclude validity of any conclusions regarding comparative differences. In practice, such procedures may be most useful in allowing practitioners to derive qualitative information—that is, by observing behavior, evaluating learning propensity, evaluating developmental capabilities, analyzing errors, and so forth. Perhaps the best recommendation for practitioners who are considering use of these types of methods would be to administer tests in a standardized manner first and then retest with any modifications or adaptations that might help illuminate the actual or true level of an individual's ability. In this way, it may be possible to evaluate the issue of validity by limiting the threats rather than adding to them.

Nonverbal Testing

Much as in the development of the Beta version of the Army examination (Yerkes, 1921), the use of nonverbal methods and tests in the evaluation of ELLs has been predicated on a simple notion: Eliminate the language barrier, and testing can proceed as usual. Nonverbal tests have in fact become quite popular in psychological practice, and various tools have been published expressly for this purpose. According to a recent survey, when evaluating the intelligence of culturally and linguistically diverse individuals, 88% of all practitioners choose to administer a nonverbal test (Sotelo-Dynega et al., 2011). Similar to the claims originally put forth by Brigham (1923), these tests offer the promise of validity based on the idea that language has been effectively removed from the testing equation. For example, according to Weiss and colleagues (2006), administration of a nonverbal cognitive assessment is still promoted as "an acceptable answer to this problem" (p. 49). This appears, however, to be an overly optimistic view.

The phrase *nonverbal testing* is itself a bit of a misnomer; what is meant is probably better characterized as *language-reduced testing* or *assessment*. This is because no matter the test, its use in any evaluation requires that the examiner and examinee be able to communicate with each other. Even tests whose developers claim that they can be administered in a completely nonverbal manner (i.e., via gestures or pantomime) first require that the examinee understand and comprehend the meaning of the gestures. This meaning must necessarily include instructions on when to start, when to stop, what is a right answer, and when to work quickly. Other testing issues (establishing rapport, explaining the purpose of testing, etc.) also need to be conveyed to the examinee. How all this is to be communicated in the absence of any verbal interaction is not clear. Even if it were possible to do so, the fact remains that the teaching of gestures is akin to the teaching of a new, albeit very brief and limited, "language." Thus, whether spoken language is used or not, administration of a test always requires some type of communication between examinee and examiner. Nonverbal testing may well reduce the language barrier, but it clearly does not eliminate it.

In a similar manner, the claim that a test's cultural fairness is increased because it is nonverbal does not mean that cultural content embedded in the test is eliminated. Given the emphasis on abilities that are less verbal, there may be some reduction in cultural content unless the use of visual stimuli includes pictures of actual objects and artifacts, which continue to embed culture even with the reduction in language. Many nonverbal tests continue to rely on visual images that remain culturally bound (Sattler, 1992). In addition, nonverbal tests are often used to derive a score that will serve as an indicator of an individual's general intelligence. Such practice, especially in the context of evaluation for a specific learning disability (SLD), is problematic for several reasons. First, it has been demonstrated that nonverbal estimates of intelligence may be no more fair or valid than those that include verbal abilities (Figueroa, 1989). Second, the range of abilities measured by a nonverbal composite is by definition likely to be narrower than that measured by verbal batteries, despite correlations with broader measures of intelligence (Flanagan, Ortiz, & Alfonso, 2007; Ortiz, 2008). Third, the majority of referrals for SLD evaluation are based on problems in language arts, particularly reading. This means that an assessment for SLD will need to include testing for those abilities most related to reading, including auditory processing (Ga) and crystallized knowledge (Gc) (Flanagan et al., 2007; Flanagan, Ortiz, Alfonso, & Mascolo, 2006). These abilities cannot be easily measured or measured at all with nonverbal tests, and such tests are therefore not useful for evaluation in a large majority of SLD evaluations. Finally, nonverbal tests are subject to the same problems with norm sample representation as those existing for verbal tests, as described earlier. That is, neither type of tests has norm samples that systematically and adequately control for the differences in acculturative experiences or language development characterizing bilingual and bicultural individuals. In sum, language-reduced tests are not as helpful in the evaluation of the abilities of individuals from diverse cultural and linguistic backgrounds as their developers often claim. Although such tests may provide better estimates of true functioning in certain areas, they do not represent a satisfactory solution with respect to validity and fairness in testing, and in the majority of cases will be inadequate to serve the purpose of SLD identification when the focus is on language-related abilities (e.g., reading, writing).

It seems likely that these problems may help explain why the empirical evidence for the predictive validity of nonverbal tests tends to be rather dubious (Figueroa, 1989; Lohman et al., 2008). In an examination of three different nonverbal tests often used to identify gifted children from culturally and linguistically diverse backgrounds, Lohman et al. (2008) noted that "one cannot assume that nonverbal tests level the playing field for children who come from different cultures or who have had different educational opportunities" (p. 292). In contrast to claims of reduced "ethnic" score differences for many nonverbal measures, this study found "large differences between the scores of ELL and non-ELL children on the three nonverbal tests"; these findings indicated that practitioners "must consider opportunity to learn not only for tests that measure verbal and quantitative abilities and achievements but also for those abilities measured by nonverbal tests" (Lohman et al., 2008, p. 292).

Despite their widespread popularity, immense intuitive appeal, and long history of clinical use with culturally and linguistically diverse individuals, nonverbal tests simply do "not fulfill a utopian vision as measures of innate ability unencumbered by culture, education, or experience" (Lohman et al., 2008; Valdés & Figueroa, 1994). This is not to say that such tests are not helpful or valuable in evaluating diverse individuals, but only that they are not the sole or definitive solution to issues of fairness and validity, as they are often purported to be. The best recommendation that can be made regarding the evidence base for the use of nonverbal tests is that they should be viewed as only one component of a broader, comprehensive evaluation—a component that assists in examining functioning in the particular areas such tests measure. Whether the obtained results are valid remains a question not adequately addressed merely by their use in practice.

Native-Language Testing

The relatively recent development of psychometrically sound, standardized tests of intelligence and cognitive abilities in languages other than English, coupled with a slight increase in the number of psychologists with sufficient competency in evaluations conducted in languages other than English, has led to a growth in approaches based on the use of the native language. Unfortunately, such practice has become identified with the inaccurate label of "bilingual assessment." Bilingual assessment implies evaluation that is to be conducted *bilingually*—that is, with the concurrent use of two languages as the situation may dictate, or as desired by the individuals, as is the custom when bilingual persons speak to each other. Native-language tests, however, are not standardized using two languages, but only one. Of course, it would probably be impossible to standardize rote transitions from one language to another because artificial and arbitrary changes by an individual would lead to considerable awkwardness in communication. Except on some tests where responses are accepted when given in either language, code switching (into or out of English) is not specified or standardized. Thus so-called "bilingual assessment" is better described as monolingual testing, even in those situations where a test is given in one language followed by retesting in another language.

Irrespective of the manner in which it may be best characterized, use of a native-language test requires that psychologists speak the language of the test (i.e., they need to be bilingual themselves). The ability to communicate with an examinee directly is an important and significant benefit to this approach and places a psychologist in a position to conduct assessment activities in a manner (i.e., bilingually) not available to a monolingual psychologist even with the aid of a translator/interpreter. This notion may partly explain why the simple hiring of a bilingual practitioner is often seen as an acceptable solution to the problem of evaluating diverse individuals. However, "mere possession of the capacity to communicate in an individual's native language does not ensure appropriate, nondiscriminatory assessment of that individual. Traditional assessment practices and their inherent biases can be easily replicated in any number of languages" (Flanagan, McGrew, & Ortiz, 2000, p. 291). Speaking the same language as an examinee and utilizing a test available in the language spoken by the examinee do not, by themselves, resolve issues of fairness or validity. Indeed, they may actually lead practitioners, and those for whom they work, into a false sense of security regarding the meaning of their obtained test results. In addition, not only are there are no truly "bilingual" tests or assessment protocols, but very little is currently known about the performance of bilingual individuals on monolingual tests administered in the primary language. Compared to the body of research on the use of tests administered in English, research on testing in the native language is a relatively new tradition, with very little empirical evidence upon which to guide appropriate activities or base standards for practice. The general question regarding how a bilingual individual who was born in or has recently moved to the United States would be expected to perform on a test administered in the native language has yet to

be answered. Such a question is bound to be complicated by various factors, such as the individual's age, his or her level and type of prior education, the current language of instruction, and the type of instructional program (Goldenberg, 2008).

Furthermore, when native-language testing is accomplished in the United States, an examinee cannot rightly be viewed as a monolingual speaker or as coming from a monocultural background. Because the norms of native-language tests often utilize monolingual speakers from other countries who are being raised by parents who speak the language and who are being educated in the native language, they do not form an adequately representative norm sample for comparisons with individuals now residing in the United States. In such cases, the experiential backgrounds of these two populations are no more similar than they are to the backgrounds of monolingual individuals. As noted by Harris and Llorente (2005), "these children indeed represent a proportion of U.S. school children who are ELLs. Realistically, however, little is known about the language abilities of these learners and the degree to which they are bilingual" (pp. 392–393). Even when test developers attempt to include bilingual speakers, they are not sampled systematically with respect to the two major variables (current proficiency in both languages and level of acculturation) that would be necessary to create representative groups. For example, despite inclusion of bilingual individuals in the developmental sample of the Wechsler Intelligence Scale for Children—Fourth Edition (WISC-IV) Spanish version (Wechsler, 2005), they are grouped primarily by country of origin, length of time in the United States, or length of schooling in the United States, all of which fail to account for the influence of cultural and linguistic differences (Harris & Llorente, 2005). In addition, it should be noted that the actual WISC-IV Spanish norms are equated to the WISC-IV English norms, and thus the Spanish version does not have actual, separate norms (Braden & Iribarren, 2007).

It would appear that until such time that a sufficient body of knowledge exists on which bilingual psychologists can base expectations of performance on native-language tests, their use will continue to provide results that are of dubious validity and extremely difficult to interpret. Accordingly, the most prudent recommendation for practice involving the use of native-language tests is similar to those offered previously: Administer tests in a standardized manner first, and then apply whatever modifications or adaptations may be appropriate and may inform the referral questions. Well-trained bilingual examiners may be limited by the tools and practices available to them, but they remain the best choice for conducting evaluations of culturally and linguistically diverse individuals. Despite the limitations inherent in all approaches, bilingual examiners have one unique and significant advantage over other examiners employing other approaches—their ability to directly communicate with and observe the behaviors of diverse examinees in a controlled setting. This advantage alone places native-language testing in front of all other approaches and represents the current "ideal" situation—not because the test results are necessarily more fair or valid, but because of the examiners' ability to engage in direct interaction with the examinees and utilize a wide variety of procedures (including authentic assessment, informal measures, error analyses, and whatever other methods may be helpful and informative in understanding and gauging the examinees' true abilities).

English-Language Testing

Given the increasingly large numbers of culturally and linguistically diverse individuals in the U.S. population, coupled with the fraction of professionals who have sufficient competency to conduct evaluations in such persons' native languages, it is not likely that all such individuals will be evaluated in their native languages or by bilingual professionals. Of the 480 practitioners surveyed by Sotelo-Dynega and colleagues (2011), only about 12% identified themselves as "bilingual/multicultural school psychologists," yet 86% reported that they evaluate students who are culturally and linguistically diverse. The reality is that the majority of diverse individuals are being evaluated by monolingual English-speaking practitioners and that these evaluations will be conducted primarily, if not exclusively, in English. Compared to the three prior methods, this particular approach would seem to be the most biased and least fair. In many ways it echoes Brigham's (1923) general comments about testing when he stated,

> If the tests used included some mysterious type of situation that was "typically American," we are indeed fortunate, for this is America, and the purpose of our inquiry is that of obtaining a measure of the character of our immigration. Inability to respond to a "typically American" situation is obviously an undesirable trait. (p. 96)

When testing adopts this type of unapologetic position and makes no concessions to the fact that a child is not a native English speaker, does not permit alteration of the content or administration of the test, and does not investigate the abilities a child may be able to demonstrate in their native language but not in English, what could be more biased? On the other hand, if we dispense with Brigham's mistaken notions about personal character, we can in fact recognize that this is also the only approach where there exists a great deal of scientific research regarding how culturally and linguistically diverse individuals actually perform on tests—tests given to them in English.

Although it certainly was not intentional, the field of psychometrics has nevertheless provided perhaps the most empirically supportable basis for evaluating the validity of bilingual individuals' test performance. The development of standardized procedures, coupled with repeated evaluation of subjects proficient enough in English to comprehend test instructions reasonably well, has established a rather extensive and cohesive database on the manner in which such examinees perform on tests administered to them in English (Brigham, 1923; Cummins, 1984; Figueroa, 1989; Goddard, 1913; Jensen, 1974, 1976; Mercer, 1979; Sanchez, 1934; Valdés & Figueroa, 1994; Vukovich & Figueroa, 1982; Yerkes, 1921). A review of this research indicates that non-native speakers of English consistently perform more poorly (about one full standard deviation or more below average) than native English speakers on tasks that rely on English-language development, skills, or proficiency, and that they perform comparably to them (at or near the normative mean) on tasks that do not require such verbal or language-based development or skill (Cummins, 1984; Figueroa, 1989; McShane, 1980; Mercer, 1979; Naglieri, 1982; Valdés & Figueroa, 1994; Vukovich & Figueroa, 1982).

On the surface, testing diverse individuals with English-language tests appears to result in highly biased estimates of ability, particularly those abilities that may rely heavily on language and acculturative knowledge development. On the other hand, if this research is viewed as illuminating the magnitude and degree to which such factors as differences in language and acculturative development actually affect test performance, it seems reasonable that it may be an effective way to develop an empirically based approach for evaluating the validity of obtained test results. Research is available that provides estimates of the degree of attenuation that may have occurred in testing as a function of the presence of the main operating variables—namely, English-language proficiency and acculturative knowledge. Whether or not the results are valid can thus be examined by comparing diverse examinees' performance to that of a group far more similar to the examinees in terms of developmental background and experience than existing norm samples are. Ideally, individuals from diverse cultural and linguistic backgrounds should rightly be evaluated by qualified, competent professionals with specific expertise in nondiscriminatory assessment and knowledge of the manner in which such differences influence test performance (Ortiz, 2008). There is nothing, however, that prevents any practitioner from evaluating such an individual in both the native language and English. And when there is no other option available but to evaluate in English, the same type of expertise, knowledge, and research base may well be applied to assist in evaluating validity—a process that is often couched in terms of determining "difference versus disorder." The potential application of this body of literature in support of an evidence-based approach using English test administration is explored further in the next section regarding integration of research into practice. For the moment, testing only in English without regard for the inherent problems in fairness and validity will certainly lead to extremely discriminatory interpretations and conclusions.

INTEGRATING RESEARCH INTO DEFENSIBLE PRACTICE

Fallacies and Misconceptions in Early Research

Although tests can be quite reliable, even perfect reliability does not guarantee validity. It is possible that something can be measured very accurately and consistently over time, but this does not ensure that the construct one believes is being measured is actually the one that is. The difference between reliability and validity is central to the issue of testing with culturally and linguistically diverse individuals. Although this notion was certainly well understood by early psychometricians and psychologists, preconceptions and the early cultural *zeitgeist* may have prevented their recognition.

A particularly stark example can be seen in the work of Henry Herbert Goddard, a leading American psychologist who translated the Binet–Simon Scale into English and promptly began using it in work with bilingual examinees and individuals from diverse cultural backgrounds. Goddard's intent was not to study bilingualism or its effect on test performance, but rather to prove an a priori conviction—that IQ was an innate, inherited trait and that it explained the division among the "haves" and "have-nots." To examine the issue, he went to Ellis Island in New York and began testing immigrants—not randomly selected ones, but those whom he already believed were intellectually inferior, primarily on the basis of their appearance. In the process of his investigation, Goddard (1913) eventually concluded that approximately 80% of all immigrants arriving from Eastern Europe were mentally defective or feeble-minded. He even developed a specific word to define their level of functioning—*moron*. The degree to which Goddard (1913) was working from preconceptions that made him oblivious to patterns in his own data can be seen in his explicit comments, such as "We picked out one young man whom we suspected was defective, and, through the interpreter, proceeded to give him the test" (p. 105); in his inability to entertain any hypothesis contrary to his own when the interpreter questioned the fairness of the testing by stating, "I could not have done that when I came to this country" (p. 105); and in his curt and decisive reply to the interpreter, "We convinced him that the boy was defective" (p. 105).

Not much later, Robert Yerkes, already an eminent American psychologist, developed the Army mental tests in response to the Department of the Army's request to help in distinguishing men who would be good officer candidates from those who could serve merely as infantrymen. In the course of his work, Yerkes (1921) did in fact recognize and acknowledge the problem posed by individuals from diverse cultural and linguistic backgrounds, which he viewed mostly as an issue of illiteracy. Because his initial (Alpha) test had components that required reading, he could not administer the test to anyone (regardless of country of origin) who could not read English. He therefore set about creating an alternative (Beta) version, which eliminated any test requiring reading and which utilized "nonverbal" demonstrations drawn on blackboards to provide presumably comprehensible instructions. He believed that the Beta test represented a valid method for evaluating the abilities of the many men he needed to test who were illiterate, at least in English, or who did not speak English. In examining his data on nearly 1.75 million American men, Yerkes noted that the average raw score on the Beta for native English speakers (even those who could not read at all in English) was a stout 101.6, which classified them as Very Superior (Grade A). In contrast, the average raw score for non-native English speakers (who also could not read in English) came in at only 77.8, which classified these individuals as Average (Grade C). For Yerkes, as well as the contingent of other notable psychologists working with him (e.g., Carl Brigham, David Wechsler, Lewis Terman), the results confirmed their own beliefs—that immigrants, particularly those from certain countries and from lower classes, were merely displaying their inherited lack of intelligence. Questions regarding the potential issues involved in testing individuals with LEP or no English at all, and with limited opportunity for learning about the cultural content embedded in the test, were not addressed, even if they hovered in the air when the pattern of results was examined. Given the atmosphere of the era, none of these psychologists were inclined to seriously abandon their causal explanations related to intelligence as an innate quality, even when the data strongly suggested otherwise.

Figure 22.1 provides an example of this tendency, using Yerkes's data, which were later reanalyzed by Brigham in *A Study of American Intelligence* (1923). The increase in mental age as time of residence in the United States increased is particularly striking. Nevertheless, this particular finding seemed to bother Brigham—perhaps subconsciously, as he first admitted—but then he dismissed the obviously correct interpretation and instead provided a convoluted hypothesis consistent with his and the prevailing beliefs. In examining the data in Figure 22.1, Brigham gave the following explanation:

Instead of considering that our curve indicates a growth of intelligence with increasing length of residence, we are forced to take the reverse of the picture and accept the hypothesis that the curve indicates a gradual deterioration in the class of immigrants examined in the army, who came to this country in each succeeding 5 year period since 1902. (pp. 110–111) . . . The average intelligence of succeeding waves of immigration has become progressively lower. (p. 155)

When combined with the data showing significantly lower raw scores on the Army Beta test between native and non-native English speakers, to which Brigham had access, it seems reasonable that the far more plausible interpretation as previously noted should also have been reached by Brigham—that the longer one lives in the United States, the more English one learns (which increases comprehension), and the more familiar one becomes with U.S. cultural artifacts (including those that appeared on the test). That such an obvious conclusion was not offered by Brigham again emphasizes the degree to which evidence indicating that testing was being affected by differences in the cultural and linguistic backgrounds of individuals went largely unappreciated. Even when deliberate attempts were made to bring the issue to light, it was often buried in obscure journals or flatly dismissed as inconsistent with scientific fact, as is evident in Terman's (1916) comments:

> The common opinion that the child from a cultured home does better in tests solely by reason of his superior home advantages is an entirely gratuitous assumption. Practically all of the investigations which have been made of the influence of nature and nurture on mental performance agree in attributing far more to original endowment than to environment. (p. 115)

George Sanchez, a Mexican American psychologist, was one of the few investigators from outside the mainstream who did manage to publish his research on the performance of bilingual individuals in scholarly journals (Sanchez, 1932, 1934). He explicitly outlined the idea that differences in language development and proficiency, as well as differing levels of experience with the cultural content embedded in the test, were in fact the variables responsible for the observed difference in test scores between native and non-native English speakers. According to Sanchez (1934), "as long as tests do not at least sample in equal degree a state of saturation [i.e., assimilation of fundamental ex-

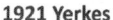

1921 Yerkes

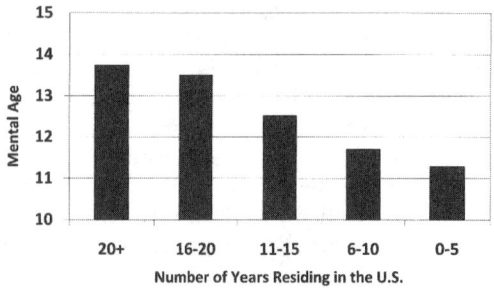

FIGURE 22.1. Mean mental age on the Binet–Simon Scale for immigrants tested with the Army Beta examination.

periences and activities] that is equal for the 'norm children' and the particular bilingual child it cannot be assumed that the test is a valid one for the child" (p. 770). Sanchez's viewpoint remained an isolated one, however. By the time the issue was being given serious considerations in the 1970s, the legacy of these early studies remained embedded in psychological science, and genetic explanations of test performance remained dominant or were replaced by ones suggesting that bilingualism itself was a handicap (Valdés & Figueroa, 1994).

One of the individuals who helped to promote and maintain notions regarding genetic explanations was Arthur Jensen (1974, 1976, 1980). Ironically, Jensen was also one of the first researchers to admit to the existence of bias (as related to validity) through an experiment of his own, which, unlike his more controversial assertions, garnered very little attention. In an investigation of the convergence of two separate measures of intelligence with Mexican and European American ("white") groups, one using a verbal modality and one using a nonverbal modality, he expected to find similar patterns of performance on the tests and equivalent degrees of difficulty among items for both groups. In fact, he did find equivalent degrees of difficulty among items for both groups, but he did not find similar patterns of performance. Instead, he found that whereas both groups did show similar score patterns on the nonverbal task, the Mexican group had significantly lower scores on the verbal task

than the European American group. The lack of concurrence between test scores on the two tasks for both groups led Jensen (1974) to the following conclusion:

> The fact that the Mexican group is very similar to the white in rank order of p values and p decrements on both the PPVT [Peabody Picture Vocabulary Test] and the Raven, yet has lower scores on the PPVT than on the Raven, suggest that some factor is operating to depress the PPVT performance more or less uniformly for all items and that this factor does not depress Raven performance, at least to the same degree. It seems plausible to suggest that this factor is verbal and may be associated with bilingualism in the Mexican group. (pp. 239–240)

Two years later, in a separate publication, Jensen (1976) offered the following comment on the result of his earlier study: "Thus, there is some evidence that a vocabulary test in English may be a biased test of intelligence for Mexican-Americans" (p. 342). Shortly thereafter, other researchers reached much the same conclusion. Although Jensen and others kept pointing to a verbal–nonverbal dichotomy in performance, the evidence began to demonstrate a pattern that was much more consistent with what Yerkes and Brigham had found originally with the Binet–Simon Scale—a more or less continuous, linear variation in decline. Table 22.1 provides a comparison of mean scores on 11 subtests from the WISC-R/WISC-III among "Hispanic" (Vukovich

TABLE 22.1. Results of Testing among Four Different Groups of Non-Native English Speakers

WISC-R/WISC-III subtest name	"Hispanic" group (Vukovich & Figueroa, 1972) Mean scaled score	"Hispanic" group (Vukovich & Figueroa, 1982) Mean scaled score	"ESL" group (Cummins, 1982) Mean scaled score	"Bilingual" group (Nieves-Brull, 2006) Mean scaled score
Information	7.5	7.8	5.1	7.2
Vocabulary	8.0	8.3	6.1	7.5
Similarities	7.6	8.8	6.4	8.2
Comprehension	7.8	9.0	6.7	8.0
Digit Span	8.3	8.5	7.3	—[a]
Arithmetic	8.7	9.4	7.4	7.8
Picture Arrangement	9.0	10.3	8.0	9.2
Block Design	9.5	10.8	8.0	9.4
Object Assembly	9.6	10.7	8.4	9.3
Picture Completion	9.7	9.9	8.7	9.5
Coding	9.6	10.9	8.9	9.6

[a]Data for this subtest were not reported in the study.

& Figueroa, 1982), "ESL" (Cummins, 1984), and "bilingual" (Nieves-Brull, 2006) groups as compared to the norm sample mean (scaled score = 10). Two things are particularly evident in the data: (1) The Verbal tests show significantly more attenuation than the Performance tests and (2) the degree of attenuation lessens across the tests and does not depress performance in a manner that can be considered equal within either the Verbal or the Performance domain. In general, it is clear that all four groups show a variable but systematic decline in performance, and not merely a difference between "verbal" and "nonverbal" tasks. Some tests that are considered verbal (e.g., Arithmetic) do not attenuate performance as much as others that are very verbal in nature (e.g., Information). Likewise, some tests that are considered nonverbal and have very low linguistic demands (e.g., Coding) have smaller adverse effects on test performance than other nonverbal ones with low linguistic demands (e.g., Picture Arrangement).

This type of declining pattern is particularly evident when scores are graphed and arranged in terms of highest mean to lowest mean. Figure 22.2 provides such an illustration and demonstrates several important dimensions relevant to the present discussion, including the fact that the change in scores does not appear to be an either–or propo-

sition, but rather a smooth, gradual decline as the tasks increase in their measurement of language skills and cultural knowledge. These graphs are particularly striking in their similarity to Yerkes's data shown in Figure 22.1—data that are from 50 to 80 years older than those illustrated. Another pattern in the data can be seen in the difference in the magnitude of the means between the 1972 and 1982 Vukovich and Figueroa groups. Although both groups show a clear and similar decline in test performance relative to increasing verbal and knowledge demands, the means for the latter group are consistently higher than those for the former and would suggest the existence of differences between them in the two principal variables (language proficiency and opportunity for learning about the culture). Personal communication with the author (D. Vukovich, September 29, 2008) has confirmed the difference in these factors and highlights the necessity to account for them in evaluations, as well as the mistakes that can occur if all "bilingual" individuals are treated as equal or as a monolithic group. In sum, these studies all point to the notion that adherence to a strict verbal–nonverbal conceptualization of test performance for culturally and linguistically diverse individuals is much too simplistic and not entirely supported by the evidence. An understanding of performance

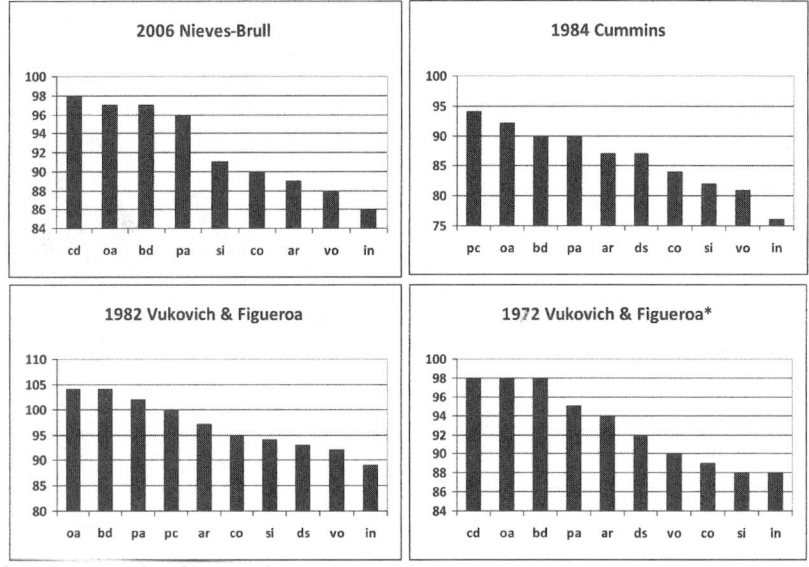

FIGURE 22.2. Comparison of mean WISC-R/WISC-III subtest scores from four investigations with "Hispanic," "ELL," and "bilingual" populations (see Table 22.1). Subtest abbreviations: pc, Picture Completion; cd, Coding; oa, Object Assembly; bd, Block Design; pa, Picture Arrangement; si, Similarities; co, Comprehension; ar, Arithmetic; vo, Vocabulary; in, Information; ds, Digit Span. *The 1972 Vukovich and Figueroa sample is reported in Vokovich and Figueroa (1982).

and the extent to which it is affected by cultural and linguistic influences instead appears to require paying attention to the unique characteristics of each subtest, as well as the construct it purports to measure.

Despite research spanning over a century thus far, as well as the robust and persistent finding regarding the pattern of performance for bilingual groups on tests given to them in English, very little of this information has found its way into actual practice. This question was raised by Valdés and Figueroa (1994), who wondered why "these and other anomalous psychometric outcomes associated with bilingual populations (such as the ubiquitous and intractable low-VIQ, high-PIQ bilingual profile) are curious in and of themselves, but not quite as perplexing as psychometricians' lack of interest about why such outcomes occur" (p. 108). Practitioners do not have the same luxury as academicians in being able to ignore such issues. Perhaps the seductive nature of the verbal–nonverbal duality has resulted in its unquestioned use among practitioners—or, more likely, there simply has not been much of an alternative. As we have noted earlier, there are few general approaches a practitioner can employ in evaluating an individual from a diverse cultural and linguistic background, and none of the methods we have discussed provide a truly satisfactory or evidence-based solution, particularly in addressing the issue of validity. Moreover, it cannot be said that any of these approaches are based on any substantive body of research, albeit nonverbal testing has relied on the general verbal–nonverbal pattern. Nevertheless, even when nonverbal methods are employed, several significant problems remain (Figueroa, 1989, 1990; Flanagan & Ortiz, 2001; Lohman et al., 2008; Ortiz, 2008), especially in cases where there is a need to measure the full range of cognitive abilities (Carroll, 1993; McGrew & Flanagan, 1998; Horn & Blankson, Chapter 3, this volume; Woodcock, 1990).

Moving toward Research-Based Practice

If currently available instruments have limitations in terms of demonstrating adequate validity, and if such tools lack evidence to support their use with various linguistic or cultural subgroups (i.e., groups that vary in terms of proficiency and experience within a larger ethnic group), and if the notion of verbal–nonverbal views of performance is greatly overgeneralized, then what is the average practitioner to do in terms of engaging in evidence-based practice? At this point in time, the answer to this question may be rather surprising. If evidence-based practice must rest on just that—evidence—then the only sufficient body of empirical research currently available to guide the practice of evaluating a wide range of cognitive abilities in individuals from diverse cultural and linguistic backgrounds is the research on the use of standardized tests administered in English. It is perhaps ironic, but the fact remains that there is a considerable amount of information (much of which has been discussed previously) regarding the performance of bilingual individuals on tests given to them in English. If this literature is combined with defensible psychometric procedures (particularly maintenance of standardization without alteration), and the main focus in evaluation is placed on examining the validity of the obtained test data (leaving interpretation to occur only if the data are deemed valid), it may be possible to conduct evaluations of diverse individuals that begin to meet the criteria for being both evidence-based and defensible. At present, only two such methods that are expressly designed to deal with the matter of validity have been proposed in the literature. Both are discussed below.

Multidimensional Assessment Model for Bilingual Individuals

It has been common practice (Ochoa et al., 2004) for practitioners to seek and find the "best" tool for use with diverse individuals as a de facto method of establishing validity. The presumption has been that if the "gold standard" is used, then what questions can there be regarding validity? This has effectively absolved practitioners from having to deal with the issue any further. As practitioners have become more sophisticated in their assessment activities, most have adopted an alternative and pragmatic approach that does not involve merely selecting the best tool, but selecting an approach that is most likely to yield valid results, regardless of the test chosen. The choice of approach involves consideration of various factors, including, at a minimum, the individual's proficiency in both his or her native language (hereafter referred to as L1) and a second language—in the United States, English (L2); the student's current grade level; the type of educational program; and the length of the student's instruction in that program. Certainly other factors can play an important role in making such decisions, but these stand out as the ones that merit foremost attention. In partial recognition of the difficulties and complexities practitioners encountered in trying to make such decisions, Ochoa and Ortiz (2005) developed the Multidimensional Assessment Model for Bilingual Individuals (MAMBI) as a guide to make the decision-making process more systematic. The MAMBI is depicted in Figure 22.3.

The MAMBI chart assists a practitioner in integrating the three major variables that affect selection of the most appropriate modality for testing: the student's current grade, type of educational program, and level of proficiency in both L1 and L2. Because the MAMBI arranges these variables in a manner that facilitates deliberate consideration, the practitioner can select an appropriate assessment modality in a manner that serves the purpose of obtaining the results likely to be the most valid ones. Again, it should be noted that validity is not a continuous variable, but rather a more direct either–or proposition. Results are valid or they are not, and notions of "greater" or "more" validity are somewhat misguided. To this end, Ochoa and Ortiz (2005) have listed four approaches to evaluation: (1) nonverbal assessment (NV in the MAMBI chart); (2) assessment primarily in L1; (3) assessment primarily in L2; and (4) bilingual assessment, using a combination of the native language and English (BL in the MAMBI chart). Note that earlier in this chapter, L1 assessment and bilingual assessment have been discussed as similar approaches, and that adaptation or modification of tests is not presented as an option within the MAMBI framework. Otherwise, the approaches listed in the MAMBI are substantially similar to those already described.

Nonverbal assessment is defined (Rhodes et al., 2005) as an approach to evaluation that is conducted primarily in a nonverbal or "language-reduced" manner, using tests that either are designed specifically to be free of oral language requirements or incorporate reductions in the need or demand for L2 proficiency. The limitations of these types of tests notwithstanding, this approach is perhaps most appropriate and best suited for individuals with very low levels (minimal or emergent) of proficiency in either L1 or L2. When communication with the individual is greatly limited, none of the other approaches are likely to prove as appropriate and are more likely to lead to problems with validity. Individuals with minimal or emergent levels of proficiency in L1 or L2 are depicted in the MAMBI chart by language profiles 1, 2, 4, and 5. In contrast, use of a nonverbal approach with those bilingual individuals who have reached high levels of cognitive academic language proficiency (CALP; Cummins, 1984) in either L1 or L2 may

not be necessary and might not support test score validity any better than other methods. These individuals will have language profile 3, 6, or 9, and the rationale is that because they have developed CALP, the attenuating influence of the linguistic demands of any given tests is reduced and becomes a lesser (but certainly not a negligible) concern in testing.

The second assessment modality described in the MAMBI is assessment that is conducted primarily in L1. Use of this approach seeks to measure an individual's abilities in L1 in cases where it is felt that measurement in L2 would be difficult or impossible, or where additional information beyond L2 testing is desired. However, this modality presents problems for practitioners who are not bilingual and who lack the capability to administer tests in examinees' L1. They may employ translators/interpreters to assist in the process, but this would represent an alternative approach—modification or adaptation of the testing protocol, which is not equivalent to L1 testing. When considering the major variables, Ochoa and Ortiz (2005) argue that L1 testing will probably be most appropriate (and most likely to produce valid test scores) for individuals who have language profile 3, 6, or 9 (i.e., where L1 is at the fluent level). Because such individuals have developed a high degree of proficiency in their native language, it would imprudent to ignore this development given that it forms a considerable part of their entire linguistic repertoire.

The third modality incorporated into the MAMBI is bilingual assessment. As discussed previously, the term *bilingual assessment* is often misunderstood and is usually applied in cases where testing actually occurs in one language only—L1. The differences between genuinely bilingual assessment and L1 assessment are that in bilingual assessment, the examiner may use both languages in working with the individual, may administer tests in either language, and makes deliberate attempts to integrate findings from performance across tests given in both languages. L1 testing often ignores English development entirely and carries out the evaluation as if the individual were a monolingual L1 speaker. Of course, bilingual assessment can be problematic because there are no actual "bilingual" tests that allow concurrent and simultaneous use of both L1 and L2. Bilingual individuals communicate with spontaneous code switching as desired or needed, and such interaction simply cannot be scripted in a way that would approach natural, conversational interaction. Given this limitation,

FIGURE 22.3. The Ochoa and Ortiz Multidimensional Assessment Model for Bilingual Individuals (MAMBI). Adapted from Rhodes, Ochoa, and Ortiz (2005, p. 171). Copyright 2005 by The Guilford Press. Adapted by permission.

Instructional program/history	Currently in a bilingual education program, in lieu of or in addition to receiving ESL services								Previously in bilingual education program, now receiving English-only or ESL services								All instruction has been in an English-only program with or without ESL services							
Current grade	K–4				5–7				K–4				5–7				K–4				5–7			
Assessment mode	NV	L1	L2	BL	NV	L1	L2	BL	NV	L1	L2	BL	NV	L1	L2	BL	NV	L1	L2	BL	NV	L1	L2	BL
Language profile 1 L1 minimal/L2 minimal	(✓)	✓		✓	(✓)	✓	✓	✓	(✓)	✓	✓	✓	(✓)	✓	✓	✓	(✓)		✓*	✓	(✓)		✓	✓
Language profile 2 L1 emergent/L2 minimal	(✓)	✓		✓	(✓)	✓	✓	✓	(✓)	✓	✓	✓	(✓)	✓	✓	✓	(✓)	✓	✓*	✓				
Language profile 3 L1 fluent/L2 minimal		(✓)				(✓)	✓			(✓)				(✓)	✓									
Language profile 4 L1 minimal/L2 emergent	(✓)	✓		✓	(✓)	✓	✓	✓	(✓)	✓	✓	✓	(✓)	✓	✓	✓	(✓)	✓	✓#	✓	(✓)	✓	✓	✓
Language profile 5 L1 emergent/L2 emergent	(✓)	✓		✓	(✓)	✓	✓	✓	(✓)	✓	✓	✓	(✓)	✓	✓	✓	(✓)	✓	✓#	✓	(✓)	✓	✓	✓
Language profile 6 L1 fluent/L2 emergent					(✓)	(✓)	✓	✓					(✓)	(✓)	✓	✓								
Language profile 7 L1 minimal/L2 fluent																								
Language profile 8 L1 emergent/L2 fluent					(✓)		✓						(✓)		✓									
Language profile 9 L1 fluent/L2 fluent					(✓)																			

CALP level 1–2 = minimal proficiency; CALP level 3 = emergent proficiency; CALP level 4–5 = fluent level of proficiency.

NV = Assessment conducted primarily in a nonverbal manner with English-language-reduced/acculturation-reduced measures.

L1 = Assessment conducted in the first language learned by the individual (i.e., native or primary language).

L2 = Assessment conducted in the second language learned by the individual, which in most cases refers to English.

BL = Assessment conducted relatively equally in both languages learned by the individual (i.e., the native language and English).

■ = Combinations of language development and instruction that are improbable or due to other factors (e.g., Saturday school, foreign-born adoptees, delayed school entry).

(✓) = Recommended mode of assessment that should take priority over other modes and that is most likely to be the most accurate estimate of the student's true abilities.

✓ = Secondary or optional mode of assessment that may provide additional valuable information, but that is likely to result in an underestimate of the student's abilities.

✓* = This mode of assessment is not recommended for students in K–2, but may be informative in 3–4; however, results are likely to be an underestimate of true ability.

✓# = This mode of assessment is not recommended for students in K–1, but may be informative in 2–4; however, results are likely to be an underestimate of true ability.

Ochoa and Ortiz (2005) recommend bilingual assessment as the testing modality primarily for individuals with language profile 9 (L1 fluent/L2 fluent) and as a secondary option for those with language profiles 1, 2, and 5, where both languages are at low and relatively similar levels of development. Individuals with these profiles have yet to develop CALP in either L1 or L2. Depending on their educational experiences, the total verbal repertoire of individuals with language profile 1, 2, or 5 may be shared across L1 and L2. Thus bilingual assessment is the most appropriate modality and the one most likely to produce valid test scores for individuals with these language profiles because it allows them to express themselves in whatever language may be necessary at any given moment or for any particular purpose.

The fourth and last assessment modality incorporated into the MAMBI is assessment in L2 (again, in the United States, English). The approach is straightforward and involves the administration of psychological tests in English. Unfortunately, the many potential problems and impediments to normal language development that occur as a function of type of educational programming and the fact that English *is* L2 and not L1 for these examinees makes this approach to assessment problematic. Consequently, L2 testing is not recommended in the MAMBI as the most appropriate approach for any of the different language profiles, albeit it could certainly be applied without issue for profile 9, in which individuals are equally and highly fluent in both languages. Thus individuals who have reached high levels of L2 proficiency can be considered viable candidates for assessment in L2 that would be considered a reasonably fair estimate of their true functioning. Research has demonstrated, however, that individuals considered to be "proficient" in English still perform at levels below those of their monolingual English-speaking peers, primarily on highly verbal tests (Aguera, 2006; Dynda, 2008; Nieves-Brull, 2006; Sotelo-Dynega, 2007; Tychanska, 2009; Vukovich & Figueroa, 1982). Practitioners are therefore cautioned not to overestimate the validity of results obtained from the use of tests administered in English, even when an individual appears to have a high degree of proficiency in English. As discussed previously, the norms of standardized tests do not provide suitable representation of the different and varied linguistic backgrounds of bilingual individuals, and thus may not be entirely appropriate for use with these populations, including those who now use English predominantly and are fluent in English. Despite the apparent limitations regarding L2 testing, there remain the substantial advantages that have been outlined earlier. Testing in English represents the only approach with a substantial body of research, and it remains accessible to all practitioners, regardless of proficiency in any language other than English. Indeed, it was the issue of difference in the evidence bases of the four approaches that led to the development of the method to be discussed below.

In sum, the MAMBI is a relatively straightforward framework that integrates several important variables affecting decisions regarding the best approach to assessment with bilingual individuals, in order to gather data most likely to be valid. Despite its attempts to simplify consideration of the pertinent variables, however, the MAMBI is not without its limitations. It does not *directly* examine the validity of results obtained from testing conducted on individuals in the manners it specifies. Of course, it is not designed to do so; rather, it is meant to offer a systematic method for selecting an assessment approach that can be defended as much more likely to produce valid results than any other approach. Other issues in assessment, particularly those related to interpretation of results, cannot be directly guided by this method. The presumption of validity remains just that—a presumption—and it is not possible to examine it within the context of this framework. Thus a practitioner's ability to generate fair and equitable estimates of actual ability is bolstered only by the systematicity inherent in the selection process provided by the MAMBI. That is, decisions are not made in a random manner, but through a careful and deliberate process that provides greater systematicity and replicability which better support defensibility. Ochoa and Ortiz (2005) recognize these limitations and caution that their recommendations regarding selection of the most appropriate assessment modality are meant only to assist in reducing, not entirely eliminating, some of the potential discriminatory aspects of assessing bilingual individuals. The degree of validity that may be expected from test results garnered from use of the MAMBI to select an assessment modality is not discernible, and practitioners should be aware of the limitations of any approach they employ, regardless of how appropriate it may appear to be.

The Culture–Language Test Classifications and Culture–Language Interpretive Matrix

We have noted that the MAMBI was designed primarily to address fundamental concerns with data validity relative to selection of assessment modality. Once the approach most likely to yield valid results has been determined, practitioners must still wrestle with the knowledge that validity has not been examined directly and that data interpretation may still prove inequitable and discriminatory. Without any confidence in the validity of obtained test results, interpretations will always be largely speculative. There is simply no way the evaluator can be certain that what has been measured is actual ability and not some other construct (e.g., level of acculturation or L2 proficiency). As noted earlier, the familiar refrain "difference versus disorder" elegantly captures the dilemma regarding test score validity, which is the heart of the matter in the evaluation of culturally and linguistically diverse individuals. If test scores are believed to be valid, low performance may then be interpreted as possibly reflecting the lack of an ability or attribute. If test scores are not believed to be valid, low performance may then be interpreted as a reflection of the influence of cultural and linguistic differences. The manner in which this fundamental question may be addressed is the purpose and intent of the Culture–Language Test Classifications (C-LTC) and the Culture–Language Interpretive Matrix (C-LIM).

The Culture–Language Test Classifications

Development of the C-LTC (Flanagan et al., 2000, 2007; Flanagan & Ortiz, 2001; McGrew & Flanagan, 1998) and the C-LIM (Flanagan & Ortiz, 2001; Flanagan et al., 2007; Ortiz, 2001, 2004; Ortiz & Flanagan, 1998) was spurred by the need to consider the "difference versus disorder" question, as well as by the wealth of research available on the performance of bilingual individuals tested in English. The C-LTC was initially developed as an extension of the Cattell–Horn–Carroll (CHC) theoretical classifications presented as the basis of the CHC cross-battery assessment and interpretive approach (Flanagan et al., 2000; McGrew & Flanagan, 1998). The C-LIM evolved shortly afterwards as a further refinement of the C-LTC designed specifically to aid in interpretation by allowing practitioners to assess whether or not what is measured is due primarily to the influence of cultural or linguistic variables (Flanagan & Ortiz, 2001; Flanagan et al., 2007; Mpofu & Ortiz, 2009; Ortiz, 2001, 2004; Ortiz & Dynda, 2010). Although the C-LTC and the C-LIM were initially linked to the CHC cross-battery approach, they can be used independently, and their utility does not depend on the use or application of any particular assessment procedure. Whereas the MAMBI

is intended to guide the selection of an appropriate test modality, the C-LTC and C-LIM are designed to evaluate whether obtained test results are either valid (permitting interpretation) or invalid (thereby precluding interpretation).

In an appeal for less discriminatory practices, Figueroa (1990a, 1990b) suggested that application of defensible theoretical frameworks in the assessment of culturally and linguistically diverse individuals was an important avenue to explore. In addition, he admonished practitioners to pay particular attention to the cultural and linguistic dimensions of tests that were often ignored or misunderstood in evaluation. In response to such issues, Ortiz and Flanagan (1998), Flanagan and Ortiz (2001), and Flanagan and colleagues (2000) developed the C-LTC, essentially a classification system for cognitive ability tests based on two critical test dimensions—degree of cultural loading and degree of linguistic demand. These two dimensions were deliberately selected because they have been identified as factors that have a significant and powerful relationship to test performance and can render results invalid for individuals who are culturally and linguistically diverse (Figueroa, 1990a, 1990b; Sandoval et al., 1998; Valdés & Figueroa, 1994). What establishes the C-LTC as an evidence-based practice is the fact that the initial and some of the subsequent test classifications were and continue to be drawn directly from actual research on bilingual persons tested in English. By using the comparative subtest means available for such groups (see Table 22.1), one can easily sort tests into categories that correspond to the three basic classification levels (low, moderate, high) used for both dimensions of the C-LTC framework. It bears repeating that the classifications are data-driven, organized by the available empirical studies on the testing of bilingual individuals in English. In cases where no such data exist, classifications have been made via an expert consensus procedure as well as by examination of task characteristics, manner of administration, and construct for which the subtest was designed to measure. Given the extent to which ability tests establish validity via correlations with other ability tests and via factor-analytic methods, test classifications based on this information also represent an application of research.

The manner in which standardized, norm-referenced tests included in the C-LTC are organized represents a departure from the more common organization related to the theoretical constructs to be measured. The C-LTC categorizes tests only by the degree to which subtest means indicate that bilingual examinees' performance is attenuated: High attenuation earns classification in the high category, moderate attenuation suggests the moderate category, and little attenuation points to the low category. Classification of tests in this manner is meant to reflect the degree of cultural loading and the extent of linguistic demand that are embedded in a particular subtest and that are responsible for the degree of test score attenuation. In effect, the organization of the C-LTC provides a unique frame of reference from which to view test performance. An example of the C-LTC for various subtests of the Woodcock–Johnson III Tests of Cognitive Abilities (WJ III COG; Woodcock, McGrew, & Mather, 2001) is presented in Figure 22.4.

As is evident in Figure 22.4, the C-LTC is organized as a matrix, with degree of cultural loading along the vertical axis and degree of linguistic demand along the horizontal axis. Each variable is subdivided into three levels (low, moderate, and high) that are intended to distinguish the classifications further. In the resulting 3×3 matrix, the nine cells contain tests that share a particular combination of cultural loading and linguistic demand. The classifications are not based on cognitive ability constructs; that is, two tests within the same cell are not there because they measure the same thing (e.g., visual processing), but rather because research has indicated that they appear to share similar levels of cultural loading and linguistic demand, as manifested in comparable subtest means. Subtests classified as high along both dimensions have relatively lower means, and

those classified as low along both dimensions have relatively higher means. A notable feature of the C-LTC is that the arrangement of the tests is dynamic and easily altered to be consistent with new research on the performance of bilingual individuals as it may emerge. Recently, for example, Kranzler, Flores, and Coady (2010) suggested that the current classifications for the WJ III COG subtests appeared somewhat inconsistent with data gathered in their study. This conclusion appears to have been based on the mistaken notion that the classifications imply statistically significant differences between subtests classified in one cell or in one category versus another. Rather, the C-LTC only provides a guide to the order in which performance may be expected to decline as a function of increasing cultural loading and linguistic demands of the tests. The C-LTC for the WJ III COG, as illustrated in Figure 22.4, thus suggests the following order from highest to lowest value for the first seven subtests of the Standard Battery: Spatial Relations, Numbers Reversed, Visual Matching, Concept Formation, Visual–Auditory Learning, Sound Blending, and Verbal Comprehension. The order of means found by Kranzler and colleagues was actually Spatial Relations, Numbers Reversed, Visual Matching, Concept Formation, Sound Blending, Visual–Auditory Learning, and Verbal Comprehension. The order of means found by Sotelo-Dynega (2007) was Sound Blending, Spatial Relations, Visual–Auditory Learning, Visual Matching, Numbers Reversed, Concept Formation, and Verbal Comprehension. Thus the lone exception to the order of classifications provided

		Degree of linguistic demand		
		Low	Moderate	High
Degree of cultural loading	Low	Spatial Relations (Gv-VZ, Sr)	Visual Matching (Gs-P,R9) Numbers Reversed (Gsm-MW)	Concept Formation (Gf-I) Analysis Synthesis (Gf-RG) Auditory Working Memory (Gsm-MM)
	Moderate	Picture Recognition (Gv-MV) Planning (Gv-SS) Pair Cancellation (Gs-R9)	Visual–Auditory Learning (Glr-MA) Delayed Recall—Visual–Auditory Learning (Glr-MA) Retrieval Fluency (Glr-FI) Rapid Picture Naming (Glr-NA)	Memory For Words (Gsm-MS) Incomplete Words (Ga-PC) Sound Blending (Ga-PC) Auditory Attention (Ga-US/U3) Decision Speed (Gs-R4)
	High			Verbal Comprehension (Gc-VL,LD) General Knowledge (Gc-KO)

FIGURE 22.4. The Culture–Language Test Classifications (C-LTC) matrix for the WJ III: Tests of Cognitive Abilities.

in the C-LTC was Visual–Auditory Learning. All other means followed precisely the order specified by the C-LTC. For various reasons (notably sample size and characteristics—subjects in the Kranzler et al. study tended to be older, with an average age of 11), whether or not the classification for the Visual–Auditory Learning subtest needs changing is not clear from the Kranzler and colleagues (2010) study. Nevertheless, the best classification for the Visual–Auditory Learning subtest will eventually be discerned by and based on additional research.

It was initially thought that the C-LTC would allow practitioners to select tests measuring a particular construct that would have the best chance of producing valid data. Naturally, this meant selecting tests that were classified as low in cultural loading and linguistic demand. As discussed previously, individuals who have had less opportunity for learning about mainstream U.S. culture, or who have a different level of English-language proficiency from that of same-age or grade-peers who are native speakers, tend to obtain lower scores than the individuals on whom virtually all tests are typically normed (Aguera, 2006; Dynda, 2008; Figueroa, 1990a, 1990b; Hamayan & Damico, 1991; Jensen, 1974; Mercer, 1979; Nieves-Brull, 2006; Sotelo-Dynega, 2007; Tychanska, 2009; Valdés & Figueroa, 1994). Consequently, scores for diverse individuals are expected to be better approximations of true ability on tests that are lower in cultural loading and linguistic demand, and poorer estimates of true ability on tests that are higher in cultural loading and linguistic demand. Unfortunately, use of the C-LTC in selecting tests for administration runs up against the very same problems identified in the use of the MAMBI. Despite using research to guide the classifications, the presumption of validity remains a question not answerable by simply selecting tests that are low in cultural content and linguistic demands. In addition, it quickly became apparent that some abilities, particularly those related to language skills and verbal ability, simply could not be measured through tests that were culturally or linguistically reduced or classified as low on both dimensions. The problem of "difference versus disorder" remained, and it was not until the development of the C-LIM (Flanagan & Ortiz, 2001; Flanagan et al., 2007) that this issue was more fully addressed.

The Culture–Language Interpretive Matrix

The classification of tests on the C-LIM according to shared levels of cultural loading and linguistic demand helped to identify tests that might result in the fairest estimates of true ability for culturally and linguistically diverse individuals. But this turned out to be only one benefit of the manner in which the tests were organized. In reviewing the decades of research on the test performance of bilingual individuals, Flanagan and colleagues (2007) realized that the arrangement of the classifications meant that tests contained in the upper left cell of the C-LIM (low cultural loading/low linguistic demand) would collectively produce a much higher aggregate score than tests classified in the lower right cell (high cultural loading/high linguistic demand). Data from numerous studies supported not only the classifications themselves, but also the nature of expected patterns of performance for diverse individuals (Aguera, 2006; Brigham, 1923; Cummins, 1984; Dynda, 2008; Figueroa, 1990a; Gould, 1996; Jensen, 1974, 1976, 1980; Nieves-Brull, 2006; Sanchez, 1932, 1934; Sotelo-Dynega, 2007; Tychanska, 2009; Valdés & Figueroa, 1994; Vukovich & Figueroa, 1982; Yerkes, 1921). This pattern is illustrated in Figure 22.5, which depicts the C-LIM.

Although placed in an orthogonal arrangement, the two dimensions in Figure 22.5 are in fact highly correlated because it is not entirely appropriate to separate the effects of culture from language and vice versa. Nevertheless, the arrows in the illustration depict the three possible ways in which the test results of diverse individuals may be attenuated. First, test performance may decrease primarily as a function of the increasing cultural loading of tests. Second, test performance may decrease largely as a function of the increasing linguistic demands of tests. And finally, test performance may decrease as a function of the combination of cultural loading and linguistic demand. In practice and research, however, there has not been significant evidence of a singular effect for either culture or language, with the exception that strong, primary language effects have been seen in culturally and linguistically diverse children who also have significant speech–language disorders (Aziz, 2010; Lella, 2010; Tychanska, 2009). Therefore, except for some specific occasions, interpretation of the pattern of test performance via the C-LIM should be limited to examination of the combined effect of both dimensions and not focused on the singular influence of either one alone. This information, coupled with knowledge regarding an individual's cultural and linguistic experience, makes it possible to accomplish defensible interpretation through analysis of the patterns formed by test data collected over the past century.

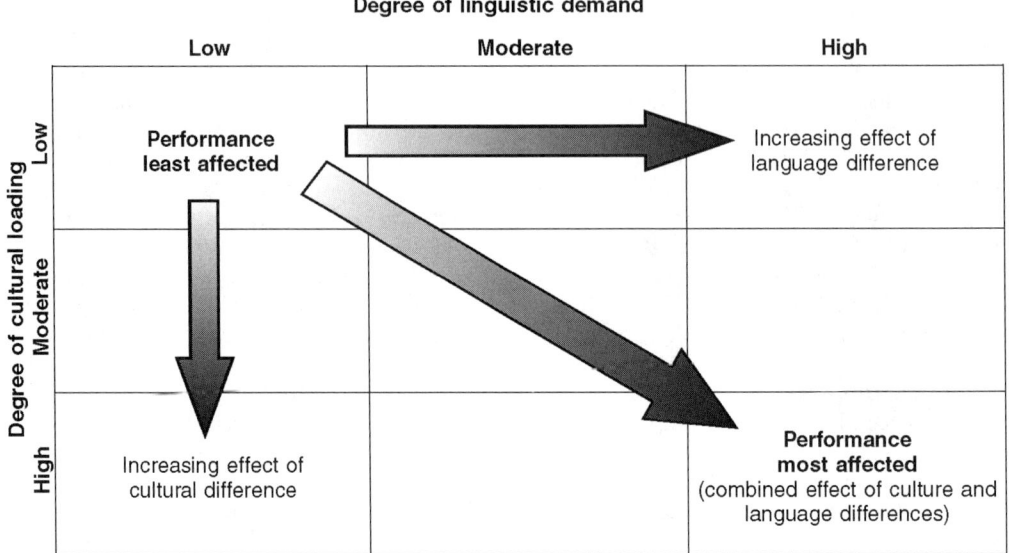

FIGURE 22.5. The Culture–Language Interpretive Matrix (C-LIM): General pattern of expected performance for culturally and linguistically diverse children. From Flanagan and Ortiz (2001). Copyright 2001 by John Wiley & Sons. Adapted by permission.

The value of understanding this declining pattern of performance lies in its empirical base, which provides predictability not only for diverse groups, but also for diverse individuals. The research on the test performance of bilingual individuals reflects a linear and continuous decline in performance on tests as a function of their cultural content and linguistic demands. For example, apart from their examination of the classification of the WJ III COG subtests, Kranzler and colleagues (2010) conducted additional analyses and concluded that a "statistically significant (decreasing) trend was observed for the effect of linguistic demand and cultural loading combined" (p. 431). Despite their concerns stemming primarily from expectations of statistically significant differences, their investigation provides a current, independent replication of the robust, linearly declining performance of bilingual examinees as subtests increase their demands for acquired cultural knowledge and developmental language proficiency.

In short, the Kranzler and colleagues (2010) study reinforces the very foundations upon which the C-LIM is built and the principles that guide examination of test score validity. To evaluate issues of validity, an individual's obtained subtest scores are classified within the cells specified by the C-LTC and are then aggregated to create values across the matrix. These mean values then permit closer examination and, more importantly, comparison against the means obtained for other bilingual examinees as reported in the literature. For example, if the pattern of aggregate scores within the matrix approximates the declining pattern of scores (in terms of both magnitude and rate of decline) derived from the literature, the results can be said to be invalid, in that they are reflecting primarily the influence of cultural and linguistic influences—not the constructs the subtests were intended to measure. Conversely, if the pattern of aggregate scores within the matrix does not approximate the pattern of scores derived from the literature (i.e., the magnitude of scores is lower than the range predicted, or there is an absence of systematic decline as linguistic and cultural demands increase), then the results can be said to be valid, in that they are reflecting the primary influence of a variable or variables other than those related to cultural or linguistic differences. Use of the term *primary* is important here because cultural and linguistic differences may never be completely absent in such cases and may well be contributory factors in almost all situations where bilingual examinees are concerned. However, identification of any potential deficits must be made on the basis of performance that cannot be attributed primarily to cultural or linguistic difference. This is where the C-LIM provides significant utility to practitioners. Failure to identify a clear pattern of decline within the expected range for bilingual individuals implies that cultural or linguistic factors cannot be viewed as the primary or only factors affecting the results (although they may be contributing to some part of the pattern), and this strongly suggests that the test results are valid.

However, an extremely important caveat in using the C-LIM is that many other variables may be affecting test score performance apart from the possibility of cognitive deficits or disorder (e.g., lack of motivation, emotional disturbance, incorrect scoring or administration). As such, the lack of a declining pattern does not automatically indicate disorder, and any diagnosis involving deficient ability must be made by excluding other potential explanations and making use of corroborating data. In any event, the C-LIM appears to provide a solid, evidence-based method for establishing test score validity and helps practitioners ask and answer the question of "difference versus disorder." Moreover, two particular advantages of the C-LIM make it exceedingly practical. First, the use of testing in English allows it to remain accessible to all practitioners; second, once applied to evaluate the validity of obtained test scores, it permits use of any interpretive method, schema, or framework with which a practitioner may already be familiar or comfortable. Thus, apart from learning how to use and apply it, the C-LIM does not require alteration of procedures that virtually every practitioner already knows and uses.

A complete discussion of the MAMBI, C-LTC, or C-LIM is beyond the scope of this chapter. The reader is referred to the original sources for better and more detailed guidance on their use and application in testing practices. In addition, despite the research base upon which these approaches have been developed, none of them should be relied upon as the only method for establishing validity and making defensible interpretations. Rather, all of these approaches are intended to supplement those assessment and evaluation practices already in use by practitioners. They are designed and intended to bring more rigor and defensibility to current testing practices, not to replace them entirely. When used in conjunction with other relevant assessment data and information (e.g., direct observations, review of records, interviews, language proficiency testing, socioeconomic status, developmental data, family history, etc.), these methods should assist in bringing assessment and testing procedures into accordance with current calls for evidence-based practice.

SUMMARY

As noted at the outset, the purpose of this chapter has been to present a discussion of the main issues facing practitioners who seek to evaluate the cognitive abilities of diverse individuals in a manner that integrates research and results in evidence-based practice. Fair and equitable assessment is accomplished via recognition of the nature and sources of potential bias, and by application of methods and procedures that are specifically designed to ensure validity. Toward that end, cognitive assessment of culturally and linguistically diverse individuals must move beyond traditional practices that lack defensibility or utility in addressing problems with validity, and must dispense with simplistic notions that recognition of a verbal–nonverbal pattern is sufficient. Integration of research into practice appears to necessitate a good grasp of the basic influences on test performance, including developmentally based cultural and linguistic differences and their relation to various aspects of tests and testing (such as norm sample representation, degree and patterns of score attenuation, and test characteristics and demands). Existing approaches lack sufficient empirical support to stand alone as viable or defensible evidence-based practice; they require supplementation via emerging methods that are designed specifically to examine issues of validity. Without application of frameworks that permit direct inspection of score validity, use of any particular approach—whether testing in an examinee's native language, testing in English, nonverbal testing, modified/adapted testing, or any combination of them—will remain limited in the extent to which the obtained results can be interpreted validly as measures or estimates of true ability. Success in these endeavors may be facilitated by emerging, research-based techniques, including the MAMBI and the C-LTC/C-LIM. Such approaches appear to hold significant promise for elevating current assessment practices to meet the call for evidence-based assessment.

Whether current practitioners and researchers realize it or not, differences in the cultural and linguistic backgrounds and experiences of diverse individuals have always posed and will continue to pose serious threats to the validity and meaning of test results. As we have discussed, the type of bias that stems from such differences is not related to any technical or psychometric flaws within the tests themselves, but primarily to violations of the assumption of comparability. Individuals whose cultural/linguistic development differs from that of their same-age or same-grade monolingual English-speaking peers cannot be held to the same expectations, as is the case when performance standards are based on mainstream, monolingual English speakers. Questions regarding validity are crucial, if not central, to the task of evaluating individuals from diverse cultural and linguistic backgrounds. And such complicated questions will not be answered via simple prescriptions. The complex nature of bilingualism and level of acculturation are such that practitioners should not expect that the question of how to conduct nondiscriminatory assessment can ever be reduced to the question of what is the "right" test to use. Sattler (1992) notes:

> Probably no test can be created that will entirely eliminate the influence of learning and cultural experiences. The test content and materials, the language in which the questions are phrased, the test directions, the categories for classifying the responses, the scoring criteria, and the validity criteria are all culture bound. (p. 579)

At the core of any evaluation lies the question of validity and this issue, more than any other, will require significant attention and scrutiny because it alone provides the defensible foundation upon which meaning can be ascribed confidently to obtained results.

REFERENCES

Aguera, F. (2006). *How language and culture impact test performance on the Differential Ability Scale in a preschool population.* Unpublished manuscript, St. John's University.

American Educational Research Association (AERA), American Psychological Association (APA), & National Council on Measurement in Education (NCME). (1999). *Standards for educational and psychological testing.* Washington, DC: AERA.

American Psychological Association (APA). (1990). *Guidelines for providers of psychological services to ethnic, linguistic, and culturally diverse populations.* Washington, DC: Author.

Aziz, N. (2010). *English language learners with global cognitive impairment: Evaluation of patterns within the Culture–Language Interpretive Matrix.* Unpublished doctoral dissertation, St. John's University.

Braden, J. P., & Iribarren, J. A. (2007). Test review: Wechsler, D. (2005). Wechsler Intelligence Scale for Children—Fourth Edition, Spanish. *Journal of Psychoeducational Assessment, 25,* 292–299.

Brigham, C. C. (1923). *A study of American intelligence.* Princeton, NJ: Princeton University Press.

Brigham, C. C. (1930). Intelligence tests of immigrant groups. *Psychological Review, 37,* 158–165.

Brody, N. (1997). Intelligence, schooling, and society. *American Psychologist, 52,* 1046–1050.

Carroll, J. B. (1993). *Human cognitive abilities.* New York: Cambridge University Press.

Cummins, J. C. (1984). *Bilingual and special education: Issues in assessment and pedagogy.* Austin, TX: PRO-ED.

Dynda, A. M. (2008). *The relation between language proficiency and IQ test performance.* Unpublished manuscript, St. John's University.

Figueroa, R. A. (1983). Test bias and Hispanic children. *Journal of Special Education, 17,* 431–440.

Figueroa, R. A. (1989). Psychological testing of linguistic-minority students: Knowledge gaps and regulations. *Exceptional Children, 56,* 145–152.

Figueroa, R. A. (1990a). Assessment of linguistic minority group children. In C. R. Reynolds & R. W. Kamphaus (Eds.), *Handbook of psychological and educational assessment of children: Intelligence and achievement* (pp. 691–696). New York: Guilford Press.

Figueroa, R. A. (1990b). Best practices in the assessment of bilingual children. In A. Thomas & J. Grimes (Eds.), *Best practices in school psychology II* (pp. 93–106). Washington, DC: National Association of School Psychologists.

Flanagan, D. P., McGrew, K. S., & Ortiz, S. O. (2000). *The Wechsler intelligence scales and Gf-Gc theory: A contemporary approach to interpretation.* Boston: Allyn & Bacon.

Flanagan, D. P., & Ortiz, S. O. (2001). *Essentials of cross-battery assessment.* New York: Wiley.

Flanagan, D. P., Ortiz, S., & Alfonso, V. C. (2007). *Essentials of cross-battery assessment* (2nd ed.). New York: Wiley.

Flanagan, D. P., Ortiz, S., Alfonso, V. C., & Mascolo, J. (2006). *The Achievement Test Desk Reference (ATDR)—Second Edition: A guide to learning disability identification.* New York: Wiley.

Goddard, H. H. (1913). The Binet tests in relation to immigration. *Journal of Psycho-Asthenics, 18,* 105–107.

Goldenberg, C. (2008). Teaching English language learners: What the research does and does not say. *American Educator, 32*(2), 8–11.

Gould, S. J. (1996). *The mismeasure of man.* New York: Norton.

Gustafsson, J.-E., & Undheim, J. O. (1996). Individual

differences in cognitive functions. In D. Berliner & R. Calfee (Eds.), *Handbook of educational psychology* (pp. 186–242). New York: Macmillan.

Hamayan, E. V., & Damico, J. S. (1991). *Limiting bias in the assessment of bilingual students.* Austin, TX: Pro-Ed.

Harris, J. G., & Llorente, A. M. (2005). Cultural considerations in the use of the Wechsler Intelligence Scale—Fourth Edition (WISC-IV). In A. Prifitera, D. H. Saklofske, & L. G. Weiss (Eds.), *WISC-IV clinical use and interpretation: Scientist-practitioner perspectives* (pp. 381–413). Burlington, MA: Elsevier.

Jensen, A. R. (1974). How biased are culture-loaded tests? *Genetic Psychology Monographs, 90,* 185–244.

Jensen, A. R. (1976). Construct validity and test bias. *Phi Delta Kappan, 58,* 340–346.

Jensen, A. R. (1980). *Bias in mental testing.* New York: Free Press.

Kranzler, J. H., Flores, C. G., & Coady, M. (2010). Examination of the cross-battery approach for the cognitive assessment of children and youth from diverse linguistic and cultural backgrounds. *School Psychology Review, 39*(3), 431–446.

Lella, S. (2010). *Evaluating speech–language and cognitive impairment patterns via the Culture–Language Interpretive Matrix.* Unpublished doctoral dissertation, St. John's University.

Llorente, E., & Sheingold, D. (2010, September 15). Minorities now nearly half of Bergen County children, and just over half in the state. *Passaic County News.*

Lohman, D. F., Korb, K., & Lakin, J. (2008). Identifying academically gifted English language learners using nonverbal tests: A comparison of the Raven, NNAT, and CogAT. *Gifted Child Quarterly, 52,* 275–296.

Lopez, E. C. (1997). The cognitive assessment of limited English proficient and bilingual children. In D. P. Flanagan, J. L. Genshaft, & P. L. Harrison (Eds.), *Contemporary intellectual assessment: Theories, tests, and issues* (pp. 503–516). New York: Guilford Press.

Lopez, E. C. (2002). Best practices in working with school interpreters to deliver psychological services to children and families. In A. Thomas & J. Grimes (Eds.), *Best practices in school psychology IV* (pp. 1419–1432). Bethesda, MD: National Association of School Psychologists.

McCallum, R. S., & Bracken, B. A. (1997). The Universal Nonverbal Intelligence Test. In D. P. Flanagan, J. L. Genshaft, & P. L. Harrison (Eds.), *Contemporary intellectual assessment: Theories, tests, and issues* (pp. 268–280). New York: Guilford Press.

McGrew, K. S., & Flanagan, D. P. (1998). *The intelligence test desk reference (ITDR): Gf-Gc cross-battery assessment.* Boston: Allyn & Bacon.

McShane, D. (1980). A review of scores of American Indian children on the Wechsler intelligence scales. *White Cloud Journal, 1,* 3–10.

Mercer, J. R. (1979). *System of multicultural pluralistic assessment: Technical manual.* New York: The Psychological Corporation.

Mpofu, E., & Ortiz, S. O. (2009). Equitable assessment practices in diverse contexts. In E. L. Grigorenko (Ed.), *Assessment of abilities and competencies in the era of globalization* (pp. 41–76). New York: Springer.

Naglieri, J. A. (1982). Does the WISC-R measure verbal intelligence for non-English speaking children? *Psychology in the Schools, 19,* 478–479.

Neisser, U., Boodoo, G., Bouchard, T. J., Boykin, A. W., Brody, N., Ceci, S. J., et al. (1996). Intelligence: Knowns and unknowns. *American Psychologist, 51,* 77–101.

Nieves-Brull, A. (2006). *Evaluation of the Culture–Language Matrix: A validation study of test performance in monolingual English speaking and bilingual English/Spanish speaking populations.* Unpublished manuscript, St. John's University.

Oakland, T. (Ed.). (1976). *Nonbiased assessment of minority group children.* Lexington, KY: Coordinating Office for Regional Resource Centers.

Oakland, T., & Laosa, L. (1976). Professional, legislative, and judicial influences on psychoeducational assessment practices in schools. In T. Oakland (Ed.), *Nonbiased assessment of minority group children.* Lexington, KY: Coordinating Office for Regional Resource Centers.

Ochoa, S. H., & Ortiz, S. O. (2005). Cognitive assessment of culturally and linguistically diverse individuals: An integrative approach. In R. L. Rhodes, S. H. Ochoa, & S. O. Ortiz (Eds.), *Assessing culturally and linguistically diverse individuals: A practical guide* (pp. 168–201). New York: Guilford Press.

Ochoa, S. H., Riccio, C. A., Jimenez, S., Garcia de Alba, R., & Sines, M. (2004). Psychological assessment of limited English proficient and/or bilingual students: An investigation of school psychologists' current practices. *Journal of Psychoeducational Assessment, 22,* 93–105.

Ormrod, J. E. (2008). *Educational psychology: Developing learners* (6th ed.). Upper Saddle River, NJ: Pearson/Merrill/Prentice Hall.

Ortiz, S. O. (2001). Assessment of cognitive abilities in Hispanic children. *Seminars in Speech and Language, 22*(1), 17–37.

Ortiz, S. O. (2004). Use of the WISC-IV with culturally and linguistically diverse populations. In D. P. Flanagan & A. S. Kaufman (Eds.), *Essentials of WISC-IV assessment* (pp. 183–215). Hoboken, NJ: Wiley.

Ortiz, S. O. (2008). Best practices in nondiscriminatory assessment. In A. Thomas & J. Grimes (Eds.), *Best practices in school psychology V* (pp. 661–678). Bethesda, MD: National Association of School Psychologists.

Ortiz, S. O., & Dynda, A. M. (2010). Diversity, fairness, utility and social issues. In E. Mpofu & T. Oakland (Eds.), *Assessment in rehabilitation and health* (pp. 37–55). Upper Saddle River, NJ: Merrill.

Ortiz, S. O., & Flanagan, D. P. (1998). Gf-Gc cross-battery interpretation and selective cross-battery assessment: Referral concerns and the needs of culturally and linguistically diverse populations. In K. S. McGrew & D. P. Flanagan, *The intelligence test desk reference (ITDR): Gf-Gc cross-battery assessment* (pp. 401–444). Boston: Allyn & Bacon.

Ortiz, S. O., & Flanagan, D. P. (2002). Best practices in working with culturally and linguistically diverse children and families, In A. Thomas & J. Grimes (Eds.), *Best practices in school psychology IV* (pp. 1351–1372). Bethesda, MD: National Association of School Psychologists.

Reynolds, C. R. (2000). Why is psychometric research on bias in mental testing so often ignored? *Psychology, Public Policy, and Law, 6*, 144–150.

Reynolds, C. R., & Kamphaus, R. W. (Eds.). (1990). *Handbook of psychological and educational assessment of children: Personality, behavior, and context.* New York: Guilford Press.

Reynolds, C. R., & Ramsay, M. C. (2003). Bias in psychological assessment: An empirical review and recommendations. In I. B. Weiner (Series Ed.) & J. R. Graham & J. A. Naglieri (Vol. Eds.), *Handbook of psychology: Vol. 10. Assessment psychology* (pp. 67–94). Hoboken, NJ: Wiley.

Rhodes, R., Ochoa, S. H., & Ortiz, S. O. (2005). *Assessing culturally and linguistically diverse students: A practical guide.* New York: Guilford Press.

Salvia, J., & Ysseldyke, J. (1991). *Assessment in special and remedial education* (5th ed.). Boston: Houghton Mifflin.

Sanchez, G. I. (1932). Group differences and Spanish-speaking children: A critical review. *Journal of Applied Psychology, 16*, 549–558.

Sanchez, G. I. (1934). Bilingualism and mental measures: A word of caution. *Journal of Applied Psychology, 18*, 756–772.

Sandoval, J. (1979). The WISC-R and internal evidence of test bias with minority groups. *Journal of Consulting and Clinical Psychology, 47*, 919–927.

Sandoval, J., Frisby, C. L., Geisinger, K. F., Scheuneman, J. D., & Grenier, J. R. (Eds.). (1998). *Test interpretation and diversity: Achieving equity in assessment.* Washington, DC: American Psychological Association.

Sattler, J. M. (1992). *Assessment of children* (3rd ed.). San Diego, CA: Author.

Sattler, J. M. (2001). *Assessment of children: Behavioral and clinical applications* (4th ed.). San Diego, CA: Author.

Smith, D. (2008, August 7). Minority children become majority. *Washington Post.*

Sotelo-Dynega, M. (2007). *Cognitive performance and the development of English language proficiency.* Unpublished doctoral dissertation, St. John's University.

Sotelo-Dynega, M., Cuskley, T., Geddes, L., McSwiggan, K., & Soldano, A. (2011). *Cognitive assessment: A survey of current school psychologists' practices.* Poster presented at the annual conference of the National Association of School Psychologists, San Francisco.

Terman, L. M. (1916). *The uses of intelligence tests.* Boston: Houghton Mifflin.

Tychanska, J. (2009). *Evaluation of speech and language impairment using the Culture–Language Test Classifications and Interpretive Matrix.* Unpublished doctoral dissertation, St. John's University.

U.S. Census Bureau. (2009). Current population survey, released 2009. Retrieved September 25, 2010 from *www.census.gov/cps.*

Valdés, G., & Figueroa, R. A. (1994). *Bilingualism and testing: A special case of bias.* Norwood, NJ: Ablex.

Vukovich, D., & Figueroa, R. A. (1982). *The validation of the system of multicultural pluralistic assessment: 1980–1982.* Unpublished manuscript, University of California at Davis, Department of Education.

Wechsler, D. (2005). *Wechsler Intelligence Scale for Children—Fourth Edition Spanish.* San Antonio, TX: The Psychological Corporation.

Weiss, L. G., Harris, J. G., Prifitera, A., Courville, T., Rolfhus, E., Saklofske, D. H., et al. (2006). WISC-IV interpretation in societal context. In L. G. Weiss, D. H. Saklofske, A. Prifitera, & J. A. Holdnack (Eds.), *WISC-IV advanced clinical interpretation* (pp. 1–58). Burlington, MA: Academic Press/Elsevier.

Woodcock, R. W. (1990). Theoretical foundations of the WJ-R measures of cognitive ability. *Journal of Psychoeducational Assessment, 8*, 231–258.

Woodcock, R. W., McGrew, K. S., & Mather, N. (2001). *Woodcock–Johnson III Tests of Cognitive Abilities.* Itasca, IL: Riverside.

Yerkes, R. M. (1921). Psychological examining in the United States Army. *Memoirs of the National Academy of Sciences, 15*, 1–890.

CHAPTER 23

Linking Cognitive Abilities to Academic Interventions for Students with Specific Learning Disabilities

Nancy Mather
Barbara J. Wendling

Both psychologists and diagnosticians need to know the research that addresses the relationships between cognitive abilities and achievement. An understanding of these relationships helps an evaluator make informed decisions regarding the choice of assessment tools, the type of diagnosis, the selection of accommodations, and the choice of instructional methodologies. In addition, cognitive assessment data are critical for the identification and understanding of specific learning disabilities (SLD). The definition of SLD indicates that a deficit exists in some aspect of basic psychological processing that is affecting learning and interfering with academic progress. Therefore, in this chapter we focus on (1) the cognitive abilities that are most commonly measured by various assessment instruments, (2) the ways these constructs relate to SLD, and (3) the possible instructional implications.

GENERAL ISSUES

Before focusing on how performance on specific cognitive abilities can provide insight into the selection of interventions, we discuss four general issues related to cognitive assessments of students with SLD: (1) the role of response to intervention (RTI) and cognitive assessments; (2) the rationale for understanding the cognitive correlates of an academic area; (3) the need for and provision of differentiated instruction; and (4) the importance of establishing a *pattern of strengths and weaknesses* (PSW) for the determination of SLD.

The Role of RTI and Cognitive Assessments

Within the last decade, the identification procedure for SLD within the U.S. public schools has changed. The reauthorization of the Individuals with Disabilities Education Improvement Act of 2004 (IDEA 2004) has eliminated the requirement of establishing an IQ–achievement discrepancy for determining the presence of SLD and now offers other alternative procedures. One alternative approach is establishing a PSW that suggests the presence of an SLD. Professionals implementing the PSW approach typically use both cognitive and academic assessments, so this group would find linking cognitive results to academic interventions to be of interest. Another alternative approach permits the use of limited response to evidence-based instruction as *part* of the process for determining SLD. This process of documenting progress on interventions has been referred to as RTI. For those embracing an RTI model, the results from cognitive assessments may seem to be irrelevant for both identification and instructional planning.

So times have changed since the publication of the first edition of this book, in which RTI was rarely mentioned. Currently, the number of districts implementing some type of RTI model increases each year. According to the Response to Intervention Adoption Survey 2010 (Spectrum K12 School Solutions, 2010), the percentage of districts responding to the survey that were piloting or implementing RTI programs increased from 24% in 2007 to over 61% in 2010. Within the context of this educational reform, professionals have to consider this question: What is the role of cognitive assessment in the identification and treatment of individuals with SLD? Is there any evidence to support the efficacy of linking cognitive assessment results to academic interventions?

As a result of the RTI movement, professionals have debated the usefulness of cognitive assessments to document the presence of SLD. Some indicate that cognitive assessments are unnecessary (e.g., Fletcher & Vaughn, 2007; Fuchs & Young, 2006; Reschly, 2005); others insist that this type of assessment is essential for an accurate diagnosis (e.g., Flanagan, Ortiz, Alfonso, & Dynda, 2006; Hale, Kaufman, Naglieri, & Kavale, 2006; Wodrich, Spencer, & Daley, 2006). This current debate is a bit reminiscent of the "reading wars" that depicted whole-language versus phonics instruction as an either–or proposition. Eventually, a compromise prevailed, and a "balanced" approach to teaching reading evolved; perhaps this will also occur in the RTI–cognitive assessment debate. In fact, most professionals supporting the role of cognitive assessment also encourage the use of RTI (e.g., Hale et al., 2006). Thus general agreement exists regarding the value of RTI as an instructional model of prevention. The disagreements arise when RTI is suggested for use as the sole identification or diagnostic model for determining the presence of SLD.

Those who argue for the elimination of cognitive testing believe that it adds little value to diagnosing SLD or to planning instruction (e.g., Gresham, 2002; Reschly, 2005; Stanovich, 1991). These beliefs may at least partially stem from the limited information gained from intelligence tests of the past, as well as the procedures that were typically used for identification, such as a determining a discrepancy between a full-scale IQ score and an achievement score. These procedures were mechanistic and placed a focus on the use of a single global score of intelligence, rather than encouraging practitioners to perform a careful analysis of the various factor, cluster, or subtest scores. Today's cognitive assessments themselves, as well as the approaches to assessment, are more theory-based and more diagnostic, helping practitioners explore and document an individual's PSW.

RTI is not a diagnostic model, but rather focuses on analysis of groups or grade levels of students and treats them in the same manner: "One size fits all" (Wodrich et al., 2006). In contrast, special education is focused on addressing the needs of a specific individual: "One size fits one." In order to implement an individualized approach, a clinician must first understand an individual's unique strengths and weaknesses. Thus most psychologists and diagnosticians are shifting their focus from the use of full-scale IQ scores to interpreting an individual's cognitive and academic profiles. For the results of cognitive tests to be useful, the focus must be on obtaining information that is relevant to academic performance and instruction. Even though a student may be deemed ineligible for certain services, all evaluations need to address the referral concerns and propose solutions. As Cruickshank (1977) noted, "Diagnosis must take second place to instruction, and must be a tool of instruction, not an end in itself" (p. 194). Within the field of SLD, the purpose of testing cognitive abilities is to determine a person's unique PSW and identify the underlying cognitive weaknesses that are often directly linked to the specific difficulties in achievement. Therefore, it is important to identify the areas of strength and weakness, in order to individualize educational planning for students who do not respond adequately to intervention (Kavale & Flanagan, 2007). From the perspective of making an accurate SLD diagnosis, understanding *why* a student is not responding adequately does indeed matter, and the results from cognitive assessments often help to provide the necessary insights.

Although these legal changes in identification procedures have created uncertainty and disequilibrium in the field, they have also led to a greater interest in understanding the relationships among cognitive abilities and achievement. Implementation of a simple discrepancy formula for SLD identification was inadequate for determining eligibility and never was sufficient for informing instructional planning. In today's educational world, professionals must assess, explore, and understand an individual's profile of cognitive, linguistic, and academic strengths and weaknesses to inform both eligibility determinations and instructional planning. So, now more than ever, a need exists for understanding how various cognitive abilities are linked to school achievement.

Understanding the Cognitive Correlates of Academic Areas

A growing body of research supports the usefulness of factor or specific ability scores in identifying the cognitive processing problems that specifically inhibit school learning (e.g., Evans, Floyd, McGrew, & Leforgee, 2002; Fiorello, Hale, & Snyder, 2006; Flanagan, Ortiz, Alfonso, & Mascolo, 2006; Gregg, Davis, Coleman, Wisenbaker, & Hoy, 2004; McGrew & Wendling, 2010). As examples in math achievement, Bull and Johnston (1997) found that processing speed was the best predictor of arithmetic competence in 7-year-olds. Also, researchers have identified fluid reasoning as an important correlate of math reasoning (e.g., Geary, Hoard, Byrd-Craven, Nugent, & Numtee, 2007; Hale, Fiorello, Kavanagh, Holdnack, & Aloe, 2007). In reading, Adams (1990) found that a child's level of phonemic awareness in kindergarten was the best predictor of reading success in elementary school. Numerous researchers have confirmed the importance of phonemic awareness to basic reading skills (e.g., Berninger et al., 2006; Cooper, 2006; Shaywitz, Morris, & Shaywitz, 2008; Torgesen, 2002; Vellutino, Tunmer, Jaccard, & Chen, 2007). Others have described the relationship between deficits in rapid automatized naming (RAN) and poor reading skills (e.g., Berninger et al., 2006; Denckla & Rudel, 1974; Swanson, Trainin, Necoechea, & Hammill, 2003; Torgesen, 1997; Wolf, Bowers, & Biddle, 2000). Still others have described the significant relationships between working memory and reading comprehension (e.g., Cooper, 2006; Swanson, 1999, 2000; Torgesen, 2002), as well as between working memory and math problem solving (Swanson, Jerman, & Zheng, 2008). Similar difficulties have been observed in both children and adults. For example, in a recent meta-analysis of reading research, Swanson and Hsieh (2009) found that the cognitive processes of phonological skills, verbal memory, naming speed, and vocabulary all made significant contributions to reading disabilities in adults.

Early identification of students at risk for academic failure continues to be a primary goal of educators, including those in RTI environments. Researchers continue to document the relationships among specific cognitive, linguistic, and academic abilities, identifying prerequisite skills and delineating early indicators of risk. Many investigators have thus encouraged assessment of cognitive abilities to identify children at risk for reading disabilities (e.g., Berninger et al., 2006; Fuchs et al., 2005; Torgesen, 2002). Several relevant cognitive abilities can be assessed before students learn to read, such as phonemic awareness and RAN; at-risk students can thereby be identified at a very young age—even before they experience reading difficulties. Exploring cognitive abilities can also help with establishing a PSW that is relevant to identifying an SLD, trying to understand why a student fails to make adequate progress, and/or planning the most effective instructional programs.

The evolution and refinement of theory- and research-based tests measuring multiple abilities have also given professionals the opportunity to gain a better understanding of an individual's unique characteristics. Hannon and Daneman (2001) described the increasing focus on theory:

> With the advent and dominance of the information-processing approach to cognition, the emphasis has switched from measurement to theory. The goal is no longer simply to quantify individual differences in intellectual tasks, but also to explain the individual differences in terms of the architecture and processes of the human information-processing system. (p. 103)

Need for and Provision of Differentiated Instruction

Responsive teaching is a simple definition of differentiated, prescriptive instruction. Because all students are not alike, a teacher plans varied approaches to address what individual students need to learn, how they will learn it, and how they will demonstrate what they have learned, thus increasing the likelihood that each student will learn as much as possible (Tomlinson, 2006). With the growing diversity of the U.S. population and the increased demand for accountability in education, the need to accommodate the individual learner has intensified in general education.

However, although the concept of meeting individual student needs is widely embraced by educators, many lack the training necessary to implement differentiated instruction (Frieberg, 2002; McNaughton, Hall, & Maccini, 2001; Whitaker, 2001). This lack of teacher preparation stems in part from the failure of teacher training programs to integrate recommended methodologies and strategies into the required courses (Elksmin, 2001; Whitaker, 2001). Thus many teachers do not accommodate the diverse needs of the students in their classrooms; they offer a uniform rather than an individualized approach to instruction (Gable, Hendrickson, Tonelson, & Van Acker, 2000).

Unfortunately, even in special education, many students with individualized education programs (IEPs) receive the same treatment goals and teaching strategies as their normally achieving peers (Reynolds & Lakin, 1987). To explore the implementation of differentiated instruction, Schumm, Moody, and Vaughn (2000) interviewed third-grade teachers who served students with SLD in inclusive classrooms. Overall, the teachers reported using whole-class instruction that included the same materials for all students, regardless of performance levels. All students were expected to read grade-level materials, even if they could not pronounce the words. Furthermore, students with SLD did not receive instruction directed at improving their word analysis skills. One teacher voiced strong opposition to providing instruction in word analysis, stating, "By the time they come to third grade they really should have those skills" (quoted in Schumm et al., 2000, p. 483). With undifferentiated instruction and minimal direct instruction in reading, the students with SLD made little academic improvement, and their attitudes toward reading declined as well.

Historically, the field of SLD has been based on the belief that children differ in their abilities and therefore should be taught and treated differently (Kavale & Forness, 1998; Whitener, 1989); this belief led to the requirement that an IEP must be developed for each child eligible for special education services. A child who has difficulty memorizing information requires a different type of instruction from that for a child who memorizes facts easily. A child who works slowly needs more time than one who works rapidly. A child who struggles to pay attention requires more novelty and structure than one who attends easily. In some cases, these marked differences in learning and behavior are neurologically based (Semrud-Clikeman et al., 2000; Shaywitz, 1998, 2003; Shaywitz et al., 2003). Clearly, for students with SLD, differential, remedial instruction that addresses the source of their problems will be more effective than global approaches that do not (Aaron, 1997).

Determining a PSW

As mentioned previously, IDEA 2004 states that a PSW suggestive of SLD is one method for determining eligibility for special education services. Helping practitioners explore significant intraindividual variations among abilities is precisely how

intelligence tests can contribute to SLD determination and educational planning. As long as interpretation is performed within the context of all data, this type of analysis is supported by the following statement from the *Standards for Educational and Psychological Testing* (American Educational Research Association [AERA], American Psychological Association [APA], & National Council on Measurement in Education [NCME], 1999):

> Because each test in a battery examines a different function, ability, skill, or combination thereof, the test taker's performance can be understood best when scores are not combined or aggregated, but rather when each score is interpreted within the context of all other scores and assessment data. For example, low scores on timed tests alert the examiner to slowed responding as a problem that may not be apparent if scores on different kinds of tests are combined. (p. 123)

Assessments should then focus on understanding a person's information-processing capabilities, including the factors that can facilitate performance. As Gardner (1999) has suggested, in the study of human cognition, awareness of distinctive strengths is of critical importance. Understanding the "constraints" (e.g., limited instruction, specific cognitive or linguistic weaknesses, limited cultural experiences, poor motivation) that affect performance, as well as the multidimensional impact of these constraints (Berninger, 1996), is also important. Because the various constraints affect different aspects of academic functioning, they can help inform the type and extent of accommodations and instruction needed. Interpreting intraindividual variations and determining how these differences affect performance then become the cornerstone for linking the results of cognitive ability tests to meaningful instructional plans. To do this in a valid manner, clinicians must know the existing research on the relationship between cognitive abilities and achievement, and must incorporate that knowledge into their decision-making process.

One basic concept underlying identification of SLD is that a student's difficulty does not extend too far into other domains. In other words, the problem is relatively specific, circumscribed, or domain-specific (Stanovich, 1999). This concept of specificity is not new. For example, Travis (1935) observed that in some students, a striking disparity exists between achievement in one area and achievement in another. For example, a student cannot read, but can comprehend material that is read aloud; or a student excels in reading and writing, but struggles with mathematical concepts and applications. These children, who do not achieve as well as would be expected in one or more areas of performance, may be regarded as having a "special defect or disability" (Travis, 1935, p. 43).

To maintain this concept of specificity, the academic problem is best described as a specific reading disability, math disability, or spelling disability that is presumably caused by weaknesses in specific cognitive or linguistic processes. The first part of an evaluation is then to determine an initial domain-specific classification (Stanovich, 1999); the next part is to identify the deficient cognitive processes that underlie the disorder (Robinson, Menchetti, & Torgesen, 2002). An SLD is caused by one or more inherent weaknesses in underlying cognitive processes (Robinson et al., 2002). The assessment process can then be viewed as an ability-oriented evaluation designed to help formulate the problem and then determine specific interventions (Fletcher, Taylor, Levin, & Satz, 1995).

COGNITIVE ABILITIES AND ACADEMIC PERFORMANCE

An important goal of education reform is to promote the early and accurate identification of at-risk students. This desire for early identification fuels the research into the causes of academic failure and seeks to determine the predictive value of specific cognitive and linguistic factors that may be considered "precursors to manifest disabilities" (Fletcher et al., 2002, p. 51). Ideally, a predictor or subset of predictors will accurately differentiate between the children who will struggle with certain academic subjects and those who will not, so that intervention efforts can be initiated early in a timely fashion (Bishop, 2003).

As noted previously, a growing body of research links certain cognitive and linguistic factors to the various domains of achievement. The relationships between certain cognitive abilities and academic performance are well established (e.g., phonemic awareness and decoding), whereas others are not (e.g., visual processing and reading). Furthermore, some important cognitive constructs are commonly measured on many intelligence tests (e.g., vocabulary and memory), whereas others are not (e.g., phonological awareness and RAN). Even though we discuss these cognitive abilities separately, Horn (1991) admonished that attempting to measure cognitive abilities in isolation "is like slicing smoke"

(p. 198). Cognitive and academic abilities are interrelated, and various combinations of abilities are employed as a person completes specific tasks.

Consider the various skills required to take notes while listening to a lecture. The note taker must pay attention, have knowledge of the topic, understand the vocabulary, use memory to hold on and paraphrase the important points, and then record thoughts in writing. A student may struggle with note taking for any or all of these reasons. In addition, the prediction of performance for students with SLD may be improved when several factors are considered (Gregg et al., 2004). For example, when combined, measures of working memory and language comprehension appear to provide the best prediction of reading comprehension ability (Daneman & Carpenter, 1980). In some circumstances, performance is influenced by something other than what a test was designed to measure. Stern (1938) noted: "It should never, of course, be supposed possible to test a definite, narrowly circumscribed separate capacity of thought with any one of these tests. Other abilities are always involved" (p. 315). He continued:

> Yet this is in no sense to be construed as a defect in the tests. On the contrary, they provide a favorable opportunity for observing the process of thinking in all its complexity. One must not be content to calculate the score for each performance. A completed test, which according to the system of scoring is thrown out as erroneous or deficient in performance, may very frequently result from the fact that *other* kinds of thinking than those expected have intervened, but which may have significance in terms of the subject's particular intellectual approach. (p. 316; emphasis in original)

Thus Stern emphasized that intelligence tests are valuable beyond the mere production of scores because careful observation during performance and analysis of the psychological processes that led to the test answer can deepen an evaluator's insight into the structure and functioning of cognitive abilities. Accordingly, we reemphasize the value of forming, exploring, confirming, or rejecting diagnostic hypotheses that are based upon test scores, as well as careful, systematic observations of behavior.

Vocabulary, Acquired Knowledge, and Language Comprehension

Unless they are designed primarily to measure nonverbal abilities, most intelligence batteries contain measures of vocabulary, acquired knowledge, and language comprehension. Often described as *crystallized intelligence*, *Gc*, *verbal or oral language abilities*, or *stores of acquired knowledge*, these abilities are highly correlated with achievement and are good predictors of academic success (Anastasi, 1988; Johnson, 1993). Because most of the measures of crystallized intelligence rely on language, crystallized intelligence can be equated with verbal intelligence (Carroll, 1993; Hunt, 2000) and is often used as a key indicator of giftedness (Benbow & Lubinski, 1996). These subtests typically measure aspects of cultural knowledge, rather than specialized knowledge specific to a domain. Because of the cultural and linguistic content of these tasks, caution must be used when testing individuals from different linguistic or cultural backgrounds, such as English-language learners (ELLs).

Verbal abilities and background knowledge have a strong and consistent relationship with reading (e.g., Cooper, 2006; Evans et al., 2002; Hammill, 2004; Kintsch & Rawson, 2005; Nation, 2007; Perfetti, Landi, & Oakhill, 2007; Shaywitz et al., 2008), mathematics (Floyd, Evans, & McGrew, 2003; Gelman & Butterworth, 2005; Swanson & Jerman, 2006), and writing (Berninger, 2009; McCloskey, Perkins, & Van Divner, 2009; McGrew & Knopik, 1993) across the lifespan. The most fully substantiated relationship is with reading comprehension and written expression. Both reading comprehension and written expression depend upon background knowledge, which enables a person to understand and create messages, interpret sentence structures, use verbal reasoning abilities, and employ a broad and deep vocabulary (McCardle, Scarborough, & Catts, 2001; Nation, Clarke, & Snowling, 2002). Words and the concepts they represent are thus the building blocks of literacy (Bell & Perfetti, 1994; Cunningham, Stanovich, & Wilson, 1990; Perfetti, Marron, & Foltz, 1996). In addition to vocabulary and background knowledge, researchers have identified other verbal abilities that are frequently weaknesses for individuals with reading comprehension difficulties: listening comprehension (Nation, Clarke, Marshall, & Durand, 2004), figurative language (Cain, Oakhill, & Lemmon, 2004), grammar (Nation & Snowling, 2000), and oral expression (Nation et al., 2004).

Unlike other cognitive abilities, crystallized intelligence has been described as a maintained ability rather than a vulnerable ability because it continues to develop until midlife and does not decline with age as significantly as other abilities (Horn, 1991). On growth curves, the rate of growth for crystallized intelligence is much greater than other abilities, and it shows a less rapid rate of decline (McGrew & Woodcock, 2001).

Reasons for Differences in Performance

Some people will demonstrate a weakness on verbal ability tests because of language impairments, whereas others will have weaknesses due to limited experiences with language and/or a lack of educational experiences and opportunities (Carlisle & Rice, 2002). In addition, tests of general knowledge, vocabulary, and language comprehension most often reflect the culture and language of the norm group. Therefore, individuals from diverse cultural and/or linguistic backgrounds or from low socioeconomic levels often obtain lower scores on measures of acquired knowledge. A child's language acquisition is influenced by the parents' attained level of education and the family's socioeconomic status, as well as by exposure to literacy and language activities (Hart & Risley, 1995).

A person's vocabulary is influenced by three main factors: (1) familiarity with words, (2) the depth of conceptual understanding of those words, and (3) the ability to retrieve words as needed (Gould, 2001). A student may understand the meaning of a word, but have difficulty using the word correctly when speaking. These word-finding or word-retrieving difficulties may also negatively influence performance on the verbal subtests found on many intelligence measures. If a person obtains a low score on a vocabulary measure, the evaluator must determine whether that low score is a result of limited verbal knowledge, limited cultural experiences, or difficulty in retrieving verbal labels (a problem more closely linked to associative memory).

Implications for Achievement

Since many academic tasks require linguistic competence, individuals with low verbal abilities are likely to encounter academic difficulties in most areas and will need increased opportunities and experiences to improve linguistic abilities, including vocabulary and world knowledge. In general, people who have difficulty understanding or using spoken language will have difficulty with the aspects of reading, writing, and mathematics that depend upon language-specific processes, such as reading comprehension, written expression, and math problem solving.

Because reading and writing share many of the same cognitive and linguistic processes, individuals frequently have difficulties in both areas. For example, a study of individuals with writing disabilities found that 75% of the sample also had reading difficulties (Katusic, Colligan, Weaver, & Barbaresi, 2009). As noted previously, both reading comprehension and written expression require vocabulary and background knowledge—in other words, a good foundation of language. Early deficits in vocabulary have been identified as a risk factor for later reading problems (Coyne, Simmons, Kame'enui, & Stoolmiller, 2004). Researchers have also established that the primary differences between individuals with good reading comprehension and those with poor reading comprehension are differences in verbal ability (Floyd, Bergeron, & Alfonso, 2006). In discussing the reasons for reading comprehension failure, Perfetti and colleagues (1996) distinguished between the processes involved in comprehension (e.g., working memory and comprehension monitoring) and knowledge—which includes word meanings or vocabulary, as well as *domain knowledge* (i.e., the concepts specific to a domain, such as physics, biology, or history). Clearly, knowledge is an important component underlying reading comprehension that contributes to individual differences in reading (Hannon & Daneman, 2001). A person's level of acquired knowledge, including domain knowledge obtained through life experiences, school, or work, is highly predictive of academic performance. Breadth and depth of knowledge and a robust oral vocabulary suggest that the person will excel on tasks involving language-learning abilities, whereas limited knowledge and a poor vocabulary suggest that the person will struggle.

In the simple view of reading (Gough & Tunmer, 1986), reading ability equals the product of decoding and linguistic comprehension. The equation used to represent this simple view is $R = D \times C$. Within this model, decoding is measured by the ability to pronounce pseudowords, and linguistic comprehension is assessed by a test of listening comprehension. If either decoding or linguistic comprehension is impaired, reading performance is compromised. Gough and Tunmer proposed that three types of reading disabilities could exist: inability to decode (dyslexia), inability to comprehend (hyperlexia), or both (the garden variety poor reader).

Therefore, individuals with specific reading disabilities, or dyslexia, typically have verbal abilities that are more advanced than their decoding skills. Essentially, what distinguishes individuals with reading disabilities from other poor readers is that their listening comprehension ability is higher than their ability to decode words (Rack, Snowling, & Olson, 1992). Listening comprehension is frequently cited as a good predictor of reading comprehension (Aaron & Joshi, 1992; Cooper, 2006; Hammill, 2004). Thus measures of verbal abilities, including listening comprehension, can be used to provide the best estimate of how much poor readers would profit from written text if their deficient decoding skills were resolved (Stanovich, 1999).

Beyond third grade, individuals with good verbal ability and good reading skills acquire knowledge and new vocabulary primarily through reading. In contrast, individuals with good verbal ability but poor reading skills are much more likely to learn new vocabulary through oral discussions (Carlisle & Rice, 2002). Unfortunately, since reading rather than listening is used to acquire more complex syntax and abstract vocabulary, poor readers tend to fall behind good readers on verbal tasks as they progress through school. Since many intelligence tests include vocabulary measures, a poor reader's relative standing on the verbal scores may decline when compared to that of normally achieving peers. As a result, poor language contributes to a lower IQ score, as well as to poor reading (Fletcher et al., 1998; Strang, 1964).

The relationship between verbal intelligence measures and reading ability is reciprocal, in that reading experience influences verbal intelligence test scores, and cognitive and academic tests assess many of the same underlying abilities (e.g., vocabulary, general information) (Aaron, 1997). Older students with reading difficulties may have depressed performance on measures of verbal intelligence or oral language because of limited experiences with text. Strang (1964) summarized this problem as follows:

> Intelligence tests are not a sure measure of innate ability to learn. They measure "developed ability," not innate or potential intelligence. Previous achievement affects the test results. The poor reader is penalized on the verbal parts of the test. The fact that his store of information is limited by the small amount of reading he has done also works against him. (p. 212)

Thus, for students with reading disabilities, lack of exposure to print contributes to reduced knowledge and vocabulary, and these deficiencies in language-based abilities are likely to increase over time (Vellutino, Scanlon, & Lyon, 2000). This phenomenon, nicknamed the "Matthew effect" from the Biblical reference that the rich get richer and the poor get poorer (Stanovich, 1986; Walberg & Tsai, 1983), alters the course of development in education-related cognitive skills (Stanovich, 1993). In other words, poor reading contributes to lowered verbal ability and knowledge. Furthermore, measures of verbal ability and listening comprehension may underestimate potential for achievement among students with attention or language-processing problems, as well as among students for whom English is a second language (Berninger & Abbott, 1994; Fletcher et al., 1998).

Verbal ability has also been identified as a strong predictor of math performance (Hale, Fiorello, Kavanagh, Hoeppner, & Gaither, 2001) and has been linked to early math achievement, especially to the development of number concepts (Carey, 2004; Gelman & Butterworth, 2005). The importance of verbal ability for math performance appears to increase with age and is most likely related to the increased linguistic demands of complex problem solving (Fuchs et al., 2006, 2008; Geary, 1994; McGrew & Wendling, 2010). Individuals with a math disability tend to score lower on verbal ability measures than typical age peers (Proctor, Floyd, & Shaver, 2005) and have limited oral language abilities (Fuchs et al., 2008). In addition, individuals with low verbal ability often experience problems in both math and reading, whereas those with more intact verbal abilities have problems that are more specific to math.

Interventions for Limited Verbal Ability

An individual with limited knowledge or vocabulary is likely to experience difficulty acquiring new knowledge or vocabulary, unless the new information is connected to prior knowledge (Beck, Perfetti, & McKeown, 1982). Instruction needs to build on prior knowledge and may need to be modified so that it occurs at the individual's language level.

The National Reading Panel (NRP, 2000) found that individuals with limited vocabulary benefit from a variety of approaches and that no one single approach is best for everyone. Some of the most effective instructional approaches for building vocabulary include both direct and indirect methods, such as reading aloud to the child, providing explicit instruction in vocabulary, and

making use of technology. Ideally, an individual's home and school environments are language-rich, with many opportunities and experiences to reinforce learning. A variety of strategies can be used to help individuals understand the nature of related words and concepts, such as semantic feature analysis, word webs, and graphic organizers. One important way language develops is through social interactions with more knowledgeable language users (Vygotsky, 1962). As teachers and students work together to attain educational goals, they can model the process of learning by talking about these processes as they perform tasks. Thus modeling and thinking aloud are useful for promoting language development.

A reciprocal relationship exists between learning to read and learning to write (Ehri, 2000), so instruction is more effective when skills are taught in an integrated manner (Clay, 1982). Reading has been referred to as "language by eye" and writing as "language by hand" (Berninger, 2000; Berninger & Graham, 1998), further connecting the two achievement domains. Individuals with limited verbal ability will struggle primarily with reading comprehension and written expression. Although these individuals may experience success with lower-level skills, such as phonemic awareness or handwriting, their limits in language will interfere with the acquisition of higher-level skills, including vocabulary, comprehension, fluency, sentence formulation, and expression. Thus instruction should focus on increasing vocabulary, as well as both declarative and procedural knowledge.

Although math is considered a less "verbal" achievement area, its demands on language and acquired knowledge are actually quite significant. Math requires knowledge of content-specific concepts and vocabulary, as well as the ability to understand story or word problems. Supporting the role of verbal ability in math, difficulty with math problem solving has been associated with deficient oral language abilities (Fuchs et al., 2008). In addition, conceptual knowledge of numbers and their relationships is an important correlate of math achievement (Hecht, Close, & Santisi, 2003). Explicit instruction, concrete examples, and guided practice are important for developing math vocabulary and concepts. The concrete–representational–abstract teaching sequence is beneficial for individuals struggling with mathematics. In this teaching sequence, the concrete level involves the use of objects or manipulative devices; the representational level involves visual representations, such as tallies or pictures; and the abstract level involves the use of actual numbers and equations.

Phonological Processing

Phonological awareness, another component of oral language, is important to an understanding of reading, writing, and even math disabilities. *Phonological awareness* refers to the ability to attend to various aspects of the sound structure of speech, whereas *phonemic awareness* refers to the understanding that words can be divided or segmented into individual speech sounds. The importance of phonological processing for promoting reading and spelling achievement has been extensively documented (e.g., Ehri, 1998; Fletcher, Lyon, Fuchs, & Barnes, 2007; Shaywitz, 2003; Snow, Burns, & Griffin, 1998; Torgesen, 1998; Uhry, 2005). In addition, phonological awareness has a reciprocal relationship with the development of reading and spelling: Learning to read and spell helps develop phonological processing. Rack and colleagues (1992) hypothesized that phonological awareness underlies the establishment of the graphemic memory store that is required for written language. Because phonological awareness abilities are known to be prerequisites for success in reading and spelling competence, they should be assessed early, especially in cases where a child is developing slowly in word identification or spelling skill.

The role of phonological processing in math achievement is not as well documented as it is for reading. Some researchers suggest that it plays a role in forming and encoding accurate phonological representations of math facts in working memory (Logie, Gilhooly, & Wynn, 1994; Swanson & Jerman, 2006). Geary (2007) found that individuals with comorbid reading and math difficulties often display phonological processing problems. Furthermore, phonological processing appears to predict math achievement (e.g., Hecht et al., 2003; McGrew & Wendling, 2010; Rasmussen & Bisanz, 2005).

Reasons for Differences in Performance

Cultural and linguistic differences have an impact on the development of phonological awareness. Individuals who have had limited exposure to the sounds of the English language, have limited oral language, have not been read to during the preschool years, and/or come from a low socioeco-nomic environment may have difficulty discriminating and manipulating speech sounds.

Implications for Achievement

A weakness in phonological processing as a common factor among individuals with early reading problems has been substantiated by an impressive body of research (e.g., Ehri, 1998; Fletcher & Foorman, 1994; Shaywitz et al., 2008; Stanovich & Siegel, 1994; Torgesen, 2002; Vellutino et al., 2007). Phonological processes are critical for the development of reading and spelling skills (Adams, 1990; Goswami & Bryant, 1990; Gough, 1996). Results from longitudinal studies suggest that 75% of children who struggle with reading in third grade will still be poor readers at the end of high school, primarily because of problems in phonological awareness (Francis, Shaywitz, Stuebing, Shaywitz, & Fletcher, 1996; Lyon, 1998). Individuals with poor phonological abilities typically make less progress in basic word-reading skills than normally achieving peers. Even spelling problems in young adults often reflect specific problems in the phonological aspects of language (Moats, 2001).

Recent findings have documented the neuroanatomical differences between the brains of poor readers and those of normally achieving readers (Shaywitz, 2003). The evolution of functional magnetic resonance imaging technology has made it possible to discover exactly which parts of the brain are engaged during phonological tasks. Good readers engage both the front and back of the brain as they perform phonological processing tasks, whereas poor readers appear to use only the front of the brain. Research has also documented that effective instruction in reading creates changes in brain behavior during reading (Shaywitz, 2003); this finding further emphasizes the extreme importance of implementing high-quality instruction at an early age.

Some children who show phonologically based reading difficulties also exhibit difficulties in the retrieval of math facts (Ashcraft, 1987, 1992; Geary, 2007; Light & DeFries, 1995). Phonological processing is a persistent weakness in individuals with math fact fluency deficits (Chong & Siegel, 2008). Speech sound processes are used when solving math computations—for example, when counting (Bull & Johnston, 1997; Geary, 1993). Several studies have implicated phonological processing as an underlying cause of individual differences in math problem solving as well (Furst & Hitch, 2000; Gathercole & Pickering, 2000; Geary & Brown, 1991; Swanson & Sachse-Lee, 2001).

Interventions for Limited
Phonological Processing

Research results indicate a causal and reciprocal relationship between phonological awareness and reading; gains in one lead to gains in the other (e.g., Castles & Coltheart, 2004; Hulme, Snowling, Caravolas, & Carroll, 2005; Muter, Hulme, Snowling, & Stevenson, 2004). Because children with poor phonological awareness can be identified before learning to read (Hulme & Snowling, 2009; Wise & Snyder, 2001), early intervention is possible. Poor phonological awareness has been described as the single best predictor of risk of early reading failure (Uhry, 2005), so early evaluation is essential. Explicit, systematic, synthetic phonics instruction involving the direct teaching of the relationships among phonemes (speech sounds) and graphemes (letters and letter strings that represent the phonemes) is most effective and results in improved word reading (Jenkins & O'Conner, 2001; NRP, 2000). Without direct systematic instruction in phonemic awareness and sound–symbol associations, individuals with phonologically based reading problems will not attain adequate reading levels (Frost & Emery, 1995).

The NRP (2000) identified phonemic awareness as one of the five key components to effective reading instruction. The most important phonological ability for reading is *blending* (the ability to push together sounds), whereas the most important ability for spelling is *segmentation* (the ability to break apart the speech sounds in a word). Explicit, sequenced, multisensory instruction at the appropriate level, delivered by highly trained teachers to groups of six or fewer, appears most effective for increasing phonological awareness (Wise & Snyder, 2001).

In general, individuals with limited phonological processing should be exposed to a language-rich environment that includes daily practice with sounds, words, and language. Reading aloud to individuals with a weakness in phonological processing and providing books on tape can be two beneficial accommodations.

Short-Term Memory
and Working Memory

Two types of memory are discussed briefly in this section: *short-term memory*, or *memory span*, and *working memory*. The relationship between short-term memory and working memory has been described in three different ways: (1) the two as similar constructs; (2) working memory as a subset of short-term memory; and (3) short-term memory as a subset of working memory (Engle, Tuholski, Laughlin, & Conway, 1999). For purposes of this discussion, we address these constructs as being related but distinct.

Short-term memory is a limited-capacity system that requires apprehending and holding information in immediate awareness. Most adults can hold seven pieces of information (plus or minus two) at one time. Short-term memory can be thought of as the "use it or lose it" memory. When new information requires a person's short-term memory, the previous information held is either stored or discarded. Common short-term auditory memory span tasks include sentence repetition tasks and repeating digits or words in serial order. Research has documented the importance of memory span to achievement (Flanagan, Ortiz, Alfonso, & Mascolo, 2006), as well as to the development of verbal abilities (Engle et al., 1999). Memory span also appears to be significantly related to reading recognition (Swanson & Saez, 2003); basic writing skills, particularly spelling (Berninger, 1996; Lehto, 1996); and math problem solving (Geary, 1993, 2007).

Working memory has been described as a brain-based function in which plans can be retained temporarily as they are being formed, transformed, or executed (Miller, Galanter, & Pribram, 1960). Similarly, Baddeley (1990) described working memory as a system for temporarily storing and manipulating information while executing complex cognitive tasks that involve learning, reasoning, and comprehension. Jensen (1998) described it as the "mind's scratchpad." More recently, working memory has been described as "a broad neuroscientific construct that refers to a dynamic system for temporary storage and manipulation of information in human cognition" (Schrank, Miller, Wendling, & Woodcock, 2010, p. 160). Thus working memory is engaged when information in short-term memory must be maintained, while other information is being manipulated or transformed in some manner. An example of a common working memory task is listening to numbers in a forward sequence and then restating the numbers in a reversed order. Working memory shows a strong connection to fluid intelligence and reasoning ability (Kane & Engle, 2002; Kyllonen & Christal, 1990), whereas memory span does not (Engle et al., 1999).

Strong connections exist between working memory and most areas of academic performance, making working memory useful in identifying individuals at risk for many types of learning problems (Gathercole & Alloway, 2008). As examples, significant correlations have been found between working memory and reading comprehension (e.g., Cain, Oakhill, & Bryant, 2004; Cooper, 2006; Fletcher et al., 2007; Hammill, 2004; Torgesen et al., 1999), language comprehension (King & Just, 1991), vocabulary acquisition (Daneman & Green, 1986; Gathercole & Baddeley, 1993), spelling (Ormrod & Cochran, 1988), math computation (Ashcraft & Kirk, 2001; Passolunghi, Mammarella, & Altoè, 2008; Swanson & Jerman, 2006; Wilson & Swanson, 2001), and math problem solving (Fuchs et al., 2008; Geary, 2007; Logie et al., 1994). Children who have both reading and math disabilities often have difficulty on tasks involving working memory (Evans et al., 2002; Floyd et al., 2003; Reid, Hresko, & Swanson, 1996; Siegel & Ryan, 1988; Wilson & Swanson, 2001), as do children who only have difficulties in math. Both verbal working memory tasks and visual–spatial working memory tasks appear to be important predictors of math ability (Wilson & Swanson, 2001). Working memory deficits have been identified as the primary characteristic of individuals with a math disability (e.g., Bull, Espy, & Wiebe, 2008; Chong & Siegel, 2008; Geary, 2003).

Reasons for Differences in Performance

Many factors can influence performance on short-term memory and working memory tasks. If an individual lacks automaticity or efficiency in performing a particular task, or has poor attention, performance on memory tasks may be impaired. Language proficiency is a factor for some types of memory span tasks, such as sentence repetition. Knowledge of syntax and vocabulary helps facilitate performance on sentence repetition tasks, placing individuals with different or limited linguistic backgrounds at a distinct disadvantage. Because most memory tasks present the stimulus briefly and only once, performance can also be affected by attention or anxiety. For example, individuals with high math anxiety demonstrate smaller working memory spans when performing math-related tasks (Ashcraft & Kirk, 2001), and stress in general has a negative impact on working memory capacity (Klein & Boals, 2001). Moreover, attention and working memory are closely related; this has been substantiated by a meta-analysis of 26 studies, which concluded that individuals with attentional problems also manifested

limits in working memory (Martinussen, Hayden, Hogg-Johnson, & Tannock, 2005). In one study, over 74% of individuals diagnosed with attention-deficit/hyperactivity disorder (ADHD) were found to have working memory deficits (Brown, Reichel, & Quinlan, 2009).

Implications for Achievement

Working memory deficits are characteristic of individuals with SLD (Swanson & Saez, 2003). Individuals with limited memory abilities may (1) appear inattentive, (2) have difficulty following directions or recalling sequences (e.g., months of the year), (3) have trouble memorizing factual information, (4) have difficulty following a lecture or a class discussion, (5) have trouble taking notes, or (6) struggle to comprehend what has been stated or read. For reading comprehension to occur, an individual must decode the words to obtain meaning. If decoding is labored, then fluency is reduced, and greater demands are placed on working memory, diminishing comprehension.

In math, weaknesses in memory span and working memory may contribute to difficulties in retrieving basic facts or solving algorithms. Individuals with math disabilities appear to have difficulty holding information in their minds while completing other processes (Geary, 1994). They may understand the rules, but forget the numerical information or have trouble following the steps of an algorithm in order. They know fewer facts and forget them more quickly than other children do. Difficulties in learning basic number facts do not necessarily mean that a person has poor memory. Limited knowledge can also result from insufficient exposure, poor instruction, or attentional weaknesses, rather than specific math disabilities (Robinson et al., 2002).

In contrast, above-average performance on memory tasks can indicate good attention. If information can be dealt with quickly, then the limited-capacity system of short-term memory will not be overloaded, and more attention can be directed to higher-level tasks. Good working memory facilitates proficiency in higher-level abilities, such as reading comprehension, math problem solving, and written expression.

Interventions for Limited Short-Term Memory and/or Working Memory

Practice, review, and specific instruction in memory strategies often benefit individuals with limited short-term memory or working memory. For example, the use of chunking strategies, mnemonics, and verbal rehearsal of information can help improve performance. The more routines are practiced, the more automatic these tasks become (Buchel, Coull, & Friston, 1999). Automaticity is especially important for activities that require rapid, efficient responses, such as pronouncing words or responding quickly to math facts.

For individuals with memory difficulties, explicit instruction in the academic area of concern is essential. Teachers are encouraged to review prerequisite information and previously learned skills, to provide distributed practice over time, and to introduce new skills carefully and systematically. Validated instructional techniques to improve academic performance include (1) providing demonstration and modeling of the skill to be learned, using a think-aloud procedure; (2) providing guided practice with immediate corrective feedback; (3) requiring independent practice to promote mastery; (4) setting goals with a student; and (5) monitoring the student's progress.

At times, accommodations may be necessary. To accommodate individuals with memory difficulties, oral directions need to be short—or, better yet, written down. In addition, oral instructions can be supported with visual cues, such as demonstrations, pictures, or graphic representations. Accommodations for memory difficulties often involve reducing the amount of information that must be memorized. For example, a teacher can provide a student with a fact chart or calculator, rather than requiring memorization of math facts; or the teacher can have the student maintain a personal dictionary of words the student commonly uses, so that the spellings do not have to be memorized.

Some students will require specific accommodations, such as the use of books on tape, permission to tape-record lectures, and/or the provision of study guides and lecture notes. In addition, individuals who struggle on tasks involving memory need to understand how their difficulties with memory affect their learning, so that they can request specific accommodations when needed.

Long-Term Retrieval and RAN

Long-term retrieval is another type of memory process that involves associative memory or the process of storing and retrieving information. Problems with this process can affect how effectively new information is stored, as well as how efficiently it is retrieved. Long-term retrieval is not to be confused with the actual information being stored or recalled, which is considered to be crystallized or verbal intelligence. Word-finding difficulties (discussed below) are related to problems with the retrieval process.

Associative memory, a narrow ability of long-term retrieval, appears to be an important ability at the early stages of reading (Evans et al., 2002; Flanagan, Ortiz, Alfonso, & Mascolo, 2006; McGrew & Wendling, 2010) and math development (Floyd et al., 2003; McGrew & Wendling, 2010). Acquisition of basic reading or math skills requires the individual to associate pairs of information, such as phonemes (speech sounds) and graphemes (a letter or letters that represent the speech sound), and to store this information for later use. This ability to form, store, and retrieve sounds and symbols, as well as to store and retrieve lexical knowledge, is important to early reading development (Cooper, 2006; Hammill, 2004; Perfetti, 2007). The acquisition of alphabetic knowledge (phoneme–grapheme correspondence) can be described as a visual–verbal paired-associate learning task (Hulme, 1981; Manis, Seidenberg, Stallings, et al., 1999). Research indicates that paired-associate learning accounts for unique variance in reading, independent of the powerful influence of phonological awareness (Hulme, Goetz, Gooch, Adams, & Snowling, 2007; Windfuhr & Snowling, 2001). These findings suggest that difficulties in recalling associations may impose an independent constraint on learning to read.

Both letter sound knowledge and letter name knowledge have also been identified as strong predictors of reading attainment (Adams, 1990; Muter, Hulme, Snowling, & Taylor, 1997). These aspects of literacy development require the ability to form associations between visual and verbal representations, store those associations, and retrieve them later as needed. In addition, several studies have reported that individuals with dyslexia have difficulties associating verbal labels with visual stimuli (Holmes & Castles, 2001; Vellutino, 1995).

The same basic memory problem that results in common features of reading disabilities, such as difficulties in retaining letter–sound correspondences and retrieving words from memory, may also contribute to the fact retrieval problems of many children with math disabilities. Conceivably, a weakness in the long-term storage and retrieval process is a core difficulty that helps explain the high comorbidity of reading and math disabilities (Robinson et al., 2002). Geary (2007) has hypothesized that individuals with both reading and math disabilities have a common memory problem that affects decoding and math fact learning. Associative memory may be that common memory deficit.

Naming facility, another narrow ability of long-term retrieval, has also been identified as a key predictor of early reading achievement (e.g., Berninger et al., 2006; Scarborough, 1998; Wolf et al., 2000). Carroll (1993) classifies naming facility as a narrow ability of long-term retrieval that is sometimes referred to as *speed of lexical access*, or the efficiency with which individuals retrieve and pronounce letters or words.

As noted earlier, this type of naming facility has been referred to as RAN (Denckla & Rudel, 1974). On RAN tasks, a person is typically shown a randomized array of several objects, colors, letters, or digits (6–8 in a row, with a total of 30–50), and is asked to name the stimuli as quickly as possible. Unlike other long-term retrieval tasks, these measures are timed, and the person is asked to name the symbols as quickly as possible. Although RAN has been the focus of extensive research in recent years, use of this type of assessment began with the original work of Geschwind (1965) and Denckla and Rudel (1974). Since these early reports, results from many studies have demonstrated a connection between deficits in RAN and subsequent poor reading skill (e.g., Hammill, 2004; Perfetti, 1994; Torgesen et al., 1999; Wagner, Torgesen, Laughon, Simmons, & Rashotte, 1993; Wolf, 2007; Wolf & Bowers, 1999). Phonemic awareness and RAN appear to account for independent variance in later reading scores and relate to distinct aspects of reading development (Manis, Seidenberg, & Doi, 1999).

To attempt to refine explanations of reading failure, Wolf and Bowers (1999) have proposed a theory referred to as the *double-deficit hypothesis*. According to this theory, three major subtypes of poor readers exist: (1) ones with phonological deficits, (2) ones with naming speed deficits, and (3) ones with a combination of the two. Wolf and Bowers have hypothesized that RAN tasks tap nonphonological skills related to reading, such as the processes involved in the serial scanning of print. Presumably, children who are slow to name symbols are slower to form orthographic representations of words (Bowers, Sunseth, & Golden, 1999)—abilities related to the visual aspects of reading. If common letter patterns are not recognized easily and quickly, orthographic pattern knowledge, and subsequently reading rate, will be slow to develop (Bowers & Wolf, 1993).

Some evidence also suggests that RAN differentially predicts reading, based upon level of reading skill. For example, Meyer, Wood, Hart, and Felton (1998) found that RAN tasks had predictive power only for poor readers. Manis, Seidenberg, and Doi (1999) and Abu-Hamour (2009) summarized what existing research suggests about RAN: (1) RAN appears to be independent of phonology and to contribute independent variance to word identification and comprehension; (2) its independent contribution appears larger with younger children and individuals with reading disabilities; (3) RAN is more closely related to reading irregular words than to reading phonically regular nonsense words; (4) it appears to be more closely related to tasks involving orthography than to tasks involving phonology; and (5) RAN is related to both the accuracy and speed of reading words, but the relationship is stronger with speeded measures. In addition, pause time is significantly correlated with both reading accuracy and reading fluency measures, whereas articulation time is not (Georgiou, Parrila, & Kirby, 2006; Georgiou, Parrila, Kirby, & Stephenson, 2008). Thus RAN tasks seem to be measuring the speed in which an individual can retrieve and name a visual symbol.

Reasons for Differences in Performance

As with other measures of memory, tasks measuring long-term retrieval may be affected by attention or anxiety. Individuals with math disabilities have difficulty learning basic facts and then, once facts are stored, have difficulty accessing them (Geary, 1993; Miller & Mercer, 1997); these problems suggest difficulties in the storage and retrieval process, which appear to be similar to the word retrieval difficulties common in individuals with reading disabilities. Another problem noted in the retrieval process is the inability to inhibit the recall of related but unnecessary information when one is trying to retrieve a specific answer. For example, an individual not only may recall 9 as the answer to 4 + 5, but may also recall 6, the number following the 4-5 sequence, or 20, the product of 4 × 5. Thinking of these extraneous facts slows down the process of getting to the correct answer and increases the chance for error.

Word retrieval difficulties can also impede the effortless retrieval of numbers, letters, and words. German (2001) has described three types of word-finding errors as "slip of the tongue" (recalling the wrong word), "tip of the tongue" (unable to recall the word), and "twist of the tongue" (mispronouncing the target word). An individual manifesting word-finding difficulties is not necessarily lacking "knowledge," but may be unable to retrieve and express that knowledge on demand. Higbee (1993) has distinguished between *available* and *accessible* information. Available information is known and stored; accessible information is available information that is retrievable. When known information cannot be recalled, a word-finding difficulty is present.

Like word retrieval difficulties, differences in performance on RAN tasks can be attributed to a variety of cognitive and linguistic processes. Wolf et al. (2000) describe serial naming speed as similar to reading because it involves a "combination of rapid, serial processing, and integration of attention, perceptual, conceptual, lexical, and motoric subprocesses" (p. 393). A person may have slow naming speed because of any one, or several of, the multiple processes underlying these tasks.

Morris and colleagues (1998) have described this specific subtype of reading disability as a "rate deficit." Students are impaired on tasks requiring rapid serial naming, but not on measures of phonological awareness. Conceivably, rapid sequential processing is common to naming speed, processing speed, and reading tasks, and slow naming speed reflects a global deficit in the rapid execution of a variety of cognitive processes (Kail, Hall, & Caskey, 1999). Whatever RAN measures, it may be partially subsumed under the rubric of processing speed (Denckla & Cutting, 1999).

Implications for Achievement

High performance on associative storage and retrieval tasks suggests that an individual will be successful in learning new information and recalling stored information. Long-term retrieval helps an individual retrieve and demonstrate knowledge. Low performance on tasks measuring this ability suggests that the individual will experience difficulty storing new information and recalling previously learned information. These individuals may have difficulty acquiring phoneme–grapheme knowledge, memorizing math facts, and completing fill-in-the-blank tests that require the precise recall of specific information.

Presently, more is known about RAN than about other associative memory abilities. The best predictive measures of early reading achievement appear to be a combination of letter identification, phonological awareness, and RAN (Adams, 1990; Bishop, 2003). In addition, children with weak-

nesses in both RAN and phonemic awareness appear to be the most resistant to reading intervention (Wolf & Bowers, 1999). One study found that low RAN scores were the single best predictor of treatment resistance among second-grade students (Vaughn, Linan-Thompson, & Hickman, 2003). Children with only naming speed deficits (no weaknesses in phonological awareness) are characterized by problems in word identification, fluency, and comprehension (Wolf et al., 2000). Although future research is likely to confirm the exact processes involved in RAN tasks, students with naming deficits appear to have a poorer prognosis for reading success than do other subgroups (Korhonen, 1991). Denckla (1979) described these students as a "hard-to-learn" group. Naming speed deficits persist into adolescence and adulthood (e.g., Denckla & Rudel, 1974; Vukovic, Wilson, & Nash, 2004), making it an important marker for identifying reading problems in older individuals.

The double-deficit theory attempts to explain two cognitive correlates of reading failure—poor phonological awareness and slow naming speed— but these are not the only tasks that differentiate poor readers from good readers. For example, Ackerman, Holloway, Youngdahl, and Dykman (2001) found that poor readers scored lower than normally achieving peers on orthographic tasks, attention ratings, and arithmetic achievement. Wolf (1999) also acknowledged the importance of using multidimensional models for explaining reading difficulties, stating that

this new conceptualization of reading disabilities was ironically, named too quickly. To be sure, double deficit captures the phenomenon of study—that is, the importance of understanding the separate and combined effects of two core deficits—but it fails miserably in redirecting our simultaneous attention as a field to the entire profile of strengths and limitations manifest in children with reading disabilities. Only when we develop truly multi-dimensional models of deficits and strengths will our diagnostic and remedial efforts be best matched to individual children. (p. 23)

Interventions for Deficits in Long-Term Retrieval and RAN

Individuals with difficulties in associative memory and retrieval will require repeated opportunities and more practice to learn new information. Carroll (1989) has suggested: "The degree of learning or achievement is a function of the ratio of the time actually spent on learning to the time needed to learn" (p. 26). In other words, students who have trouble retaining associations require more time to learn. The strategies that may be most useful include limiting the amount of information presented at one time, and using multisensory and meaning-based instructional approaches that help a person make connections and retain new learning. Examples of approaches include verbal rehearsal, active learning, use of manipulatives, and real-life projects. Smith and Rivera (1998) found that demonstration plus a permanent model was an effective strategy for helping children master computational mathematics, especially learning math skills and organizing and remembering the sequences of multistep algorithms. In addition, techniques that activate the emotional center of the brain by using humor, dramatizations, or movement can enhance learning (Leamnson, 2000). The most effective strategies help a learner form associations between new and learned information by activating prior knowledge, so that the learning of new information occurs in the context of what the learner already knows (Marzano, 1992).

Another helpful method to facilitate recall is instruction in the use of mnemonic strategies. For example, the *keyword* method involves associating new words with visual images, to help students recall word meanings and learn new vocabulary (Mastropieri, 1988). Three steps are used: *recoding*, *relating*, and *retrieving*. For recoding, students change the new vocabulary word into a known word, the keyword, which has a similar sound and is easily pictured. For relating, students associate the keyword with the definition of the new vocabulary word through a mental image or a sentence. For retrieving, students think of the keyword, remember the association, and then retrieve the definition. A more specific program that addresses the challenges imposed by RAN deficits is RAVE-O (Reading through Automaticity, Vocabulary, Engagement, and Orthography) (Wolf, 2010). This program emphasizes expansion of vocabulary and building fluency through rapid recognition of the most frequent orthographic multiletter patterns in the language.

Visual Processing

Visual–spatial tasks, because they are inherently less verbal in nature, are commonly included in intelligence tests. Carroll (1993) described broad *visual–spatial ability* as including the narrow abilities of *spatial relations*, *visualization*, *visual memory*, *closure speed*, *spatial scanning*, and a number of others that are not typically included on intelligence tests. Thus a wide range of these abilities exists, and they emphasize the processes of image generation, storage, retrieval, and transformation (Lohman, 1994).

Results from current research do not indicate a strong relationship between visual–spatial abilities and academic performance (Ackerman et al., 2001; Flanagan, Ortiz, Alfonso, & Mascolo, 2006; McGrew & Flanagan, 1998; McGrew & Wendling, 2010; Nation et al., 2002; Swanson & Berninger, 1995). This is not to say that such abilities are unimportant to academic success. Clearly, spelling involves a visual component of retrieving a mental image of the word to spell, but the visual–spatial tasks on intelligence measures have little relationship with spelling competence (Liberman, Rubin, Duques, & Carlisle, 1985; Sweeney & Rourke, 1985; Vellutino, 1979). This lack of correlation may be due to the types of visual–spatial tasks traditionally included on intelligence tests, such as manipulating patterns, assembling objects, or noting visual details in pictures, that differ from the visual–orthographic processing abilities that are required for efficient reading and spelling. Visual–spatial abilities are often three-dimensional in nature, and should therefore not be confused with the orthographic processing abilities that include the visual representations of the writing system (Berninger, 1990). A better measure of orthographic processing abilities appears to be perceptual speed tasks that involve the rapid processing of symbols such as letters (see "Processing Speed," below).

Visual–spatial thinking abilities do appear, however, to be related to math achievement (Geary, 1994, 2007; Hegarty & Kozhevnikov, 1999; Rourke, 1993; Strawser & Miller, 2001). Estimation skills, representations of magnitude, and visualizing a mental number line are dependent on visual–spatial systems (Dehaene, Spelke, Pinel, Stanescu, & Tsivkin, 1999; Pinel, Piazza, Le Bihan, & Dehaene, 2004; Zorzi, Priftis, & Umiltá, 2002). Visual processing is frequently a weakness in individuals with math disabilities (Hale et al., 2008; McLean & Hitch, 1999; Proctor et al., 2005), and difficulties in visual memory and visual–spatial working memory have been noted (Fletcher, 1985; McLean & Hitch, 1999). Geary (1993) identified a visual–spatial disorder subtype of math disability, characterized by difficulties with spatial representations (e.g., alignment) as well as place value errors. Rourke and Finlayson (1978) found that students with math disabilities scored lower on measures of visual-perceptual and visual–spatial ability than did students who had comorbid math and reading disabilities. Several researchers have found a relationship between math and specific spatial abilities (Assel, Landry, Swank, Smith, & Steelman, 2003; Osmon, Smertz, Braun, & Plambeck, 2006). Still others have suggested that visual–spatial abilities are related to performance on higher-level mathematics, but not to basic math skills (Flanagan, Ortiz, Alfonso, & Mascolo, 2006).

Reasons for Differences in Performance

Visual processing tasks can measure an array of narrow abilities, so identifying the specific weakness(es) is an important prerequisite to understanding performance. For example, an individual may have strengths in visual memory of objects, but weaknesses in spatial relations. Other factors, such as speed (on timed visual–spatial tasks), attention, motivation, and working memory, can influence performance. Problems in visual–motor coordination can also affect performance on timed visual–spatial tasks that involve the use of manipulatives, such as moving and assembling blocks or puzzle pieces, or drawing with a pencil.

Implications for Achievement

Except for math, research has not documented a significant relationship between visual processing and reading or writing achievement. Therefore, it would be erroneous to conclude that a student with high scores on visual–spatial tasks would benefit from a sight word approach to teaching reading, or that a student with low scores would benefit from a phonics approach to reading instruction. Many individuals, including those in clinical groups, demonstrate average scores on visual–spatial tasks with simultaneous low achievement. For example, visual processing scores do not differentiate between college students with and without SLD (McGrew & Woodcock, 2001). In many children with reading disabilities, visual–spatial skills are better developed than other abilities (Fletcher et al., 1995). Furthermore, in a recent review of over 6,000 clinical cases representing 21 different clinical groups, visual processing was generally not impaired (Schrank et al., 2010). For example, individuals with autism or Asperger syndrome were found to have little difficulty with visual–spatial tasks, which is consistent with other research (Corbett, Carmean, & Fein, 2009). These findings provide further evidence that visual processing abilities remain relatively intact in clinical groups, and therefore are not good predictors of academic performance in reading or writing.

Although much of the emphasis in the field of SLD has been placed on students who struggle with the acquisition and use of spoken and written language, a smaller subset of students evidence symptoms characteristic of what have been referred to as *nonverbal learning disorders* (NLD). Two major characteristics of NLD are poor spatial organization and inattention to visual details—abilities related to visual–spatial thinking. In addition, many students with NLD are poorly organized and appear unfocused. Although they may be described as inattentive and distractible, these observed behaviors result from a reduced capacity for self-directed behavior, rather than from poor attention (Fletcher et al., 1995). A student with NLD often has strengths in word decoding, spelling, and rote memory, but encounters extreme difficulty with reading comprehension, computational arithmetic, and mathematical problem solving (Rourke, 1995). The student may also have social difficulties, find reasoning difficult, and struggle to acquire new skills, particularly motor skills. Difficulties in dealing with novel and complex materials are especially evident. Since a large proportion of the communication in an average conversation is nonverbal in nature, a student with NLD may also miss information about what is being communicated, and then may be unsure of how to respond (Rothenberg, 1998). Because a student with NLD has early strengths in the development of general declarative knowledge and vocabulary, identification of problems tends to occur in later grades. As the student moves through school, tasks that require higher-level spatial–analytic abilities (such as writing compositions and problem solving) become increasingly difficult. Thus, when considered in an educational setting, measures of visual–spatial thinking may be most useful for documenting strengths and identifying students with NLD.

Interventions for Limited Visual Processing

In general, students with visual processing deficits benefit when interventions are highly concrete and as verbal as possible. The most effective methods are highly structured and provide external guidance—methods employed in explicit instruction. The guiding principles for treating children with NLD are that interventions should be verbal, highly concrete, and systematic, and should reinforce organization and structure (Fletcher et al., 1995). Expectations may need to be simplified, broken down, or modified. Because verbal abilities are typically unimpaired, teaching a student how to use self-talk to reinforce routines or procedures can help with the completion of simple as well as more complex tasks. Rourke (1995) recommends using a "part-to-whole" verbal teaching approach by presenting information in a logical sequence, one step at a time, so that the student can pay attention to details.

Teaching specific learning strategies, such as the use of imagery, graphic organizers, and puzzles, may significantly improve less skilled individuals' performances on visual–spatial tasks. Another strategy, verbal labeling, uses language to describe visual forms as they are manipulated and represented spatially (Kibel, 1992). For individuals with strengths in visual–spatial abilities, teachers may enhance the students' performance by instruction with pictures, diagrams, or graphic organizers. These individuals often excel in tasks such as visualizing and drawing three-dimensional objects.

Processing Speed

One commonly identified characteristic of intelligent behavior is mental quickness (Nettelbeck, 1994). *Processing speed* is the ability to perform simple cognitive tasks quickly and fluently over a sustained period of time. McGrew and Flanagan (1998) define processing speed as the ability to perform cognitive tasks automatically, especially when under pressure to maintain focused attention and concentration; they state that "attentive speediness" encapsulates the essence of processing speed. From an information-processing perspective, speediness and automaticity of processing underlie efficient performance (Kail, 1991; Lohman, 1989). Processing information quickly frees up limited resources so that higher-level thinking can occur. A processing speed deficit may be characterized as a domain-general deficit because it underlies performance in many areas and is not specific to one area or disability. For example, slow processing speed characterizes both individuals with dyslexia and those with ADHD (Eden & Vaidya, 2008), although children with reading disabilities appear to have greater deficits than those with ADHD (Shanahan et al., 2006).

Perceptual speed is a narrow ability of processing speed; Carroll (1993) describes it as the ability to search for and compare visual symbols. This ability is strongly related to reading achievement (McGrew, Flanagan, Keith, & Vanderwood, 1997; McGrew & Wendling, 2010), math achievement (Fiorello & Primerano, 2005; Floyd et al., 2003; McGrew & Hessler, 1995; McGrew & Wendling, 2010), and writing achievement (McGrew & Knopik, 1993; Williams, Zolten, Rickert, Spence, & Ashcraft, 1993). Thus the ability to process symbols rapidly is strongly related to academic performance.

Speed of processing has been identified as a primary process in reading (Joshi & Aaron, 2000), and many researchers have emphasized the importance of speed constructs in early reading acquisition (e.g., Berninger et al., 2006; Kintsch & Rawson, 2005; Shaywitz et al., 2008; Torgesen et al., 1999). In studies investigating the differences between normally achieving readers and those with reading disabilities, processing speed was slower for students with reading disabilities (Kruk & Willows, 2001), and was deficient on both linguistic and nonlinguistic tasks (Shanahan et al., 2006). Research results have indicated a relationship between perceptual speed and word reading (e.g., Berninger, 1990; Urso, 2008), as well as basic writing skills and composition (Berninger, 2009).

In the area of math, as noted previously, processing speed was found to be the best predictor of arithmetic competence in 7-year-olds (Bull & Johnston, 1997). Various researchers have identified speed-related issues for individuals with math disabilities: counting speed (Geary, 1993, 2007), numerical processing fluency (Swanson & Jerman, 2006), and efficiency in executing simple cognitive tasks during math fact tasks (Fuchs et al., 2006).

Reasons for Differences in Performance

When a clinician is examining a person's performance on processing speed tasks, several additional factors need to be considered. Because most tasks used to measure processing speed are visual in nature (often involving rapid searching of symbols or shapes), the individual's vision and visual processing may be a factor. Motivation and attention are factors to consider as well. Processing speed tasks are typically timed and clerical in nature. Some individuals may have difficulty maintaining attention, and some may not be motivated to complete a relatively simple task. Personality style can also affect performance on speeded tasks, as can cultural differences. Some cultures do not value speeded performance as an important behavioral attribute. In general, individuals who are reflective will work more slowly, carefully reviewing their options before responding. Some gifted individuals exhibit a relative weakness on speeded tasks because they reflect and check answers before making a decision. In contrast, individuals who are impulsive may work quickly and carelessly.

Implications for Achievement

Limited processing speed suggests that a person may process information slowly, thus creating a "bottleneck" that affects new learning in particular. When information is well known, it can be processed more automatically; when information is new, the processing is more effortful. Schneider and Shiffrin (1977) made a distinction between *automatic* and *conceptual* processing. The automatic processes require little attentional resources, whereas the conceptual processes are controlled and require the application of knowledge and strategies. Processing speed appears to be most closely related to the lower-order academic tasks that become increasingly automatic with repeated practice, such as reading words quickly, knowing multiplication facts, or spelling words with accuracy. Two consistent findings have emerged from the research on individuals with SLD: (1) Individuals both with and without SLD exhibit a range of responses on a variety of speeded tasks, and the intercorrelations between different speeded tasks often differ for both groups; and (2) individuals with SLD typically obtain lower scores than normally achieving individuals on a variety of speeded tasks (Ofiesh, Mather, & Russell, 2005).

Thus the issue of extended time has particular relevance for students with SLD. In considering the provision of time accommodations on exams, Kelman and Lester (1997) advise educational authorities to consider whether or not speed is a genuine academic virtue in the particular context. If not, the test should be untimed. In the very few cases where speed is judged to be necessary, no one should be provided with accommodations.

Interventions for Limited Processing Speed

Individuals with limited processing speed often require specific accommodations, particularly when an academic area is compromised as well. These individuals may need extended time, as well as shortened directions and assignments. In addition, copying activities should be limited or eliminated. It may be necessary to increase "wait" time so that an individual has more time to think and to respond. In order to suggest appropriate interventions or accommodations, it is important to determine first whether the person's processing speed deficit is due to limits in speed or accuracy or both. For example, some individuals work slowly but accurately, whereas others may work quickly but inaccurately. If the person's performance is slow and accurate, he or she may benefit from extra time or shorter assignments. If the person works quickly but inaccurately, extra time may not be appropriate. More time will not benefit an individual who does not understand the task or one who has attentional problems.

Use of explicit instruction in the relevant academic area is also recommended, as it scaffolds instruction for the individual learner to ensure a successful learning experience. Instructional interventions designed to increase rate and fluency in the academic area of concern may be of benefit. For example, repeated practice to build automaticity, speed drills, and computer programs that focus on rate or making decisions quickly may improve the performance of individuals with slow processing speed (Klingberg, 2009; Mahncke, Bronstone, & Merzenich, 2006).

Fluid Reasoning

Fluid reasoning involves the ability to solve novel problems via inductive or deductive reasoning and to transfer or generalize learning. Intelligence tests typically include fluid reasoning tasks, such as matrices, sequences, or analogies. Research has documented the relationship between fluid reasoning and reading comprehension (Floyd et al., 2006; McGrew, 1993; Nation et al., 2002), math achievement (Fiorello & Primerano, 2005, Flanagan, Ortiz, Alfonso, & Mascolo, 2006; Floyd et al., 2003; Fuchs et al., 2006; Geary, 1993, 2007; Hale et al., 2007; Rourke & Conway, 1997), and writing achievement (Floyd, McGrew, & Evans, 2008).

Some individuals with SLD tend to have great difficulties in abstracting principles from experiences (Geary, 1993; Swanson, 1987), and some appear to struggle with making generalizations (Ackerman & Dykman, 1995). Unfortunately, little is known about the breadth, depth, and developmental course of children's generalization capabilities (Pressley & Woloshyn, 1995), but a growing body of research indicates that poor inferential reasoning is one cause of reading comprehension problems (Wise & Snyder, 2001). For individuals with math disabilities, research indicates that fluid reasoning is frequently impaired (Geary, 2007; Proctor et al., 2005). These inferential reasoning difficulties then interfere with an individual's ability to "classify an event as belonging to a category" (Bruner, 1971, p. 93), and thereby affect success at mathematical problem solving. A deficit in fluid reasoning may affect the development of other cognitive abilities, especially in the domain of acquired knowledge (Blair, 2006).

Reasons for Differences in Performance

Performance on fluid reasoning tasks may vary for a number of reasons. One reason for variation is how effectively an individual uses strategies. Results from one study indicated that high achievers are more attentive and use more effective strategies (e.g., talking through a task) that help them learn and practice the task at hand, whereas low achievers use less effective strategies for task completion (e.g., guessing, carelessness, attending to inappropriate contextual clues) (Anderson, Brubaker, Alleman-Brooks, & Duffy, 1985). Another reason for differences in performance is mental flexibility, or the ability to shift cognitive gears. Individuals who have mental flexibility are able to anticipate what is expected on a task and change the approach when needed, resulting in more successful outcomes (Kronick, 1988). In contrast, individuals with rigid cognitive styles may be unable to use their knowledge except when the context closely resembles the original learning situation (Westman, 1996). Performance can also vary, depending on the type of reasoning task. Some tasks require reasoning with language (e.g., analogies), whereas others require nonverbal problem solving (e.g., matrices).

Implications for Achievement

It is likely that individuals with limited fluid reasoning may require instruction at a reduced level of difficulty—in other words, a modification to instruction rather than an accommodation. These individuals experience difficulty with higher-level thinking tasks and may struggle with comprehending what they read, solving math problems, or expressing themselves in writing. They may display rigidity when attempting new things and continue to apply a strategy that does not work. Even after learning a skill, they may not be able to apply that skill in a new context.

On the other hand, individuals with high performance on fluid reasoning tasks are likely to succeed in higher-level thinking tasks, such as those involved in reading comprehension, math reasoning, or written expression. They will typically display mental flexibility when approaching problem-solving tasks, shift strategies to accomplish their goals, and demonstrate self-regulation.

Interventions for Limited Fluid Reasoning

Providing opportunities for individuals to develop their metacognitive skills and higher-order thinking skills is important. Such opportunities may include engaging in reflective discussions about lessons, comparing and contrasting concepts, or using thought journals. Teaching students to use self-questioning techniques, identify main ideas and themes, classify and categorize objects, attend to organizational cues, and implement strategies can lead to significant gains in inferential skills. Strategy instruction has proven to be effective in improving the performance and achievement of students with SLD (e.g., Deshler, Ellis, & Lenz, 1996; Pressley & Woloshyn, 1995; Swanson, 2001). This type of instruction appears to be more effective for higher-order, conceptual tasks than for lower-order tasks (Deshler et al., 1996), but the strategies must be taught explicitly (Klauer, Willmes, & Phye, 2002).

Higher-level thinking skills (e.g., analyzing, comparing, evaluating, synthesizing) require the brain to use multiple and complex systems of retrieval and integration (Lowery, 1998). Experiential learning appears to activate the area of the brain responsible for higher-order thinking (Sousa, 1998). Therefore, instruction that combines physical activities with problem-solving tasks can help connect the motor cortex with the frontal lobes, where thinking occurs, and can thus increase memory and learning (Kandel & Squire, 2000). Learning can be demonstrated in multiple ways, such as dramatizations, experiments, visual displays, music, or inventions. Effective instructional principles, such as activating prior knowledge, actively engaging learners, and explicit instruction are recommended.

CONCLUSION

Cognitive assessment is not only relevant, but essential, for the accurate identification of individuals with SLD. As research continues to increase our knowledge of the relationships among cognitive abilities and achievement, more and more evaluators are taking advantage of that knowledge and applying it to their evaluation practices.

Interestingly, the research on cognitive–achievement relationships connects comprehensive evaluations to RTI in a way suggesting that they both provide useful data. Advocates of RTI talk about cognitive markers when discussing the need for early screening to identify children at risk for academic difficulties. For example, phonemic awareness and RAN are often mentioned as predictors of early reading skill; processing speed and memory span are predictors of math achievement. When an evaluator is establishing a PSW that suggests the presence of an SLD, the focus is on a child who is experiencing academic difficulties. RTI allows for early identification and intervention of such a child. Comprehensive evaluation enables us to understand why that child is struggling or making insufficient progress. If a student fails to respond to intervention, and the results of a comprehensive evaluation indicate that the student has a processing deficit that affects academic performance, both the definitional criteria for SLD and the SLD eligibility criterion of limited response to evidence-based instruction have been addressed, resulting in a balanced model that promotes diagnostic accuracy (Hale et al., 2006).

In discussing the assessment of intellectual functioning, Wasserman (2003) has indicated that one of applied psychology's biggest failures of the last century was that intellectual assessments were not systematically linked to effective interventions.

Fortunately, progress is being made to correct this. First, research continues to identify and clarify the cognitive correlates and predictors of achievement. Second, most modern intelligence tests measure a broad array of abilities that reflect the findings of current research. Third, U.S. law now requires that instruction be designed to acknowledge and address individual differences. Finally, the principles of effective instruction are known, and educators are responsible for implementing evidence-based instruction. Ultimately, all psychologists and educators share the same goal: to provide the best educational experiences and opportunities for each and every child.

REFERENCES

Aaron, P. G. (1997). The impending demise of the discrepancy formula. *Review of Educational Research, 67,* 461–502.

Aaron, P. G., & Joshi, M. R. (1992). *Reading problems:* *Consultation and remediation.* New York: Guilford Press.

Abu-Hamour, B. (2009). *The relationships among cognitive ability measures and irregular word, non-word, and word reading.* Unpublished doctoral dissertation, University of Arizona, Tucson.

Ackerman, P. T., & Dykman, R. A. (1995). Reading-disabled students with and without comorbid arithmetic disability. *Developmental Neuropsychology, 11,* 351–371.

Ackerman, P. T., Holloway, C. A., Youngdahl, P. L., & Dykman, R. A. (2001). The double-deficit theory of reading disability does not fit all. *Learning Disabilities Research and Practice, 16,* 152–160.

Adams, M. J. (1990). *Beginning to read: Thinking and learning about print.* Cambridge, MA: MIT Press.

American Educational Research Association (AERA), American Psychological Association (APA), & National Council on Measurement in Education (NCME). (1999). *Standards for educational and psychological testing.* Washington, DC: AERA.

Anastasi, A. (1988). *Psychological testing* (6th ed.). New York: Macmillan.

Anderson, L. M., Brubaker, N. L., Alleman-Brooks, J., & Duffy, G. S. (1985). A qualitative study of seatwork in first-grade classrooms. *Elementary School Journal, 86,* 123–140.

Ashcraft, M. H. (1987). Children's knowledge of simple arithmetic: A developmental model and simulation. In J. Bisanz, C. J. Brainerd, & R. Kail (Eds.), *Formal methods in developmental psychology: Progress in cognitive developmental research* (pp. 302–338). New York: Springer-Verlag.

Ashcraft, M. H. (1992). Cognitive arithmetic: A review of data and theory. *Cognition, 44,* 75–106.

Ashcraft, M. H., & Kirk, E. P. (2001). The relationships among working memory, math anxiety, and performance. *Journal of Experimental Psychology: General, 130,* 224–237.

Assel, M. A., Landry, S. H., Swank, P., Smith, K. E., & Steelman, L. M. (2003). Precursors to mathematical skills: Examining the roles of visual–spatial skills, executive processes, and parenting factors. *Applied Developmental Science, 7,* 27–38.

Baddeley, A. D. (1990). *Human memory: Theory and practice.* Boston: Allyn & Bacon.

Beck, I. L., Perfetti, C. A., & McKeown, M. G. (1982). The effects of long-term vocabulary instruction on lexical access and reading comprehension. *Journal of Educational Psychology, 74,* 506–521.

Bell, L. C., & Perfetti, C. A. (1994). Reading skill: Some adult comparisons. *Journal of Educational Psychology, 86,* 244–255.

Benbow, C. P., & Lubinski, D. (Eds.). (1996). *Intellectual talent: Psychometric and social issues.* Baltimore: Johns Hopkins University Press.

Berninger, V. W. (1990). Multiple orthographic codes: Key to alternative instructional methodologies for developing orthographic phonological connections underlying word identification. *School Psychology Review, 19,* 518–533.

Berninger, V. W. (1996). *Reading and writing acquisition: A developmental neuropsychological perspective.* Boulder, CO: Westview Press.

Berninger, V. W. (2000). Development of language by hand and its connections to language by ear, mouth, and eye. *Topics in Language Disorders, 20,* 65–84.

Berninger, V. W. (2009). Highlights of programmatic, interdisciplinary research on writing. *Learning Disabilities Research and Practice, 24,* 69–80.

Berninger, V. W., & Abbott, R. D. (1994). Redefining learning disabilities: Moving beyond aptitude–achievement discrepancies to failure to respond to validated treatment protocols. In G. R. Lyon (Ed.), *Frames of reference for the assessment of learning disabilities: New views on measurement issues* (pp. 163–183). Baltimore: Brookes.

Berninger, V. W., Abbott, R. D., Thomson, J., Wagner, R., Swanson, H. L., Wijsman, E., et al. (2006). Modeling developmental phonological core deficits within a working-memory architecture in children and adults with developmental dyslexia. *Scientific Studies in Reading, 10,* 165–198.

Berninger, V. W., & Graham, S. (1998). Language by hand: A synthesis of a decade of research on handwriting. *Handwriting Review, 12,* 11–25.

Bishop, A. G. (2003). Prediction of first-grade reading achievement: A comparison of fall and winter kindergarten screenings. *Learning Disability Quarterly, 26,* 189–200.

Blair, C. (2006). How similar are fluid cognition and general intelligence?: A developmental neuroscience perspective on fluid cognition as an aspect of human cognitive ability. *Behavioral and Brain Sciences, 29,* 109–160.

Bowers, P. G., Sunseth, K., & Golden, J. (1999). The route between rapid naming and reading progress. *Scientific Studies of Reading, 3,* 31–53.

Bowers, P. G., & Wolf, M. (1993). Theoretical links between naming speed, precise timing mechanisms, and orthographic skill in dyslexia. *Reading and Writing: An Interdisciplinary Journal, 5,* 69–85.

Brown, T. E., Reichel, P. C., & Quinlan, D. M. (2009). Executive function impairments in high IQ adults with ADHD. *Journal of Attention Disorders, 13,* 161–167.

Bruner, J. S. (1971). *The relevance of education.* New York: Norton.

Buchel, C., Coull, J. T., & Friston, K. J. (1999). The predictive value of changes in effective connectivity for human learning. *Science, 283,* 1538–1541.

Bull, R., Espy, K. A., & Wiebe, S. A. (2008). Short-term memory, working memory, and executive functioning in preschoolers: Longitudinal predictors of mathematical achievement at age 7 years. *Developmental Neuropsychology, 33,* 205–228.

Bull, R., & Johnston, R. S. (1997). Children's arithmetical difficulties: Contributions from processing speed, item identification, and short-term memory. *Journal of Experimental Child Psychology, 65,* 1–24.

Cain, K., Oakhill, J., & Bryant, P. (2004). Children's reading comprehension ability: Concurrent prediction by working memory, verbal ability, and component skills. *Journal of Educational Psychology, 96,* 31–42.

Cain, K., Oakhill, J., & Lemmon, K. (2004). Individual differences in the inference of word meanings from context: the influence of reading comprehension, vocabulary knowledge, and memory capacity. *Journal of Educational Psychology, 96,* 671–681.

Carey, S. (2004). Bootstrapping and the origin of concepts. *Daedalus, 133,* 59–68.

Carlisle, J. F., & Rice, M. S. (2002). *Improving reading comprehension: Research-based principles and practices.* Baltimore: York Press.

Carroll, J. B. (1989). Factor analysis since Spearman: Where do we stand? What do we know? In R. Kanfer, P. L. Ackerman, & R. Cudeck (Eds.), *Abilities, motivation, and methodology* (pp. 43–67). Hillsdale, NJ: Erlbaum.

Carroll, J. B. (1993). *Human cognitive abilities: A survey of factor-analytic studies.* New York: Cambridge University Press.

Castles, A., & Coltheart, M. (2004). Is there a causal link from phonological awareness to success in learning to read? *Cognition, 91,* 77–111.

Chong, S. L., & Siegel, L. S. (2008). Stability of computational deficits in math learning disability from second through fifth grades. *Developmental Neuropsychology, 33,* 300–317.

Clay, M. M. (1982). *Observing the young reader.* Auckland, New Zealand: Heinemann.

Cooper, K. L. (2006). *A componential reading comprehension task for children.* Unpublished doctoral dissertation, University of New England.

Corbett, B. A., Carmean, V., & Fein, D. (2009). Assessment of neuropsychological functioning in autism spectrum disorders. In S. Goldstein, J. A. Naglieri, & S. Ozonoff (Eds.), *Assessment of autism spectrum disorders* (pp. 253–289). New York: Guilford Press.

Coyne, M. D., Simmons, D. C., Kame'enui, E. J., & Stoolmiller, M. (2004). Teaching vocabulary during shared storybook readings: An examination of differential effects. *Exceptionality, 12,* 145–162.

Cruickshank, W. M. (1977). Least-restrictive placement: Administrative wishful thinking. *Journal of Learning Disabilities, 10,* 193–194.

Cunningham, A. E., Stanovich, K. E., & Wilson, M. R. (1990). Cognitive variation in adult college students differing in reading ability. In T. H. Carr & B. A. Levy (Eds.), *Reading and its development: Component skills approaches* (pp. 129–159). San Diego, CA: Academic Press.

Daneman, M., & Carpenter, P. A. (1980). Individual differences in working memory and reading. *Journal of Verbal Learning and Verbal Behavior, 19,* 450–466.

Daneman, M., & Green, I. (1986). Individual differences in comprehending and producing words in context. *Journal of Memory and Language, 25,* 1–18.

Dehaene, S., Spelke, E., Pinel, P., Stanescu, R., & Tsivkin, S. (1999). Sources of mathematical thinking: Behavioral and brain-imaging evidence. *Science, 284,* 970–974.

Denckla, M. B. (1979). Childhood learning disabilities. In K. M. Heilman & E. Valenstein (Eds.), *Clinical neuropsychology* (pp. 535–573). New York: Oxford University Press.

Denckla, M. B., & Cutting, L. E. (1999). History and significance of rapid automatized naming. *Annals of Dyslexia, 49,* 29–42.

Denckla, M. B., & Rudel, R. (1974). Rapid automatized naming of pictured objects, colors, letters and numbers by normal children. *Cortex, 10,* 186–202.

Deshler, D. D., Ellis, E. S., & Lenz, B. K. (1996). *Teaching adolescents with learning disabilities: Strategies and methods* (2nd ed.). Denver, CO: Love.

Eden, G. F., & Vaidya, C. (2008). ADHD and dyslexia: Neural basis and treatment. *Annals of the New York Academy of Sciences, 1145,* 316–327.

Ehri, L. C. (1998). Grapheme–phoneme knowledge is essential for learning to read words in English. In J. L. Metsala & L. C. Ehri (Eds.), *Word recognition in beginning literacy* (pp. 3–40). Mahwah, NJ: Erlbaum.

Ehri, L. C. (2000). Learning to read and learning to spell: Two sides of a coin. *Topics in Language Disorders, 20,* 19–36.

Elksmin, L. K. (2001). Implementing case method of instruction in special education teacher preparation programs. *Teacher Education and Special Education, 24,* 95–107.

Engle, R. W., Tuholski, S. W., Laughlin, J. E., & Conway, A. R. A. (1999). Working memory, short-term memory, and general fluid intelligence: A latent-variable approach. *Journal of Experimental Psychology: General, 128,* 309–331.

Evans, J. J., Floyd, R. G., McGrew, K. S., & Leforgee,

M. H. (2002). The relations between measures of Cattell–Horn–Carroll (CHC) cognitive abilities and reading achievement during childhood and adolescence, *School Psychology Review, 31,* 246–262.

Fiorello, C. A., Hale, J. B., & Snyder, L. E. (2006). Cognitive hypothesis testing and response to children with reading problems. *Psychology in the Schools, 43*(8), 835–853.

Fiorello, C. A., & Primerano, D. P. (2005). Research into practice: Cattell–Horn–Carroll cognitive assessment in practice: Eligibility and program development issues. *Psychology in the Schools, 42*(5), 525–536.

Flanagan, D. P., Ortiz, S. O., Alfonso, V. C., & Dynda, A. M. (2006). Integration of response to intervention and norm-referenced tests in learning disability identification: Learning from the Tower of Babel. *Psychology in the Schools, 43,* 807–825.

Flanagan, D. P., Ortiz, S. O., Alfonso, V. C., & Mascolo, J. T. (2006). *The achievement test desk reference (ATDR-2)* (2nd ed.). Hoboken, NJ: Wiley.

Fletcher, J. M. (1985). Memory for verbal and nonverbal stimuli in learning disabilities subgroups: Analysis by selective reminding. *Journal of Experimental Child Psychology, 40,* 244–259.

Fletcher, J. M., & Foorman, B. R. (1994). Issues in the definition and measurement of learning disabilities: The need for early intervention. In G. R. Lyon (Ed.), *Frames of reference for the assessment of learning disabilities: New views on measurement issues* (pp. 185–200). Baltimore: Brookes.

Fletcher, J. M., Foorman, B. R., Boudousquie, A., Barnes, M. A., Schatschneider, C., & Francis, D. J. (2002). Assessment of reading and learning disabilities: A research-based intervention oriented approach. *Journal of School Psychology, 40,* 27–63.

Fletcher, J. M., Francis, D. J., Shaywitz, S. E., Lyon, G. R., Foorman, B. R., Stuebing, K. K., et al. (1998). Intelligent testing and the discrepancy model for children with learning disabilities. *Learning Disabilities Research and Practice, 13,* 186–203.

Fletcher, J. M., Lyon, G. R., Fuchs, L. S., & Barnes, M. A. (2007). *Learning disabilities: From identification to intervention.* New York: Guilford Press.

Fletcher, J. M., Taylor, H. G., Levin, H. S., & Satz, P. (1995). Neuropsychological and intellectual assessment of children. In H. Kaplan & B. Sadock (Eds.), *Comprehensive textbook of psychiatry* (pp. 581–601). Baltimore: Williams & Wilkins.

Fletcher, J. M., & Vaughn, S. (2007). Response to intervention: Preventing and remediating academic difficulties. *Child Development Perspectives, 3,* 30–37.

Floyd, R. G., Bergeron, R., & Alfonso, V. C. (2006). Cattell–Horn–Carroll cognitive ability profiles of poor comprehenders. *Reading and Writing*, 19(5), 427–456.

Floyd, R. G., Evans, J. J., & McGrew, K. S. (2003). Relations between measures of Cattell–Horn–Carroll (CHC) cognitive abilities and mathematics achievement across the school-age years. *Psychology in the Schools*, 60, 155–171.

Floyd, R. G., McGrew, K. S., & Evans, J. J. (2008). The relative contributions of the Cattell–Horn–Carroll (CHC) cognitive abilities in explaining writing achievement during childhood and adolescence. *Psychology in the Schools*, 45, 132–144.

Francis, D. J., Shaywitz, S. E., Stuebing, K. K., Shaywitz, B. A., & Fletcher, J. M. (1996). Developmental lag versus deficit models of reading disability: A longitudinal, individual growth curves study. *Journal of Educational Psychology*, 88, 3–17.

Frieberg, H. (2002). Essential skills for new teachers. *Educational Leadership*, 59, 56–60.

Frost, J. A., & Emery, M. J. (1995, August). *Academic interventions for children with dyslexia who have phonological core deficits.* Reston, VA: Council for Exceptional Children. (ERIC Digest No. 539)

Fuchs, L. S., Compton, D. L., Fuchs, D., Paulsen, K., Bryant, J. D., & Hamlett, C. L. (2005). The prevention, identification, and cognitive determinants of math difficulty. *Journal of Educational Psychology*, 97, 493–513.

Fuchs, L. S., Fuchs, D., Compton, D. L., Powell, S. R., Seethaler, P. M, Capizzi, A. M., et al. (2006). The cognitive correlates of third-grade skill in arithmetic, algorithmic computation, and arithmetic word problems. *Journal of Educational Psychology*, 98, 29–43.

Fuchs, L. S., Fuchs, D., Stuebing, K., Fletcher, J. M., Hamlett, C. L., & Lambert, W. (2008). Problem solving and computational skill: Are they shared or distinct aspects of mathematical cognition? *Journal of Educational Psychology*, 100, 30–47.

Fuchs, D., & Young, C. L. (2006). On the irrelevance of intelligence in predicting responsiveness to reading instruction. *Exceptional Children*, 73, 8–30.

Furst, A., & Hitch, G. J. (2000). Separate roles for executive and phonological components in mental arithmetic. *Memory and Cognition*, 28, 774–782.

Gable, R. A., Hendrickson, J. M., Tonelson, S. W., & Van Acker, R. (2000). Changing disciplinary and instructional practices in the middle school to address IDEA. *Clearing House*, 73, 205–208.

Gardner, H. (1999). *Intelligence reframed: Multiple intelligences for the 21st century.* New York: Basic Books.

Gathercole, S. E., & Alloway, T. P. (2008). Working memory and classroom learning. In S. K. Thurman & C. A. Fiorello (Eds.), *Applied cognitive research in K–3 classrooms* (pp. 17–40). New York: Routledge.

Gathercole, S. E., & Baddeley, A. D. (1993). Phonological working memory: A critical building block for reading development and vocabulary acquisition. *European Journal of Psychology*, 8, 259–272.

Gathercole, S. E., & Pickering, S. J. (2000). Working memory deficits in children with low achievements in the national curriculum at 7 years of age. *British Journal of Educational Psychology*, 70, 177–194.

Geary, D. C. (1993). Mathematical disabilities: Cognitive, neuropsychological, and genetic components. *Psychological Bulletin*, 114, 345–362.

Geary, D. C. (1994). *Children's mathematical development: Research and practical applications.* Washington, DC: American Psychological Association.

Geary, D. C. (2003). Learning disabilities in arithmetic: Problem solving differences and cognitive deficits. In H. L. Swanson, K. Harris, & S. Graham (Eds.), *Handbook of learning disabilities* (pp. 199–212). New York: Guilford Press.

Geary, D. C. (2007). An evolutionary perspective on learning disabilities in mathematics. *Developmental Neuropsychology*, 32, 471–519.

Geary, D. C., & Brown, S. C. (1991). Cognitive addition: Strategy choice and speed-of-processing differences in gifted, normal, and mathematically disabled children. *Developmental Psychology*, 27, 398–406.

Geary, D. C., Hoard, M. K., Byrd-Craven, J., Nugent, L., & Numtee, C. (2007). Cognitive mechanisms underlying achievement deficits in children with mathematical learning disability. *Child Development*, 78, 1343–1359.

Gelman, R., & Butterworth, B. (2005). Number and language: How are they related? *Trends in Cognitive Sciences*, 9, 6–10.

Georgiou, G., Parrila, R., & Kirby, J. (2006). Rapid naming speed components and early reading acquisition. *Scientific Studies of Reading*, 2, 199–220.

Georgiou, G., Parrila, R., Kirby, J., & Stephenson, K. (2008). Rapid naming components and their relationship with phonological awareness, orthographic knowledge, speed of processing, and different reading outcomes. *Scientific Studies of Reading*, 12, 325–350.

German, D. J. (2001). *It's on the tip of my tongue.* Chicago: Word Finding Materials.

Geschwind, N. (1965). Disconnection syndrome in animals and man (Parts I, II). *Brain*, 88, 237–294, 585–644.

Goswami, U., & Bryant, P. (1990). *Phonological skills and learning to read.* Hove, UK: Erlbaum.

Gough, P. B. (1996). How children learn to read and why they fail. *Annals of Dyslexia*, 46, 3–20.

Gough, P. B., & Tunmer, W. E. (1986). Decoding, reading, and reading disability. *Remedial and Special Education*, 7, 6–10.

Gould, B. W. (2001). Curricular strategies for written expression. In A. M. Bain, L. L. Bailet, & L. C. Moats (Eds.), *Written language disorders: Theory into practice* (2nd ed., pp. 185–220), Austin, TX: PRO-ED.

Gregg, N., Davis, M., Coleman, C., Wisenbaker, J., & Hoy, C. (2004). *Implications for accommodation decisions at the postsecondary level.* Unpublished manuscript, University of Georgia.

Gresham, F. M. (2002). Responsiveness to intervention: An alternative approach to the identification of learning disabilities. In R. Bradley, L. Danielson, & D. Hallahan (Eds.), *Identification of learning disabilities: Research to practice* (pp. 467–519). Mahwah, NJ: Erlbaum.

Hale, J. B., Fiorello, C. A., Dumont, R., Willis, J. O., Rackley, C., & Elliott, C. (2008). Differential Ability Scales—Second Edition (neuro)psychological predictors of math performance for typical children and children with math disabilities. *Psychology in the Schools, 45*(9), 838–858.

Hale, J. B., Fiorello, C. A., Kavanagh, J. A., Hoeppner, J. B., & Gaither, R. A. (2001). WISC-III predictors of academic achievement for children with learning disabilities: Are global and factor scores comparable? *School Psychology Quarterly, 16*, 31–35.

Hale, J. B., Fiorello, C. A., Kavanagh, J. A., Holdnack, J. A., & Aloe, A. M. (2007). Is the demise of IQ interpretation justified?: A response to special issue authors. *Applied Neuropsychology, 14*, 37–51.

Hale, J. B., Kaufman, A. S., Naglieri, J. A., & Kavale, K. A. (2006). Implementation of IDEA: Response to intervention and cognitive assessment methods. *Psychology in the Schools, 43*, 753–770.

Hammill, D. (2004). What we know about the correlates of reading. *Exceptional Children, 70*, 453–468.

Hannon, B., & Daneman, M. (2001). A new tool for measuring and understanding individual differences in the component processes of reading comprehension. *Journal of Educational Psychology, 93*(1), 103–128.

Hart, B., & Risley, T. R. (1995). *Meaningful differences in the everyday experience of young American children.* Baltimore: Brookes.

Hecht, S., Close, L., & Santisi, M. (2003). Sources of individual differences in fraction skills. *Journal of Experimental Child Psychology, 86*, 277–302.

Hegarty, M., & Kozhevnikov, M. (1999). Types of visual–spatial representations and mathematical problem-solving. *Journal of Educational Psychology, 91*, 684–689.

Higbee, K. L. (1993). *Your memory, how it works and how you improve it.* New York: Paragon House.

Holmes, V. M., & Castles, A. E. (2001). Unexpectedly poor spelling in university students. *Scientific Studies of Reading, 5*, 319–350.

Horn, J. L. (1991). Measurement of intellectual capabilities: A review of theory. In K. S. McGrew, J. K. Werder, & R. W. Woodcock, *WJ-R technical manual* (pp. 197–232). Chicago: Riverside.

Hulme, C. (1981). *Reading retardation and multisensory teaching.* London: Routledge & Kegan Paul.

Hulme, C., Goetz, K., Gooch, D., Adams, J., & Snowling, M. (2007). Paired-associate learning, phoneme awareness, and learning to read. *Journal of Exceptional Child Psychology, 96*, 150–166.

Hulme, C., & Snowling, M. (2009). *Developmental cognitive disorders.* Oxford: Blackwell/Wiley.

Hulme, C., Snowling, M., Caravolas, M., & Carroll, J. (2005). Phonological skills are (probably) one cause of success in learning to read: A comment on Castles and Coltheart. *Scientific Studies of Reading, 9*, 351–365.

Hunt, E. (2000). Let's hear it for crystallized intelligence. *Learning and Individual Differences, 12*, 123–129.

Individuals with Disabilities Education Improvement Act of 2004 (IDEA 2004) Pub. L. No. 108-446, 20 U.S.C 1400 (2004).

Jenkins, J., & O'Conner, R. E. (2001, August). *Early identification and intervention for young children.* Paper presented at the U.S. Department of Education LD Summit, Washington, DC.

Jensen, A. R. (1998). *The g factor: The science of mental ability.* Westport, CT: Praeger.

Johnson, D. J. (1993). Relationship between oral and written language. *School Psychology Review, 22*, 595–609.

Joshi, M. R., & Aaron, P. G. (2000). The component model of reading: Simple view of reading made a little more complex. *Reading Psychology, 21*, 85–97.

Kail, R. (1991). Developmental change in speed of processing during childhood and adolescence. *Psychological Bulletin, 109*, 490–501.

Kail, R., Hall, L. K., & Caskey, B. J. (1999). Processing speed, exposure to print, and naming speed. *Applied Psycholinguistics, 20*, 303–314.

Kandel, E. R., & Squire, L. R. (2000). Neuroscience: Breaking down scientific barriers to the study of brain and mind. *Science, 290*, 1113–1120.

Kane, M. J., & Engle, R. W. (2002). The role of prefrontal cortex in working-memory capacity, executive attention, and general fluid intelligence: An individual differences perspective. *Psychonomic Bulletin and Review, 9*, 637–671.

Katusic, S. K., Colligan, R. C., Weaver, A. L., & Barbaresi, W. J. (2009). The forgotten learning disability: Epidemiology of written-language disorder in a population-based birth cohort (1976–1982), Rochester, Minnesota. *Pediatrics, 123*(5), 1306–1313.

Kavale, K. A., & Flanagan, D. P. (2007). Ability–achievement discrepancy, response to intervention, and assessment of cognitive abilities/processes in specific learning disability identification: Toward a contemporary operational definition. In S. R. Jimerson, M. K. Burns, & A. M. VanDerHeyden (Eds.), *Handbook of response to intervention: The science and practice of assessment and intervention* (pp. 130–147). New York: Springer.

Kavale, K. A., & Forness, S. R. (1998). The politics of learning disabilities. *Learning Disability Quarterly, 21,* 245–273.

Kelman, M., & Lester, G. (1997). *Jumping the queue: An inquiry into the legal treatment of students with learning disabilities.* Cambridge, MA: Harvard University Press.

Kibel, M. (1992). Linking language to action. In T. R. Miles & E. Miles (Eds.), *Dyslexia and mathematics* (pp. 42–57). London: Routledge.

King, J., & Just, M. A. (1991). Individual differences in syntactic processing: The role of working memory. *Journal of Memory and Language, 30,* 580–602.

Kintsch, W., & Rawson, K. A. (2005). Comprehension. In M. J. Snowling & C. Hulme (Eds.), *The science of reading: A handbook* (pp. 209–226). Oxford: Blackwell.

Klauer, K. J., Willmes, K., & Phye, G. D. (2002). Inducing inductive reasoning: Does it transfer to fluid intelligence? *Contemporary Educational Psychology, 27,* 1–25.

Klein, K., & Boals, A. (2001). The relationship of life stress and working memory. *Applied Cognitive Psychology, 15,* 565–579.

Klingberg, T. (2009). *The overflowing brain: Information overload and the limits of working memory* (N. Betteridge, Trans.). New York: Oxford University Press.

Korhonen, T. T. (1991). Neuropsychological stability and prognosis of subgroups of children with learning disabilities. *Journal of Learning Disabilities, 24,* 48–57.

Kronick, D. (1988). *New approaches to learning disabilities: Cognitive, metacognitive, and holistic.* Philadelphia: Grune & Stratton.

Kruk, R. S., & Willows, D. M. (2001). Backward pattern masking of familiar and unfamiliar materials in disabled and normal readers. *Cognitive Neuropsychology, 18*(1), 19–37.

Kyllonen, P. C., & Christal, R. E. (1990). Reasoning ability is (little more than) working memory capacity?! *Intelligence, 14,* 389–433.

Leamnson, R. (2000). Learning as biological brain change. *Change, 32*(6), 34–40.

Lehto, J. (1996). Working memory capacity and summarizing skills in ninth graders. *Scandinavian Journal of Psychology, 37*(1), 84–92.

Liberman, I. Y., Rubin, H., Duques, S., & Carlisle, J. (1985). Linguistic abilities and spelling proficiency in kindergartners and adult poor spellers. In D. B. Gray & J. F. Kavanaugh (Eds.), *Biobehavioral measures of dyslexia* (pp. 163–176). Parkton, MD: York Press.

Light, J. G., & DeFries, J. C. (1995). Comorbidity of reading and mathematics disabilities: Genetic and environmental etiologies. *Journal of Learning Disabilities, 28,* 96–106.

Logie, R. H., Gilhooly, K. J., & Wynn, C. (1994). Counting on working memory in arithmetic problem solving. *Memory and Cognition, 21,* 11–22.

Lohman, D. F. (1989). Human intelligence: An introduction to advances in theory and research. *Review of Educational Research, 59,* 333–373.

Lohman, D. F. (1994). Spatial ability. In R. J. Sternberg (Ed.), *Encyclopedia of human intelligence* (pp. 1000–1007). New York: Macmillan.

Lowery, L. (1998). How new science curriculums reflect brain research. *Educational Leadership, 56*(3), 26–30.

Lyon, G. R. (1998). Why reading is not natural. *Educational Leadership, 3,* 14–18.

Mahncke, H. W., Bronstone, A., & Merzenich, M. M. (2006). Brain plasticity and functional losses in the aged: Scientific bases for a novel intervention. In A. R. Møller (Ed.), *Progress in brain research: Vol. 157. Reprogramming the brain* (pp. 81–109). Amsterdam: Elsevier.

Manis, F. R., Seidenberg, M. S., & Doi, L. M. (1999). See Dick RAN: Rapid naming and the longitudinal prediction of reading subskills in first and second graders. *Scientific Studies of Reading, 3,* 129–157.

Manis, F. R., Seidenberg, M. S., Stallings, L., Joanisse, M., Bailey, C., Freedman, L., et al. (1999). Development of dyslexic subgroups: A one-year follow up. *Annals of Dyslexia, 49,* 105–134.

Martinussen, R., Hayden, J., Hogg-Johnson, S., & Tannock, R. (2005). A meta-analysis of working memory impairments in children with attention-deficit/hyperactivity disorder. *Journal of the American Academy of Child and Adolescent Psychiatry, 44,* 377–384.

Marzano, R. J. (1992). *A different kind of classroom: Teaching with dimensions of learning.* Alexandria, VA: Association for Supervision and Curriculum Development.

Mastropieri, M. A. (1988). Using the keyboard (sic) method. *Teaching Exceptional Children, 20*(2), 4–8.

McCardle, P., Scarborough, H. S., & Catts, H. W. (2001). Predicting, explaining, and preventing children's reading difficulties. *Learning Disabilities Research and Practice, 16,* 230–239.

McCloskey, G., Perkins, L. A., & Van Divner, B. (2009). *Assessment and intervention for executive function difficulties.* New York: Routledge.

McGrew, K. S. (1993). The relationship between the WJ-R Gf-Gc cognitive clusters and reading achievement across the lifespan. *Journal of Psychoeducational Assessment, Monograph Series: WJ R Monograph,* 39–53.

McGrew, K. S., & Flanagan, D. P. (1998). *The intelligence test desk reference (ITDR): Gf-Gc cross-battery assessment.* Needham Heights, MA: Allyn & Bacon.

McGrew, K. S., Flanagan, D. P., Keith, T. Z., & Vanderwood, M. (1997). Beyond *g*: The impact of Gf-Gc specific cognitive abilities research on the future use and interpretation of intelligence tests in the schools. *School Psychology Review, 26*, 177–189.

McGrew, K. S., & Hessler, G. L. (1995). The relationship between the WJ-R Gf-Gc cognitive clusters and mathematics achievement across the life-span. *Journal of Psychoeducational Assessment, 13*, 21–38.

McGrew, K. S., & Knopik, S. N. (1993). The relationship between the WJ-R Gf-Gc cognitive clusters and writing achievement across the life span. *School Psychology Review, 22*, 687–695.

McGrew, K. S., & Wendling, B. J. (2010). CHC cognitive–achievement relations: What we have learned from the past 20 years of research. *Psychology in the Schools, 47*, 651–675.

McGrew, K. S., & Woodcock, R. W. (2001). *Woodcock–Johnson III technical manual.* Itasca, IL: Riverside.

McLean, J. F., & Hitch, G. J. (1999). Working memory impairments in children with specific arithmetic learning difficulties. *Journal of Experimental Child Psychology, 74*, 240–260.

McNaughton, D. B., Hall, T. E., & Maccini, P. (2001). Case-based instruction in teacher education. *Journal of Teacher Education, 24*, 84–94.

Meyer, M. S., Wood, F. B., Hart, L. A., & Felton, R. H. (1998). Selective predictive value of rapid automatized naming in poor readers. *Journal of Learning Disabilities, 31*, 106–117.

Miller, G., Galanter, E., & Pribram, K. (1960). *Plans and the structure of behavior.* New York: Holt.

Miller, S. P., & Mercer, C. L. (1997). Educational aspects of mathematics disabilities. *Journal of Learning Disabilities, 30*, 47–56.

Moats, L. C. (2001). Spelling disability in adolescents and adults. In A. M. Bain, L. L. Bailet, & L. C. Moats (Eds.), *Written language disorders: Theory into practice* (2nd ed., pp. 43–75). Austin, TX: PRO-ED.

Morris, R. D., Stuebing, K. K., Fletcher, J. M., Shaywitz, S. E., Lyon, G. R., Shankweiler, D. P., et al. (1998). Subtypes of reading disability: Variability around a phonological core. *Journal of Educational Psychology, 90*, 347–373.

Muter, V., Hulme, C., Snowling, M. J., & Taylor, S. (1997). Segmentation, not rhyming predicts early progress in learning to read. *Journal of Experimental Child Psychology, 65*, 370–398.

Muter, V., Hulme, C., Snowling, M. J., & Stevenson, J. (2004). Phonemes, rimes, vocabulary, and grammatical skills as foundations of early reading development: Evidence from a longitudinal study. *Developmental Psychology, 40*, 665–681.

Nation, K. (2007). Children's reading comprehension difficulties. In M. J. Snowling & C. Hulme (Eds.), *The science of reading: A handbook* (pp. 248–265). Oxford: Blackwell.

Nation, K., Clarke, P., Marshall, C. M., & Durand, M. (2004). Hidden language impairments in children: Parallels between poor reading comprehension and specific language impairment? *Journal of Speech, Language, and Hearing Research, 47*, 199–211.

Nation, K., Clarke, P., & Snowling, M. J. (2002). General cognitive ability in children with reading comprehension difficulties. *British Journal of Educational Psychology, 72*, 549–560.

Nation, K., & Snowling, M. J. (2000). Factors influencing syntactic awareness in normal readers and poor comprehenders. *Applied Psycholinguistics, 21*, 229–241.

National Reading Panel (NRP). (2000). *Report of the National Reading Panel: Teaching children to read: An evidence-based assessment of the scientific research literature on reading and its implications for reading instruction.* Washington, DC: National Institute of Child Health and Human Development.

Nettelbeck, T. (1994). Speediness. In R. J. Sternberg (Ed.), *Encyclopedia of human intelligence* (pp. 1014–1019). New York: Macmillan.

Ofiesh, N., Mather, N., & Russell, A. (2005). Using speeded cognitive, reading, and academic measures to determine the need for extended test time among university students with learning disabilities. *Journal of Psychoeducational Assessment, 23*, 35–52.

Ormrod, J. E., & Cochran, K. F. (1988). Relationship of verbal ability and working memory to spelling achievement and learning to spell. *Reading Research and Instruction, 28*, 33–43.

Osmon, D. C., Smertz, J. M., Braun, M. M., & Plambeck, E. (2006). Processing abilities associated with math skills in adult learning disability. *Journal of Clinical and Experimental Neuropsychology, 28*, 84–95.

Passolunghi, M. C., Mammarella, I. C., & Altoè, G. (2008). Cognitive abilities as precursors of the early acquisition of mathematical skills during first through second grades. *Developmental Neuropsychology, 33*, 229–250.

Perfetti, C. A. (1994). Reading. In R. J. Sternberg (Ed.), *Encyclopedia of human intelligence* (pp. 923–930). New York: Macmillan.

Perfetti, C. A. (2007). Reading ability: Lexical quality to comprehension. *Scientific Studies of Reading, 11*, 357–383.

Perfetti, C. A., Landi, N., & Oakhill, J. (2007). The acquisition of reading comprehension skill. In M. J.

Snowling & C. Hulme (Eds.), *The science of reading: A handbook* (pp. 227–247). Oxford, UK: Blackwell.

Perfetti, C. A., Marron, M. A., & Foltz, P. W. (1996). Sources of comprehension failure: Theoretical perspectives and case studies. In C. Cornoldi & J. Oakhill (Eds.), *Reading comprehension difficulties: Processes and intervention* (pp. 137–165). Mahwah, NJ: Erlbaum.

Pinel, P., Piazza, D., Le Bihan, D., & Dehaene, S. (2004). Distributed and overlapping cerebral representations of number, size, and luminance during comparative judgments. *Neuron, 41,* 1–20.

Pressley, M., & Woloshyn, V. (Eds.). (1995). *Cognitive strategy instruction that really improves children's academic performance.* Cambridge, MA: Brookline Books.

Proctor, B. E., Floyd, R. G., & Shaver, R. B. (2005). Cattell–Horn–Carroll broad cognitive ability profiles of low math achievers. *Psychology in the Schools, 42*(1), 1–12.

Rack, J. P., Snowling, M., & Olson, R. (1992). The nonword reading deficit in developmental dyslexia: A review. *Reading Research Quarterly, 27,* 28–53.

Rasmussen, C., & Bisanz, J. (2005). Representation and working memory in early arithmetic. *Journal of Experimental Child Psychology, 91,* 137–157.

Reid, D. K., Hresko, W. P., & Swanson, H. L. (1996). *Cognitive approaches to learning disabilities.* Austin, TX: PRO-ED.

Reschly, D. J (2005). Learning disabilities identification: Primary intervention, secondary intervention, and then what? *Journal of Learning Disabilities, 38,* 510–515.

Reynolds, M. C., & Lakin, K. C. (1987). Noncategorical special education for mildly handicapped students. A system for the future. In M. C. Wang, M. C. Reynolds, & H. J. Walberg (Eds.), *The handbook of special education: Research and practice* (Vol. 1, pp. 331–356). Oxford, UK: Pergamon Press.

Robinson, C. S., Menchetti, B. M., & Torgesen, J. K. (2002). Toward a two-factor theory of one type of mathematics disabilities. *Learning Disabilities Research and Practice, 17,* 81–90.

Rothenberg, S. (1998). Nonverbal learning disabilities and social functioning: How can we help? *Journal of the Learning Disabilities Association of Massachusetts, 8*(4), 10.

Rourke, B. P. (1993). Arithmetic disabilities, specific and otherwise: A neuropsychological perspective. *Journal of Learning Disabilities, 26,* 214–226.

Rourke, B. P. (1995). *Syndrome of nonverbal learning disabilities: Neurodevelopmental manifestations.* New York: Guilford Press.

Rourke, B. P., & Conway, J. A. (1997). Disabilities of arithmetic and mathematical reasoning: Perspectives from neurology and neuropsychology. *Journal of Learning Disabilities, 30,* 34–46.

Rourke, B. P., & Finlayson, M. A. L. (1978). Neuropsychological significance of variations in patterns of academic performance: Verbal and visual–spatial abilities. *Journal of Abnormal Child Psychology, 6,* 121–133.

Scarborough, H. S. (1998). Predicting the future achievement of second graders with reading disabilities: Contributions of phonemic awareness, verbal memory, rapid naming, and IQ. *Annals of Dyslexia, 48,* 115–136.

Schneider, W., & Shiffrin, R. M. (1977). Controlled and automatic human information processing: Detection, search, and attention. *Psychological Review, 84,* 1–66.

Schrank, F. A., Miller, D. C., Wendling, B. J., & Woodcock, R. W. (2010). *Essentials of the WJ III cognitive abilities assessment* (2nd ed.). Hoboken, NJ: Wiley.

Schumm, J. S., Moody, S. W., & Vaughn, S. (2000). Grouping for reading instruction: Does one size fit all? *Journal of Learning Disabilities, 33,* 477–488.

Semrud-Clikeman, M., Steingard, R. J., Filipeck, P., Biederman, J., Bekken, K., & Renshaw, P. F. (2000). Using MRI to examine brain–behavior relationships in males with attention deficit disorder with hyperactivity. *Journal of the American Academy of Child and Adolescent Psychiatry, 39,* 477–484.

Shanahan, M. A., Pennington, B. F., Yerys, B. E., Scott, A., Boada, R., Willcutt, E. G., et al. (2006). Processing speed deficits in attention deficit/hyperactivity disorder and reading disability. *Journal of Abnormal Child Psychology, 34,* 585–602.

Shaywitz, S. E. (1998). Dyslexia. *New England Journal of Medicine, 338,* 307–312.

Shaywitz, S. E. (2003). *Overcoming dyslexia: A new and complete science-based program for overcoming reading problems at any level.* New York: Knopf.

Shaywitz, S. E., Morris, R., & Shaywitz, B. A. (2008). The education of dyslexic children from childhood to young adulthood. *Annual Review of Psychology, 59,* 451–475.

Shaywitz, S. E., Shaywitz, B. A., Fulbright, R. K., Skudlarski, P., Mencl, W. E., Constable, R. T., et al. (2003). Neural systems for compensation and persistence: Young adult outcome of childhood reading disability. *Biological Psychiatry, 54,* 25–33.

Siegel, L. S., & Ryan, E. B. (1988). Development of grammatical sensitivity, phonological, and short-term memory in normally achieving and learning disabled children. *Developmental Psychology, 24,* 28–37.

Smith, D. D., & Rivera, D. P. (1998). Mathematics. In B. Wong (Ed.), *Learning about learning disabilities* (2nd ed., pp. 346–374). San Diego, CA: Academic Press.

Snow, C., Burns, S., & Griffin, P. (1998). *Preventing reading difficulties in young children*. Washington, DC: National Academy Press.

Sousa, D. (1998). Brain research can help principals reform secondary schools. *NASSP Bulletin, 82*, 21–28.

Spectrum K12 School Solutions. (2010). Response to intervention adoption survey 2010. Available at *www.spectrumK12.com/rti/the_rti_corner/rti_adoption_report*.

Stanovich, K. E. (1986). Matthew effects in reading: Some consequences of individual differences in the acquisition of literacy. *Reading Research Quarterly, 21*, 360–407.

Stanovich, K. E. (1991). The psychology of reading: Evolutionary and revolutionary developments. *Annual Review of Applied Linguistics, 12*, 3–30.

Stanovich, K. E. (1993). The construct validity of discrepancy definitions of reading disability. In G. R. Lyon, D. B. Gray, J. F. Kavanagh, & N. A. Krasnegor (Eds.), *Better understanding learning disabilities: New views from research and their implications for education and public policies* (pp. 273–307). Baltimore: Brookes.

Stanovich, K. E. (1999). The sociopsychometrics of learning disabilities. *Journal of Learning Disabilities, 32*, 350–361.

Stanovich, K. E., & Siegel, L. S. (1994). Phenotypic performance profile of children with reading disabilities: A regression-based test of the phonological–core variable–difference model. *Journal of Educational Psychology, 86*, 24–53.

Stern, W. (1938). *General psychology from the personalistic standpoint*. New York: Macmillan.

Strang, R. (1964). *Diagnostic teaching of reading*. New York: McGraw-Hill.

Strawser, S., & Miller, S. P. (2001). Math failure and learning disabilities in the postsecondary student population. *Topics in Language Disorders, 21*, 68–84.

Swanson, H. L. (1987). Information-processing theory and learning disabilities: An overview. *Journal of Learning Disabilities, 20*, 3–7.

Swanson, H. L. (1999). Reading research for students with LD: A meta-analysis of intervention outcomes. *Journal of Learning Disabilities, 32*, 504–532.

Swanson, H. L. (2000). Are working memory deficits in readers with learning disabilities hard to change? *Journal of Learning Disabilities, 33*, 551–566.

Swanson, H. L. (2001). Searching for the best model for instructing students with learning disabilities. *Focus on Exceptional Children, 34*, 1–15.

Swanson, H. L., & Berninger, V. (1995). The role of working memory in skilled and less skilled readers' comprehension. *Intelligence, 21*, 83–108.

Swanson, H. L., & Hsieh, C. J. (2009). Reading disabilities in adults: A selective meta-analysis of the literature. *Review of Educational Research, 79*, 1362–1390.

Swanson, H. L., & Jerman, O. (2006). Math disabilities: A selective meta-analysis of the literature. *Review of Educational Research, 76*, 249–274.

Swanson, H. L., Jerman, O., & Zheng, X. (2008). Growth in working memory and mathematical problem solving in children at risk and not at risk for serious math difficulties. *Journal of Educational Psychology, 100*, 343–379.

Swanson, H. L., & Sachse-Lee, C. (2001). Mathematical problem solving and working memory in children with learning disabilities: Both executive and phonological processes are important. *Journal of Experimental Child Psychology, 79*, 294–321.

Swanson, H. L., & Saez, L. (2003). Memory difficulties in children and adults with learning disabilities. In H. L. Swanson, K. R. Harris, & S. Graham (Eds.), *Handbook of learning disabilities* (pp. 182–198). New York: Guilford Press.

Swanson, H. L., Trainin, G., Necoechea, D. M., & Hammill, D. D. (2003). Rapid naming, phonological awareness, and reading: A meta-analysis of the correlation evidence. *Review of Educational Research, 73*, 407–440.

Sweeney, J. E., & Rourke, B. P. (1985). Spelling disability subtypes. In B. P. Rourke (Ed.), *Neuropsychology of learning disabilities: Essentials of subtype analysis* (pp. 133–144). New York: Guilford Press.

Tomlinson, C. A. (2006). *An educator's guide to differentiating instruction*. Boston: Houghton Mifflin.

Torgesen, J. K. (1997). The prevention and remediation of reading disabilities: Evaluating what we know from research. *Journal of Academic Language Therapy, 1*, 11–47.

Torgesen, J. K. (1998). Catch them before they fall: Identification and assessment to prevent failure in young children. *American Educator, 22*, 32–39.

Torgesen, J. K. (2002). The prevention of reading difficulties. *Journal of School Psychology, 40*(1), 7–26.

Torgesen, J. K., Wagner, R. K., Rashotte, C. A., Rose, E., Lindamood, P., Conway, T., et al. (1999). Preventing reading failure in young children with phonological processing disabilities: Group and individual responses to instruction. *Journal of Educational Psychology, 91*, 579–593.

Travis, L. E. (1935). Intellectual factors. In G. M. Whipple (Ed.), *The thirty-fourth yearbook of the National Society for the Study of Education: Educational diagnosis* (pp. 37–47). Bloomington, IL: Public School Publishing Company.

Uhry, J. K. (2005). Phonological awareness and reading: Theory, research, and instructional activities. In J. R. Birsh (Ed.), *Multisensory teaching of basic language skills* (2nd ed., pp. 83–111). Baltimore: Brookes.

Urso, A. (2008). *Processing speed as a predictor of poor reading.* Unpublished doctoral dissertation, University of Arizona, Tucson.

Vaughn, S., Linan-Thompson, S., & Hickman, P. (2003). Response to instruction as a means of identifying students with reading/learning disabilities. *Exceptional Children, 69,* 391–409.

Vellutino, F. R. (1979). *Dyslexia: Theory and research.* Cambridge, MA: MIT Press.

Vellutino, F. R. (1995). Semantic and phonological coding in poor and normal readers. *Journal of Exceptional Child Psychology, 59,* 76–123.

Vellutino, F. R., Scanlon, D. M., & Lyon, G. R. (2000). Differentiating between difficult-to-remediate and readily remediated poor readers: More evidence against the IQ–achievement discrepancy definition of reading disability. *Journal of Learning Disabilities, 33,* 223–238.

Vellutino, F. R., Tunmer, W. E., Jaccard, J. J., & Chen, S. (2007). Components of reading ability: Multivariate evidence for a convergent skills model of reading development. *Scientific Studies of Reading, 11*(1), 3–32.

Vukovic, R. K., Wilson, A.M., & Nash, K. K. (2004). Naming speed deficits in adults with reading disabilities: A test of the double-deficit hypothesis. *Journal of Learning Disabilities, 37,* 440–450.

Vygotsky, L. S. (1962). *Thought and language.* Cambridge, MA: MIT Press.

Wagner, R. K., Torgesen, J. K., Laughon, P., Simmons, K., & Rashotte, C. A. (1993). The development of young readers' phonological processing abilities. *Journal of Educational Psychology, 85,* 83–103.

Walberg, H. J., & Tsai, S. (1983). Matthew effects in education. *American Educational Research Journal, 20,* 359–373.

Wasserman, J. D. (2003). Assessment of intellectual functioning. In J. R. Graham & J. A. Naglieri (Eds.), *Handbook of psychology* (pp. 417–442). New York: Wiley.

Westman, J. C. (1996). Concepts of dyslexia. In L. R. Putnam (Ed.), *How to become a better reading teacher:* *Strategies for assessment and intervention* (pp. 65–73). Englewood Cliffs, NJ: Merrill.

Whitaker, S. D. (2001). Supporting beginning special education teachers. *Focus on Exceptional Children, 34,* 1–18.

Whitener, E. M. (1989). A meta-analytic review of the effect on learning of the interaction between prior achievement and instructional support. *Review of Educational Research, 59,* 65–86.

Williams, J., Zolten, A. J., Rickert, V. I., Spence, G. T., & Ashcraft, E. W. (1993). Use of nonverbal tests to screen for writing dysfluency in school-age children. *Perceptual and Motor Skills, 76,* 803–809.

Wilson, K. M., & Swanson, H. L. (2001). Are mathematics disabilities due to a domain-general or a domain-specific working memory deficit? *Journal of Learning Disabilities, 34,* 237–248.

Windfuhr, K. L., & Snowling, M. J. (2001). The relationship between paired associate learning and phonological skills in normally developing readers. *Journal of Experimental Child Psychology, 80,* 160–173.

Wise, B. W., & Snyder, L. (2001, August). *Judgments in identifying and teaching children with language-based reading difficulties.* Paper presented at the U.S. Department of Education LD Summit, Washington, DC.

Wodrich, D. L., Spencer, M. L. S., & Daley, K. B. (2006). Combining use of RTI and psychoeducational testing: What we must assume to do otherwise. *Psychology in the Schools, 43,* 798–806.

Wolf, M. (1999). What time may tell: Towards a new conceptualization of developmental dyslexia. *Annals of Dyslexia, 49,* 3–27.

Wolf, M. (2007). *Proust and the squid: The story and science of the reading brain.* New York: HarperCollins.

Wolf, M. (2010). *RAVE-O: Retrieval through automaticity, vocabulary, elaboration, and orthography.* Longmont, CO: Sopris.

Wolf, M., & Bowers, P. G. (1999). The double-deficit hypothesis for the developmental dyslexias. *Journal of Educational Psychology, 91,* 415–438.

Wolf, M., Bowers, P. G., & Biddle, K. (2000). Naming speed processes, timing, and reading: A conceptual review. *Journal of Learning Disabilities, 33,* 387–407.

Zorzi, M., Priftis, K., & Umiltá, C. (2002). Neglect disrupts the mental number line. *Nature, 417,* 138–139.

PART V

ASSESSMENT OF INTELLIGENCE AND COGNITIVE FUNCTIONING IN DIFFERENT POPULATIONS

CHAPTER 24

Cognitive Assessment in Early Childhood
Theoretical and Practice Perspectives

Laurie Ford
Michelle L. Kozey
Juliana Negreiros

It is an exciting time for both researchers and clinicians working in the area of cognitive assessment. Earlier chapters in this book point to the rich history of cognitive and intellectual assessment, and the movement to contemporary ways of assessing cognitive abilities. Advances in cognitive theory, psychometrics, and the development of the tests themselves have resulted in more sophisticated ways to assess the cognitive abilities of school-age students and adults. Much of this work has been applied to and informs assessment in early childhood. However, the cognitive assessment of very young children is a unique and specialized endeavor. Best practice in the contemporary assessment of children in the early years requires knowledge not only of the contemporary theory, tests, and practices highlighted in other chapters of this book, but also a solid and fluent understanding of early child development, awareness of the different measures currently available to assess cognitive abilities in young children, and specific knowledge of considerations unique to the cognitive assessment of this population. It is our hope that the readers of this chapter will gain a better understanding of both theoretical and practical considerations for conducting a cognitive assessment with children during their early years.

Consistent with the terms used in the preschool assessment chapter in an earlier edition of this text (Ford & Dahinten, 2005), we use the terms *cognitive abilities* and *cognitive assessment* relatively interchangeably with *intelligence* and *intellectual assessment*, respectively, despite acknowledged differences between these terms. Although the terms *intelligence* and *intelligence testing* are commonly used with school-age children and adults (and indeed *intellectual assessment* has been selected for the title of this book), most professionals working with young children prefer the broader term *cognitive ability* to *intelligence*, given the many misunderstandings and potential misuses of the term *intelligence*. The best word or phrase to capture the age range of focus also may prove confusing. *Infancy and toddlerhood* refer to the ages between birth and 2 years, whereas the *preschool years* typically begin between 2 and 3 years and extend to the beginning of school, usually about 5 or 6 years. At this time, most children enter school for their primary years, which typically include kindergarten, grade 1, and grade 2 (approximately ages 5–6 through 8 years). However, students with developmental delays at ages 6, 7, and 8 may demonstrate many characteristics of preschool-age children. As a result, the cognitive assessment procedures discussed in this chapter apply to children from birth through primary years.

THEORETICAL FOUNDATIONS

Historical Perspectives

During the 20th century, many cognitive theories were generated to explain how individuals' cognitive abilities develop throughout the lifespan. Several of these theories (e.g., those of Piaget, Gesell, and Vygotsky) place considerable emphasis on children in the early years. A comprehensive review of these early cognitive theories is beyond the scope of this chapter. However, for a clinician assessing any young child, a good working understanding of cognitive development will facilitate success not only in selecting appropriate measures, but also in interacting with the child during the test session, and (perhaps most importantly) in adequately interpreting the information gained from any assessment. An overview of cognitive-developmental theories widely referenced in the early childhood literature is provided in Table 24.1, and a basic overview of the work of two of the more influential theorists is given below.

Most clinicians have some sense of the more readily observable domains of development, such as social, language, and motor development. Many know that it is typical for a child to begin walking at about 1 year of age, to combine two or more words at about 18–24 months, and to play alongside other peers at 3–4 years of age; they also know that frequent tantrums may be common to age 6 (and sometimes beyond!). However, some professionals have less training and experience in cognitive development and the impact of cognitive development on other domains of development. Indeed, most behavioral, social, and language concerns are linked with cognitive development (Spritz & Sandberg, 2010). Those who are unfamiliar with the development of young children may consider behavior that is different from the norms for older children as "abnormal" and may misidentify typical development as learning concerns (Spritz & Sandberg, 2010; Vig & Sanders, 2007).

The work of Piaget (1967/1971) and Vygotsky (1978) has had a significant impact on our understanding of early child development. Piaget defined intelligence as a form of *adaptation* to the environment. Through direct experiences and interactions with the world, children are able to build schemes (or mental structures) that facilitate their adaptation to the environment, and knowledge is constructed and organized through the two complementary mechanisms of *assimilation* and *accommodation*. Because individuals progressively adapt to the environment in more complex ways, both of these mechanisms are used throughout life (Huitt & Hummel, 2003). Piaget stressed that child development occurs through six stages, which often are condensed into four stages (*sensorimotor, preoperational, concrete operational,* and *formal operational*). Through this process, the brain and nervous system mature, physical operations develop into mental operations, and children are exposed to experiences that enhance their adaptation to the environment. Between birth and 2 years, infants and toddlers rely on their senses and motor abilities to learn and act upon the world (sensorimotor stage). Their physical interactions and experiences initiate the development of new intellectual abilities, and at the end of this stage, language (symbolic ability) develops. As children progress to the preoperational stage (ages 2–7), their intellectual abilities are demonstrated through the use of symbols, language, memory, and imagination, characterized by egocentric thinking and often by illogical and irreversible reasoning (Piaget, 1969).

Vygotsky (1978) offered an alternative view of early development from a sociocultural perspective, with a strong focus on language as a social and communicative central process for cognitive development. He theorized that children construct meaning through their social interactions with other individuals. The construction of knowledge occurs socially rather than individually and in two ways: at the social level (between people) and later at the individual level (inside a child). As children mature, they learn to speak and engage in social dialogue with other individuals; this language begins to shape the children's actions and to increase their self-controlling behavior. Central to Vygotsky's work is the concept of the *zone of proximal development* (ZPD). The ZPD is "the distance between the actual developmental level, as determined by independent problem solving, and the level of potential development, as determined through problem solving under adult guidance or in collaboration with more capable peers" (Vygotsky, 1978, p. 86). The goal in the learning process is for the child to achieve the higher level of potential development. For this to happen, guidance provided by adults or more advanced peers is needed. The idea is that children who belong to the same age group do not necessarily have the same ZPD, and this is an important consideration when asking children to perform tasks with a focus on *scaffolding* strategies (a method that decreases the amount of direct instruction given to the children as they learn new tasks). In contrast to Piaget, Vygotsky proposed no universal stages of cognitive development; he believed that individual sociocultural histories and interaction with contexts shape children's learning (Zembar & Blume, 2009).

These two theories are among the most widely cited in the early child development literature. Along with an understanding and application of neo-Piagetian (Case, 1992; Case & Okamoto, 1996), maturation (Gesell & Amatruda, 1941), structural cognitive (Feurestein, 1990), social-cognitive (Bruner, 1960, 1990), Reggio Emilia (Malaguzzi, 1998), and attachment (Ainsworth, Blehar, Waters, & Wall, 1978; Bowlby, 1969/1999) theories and models, they provide an important foundation for the assessment of young children.

Cattell–Horn–Carroll Theory and Early Childhood Assessment

The theoretical models highlighted above have influenced thinking about cognitive development in young children, and the development of many early childhood cognitive measures has been in turn been influenced by these theories. Most of the cognitive tests given to young children, including those reviewed in this chapter, utilize downward extensions of the theoretical frameworks used in the interpretation of tests with older individuals. Although most contemporary cognitive assessment measures now have strong and well-articulated theoretical foundations with school-age children and adults, little empirical evidence is provided on the application of these models to the early childhood components of these the tests.

The work of Horn and Cattell (1966) and of Carroll (1993), detailed in other chapters of this book, has revolutionized our approach to cognitive testing and interpretation. However, surprisingly little work has been done to examine the validity of the Cattell–Horn–Carroll (CHC) model with preschool-age children. Evidence from factor-analytic studies indicates that there are typically fewer factors for younger children than for older populations (Hunt, 2008; Morgan, 2008; Morgan, Rothlisberg, McIntosh, & Hunt, 2009; League, 2000; Teague, 1999; Tusing, 1998; Tusing & Ford, 2004). The results of key studies examining the application of the CHC model in the early years are highlighted in Table 24.2.

Early work asserted that cognitive abilities in young children are less differentiated than in older children (Garrett, 1946). Although they are not as differentiated as in older populations, contemporary perspectives on cognitive develop-

ment support greater differentiation of cognitive abilities in young children than was once believed (Chen & Siegler, 2000; Grannot, 1998; Holler & Greene, 2010; Sandberg & McCullough, 2010). While the five, six, or seven factors evidenced in many measures for school-age and adult populations have not been demonstrated in cognitive measures in early childhood, recent psychometric studies have identified latent factors including crystallized abilities or general knowledge, short-term memory, auditory processing, visual processing, and in some studies fluid reasoning (Hooper, 2000; Hooper, Molnar, Beswick, & Jacobi-Vessels, 2007; Hunt, 2008; League, 2000; Morgan, 2008; Morgan et al., 2009; Stone, Gridley, & Gyurke, 1991; Teague, 1999; Tusing, 1998; Tusing & Ford, 2004). The majority of the work in this area uses confirmatory-factor-analytic approaches, given the strong support for CHC theory. Given that many of the tests and subtests in current measures were developed as downward extensions of their school-age counterparts, perhaps the tasks need to be different and not just more child-friendly versions of the tasks to capture a broader range of abilities. Finally, perhaps exploratory analysis following procedures similar to Carroll's, now that we have datasets with improved early childhood measures, would allow us to better understand the application of the CHC model to measures of cognitive abilities in early childhood.

PERSPECTIVES ON PRACTICE

Historical and Legislative Perspectives

In addition to advances in understandings of early development, practices related to the cognitive assessment of young children have evolved partially as a direct function of demands imposed by U.S. federal policy, regulations, and laws. Indeed, legislative changes have frequently been linked to advances in assessment measures and practice guidelines for young children. In the past 40 years, programs and legislation related to early assessment and intervention services have become more widespread, have been extended to a greater age range of children, and have become more detailed in their requirements regarding eligibility (Anastasi & Urbina, 1997; Nuttall, Romero, & Kalesnik, 1992). Whereas initial early childhood programs focused upon serving children with significant socioeconomic disadvantage (e.g., Head Start in the 1960s; see Peterson, 1987), subsequent and most

TABLE 24.1. Key Cognitive and Developmental Theories Relevant to Early Childhood Cognitive Assessment

Paradigm	Theory	Key figures	Key messages	Common terms	Key reference
Cognitive	Maturation model	Arnold Gesell	• Recognizes the importance of both nature and nurture • Development occurs in a specific order, time, and sequence and thus is predictable.	Development preprogrammed; maturation; growth	Gesell and Amatruda (1941)
Cognitive	Theory of cognitive development	Jean Piaget	• Intelligence as a form of adaptation to the environment • Children learn experiencing cognitive disequilibrium • Thought and problem-solving skills are developed through direct interaction with the environment through the processes of assimilation and accommodation	Equilibration; adaptation; schema; assimilation; accommodation; stages of cognitive development	Piaget (1967/1971)
Cognitive	Information processing	Alexander Luria	• Brain is organized into functional units that provide for basic psychological processes including attention/cortical arousal, simultaneous and successive processes (receiving, analyzing, and storing information), and self-monitoring and control of cognitive activities	Functional units; central executive; encoding; sensory registers; working memory; long-term storage	Luria (1973)
Cognitive	Structural cognitive modifiability	Reuven Feuerstein	• Recognized the importance of both nature and nurture • Intelligence can be modified through mediated interventions • Explored the aspects of shaping environments to promote individuals' modifiability	Mediated learning experience; modifiability; cognitive map; dynamic assessment; learning propensity assessment device; shaping modifying environments	Feuerstein (1990)
Cognitive	Neo-Piagetian theories of development	Juan Pascual-Leone, Andrea Demetriou, Robbie Case	• Explored the patterns of developmental changes through aspects of cognition (Pascal) • Investigated cognitive development based on individual differences and its underlying cognitive mechanisms • Integration of cognitive, developmental, and information processing approaches to development	Theory of constructive operators; metaconstructs; processing potentials; domain specificity; hypercognition; central conceptual structures; executive control structures	Pascual-Leone and Goodman (1979) Demetriou, Doise, and van Lieashout (1998) Case (1992)

Category	Theory	Theorist	Description	Key concepts	Reference
Constructivist	Social development theory	Lev Vygotsky	• Emphasis on the role of social interaction in the development of cognition • Development must be considered in the social and cultural context in which it is embedded • Cognitive processes, including language, thought, and reasoning, develop through social interaction	Zone of proximal development; elementary mental functions; scaffolding; guided participation; role of culture in learning; more knowledgeable others	Vygotsky (1978)
Constructivist	Theory on constructivism	Jerome Bruner	• Learning is a process in which new ideas or concepts are developed based on the learner's current and past knowledge • Interpersonal communication (language) is necessary for development and the ability to deal with abstract concepts • Development occurs through social interaction and active intervention of adults • Organized instruction allows learners at all ages to learn any material	Constructivism; discovery learning; instructional scaffolding; cognitive structures	Bruner (1960, 1990)
Constructivist	Reggio Emilia approach	Loris Malaguzzi	• More of a philosophical approach with roots in sociocultural and constructivist approaches and theory than a specific theory of development • Environment is at the center of development • Children have some control over the course of learning • Learning occurs through senses (seeing, hearing, listening, touching, and moving)	Collective responsibility; the hundred languages of children; project-based learning	Edwards, Gandini, and Forman (1998)
Cognitive-developmental	Attachment theory	John Bowlby, Mary Ainsworth	• Early attachments with significant others shape relationships for the remainder of individuals' lives • Developmental sequence of attachment relationships during the first 3 years of life has a significant impact on later development • Goal of attachment is to move from a totally dependent relationship with an attachment figure in infancy to a more interdependent partnership	Strange Situation; phases of attachment (secure, ambivalent, insecure, avoidant)	Bowlby (1969/1999); Ainsworth, Blehar, Waters, and Wall (1978)

TABLE 24.2. Summary of Selected CHC Factor-Analytic Studies with Early Childhood Populations

Citation	Measures	CHC abilities	Age range	Key findings
Gyurke, Stone, and Beyer (1990)	WPPSI-R	Not fully addressed due to time of publication, but crystallized abilities and visual processing abilities were highlighted.	3:0–7:3	A comparison of underlying theory and goodness-of-fit statistics for the analyses provided support for the two-factor solution as best representing the scale's underlying structure.
Hunt (2008)	KABC-II, WJ III COG	Gc, Glr, Gv, Gsm	4:0–5:11	A two-model Gf-Gc model was the best-fitting model, but the three-tiered CHC model also fit data for KABC-II. WJ-III COG was represented by an alternative CHC model where Gf factor and subtests were removed, meaning that all CHC constructs on the WJ III COG could reliably be identified among young children. Overall, results confirmed that multiple CHC abilities can be assessed, implying that clinicians can use these measures in preschool-age populations.
League (2000)	WJ III COG, WPPSI-R	Gc, Gv, Gs, Gsm	3:0–5:11	A two-factor structure representing verbal and nonverbal abilities was supported for the WPPSI-R. A three- or four-factor structure, including Gc, Gv, Gs, and Gsm, was supported for the WJ III COG dataset. A two-factor structure representing verbal and nonverbal abilities was supported for the combined dataset.
Morgan, Rothlisberg, McIntosh, and Hunt (2009); Morgan (2008)	KABC-II	Gc, Gv, Glr, Gsm	4:0–5:11	Confirmatory factor analysis suggested that a broad-factor-plus-g CHC model was the best fitting model to explain the KABC-II. Models 2 and 3 were better representations of data than model 1; preschoolers' intelligence was most similar to hierarchical CHC theory (i.e., including global intelligence score).
Stone, Gridley, and Gyurke (1991)	WPPSI-R	Not fully addressed due to time of publication, but crystallized abilities and visual processing abilities were highlighted.	3:0–7:3	Goodness-of-fit statistics revealed that a two-factor solution was the best model for both samples. Support for the interpretation of two consistent factors was found across the WPPSI-2 age range.
Teague (2002)	DAS, WJ III COG	Gc, Gv, Glr/Gsm, Ga, Gs	3:0–5:11	The DAS measured verbal–nonverbal and multiple Gf-Gc abilities. A seven-factor Gf-Gc model was not supported for the WJ III COG. Joint analyses examining the DAS and WJ III COG with the seven Gf-Gc abilities failed to support the seven factors, with four factors providing the best fit.
Tusing (1998)	WJ-R, DAS	Gc, Ga, Gv, Gsm, Glr	4:0–5:11	Confirmatory factor analyses supported a four-factor interpretation (Ga, Gv, Gsm, Glr) of the WJ-R and a two-factor interpretation (Nonverbal Ability, Verbal Ability) of the DAS. Joint confirmatory factor analysis of the combined group of subtests supported a hierarchical representation of the abilities measured by both tests, which was likened to Vernon's (1950) theory of intelligence and modern Gf-Gc.
Tusing and Ford (2004)	WJ-R, DAS	Gc, Ga, Gsm, Glr, Gf, Gv, Gq	4:0–5:11	Five broad-ability factors were reliably identified (Gc, Glr, Gsm, Ga, nonverbal ability). Gq and Gf could not be significantly distinguished in this sample.

contemporary early childhood programs and mandates have been expanded to serve primarily young children with special needs, with an increased focus on family-centered service provision (e.g., the 1972 Economic Opportunity Amendment, the 1968 Handicapped Children's Early Education Assistance Act). These legislative and program expansions and diversifications were accompanied by a need to better understand and measure the development of young children; Head Start alone accounted in part for the creation of more than 200 childhood screening, monitoring, and general assessment instruments between the 1960s and 1980s (Kelley & Surbeck, 2007).

Practices in cognitive and developmental assessment of young children were similarly influenced by subsequent developments in special education law (for more detailed reviews, see Jacob & Decker, 2007; Kelley & Surbeck, 2007). Beginning with the 1975 Education for All Handicapped Children Act (EHA) and the 1986 EHA Amendments (the Infants and Toddlers with Disabilities Act), a free, appropriate public education for children with disabilities between the ages of 3 and 21 was mandated, followed by requirements for state provision of special education services for children ages 3–5 (Yell, 1998). Part H of the 1986 EHA Amendments also granted the first major financial incentives for state provision of early intervention services for very young children (birth through 3 years), which were to feature the involvement of multidisciplinary professionals and the development of individual family service plans.

Collectively, policy and legislative changes during these periods were accompanied by a need for new measures to evaluate the efficacy of early intervention programs and evaluate the development of young children, with an emphasis on cognitive testing (see Ford & Dahinten, 2005; Yell, 1998). As noted above, many new preschool-specific measures were created in this era, such as the Wechsler Preschool and Primary Scales of Intelligence (Wechsler, 1967), the Bayley Scales of Infant Development (Bayley, 1969), the Stanford–Binet Intelligence Scale: Fourth Edition (Thorndike, Hagen, & Sattler, 1986), the Kaufman Assessment Battery for Children (K-ABC; Kaufman & Kaufman, 1983), and the Battelle Developmental Inventory (Newborg, Stock, Wnek, Guidubaldi, & Svinicki, 1984). However, many of these tests had serious technical flaws and sociocultural biases (see Bracken, 1987, 1988).

As special education mandates were extended to identify and serve younger children, demand has continued for more reliable, valid, and sensitive measures specific to young children, along with practice guidelines and additional training specific to the assessment of young children (Yell, 1998). Early special education legislation was reauthorized and renamed in the 1990s and again in 2004, and is currently known as the Individuals with Disabilities Education Improvement Act of 2004 (IDEA 2004). Within this framework, the provision of special education to children ages 3 and older is mandated under Part B, and the provision of services specific to infants and toddlers is detailed in Part C. Part C currently mandates state-provided, multidisciplinary "child find" (early identification) and intervention services for children from birth to 3 years with either a developmental delay, or a diagnosed physical or mental condition associated with a high probability of developmental delay. Whereas Part B of the IDEA 2004 legislation was reauthorized in 2009, Part C and related implementation guidelines proposed in 2007 (U.S. Department of Education, 2007) were subsequently withdrawn and remain under review at this writing (National Early Childhood Technical Assistance Center [NECTAC], 2011).

Several notable trends or features of federal legislation have had significant consequences for the assessment of young children. First, "developmental delay" was added as a disability category in 1990 for children ages 3 through 5; in the 1997 reauthorization under Part C, it was extended downward to birth, and upward for the optional inclusion of children up to 9 years. Under Part C, young children with delays in physical, cognitive, communication, social, emotional, or adaptive development are now eligible for early intervention services from birth to age 3, with a right to special education services during the 3- to 9-year range. Use of the term *developmental delay*, what constitutes a developmental delay, and specific assessment and eligibility criteria frequently differ across state special education agencies, as well as across school districts or infant–toddler versus preschool programs within the same state. Furthermore, one-fifth of states have narrowed their eligibility criteria over the past 10 years (NECTAC, 2011).

Other challenges in the area of early childhood assessment are related to the paradoxical combination of child find (early identification) requirements and funding arrangements for IDEA 2004 Part C. In contrast to Part B special education services for preschool children, Part C state funding for services for infants and toddlers is time-limited and subject to renewal approximately every 4–5 years (Jacob & Decker, 2007). Data presented by the IDEA Infant and Toddler Coordinators Association (2011) suggest that the number of children served under Part C has increased by 55% between 1999 and 2005, whereas the funding per child has decreased by 24%. Finally, most jurisdictions require financial contributions for services from multiple sources, including parents, insurance, Medicaid, or educational institutions. All of these financial contributions may affect clinicians' ability to conduct contemporary, comprehensive, or more frequent evaluations, which are often needed with young children. These legislative requirements have had and probably will continue to have a significant impact on the practice of cognitive assessment with children in the early years.

What's Special about Cognitive Assessment with Young Children?

Overview

Examiners new to testing young children often mistakenly rely upon tests and procedures more appropriate to older children (Bagnato, Neisworth, & Munson, 1997; Ford & Dahinten, 2005; McLean, Bailey, & Wolery, 1996). Clinicians must recognize that the process of cognitive assessment with this age group is unique because the behavior of young children is so different from that of school-age children and adults. Even for an examiner who is experienced in cognitive assessment but inexperienced in early childhood assessment, the unique characteristics and behaviors of young children can make cognitive assessment challenging.

Cognitive assessment of young children is both special because of, and complicated by, the complex nature of development in early childhood. Developmental change can be highly idiographic, and changes in cognitive development occur more rapidly during the early years. Furthermore, there is considerable overlap in growth across domains of development (e.g., cognitive, social, motor, and language), which means that examiners must have knowledge of both early cognitive development and the relationship among cognitive, physical, social, emotional, behavioral, and language development. Behavior that is generally considered atypical or extreme in a school-age student may be the norm in the early years. A young child's spontaneity, attention, focus, compliance, activity level, wariness of strangers, adjustment to new environments, language, articulation, and other developmental characteristics pose unique challenges for even the most experienced examiner. However, with a strong and flexible understanding of developmental considerations in the predictable sequence of development in young children, reliable and valid assessment information may be obtained. Given the interplay among children, adults (including examiners and caregivers), and the environment, ecological frameworks with roots in Bronfenbrenner's (1977, 1979) model are supported by most who work with young children and publish in the area of early childhood assessment (e.g., Bracken & Nagle, 2007; Brassard & Boehm, 2007; Lichtenstein & Ireton, 1984; McLean, Wolery, & Bailey, 2004; Mowder, Rubinson, & Yasik, 2008; Shepard, Kagan, & Wurtz, 1998). Ecological models provide a helpful framework for professionals assessing children in early childhood. Details of these models are beyond the scope of this chapter; however, Brassard and Boehm (2007) provide an excellent synthesis of the research in this area and describe an ecocultural model for the assessment of young children. The following paragraphs highlight specific examinee (child), examiner (adult), and environment considerations in the cognitive assessment of children in their early years.

The Child

The examiner must be comfortable with the young child and his or her behaviors, and keep in mind the idiographic nature of child development. Children in their early years are often reported by psychologists as "untestable" when the examiners attempt to administer traditional, standardized measures (Bagnato & Neisworth, 1994; Dudley, 2000). Short attention span, limited degree of focus, high activity level, separation difficulty, anxiety, and a general lack of concern about pleasing the examiners through their responses, are common characteristics reported by examiners testing young children. Although such behaviors may make standardized, norm-referenced cognitive assessment a challenge, they are common for a young child to display in a novel situation, such as standardized testing. Many children of this age also have limited experience working directly with unfamiliar adults, and a new adult's asking such a child to do unfamiliar tasks in an unfamiliar environment may prove challenging for both.

Language and motor development may have an impact on the assessment of cognitive abilities as well. The language abilities of young children— including their ability to comprehend directions, the intelligibility of their speech, and their ability to express themselves verbally—can all affect assessment. Furthermore, perceptual–motor skills such as pointing or drawing are included in many early childhood cognitive measures, but may not be developed adequately for a given child to respond as needed for the tasks' demands. Subsequently, interpretation of any cognitive test results must take into consideration the possibility of confounding language or motor delays.

Developing familiarity with a child of any age through observation and relationship-building activities is important in assessment. With a young child, however, it is critical to spend time with and/or observe the child before the testing, to reduce separation or "warm-up" concerns. When possible, the examiner should spend time with the child in the company of his or her parent/caregiver or teacher in the location where testing will occur. Examples include working with the child in his or her preschool classroom, playing cars in a waiting area, reading a book in the testing room, or getting to know the child in other ways. It is essential to let the child know that familiar adults are nearby and will be available when the testing is completed (Ford & Dahinten, 2005).

The Examiner

The examiner's background in child development and familiarity with the tests will influence the information gained from any assessment (Flanagan, Mascolo, & Genshaft, 2000; Ford & Dahinten, 2005). One of the more common challenges faced by examiners is the lack of opportunity for supervised training in the assessment of young children. In spite of the need for psychologists with preparation and skill in the assessment of this population (which arose with the passage of amendments to federal law in the 1980s and continues today), few training programs in school or child clinical psychology have historically offered supervised training in the psychological, developmental, or educational assessment of young children, and often do not emphasize the use of standardized, norm-referenced cognitive assessment procedures with these children (Alfonzo, Oakland, LaRocca, & Spanakos, 2000; Dudley, 2000; Ford & Dahinten, 2005; Ford & Rivera, 1995; Percy, Ford, & Negreiros, 2010). Many interested examiners attempt to gain training largely through workshop and inservice training on new tests. These trainings, however, often focus on tests that span the age range, with no specific training in early child-

hood assessment. Familiarity with test procedures is important, but it is equally critical that examiners have experience in working directly with young children and seek opportunities for supervision as they begin to work with this age group.

A manner that is friendly and engaging, yet firm, consistent, and professional, facilitates a successful testing session. The examiner's language should be developmentally appropriate for the age of the child, and examiners should be conscious of how their own verbalizations impact session behavior management. The use of "baby talk" or sing-song, game-like approaches should be avoided, as such language and behavior may work against optimal testing. Although standardized testing can be fun and enjoyable for all, it requires the child to comply with a series of instructions and requests from the examiner. If the child views the test session as a game in which he or she can do what he or she prefers, the child may be less likely to comply with the examiner's requests (Ford & Dahinten, 2005).

Examiners should also be aware of how their language usage fits with the temperament and arousal level of a particular child. Some children respond well to a "chatty" examiner, while others, especially those with language delays, may be overwhelmed by a lot of questions and verbal praise. Familiarity with a wide array of standardized assessment instruments coupled with other formal and informal procedures will help the examiner tailor the assessment to the unique needs of each child. For example, if a child is initially shy and hesitant to provide a verbal response, the examiner can begin with a test or subtest that involves manipulating materials such as blocks or formboards, or that requires limited or no verbal response (e.g., allows pointing to responses). Many children become less hesitant and more verbal and engaged as the session progresses.

An examiner new to testing young children may find a greater need to make accommodations, such as adjusting the order of test/subtest administration and the pace of administration, or taking more frequent breaks. Examiners should carefully review in advance the guidelines on the accommodations that are allowable for a given test at the younger ages specified in most test manuals; once the test session begins, there is little time or opportunity for review, given the pace needed to keep the examinee engaged.

There may be a need to adjust the pace within and across assessment sessions. Many young children respond to a brisk, quick pace, while others respond better to a slower pace. Some children are easily distracted, while others fatigue quickly. The examiner should watch the child for signs of fatigue and carefully monitor the need for breaks, as many children will not ask for a break on their own. Although young children typically need more frequent breaks than do older children and adults during the testing sessions, the breaks can be much shorter. In most cases, several short breaks may prove more helpful than one longer break. Breaks with a clear beginning and end, such as taking a short walk, getting a drink of water or snack, tossing a ball, or stretches, are desirable (Ford & Dahinten, 2005). Ultimately, the pace of the testing session must be adjusted to the needs of the child, not the examiner.

Young children often require more praise and reinforcement than do older students. Whereas verbal praise may be sufficient for most children at this early age, some may require additional reinforcement through a soft touch on the hand or tangible reinforcers (e.g., stickers and stamps). The latter practices are appropriate with young children, given their likely lack of familiarity with testing situations, or with seatwork in very structured environments. However, the examiner must be careful not to praise the child's correct responses, but rather to praise his or her effort and engagement with the task. The ultimate goal is a positive and engaging experience for the child.

The Testing Environment

The testing space often creates additional assessment challenges. Although a colorful and engaging testing room is useful in attracting young children to the testing situation, such attractions may serve as distractions once the assessment begins. In other cases, an examiner may attempt to test a child in a corner of a child care center or preschool, due to the familiarity of these settings for the examinee. However, environmental distractions (e.g., other materials and happenings in the center) often interfere with the assessment and should be minimized. Windows, shades, and doors should be closed to limit visual and auditory distractions, and the child should be positioned so that he or she is not looking at a window or door.

The physical set-up of the testing furniture and materials should also be tailored to the needs of young children. The examinee should be sitting at a table and a chair appropriate for his or her size, so that feet are on the ground and arms are able to rest comfortably on the table. Because of difficulty with positioning and management of movement,

testing should not be conducted by sitting on the floor. In the case of an extremely active child, it may be helpful to position the table, child, and examiner in a manner that restricts child movement and facilitates behavior management—for example, seating the child in a corner of the room, with a table at an angle in front of him or her, and the examiner on the corner next to the child. Materials not in immediate use, such as pencils, response booklets, manipulatives for later items, or additional easel books, should be out of the child's reach (and, if possible, out of sight).

It is typical to test an infant or toddler with a parent or other adult caregiver in the room, but a caregiver should typically not be present in the room during testing for most early childhood cognitive measures. Although it is not optimal, a parent may remain in the testing room if separation problems do occur, in order to help the child adjust to the test situation and to increase his or her comfort with the examiner. If a parent remains in the room, the child should sit on his or her own chair with the parent to one side and slightly behind the child, to limit parent–child interaction. In the latter situation, the examiner must clearly explain the reasons for and importance of standardized procedures to the parent, and firmly instruct the parent not to provide any prompting or assistance on any items, even if the parent believes the child knows the correct response when the child has not responded. Letting the parent know that some items will be easy, that others will be difficult, and that the child is not expected to know all the answers is likely to help put the parent at ease.

CONSIDERATIONS IN SELECTING COGNITIVE MEASURES FOR YOUNG CHILDREN

A multimodal, multidomain approach, with information gathered from multiple sources in a multi- or interdisciplinary manner, is considered best practice for the assessment of children in early childhood—even when assessment covers only one domain, such as cognitive abilities. Debates have occurred in the literature over the past 20 years regarding the use of standardized, norm-referenced measures in the cognitive assessment of young children, in large part because of concerns about their ability to predict future performance and about their developmental and ecological validity (Bagnato & Neisworth, 1994; Epstein, Schweinhart, DeBruin-Parecki, & Robin, 2004;

Greenspan & Meisels, 1996; Lidz, 2003; Meisels & Atkins-Burnett, 2000; Rock & Stenner, 2005; Vig & Sanders, 2007). Many researchers in the field stress the importance of informal and play-based approaches, along with standardized tests, as part of a more holistic approach to assessment (Bracken, 1994; Epstein et al., 2004; Gyurke, 1994; Lidz, 2003; Linder, 2008; Vig & Sanders, 2007). Early childhood and professional organizations likewise support the use of more holistic, developmentally appropriate, and ecologically valid approaches to the assessment of young children (e.g., the Division for Early Childhood within the Council for Exceptional Children, the National Association for the Education of Young Children, the National Association of School Psychologists, the National Institute for Early Education Research, and Zero to Three). However, when the reason for the referral and the context and purpose of the assessment call for standardized testing, and when details of the tests themselves are used carefully by an examiner with supervised training and experience in the cognitive assessment of young children, standardized, norm-referenced measures can provide valuable information for both diagnosis and program planning that may be integrated with other sources of assessment data.

A detailed examination of the technical characteristics of all the major early childhood measures of cognitive abilities is beyond the scope of this chapter. However, the following section of the chapter provides an overview and brief review/critique of the most widely used early childhood measures. The measures reviewed were chosen on the basis of their frequency of use by psychologists that assess young children, and their status as contemporary or current measures (i.e., developed or revised in the last 10 years, with one exception). All cognitive measures included have some version of the test available for use with school-age students, and many are either appropriate for use with adults or have adult versions. Readers are referred to chapters elsewhere in this text, where the full batteries of most of the cognitive measures described below are discussed in greater detail. A summary of key features of the measures reviewed in this chapter is provided in Table 24.3.

In addition to cognitive measures, measures with separate sections for assessment of multiple domains (e.g., cognitive, language, motor, and adaptive development), are not common for school-age populations and adults, but are often used in early childhood. Such multidomain measures typically span the full early childhood range (birth to early primary grades). Given their widespread use, a brief review of these measures is also provided, and Table 24.4 summarizes their key features. For more detailed reviews, the reader is referred to Alfonzo and Flanagan (1999, 2007, 2009), Bracken (1987), Bradley-Johnson (2001), Flanagan and Alfonzo (1995), Ford, Kozey, and Negreiros (2011), Kozey, Ford, Merkel, and Morgan (2005), Lichtenberger (2005), and Tusing, Maricle, and Ford (2003).

The nature of early childhood, including the rapid and uneven periods of development and other child characteristics highlighted earlier, makes reliable and valid assessment of this population difficult (Nagle, 2000, 2007). Several studies have critiqued the technical adequacy of early childhood cognitive measures over the years (see Alfonzo & Flanagan, 1999, 2007, 2009; Bracken, 1987; Bracken, Keith, & Walker, 1998; Bradley-Johnson, 2001; Kozey et al., 2005). Attempts have been made to establish and apply common evaluation criteria to cognitive measures for young children, and variations on the criteria established by Bracken (1987) are commonly used in most research in this area to establish the psychometric quality of such measures. Areas of review typically include reliability, validity, test floors and ceilings, item gradients, and recency and nature of normative data (see Alfonzo & Flanagan, 2009, for a more comprehensive review). Others have pointed to a need to examine the language demands, particularly the use of basic concepts, in early childhood cognitive measures (Flanagan, Alfonzo, Kaminer, & Rader, 1995). More recently, culture and linguistic considerations have been added as important aspects of a comprehensive review (Flanagan, Ortiz, & Alfonzo, 2007).

Historically, the ceiling problems of infant/toddler tests and floor problems of preschool tests presented examiners with challenges in assessing young children with developmental delays. Floor and ceiling problems are significant concerns with early childhood measures, due to their limited distribution of scores at the top and bottom of a scale (Rock & Stenner, 2005). However, recent revisions of several measures for young children have attempted to address these concerns—either by extending the age ranges of the tests as a whole, or by expanding the age range for some factors or clusters on the tests.

Although the tests presented in the remainder of this chapter all have limitations in addition to their strengths, they represent the best and most widely used measures of cognitive abilities or intelligence for young children at the present time. The

TABLE 24.3. Overview of Widely Used Early Childhood Cognitive Assessment Measures

Cognitive measure	Author(s) (date); current publisher	Early childhood coverage and age groupings	Average time	CHC abilities[a]	Primary available scores	Brief technical considerations
Differential Ability Scales—Second Edition (DAS-II)	Elliott (2007); Pearson	2:6–17:11 (full battery), 2:5–3:5 (Early Years Lower Level), 3:6–6:11 (Early Years Upper Level)	20–40 minutes (core), up to 70 minutes (with diagnostic tests)	Crystallized intelligence/knowledge (Gc), fluid intelligence/reasoning (Gf), visual–spatial abilities (Gv), short-term memory (Gsm), long-term storage and retrieval (Glr), cognitive processing speed (Gs), auditory processing (Ga), quantitative knowledge (Gq)	Standard scores: General Conceptual Ability (GCA), Special Nonverbal Composite, Verbal, Nonverbal Reasoning, Spatial, Working Memory, Processing Speed, School Readiness. Subtests are T scores.	• Very developmentally appropriate items and levels • Generally strong internal consistency • Test–retest values for at least half of the core and diagnostic subtests are limited • A few core and almost all diagnostic subtests have test floors above prescribed aged range
Kaufman Assessment Battery for Children—Second Edition (KABC-II)	Kaufman and Kaufman (2004); Pearson	3:0–18:11 (full battery), 3:0–3:11 (5 core subtests), 4:0–6:11 (10 core subtests)	25–60 minutes (Luria), 30–75 minutes (CHC)	Crystallized intelligence/knowledge (Gc), visual–spatial abilities (Gv), short-term memory (Gsm), long-term storage and retrieval (Glr), fluid intelligence/reasoning (Gf)	Standard scores: Mental Processing Index (MPI), Fluid–Crystallized Index (FCI), Nonverbal Index (NVI), Knowledge, Sequential, Simultaneous, Learning. Subtests are scaled scores.	• Cluster and index scores are generally reliable • Preschool portion of norm sample is small • Many subtests have less than adequate internal and test–retest reliability • Test floors vary as a function of age, and should be reviewed carefully prior to subtest use and interpretation
Leiter International Performance Scale—Revised (Leiter-R)	Roid and Miller (1997); Stoelting	2:0–20:11 (full battery), 2:0–3:11, 20 min 4:0–5:11, 20 min 6:0+, 40 min	40 minutes per battery (80 minutes total)	Visual–spatial abilities (Gv), short-term memory (Gsm), long-term storage and retrieval (Glr), fluid intelligence/reasoning (Gf)	Standard scores: Full Scale IQ (for Visualization and Reasoning battery only), Brief IQ, Fluid Reasoning, Fundamental Visualization, Memory Screener, Recognition Memory. Subtests are scaled scores.	• Strong factor-analytic basis for test content • Inclusion of preschool children in several clinical studies • Norms are dated • Reliability data and test floors are variable at preschool ages
NEPSY-II	Korkman, Kirk, and Kemp (2007); Pearson	3:0–16:11 (full battery), 3:0–4:11 (18 subtests), 5:0–16:11 (26 subtests)	45–90 minutes (3–4 years), 60–180 minutes (5 years)	Not available	No domain or cluster scores (all scores are subtest-specific). Subtests provide scaled, base rate, and cumulative percentage scores. Additional contrast and processing scores available.	• Multiple processing scores available • Generally adequate subtest internal consistency • Preschool portion of norm sample is small, with norm table intervals that are larger than desirable • Select subtests have inadequate test floors at both 3- and 5-year levels

Test	Author/Publisher	Age range	Administration time	Broad (CHC) abilities measured	Standard scores	Comments
Reynolds Intellectual Assessment Scales (RIAS)[b]	Reynolds and Kamphaus (2003); Psychological Assessment Resources	3:0–94 (full battery)	20–25 minutes (basic scales), 10 minutes (memory tests)	Crystallized intelligence/knowledge (Gc), fluid intelligence/reasoning (Gf), visual–spatial abilities (Gv), short-term memory (Gsm), long-term storage and retrieval (Glr)	Standard scores: Composite Intelligence Index (CIX), Verbal Intelligence Index (VIX), Nonverbal Intelligence Index (NIX), Reynolds Intellectual Screening Test (RIST), Composite Memory Index (CMX). Subtests are T scores.	• Age range extends down to preschool age for all subtests in the battery • Limited external information available on its use with preschool-age children at the present time
Stanford–Binet Intelligence Scales for Early Childhood, Fifth Edition (Early SB5)	Roid (2003, 2005); Riverside, PRO-ED)	2:0–80+ (full SB5 battery), 2:0–7:3 (Early SB5)	50 minutes	Crystallized intelligence/knowledge (Gc), fluid intelligence/reasoning (Gf), visual–spatial abilities (Gv), short-term memory (Gsm), quantitative knowledge (Gq)	Standard scores: Full Scale IQ (FSIQ), Nonverbal IQ (NVIQ), Verbal IQ (VIQ), Knowledge, Fluid Reasoning, Visual–Spatial Processing, Working Memory, Quantitative Reasoning. Subtests are scaled scores.	• Large number of preschool children in standardization sample • Consistently adequate to good internal consistency at subtest level • Test–retest sample is lacking; select subtests have inadequate stability • Three cluster scores have inadequate test floors at lower ages; most subtests do not have adequate test floor until 3-year level
Wechsler Preschool and Primary Scale of Intelligence—Third Edition (WPPSI-III)	Wechsler (2002); Pearson	2:6–7:3 (full battery), 2:6–3:11 (lower level), 4:0–7:3 (upper level)	45 minutes (lower level), 60 minutes (upper level)	Crystallized intelligence/knowledge (Gc), visual–spatial abilities (Gv), fluid intelligence/reasoning (Gf), cognitive processing speed (Gs)	Standard scores: Full Scale IQ (FSIQ), Verbal IQ (VIQ), Performance IQ (PIQ), Processing Speed IQ (PSIQ). Subtests are scaled scores.	• Consistently adequate to good internal consistency at subtest level • Large number of clinical studies specific to preschool age range • Test–retest sample is lacking, and core Performance tests have inadequate stability values • Processing Speed and supplemental Verbal subtests have very poor test floors
Woodcock–Johnson III Tests of Cognitive Abilities—Normative Update (WJ III COG NU)	Woodcock, McGrew, and Mather (2001, 2007); Riverside	2:0–80+ (full battery), 2:0–5:11 (Early Development tests)	30–60 minutes (Early Development tests)	Crystallized intelligence/knowledge (Gc), visual–spatial abilities (Gv), short-term memory (Gsm), cognitive processing speed (Gs), long-term storage and retrieval (Glr), auditory processing (Ga)	Standard scores: General Intellectual Ability—Early Development (GIA-EDev). Individual tests are standard scores.	• Wide range of cognitive abilities evaluated • Low number of basic concepts in test directions • Test–retest data are lacking • Test floors are inadequate for approximately half the Early Development tests until the 3–4 level

[a] Based on respective test manuals and Flanagan, Ortiz, and Alfonso (2007).
[b] Not included in chapter reviews, due to limited research on the RIAS with early childhood populations at the present time.

TABLE 24.4. Overview of Widely Used Early Childhood Multidomain Assessment Measures

Multidomain measure	Author(s) (date); current publisher	Early childhood age coverage	Average time	Developmental domains covered by the test	Primary scores available	Technical highlights
Battelle Developmental Inventory, Second Edition (BDI-2)	Newborg (2004); Riverside	Birth–7:11	60–90 minutes	Adaptive (Self-Care, Personal Responsibility); Communication (Receptive and Expressive); Motor (Fine, Gross, and Perceptual–Motor); Personal (Adult Interaction, Peer Interaction, Self-Concept and Social Role); Cognitive (Attention and Memory, Reasoning and Academic Skills, Perception and Concepts)	Standard scores for composites. Scaled scores for subdomains.	• Very large standardization sample • Internal consistency of domain scores is consistently adequate • Generally adequate test floors • Internal consistency of some subdomains is inadequate, and test-retest data are lacking • "Birthday effects" are reported at 23- to 24-month shift
Bayley Scales of Infant–Toddler Development, Third Edition (Bayley-III)	Bayley (2005); Pearson	0:1–3:6	50–90 minutes	Cognitive, Language (Receptive and Expressive), Motor (Fine and Gross), Adaptive, Social-Emotional	Standard scores for composites. Scaled scores for subscales.	• Internal consistency of domain scores is consistently adequate • Internal consistency of Receptive Language, Fine Motor, and (to a lesser degree) Expressive Language subdomains are variably adequate below 16 months • Test–retest data are lacking, although stability appears to be adequate above the 19-month level • Test floors are psychometrically adequate
Merrill–Palmer—Revised Scales of Development (M-P-R)	Roid and Sampers (2004); Stoelting	0:1–6:6	30–40 minutes (Cognitive portion)	Cognitive Development, Language/Communication, Motor Development, Social-Emotional Development, Self-Help/Adaptive Behavior	Standard scores for domains.	• Internal consistency is generally adequate for domains and subscales • Documented validity with special populations • Age of norm data is unclear • Test–retest data are inadequate, and information on test floors is lacking
Mullen Scales of Early Learning: AGS Edition (MSEL)	Mullen (1995); Pearson	Birth–5:9	15–60 minutes	Motor (Fine and Gross), Language (Receptive and Expressive), Visual Reception	Standard score for Early Learning Composite. Domain and subdomain scores are T scores.	• Internal consistency is inadequate for most subscales • Test–retest data are lacking • Large "birthday effects" are reported • Norms extremely dated • Use for diagnostic decisions not recommended

examiner is encouraged to review not only the information provided here, but also the information highlighted in the specific test chapters in this text and the manuals of the instruments themselves, to determine which tool is most appropriate for the age of the child, the reason for referral, and the unique characteristics of the testing situation.

REVIEW AND CRITIQUE OF WIDELY USED COGNITIVE MEASURES

Differential Ability Scales— Second Edition

Overview and Key Features

The Differential Ability Scales—Second Edition (DAS-II; Elliott, 2007) is an updated version of the Differential Ability Scales (DAS; Elliott, 1990), one of the most widely used measures of cognitive abilities in young children for the past 20 years. The DAS-II measures cognitive abilities in children ages 2 years, 6 months through 17 years, 11 months (2:6 through 17:11). The battery has strong developmental focus in its approach, with tests divided into two levels, a School-Age battery (7:0–17:11) and an Early Years battery (2:6–6:11). The batteries are co-normed at ages 5:0–8:11, allowing examiners to conduct out-of-level testing with high-functioning preschool children or low-functioning young school-age children.

The DAS-II Early Years battery is further subdivided into Lower Level (ages 2:5–3:5) and Upper Level (ages 3:5–6:11) sets of subtests. At the Early Years Lower Level, four core subtests yield a General Conceptual Ability (GCA) score, along with Verbal and Nonverbal composite scores; three supplementary diagnostic subtests are available to measure short-term verbal and visual memory, and early number concepts. At the Early Years Upper Level, global scores include both a GCA and Special Nonverbal Composite, as well as six core subtests that yield Verbal, Nonverbal Reasoning, and Spatial composite scores. A total of 11 supplemental subtests are available and provide three diagnostic composite scores (School Readiness, Working Memory, and Processing Speed) at the Early Years Upper Level. Subtest-level diagnostic indicators of short- and long-term memory are available, but are not associated with cluster scores.

The aim of both the DAS and the DAS-II has been to provide a strong measure of general intelligence, driven by a hierarchical but integrative and nonspecific view of cognitive processing (Beran,

2007; Davis & Finch, 2010). While not specifically designed with CHC as its underlying theory, the DAS-II is readily interpretable from a CHC perspective, and numerous authors (e.g., Dumont, Willis, & Elliott, 2008; Flanagan et al., 2007) have adopted this approach to DAS-II interpretation as well as providing CHC content analyses. At the Early Years Lower Level, the core Verbal tests are associated with crystallized abilities (Gc); the core Nonverbal tests with fluid reasoning (Gf) and visual–spatial processing (Gv); and the diagnostic tests with verbal short-term memory (Gsm), short-term visual memory (Gv), and quantitative knowledge (Gq). The Early Years Upper Level core subtests provide separate indicators of Gc, Gf, and Gv, while the Early Years Upper Level diagnostic subtests provide estimates of Gsm, Gv, and Gq, as well as processing speed (Gs), auditory processing (Ga), and long-term storage and retrieval (Glr).

Compared to most cognitive tests for young children, the DAS-II is extremely efficient. Test items are organized into blocks or item sets within subtests based on Rasch scaling. Total testing time in the earlier years varies from 20 to 40 minutes for core subtests, and can last up to 70 minutes, depending upon the age level and number of diagnostic tests given.

Strengths, Limitations, and Special Considerations

The DAS-II has been well tailored to be developmentally appropriate for use with young children. In addition to being time-efficient, it easily maintains child interest by the inclusion of and rotation through multiple sets of activities for a given subtest. The DAS-II materials also are very appealing to most young children, and often resemble common toy or game pieces. Test manipulatives include colorful pictures, rubber toys, wooden puzzle boards, stacking blocks, and building shapes. The subtests provide both teaching and practice items, which are important in helping young children make transitions to new tasks and ensuring that scores reflect performance rather than poor comprehension of directions.

Only a few, relatively minor limitations have been reported with regard to the use of the DAS-II (Marshall, McGoey, & Moschos, 2011). Examiners must be very fluent with the test procedures, due to the tendency of the DAS-II to rapidly switch materials and activities within and across subtests, and to the number of booklets and manipulatives used. Clinicians need to determine whether children have adequate knowledge of basic concepts in order to complete the memory tasks, as they require familiarity with the concepts of *forward* and *backward*, as well as basic number sense and knowledge of body parts.

Across its overall age range, the DAS-II has been lauded for its solid technical characteristics; however, our review in preparing this chapter indicates that its psychometric properties, though generally strong, are somewhat variable across the early childhood range. For these years, the standardization sample is adequately large (1,280 children from 2:6 to 8:11); includes an adequate number of children per 1-year age interval (>176 for the full preschool age range); is representative; and offers normative data in 3-month intervals for the entire preschool age range. For this age range, the internal-consistency coefficients are consistently high for composite scores (.85–.96) and generally adequate to good for most subtests, with a few exceptions (Verbal Comprehension, .74–.89; Matrices, .75–.87; Recognition of Pictures, .73–.85; and Recall of Objects—Immediate, .74–.81).

The test–retest stability of the DAS-II composite scores exceeds the minimum .80 standard, except for the Nonverbal Reasoning Ability score (.73–.77) at the Early Years Upper Level. However, a number of the subtest stability values are slightly below the .80 typically recommended. At the Early Years Lower Level, two of four core subtests have inadequate test–retest reliability (Verbal Comprehension, .78; Picture Similarities, .67), as do all three diagnostic tests (Recall of Digits—Forward, .76; Recognition of Pictures, .73; Early Number Concepts, .79). At the Early Years Upper Level, three of six core subtests have inadequate stability (Verbal Comprehension, .78; Picture Similarities, .67; Matrices, .63–.69), as do three or four of 11 diagnostic tests, either across part or all of the preschool age ranges reported (Matching Letter-Like Forms, .56–.69; Recognition of Pictures, .65–.73; Recall of Objects—Immediate, .54–.80; Recall of Objects—Delayed, .72). Several core subtest floors are slightly above their recommended age range and thus considered inadequate (Early Years Lower Level: Picture Similarities, 2:9; Early Years Upper Level: Copying of Designs, 3:6; and Matrices, 4:3). With the exception of the Rapid Naming subtest, all of the diagnostic subtests have floors above their prescribed age level (2:9–6:6).

Readers are referred to the DAS-II manual (Elliott, 2007), which includes detailed descriptions of numerous validity studies, including the results of concurrent, confirmatory-factor-analytic,

and special-population studies. The Early Years Battery scores are strongly correlated with scores on other cognitive, developmental, and achievement test batteries, such as the Wechsler Preschool and Primary Scale of Intelligence—Third Edition (WPPSI-III); the Bayley Scales of Infant and Toddler Development, Third Edition (Bayley-III); the Bracken Basic Concepts Scale—Revised; and Ready to Learn. The factor structure across the different age groupings is supported, with the diagnostic subtests having relatively high levels of specificity. Clinically, the DAS-II is viewed as a valid tool for use with school-age children with a wide range of special needs, including attention and various learning problems. However, more special-population data with younger children are recommended: Special-population studies that included preschoolers were restricted to children with intellectual disabilities, language disorders, and identification as developmentally at risk, and disaggregation of data by age is not available. Overall, the DAS-II has been identified as particularly appropriate for use with children who have language and communication challenges (Beran, 2007; Marshall et al., 2011). Spanish and American Sign Language translations are available for the nonverbal tests, and the SNC is frequently used with students who are English-language learners, are deaf or hard of hearing, or have speech and language impairments.

Overall, the DAS-II has a number of strengths and is considered an adequate measure to assess the cognitive abilities of young children. Although users should be aware of some of the challenges with the floors of some subtests, it is still a very popular and useful test with young children and continues to be one of the best-rated of the cognitive measures available for this age group.

Kaufman Assessment Battery for Children—Second Edition

Overview and Key Features

The Kaufman Assessment Battery for Children—Second Edition (KABC-II; Kaufman & Kaufman, 2004) is an individually administered instrument, designed to assess the processing and cognitive abilities of children and adolescents ages 3:0–18:11. The KABC-II is a significant revision of the K-ABC (Kaufman & Kaufman, 1983), and includes a wider age range, 10 new subtests, and expanded interpretive features that incorporate both neuropsychological and psychometric theories.

The KABC-II assesses one to five different processing and cognitive domains, depending on the interpretive approach chosen and the age of the child (Kaufman, Lichtenberger, Fletcher-Janzen, & Kaufman, 2005). The KABC-II consists of 18 subtests, with 5 and 10 core subtests used to assess preschool children at the 3-year age level and the 4- to 6-year age level, respectively.

Unique to the KABC-II is its grounding in both Lurian neuropsychological theory processing (Luria, 1973) and CHC theory (Carroll, 1993), which allows for alternative theoretical interpretation of the scales (see Kaufman Singer et al., Chapter 11, this volume). Depending on the interpretive approach, the KABC-II provides two different overall scores: the Mental Processing Index (MPI) with the Luria neuropsychological interpretation, or the Fluid–Crystallized Index (FCI) with the CHC approach. Both Hunt (2008) and Morgan and colleagues (2009) provide support for the four CHC factors (Glr, Gsm, Gv, and Gc) identified by the test authors at the preschool level, suggesting that the CHC theory provides a meaningful interpretation of young children's cognitive abilities. In addition, a Nonverbal Index is available and may be used to represent the cognitive level of functioning of children with oral communication difficulty. At age 3, only a choice of one scale that assesses global ability is available (either five subtests [MPI] or seven subtests [FCI]), and at ages 4–6, the Planning or Fluid Reasoning scale is excluded. Time administration increases with age; the manual estimates that at the 3-year level it takes approximately 25–35 minutes to administer the core battery and 35–55 minutes to administer the core and supplemental subtests, increasing to 75 minutes in the primary age range.

Strengths, Limitations, and Special Considerations

The KABC-II offers flexibility for the examiner to choose between two theories; it also permits the assessment of children with communication impairments or with English as a second language, particularly with the optional Nonverbal Index. The KABC-II authors assert that this is also a culturally fair assessment because examiners can opt to conduct the assessment without including measures of acquired knowledge (a consideration for ELLs). Similarly, the sample and teaching items can be provided in a child's native language, and most of the subtests rely on a visual and auditory rather than a verbal format, increasing the opportunities for the child to understand the task (Branden & Ouzts, 2005; Kaufman et al., 2005). Other positive features include the appealing, colorful, and child-friendly materials; the time-efficient nature of the battery; and out-of-level norms for preschool children, which allow for enhanced score interpretation. In contrast, the most common criticism is that even though examiners are allowed to choose between the Lurian and CHC frameworks, no evidence is provided to support the choice of one model over the other. Furthermore, the implications for use with culturally and linguistically diverse populations could use further evidence to support the information provided by the test authors.

Psychometrically, the KABC-II's technical proprieties are rated as adequate to good across the full age range of the test (see Branden & Ouzts, 2005, and Lichtenberger, Sotelo-Dynega, & Kaufman, 2009, for detailed reviews), but there is greater variability with the technical properties at the preschool level. The standardization sample for children in this age range is relatively recent (2001), is representative of the U.S. population, and has at least 200 children per 1-year age interval; however, its total number of young children is smaller than seen with other batteries (850 preschoolers in an overall norm sample of 3,025), and norm tables are divided into 3- and 4-month intervals. KABC-II internal-consistency coefficients were strong for the cluster and index scores (.85–.97), but varied from inadequate to good for the subtests (.57 .93) Of greatest concern were the Gestalt Closure (.71–.76), Face Recognition (.65–.81), and Hand Movements (.57–.75) subtests.

Stability of test scores is difficult to assess, as the test–retest sample size is low (47–62 children), and the test–retest age range (3–5 years) does not cover the 6-year level. Whereas the MPI and FCI test–retest coefficients are .86 and .90, 9 of the 12 subtests designed for preschool-age children have adjusted test–retest coefficients lower than .80. The KABC-II test floor adequacy increases with age. At the 3-year level, four of the seven core test floors are inadequate (Word Order, 3:3, Conceptual Thinking, 5:3, Face Recognition, 4:6; Riddles, 3:6); at the 4- to 5-year level, 5 of the 10 core tests have inadequate floors (Number Recall, 4:6; Conceptual Thinking, 5:3; Face Recognition, 4:6; Pattern Reasoning, 6:0; Rebus, 4:9). The two subtests that measure planning or fluid reasoning at 6 years also have inadequate floors until after their prescribed age range (Rover, 6:4; Story Completion, 7:0).

The examiner's manual provides detailed descriptions of empirical research regarding construct, content, and concurrent validity. For example, to support the concurrent validity for ages 3–5 years, scores on the KABC-II were compared to scores on the original K-ABC and the WPPSI-III. Although data are available for several special-population studies with school-age children, there appears to be limited evidence regarding its clinical utility and predictive validity with preschoolers specifically. According to the manual, children as young as 3:10 and 4:3 were included in studies of KABC-II differences related to intellectual disabilities and autism, respectively, but no breakdown of age-related differences is available for these two studies. Nor are other studies of preschoolers with important areas of disability or educational challenges, such as language/communication disorders and other disabilities, reported.

When using the KABC-II with very young children, examiners must carefully inspect the technical features of subtests at the lower end of its prescribed age range. Nonetheless, its child-friendly features, the developmental sequencing of the tasks, and the reduced language demands throughout much of the test make the KABC-II a valuable tool for psychologists assessing cognitive abilities of preschoolers.

Leiter International Performance Scales—Revised

Overview and Key Features

The Leiter International Performance Scales—Revised (Leiter-R; Roid & Miller, 1997) is an individually administered measure of nonverbal intellectual ability, with a secondary focus on the assessment of memory and attention. The Leiter-R is a revision of one of the oldest nonverbal batteries, the Leiter International Performance Scale (Leiter, 1979), which was initially developed by Leiter in the 1930s and has long been used with individuals with significant language limitations. The Leiter-R continues as a measure for use with special populations; it has been most frequently utilized with children with significant communication impairments, those with hearing impairments, and ELLs, but also children with brain injury, motor impairments, attention-deficit/hyperactivity disorder (ADHD), and specific types of learning disabilities. Although the Leiter-R is older (1997) than other measures highlighted in this chapter, it has been the primary nonverbal option available to clinicians working with young

children, and for this reason it is included in our review. It is designed for children and adolescents ages 2:0–20:11, but some of the tasks said to be appropriate for younger children have been criticized by some as too difficult for very young children with delays (Vig & Sanders, 2007).

The Leiter-R is divided into two domains: the Visualization and Reasoning (VR) battery and the Attention and Memory (AM) battery. The VR battery was designed to assess more traditional aspects of intelligence, such as nonverbal reasoning and problem solving, as well as visual–spatial abilities. Associated subtests are used to calculate four index scores at the preschool age (Full Scale IQ, IQ Screener, Fluid Reasoning, and Fundamental Visualization). The AM battery was designed to assess nonverbal memory and attention abilities. The test ages for the 10 AM subtests vary significantly across the preschool range; Memory Screener and Memory Recognition scores are available for children 2 years and older, while the Associative Memory, Memory Span, and Attention and Memory Process scores are only available for children 6 years of age and older.

The Leiter-R has a strong theoretical foundation; it is grounded in Carroll's (1993) and Gustafsson's (1984) hierarchical factor models of cognitive abilities and emphasizes developmentally appropriate measurement of g. CHC analyses (Flanagan et al., 2007) of the Leiter-R indicate that the test content of the VR battery at the preschool level selectively measures fluid reasoning (Gf, primarily induction) and visual–spatial processing (Gv, primarily visualization). Similarly, CHC analyses of the AM battery indicate that it assesses a combination of visual–spatial processing (Gv, primarily visual memory), processing speed (Gs), short-term memory (Gsm), and long-term memory and retrieval (Glr). The two batteries may be administered independently. The full VR and AM require roughly 40 minutes each to administer, while the screeners demand approximately 25 minutes each.

Strengths, Limitations, and Special Considerations

The greatest strengths of the Leiter-R are the test instructions and teaching items that are truly nonverbal. Directions are given largely through pantomime, and examiners are encouraged to find "creative" ways to communicate with examinees by using hand, head, and facial gestures, with verbalizations minimized or eliminated. The test kit contains a number of engaging materials, such as colorful pictures, chips, and cards; subtest activities and response formats variably involve organizing manipulatives, ordering the cards, and pointing, and typically maintain the interest of most young children. Other positive features include the provision of growth scores and four optional rating scales (examiner, parent, and teacher, with a self-report for children ages 9 and older), which can be used to obtain more in-depth behavioral information.

The strong nonverbal characteristics of the Leiter-R also constitute a limitation. Each subtest has unique pantomime instructions, necessitating extensive examiner practice and supervision prior to test administration (Marco, 2001; Stinnett, 2003). Some of the manual's instructions (particularly clarifications regarding procedures for when a child does not respond as expected) are vague and may result in significant variability both across examiners and within one examiner's administrations. Furthermore, since the typical clinician will use the Leiter-R on limited occasions, gains in fluency and accuracy of administration may be easily lost. The latter can be problematic with a number of subtests, such as Visual Coding and Attention Divided, which are challenging to teach. Bracken and Naglieri (2003) also have suggested that the Leiter-R's content may be largely nonverbal, but its stimulus may strongly reflect U.S. mainstream culture, and thus it should be used cautiously with recent immigrants.

Overall, the Leiter-R's authors have been applauded for the overall quality of its psychometric properties, as well as the rigorous efforts expended in test construction (e.g., use of factor analysis to develop the two batteries, and of item response theory and Rasch scaling for item and norm creation). In references to its utility and in findings from our own analysis, however, the technical properties of the Leiter-R vary considerably at younger ages. The two separate standardization samples for the VR and AM batteries both adequately represent the U.S. population, but the norms are becoming dated. The AM battery norms were derived from a very small sample of 369 children between the ages of 2 and 6 years, with a limited number of children per 1-year age interval for this age range (e.g., 44–86). For the 2- to 6-year age range, internal-consistency coefficients vary from inadequate to good, with several subtests from both the VR and AM batteries having values well below the acceptable .80 standard (e.g., Sequential Order, Repeated Patterns, Associated Pairs, Delayed Pairs, Attention Divided).

The test–retest stability properties are somewhat difficult to interpret, as values were only provided collectively for the age range of 2–5 years, with no reference to the test–retest reliability intervals. Of most concern are the test floors, which are well above the recommended age ranges for several cluster scores (e.g., Fluid Reasoning, 2:6; Fundamental Visualization, 2:6; and Memory Screener, 3:2). For the individual subtests, test floors range from 3:6 to no floor below 6:11, with the exception of four subtests from the VR battery whose floors approach but still do not meet their prescribed age range (Figure Ground, 2:4; Form Completion, 3:0; Matching, 2:10; and Picture Context, 3:0).

The majority of the validity data supporting the Leiter-R are derived from studies presented in the manual and a select number of papers published shortly after the release of the Leiter-R. Almost all of the concurrent validity data are for school-age children. Across the school-age range, critics suggest that the test may have more limited efficacy with children who are gifted or who have attention/learning problems (Stinnett, 2003). However, a number of independent studies support its use for children with autism (e.g., Tsatsanis et al., 2003) and Spanish-speaking populations (e.g., Cathers-Schiffman & Thompson, 2007). Notably, the Leiter-R is one of the few batteries to routinely include children as young as 2 years in its validation studies of clinical groups, including children with language, hearing, motor, and cognitive delays, as well as ELLs.

Historically, the Leiter-R has been one of the few measures of nonverbal cognitive abilities that may be used with young children. However, given the complications with the administration procedures, datedness of the norms, and concerns with technical properties across the early childhood range, practitioners are strongly encouraged to carefully consider its use with children who either have significant delays or are below 4:0 years of age, particularly with the AM battery. Although the Leiter-R was once thought to be a strong measure for young children, more recently developed tests may be preferred.

NEPSY-II

Overview and Key Features

The NEPSY-II (Korkman, Kirk, & Kemp, 2007)—a revised version of the NEPSY (Korkman, Kirk, & Kemp, 1998), whose title represents the incorporation of neuropsychology (NE) with psychology (PSY)—is an individually administered battery, designed as a developmentally appropriate set of neuropsychological measures for children ages 3:0 through 16:11. The battery is theoretically driven by the principles of Luria (1973). Reflecting its neuropsychological roots, some of the subtests evaluate more basic and specific neurocognitive skills, but many of its subtests require the examinee to utilize multiple neurocognitive abilities in an integrated and concerted fashion (D'Amato & Titley, 2010). The NEPSY-II offers measures of six different functional domains: Language, Memory and Learning, Visuospatial Processing, Sensorimotor, and Executive Function and Attention (all of which were retained from the previous edition), and the newly added domain of Social Perception. The CHC content of the NEPSY-II is not available in Flanagan, Ortiz, and Alfonzo (2007), but classifications of the original NEPSY are included. However, given the neuropsychological nature of the NEPSY-II, categorization of the CHC abilities measured may not be a primary need for many users.

Whereas the full NEPSY-II consists of 32 different subtests that can be selectively and flexibly administered (depending upon referral concerns), only 18 and 26 subtests of these subtests are available for use with children ages 3–4 years and 5–6:11 years, respectively. Domain scores were eliminated altogether from the NEPSY-II. Consequently, available scores and interpretation are at the subtest level; the focus is on profile analysis of subtest primary, process, contrast, and behavioral observation rating scores, which are variably converted to scaled scores, percentile ranks, and ratings linked to cumulative population percentages and base rates consistent with approaches used in neuropsychological assessment. Administration time varies by both age and the number of subtests selected; the manual estimates a more comprehensive administration as requiring 45–90 minutes at ages 3–4, and 60–180 minutes at ages 5–16.

Strengths, Limitations, and Special Considerations

Although the NEPSY-II is one of the primary neuropsychological batteries for use with children, it has multiple purposes: It may be selectively used for the evaluation of cognitive abilities and for diagnostic purposes, as well as for general and comprehensive neuropsychological assessment (D'Amato & Titley, 2010). To assist with subtest selection, the manual lists suggested "referral batteries" for different types of referral concerns. The NEPSY-II

is unique in its inclusion of measures of Executive Function and Attention designed for young children, which are thought to have high diagnostic utility across clinical groups. The NEPSY-II protocol also includes several options for detailed qualitative assessment, such as a clinical history section, as well as behavioral, error, and strategy/process observation ratings for each subtest.

Although the flexibility, breadth, and neuropsychological features of the NEPSY-II allow for more comprehensive assessment, these characteristics also present practical challenges for examiners. Due to the number of subtests, competency with the NEPSY-II requires more training and supervised practice than many of the other measures highlighted in this chapter (Napolitano, 2010). The complexity of administration is further amplified by the highly variable start, basal, and ceiling rules, and differences in timing across subtests. In addition, many preschool children or school-age children with delays may have difficulty with the complexity of and basic concepts contained within the instructions of some of the tasks (e.g., the Arrows subtest).

The technical properties of the NEPSY-II are adequate to very good across its upper age range (see Brooks, Sherman, & Strauss, 2010, and Davis & Mathews, 2010, for detailed reviews). However, our analysis indicates that there remain concerns with the technical properties of the NEPSY-II with younger children, although these are much improved over the first edition. In particular, the number of children ages 3–7 (500) and the size of the age intervals within the norm tables (6 months) are not considered adequate for the assessment of young children. For three of the tests at the lower preschool level (Imitating Hand Positions, Manual Motor Sequences, and Oromotor Sequences), and three of the tests at the upper preschool level (Design Fluency, Repetition of Nonsense Words, and Route Finding), the norms were not updated from the prior edition, although the content of these measures is thought to be relatively insulated from the Flynn effect (D'Amato & Titley, 2010). For the preschool range, a few of the subtests have internal reliabilities (split-half or alpha) below .80 and often below .70 (e.g., most of the Attention and Executive Function subtests, Body Part Naming, Word Generation, Memory for Faces, Narrative Memory, Visuomotor Precision, Affect Recognition, and Theory of Mind).

Not unsurprisingly, the test–retest stability of scores for the Memory and Learning domain was lower than .80 across most ages (Napolitano,

2010). At the 3- to 6-year level, lower reliabilities are reported for many of the Memory and Learning and almost all of the Visuospatial Processing subtests, as well as the Affect Recognition, Imitating Hand Positions, Design Copying, and Arrows subtests. Finally, several subtests have inadequate test floors at the prescribed 3-year (e.g., Statue, Body Part Naming, Narrative Memory, Sentence Repetition, Word Generation, Imitating Hand Positions, Affect Recognition, and Design Copying) and 5- to 6-year (e.g., Auditory Attention, Memory for Faces, Memory for Names—Delayed, and Arrows) levels.

The NEPSY-II manual details ample evidence of content, concurrent, and construct validity against contemporary tests of intelligence, such as the DAS-II (Elliott, 2007), the Children's Memory Scale (CMS; Cohen, 1997), and the Wechsler Intelligence Scale for Children—Fourth Edition (WISC-IV; Wechsler, 2003a), as well as other widely used academic, neuropsychological, and behavioral measures (see Brooks et al., 2010; D'Amato & Titley, 2010; Davis et al., 2010; Napolitano, 2010). Numerous special-population studies also are available in the manual, and Brooks et al. suggest that the Executive Function and Attention and the Language subtests may be the most consistent identifiers of clinical problems. Only 22 of the 32 subtests were administered in the clinical studies, however; these studies also frequently lacked children with neurological problems, and the inclusion of preschool children in these studies is very limited. Several authors (Brooks et al., 2010; D'Amato & Titley, 2010) note that the manual lacks adequate factor-analytic data to support the current six-factor domain structure of the NEPSY-II across its larger age range, and the intracorrelations between the subtests of a given domain are frequently low (one of the likely reasons for the elimination of domain scores). The test authors do not view this as overly problematic, as the latter can be accounted for by the possibility that the subtests within a given domain have high specificity, and thus measure significantly different aspects of a related construct. Limited information is provided about how these issues relate to preschool children.

Because the NEPSY-II is a neuropsychological instrument, its use should be accompanied by more advanced training that includes knowledge of both general neuropsychology and the administration and interpretation of neuropsychological tests. For those working with young children, this is in addition to the need for experience in cognitive assessment during early childhood. The NEPSY-II kit does provide a training CD that covers test administration; however, training in the interpretation of neuropsychological measures is needed to interpret them appropriately (Brooks et al., 2010), and unique issues in the assessment of young children are not addressed. Nonetheless, as the practice of and training for early childhood and development assessment become increasingly complex and integrated with neuropsychological approaches to assessment, the NEPSY-II holds significant promise for the evaluation of young children by a well-trained and experienced examiner.

Stanford–Binet Intelligence Scales for Early Childhood, Fifth Edition

Overview and Key Features

The Stanford–Binet Intelligence Scales for Early Childhood, Fifth Edition (Early SB5; Roid, 2005) battery is an economical version of the Stanford–Binet Intelligence Scales, Fifth Edition (SB5; Roid, 2003) battery, which is an individually administered measure of cognitive abilities and development used for the identification of developmental disabilities and exceptionality. The Early SB5 battery is designed for use with children ages 2:0–7:3, and is accompanied by several additional features specific to the assessment of young children. The SB5 and the Early SB5 are intended to evaluate 5 of 10 factors within the CHC model of cognitive abilities (Roid, 2003, 2005; Roid & Barram, 2004). In principle, the Early SB5 assesses the highest three g-loaded CHC factors (fluid reasoning, Gf; knowledge, Gc; and quantitative reasoning, Gq) and the three CHC factors most predictive of academic achievement (Gc, Gq, and short-term memory and reasoning, Gsm), plus visual–spatial processing, Gv.

The 10 SB5 subtest scores provide standardized Verbal and Nonverbal domain scores in five areas: Knowledge, Fluid Reasoning, Visual–Spatial Processing, Working Memory, and Quantitative Reasoning. A Full Scale IQ (FSIQ), Verbal IQ (VIQ), and Nonverbal IQ (NVIQ) as well as an Abbreviated Battery IQ (ABIQ) provide estimates of overall intelligence, along with "change-sensitive scores" that can be used to monitor growth and response to interventions over time. Both the Early SB5 and the SB5 are designed to make test administration as efficient as possible. Two "routing subtests" that tap the g-loaded domains of Knowledge and Fluid Reasoning are used to determine a developmentally appropriate start point for each child, theoretically minimizing the administration of unnecessary items or start point reversals. Overall testing times with young children are commonly reported as 15 and 50 minutes for the ABIQ and the full battery, respectively (Roid, 2005; Sink & Eppler, 2007).

Strengths, Limitations, and Special Considerations

Both the Early SB5 and the SB5 have several unique features that make them very useful in the assessment of young children (Alfonso & Flanagan, 2007; Ford & Dahinten, 2005). First, the shorter administration time of the SB5 tests is developmentally appealing and engaging for use with young children. Similarly, its relatively stringent ceiling rules (typically two items within a "testlet" of three to six items) help to minimize both testing time and potential frustration in young children (Vig & Sanders, 2007). Second, the content and materials of the Early SB5 are typically appealing to young children, especially the toy-like quality of the manipulatives (including cubes, rubber animals, colorful pictures, and various puzzles). The interest and attention of young examinees are also easily maintained by the spiraling administration sequence: Test items for the various CHC abilities are grouped into approximately five ability levels or testlets, and a child is administered a brief series of items for four different cognitive factors before advancing to the next level of the test.

Although the Early SB5 is relatively popular with most clinicians and is generally viewed as having few practical limitations, use and control of the materials with younger children may be somewhat challenging for examiners who are unfamiliar with the manipulatives or less skilled at behavior management. In addition, although the Nonverbal subtests are presented as appropriate for nonverbal assessment (e.g., with ELLs, children with hearing impairments, and young children with communication disorders or delayed language development) (Roid, 2003, 2005), both Bain and Allin (2005) and Alfonso and Flanagan (2007) rate the Early SB5 subtests (including the Nonverbal subtests) as having relatively high language demands.

Both our review and results from the comprehensive reviews by Alfonso and Flanagan (2007, 2009) indicate that the SB5 and Early SB5 have perhaps the strongest psychometric properties of all the available cognitive batteries intended for use with young children. For children 2–7 years of age, the SB5 normative sample is recent, relatively

large (1,280 children in this age group overall, with 175–352 per 1-year age interval), and representative of the U.S. population; across this age range, its norm tables are divided into 3- to 4-month intervals. For ages 2:0–6:11, all of the SB5 cluster scores have adequate to good internal-consistency values, as do almost all of its subtests, with a few minor exceptions (Nonverbal Knowledge, Verbal Visual–Spatial Processing, and Nonverbal Quantitative Reasoning have approximately one age interval each with internal-reliability values just below the .80 level).

The stability of the Early SB5 scores is, however, of greater concern. The test–retest samples were somewhat limited in size for the age ranges analyzed ($n = 96$ for children 2–5 years, $n = 86$ for children and adolescents 6–20 years); all of the cluster scores were adequately stable over a relatively short test–retest interval (mean time interval of 8 days or less for both age samples), but a few subtests had inadequate stability at ages 2–5 (Nonverbal Fluid Reasoning, both Visual–Spatial Processing subtests, and Verbal Quantitative Reasoning) and at ages 6+ (Nonverbal Fluid Reasoning and Verbal Visual–Spatial Processing). In addition, three of the cluster scores lack an adequate test floor (Fluid Reasoning, 3:0; Working Memory, 2:4; Quantitative Reasoning, 3:4). With the exception of the two Knowledge subtests and the Verbal Visual–Spatial Processing subtest, almost all of the remaining subtests do not have an adequate test floor until the 3:0–3:8 age level. In particular, the test floors for a raw score of 1 are even higher for the Verbal Fluid Reasoning (4:6) and Verbal Quantitative Reasoning (4:0) subtests.

Extensive validity evidence is primarily documented in the SB5 and secondarily the Early SB5 (Roid, 2003, 2005) manuals, as well as in the review by Flanagan and Alfonso (1995), who characterize the validity properties of the SB5 as impressive overall. Clear evidence related to content, criterion, and construct validity is also available, with notable studies of age-related growth curve patterns and factor structure (including Rasch modeling) that have been similarly commended by other authors (Bain & Allin, 2005; Johnson & D'Amato, 2004; Vacca, 2007). However, the five-factor structure and factor loadings of the individual subtests have been questioned for younger children, and an alternative four-factor structure has been suggested (Alfonso & Flanagan, 2007, 2009). Available predictive validity data are restricted to school-age children, but clinical utility with younger children appears to be relatively well demonstrated by a series of special-population studies that included children as young as 2 years of age with intellectual disabilities, developmental delay, autism, language and motor disorders, or ELL status. As with many other batteries, though, discriminative validity data disaggregated by age are not available.

Compared to other available measures, the Early SB5 is a popular and widely respected measure of cognitive development in preschool children. It is appealing to young children, and efficiently provides information to examiners about specific cognitive abilities that are thought to be most important to early cognitive development and schooling. However, reviews of its psychometric characteristics suggest that the Early SB5 may be most appropriate for use with children who are 4–5 years of age or older (Vig & Sanders, 2007), and caution should be exercised with its application in identifying very young children with delays.

Wechsler Preschool and Primary Scale of Intelligence—Third Edition

Overview and Key Features

The Wechsler Preschool and Primary Scale of Intelligence—Third Edition (WPPSI-III; Wechsler, 2002) is an individually administered test of intelligence and the most recent version of the downward extension of the traditional Wechsler scales, widely used with school-age children and adults. The WPPSI-III is designed for use with children ages 2:6–7:3, four core subtests are administered at the "lower" (2:6–3:11) age level, and seven core tests are typically given at the "upper" (4:0–7:3) age level.[1] The WPPSI-III continues to be driven by a clinical approach to cognitive assessment, without a strong link to any particular contemporary theory of cognitive abilities. Scores and related interpretation emphasize overall intelligence (Full Scale IQ or FSIQ), verbal abilities (Verbal IQ or VIQ), and nonverbal abilities (Performance IQ or PIQ). A General Language Composite score with special utility for younger children can be calculated at both age levels, utilizing a combination of VIQ and supplemental tests. At the 4:0–7:3 level, a Processing Speed IQ (PSIQ) and several new PIQ subtests have been introduced in the WPPSI-III, as part of an attempt to integrate a more "developmentally appropriate structure based on contemporary developmental theory" (Wechsler, 2002, p. 1).

In reviews of the test content of the WPPSI-III indexes and subtests from a CHC perspective, most indexes and subtests are thought to measure more than one broad ability and multiple narrow abilities, respectively. At the lower age level, the VIQ index is characterized as consistently evaluating crystallized intelligence/knowledge (Gc), and the PIQ is characterized as measuring exclusively visual–spatial abilities (Gv); there is no measure of nonverbal, abstract, or fluid reasoning (Flanagan et al., 2007; Lichtenberger & Kaufman, 2004). At the upper age level, the VIQ again is primarily a measure of Gc, but the PIQ is thought to measure a combination of Gc, Gv, and fluid intelligence/reasoning (Gf). The PSIQ is categorized as consistently measuring processing speed (Gs).

The WPPSI-III provides a relatively efficient measurement of two important aspects of general intelligence. With the changes in the number of core subtests, as well as reductions in time limits for some items, administration times are now more efficient than for the WPPSI-R and are estimated at 45 and 60 minutes for the upper and lower age levels, respectively (Hamilton & Burns, 2003; Wechsler, 2002). Administration of the WPPSI-III can also be expanded for diagnostic purposes with the use of several supplementary subtests (one and five at the lower and upper age levels, respectively). The assessment of memory abilities has been eliminated from the current edition, but the test manual recommends that if memory must be assessed, it can be accomplished through the supplemental administration of the CMS (Cohen, 1997).

Strengths, Limitations, and Special Considerations

The WPPSI-III reflects several notable changes, which have been well received by clinicians and reviewers alike: an expanded age range, the addition of seven new subtests, and the inclusion of practice and teaching items on all subtests (Hamilton & Burns, 2003). Test materials now include updated puzzle pieces at the lower age level, and colorful pictures and stackable cubes across the test age range. The addition of "bidirectional" base rate tables allows for better interpretation with both low- and high-functioning populations (Hamilton & Burns, 2003). A new feature of the WPPSI-III is the opportunity to compare WPPSI-III findings with co-normed Wechsler Individual Achievement Test—Second Edition (Wechsler, 2001) data.

Limitations of the WPPSI-III are primarily associated with the instructions, the child response formats, and some of its psychometric features.

Despite an attempt to make the WPPSI-III more developmentally appropriate, the language demands for many of the subtests, particularly at the 4:0–7:3 level, are rather high. Out of all of the major cognitive batteries, the WPPSI-III requires the greatest knowledge of basic concepts for children simply to comprehend test directions (i.e., it has a high frequency and number of difficult basic concepts, such as *the same*, *missing*, or *together*) (Merkel, Kozey, Swart, & Ford, 2005). Automated or random response patterns are not uncommon with the Picture Concepts or Matrix Reasoning subtests, due to their multiple-choice format with pointing responses (Vig & Sanders, 2007). Similarly, some children have difficulty with the Coding and Symbol Search subtests because the paper-and-pencil response format is easily affected by poor fine motor skills instead of cognitive aspects of processing speed. The retention of the ceiling rules requiring more errors before a subtest is discontinued (e.g., four to five consecutive errors) may produce frustration in younger children as well.

Prior editions of the WPPSI were heavily criticized for their psychometric limitations (Bracken, 1987; Flanagan & Alfonso, 1995). Our own review and ratings by others (Gordon, 2004; Madle, 2005; McCurdy & Johnsen, 2005) indicate significant improvements to the technical characteristics of the WPPSI-III, but a few areas of concern remain. The standardization sample is fairly recent, is large (N = 1,700, with at least 100–200 children per 1-year age group), and provides norm table data in 3-month age intervals until 6 years of age, although Madle (2005) suggests that the southern United States was overrepresented in the standardization sample. Internal consistency was .89 and above for index scores, and .79 and above for all subtests.

The stability of the WPPSI-III scores is somewhat difficult to interpret, given the inadequate sample size (N = 157) that is not broken down clearly by age. Test–retest values for the Verbal tests all were rated as at least .80 across three different age groups, but were well below the acceptable rating of .80 for children ages 4:0+ on the core Performance subtests of Block Design (.69–.77), and Picture Concepts (.75). There are several concerns with the WPPSI-III subtest floors. Three of the five subtests in the lower age range do not provide an adequate floor, using a raw score of 1 until the 3-year level (Receptive Vocabulary, 3:0; Picture Naming, 3:0; and Object Assembly, 3:6). For a large portion of the upper age range, lower-

functioning and typically functioning children cannot be distinguished on Processing Speed and supplemental Verbal tests, due to inadequate test floors (Picture Concepts, 4:6; Coding, 5:0; Symbol Search, 6:0; Word Reasoning, 5:6; Comprehension, 6:0, and Similarities, 6:4).

The validity of the WPPSI-III as an instrument for use with young children has several lines of support. Factor-analytic work similarly supports a two- and three-factor structure for the lower and upper age levels, respectively, although the relative factor loadings of the Matrix Reasoning and Picture Concepts subtests are somewhat unclear; findings also yield a pattern of subtest factor loadings and structure similar to those found for the WISC-IV (Gordon, 2004; Wechsler, 2002). Strong correlations are reported with the WISC-IV, and other measures of early childhood cognitive abilities, including the WPPSI-R, the Bayley Scales of Infant Development—Second Edition (BSID-II), and the original DAS (see Coalson & Spruill, 2007, for a detailed review; see also Wechsler, 2002). Details are provided in the technical manual for 10 different special-population studies, which vary in their quality of sample size and rigor. Results collectively suggest that the WPPSI-III may be appropriate to identify children with limited English proficiency, language disorders, and autism, as well as children with intellectual disabilities/developmental delays at select ages (Madle, 2005). Caution is recommended in its use to identify children with extremely low functioning (due to floor inadequacies) or children with ADHD (Coalson & Spruill, 2007).

Overall, the WPPSI-III is a significant improvement over previous versions. In spite of some problems with floors for a number of subtests, the WPPSI-III is a valuable addition to early childhood cognitive measures because of its more efficient testing times, engaging materials, and improved psychometric properties.

Woodcock–Johnson III Tests of Cognitive Abilities, Normative Update

Overview and Key Features

The Woodcock–Johnson III Tests of Cognitive Abilities—Normative Update (WJ III COG NU; Woodcock, McGrew, & Mather, 2001b, 2007b) and the accompanying WJ III Diagnostic Supplement to the Tests of Cognitive Abilities, Normative Update (WJ III DS NU; Woodcock, McGrew,

Mather, & Schrank, 2003, 2007) are collections of individually administered, stand-alone tests of cognitive abilities, normed for ages 2:0–80+. Although the WJ III COG NU and the WJ III DS NU have 20 and 11 tests, respectively, only a select portion of them are appropriate for use with young children (see Tusing et al., 2003). A subset of six tests from the WJ III COG NU and WJ III DS NU can be combined to create a General Intellectual Ability—Early Development (GIA-EDev) score, which was designed specifically for use with young children or individuals of any age who function at a very low level. The GIA-EDev provides a weighted estimate of general cognitive ability; it is most strongly influenced by contributing tests that are thought to have the highest impact upon general intelligence. In addition, two indicators of early achievement, Preacademic Skills and Preacademic Knowledge and Skills, can be obtained from the WJ III Tests of Achievement Normative Update (WJ III ACH NU; Woodcock, McGrew, & Mather, 2001a, 2007a).

The structure and interpretation of the WJ III COG NU is driven by the CHC model of cognitive abilities (McGrew, 2005). The GIA-EDev measures six of the seven CHC broad abilities that are thought to be most central for understanding young children's cognitive strengths and weaknesses (Ford, 2003; Schrank, Mather, McGrew, & Woodcock, 2003). Three of the six tests in the GIA-EDev are located in the WJ III COG NU, and three are located in the WJ III DS NU. Included are measures of crystallized abilities (Gc; Verbal Comprehension), visual–spatial processing (Gv; Visual Closure), auditory processing (Ga; Incomplete Words), processing speed (Gs; Visual Matching), short-term memory (Gsm; Memory for Words), and long-term storage and retrieval (Glr; Memory for Names). The CHC broad ability of fluid reasoning (Gf) is not included in the GIA-EDev.

In terms of administration, the GIA-EDev test materials exclusively use an easel format (and, in the case of the auditory tests, recorded tracks from an audio player). Depending upon the age and ability of the child, the individual tests require 5–10 minutes each to administer. Total administration time thus can vary from approximately 30 to 60 minutes. Additional tests from the WJ III COG NU may be administered with some caution, depending on the age of the child. A review in the technical manual reveals the age at which each test was standardized, for those considering tests beyond those included in the GIA-EDev.

Strengths, Limitations, and Special Considerations

In the early childhood context, most of the strengths associated with the WJ III COG NU are its theoretically driven assessment of a wide range of cognitive abilities, within the larger context of superior test construction theory and development. In comparison to other measures available for use in early childhood, the GIA-EDev evaluates a significantly wider range of cognitive abilities (six of seven CHC factors) (Ford, Kozey, & Merkel, 2006). The WJ III COG NU also has an interpretive advantage through the provision of relative proficiency index (RPI) scores, which offer information about a child's rate of success on a task compared to same-age peers (and thus the degree of difficulty that a child may experience with a task, regardless of the number of items with which he or she is successful). For example, an RPI score of 50/90 indicates that a child is only performing with 50% success on those tasks, when typical age-mates would perform with 90% success. The RPI is an extremely useful feature for assessing young children. Finally, the WJ III DS manual offers a full chapter on the use of the WJ III DS with young children (Ford, 2003).

Other preschool-friendly features of the WJ III GIA-EDev tests are their relatively limited demands on language and fine motor abilities, which are often delayed in young children with developmental challenges. Analyses by Merkel and colleagues (2005) indicate that the WJ III GIA-EDev tests require knowledge of only 11 basic language concepts that are typically understood by most children; this is substantially less than the total number, frequency, and related difficulty of linguistic concepts required for most other early childhood measures of intelligence. Similarly, the response formats of the WJ III GIA-EDev tests generally minimize fine motor and visual–motor coordination demands (except for the Visual Matching and Memory for Names tests, which require pointing).

It has been suggested that the WJ III easel format and lack of appealing manipulatives may not be developmentally appropriate for young children. However, the corner seating arrangement used with the WJ III easels allows for closer physical proximity between examiner and examinee, and thus may facilitate the management of child behavior during testing. Similarly, the consistency of the easel presentation may help children who are slow to acclimatize to tasks, or children who have difficulties shifting between different activities.

An in-depth review of the technical properties of the WJ III COG and WJ III ACH during the preschool years can be found in Tusing and colleagues (2003). Our more recent data indicate that the psychometric properties of the WJ III NU GIA-EDev tests are somewhat variable. The related standardized sample was large (> 1,153 for ages 2–5), recent, and representative, and the computerized scoring software provides norms based on monthly age intervals. The internal consistency of the WJ III NU GIA-EDev global score exceeds .90 for ages 2 through 6 years; the reliability of the individual tests is generally adequate, either approaching or above the .80 level, except for Visual Closure (.69–.82).

The stability of the WJ III NU GIA-EDev scores and individual tests is somewhat difficult to determine, as the shortest test–retest interval was listed as "less than 1 year," with data amalgamated across the 2- to 7-year age range. While three of the six individual tests are reported to have adequate test–retest properties, the manuals do not provide a stability statistic for the GIA-EDev score itself, or for the Verbal Comprehension and Visual Matching tests at less than a 1-year interval. As with many tests reviewed here, the early development test floors are also problematic; the GIA-EDev score itself was found to be adequate only at the age of 2:4, and some of the individual tests did not demonstrate an adequate floor until the 4-year level (Visual Closure, 2:5; Verbal Comprehension, 2:7; Memory for Sentences, 2:9; Memory for Names, 3:6, Incomplete Words, 4:1, and Visual Matching, 4:4).

The WJ III COG and DS NU, and in particular the GIA-EDev tests, offer options to evaluate a wider array of cognitive abilities in young children. However, many of the tests can be used with children as young as 24 months, this does not necessarily mean that they are appropriate for 2- or 3-year-old children with developmental delays. Examiners using the WJ III need to carefully consider a child's age and developmental level, as well as the psychometric properties of the tests being considered for use.

The appeal of the WJ III NU GIA-EDev is that it provides a downward extension of tests, appropriate for use with young children, for users of the WJ III NU. Few if any new administration procedures must be used, and this makes administration easier for the examiner. Although the WJ III NU offers 50 tests across the COG and ACH batteries, only a small portion of those are appropriate for use in early childhood. As a result, some caution is advised in using the WJ III COG with young children; examiners are encouraged to select the most appropriate tests for a child's age and referral question.

REVIEW AND CRITIQUE OF MULTIPLE-DOMAIN MEASURES

Battelle Developmental Inventory, Second Edition

Overview and Key Features

The Battelle Developmental Inventory, Second Edition (BDI-2; Newborg, 2004) can be used as an individually administered measure of development, a developmental screener, or a diagnostic tool to assess infants and children from birth to age 7:11. The BDI-2 provides an overall Developmental Quotient score, as well as a series of standardized domain scores. The BDI-2 evaluates five domains, which in turn are subdivided into 13 subdomains: (1) Personal Social domain (Adult Interaction, Peer Interaction, and Self-Concept and Social Role); (2) Adaptive domain (Personal Responsibility and Self-Care); (3) Motor domain (Fine Motor, Perceptual Motor, and Gross Motor); (4) Communication domain (Receptive and Expressive Communication); and (5) Cognitive domain (Attention and Memory, Reasoning and Academic Skills, and Perception and Concepts). A screening version and related Screening Quotient are available; as noted by Bliss (2007), however, it consists of items that had the highest factor loadings on the Developmental Quotient and the highest difficulty ratings, but was not standardized separately. Theoretically, the BDI-2 focuses on the attainment of developmental milestones, with significant similarities present between its content and the curriculum of many early childhood education programs.

The administration of specific subdomains varies according to the age of the child (e.g., self-care items are meant for children age 5:11 and younger; Athanasiou, 2007). Whereas the administration time of the entire battery is approximately 60 minutes for children younger than 2 years and older than 5 years, it takes approximately 90 minutes to administer the test to children between 2 and 5 years of age. Similarly, the administration time for the screening test varies between 10 and 30 minutes, according to the age of the child.

Strengths, Limitations, and Special Considerations

Overall, the BDI-2 is a valuable tool for the evaluation of child development. In particular, its large age range allows clinicians to monitor and document progress over time (Brassard & Boehm, 2007). Among the major multidomain batteries, the BDI-2 most readily allows for a multidisciplinary and team-based approach to assessment. The examiner's manual provides detailed instructions on test procedures, as well as information on developmental milestones; this is appropriate, given that it can be administered by adequately trained individuals other than psychologists. Item scoring methods are somewhat flexible, and behaviors may be scored from a variety of sources other than direct testing. The manual also includes recommendations for interpretation and communication of results, as well as suggestions for modifications to test administration when children with diverse needs are assessed.

A few general limitations of the BDI-2 should be noted. Prior to assessment, examiners need to be aware that the basic test kit does not include the child-friendly toy manipulatives, which need to be ordered separately (either as a full set or as a partial set specific to certain ages). Some of the item scoring criteria have been criticized as being vague and somewhat subjective (Athanasiou, 2007). Bradley-Johnson and Johnson (2007) expressed concerns that it is unclear whether some items can be scored on the basis of observation, direct testing, or interviews, and highlighted the absence of interrater reliabilty data. A Spanish translation/adaptation is available, but some have questioned whether the content of the BDI-2 has been adequately evaluated for cultural bias and fairness, and there is a lack of normative and technical data for the translated version (Athanasiou, 2007; Barton & Spiker, 2007).

It appears from our data and other reviews that the technical properties of the revised BDI-2 are greatly improved over those of its predecessor (Athanasiou, 2007; Barton & Spiker, 2007; Bradley-Johnson & Johnson, 2007). Of all the measures discussed in this chapter, the BDI-2 has one of the best available standardization samples; however, children with documented disabilities, or those referred for or receiving support services for more than 50% of the day, were excluded from the norm sample (Barton & Spiker, 2007). The normative sample is recent (2003), large in size (*N* = 2,500, with at least 125 children per a maximum of 6-month age intervals), and representative of the U.S. population. Moreover, the age divisions of the normative tables are more than adequate. Domain scores generally displayed good (.90 or above) internal-consistency coefficients, with one exception (Adaptive domain, .79 at the 12- to 17-month level). The internal consistency of the subdomains was generally either adequate or approaching adequate, with the more notable exceptions of the Motor subscales (.75–.97); the Cognitive Perception and Concepts subdomain (.58–.75 over the 6- to 23-month range); and, rather unexpectedly, the Cognitive Attention and Memory subdomain (.70–.79 over the 42- to 71-month range).

As noted by Bradley-Johnson and Johnson (2007), only available data on the test–retest stability of the BDI-2 are for children ages 2:0–2:11 and 4:0–4:11. For the older ages, the available domain values are all relatively stable (>.80), as are most of the subdomain scores, with the exception of the Cognitive Attention and Memory subscale (.74–.77). Floors are adequate for the global Cognitive score, the Cognitive Attention and Memory test, and the Cognitive Perception and Concepts test at <1, 2, and 3 months, respectively; the Cognitive Reasoning and Academic Skills test floor is also adequate at 24 months. Examiners should be aware of the "birthday effects" reported by Bradley-Johnson and Johnson (2007); that is, significant changes in scores occur if a child's age changes by a day, particularly at the shift between the 23- and 24-month norm tables.

Detailed information and reviews about content and criterion-related validity are provided in the examiner's manual, Barton and Spiker (2007), and Bliss (2007). However, the BDI-2 has been criticized for its notable lack of predictive validity and longitudinal evidence (Barton & Spiker, 2007). Given the tendency of the first edition to overrefer children, more information about the predictive validity, sensitivity, and specificity of the BDI-2 is needed (Brassard & Boehm, 2007).

Overall, the BDI-2 is a useful assessment tool to identify developmental strengths of infants and young children. Although it has been suggested that the BDI-2 can be used to detect children who have disabilities or delays, the standardization sample excluded children with special needs and those from linguistically and culturally diverse backgrounds (Athanasiou, 2007), and more detailed information on its predictive validity, sensitivity, and specificity is needed. As such, examiners are cautioned about use of the BDI-2, particularly the Cognitive domain in isolation, as a stand-alone tool for diagnostic decision making.

Bayley Scales of Infant and Toddler Development, Third Edition

Overview and Key Features

The Bayley Scales of Infant and Toddler Development, Third Edition (Bayley-III; Bayley, 2005) is an individually administered developmental assessment for infants and toddlers ages 1 through 42 months. Rather than to assess intelligence or to predict academic achievement, the Bayley-III is used to identify young children with developmental strengths and delays, and to determine whether more in-depth evaluation is necessary. The full Bayley-III evaluates five domains (Cognitive, Language, Motor, Social-Emotional, and Adaptive Behavior), some of which are further subdivided into subdomains (Receptive and Expressive Communication, Fine and Gross Motor). The Cognitive, Language, and Motor scales are examiner-administered, with direct testing and some limited observation; the Social-Emotional and Adaptive Behavior scales consist of parent questionnaires. Both standard and growth scores are provided at the domain level, and the latter reportedly can be used to monitoring developmental change. The Bayley-III focuses on research-based developmental milestones, and is theoretically eclectic, with play and information-processing theories obvious influences (Albers & Grieve, 2007; Tobin & Hoff, 2007). The Social-Emotional questionnaire is modeled upon work by Greenspan (2004), while the Adaptive Behavior questionnaire's content is derived from that of Harrison and Oakland (2003). The Bayley-III must be administered by a trained and qualified examiner, typically a psychologist. The administration time varies between 50 minutes (12 months or younger) and 90 minutes (13 months or older). A short version (the Bayley-III Screening Test) is available that assesses the Cognitive, Language, and Motor domains, and that can be administered in 15–25 minutes.

Strengths, Limitations, and Special Considerations

The Bayley-III materials are extremely child-friendly and include sorting shapes, animal figures, puzzles, and a wide assortment of typical toys popular with young children. Testing procedures frequently allow for demonstrations and repeated trials of an item; these allow an examiner to verify responses as intentional, or provide a child with the opportunity for a second attempt. A training video and separate scoring DVD are available to help examiners learn the Bayley-III testing and scoring procedures. Finally, an effort was made to reduce confounding motor or language demands by separating the Mental Scale used in previous editions into the Cognitive and Language domains (Tobin & Hoff, 2007).

Among the Bayley-III's disadvantages, the number of items that require verbatim directions from the examiner is high, and thus prior review and rehearsal are necessary. The kit is heavy, with poor internal organization of the many manipulatives within the kit. Examiners must carefully organize materials and be extremely familiar with the items prior to testing; otherwise, time and the child's attention are easily lost in fumbling between activities. Examiners must carefully monitor and control presentation of a few of the items (e.g., the rubber glitter bracelet, which is tagged as not suitable for very young children). A large number of the items are timed (Bradley-Johnson & Johnson, 2007), which can be problematic in testing young children who have delays or are not initially cooperative.

Although the Bayley-III has received some extremely positive reviews regarding the technical properties of its examiner-administered scales, our data suggest that the psychometric characteristics of the Bayley-III Cognitive, Language, and Motor scales vary from inadequate to good. The standardization sample is recent (2003–2004), adequately large (>1,700, with at least 100 children per 1-year interval), and representative, and normative data are provided at appropriately small age intervals. For the full age range of the test, internal-consistency coefficients are largely adequate (>.79) for the three primary domain scores (Cognitive, Language, and Motor). Although the internal consistency of the Gross Motor subscale is consistently adequate (>.80), the Receptive Communication, Fine Motor, and (to a lesser degree) Expressive Communication subscales have more variable reliability (.71–.96, .72–.95, and .71–.97, respectively). However, the latter is exclusively observed in the age range below 16 months, and thus all subscales can be said to have adequate internal consistency above the 16 month level.

Stability of the Bayley-III scores is difficult to determine, as complete test–retest data are not provided for the full age range of the test (e.g., four samples of truncated age ranges were collected at 2–4, 9–13, 19–26, and 33–42 months); nor are full data given on the demographic composition of the test–retest sample. Bradley-Johnson and Johnson (2007) have also criticized the test–retest interval as being potentially too short (2 days in some cases). Stability of the Bayley-III scores also appears to be a function of age: At least half of the domain/subscale coefficients are inadequate for ages 2–5 and 9–13 months, while all of the domain/subscale coefficients are at least adequately stable at ages 19–26 and 33–42 months, with the exception of the Fine Motor subscale at 19–26 months (.71). For ages 24 months+, the Bayley-III has adequate test floors for all of the Cognitive, Language, and Motor scales; other reviews suggest that the floors have been adequately extended to allow for the assessment of low-functioning infants and toddlers (Bradley-Johnson & Johnson, 2007; Brassard & Boehm, 2007; Tobin & Hoff, 2007).

Readers are referred to the manual for a detailed description of numerous validity studies. The Bayley-III test content, construct validity, and concurrent validity are generally perceived as well established, at least for the Cognitive, Language, and Motor scales; however, concerns have been raised about its clinical/treatment utility (Albers & Grieve, 2007; Anderson, De Luca, Hutchinson, Roberts, & Doyle, 2010), and predictive validity (Brassard & Boehm, 2007; Tobin & Hoff, 2007; Venn, 2007). Scores from the Bayley-III have been correlated with those from other infant–toddler and preschool measures, such as the BSID-II, WPPSI-III, Preschool Language Scales—Fourth Edition (PLS-4), Peabody Developmental Motor Scales—Second Edition (PDMS-2), and Adaptive Behavior Assessment System—Second Edition—Preschool (ABAS-II-P). In addition to inclusion of special populations within the normative sample, several clinical studies have been conducted with such populations (including children with developmental delay, language and motor disorders, Down syndrome, autism spectrum diagnoses, and perinatal conditions), although these latter studies have been criticized for their small sizes and nonrandom selection procedures (Brassard & Boehm, 2007). The technical manual data suggest that the Bayley-III is sensitive to performance differences between children from the normative sample and the various special populations, but concerns have been raised about the ability of the Bayley-III to accurately estimate developmental delay and correctly identify which children are eligible for early intervention services, at least in contexts where

premature birth is a factor (Anderson et al., 2010; Msall, 2010). In the Anderson and colleagues study, children with delays scored within the average range, but significantly lower than controls, who scored between 0.55 and 1.23 standard deviations above the normative standard score mean. Examiners similarly be familiar with the technical report on scores differences between the Bayley-III and the BSID-II, issued by the publisher (Pearson, 2008).

Overall, the Bayley-III is a child-friendly instrument that can be used from birth into the preschool years. Its technical characteristics are among the best available for the multidomain measures. Furthermore, its long tradition of previous research and clinical use make it a very desirable choice for developmental assessments with infants, toddlers, and young preschool-age children.

Merrill–Palmer—Revised Scales of Development

Overview and Key Features

The Merrill–Palmer—Revised Scales of Development (M-P-R; Roid & Sampers, 2004) is an individually administered, norm-referenced measure designed to assess cognitive and other primary developmental abilities in children ages 0:1–6:6. The M-P-R evaluates multiple areas of development with a combination of (1) examiner scales, which involve direct testing and ratings of test session behavior, optional social-emotional problem indicators, and observed language skills; and (2) parent rating forms. Two examiner-administered batteries include a formal Cognitive battery, which has three subscales (Cognitive, Language, and Fine Motor skills) that are used to calculate a Developmental Index (DI). The Gross Motor battery evaluates general gross motor development and atypical movement. An Expressive Language scale is derived from examiner and parental ratings, as is the Social-Emotional scale (Examiner Observation Form/Test-Session Behavior, the Social-Emotional Developmental Scale—Parent Report, the Social/Emotional Temperament Scale—Parent Report, and the Social-Emotional Problem Indicators). The Self-Help/Adaptive scale is based exclusively upon parent reports. The administration time for the Cognitive battery is approximately 30–45 minutes.

The M-P-R battery is based theoretically on a combination of CHC theory and an exploratory play model (Loew, 2007). Exploratory factor analysis from the Try Out Edition generated five CHC factors (Gf, Gc, Gsm, Gs, and Gv) for subtest items in ages 3–5. Although independent analyses of the CHC content of the M-P-R are not readily available, several authors have associated the content of the Cognitive scale with fluid reasoning (Gf) and crystallized abilities (Gc) (Bradley-Johnson & Johnson, 2007), or, alternatively, visual–spatial processing (Gv) (Loew, 2007). However, the linkage between either exploratory play or CHC theory and development of the test content is unclear in the manual, and the inclusion of multiple abilities within the same (sub)scale does not allow for clear interpretation from a CHC perspective.

Strengths, Limitations, and Special Considerations

The M-P-R has several positive features. Its primary advantage is its suitability for use with children who have language delays, as it does not require any vocal responses until after 24 months, and the directions are intentionally brief (Bradley-Johnson & Johnson, 2004). Child attention is promoted with the use of toys and manipulatives, although Spenciner and Appl (2007) have expressed concerns that some of the toys are developmentally inappropriate and can be a choking hazard for younger children. Frustration is minimized by ceiling rules, which are based on total rather than cumulative errors. Spanish instructions for the Cognitive and Gross Motor batteries are available, and the parent forms (except for the Expressive Language scale) are also available in Spanish.

Several limitations have been reported for the M-P-R. Directions for the examiner scales have been heavily criticized as verbal and overly complex, requiring substantial rehearsal prior to use and ongoing reviews between administrations (Bradley-Johnson & Johnson, 2007). Numerous authors also have commented upon the limited interrater reliability data. The parent forms are essential for the assessment of infants, but are likely to be inappropriate and cumbersome for many parents with low literacy levels or English skills (Loew, 2007).

The technical properties of the M-P-R are variable. The standardization sample is adequately large (1,068 participants, including over 200 atypical children) and roughly representative, with appropriately small norm table intervals. However, the age of the M-P-R normative data is unclear, as data reportedly were collected over a nonspecified 6-year period (Bradley-Johnson & Johnson, 2007).

Internal consistency is good (>.90) for the DI, Gross Motor, and total Language scores; at least adequate (>.80) for the Cognitive, Receptive and Expressive Language, and Fine Motor scores.

While the test–retest values for the DI and six other scores all exceed .80, the stability of the M-P-R scores is undetermined, given the small test–retest sample size (41) and the lack of disaggregation of test–retest data by age. Test floors of the M-P-R have been characterized as adequate (Bradley-Johnson & Johnson, 2007; Brassard & Boehm, 2007), but there is an absence of detailed data on this psychometric aspect of the M-P-R in the manual. Finally, Rasch-based growth scores are provided for the DI and other subscales, but are noticeably absent for the Cognitive scale (Bradley-Johnson & Johnson, 2007).

Various validity data are available in the examiner's manual, and are reviewed in detail by Loew (2007) and Bradley-Johnson and Johnson (2007). Of particular note, the M-P-R DI demonstrates strong correlations with the BSID-II Mental Scale, the Leiter-R, and the ABIQ of the SB5. The manual also provides evidence of utility with special populations; in particular, the M-P-R reportedly effectively identifies children with severe intellectual disabilities and gross motor delays. Clinically, the M-P-R is thought to have utility for the evaluation of children with autism and hearing impairments, as well as children from culturally and linguistically diverse backgrounds, due to the minimization of spoken language (Floyd, 2004).

Mullen Scales of Early Learning: AGS Edition

Overview and Key Features

The Mullen Scales of Early Learning: AGS Edition (MSEL; Mullen, 1995) is a comprehensive measure of cognitive functioning for infants and preschool children from birth to 68 months (5:8). An Early Learning Composite can be used to represent the child's general cognitive ability. The MSEL further assesses a child's abilities across visual, motor, and linguistic domains, using five scales: Gross Motor (administered to children from birth through 33 months) and four "cognitive" scales, Visual Reception, Fine Motor, Receptive Language, and Expressive Language (administered to children from birth to 68 months). The Visual Reception scale includes items that assess memory and visual discrimination. The administration time of the entire battery ranges from 15–30 minutes for 1-year-olds to 60 minutes for 5-year-olds.

The MSEL was based on two theoretical foundations: the theory that a child's intelligence should be conceptualized as interrelated but functionally different cognitive abilities (Mullen, 1995); and the author's own information-processing model, which targets intrasensory and intersensory learning and posits gross motor development as the prerequisite for other types of development. CHC theory was not an influence in the development of the MSEL, but the author acknowledges the possible existence of a general intelligence factor (g) and indicates that most cognitive theories emphasize a number of narrow abilities represented on the MSEL. Although there are no formal CHC analyses of the MSEL, a review of items and tasks indicates that the Visual Reception and Fine Motor scales measure aspects of visual–spatial reasoning (Gv), and that the Receptive Language and Expressive Language scales measure aspects of auditory processing (Ga) and crystallized abilities (Gc). Although there may be some face validity to this approach, a lack of clear theoretical underpinning makes interpretation of the MSEL difficult.

Strengths, Limitations, and Special Considerations

The MSEL has long had a great deal of appeal to those working in early childhood education. Information can be gathered in a somewhat flexible manner, using both direct testing and interviews. The materials are attractive and engaging, with a developmentally appropriate feel about them; however, many of them are now becoming dated, and many are not very durable. Materials must be supplemented with items supplied by the examiner (e.g., coins, sitting/stepping bench, a 10-foot tape, etc.), but this list is not specified in the manual (Chittooran, 2001; Kessler, 2001). Several of the subtests do not require a verbal response, which can be useful with children with language delays, although the test does not provide a nonverbal score. None of the subtest activities are timed, allowing children to work to work at their own pace (Bradley-Johnson & Johnson, 2007).

The MSEL has several other significant limitations that primarily relate to the age of the measure, its norms, and its technical characteristics, which are not as strong as those for many of the other instruments reviewed in this chapter. The standardization sample is substantially out of date

(initially collected between 1981 and 1989, published in 1995) and should not be used to make current diagnostic decisions. Based upon our own data and two reviews (Bradley-Johnson, 2001; Bradley-Johnson & Johnson, 2007), the internal consistency is adequate across the test age range for the Early Learning Composite, but related values are inadequate for all of the subscales fairly consistently across the test age ranges (Gross Motor, .63–.92; Fine Motor, .63–.83; Visual Reception, .31–.85; Receptive Language, .45–.86; Expressive Language, .73–.91).

The stability of MSEL scores is undetermined, as data are not available for the Early Learning Composite, are not disaggregated by age for data on the five subscales, and were derived from a relatively small number of children; subscale test–retest coefficients are adequate (>.80) for ages 0–24 months, but inadequate (<.80) for ages 24–56 months. Although some reviews report that test floors are generally thought adequate, analyses indicate that raw scores of 0, 1, and 2 consistently produce the same T score. Examiners also should be aware of the "birthday effects" reported by Bradley-Johnson and Johnson (2007), where changes in a child's age by 1 day are associated with changes in T scores that are roughly equivalent to 1.5 standard deviations.

Concerns related to the validity and clinical utility of the MSEL are noted as well. Unfortunately, most concurrent validity data relate the Mullen to other very dated measures, such as the first editions of the BSID and the Peabody Motor Scales. Of greater concern, though, is that this instrument is often used with special populations (e.g., as children with autism), due to its nonverbal considerations and emphasis on both cognitive and communication delays. However, children with special needs were excluded from the standardization sample, and there is an absence of predictive validity data in general for this measure (Bradley-Johnson & Johnson, 2007). For these reasons, Chittooran (2001) and Kessler (2001) caution against its use with exceptional children.

Overall, the MSEL was a pioneer in its era, but it is currently superseded in quality by more current instruments. Due to difficulties in interpreting its results according to contemporary theoretical frameworks, the age of its norms, various psychometric challenges, and debate over its utility in making diagnostic decisions with clinical populations, examiners should be cautious about selecting the MSEL over other available options.

SUMMARY AND FUTURE DIRECTIONS

The number of reliable and valid early childhood cognitive measures continues to grow. Currently, all major cognitive assessment batteries have versions, tests, or subtests available for use with young children. Multidomain measures that are designed to address the unique and interdisciplinary nature of early childhood continue to improve as well. However, although we have come a very long way and we have many more measures to select from, more work is needed to improve the cognitive tools we use with young children.

We often quote Meisels and Atkins-Burnett (2000) in our own workshops and training in early childhood assessment: "Early childhood assessment is a field in transition. Dominated from its inception by psychometric models and measurement strategies used with older children, it is only now beginning to forge a methodology that is unique to young children" (p. 231). Today—nearly 50 years since the beginnings of Head Start and the first legislation expanding assessment practices with young children; over 25 years since the inclusion of infants, toddlers, and preschool children with special needs in U.S. special education legislation; and over 10 years since this passage was written—early childhood assessment still appears to be "in transition." Many gains have been made, but more needs to be done. The psychometric advances in testing over the last 20 years are undeniable, and are clearly evidenced in many of our early cognitive measures. With the downward extension of many cognitive measures historically used with school-age children, test floors have improved at the upper preschool ages. This has helped increase the number of options available when testing preschool and primary-age students. However, there continue to be concerns with test floors, and in turn with both the sensitivity and specificity of many early childhood cognitive measures, at their youngest ages. Young children are not adequately represented in standardization samples at all ages, and there are limited clinical or special-population studies examining the utility of cognitive measures for young children with special learning and developmental needs.

McGrew and Flanagan (1998) pointed to a "theory-to-practice deficit" in cognitive assessment. As indicated by other chapters in this book, that gap appears to have diminished considerably in contemporary cognitive assessment of school-age children and adults. Additional research is needed to improve the application of contemporary intellectual theory to the measurement of cognitive abilities in young children, however. Surprisingly few studies have examined the application of the most widely used model, CHC theory, with early childhood populations. Although some research has been done, there is still a need to better understand the nuances of the CHC model with preschool children (Ford & Dahinten, 2005; Morgan et al., 2009; Tusing & Ford, 2004; Tusing et al., 2003). With our new and revised measures, we appear to be closing the gap. It our hope that by the publication of the fourth edition of *Contemporary Intellectual Assessment*, the transition will be over, and early childhood assessment will have hit its school-age years with a solid foundation of the assessment "readiness skills" (e.g., adequate floors, sample size, theoretical foundations, developmentally appropriate interpretive frameworks) it needs to thrive. Our young children will be the ultimate winners when the best assessment tools are in the hands of examiners who understand the unique needs of young children and have the skills to interpret their findings. The future looks bright. This is indeed an exciting time to be a psychologist working with young children.

ACKNOWLEDGMENTS

We would like to acknowledge and thank Calli Craft, Sara Greflund, Reky Groendal, Carla Lehouhllier, Marita Partanen, Suretha Swart, and Julia Wallis for their assistance with the data analysis provided as a part of this chapter.

NOTE

1. The WPPSI-III is the only one of the major cognitive batteries used with young children with Canadian norms (Wechsler, 2003b). A French-language version of the Canadian WPPSI-III is also available with Canadian norms for Francophone children (Wechsler, 2004).

REFERENCES

Ainsworth, M., Blehar, M. C., Waters, C., & Wall, S. (1978). *Patterns of attachment: A psychological study of the Strange Situation.* New York: Erlbaum.

Albers, C., & Grieve, A. (2007). Test review: Bayley, N. (2006). Bayley Scales of Infant and Toddler Development. *Journal of Psychoeducational Assessment, 25,* 180–198.

Alfonzo, V. C., & Flanagan, D. P. (1999). Assessment of cognitive abilities in preschoolers. In E. V. Nuttall, I. Romero, & J. Kalisnik (Eds.), *Assessing and screening preschoolers: Psychological and educational dimensions* (pp. 186–217). Boston: Allyn & Bacon.

Alfonso, V. C., & Flanagan, D. P. (2007). Best practices in the use of the Stanford–Binet Intelligence Scales, Fifth Edition (SB5) with preschoolers. In B. Bracken & R. J. Nagle (Eds.), *Psychoeducational assessment of preschool children* (4th ed., pp. 267–296). Mahwah, NJ: Erlbaum.

Alfonso, V. C., & Flanagan, D. P. (2009). Assessment of preschool children. In B. A. Mowder, F. Rubinson, & A. Yasik (Eds.), *Evidence-based practice in infant and early childhood psychology* (pp. 129–166). Hoboken, NJ: Wiley.

Alfonso, V. C., Oakland, T. D., LaRocca, R., & Spanakos, A. (2000). The course on individual cognitive assessment. *School Psychology Review, 29*, 52–64.

Anastasi, A., & Urbina, S. (1997). *Psychological testing* (7th ed.). Upper Saddle River, NJ: Prentice-Hall.

Anderson, P. J., De Luca, C., Hutchinson, E., Roberts, G., & Doyle, L. W. (2010). Underestimation of developmental delay by the new Bayley-III Scale. *Archives of Pediatrics and Adolescent Medicine, 164*, 352–356.

Athanasiou, M. (2007). Review of the Battelle Developmental Inventory—Second Edition. In K. F. Geisinger, R. A. Spies, J. F. Carlson, & B. S. Plake (Eds.), *The seventeenth mental measurements yearbook*. Retrieved from Mental Measurements Yearbook with Tests in Print database.

Bagnato, S. J., & Neisworth, J. T. (1994). A national study of the social and treatment "invalidity" of intelligence testing for early intervention. *School Psychology Quarterly, 9*, 81–108.

Bagnato, S. J., Neisworth, J. T., & Munson, S. M. (1997). *LINKing assessment and early intervention: An authentic curriculum-based approach.* Baltimore: Brookes.

Bain, S. K., & Allin, J. D. (2005). Test review: Stanford–Binet Intelligence Scales, Fifth Edition. *Journal of Psychoeducational Assessment, 23*, 87–95.

Barton, L. R., & Spiker, D. (2007). Review of Battelle Developmental Inventory—Second Edition. In K. F. Geisinger, R. A. Spies, J. F. Carlson, & B. S. Plake (Eds.), *The seventeenth mental measurements yearbook*. Retrieved from Mental Measurements Yearbook with Tests in Print database.

Bayley, N. (1969). *Bayley Scales of Infant Development.* New York: Psychological Corporation.

Bayley, N. (2005). *Bayley Scales of Infant and Toddler Development, Third Edition.* San Antonio, TX: Harcourt Assessment.

Beran, T. N. (2007). Review of Differential Ability Scales (2nd ed.). *Canadian Journal of School Psychology, 22*, 128–132.

Bliss, S. (2007). Review of the Battelle Developmental Inventory—Second Edition. *Journal of Psychoeducational Assessment, 25*, 409–415.

Bowlby, J. (1999). *Attachment: Attachment and loss* (2nd ed., Vol. 1). New York: Basic Books. (Original work published 1969)

Bracken, B. A. (1987). Limitations of preschool instrumentations and standards for minimal levels of technical adequacy. *Journal of Psychoeducational Assessment, 5*, 313–326.

Bracken, B. A. (1988). Ten psychometric reasons why similar tests produce dissimilar results. *Journal of School Psychology, 26*, 155–166.

Bracken, B. A. (1994). Advocating for effective preschool assessment practices: A comment on Bagnato and Neisworth. *School Psychology Quarterly, 9*, 103–108.

Bracken, B. A., Keith, L. K., & Walker, K. C. (1998). Assessment of preschool behavior and social-emotional functioning: A review of thirteen third party instruments. *Journal of Psychoeducational Assessment, 16*(2), 153–169. (Reprinted from *Rehabilitation and Exceptionality, 1*, 331–346.)

Bracken, B. A., & Nagle, R. (Eds.). (2007). *Psychoeducational assessment of preschool children* (4th ed.). Mahwah, NJ: Erlbaum.

Bracken, B. A., & Naglieri, J. (2003). Assessing diverse populations with non-verbal tests of general intelligence. In C. R. Reynolds & R. W. Kamphaus (Eds.), *Handbook of psychological and educational assessment of children: Intelligence, aptitude, and achievement* (2nd ed. pp. 243–274). New York: Guilford Press.

Bradley-Johnson, S. (2001). Cognitive assessment for the youngest children: A critical review of tests. *Journal of Psychoeducational Assessment, 19*, 19–44.

Bradley-Johnson, S., & Johnson, C. M. (2007). Infant and toddler cognitive assessment. In B. A. Bracken & R. J. Nagle (Eds.), *Psychoeducational assessment of preschool children* (4th ed., pp. 325–357). Mahwah, NJ: Erlbaum.

Branden, J. P., & Ouzts, S. M. (2005). Review of Kaufman Assessment Battery for Children, Second Edition. In R. A. Spiers & B. S. Plack (Eds.), *The sixteenth mental measurements yearbook*. Retrieved from Mental Measurements Yearbook with Tests in Print database.

Brassard, M. R., & Boehm, A. E. (2007). *Preschool assessment: Principles and practices.* New York: Guilford Press.

Bronfenbrenner, U. (1977). Toward an experimental ecology of human development. *American Psychologist, 32*, 513–531.

Bronfenbrenner, U. (1979). *The ecology of human development*. Cambridge, MA: Harvard University Press.

Brooks, B. L., Sherman, E. M. S., & Strauss, E. (2010). Test review: NEPSY-II: A Developmental Neuropsychological Assessment, Second Edition. *Child Neuropsychology, 16*, 80–101.

Bruner, J. (1960). *The process of education*. Cambridge, MA: Harvard University Press.

Bruner, J. (1990). *Acts of meaning*. Cambridge, MA: Harvard University Press.

Carroll, J. B. (1993). *Human cognitive abilities: A survey of factor-analytical studies*. New York: Cambridge University Press.

Case, R. (1992). *The mind's staircase: Exploring the conceptual underpinnings of children's thought and knowledge*. Hillsdale, NJ: Erlbaum.

Case, R., & Okamoto, Y. (1996). The role of central conceptual structures in the development of children's thought. *Monographs of the Society for Research in Child Development, 61*(1–2, Serial No. 246).

Cathers-Schiffman, T. A., & Thompson, M. S. (2007). Assessment of English- and Spanish-speaking students with the WISC-III and the Leiter-R. *Journal of Psychoeducational Assessment, 25*, 41–52.

Chen, Z., & Siegler, R. S. (2000). Across the great divide: Bridging the gap between understanding of toddlers' and older children's thinking. *Monographs of the Society for Research in Child Development, 65*(2).

Chittooran, M. (2001). Review of the Mullen Early Scales of Learning. In J. J. Kramer & J. C. Conoley (Eds.), *The eleventh mental measurements yearbook*. Retrieved from Mental Measurements Yearbook with Tests in Print database.

Coalson, D., & Spruill, J. (2007). Cognitive assessment with the Wechsler Preschool and Primary Scale of Intelligence—Third Edition. In B. Bracken & R. J. Nagle (Eds.), *Psychoeducational assessment of preschool children* (4th ed., pp. 241–265). Mahwah, NJ: Erlbaum.

Cohen, M. J. (1997). *Children's Memory Scale*. San Antonio, TX: Psychological Corporation.

D'Amato, R. C., & Titley, J. E. (2010). Review of NEPSY-II-Second Edition. In R. A. Spies, J. F. Carlson, & K. F. Geisinger (Eds.), *The eighteenth mental measurements yearbook*. Retrieved from Mental Measurements Yearbook with Tests in Print database.

Davis, A., & Finch, W. (2010). Test review of the Differential Ability Scales, Second Edition. In K. F. Geisinger, R. A. Spies, & J. F. Carlson (Eds.), *The eighteenth mental measurements yearbook*. Retrieved from Mental Measurements Yearbook with Tests in Print database.

Davis, J. L., & Mathews, R. N. (2010). NEPSY-II review. *Journal of Psychoeducational Assessment, 28*, 175–182.

Demetriou, A., Doise, W., & van Lieashout, C. F. M. (1998). *Life-span developmental psychology*. London: Wiley.

Dudley, L. (2000). *A national investigation of the use of play as an assessment procedures with preschool children*. Unpublished doctoral dissertation, University of South Carolina.

Dumont, R., Willis, J. O., & Elliott, C. D. (2008). *Essentials of DAS-II assessment*. Hoboken, NJ: Wiley.

Edwards, C., Gandini L., & Forman, G. (1998). *The hundred languages of children*. Reggio Emilia, Italy: Reggio Emilia.

Elliott, C. D. (1990). *Differential Ability Scales*. San Antonio, TX: Psychological Corporation.

Elliott, C. D. (2007). *Differential Ability Scales—Second Edition*. San Antonio, TX: Harcourt Assessment.

Epstein, A. S., Schweinhart, L. J., DeBruin-Parecki, A., & Robin, K. B. (2004). *Preschool assessment: A guide to developing a balanced approach* (NIEER Policy Brief, Issue 7). New Brunswick, NJ: National Institute for Early Childhood Research.

Feuerstein, R. (1990). The theory of structural modifiability. In B. Presseisen (Ed.), *Learning and thinking styles: Classroom interaction*. Washington, DC: National Education Association.

Flanagan, D. P., & Alfonso, V. C. (1995). A critical review of the technical characteristics of new and recently revised intelligence tests for preschool children. *Journal of Psychoeducational Assessment, 13*, 66–90.

Flanagan, D. P., Alfonso, V. C., Kaminer, T., & Rader, D. E. (1995). Incidence of basic concepts in the directions of new and recently revised intelligence tests for preschoolers. *School Psychology International, 16*, 345–364.

Flanagan, D. P., Mascolo, J., & Genshaft, J. (2000). A conceptual framework for interpreting intelligence tests for preschoolers. In B. A. Bracken (Ed.), *Psychoeducational assessment of preschool children* (3rd ed., pp. 428–473). Boston: Allyn & Bacon.

Flanagan, D. P., Ortiz, S., & Alfonso, V. C. (2007). *Essentials of cross-battery assessment* (2nd ed.). Hoboken, NJ: Wiley.

Floyd, R. (2004). No evidence for ethnic and racial bias in the Tryout Edition of the Merrill–Palmer Scale—Revised. *Psychological Reports, 94*, 217–220.

Ford, L. (2003). Assessing young children. In R. W. Woodcock, K. S. McGrew, N. Mather, & F. J. Schrank, *Manual for the Woodcock–Johnson Third Edition: Diagnostic Supplement* (pp. 37–46). Itasca, IL: Riverside.

Ford, L., & Dahinten, S. (2005). The use of intelligence tests in the assessment of preschoolers. In D. P. Flanagan & P. L. Harrison (Eds.), *Contemporary intellectual assessment: Theories, tests, and issues* (2nd ed., pp. 487–503). New York: Guilford Press.

Ford, L., Kozey, M., & Merkel, C. (2006). *Use of the*

Woodcock–Johnson III with young children. Poster session presented at the annual meeting of the National Association of School Psychologists, Anaheim, CA.

Ford, L., Kozey, M., & Negreiros, J. (2011). *Revisiting the technical characteristics of widely used measures of early childhood cognitive abilities.* Manuscript under review.

Ford, L., & Rivera, B. D. (1995, March). *School psychologist and early childhood special educator training in culturally and linguistically diverse infants, toddlers, and young children.* Paper presented at the annual meeting of the National Association of School Psychologists, Chicago.

Garrett, H. E. (1946). A developmental theory of intelligence. *American Psychologist, 1*, 372–378.

Gesell, A., & Amatruda, C. S. (1941). *Developmental diagnosis: Normal and abnormal child development, clinical methods and pediatric applications.* New York: Hoeber.

Gordon, B. (2004). Test review: The Wechsler Preschool and Primary Scale of Intelligence, Third Edition. *Canadian Journal of School Psychology, 19*, 205–220.

Grannot, N. (1998). We learn, therefore we develop: Learning verses development—or developing learning? In M. C. Smith & T. Pourchot (Eds.), *Adult learning and development: Perspectives from educational psychology* (pp. 15–34). Mahwah, NJ: Erlbaum.

Greenspan, S. (2004). *The Greenspan Social Emotional Growth Chart: A screening questionnaire for infants and young children.* San Antonio, TX: Harcourt Assessment.

Greenspan, S. I., & Meisels, S. J. (1996). Toward a new vision for the developmental assessment of infants and young children. In S. J. Meisels & E. Fenichel (Eds.), *New visions for the developmental assessment of infants and young children* (pp. 11–26). Washington, DC: Zero to Three.

Gustafsson, J. E. (1984). A unifying model for the structure of intellectual abilities. *Intelligence, 8*, 179–203.

Gyurke, J. S. (1994). A reply to Bagnato and Neisworth: Intelligent versus intelligence testing of preschoolers. *School Psychology Quarterly, 9*, 109–112.

Gyurke, J., Stone, B., & Beyer, M. (1990). A confirmatory factor analysis of the WPPSI—R. *Journal of Psychoeducational Assessment, 8*, 15–21.

Hamilton, W., & Burns, T. G. (2003). Wechsler, D., WPPSI-III. *Applied Neuropsychology, 10*, 188–190.

Harrison, P. L., & Oakland, T. (2003). *Adaptive Behavior Assessment System—Second Edition.* San Antonio, TX: Psychological Corporation.

Holler, K. A., & Greene, S. M. (2010). Developmental changes in children's executive functioning. In E. H. Sandberg & B. L. Spritz (Eds.), *A clinician's guide to normal cognitive development in childhood* (pp. 215–238). New York: Routledge.

Hooper, S. R. (2000). Neuropsychological assessment of the preschool child. In B. A. Bracken (Ed.), *Psychoeducational assessment of preschool children* (3rd ed., pp. 383–398). Boston: Allyn & Bacon.

Hooper, S. R., Molnar, A., Beswick, J., & Jacobi-Vessels, J. (2007). Neuropsychological assessment of the preschool child: Expansion of the field. In B. A. Bracken & R. J. Nagle (Eds.), *Psychoeducational assessment of preschool children* (4th ed., pp. 435–364). Mahwah, NJ: Erlbaum.

Horn, J. L., & Cattell, R. B. (1966). Refinement and test of the theory of fluid and crystallized general intelligences. *Journal of Educational Psychology, 57*, 253–270.

Huitt, W., & Hummel, J. (2003). Piaget's theory of cognitive development. *Educational Psychology Interactive.* Valdosta, GA: Valdosta State University.

Hunt, M. S. (2008). A joint confirmatory factor analysis of the Kaufman Assessment Battery for Children, Second Edition, and the Woodcock–Johnson Tests of Cognitive Abilities, Third Edition, with preschool children. *Dissertation Abstracts International, 68*(11), 4605A. (UMI No. 3288307)

IDEA Infant and Toddler Coordinators Association. (2011). IDEA Part C Early Intervention: Twenty years of making a difference for young children and their families. Retrieved from *www.ideainfanttoddler. org.*

Jacob, S., & Decker, D. (2007). Ethical and legal issues in the education of pupils with disabilities under IDEA. In S. Jacob & T. Hartshorne (Eds.), *Ethics and the law for school psychologists* (5th ed., pp. 117–174). Hoboken, NJ: Wiley.

Johnson, J., & D'Amato, R. C. (2005). Review of the Stanford–Binet Intelligence Scales for Children, Fifth Edition. In R. A. Spies & B. S. Plake (Eds.), *The sixteenth mental measurements yearbook.* Retrieved from Mental Measurements Yearbook with Tests in Print database.

Kaufman, A. S., & Kaufman, N. L. (1983). *Kaufman Assessment Battery for Children (K-ABC).* Circle Pines, MN: American Guidance Service.

Kaufman, A. S., & Kaufman, N. L. (2004). *Kaufman Assessment Battery for Children—Second Edition (KABC-II).* Circle Pines, MN: American Guidance Service.

Kaufman, A. S., Lichtenberger, E. O., Fletcher-Janzen, E., & Kaufman, N. L. (2005). *Essentials of KABC-II assessment.* Hoboken, NJ: Wiley.

Kelley, M., & Surbeck, E. (2007). History of preschool assessment. In B. A. Bracken & R. Nagle (Eds.), *Psychoeducational assessment of preschool children* (4th ed., pp. 3–28). Mahwah, NJ: Erlbaum.

Kessler, C. (2001). Review of the Mullen Early Scales of Learning. In J. J. Kramer & J. C. Conoley (Eds.), *The eleventh mental measurements yearbook*. Retrieved from Mental Measurements Yearbook with Tests in Print database.

Korkman, M., Kirk, U., & Kemp, S. (1998). *NEPSY: A developmental neuropsychological assessment*. San Antonio, TX: Psychological Corporation.

Korkman, M., Kirk, U., & Kemp, S. (2007). *NEPSY—Second Edition (NEPSY-II)*. San Antonio, TX: Harcourt Assessment.

Kozey, M., Ford, L., Merkel, C., & Morgan, J. (2005, March). *Contemporary perspective and critical review of cognitive measures for young children*. Paper presented at the annual meeting of the National Association of School Psychologists, Atlanta, GA.

League, S. (2000). *A joint factor analysis with the Woodcock–Johnson Tests of Cognitive Abilities—Third Edition and the Wechsler Preschool and Primary Scales of Intelligence—Revised*. Unpublished doctoral dissertation, University of South Carolina.

Leiter, R. G. (1979). *Leiter International Performance Scale*. Wood Dale, IL: Stoelting.

Lichtenberger, E. O. (2005). General measures of cognition for the preschool child. *Mental Retardation and Developmental Disabilities Research Reviews, 11*, 197–208.

Lichtenberger, E. O., & Kaufman, A. S. (2004). *Essentials of WPPSI-III assessment*. Hoboken, NJ: Wiley.

Lichtenberger, E. O., Sotelo-Dynega, M., & Kaufman, A. S. (2009). The Kaufman Assessment Battery for Children Second Edition. In J. A. Naglieri & S. Goldstein (Eds.), *Practitioner's guide to assessing intelligence and achievement* (pp. 61–93). Hoboken, NJ: Wiley.

Lichtenstein, R., & Ireton, H. (1984). *Preschool screening*. Orlando, FL: Grune & Stratton.

Lidz, C. S. (2003). *Early childhood assessment*. New York: Wiley.

Linder, T. (2008). *Transdisciplinary play-based assessment* (2nd ed.). Baltimore: Brookes.

Loew, S. (2007). Review of the Merrill–Palmer—Revised Scales of Development. In K. F. Geisinger, R. A. Spies, J. F. Carlson, & B. S. Plake (Eds.), *The seventeenth mental measurements yearbook*. Retrieved from Mental Measurements Yearbook with Tests in Print database.

Luria, A. R. (1973). *The working brain: An introduction to neuropsychology* (B. Haigh, Trans.). London: Penguin.

Madle, R. (2005). Review of the Wechsler Preschool and Primary Scale of Intelligence—Third Edition. In B. Plake, J. C. Impara, & R. Spies (Eds.), *The sixteenth mental measurements yearbook*. Retrieved from Mental Measurements Yearbook with Tests in Print database.

Malaguzzi, L. (1998). History, ideas and basic philosophy: An interview with Lella Gandini. In C. Edwards, L. Gandini, & G. Forman (Eds.), *The hundred languages of children: The Reggio Emilia approach—Advanced reflections* (pp. 49–98). Stamford, CT: Ablex.

Marco, G. (2001). Review of the Leiter—Revised. In B. Plake & J. C. Impara (Eds.), *The fourteenth mental measurements yearbook*. Retrieved from Mental Measurements Yearbook with Tests in Print database.

Marshall, S., McGoey, K., & Moschos, S. (2011). Test review: C. D. Elliott, Differential Ability Scales—Second Edition. *Journal of Psychoeducational Assessment, 29*, 89–93.

McCurdy, M., & Johnsen, L. (2005). Review of the Wechsler Preschool and Primary Scale of Intelligence—Third Edition. In B. Plake, J. C. Impara, & R. Spies (Eds.), *The sixteenth mental measurements yearbook*. Retrieved from Mental Measurements Yearbook with Tests in Print database.

McGrew, K. S. (2005). The Cattell–Horn–Carroll theory of cognitive abilities: Past, present, and future. In D. P. Flanagan & P. L. Harrison (Eds.), *Contemporary intellectual assessment: Theories, tests, and issues* (2nd ed., pp. 136 – 181). New York: Guilford Press.

McGrew, K. S., & Flanagan, D. P. (1998). *The intelligence test desk reference (ITDR): Gf-Gc cross-battery assessment*. Boston: Allyn & Bacon.

McLean, M., Bailey, D. B., & Wolery, M. (1996). *Assessing infants and preschoolers with special needs* (2nd ed.). Englewood Cliffs, NJ: Merrill.

McLean, M., Wolery, M., & Bailey, D. B. (2004). *Assessing infants and preschoolers with special needs* (3rd ed.). Upper Saddle River, NJ: Merrill/Prentice Hall.

Meisels, S. J., & Atkins-Burnett, S. (2000). The elements of early childhood assessment. In J. P. Shonkoff & S. J. Meisels (Eds.), *Handbook of early childhood intervention* (2nd ed., pp. 231–257). New York: Cambridge University Press.

Merkel, C., Kozey, M., Swart, S., & Ford, L. (2005, March). *Basic concepts and their impact on cognitive measures for young children*. Poster presented at the annual meeting of the National Association of School Psychologists, Atlanta, GA.

Morgan, K. E. (2008). The validity of intelligence tests using the Cattell–Horn–Carroll model of intelligence with a preschool population. *Dissertation Abstracts International, 69*.

Morgan, K. E., Rothlisberg, B. A., McIntosh, D. E., & Hunt, M. S. (2009). Confirmatory factor analysis of the KABC-II in preschool children. *Psychology in the Schools, 46*, 515–526.

Mowder, B., Robinson, F., & Yasik, A. (Eds.). (2008). *Evidence based practice in infant and early childhood psychology*. Hoboken, NJ: Wiley.

Msall, M. (2010). Measuring outcomes after extreme prematurity with the Bayley-III Scales of Infant and Toddler Development: A cautionary tale from Australia. *Achieves of Pediatrics and Adolescent Medicine, 164,* 391–393.

Mullen, E. M. (1995). *Mullen Scales of Early Learning: AGS Edition.* Circle Pines, MN: American Guidance Service.

Nagle, R. J. (2000). Issues in preschool assessment. In B. A. Bracken (Ed.), *The psychoeducational assessment of preschool children* (3rd ed., pp. 19–32). Boston: Allyn & Bacon.

Nagle, R. J. (2007). Issues in preschool assessment. In B. A. Bracken & R. J. Nagle (Eds.), *Psychoeducational assessment of preschool children* (4th, ed., pp. 29–48). Mahwah, NJ: Erlbaum.

Napolitano, S. (2010). Test review of NEPSY-II-Second Edition. In R. A. Spies, J. F. Carlson, & K. F. Geisinger (Eds.), *The eighteenth mental measurements yearbook.* Retrieved from Mental Measurements Yearbook with Tests in Print database.

National Early Childhood Technical Assistance Center. (2011). Individuals with Disabilities Act: Part C regulations. Retrieved January 27, 2011, from *www.nectac.org/partc/partc.asp.*

Newborg, J. (2004). *The Battelle Developmental Inventory—Second Edition.* Itasca, IL: Riverside.

Newborg, J., Stock, J. R., Wnek, L., Guidubaldi, J., & Svinicki, J. (1984). *Battelle Developmental Inventory (BDI).* Allen, TX: DLM.

Nuttall, E. V., Romero, I., & Kalesnik, J. (1992). *Assessing and screening preschoolers: Psychological and educational dimensions.* Boston: Allyn & Bacon.

Pascual-Leone, J., & Goodman, D. (1979). Intelligence and experience: A neo-Piagetian approach. *Instructional Science, 8,* 301–367.

Pearson. (2008). *Bayley-III technical report: Factors contributing to differences between Bayley-II and BSID-II scores.* San Antonio, TX: Author.

Percy, A., Ford, L., & Negreiros, J. (2010, June). *Examining cognitive assessment training in Canadian school and clinical psychology programs.* Poster presented at the annual meeting of the Canadian Psychological Association, Winnipeg.

Peterson, N. L. (1987). *Early intervention for handicapped and at-risk children: An introduction to early childhood-special education.* Denver, CO: Love.

Piaget, J. (1969). *Collected psychological works.* Moscow: Prosveshchenie.

Piaget, J. (1971). *Biology and knowledge: An essay on the relation between organic regulations and cognitive processes.* Chicago: University of Chicago Press. (Original work published 1967)

Reynolds, C. R., & Kamphaus, R. W. (2003). *Reynolds Intellectual Assessment Scales.* Lutz, FL: Psychological Assessment Resources.

Rock, D. A., & Stenner, A. (2005). Assessment issues in the testing of children at school entry. *The Future of Children, 15,* 15–34.

Roid, G. H. (2003). *Stanford–Binet Intelligence Scales, Fifth Edition* Itasca, IL: Riverside.

Roid, G. H. (2005). *Stanford–Binet Intelligence Scales for Early Childhood, Fifth Edition (Early SB5).* Austin, TX: PRO-ED.

Roid, G. H., & Barram, R. A. (2004). *Essentials of Stanford–Binet Intelligence Scales (SB5) assessment.* Hoboken, NJ: Wiley.

Roid, G. H., & Miller, L. J. (1997). *Leiter International Performance Scale—Revised.* Wood Dale, IL: Stoelting.

Roid, G. H., & Sampers, J. L. (2004). *Merrill–Palmer—Revised Scales of Development examiner's manual.* Wood Dale, IL: Stoelting.

Sandberg, E. H., & McCullough, M. B. (2010). The development of reasoning skills. In E. H. Sandberg & B. L. Spritz (Eds.), *A clinician's guide to normal cognitive development in childhood* (pp. 179–198). New York: Routledge.

Schrank, F. A., Mather, N., McGrew, K. S., & Woodcock, R. W. (2003). *Manual: Woodcock–Johnson III Diagnostic Supplement to the Tests of Cognitive Abilities.* Itasca, IL: Riverside Publishing.

Shepard, L., Kagan, S., & Wurtz, E. (1998). *Principles and recommendations for early childhood assessments.* Washington, DC: National Education Goals Panel.

Sink, C. A., & Eppler, C. (2007). Review of the Stanford–Binet Intelligence Scales for Early Childhood, Fifth Edition. In K. F. Geisinger, R. A. Spies, J. F. Carlson, & B. S. Plake (Eds.), *The seventeenth mental measurements yearbook.* Retrieved from Mental Measurements Yearbook with Tests in Print database.

Spenciner, L. J., & Appl, D. J. (2007). Review of the Merrill–Palmer—Revised Scales of Development. In K. F. Geisinger, R. A. Spies, J. F. Carlson, & B. S. Plake (Eds.), *The seventeenth mental measurements yearbook.* Retrieved from Mental Measurements Yearbook with Tests in Print database.

Spritz, B. L., & Sandberg, E. H. (2010). The case for children's cognitive development: A clinical developmental perspective. In E. H. Sandberg & B. L. Spritz (Eds.) *A clinician's guide to normal cognitive development in childhood* (pp. 3–19). New York: Routledge.

Stinnett, T. (2003). Review of the Leiter—Revised. In B. Plake & J.C. Impara (Eds.), *The fourteenth mental measurements yearbook.* Retrieved from Mental Measurements Yearbook with Tests in Print database.

Stone, B. J., Gridley, B. E., & Gyurke, J. S. (1991). Confirmatory factor analysis of the WPPSI-R at the extreme end of the age range. *Journal of Psychoeducational Assessment, 9,* 263–270.

Teague, T. (1999). *Confirmatory factor analysis of the Woodcock–Johnson Third Edition and the Differential Ability Scales with preschool children.* Unpublished doctoral dissertation, University of South Carolina.

Teague, T. L. (2002). Joint factor-analytic investigation of the Differential Ability Scales and the Woodcock–Johnson Tests of Cognitive Abilities—Third Edition with preschool-age children. *Dissertation Abstracts International Section, 62*(7), 2338A.

Thorndike, R. L., Hagen, E. P., & Sattler, J. M. (1986). *Stanford–Binet Intelligence Scale: Fourth Edition.* Chicago: Riverside.

Tobin, R., & Hoff, K. E. (2007). Review of the Bayley Scales of Infant and Toddler Development—Third Edition. In K. F. Geisinger, R. A. Spies, J. F. Carlson, & B. S. Plake (Eds.), *The seventeenth mental measurements yearbook.* Retrieved from Mental Measurements Yearbook with Tests in Print database.

Tsatsanis, K. D., Dartnall, N., Cicchetti, D., Sparrow, S., Klin, A., & Volkmar, F. (2003). Concurrent validity and classification accuracy of the Leiter and Leiter-R in low-functioning children with autism. *Journal of Autism and Developmental Disorders, 33,* 23–30.

Tusing, M. B., & Ford, L. (2004). Examining preschool cognitive abilities using a CHC framework. *International Journal of Testing, 4,* 91–114.

Tusing, M. E. (1998). *Validation studies with the Woodcock–Johnson Psycho-Educational Battery—Revised Tests of Cognitive Ability (Early Development Scale) and the Differential Ability Scales: Preschool Level.* Unpublished doctoral dissertation, University of South Carolina.

Tusing, M. E., Maricle, D., & Ford, L. (2003). Assessment of young children with the WJ III. In F. Schrank, & D. P. Flanagan (Eds.), *The Woodcock–Johnson III: Clinical use and interpretation.* San Diego, CA: Academic Press.

U.S. Department of Education. (2007, May 9). Early intervention program for infants and toddlers with disabilities: Proposed rule. *Federal Register, 72,* 14–18.

Vacca, J. J. (2007). Review of the Stanford–Binet Intelligence Scales for Early Childhood, Fifth Edition. In K. F. Geisinger, R. A. Spies, J. F. Carlson, & B. S. Plake (Eds.), *The seventeenth mental measurements yearbook.* Retrieved from Mental Measurements Yearbook with Tests in Print database.

Venn, J. (2007). Review of the Bayley Scales of Infant and Toddler Development—Third Edition. In K. F. Geisinger, R. A. Spies, J. F. Carlson, & B. S. Plake (Eds.), *The seventeenth mental measurements yearbook.* Retrieved from Mental Measurements Yearbook with Tests in Print database.

Vernon, P. E. (1950). *The structure of human abilities.* London: Methuen.

Vig, S., & Sanders, M. (2007). Cognitive assessment. In M. R. Brassard & A. E. Boehm, *Preschool assessment: Principles and practices* (pp. 383–419). New York: Guilford Press.

Vygotsky, L. (1978). *Mind in society: The development of higher psychological processes.* Boston: Harvard University Press.

Wechsler, D. (1967). *Wechsler Intelligence Scale for Children.* San Antonio, TX: Psychological Corporation.

Wechsler, D. (2001). *Wechsler Individual Achievement Test—Second Edition.* San Antonio, TX: Psychological Corporation.

Wechsler, D. (2002). *Wechsler Preschool and Primary Scale of Intelligence—Third Edition.* San Antonio, TX: Psychological Corporation.

Wechsler, D. (2003a). *Wechsler Intelligence Scale for Children—Fourth Edition.* San Antonio, TX: Psychological Corporation.

Wechsler, D. (2003b). *The Wechsler Preschool and Primary Scale of Intelligence Scale—Third Edition, Canadian.* San Antonio, TX: Psychological Corporation.

Wechsler, D. (2004). *Échelle D'intelligence De Wechsler Pour La Période Préscolaire Et Primaire—Troisième Édition—Version Pour Francophones Du Canada.* Toronto: Harcourt.

Woodcock, R. W., McGrew, K. S., & Mather, N. (2001a, 2007a). *Woodcock–Johnson III Tests of Academic Achievement—Normative Update.* Rolling Meadows, IL: Riverside.

Woodcock, R. W., McGrew, K. S., & Mather, N. (2001b, 2007b). *Woodcock–Johnson III Tests of Cognitive Abilities: Normative Update.* Rolling Meadows, IL: Riverside.

Woodcock, R. W., McGrew, K. S., Mather, N., & Schrank, F. A. (2003, 2007). *Woodcock–Johnson III Diagnostic Supplement—Normative Update.* Rolling Meadows, IL: Riverside.

Yell, M. L. (1998). *The law and special education.* Upper Saddle River, NJ: Merrill.

Zembar, M. J., & Blume, L. B. (2009). *Middle childhood development: A contextual approach.* Columbus, OH: Prentice Hall.

Use of Intelligence Tests in the Identification of Giftedness

David E. McIntosh
Felicia A. Dixon
Eric E. Pierson

This chapter begins by providing a brief historical overview of giftedness, with an emphasis on identifying the major figures in the field. The theoretical formulation of intelligence and the conceptual links between intelligence and giftedness are also discussed from a historical perspective. The evolution of multitrait theories of intelligence, the impact of advances in psychometrics on gifted assessment, and the increase in the number of theory-based cognitive measures are examined. The refinement of theory of intelligence centering on the Cattell–Horn–Carroll (CHC) model is discussed.

A significant portion of the chapter focuses on the definition of *giftedness*. The distinction between the terms *gifted* and *talented* is made. The most recent definition of *gifted and talented* provided by the U.S. Department of Education (1993) is presented and discussed. Renzulli's (1978) multitrait definition, Tannenbaum's (1983) conception of giftedness as a psychosocial construct, Sternberg's implicit theory of giftedness (Sternberg & Zhang, 1995), and the differentiated model of giftedness and talent (Gagné, 2004) are reviewed. The implicit links among definitions, cognitive theory, and cognitive assessment are explored.

The issues of multiple intelligences versus many factors of intelligence are also considered. Specifically, Sternberg's triarchic theory of intelligence (Sternberg, Chapter 6, this volume; Sternberg & Williams, 2002) and Gardner's theory of multiple intelligences (Chen & Gardner, Chapter 5, this volume; Gardner, 1999) are reviewed. An extensive review of factor-analytic research is provided, exploring the multidimensional abilities of gifted children with commonly used measures of intelligence. Although factor-analytic research with gifted samples has for the most part supported Kaufman's (1975, 1979) two-factor model, there is a growing body of confirmatory-factor-analytic research studying more complex models of intelligence. The methodological and statistical issues contributing to differences across studies are also examined.

The process of gifted identification is then reviewed. Clark's (1997) and Borland's (1989) recommended approaches for identification are discussed. The importance of demonstrating links among a school's definition of giftedness, the identification process, and educational programming is considered. In addition, important issues to consider during the identification of cognitively gifted minority children are explored within the chapter. Alternative approaches are provided for identifying gifted children with learning disabilities.

A major portion of the chapter focuses on discussing special issues related to the intellectual assessment of gifted children. The importance of considering the theoretical differences among intelligence measures, and the importance of using theory-based measures, are discussed. The need for a better understanding of the relationships between screening procedures and the final decision outcomes based upon intelligence tests is emphasized. Implications of using a single composite IQ score and setting specific IQ "cutoff" scores when making identification decisions are examined. The chapter concludes with specific recommendations on the effective use of intelligence measures in the identification of giftedness.

HISTORICAL OVERVIEW OF INTELLIGENCE AND GIFTEDNESS

Although America's interest in giftedness has been magnified since the late 1800s, giftedness has been of general interest to virtually all societies in recorded history (Colangelo & Davis, 1997). However, until Francis Galton (1822–1911) established the conceptual link between intelligence and giftedness, there had been little research studying intellectual differences among humans (Clark, 1997). Using the work of his cousin Charles Darwin (1859) as a basis, Galton developed the theory of *fixed intelligence*, which essentially ignored the effects of the environment and emphasized the hereditary basis of intelligence. This theory of fixed intelligence dominated the literature for nearly half a century. Not until the mid-1950s, when research conducted by Jean Piaget, Maria Montessori, Beth Wellman, G. Stanley Hall, Arnold Gesell, and others was published, did researchers begin to question the fixed-intelligence model and begin to consider an interactive view of intelligence.

Along with the theoretical formulation of intelligence came the need to develop ways to assess intelligence. Interestingly, although Francis Galton was credited with developing the first intelligence test, Alfred Binet is more widely known for developing the first intelligence test in 1905, with the specific goal of differentially placing children in special education or regular classrooms. Binet has also been credited with establishing the concepts of *mental age* and *intelligence quotient* (IQ). As Colangelo and Davis (1997) deftly point out, it was Binet's concept of mental age that had implications for the identification of giftedness. Essentially, the concept of mental age implied that children demonstrate growth in intelligence; therefore, children may be behind, consistent with, or ahead of their peers intellectually (Colangelo & Davis, 1997). Consequently, some children identified will demonstrate advanced levels of intelligence.

In 1916, Lewis Terman published the famous Stanford–Binet Intelligence Scale, which has seen four revisions to date. Not only was Terman recognized for developing one of the most popular measures of intelligence, but he was also instrumental in one of the most significant longitudinal studies on giftedness of the 20th century, earning him distinction as the "father of gifted education" (Clark, 1997; Colangelo & Davis, 1997). Soon after the development of the Stanford–Binet Intelligence Scale, the popularity of intelligence testing soared. In fact, it soared so greatly that many schools based educational placement decisions solely on IQ scores. Unfortunately, many schools continue to identify gifted students by using a single measure of cognitive ability. The benefits and limitations of such an approach are discussed later.

Another landmark event that was instrumental in the public's interest in giftedness occurred in 1957, when the Soviet Union launched the world's first human-made satellite, Sputnik. The fact that the Soviets had both the scientific and technological power to accomplish this feat was viewed by some Americans as a shocking defeat to U.S. education. The results were an increase in the focus on educating gifted children in more advanced classes, especially in science and mathematics, and a call to action for a "total talent mobilization" (Davis & Rimm, 1998). In the United States, Sputnik was a wake-up call; new programs and schools were designed for high-ability students, with the purpose of keeping ahead globally. Modern societal concerns about annual academic progress and "failing schools" echo these historic concerns.

Over the last 30 years, new theories of intelligence, advances in psychometrics, and advances in technology have resulted in a renewed focus on the identification of gifted individuals. The focus on neurobiological data and mental processes has resulted in the development of new theories of intelligence. Gardner (1983, 1993, 1999; see also Chen & Gardner, Chapter 5, this volume) has proposed a theory of *multiple intelligences*, which focuses on eight areas of intellect (with a ninth one, *existential*, proposed): *linguistic, musical, logical–mathematical, spatial, bodily–kinesthetic, interpersonal, intrapersonal,* and *naturalistic.* The significance of his theory lies not so much in the eight identified areas of intellect as in the underlying assumptions that form the basis of his theory. To be specific, Gardner has emphasized the neurobiological influences on intelligence and the importance of better understanding the interaction between genetics and environment in the development of intelligence. Likewise, the *triarchic theory* of intelligence developed by Sternberg (1985; see also Sternberg, Chapter 6, this volume) and Sternberg and Williams (2002) has focused on better understanding three kinds of mental processes related to giftedness: *analytic, synthetic,* and *practical.* The difficulty with these theories of intelligence has been in determining how to assess and apply the various constructs presented by the authors. However, there have been several attempts to apply Gardner's multiple-intelligences theory and Sternberg's triarchic theory within school settings, with varying results (Coleman & Cross, 2005).

There has also been a renewed interest in the use of Luria's theory of neuropsychology in the development of cognitive tests (Kaufman & Kaufman, 2004; Naglieri & Das, 1997). Although many psychologists and neuropsychologists find this theory clinically helpful in understanding patterns of deficits in individuals, it is important to recognize that Luria's theory was drawn from a tradition of analyzing individuals with head injury. Most often, people reflect upon Luria's work with individuals with head trauma. However, Luria also wrote and studied individuals with amazing talents and abilities in memory (Luria, 1987). Those working with gifted and talented students may want to consider possible applications of this theory in contrast to the dominant CHC theory.

Long before Gardner and Sternberg developed their theories, L. L. Thurstone (1938) proposed his theory of *primary mental abilities.* According to Thurstone's theory, seven primary intelligence factors or abilities were measured in tests of intelligence: (1) *word fluency,* the ability to think of a lot of words, given a specific stimulus; (2) *verbal comprehension,* the ability to derive meaning from words; (3) *number* or *numerical ability,* the ability involved in all arithmetic tasks; (4) *memory,* the ability to use simple or rote memory of new material, both in verbal and in pictorial form; (5) *induction,* the ability to examine verbal, numerical, or pictorial material and derive from it a generalization, rule, concept, or principle; (6) *spatial perception,* the ability to see objects in space and to visualize varying arrangements of those objects; and (7) *perceptual speed,* the ability to discern minute aspects of elements of pictures, letters, and words as rapidly as possible. Feldhusen (1998) has suggested that close examination of these seven abilities reveals some parallels to the currently popular multiple intelligences of Gardner in the types of abilities mentioned. Thurstone's theory of primary mental abilities proposed that students'

achievement in school could best be understood by their relative amount of ability in these seven areas. The end of the 1990s and the beginning of the new century saw a consolidation of theory that resembles the model originally proposed by Thurstone. Specifically, this period saw the consolidation of Gf-Gc theory and the work of Carroll into the CHC model of intelligence (Schneider & McGrew, Chapter 4, this volume; Strauss, Sherman, & Spreen, 2006). Similar to Thurstone's model, CHC theory suggests that intelligence can be thought of as having seven primary ability areas: Gf (*fluid intelligence*), Gc (*crystallized intelligence*), Gsm (*short-term memory*), Gv (*visual processing*), Ga (*auditory processing*), Glr (*long-term storage and retrieval*), and Gs (*processing speed*).

Advances in psychometrics and technology have led to the development of cognitive measures that are theory-driven and reflect the multitrait nature of intelligence. In the past, cognitive measures were developed with little or no consideration of intelligence theory. Consequently, there was an overreliance on the unitary construct of intelligence, g (Flanagan & Ortiz, 2002). Following the convergence of theories surrounding the development of the CHC theory, many of the most commonly administered tests related to gifted assessments in the past (the Stanford–Binet and the Wechsler series) have been aligned with CHC theory by the test publishers (O'Donnell, 2009; Strauss et al., 2006). In addition, an increasing number of published theory-based cognitive measures now exist: the Woodcock–Johnson III (WJ III; Woodcock, McGrew, & Mather, 2001) and the Cognitive Assessment System (CAS; Naglieri & Das, 1997), for example. These are discussed in more detail later.

While current trends in test publishing and research have moved toward an increased emphasis on instruments built around theories of intelligence, it is important to keep in mind that earlier measures used with the assessment of giftedness had as their primary goal the classification of individuals along a unitary dimension of intelligence. As a result of changes in how estimates of IQ are obtained and in the nature of the tests, a child who was classified as gifted in the 1930s–1970s may look very different intellectually from what a psychologist looking at a gifted child in the current decade would see.

There is a renewed interest in providing gifted students with specific programming to meet their educational needs. At the heart of this renewed interest is an often hotly debated issue: How should children be identified for these special programs? What should guide the process of identification? Central to this issue is the importance of establishing a clear definition of *giftedness* to guide the development of services for the population defined.

THE ISSUE OF DEFINITION

The terms *gifted* and *talented* have been used in a variety of ways to describe individuals who perform at a superior intellectual level. *High-ability* or *high-functioning* have been terms frequently used in order to avoid using either *gifted* or *talented* because these terms have been problematic over the years. Borland (1989) has stated that there is a rupture between the word *gifted* in its various usages and a clearly and consensually defined group of children in schools. Hence the dichotomy between what the term actually means and how it is frequently used has caused some confusion about how to regard the dimensions of giftedness. Similarly, people have often disagreed over what *gifted* and *talented* mean in terms of individual characteristics, behaviors, and need for services.

Tannenbaum (1997) has defined *giftedness* as potential for becoming acclaimed producers. Gagné (1999) has differentiated between *gifts*, which he calls *aptitudes*, and *talents*, which he calls *expressions of systematically developed abilities or skills* in at least one field of human activity. According to Gagné, catalysts—environmental, intrapersonal, and motivational—transform intellectual, creative, socioaffective, and sensory–motor gifts (abilities, aptitudes) into talents (performances) in the academic, technical, artistic, interpersonal, and athletic areas (see also Davis & Rimm, 1998). Cox, Daniel, and Boston (1985) have avoided the term *gifted*, preferring to call these students *able learners*. Renzulli and Reis (1997) prefer *gifted behaviors*, which can be developed in certain students at certain times and in certain circumstances. Treffinger (1995) likes the term *talent development*, calling the shift a fundamentally new orientation to the nature of the field. Best-selling authors (e.g., Coyle, 2009; Gladwell, 2008) embrace talents and gifts in their current books, defining these constructs outside the cognitive dimensions present in most of the previous definitions: "[Talent is] the possession of repeatable skills that don't depend on physical size" (Coyle, 2009, p. 11), and "Outliers are those who have been given opportunities— and who have had the strength and presence of

mind to seize them" (Gladwell, 2008, p. 267). For Gladwell, at least, the gift is the opportunity as much as (or even more than) the innate traits. Many others have used the terms *gifted* and *talented* synonymously. If one standard definition were always used, the confusion would be nonexistent. This confusion in definitions has indeed been a major issue to both those concerned with studying gifted individuals and those concerned with educating them.

The definition of *gifted and talented* provided by the U.S. Department of Education (1993) is as follows:

> Children and youth with outstanding talent perform or show the potential for performing at remarkably high levels of accomplishment when compared with others of their age, experience, or environment. These children and youth exhibit high capability in intellectual, creative, and/or artistic areas, possess an unusual leadership capacity, or excel in specific academic fields. They require services or activities not ordinarily provided by the schools. Outstanding talents are present in children and youth from all cultural groups, across all economic strata, and in all areas of human endeavor. (p. 26)

Although this definition has served the purpose of informing schools of what areas should be considered in serving gifted students, it really does not inform anyone of specific ways to find these people and is perhaps too broad for most school corporations to operationalize effectively. In contrast, it does demonstrate the current trend in widening the perspective in order to allow more people to be served. Indeed, multitrait definitions tend to be the norm today.

Renzulli (1978) has proposed a multitrait definition of giftedness that focuses on three interlocking clusters of traits: above-average, but not necessarily superior, ability; motivational traits that Renzulli calls *task commitment*; and creativity. According to Renzulli, "it is the interaction among the clusters that . . . [is] the necessary ingredient for creative/productive accomplishment" (p. 182). The form of giftedness characterized by high scores on standardized tests and model classroom behavior has been termed *schoolhouse giftedness* by Renzulli and Reis (1997).

Tannenbaum (1983) has defined *giftedness* as a psychosocial construct. He states that gifted individuals are those "with the potential for becoming critically acclaimed performers or exemplary producers of ideas in spheres of activity that enhance the moral, physical, emotional, social, intellectual, or aesthetic life of humanity" (p. 86). The key to this definition is the focus on the gifted individual as a producer of ideas.

Sternberg and Zhang (1995) have developed an implicit theory of giftedness that embodies five criteria: *excellence, rarity, productivity, demonstrability,* and *value.* Stating that implicit theories are relativistic because what is perceived as giftedness is based on the values of the particular time period or place in existence, Sternberg and Zhang have argued for the need for implicit theories to fill in the gaps left by explicit theories (i.e., those that specify the content of what it means to be gifted). "The problem is that in the science of understanding human gifts, we do not have certainties. There are no explicit theories known to be totally and absolutely correct, nor are there likely to be any in the foreseeable future" (p. 91).

In contrast to multitrait or all-encompassing definitions of giftedness are the definitions centering around the cognitive aspects of reasoning and judgment that can be found in a test score. To this end, the Binet–Simon test (Binet & Simon, 1905) was developed as an early paper-and-pencil test that attempted to measure intelligence. A revision of this test later became known as the Stanford–Binet Intelligence Scale (Terman, 1916), and this IQ-based definition is still widely accepted today (Coleman & Cross, 2005). Terman (1925a), the father of the gifted movement in this country, was perfectly content with defining giftedness as the possession of a very high IQ.

Using the Stanford–Binet to identify a population of gifted children, Lewis Terman and his research team were interested in investigating intelligence and achievement in a group of high-functioning children in the 1920s. Terman (1925b) wrote the following about gifted children:

> When the sources of our intellectual talent have been determined, it is conceivable that means may be found which would increase our supply. When the physical, mental and character traits of gifted children are better understood, it will be possible to set about their education with better hope of success. . . . In the gifted child, Nature has moved far back the usual limits of educability, but the realms thus thrown open to the educator are still *terra incognita.* It is time to move forward, explore, and consolidate. (pp. 16–17)

Specifically, Terman's team asked the following questions: Do precocious children become exceptional adults? Do high-IQ adults exhibit a disproportionate degree of mental health problems? Are brilliant children also physically superior? Does having a high IQ correlate with excellent school performance? Can gifted children be expected to display exceptional adult career achievements as eminent scientists, scholars, artists, and leaders? If high-ability children become extraordinary adults, what can be learned from the personal and educational antecedents that seem to nurture their development? (Sabotnik & Arnold, 1994). Terman's group's research focused on the lives of those high-functioning individuals who had scored in the top 1% on the Stanford–Binet Intelligence Scale, and on what could be learned about their lives to create educational opportunities that would serve similar people. They concluded from their research that superior children apparently became superior adults (Oden, 1968).

Leta Hollingworth's work with high-IQ students (i.e., children with IQs over 180) at the Speyer School in New York City was also important in informing researchers about the impact of an enrichment program for gifted students on their adult achievement and values (Hollingworth, 1942). In 1981, several adults who had formerly attended the school were interviewed concerning the school's impact on their lives (White & Renzulli, 1987). Among those interviewed, three were from the group in Hollingworth's early study. They stated that the school provided lifelong love for learning, pleasure in independent work, and joy in interacting with similar high-ability students (Sabotnik & Arnold, 1994). Hence both Terman's and Hollingworth's noteworthy research depended in large part on the IQ score measured for each individual and on what these high-ability individuals became later in life.

On the contrary, Simonton (2008) used Winner's (1996) definition of giftedness—"A gifted child or adolescent is someone who masters a particular domain at a faster rate than the average youth" (p. 253)—in his historiometric study of 291 eminent African Americans. Multiple-regression analyses indicated that adulthood eminence and creative achievement were positively correlated with early giftedness. Simonton offered two main implications, one theoretical and one practical, for this study. Theoretically, his inquiry established an impressive developmental continuity across the lifespan: Precocious development in childhood and adolescence predicts the magnitude of eminence and achievement in adulthood. Practically, his study indicated that giftedness must not be evaluated according to a "one-size-fits-all" procedure, but rather according to the occurrence of precocious behaviors that are specific to a given culture and achievement domain. The variety of gifts manifested in these precocious individuals would not have been identified by a score on a standard intelligence test.

Gridley, Norman, Rizza, and Decker (2003) have proposed a definition of giftedness based on the CHC theory of intelligence. This theory combines Cattell and Horn's model of Gf (fluid) and Gc (crystallized) intelligence with Carroll's standard multifactorial model. Carroll's model (see also Carroll, Appendix, this volume) suggests that cognitive abilities exist at three levels or *strata*: (1) a lowest or first stratum composed of numerous narrow abilities; (2) a second stratum consisting of about 8–10 broad abilities; and (3) a third stratum comprising a single general intellectual ability, commonly called *g*. Gridley and colleagues' definition is as follows:

> Intellectually gifted students are those who have demonstrated 1) Superior potential or performance in general intellectual ability (Stratum III) and/or 2) Exceptional potential or performance in specific intellectual abilities (Stratum II) and/or 3) Exceptional general or specific academic aptitudes (Strata I and II). (p. 291)

The practicality of Gridley and colleagues' definition is that it suggests that giftedness can be measured by a test. The authors state that they do not "focus on the genetic causes of gifts, but rather . . . on gifts as intellectual abilities and talents as special academic aptitudes being of equal value in their need for nurturing and development" (pp. 290–291).

Most professionals regard giftedness in school as an academic need to be served (e.g., Coleman & Cross, 2005; Rizza, McIntosh, & McCunn, 2001). In order to be served appropriately, students must be identified, and standardized tests are the major methods used for identification purposes. Although a standardized test is available to measure each dimension in the federal definition, most programs for gifted individuals are particularly interested in intelligence tests because most gifted programs focus on serving students of high cognitive ability.

Gallagher (1995) has stated that IQ tests are merely one measure of the development of intellectual abilities at a given time. They give an indication of a child's current development, so that children can be compared to one another on such characteristics as their store of knowledge, reasoning ability, and ability to associate concepts—all of which are important predictors of academic success. IQ tests still remain the single most effective predictors of academic success that we have today. There is evidence (Rindermann, 2007) to suggest that one of the reasons why measures of intelligence are such good predictors of academic success is that they measure a single innate construct overlapping with academic achievement. Pyryt (1996) agrees with this focus on the best measures currently available, stating that IQ tests are very useful for making legal decisions regarding the eligibility for participation in gifted programs. IQ tests still serve as important tools for recognizing the special education needs of intellectually gifted students.

The modern IQ test, with its age-based normative comparison, allows for students' level of giftedness to be classified by a method such as that suggested by Gagné (2004) and encouraged by Baer and Kaufman (2004). It is important to recognize that this classification system may be difficult to implement, as the item ceilings for different measures of intelligence may limit the ability of individuals to be classified at the highest level or to maintain a high level of classification at different ages.

Recently, Zhu, Cayton, Weiss, and Gabel (2008) published an extended set of normative tables for use in assessing gifted children. These tables are designed for use with children who reach the ceiling of the traditional normative set for their age on one or more subtests of the Wechsler Intelligence Scale for Children—Fourth Edition (WISC-IV; Wechsler, 2003). The use of these extended tables is designed to help differentiate between gifted and highly gifted individuals. Given the frequency of individuals with IQ scores above 150, the degree to which clinicians will need to resort to these tables is limited. In addition, the tables are believed to be more beneficial in tracking progress or growth of gifted children, as they should be more sensitive to performance above the original ceiling of the test.

THE ISSUE OF ONE VERSUS MANY FACTORS IN INTELLIGENCE

Defining Intelligence(s)

The IQ score, a unidimensional construct used for many purposes, has been historically very important in identifying and understanding giftedness. In fact, as noted earlier, the idea that a child is intellectually precocious has often been synonymous with a high IQ score. Those arguing against the idea of an IQ score have stated that this measure leads to a narrow view of intelligence that is tied to the skills most valued in schools—linguistic and logical–mathematical skills (Ramos-Ford & Gardner, 1997). In addition, Ramos-Ford and Gardner note that a majority of children are still admitted to specialized educational programs for gifted students on the basis of an IQ score of 130, or two standard deviations above the mean on an intelligence test. A score of 129, virtually the same score, will keep another student out of such a program. This cutoff score process is problematic and all too prevalent in school programming for gifted students.

Arguing for a theory of multiple intelligences, Gardner (1999) has defined *intelligence* as an ability or set of abilities that permits an individual to solve problems or fashion products that are of consequence in a particular cultural setting. Ramos-Ford and Gardner (1997) conclude that "A multiple intelligences approach to assessment and instruction strives toward identifying and supporting the 'gifts' in every individual" (p. 65).

Sternberg's triarchic theory of intelligence suggests that intelligence includes "applying component processes to novel tasks for the purposes of adaptation to, shaping of, and selection of environments" (Sternberg & Williams, 2002, p. 148). Sternberg has described both his triarchic theory of intelligence and Gardner's theory of multiple intelligences by using a systems metaphor. Sternberg's metaphor suggests that to understand the various aspects of intelligence working together as a system, one needs to understand the integration within the system itself (Sternberg & Williams, 2002). Although these theories have gained popularity in recent years, they lack empirical data to support their effectiveness (Sternberg & Williams, 2002).

Sternberg and Williams (2002) state, "Perhaps the most difficult challenge in the study of intelligence is figuring out the criteria for labeling a thought process or a behavior as intelligent" (p. 1). One must establish criteria to use in trying to decide what constitutes intelligence. Early experts suggested that intelligence is based on adaptation to the environment (e.g., Colvin, 1921; Pintner, 1921; all cited in Sternberg & Kaufman, 2001). Later, Boring (1923, cited in Sternberg & Kaufman, 2001) suggested that intelligence could and should be defined operationally as that which intelligence tests test. Current definitions by both experts and laypersons suggest that adaptation to the environment, whether with practical problem-solving ability or academic skills, is still the essential theme in defining intelligence. Sternberg and Williams have further suggested three criteria to understand the mental processes and behaviors that can be labeled intelligent: correlation of a target thought or behavior with cultural success, or *cultural adaptation*; mental skills development, or *cultural and biological adaptation*; and evolutionary origins and development, or *biological adaptation*.

With these emphases in mind, then, individuals who are called gifted will be those who can best adapt to their environments, and the purpose of finding these individuals through identification processes in schools will be to maximize their abilities in doing so.

Factor-Analytic Research

Extensive factor-analytic research has been conducted with the goal of exploring the multidimensional nature of intellectual abilities among gifted children. The majority of this research has used the Wechsler Intelligence Scale for Children—Revised (WISC-R; Wechsler, 1974) (Brown & Yakimowski, 1987; Macmann, Plasket, Barnett, & Siler, 1991; Mishra, Lord, & Sabers, 1989; Reams, Chamrad, & Robinson, 1990; Watkins, Greenwalt, & Marcell, 2002) or the WISC-III (Wechsler, 1991). In general, factor-analytic studies have consistently found support for the Verbal Comprehension and Perceptual Organization two-factor model (Karnes & Brown, 1980; Sapp, Chissom, & Graham, 1985; Watkins et al., 2002) proposed by Kaufman (1975, 1979). Among the two-factor models, the Verbal Comprehension factor was typically composed of the Similarities, Vocabulary, Comprehension, and Information subtests. More variability was displayed across studies in the composition of the Perceptual Organizational factor. The majority of the studies found that the Block Design and Object Assembly subtests loaded on the Perceptual Organizational factor, while the Picture Completion and Picture Arrangement subtests were found to load inconsistently across studies on this factor.

Although factor-analytic studies generally have supported a two-factor model, there has been varying support for a three-factor model (Brown, Hwang, Baron, & Yakimowski, 1991; Brown & Yakimowski, 1987; Karnes & Brown, 1980; Macmann et al., 1991). The specific composition of the third factor has varied significantly across studies.

For example, several studies found that the Information, Arithmetic, and Coding subtests primarily composed the third factor (Brown & Yakimowski, 1987; Brown et al., 1991), whereas Sapp and colleagues (1985) found that the Information, Arithmetic, Vocabulary, and Block Design subtests primarily composed the third factor. In addition, Karnes and Brown (1980) noted that the Arithmetic and Picture Completion subtests composed the third factor (Freedom from Distractibility).

Only limited factor-analytic research has been conducted among gifted children with cognitive measures other than the WISC (Cameron et al., 1997). Cameron and colleagues (1997) conducted a confirmatory factor analysis using the Kaufman Assessment Battery for Children (K-ABC; Kaufman & Kaufman, 1983). Although they compared four models of intelligence, they determined that Horn and Cattell's theory of fluid–crystallized intelligence provided the broadest understanding of the cognitive functioning of children referred for gifted services (Cameron et al., 1997).

The factor structures of cognitive measures have also been studied among gifted ethnic minorities (Greenberg, Stewart, & Hansche, 1986; Masten, Morse, & Wenglar, 1995; Mishra et al., 1989). Factor-analytic research conducted by Greenberg and colleagues (1986) supported the WISC-R Verbal Comprehension and Perceptual Organizational two-factor model with a sample of gifted black children. Another study, which examined the factor structure of the WISC-R with Mexican American children referred for intellectually gifted assessment (Masten et al., 1995), was unable to adequately replicate the factor structure proposed by Kaufman (1975). In contrast, the cognitive constructs of gifted Navajo children were similar to the Freedom from Distractibility and Perceptual Organization factors identified based upon the standardization sample of the WISC-R (Mishra et al., 1989).

The variability in results among factor-analytic studies appears to stem primarily from methodological and statistical differences. Macmann and colleagues (1991) noted that restriction in variance due to sample selection might have contributed to differences in the composition of factors. There also appears to be great disparity across studies related to sample sizes. Although the majority of studies used large samples (e.g., Macmann et al., 1991; Watkins et al., 2002), several studies used samples with fewer than 150 participants. Factor-analytic research using gifted ethnic minorities utilized the smallest samples, with some

using fewer than 100 participants (e.g., Masten et al., 1995; Mishra et al., 1989).

A lack of consistency across studies in the criteria used for determining giftedness has also made it difficult to compare factors across studies. The criteria for inclusion ranged from a WISC Full Scale IQ of 120 and higher to 130 and higher. In addition, it was not uncommon for the criteria for inclusion to include participants with a WISC Full Scale IQ, Verbal IQ, and/or Performance IQ of 130 or higher. Gifted eligibility for some studies included children who did not meet the stated IQ criteria but did demonstrate advanced academic performance. The study conducted by Brown and Yakimowski (1987) demonstrates how selection criteria can influence the composition and the number of factors identified. They studied the WISC-R scores for three different groups of children: children who scored in the average range (IQ score between 85 and 115), children who scored 120 or higher (high-IQ group), and children in gifted programs (gifted group). The average group displayed the two-factor model commonly associated with the WISC-R; however, a four-factor solution was identified for the gifted group, and a five-factor solution was identified for the high-IQ group. The additional factors suggested that children in the high-IQ and gifted groups processed information differently from the children with average cognitive abilities (Brown & Yakimowski, 1987). Thus the composition of the sample appears to have had an influence on the number and types of factors generated.

The use of different combinations of WISC subtests in factor analyses also contributed to the different composition of the factors and to whether two- or three-factor models were generated. The 10 regularly administered WISC-R subtests were consistently utilized in the factor analyses, while the Digit Span and Mazes subtests were often excluded. Studies that included the Digit Span subtest found it to load consistently on the same factor with the Arithmetic subtest (Brown & Yakimowski, 1987; Watkins et al., 2002).

The type of extraction method used, the criteria used to determine the number of factors to interpret, and the criteria used to determine the composition of factors also varied greatly across studies. The type of extraction method used (e.g., maximum-likelihood, principal-components, principal-axis) could have influenced the number of factors generated and the composition of those factors. In addition, a vast array of criteria was used across studies for determining the number of factors to interpret. Specifically, the scree test, the chi-square statistic, eigenvalues greater than 1.0, and various combinations of these techniques were used by researchers for making this determination. Differences were also found across studies in the type of rotation methods (e.g., varimax, oblique), resulting in differences among factors. There were considerable differences in the criteria used to determine whether a subtest loaded on a specific factor. Although some studies failed to indicate the criteria used for identifying significant factor loadings, the studies that did provide criteria for significant loadings tended to range from .30 to .50. Given these differences in methodology and statistical techniques across the factor-analytic studies, it is not surprising to find some differences in the cognitive constructs of gifted children on intelligence measures.

Some of the consistency of the findings related to the structure of intelligence in gifted samples may also reflect the structure of the instruments that were used to assess it. The WISC-R and WISC-III were not closely tied to any theory of intelligence (O'Donnell, 2009). As a result, much of the structure of the WISC at that time focused narrowly on measures of Gf and Gc and underrepresented other abilities. Consequently, even if the individuals had possessed differing factor structures in these areas, they were not measured and would not emerge in the analysis.

These earlier factor-analytic structures were important in helping to improve our understanding of the continuity and similarity for the structure of intelligence in gifted samples with the rest of the population. It is important to recognize that studies using an exploratory approach are apt to dismiss more complex models in favor of simpler parsimonious models (two- or four-factor models vs. a seven- or eight-factor model). In part, the exploratory approach may sometimes hide existing factors. These occasions are more likely to occur when sample size is relatively limited and when the variance of the sample is limited, both of which have occurred in the past in the gifted literature. From a statistical viewpoint, then, the inclusion of individuals who may not have met all previous gifted criteria may actually have improved the ability of the models to fit because it added needed variance to the samples.

In summary, factor-analytic research using gifted samples has for the most part confirmed the presence of Kaufman's two-factor model. In addition, the WISC-R/WISC-III subtests that compose the Verbal Comprehension factor have been replicated across numerous studies, suggesting significant stability of this factor with gifted children. Less stability has been shown in the composition of the Perceptual Organization factor, and even less stability has been shown related to a third factor. Although the majority of the research has been exploratory, a few confirmatory-factor-analytic studies have been published (Brown et al., 1991; Cameron et al., 1997). However, there is a continued need to study hierarchical models of intelligence with gifted samples. There is also a need to demonstrate the utility of considering multiple cognitive constructs in identifying giftedness.

THE ISSUE OF IDENTIFICATION

The Process of Identification as Related to the Definition

Several authors previously mentioned have discussed the importance of cognitive ability measures for the identification process. A very controversial part of serving gifted students is the process of locating the population to be served—a process known as *identification*. Clark (1997) has suggested the following considerations in a comprehensive identification program:

- Evidence that students demonstrate extraordinary ability in relationship to their age-level peers.
- Evidence of the range of capabilities and needs.
- Processes that measure potential as well as achievement.
- Methods that seek out and identify students from varying linguistic, economic, and cultural backgrounds, and special populations.
- Implications for educational planning.

This comprehensive list of services has opened the door to much controversy as to what a school should do for this special population. Borland (1989) has cautioned that defining the target population is the first and most important step in programming for gifted students. In other words, if a school selects a narrow definition or one based exclusively on cognitive ability, then the school's program should reflect this definition. On the other hand, if the school chooses to adopt the U.S. Department of Education (1993) definition, then a very comprehensive array of services should be available. A major issue in identification of gifted and talented youth has been the validity of the identification process with respect to program goals and services

(Feldhusen & Jarwan, 1993). Since placement decisions are the goal of identification, all measures used are very important.

Identification generally begins with a screening procedure, in which students are selected first on the basis of their performance on a group achievement test. Students who score the highest on this general group test, according to the school's criteria, form a talent pool. Next, the talent pool's members take a more selective test (perhaps a more precise instrument with a lower standard error of measurement). High-ability students often score very highly on group tests, and a *ceiling effect* may occur, in which their scores cluster near the very top of possible scores on the test. It is sometimes incorrectly assumed that all of these children are equally talented and need a similar program. However, this is not always the case. More precise tests that address this ceiling effect are preferred, so that those identified for the program are truly those students most capable (if that is the definition of the target population for the specific school's program). After this second screening step, all measures to be considered in identification are added, and the top students are identified for the program. One approach to addressing the ceiling effect common with group measures may be to use individually administered intelligence tests, such as the WISC-IV (Wechsler, 2003), the Stanford–Binet Intelligence Scales, Fifth Edition (SB5; Roid, 2003), or the WJ III (Woodcock et al., 2001). However, whatever test is administered, the ceiling effect must be considered in selecting tests that truly measure the abilities to be served. Another strategy that has received some popularity over the years is the use of out-of-age tests with students believed to be gifted. The higher ceilings of these instruments allow for students to be challenged and fit with a historical definition of advanced mental age. One problem with this approach is that because the tests were given to children not in the normative sample, age-based norms cannot be used, and comparisons cannot be made. As a result, application of a proportion estimate such as that suggested in Gagné's (2004) classification system are inappropriate.

Although the use of the extended normative tables for the WISC-IV published by Zhu et al. (2008) may be desired by some who work regularly with highly gifted samples, there remain several questions that are not explained in the technical report regarding the use of these norms. One concern is how individuals who are repeatedly measured will perform. It is important to recognize that classic test theory predicts a probable drop in measured performance for individuals who are highly gifted, due to measurement error on reevaluation (Ziegler & Ziegler, 2009). The extended normative dataset will not change and may in fact increase the likelihood of an observed drop in performance because scaled and standard scores at some ages will be further away from the mean. There is no evidence from the Zhu et al. study that individuals were administered repeated measurements. The authors reasoned that the use of the same standardization sample allows for the extended normative set to match the other psychometric statistics, including test–retest reliability, for the WISC-IV.

Additional concerns about the use of the Zhu et al. (2008) extended normative tables arise because of the limited description of how participants were recruited or selected for participation in the study. The demographic data reported for the sample in the technical report are limited to age and gender. It does not report how the individuals were identified as gifted. As a result, questions about the appropriateness of the use of these tables with minority students may arise. As observed by Zhu and colleagues, this normative data may be helpful, but further validity studies are needed. Finally, the clinical choice to use the WISC-IV and its extended normative tables does not remove the question of whether or not it adequately assesses all of the suspected areas of gifted abilities (or intelligence) in children.

Identification of Gifted Minority Students

A major issue in identification of gifted students relates to the representation of minority students in gifted programs. According to Ford and Harris (1999), projections are that minority students will account for almost half (46%) of all public school students by the year 2020. This increase in minority students at the national level has not been reflected in gifted education. In fact, according to Gallagher (2002), national surveys indicate that only 10% of students performing at the highest levels are culturally, linguistically, and ethnically diverse students, even though these diverse students represent 33% of the school population. A major focus of attention in gifted education is the goal of parity in gifted programs among all members of society, but this parity has not been easy to achieve. Although the Jacob Javits Act of 1988 has helped initiate programs for gifted racial minority students from economically disadvantaged areas, the problem of finding and/or developing useful tools to identify these students still exists. Efforts to find more valid, reliable, and useful instruments to assess giftedness and potential among minority students, and to increase teacher training in identification and assessment so as ultimately to increase the referral of minority students to gifted services, are paramount in helping to find and serve these underrepresented students (Ford & Harris, 1999).

In July 1997, the National Association for Gifted Children (NAGC) adopted a policy statement on testing and assessment of gifted students, in which it called for more equitable identification and assessment instruments and procedures. The notions of fairness and accountability underlie the proposal. In this position paper on the use of tests in the identification and assessment of gifted students, the following issues were addressed:

> Given the limitations of all tests, no single measure should be used to make identification and placement decisions. That is, no single test or instrument should be used to include a child in or exclude a child from gifted education services. The most effective and equitable means of serving gifted students is to assess them—to identify their strengths and weaknesses, and to prescribe services based on these needs. Testing situations should not hinder students' performance. Students must feel comfortable, relaxed, and have a good rapport with the examiner. Best practices indicate that multiple measures and different types of indicators from multiple sources must be used to assess and serve gifted students. Information must be gathered from multiple sources (caregivers/families, teachers, students, and others with significant knowledge of the students), in different ways (e.g., observations, performances, products, portfolios, interviews) and in different contexts (e.g., in-school and out-of-school settings). (NAGC, 1997, p. 52)

This call for a different, more inclusive way to find and serve gifted minority students is a call for diversity in programs that have typically been labeled "elitist" by many. To widen the representation, school personnel must be educated to use multiple measures to find these underrepresented students. A change in identification practices must encourage the examination of gifted individuals in cultural and environmental contexts, and must provide a basis for recognizing talents without penalizing students for certain learning styles and expressions (Frasier et al., 1995).

Assessments used to identify gifted and talented students may represent a clash between cultures, in which the mainstream culture is unable to recognize or underestimates the abilities of underrepresented minority students (Briggs & Reis, 2004). One issue that has prevented the identification of gifted minority students is that of test bias. Reynolds and Kaiser (1990), in discussing the issue of content validity and its relation to test bias, have stated:

> An item or subscale of a test is considered to be biased in content when it is demonstrated to be relatively more difficult for members of one group than for members of another in a situation where the general ability level of the groups being compared is held constant and no reasonable theoretical rationale exists to explain groups' differences on the item (or subscale) in question. (p. 625)

Items on tests often tap experiences that are relevant to middle-class students. Those from impoverished families may simply not comprehend such items, and therefore may miss questions because of environmental deficiencies rather than actual lack of intelligence. Such problems point to the bias that underlies *content validity* in both achievement and intelligence tests.

In addition, bias in *construct validity* is of concern. The fact that different groups define giftedness and intelligent behaviors in a variety of ways makes the measurement of these constructs difficult and often invites bias. Again, if the construct in question is always defined in middle-class terms, impoverished students may not be found and served.

Finally, bias is also seen in terms of *predictive validity*—the extent to which an instrument predicts the future success of a person in various situations. If teachers read the results of an intelligence test and therefore judge a person's future worth on the basis of these results, the student may not fare well. In fact, teachers' expectations may diminish because of perceived deficiencies that may not be accurate indicators of a student's ability. For these reasons, assessment issues with minority students are of major concern in the identification of students for programs.

Ford and Harris (1999) have suggested the following options when evaluators are considering how best to assess ability and potential in linguistically, racially, and culturally diverse students:

- Adapt instruments (e.g., modify the instruments in terms of their language demands).
- Renorm the selected instruments based on local norms and needs.

- Modify predetermined cutoff scores for minority students.
- Use an alternative nonverbal cognitive measure thought to assess the same construct.

The issue of diversity in membership in gifted programs is currently a major issue. Educators must understand its importance and must respond to the need for alternative identification tools if they desire to provide high-quality education for all.

Identification of Gifted Students with Learning Disabilities

Another group of students who are often missed in the identification process is the group of those who are gifted but have learning disabilities. Although this description seems to be an oxymoron, Davis and Rimm (1985) stated that estimates of the number of such students in U.S. schools range from 120,000 to 180,000. Identification of students with both talents and disabilities is problematic and challenges educators (Olenshak & Reis, 2002; Sternberg & Grigorenko, 1999). Historically, most school personnel have relied on discrepancy formulas between intelligence and ability test scores; analyses of intelligence test results for differences across subtests (*scatter*); and multidimensional approaches that incorporate qualitative data, such as structured interviews and observations (Lyon, Gray, Kavanagh, & Krasnegor, 1993). With the Individuals with Disabilities Education Improvement Act of 2004 (IDEA 2004) revisions and the filtered changes enacted through different states to comply with this law, the use of dynamic and locally normed assessment strategies is increasingly becoming the standard (Reynolds & Shaywitz, 2009). As a result, the provision of special education services to children who have learning disabilities and are also gifted is likely to increase the delay in identification, with the exception of those individuals with severe disabilities or multiple areas of disability.

Furthermore, the identification of these students is complicated because their gifted abilities often mask their disabilities, or, conversely, their disabilities may disguise their giftedness (Volker, Lopata, & Cook-Cottone, 2006). These problems may exclude students from inclusion in either programs for gifted individuals or programs for those with learning disabilities (Baum et al., 1991; Olenshak & Reis, 2002). This is also true for students with other exceptionalities, such as attention-deficit/hyperactivity disorder and Asperger syndrome. Astute educators are aware of these major issues in

identification and search for ways to include rather than exclude all gifted students. As a result of the tendency for gifted students to exhibit higher levels of functioning globally when compared with other students, even in areas of suspected disability, it may be more beneficial for psychologists and committees to take an ipsative approach to analyzing test data. This method is consistent with that recommended by Volker et al. (2006); it is also a pattern approach consistent with IDEA 2004.

Identification of Gifted English-Language Learners

English-language learners (ELLs) are underrepresented in programs that serve gifted students (Lohman, Korb, & Lakin, 2008). Indeed, according to Plucker, Rapp, and Martinez (2009), the lack of attention to giftedness in underrepresented populations such as ELLs is a critical weakness in the identification literature because of the concomitant rapid increase in the number of ELLs in the United States. For example, in 1979, approximately 1 in 10 school-age children spoke a language other than English at home; by 2003, the proportion had risen to nearly 1 in 5 (9.9 million) children (National Center for Education Statistics, 2005). Plucker and his colleagues state that between the 1989–1990 and 2004–2005 school years, ELL enrollment in public schools more than doubled from 2,030,451 students to 5,119,561 (National Center for Education Statistics, 2008).

This problem of identifying a rapidly growing population provides challenges for administrators seeking unbiased identification methods. Coleman and Cross (2005) argue that the identification of culturally different gifted students is a perplexing problem because their average performance on aptitude and achievement tests tends to be one standard deviation below the mean when general norms are used. Ortiz and Dynda (2005) state that if there is to be any validity to conclusions drawn by practitioners, four issues concerning test bias must be understood: (1) acknowledging the cultural content embedded in any given test; (2) understanding the linguistic demands inherent in any given test; (3) appreciating meaningful differences in norm sample representation for diverse individuals; and (4) recognizing the limitations of "nonverbal" assessment. (See also Ortiz, Ochoa, & Dynda, Chapter 22, this volume.)

Administrators of gifted programs in schools have looked for a suitable means for identifying ELL students that would increase representation of these learners without relying solely on language as the major requisite for testing. Nonverbal tasks have long been present in intelligence tests, providing one indicator of ability for students who are native speakers of the language, while perhaps serving as the only indicator of ability for examinees who are not fluent speakers of the language (Lohman et al., 2008). Nevertheless, finding the right test and using the appropriate norm group for comparisons are essential aspects of identifying gifted ELL students.

Multiple Means of Assessment

For all these reasons, multiple means of assessing students are often used. Test scores are one determinant. Others include nominations by teachers, students, parents, and peers. In addition, checklists often tap areas of strength in students. Performance assessments, such as portfolios and auditions, are often valuable in the identification of gifted and talented students for programs. Of course, the parameters of the program must be considered in the design of any identification criteria. In addition, determining a reasonable formula that takes into account all the criteria and determines the students who then emerge as those who qualify for the program is a difficult and challenging problem for educators who manage gifted programs in schools.

SPECIAL ISSUES
Competing Theoretical Approaches

Although a lack of consideration of theory when evaluators are selecting cognitive measures is a concern in intellectual assessment with all children (Flanagan & Ortiz, 2002), an atheoretical approach appears to predominate within the schools when cognitive measures to identify gifted children are being chosen. This pattern is not unique to school professionals and reflects the greater historical need for these instruments to be able to differentiate between those who will succeed and those who will not despite educative efforts (Strauss et al., 2006). The selection of cognitive measures is often based upon ease of administration, cost, and familiarity with the test. In addition, many current psychologists choose to employ theory-based instruments. Examples include the WJ III (Woodcock et al., 2001), the SB5 (Roid, 2003), the WISC-IV (Wechsler, 2003), and the CAS (Naglieri & Das, 1997). All but the last is based upon or mapped onto the CHC theory of intelligence, and the CAS is based upon the *plan-*

ning, attention, simultaneous, sequential (PASS) model. More recently, the Kaufman Assessment Battery for Children—Second Edition (Kaufman & Kaufman, 2004) draws upon the theoretical model of Luria's neuropsychological theory and CHC theory. The Reynolds Intellectual Assessment Scales (RIAS; Reynolds & Kamphaus, 2003) battery, although it follows the historical appearance of an atheoretical verbal–performance measure, was developed through a careful analysis of Carroll's work.

Although the current advances in instrument development have led to a plethora of choices, this plethora can create additional confusion when evaluators are trying to select a measure for identifying cognitively gifted children. The problem is that different measures of intelligence, regardless of theory, assess different skills; the result is that some children are not offered opportunities to participate in gifted programs (Simpson, Carone, Burns, Seidman, & Sellers, 2002; Tyler-Wood & Carri, 1991). The implications of using a specific measure of intelligence should be considered prior to its selection. For example, subtests on the RIAS were selected to focus primarily on intelligence as a problem-solving and reasoning ability that generalizes across areas, whereas the WJ III may assess this problem-solving ability in specific ability areas (auditory processing). Characteristics of the gifted children identified, available programming that addresses the specific characteristics of the children identified, and the extent to which nonmodal gifted children (e.g., children from impoverished backgrounds, gifted children with disabilities) are excluded should all be considered when a specific measure of intelligence is chosen. Therefore, it is essential that the theoretical differences in intelligence measures be considered—and, more important, that theory-based measures be utilized during the identification process. This view is consistent with that of Flanagan and Ortiz (2002), who advocate theory as the center of all intellectual assessment activities. The process of identifying cognitively gifted children is complex enough without starting the identification process with an atheoretical or outdated measure of intelligence.

Linking Screening Procedures with Intelligence Measures

The majority of schools have developed some type of system for identifying gifted children, albeit some systems are better than others. Usually included within the system is a procedure for screening children and thus reducing the number who are eventually referred for more comprehensive testing. Unfortunately, the comprehensive testing typically includes the administration of a single standardized measure of intelligence. And in any case, many evaluators fail to study the accuracy of screening procedures related to the final decision on whether children receive gifted programming, which is often based upon individualized measures of intelligence.

Although many would consider screening to be the crucial point in the identification process, predictive validity must be established between the screening procedure and the intellectual measure(s) used to ensure the accuracy and utility of the identification process. The difficulty with demonstrating predictive validity is that screening procedures can vary from teacher nominations to the use of group intelligence tests (Coleman & Cross, 2005). Considering the wide variety of screening methods used, relationships between screening procedures and intellectual measures can range from very low to very high. The use of screening processes and tools to identify gifted and talented abilities unlikely to be identified through the use of a standardized intelligence test also need to be selected. To be clear, a screening procedure that is more highly related to a selected intelligence test will result in a higher level of agreement at different points in the identification process. However, those who are gifted and talented in such domains as leadership or music may not be identified as such on an IQ measure. Coleman and Cross (2005) recommend using a fairly liberal screening threshold, to avoid missing children who may qualify for gifted programming. This approach seems advisable, given the lack of research exploring the relationships between many of the screening procedures used and the final decision outcomes based upon intelligence tests. This process is consistent with Gagné's (2004) suggestion that those in the top 10% be considered gifted.

Use of a Single Test Composite Score

The use of a single cognitive test composite score as the primary criterion for determining giftedness is highly common within schools. In the past, the WISC-R (Wechsler, 1974) and the fourth edition of the Stanford–Binet (SB-IV; Thorndike, Hagen, & Sattler, 1986) were the most commonly used cognitive measures in the schools (Coleman & Cross, 2005). Coleman and Cross (2005) also note that one of these measures was commonly used as the final decision criterion for determining giftedness. In fact, school districts and states have defined giftedness solely on the basis of WISC IQ cutoff scores (Fox, 1981; Karnes, Edwards, & McCallum, 1986). Others have suggested that the use of strict IQ cutoff scores is too restrictive and does not consider other characteristics of giftedness (Renzulli & Delcourt, 1986; Renzulli, Reis, & Smith, 1981). However, because of the overwhelming use of intelligence tests, there is a need to discuss the implications of using a single IQ score for making decisions on giftedness.

Implications of Using Cutoff Scores

One of the crucial decisions made by any school system is where to set the IQ "cutoff" score. It is clear from reviewing the literature that there is little, if any, consensus on where the cutoff score should be set. This makes it extremely difficult not only to evaluate decision outcomes across studies, but also to interpret research on giftedness in general. In the literature, the inconsistency is quite evident. For example, Karnes and Brown (1980) used a cutoff score of 119; Hollinger (1986) used a cutoff score of 130; and Fishkin, Kampsnider, and Pack (1996) used a cutoff score of 127. However, most studies use an overall IQ score that is at least two standard deviations above the mean. Currently, this would translate into a WISC-IV and an SB5 Full Scale IQ of 130. It should be noted that the SB5 has a standard deviation of 15. It is also important to understand that the historic method of calculating IQ used in early work on giftedness was built around a mental age formula; as a result, gifted individuals might obtain an IQ of 200, but today that is not possible. The point of this lengthy review of cutoff scores is that regardless of where a school system sets a cutoff score, it is still too rigid an approach.

Many school systems fail to understand the basic psychometric process of how scores are derived, or the pitfalls of placing so much weight on a single score. To be specific, when placement decisions are being made, it is important to consider the standard error of measurement (SEM), which allows an evaluator to estimate a range of scores based upon the obtained score. For example, suppose a child obtains a Full Scale IQ of 129 on a test with an SEM of ±4 points. The examiner can be 68% confident that the next time the child is administered the same test, the child's score will fall somewhere within the range from 125 to 133. Therefore, if the criterion for placement into a gifted program is rigidly set at 130, this child will be denied services. However, if the child is later administered the same intelligence test and obtains a Full Scale IQ score of 131, the child will then be recommended for gifted services. A more sound approach would be to base decisions regarding eligibility and the test scores in the context of the child's history, academic progress, and behavior. Repeated assessments over time will truly differentiate the groups.

It also is important to note that many test manuals now report confidence intervals using the method of regression to the mean, instead of rigidly applying the ±1 *SEM*. Although many might suggest that in considering the *SEM*, all that is being proposed is to lower the cutoff score, in fact this is not what is being proposed. What is being suggested is to allow for flexibility in making identification decisions, even when cutoff scores are being used. Therefore, identification decisions should be made with a proper understanding of the underlying psychometric characteristics of standardized intelligence tests, and also with consideration of other performance variables (e.g., academic achievement).

Furthermore, it is important to recognize that children with an estimated IQ in the range of 131–134 may quite possibly obtain scores in the range of 128–131 if reassessed. The children would be less likely to obtain scores of 133–135, as these would be further from the mean.

Recent updates and versions of testing manuals also indicate that contemporary assessment tools may produce lower IQ estimates for gifted samples than previous test versions have produced. As part of the development phase for tests, many test publishers use gifted samples to help validate the cognitive measures. While measures such as the WISC-IV, the SB5, the WJ III Normative Update, and the KABC-II all show significant differences between matched samples and gifted samples, the average scores for gifted students may fall in the high average range (WJ III, WISC-IV, KABC-II). It is important to recognize that the developers of these tests used different methods to identify students, including previous test results, history of services, or independent determination by a school. This pattern of results is consistent with the Flynn effect and suggests that high-ability students are not immune to this phenomenon. Examiners identifying gifted students through the use of an IQ test are advised to use a new instrument in tandem with estimates from an instrument that has been available for 5 years or more and with which the examiners are well familiar.

The recent work of Ziegler and Ziegler (2009) adds a further wrinkle to the use of cutoff scores from a single test or even from multiple tests. An analysis of the fundamental basis of measurement error and estimation of the construct of intelligence led these authors to note that high levels of cognitive abilities (greater than 130) are likely to be underestimated by measures of intelligence. This prediction appears to be supported by the data from the previously discussed studies. What is advocated as a result is a low-threshold test that will catch all potentially gifted students, followed by an intelligence test that will underestimate but have a lower error rate as a result of a previous screen (Ziegler & Ziegler, 2009).

Beyond the Composite IQ Score

Interpretation of intelligence test results beyond the full test's composite score is also a recommended practice in identifying gifted children. Depending on an intelligence test's theoretical model, it can provide a multiple-cluster (e.g., verbal ability, thinking ability) index (e.g., Verbal Comprehension Index, Perceptual Reasoning Index) or composite scores (e.g., Verbal IQ, Nonverbal IQ) beyond the global composite score. Ignoring a child's performance on these other indices may preclude him or her from receiving gifted services. As an example, if a child attains a WISC-IV Full Scale IQ of 127, a Verbal Comprehension Index of 142, a Perceptual Reasoning Index of 117, a Working Memory Index of 121, and a Processing Speed Index of 100, the child may be overlooked for gifted services if the sole criterion is the Full Scale IQ. Here is a child who obviously displays verbal abilities within the gifted range, and the Full Scale IQ fails to account for these specific cognitive skills.

Moreover, it is important to consider the demands and skills required by specific subtests that contribute to index, cluster, or composite scores. In the aforementioned example, the child's lowest WISC-IV index score is in Processing Speed. The subtests that contribute to the Processing Speed Index rely on speed, short-term visual memory, cognitive flexibility, and concentration. Although this child demonstrates an average level of processing speed (which is considerably lower than his or her Verbal Comprehension Index score), the score may be more a function of how the child has approached each specific subtest contributing to the Processing Speed Index.

Many gifted children have learned to sacrifice speed for accuracy and perform less well on speed-related tasks than on others. Kaufman (1992) has noted that the highly reflective and perfectionistic nature of many gifted children affects their performance on measures of intelligence where speed is rewarded. Also, variances between composite scores are fairly common among gifted individuals (Malone, Brock, Brounstein, & Shaywitz, 1991). Another theoretical interpretation of this discrepancy would argue that the Processing Speed Index is a much lower g-loaded index of ability, and therefore less indicative of intelligence and more indicative of motoric speed (Reynolds & Kamphaus, 2003). The key issue here is not to rely solely on the overall composite score in understanding the cognitive skills of gifted children, but to encourage professionals to evaluate the clinical, emotional, and behavioral data leading to a performance estimate.

McGrew, Schrank, and Woodcock (2007) indicate that samples of gifted students tend to perform better on tasks of Gc and Gf than on tasks of long-term retrieval (Glr), working memory (Gsm), or visual–spatial thinking. Results from the KABC-II manual suggest that gifted students perform best on tasks designed to measure Gc (Kaufman & Kaufman, 2004).

Lack of Ceilings

With many measures of intelligence, there are not enough items at the upper end of subtests to fully discriminate the cognitive abilities of gifted individuals. Although individual items used within specific subtests are selected for their ability to discriminate between children at different levels of cognitive ability, for many subtests it is difficult to establish a ceiling, which makes it difficult to obtain an accurate estimate of cognitive ability with gifted children. When gifted children are assessed, it is common for them not to obtain a ceiling on several subtests of a specific cognitive measure. When this occurs, the overall test composite score is likely to be an underestimate of their true level of cognitive functioning. Many would suggest that this does not matter because their level of cognitive functioning is so high that they would qualify for gifted services anyway. Here the issue is not so much one of identification as of matching children with appropriate gifted programming. It is important to accurately assess the unique cognitive skills of even highly gifted students, to meet their educational needs and interests.

Recommendations on the Effective Use of Intelligence Tests

A few general recommendations on the use of intelligence tests in the identification of giftedness

are warranted. First, it is recommended that school systems develop an operational definition of giftedness that incorporates the term *cognitively gifted*. The use of this term is suggested if a school system's primary criterion for placement in its gifted program is based upon an individualized measure of intelligence. If other measures (e.g., rating scales, nominations, achievement tests) or characteristics (e.g., leadership skills, motivation) are considered along with results on an intelligence test, the definition should address the role of the intelligence test in relation to the other measures and characteristics tapped during the identification process. Second, it is recommended that the school system develop specific procedures related to the referral, screening, testing, and placement of gifted children. Again, if the school's primary identification criterion is based upon an individualized measure of intelligence and the goal is to identify cognitively gifted children, then the screening measure should be highly correlated with the selected intelligence test.

Third, it is recommended that school systems become thoroughly aware of the specific advantages and limitations of using standardized intelligence tests to identify giftedness. Coleman and Cross (2005) note that intelligence tests are highly reliable, are individually administered, allow the examiner to observe a child's behavior directly, and allow for a broader sampling of behavior than screening or group intelligence tests do. Other advantages of intelligence tests are their abilities to identify exceptionally gifted individuals with special educational needs (Gross, 1993); children who do not display the stereotypical high verbal ability, high achievement, and high motivation often associated with giftedness (Pyryt, 1996); and children who are "twice exceptional" (e.g., children identified as gifted and with learning disabilities). As for limitations, this chapter has primarily focused on assisting schools in making informed decisions regarding the use and limitations of intelligence tests with gifted students.

Fourth, it is recommended that school systems use theory as a primary guide in selecting intelligence tests. As Flanagan and Ortiz (2002) astutely note, the use of a modern and valid theory of intelligence at the beginning of the assessment process is critical in facilitating accurate measurement and interpretation. Given the recent theoretical advances in intelligence testing, there is no excuse for ignoring theory and blindly selecting intelligence tests to identify giftedness. To be specific, understanding that one measure of intelligence assesses the constructs of verbal comprehension and perceptual organization while another assesses verbal ability, working memory, and processing speed is important to consider when evaluators are choosing intelligence measures for making identification decisions. Also, it is important to understand how these psychological constructs are measured. Do the specific constructs use speeded tasks, visual tasks, or verbal tasks? Without an understanding of the underlying theory behind the aforementioned constructs, it will be difficult to interpret an individual's results on an intellectual measure. Also, if a cognitive measure is primarily found to assess verbal ability, it is likely that only gifted children with strong verbal skills will be identified, while children with excellent perceptual organization skills, strong speed-of-information-processing skills, or excellent working memory skills will be missed during the identification process.

Last, it is recommended that school systems consider using a cross-battery approach when assessing for giftedness. Specifically, the CHC cross-battery approach (Flanagan, Alfonso, & Ortiz, Chapter 19, this volume; Flanagan, Ortiz, Alfonso, & Mascolo, 2002; McGrew & Flanagan, 1998) should be considered. This approach is a method for utilizing separate batteries of tests and ensuring a broader range of theoretical constructs in the assessment of children. Although research is needed to support using the CHC cross-battery approach in the identification of gifted children, it does demonstrate how multiple batteries can be used to decrease the reliance on a single measure of cognitive ability.

SUMMARY

This chapter has explored some of the central issues related to using intelligence tests in the identification of giftedness. Although identification of giftedness is complex and has been richly debated, our goal has been to advocate for school systems' making informed decisions about the role of intelligence tests in the identification process. Although many strategies exist for identifying gifted and talented children for services, it appears that the use of a specific measure of cognitive ability dominates the identification process within the schools. It is important to design programs that begin with a definition of giftedness and build from there. The definition precedes and guides the identification process, and provides the rationale for what instruments to use in order to find

and then to serve the appropriate students. This chapter has focused on the need for precision in choosing effective theory-driven intelligence tests for the identification process. Many programs for gifted students are focused on cognitive ability, and yet misuse test data in making critical decisions. The current availability of cognitive assessments for identifying superior cognitive ability is better now than ever before. It remains to be seen whether those who administer the programs will choose instruments wisely, in order to obtain the information needed to identify those students who are in need of a different type of program because of their demonstrated cognitive ability.

REFERENCES

Baer, J., & Kaufman, J. (2004). Considering the DMGT: Something old, something new. *High Ability Studies, 15*(2), 149–150.

Baum, S., Owen, S. V., & Dixon, J. (1991). *To be gifted and learning disabled: From definitions to practical intervention strategies.* Mansfield Center, CT: Creative Learning Press.

Binet, A., & Simon, T. (1905). New methods for the diagnosis of intelligence in the child. *L'Année Psychologique, 11*, 191–244.

Borland, J. H. (1989). *Planning and implementing programs for the gifted.* New York: Teachers College Press.

Briggs, C. J., & Reis, S. M. (2004). An introduction to the topic of cultural diversity and giftedness. In C. Tomlinson, D. Ford, S. Reis, C. Briggs, & C. Strickland (Eds.), *In search of the dream: Designing schools and classrooms that work for high potential students from diverse cultural backgrounds* (pp. 5–32). Washington, DC: National Association for Gifted Children.

Brown, S. W., Hwang, M. T., Baron, M., & Yakimowski, M. E. (1991). Factor analysis of responses to the WISC-R for gifted children. *Psychological Reports, 69*, 99–107.

Brown, S. W., & Yakimowski, M. E. (1987). Intelligence scores of gifted students on the WISC-R. *Gifted Child Quarterly, 31*, 130–134.

Cameron, L. C., Ittenbach, R. F., McGrew, K. S., Harrison, P. L., Taylor, L. R., & Hwang, Y. R. (1997). Confirmatory factor analysis of the K-ABC with gifted referrals. *Educational and Psychological Measurement, 57*, 823–840.

Clark, B. (1997). *Growing up gifted.* Upper Saddle River, NJ. Prentice Hall.

Colangelo, N., & Davis, G. A. (1997). Introduction and overview. In N. Colangelo & G. A. Davis (Eds.),

Handbook of gifted education (2nd ed., pp. 3–9). Boston: Allyn & Bacon.

Coleman, L. J., & Cross, T. L. (2005). *Being gifted in school* (2nd ed.). Waco, TX: Prufrock Press.

Cox, J., Daniel, N., & Boston, B. O. (1985). *Educating able learners*. Austin: University of Texas Press.

Coyle, D. (2009). *The talent code: Greatness isn't born. It's grown. Here's how.* New York: Bantam.

Darwin, C. (1859). *On the origin of species*. London: Murray.

Davis, G. A., & Rimm, S. (1985). *Education of the gifted and talented*. Englewood Cliffs, NJ: Prentice-Hall.

Davis, G. A., & Rimm, S. (1998). *Education of the gifted and talented* (4th ed.). Boston: Allyn & Bacon.

Feldhusen, J. F. (1998). A conception of talent and talent development. In R. C. Friedman & K. B. Rogers (Eds.), *Talent in context: Historical and social perspectives on giftedness* (pp. 193–209). Washington, DC: American Psychological Association.

Feldhusen, J. F., & Jarwan, F. A. (1993). Identification of gifted and talented youth for educational programs. In K. A. Heller, F. J. Monks, & A. H. Passow (Eds.), *International handbook of research and development of giftedness and talent* (pp. 233–251). New York: Pergamon Press.

Fishkin, A. S., Kampsnider, J. J., & Pack, L. (1996). Exploring the WISC-III as a measure of giftedness. *Roeper Review, 18,* 226–231.

Flanagan, D. P., & Ortiz, S. O. (2002). Best practices in intellectual assessment: Future directions. In A. Thomas & J. Grimes (Eds.), *Best practices in school psychology IV* (pp. 1351–1372). Bethesda, MD: National Association of School Psychologists.

Flanagan, D. P., Ortiz, S. O., Alfonso, V. C., & Mascolo, J. (2002). *The achievement test desk reference (ATDR): Comprehensive assessment and learning disabilities.* Boston: Allyn & Bacon.

Ford, D. Y., & Harris, J. J. (1999). *Multicultural gifted education*. New York: Teachers College Press.

Fox, L. H. (1981). Identification of the academically gifted. *American Psychologist, 36,* 1103–1111.

Frasier, M. M., Hunsaker, S. L., Lee, J., Finely, V. S., Frank, E., Garcia, J. H., et al. (1995). *Educators' perceptions of barriers to the identification of gifted children from economically disadvantaged and limited English proficient backgrounds* (Report No. RM95216). Storrs: University of Connecticut, National Research Center on the Gifted and Talented.

Gagné, F. (1999). My convictions about the nature of abilities, gifts, and talents. *Journal for the Education of the Gifted, 22,* 109–136.

Gagné, F. (2004). Transforming gifts into talents: The DMGT as a developmental theory. *High Ability Studies, 15*(2), 119–147.

Gallagher, J. J. (1995). Education of gifted students: A civil rights issue? *Phi Delta Kappan, 76*(5), 408–410.

Gallagher, J. J. (2002). *Society's role in educating gifted students: The role of public policy* (Report No. RM02162). Storrs: University of Connecticut, National Research Center on the Gifted and Talented.

Gardner, H. (1983). *Frames of mind: The theory of multiple intelligences*. New York: Basic Books.

Gardner, H. (1993). *Multiple intelligences: The theory in practice*. New York: Basic Books.

Gardner, H. (1999). Are there additional intelligences?: The case for naturalist, spiritual, and existential intelligences. In J. Kane (Ed.), *Education, information, and transformation* (pp. 111–131). Upper Saddle River, NJ: Prentice Hall.

Gladwell, M. (2008). *Outliers: The story of success*. New York: Little, Brown.

Greenberg, R. D., Stewart, K. J., & Hansche, W. J. (1986). Factor analysis of the WISC-R for white and black children evaluated for gifted placement. *Journal of Psychoeducational Assessment, 4,* 123–130.

Gridley, B. E., Norman, K. A., Rizza, M. G., & Decker, S. L. (2003). Assessment of gifted children with the Woodcock–Johnson III. In F. A. Schrank & D. P. Flanagan (Eds.), *WJ III clinical use and interpretation: Scientist-practitioner perspectives* (pp. 285–317). San Diego, CA: Academic Press.

Gross, M. U. M. (1993). Nurturing the talents of exceptionally gifted individuals. In K. A. Heller, F. J. Monks, & A. H. Passow (Eds.), *International handbook of research and development of giftedness and talent* (pp. 473–490). New York: Pergamon Press.

Hollinger, C. L. (1986). Beyond the use of full scale IQ scores. *Gifted Child Quarterly, 30,* 74–77.

Hollingworth, L. S. (1942). *Children above 180 IQ*. Yonkers, NY: World Book.

Karnes, F. A., & Brown, K. E. (1980). Factor analysis of the WISC-R for the gifted. *Journal of Educational Psychology, 72,* 197–199.

Karnes, F. A., Edwards, R. P., & McCallum, R. S. (1986). Normative achievement assessment of gifted children: Comparing the K-ABC, WRAT, and CAT. *Psychology in the Schools, 23,* 346–352.

Kaufman, A. S. (1975). Factor structure of the WISC-R at eleven age levels between 6½ to 16½ years. *Journal of Consulting and Clinical Psychology, 43,* 135–147.

Kaufman, A. S. (1979). WISC-R research: Implications for interpretation. *School Psychology Digest, 18,* 5–27.

Kaufman, A. S. (1992). Evaluation of the WISC-III and WPPSI-R for gifted children. *Roeper Review, 14,* 154–158.

Kaufman, A. S., & Kaufman, N. L. (1983). *Kaufman Assessment Battery for Children*. Circle Pines, MN: American Guidance Service.

Kaufman, A. S., & Kaufman, N. L. (2004). *Kaufman Assessment Battery for Children—Second Edition Manual*. Circle Pines, MN: American Guidance Service.

Lohman, D. F., Korb, K. A., & Lakin, J. M. (2008). Identifying academically gifted English-language learners using nonverbal tests: A comparison of the Raven, NNAT, and CogAT. *Gifted Child Quarterly, 52*, 275–296.

Luria, A. R. (1987). *The mind of a mnemonist: A little book about a vast memory*. Cambridge, MA: Harvard University Press.

Lyon, G. R., Gray, D. B., Kavanagh, J. F., & Krasnegor, N. A. (Eds.). (1993). *Better understanding learning disabilities: New views from research and their implications for education and public policies*. Baltimore: Brookes.

Macmann, G. M., Plasket, C. M., Barnett, D. W., & Siler, R. F. (1991). Factor structure of the WISC-R for children of superior intelligence. *Journal of School Psychology, 29*, 19–36.

Malone, P. S., Brock, V., Brounstein, P. J., & Shaywitz, S. S. (1991). Components of IQ scores across levels of measured ability. *Journal of Applied Social Psychology, 21*, 15–28.

Masten, W. G., Morse, D. T., & Wenglar, K. E. (1995). Factor structure of the WISC-R for Mexican-American students referred for intellectually gifted assessment. *Roeper Review, 18*(2), 130–131.

McGrew, K. S., & Flanagan, D. P. (1998). *The intelligence test desk reference (ITDR): Gf-Gc cross battery assessment*. Boston: Allyn & Bacon.

McGrew, K. S., Schrank, F. A., & Woodcock, R. W. (2007). *Technical manual: Woodcock–Johnson III Normative Update*. Rolling Meadows, IL: Riverside.

Mishra, S. P., Lord, J., & Sabers, D. L. (1989). Cognitive processes underlying WISC-R performance of gifted and learning disabled Navajos. *Psychology in the Schools, 26*, 31–36.

Naglieri, J. A., & Das, J. P. (1997). *Das–Naglieri Cognitive Assessment System*. Itasca, IL: Riverside.

National Association for Gifted Children (NAGC). (1997). *The use of tests in the identification and assessment of gifted students*. Washington, DC: Author.

National Center for Education Statistics. (2005). *The condition of education 2005* (NCES Publication No. 2005-094). Washington, DC: U.S. Government Printing Office.

National Center for Education Statistics. (2008). Elementary and secondary enrollment of ELL students in U.S.: 1989–90 to 2004–2005. Retrieved from *www.ncela.gwu.edu/expert/faq/08leps.html*.

Oden, M. H. (1968). The fulfillment of promise: 40 year follow-up of the Terman gifted group. *Genetic Psychology Monographs, 77*, 3–93.

O'Donnell, L. (2009). The Wechsler Intelligence Scale for Children—Fourth Edition. In J. A. Naglieri & S. Goldstein (Eds.), *Practitioner's guide to assessing intelligence and achievement* (pp. 153–190). Hoboken, NJ: Wiley.

Olenshak, F. R., & Reis, S. M. (2002). Gifted students with learning disabilities. In M. Neihart, S. M. Reis, N. Robinson, & S. Moon (Eds.), *The social and emotional development of gifted children* (pp. 177–191). Waco, TX: Prufrock Press.

Ortiz, S. O., & Dynda, A. M. (2005). Use of intelligence tests with culturally and linguistically diverse populations. In D. P. Flanagan & P. T. Harrison (Eds.), *Contemporary intellectual assessment* (2nd ed., pp. 545–556). New York: Guilford Press.

Plucker, J. A., Rapp, K. E., & Martinez, R. S. (2009). Identifying gifted and talented English-language learners: A case study. *Journal for the Education of the Gifted, 32*, 368–393.

Pyryt, M. C. (1996). IQ: Easy to bash, hard to replace. *Roeper Review, 18*, 255–258.

Ramos-Ford, V., & Gardner, H. (1997). Giftedness from a multiple intelligences perspective. In N. Colangelo & G. Davis (Eds.), *Handbook of gifted education* (2nd ed., pp. 54–66). Boston: Allyn & Bacon.

Reams, R., Chamrad, D., & Robinson, N. (1990). The race is not necessarily to the swift: Validity of the WISC-R bonus points for speed. *Gifted Child Quarterly, 34*, 108–110.

Renzulli, J. S. (1978). What makes giftedness: Reexamining a definition. *Phi Delta Kappan, 60*, 18–24.

Renzulli, J. S., & Delcourt, M. A. (1986). The legacy and logic of research on the identification of gifted persons. *Gifted Child Quarterly, 30*, 20–23.

Renzulli, J. S., & Reis, S. M. (1997). *The schoolwide enrichment model: A how-to guide for educational excellence*. Mansfield Center, CT: Creative Learning Press.

Renzulli, J. S., Reis, S. M., & Smith, L. H. (1981). *The revolving door identification model*. Mansfield Center, CT: Creative Learning Press.

Reynolds, C. R., & Kaiser, S. M. (1990). Bias in assessment of attitude. In C. R. Reynolds & R. W. Kamphaus (Eds.), *Handbook of psychological and educational assessment of children: Intelligence and achievement* (pp. 611–653). New York: Guilford Press.

Reynolds, C. R., & Kamphaus, R. W. (2003). *Reynolds Intellectual Assessment Scales*. Lutz, FL: Psychological Assessment Resources.

Reynolds, C. R., & Shaywitz, S. E. (2009). Response to intervention: Ready or not? Or, from wait-to-fail to watch-them-fail. *School Psychology Quarterly, 24*(2), 130–145.

Rindermann, H. (2007). The g-factor of international

cognitive ability comparisons: The homogeneity of results in PISA, TIMSS, PIRLS and IQ-tests across nations. *European Journal of Personality, 21*(5), 667–706.

Rizza, M. G., McIntosh, D. E., & McCunn, A. (2001). Profile analysis of the Woodcock–Johnson III Tests of Cognitive Abilities with gifted students. *Psychology in the Schools, 38,* 447–455.

Roid, G. H. (2003). *Stanford–Binet Intelligence Scales, Fifth Edition.* Itasca, IL: Riverside.

Sabotnik, R. F., & Arnold, K. D. (1994). *Beyond Terman: Contemporary longitudinal studies of giftedness and talent.* Norwood, NJ: Ablex.

Sapp, G. L., Chissom, B., & Graham, E. (1985). Factor analysis of the WISC-R for gifted students: A replication and comparison. *Psychological Reports, 57,* 947–951.

Simonton, D. K. (2008).Childhood giftedness and adult genius: A historimetric analysis of 291 eminent African Americans. *Gifted Child Quarterly, 52,* 243–255.

Simpson, M., Carone, D. A., Jr., Burns, W. J., Seidman, D. M., & Sellers, A. (2002). Assessing giftedness with the WISC-III and the SB-IV. *Psychology in the Schools, 39,* 515–524.

Sternberg, R. J. (1985). *Beyond IQ: A triarchic theory of human intelligence.* Cambridge, UK: Cambridge University Press.

Sternberg, R. J., & Grigorenko, E. L. (1999). *Our labeled children.* Reading, MA: Perseus Books.

Sternberg, R. J., & Kaufman, J. D. (2001). *The evolution of intelligence.* Mahwah, NJ: Erlbaum.

Sternberg, R. J., & Williams, W. (2002). *Educational psychology.* Boston: Allyn & Bacon.

Sternberg, R. J., & Zhang, L. (1995). What do we mean by giftedness?: A pentagonal implicit theory. *Gifted Child Quarterly, 39,* 88–94.

Strauss, E., Sherman, E. S., & Spreen, O. (2006). *A compendium of neuropsychological tests: Administration, norms, and commentary* (3rd ed.). New York: Oxford University Press.

Tannenbaum, A. J. (1983). *Gifted children: Psychological and educational perspectives.* New York: Macmillan.

Tannenbaum, A. J. (1997). The meaning and making of giftedness. In N. Colangelo & G. Davis (Eds.), *Handbook of gifted education* (2nd ed., pp. 27–42). Boston: Allyn & Bacon.

Terman, L. M. (1916). *The measurement of intelligence.* Boston: Houghton Mifflin.

Terman, L. M. (1925a). *Genetic studies of genius: Mental and physical traits of a thousand gifted children* (Vol. 1). Stanford, CA: Stanford University Press.

Terman, L. M. (1925b). *Genetic studies of genius: Mental and physical traits of a thousand gifted children* (Vol. 4). Stanford, CA: Stanford University Press.

Thorndike, R. L., Hagen, E. P., & Sattler, J. M. (1986). *Stanford–Binet Intelligence Scale: Fourth Edition.* Chicago: Riverside.

Thurstone, L. L. (1938). *Primary mental abilities.* Chicago: University of Chicago Press.

Treffinger, D. J. (1995). Talent development: An emerging view. *Understanding Our Gifted, 7*(4), 3.

Tyler-Wood, R., & Carri, L. (1991). Identification of gifted children: The effectiveness of various measures of cognitive ability. *Roeper Review, 14,* 63–64.

U.S. Department of Education. (1993). *National excellence: A case for developing America's talent.* Washington, DC: U.S. Government Printing Office.

Volker, M. A., Lopata, C., & Cook-Cotone, C. (2006). Assessment of children with intellectual giftedness and reading disabilities. *Psychology in the Schools, 43*(8), 855–869.

Watkins, M. W., Greenwalt, C. G., & Marcell, C. M. (2002). Factor structure of the Wechsler Intelligence Scale for Children—Third Edition among gifted students. *Educational and Psychological Measurement, 62,* 164–172.

Wechsler, D. (1974). *Wechsler Intelligence Scale for Children—Revised.* New York: Psychological Corporation.

Wechsler, D. (1991). *Wechsler Intelligence Scale for Children—Third Edition.* San Antonio, TX: Psychological Corporation.

Wechsler, D. (2003). *Wechsler Intelligence Scale for Children—Fourth Edition.* San Antonio, TX: Psychological Corporation.

White, W. L., & Renzulli, J. S. (1987). A forty year follow-up of students who attended Leta Hollingworth's School for Gifted Children. *Roeper Review, 10*(2), 89–94.

Winner, E. (1996). *Gifted children: Myths and realities.* New York: Basic Books.

Woodcock, R. W., McGrew, K. S., & Mather, N. (2001). *Woodcock–Johnson III.* Itasca, IL: Riverside.

Zhu, J., Cayton, T., Weiss, L., & Gabel, A. (2008). *Wechsler Intelligence Scale for Children—Fourth Edition: WISC-IV extended norms* (Tech. Rep. No. 7). San Antonio, TX: Pearson.

Ziegler, A., & Ziegler, A. (2009). The paradoxical attenuation effect in tests based on classic test theory: Mathematical background and practical implications for the measurement of high abilities. *High Ability Studies, 20*(1), 5–14.

CHAPTER 26

Use of Ability Tests in the Identification of Specific Learning Disabilities within the Context of an Operational Definition

Dawn P. Flanagan
Vincent C. Alfonso
Jennifer T. Mascolo
Marlene Sotelo-Dynega

There are no rules for converting concepts to operational definitions. Therefore, operational definitions are judged by *significance* (i.e., is it an authoritative marker of the concept?) and *meaningfulness* (i.e., is it a rational and logical marker of the concept?).
—KAVALE, SPAULDING, AND BEAM (2009, p. 41)

Historically, identification of specific learning disabilities (SLD) has almost always included a consideration of an individual's overall cognitive ability, as well as his or her unique pattern of strengths and weaknesses (Flanagan, Kaufman, Kaufman, & Lichtenberger, 2008; Kavale & Flanagan, 2007; Kavale & Forness, 2000). Only recently have intelligence tests and tests of specific cognitive abilities and neuropsychological processes come under harsh attack as useful tools in the identification of SLD (Mather & Kaufman, 2006; Reynolds & Shaywitz, 2009a, 2009b). Although "IQ" tests have always had their critics, it was not until the reauthorization of the Individuals with Disabilities Education Improvement Act of 2004 (IDEA 2004) and its attendant regulations (U.S. Department of Education, 2006) that such criticism became more widespread (Flanagan et al., 2008).

It is beyond the scope of this chapter to review all the issues surrounding the debate about the utility (or lack thereof) of cognitive and neuropsychological tests in the identification of SLD. The interested reader is referred to Flanagan and Alfonso (2011) and Flanagan and colleagues (2008) for a comprehensive treatment of these issues. Based on our review of the literature and our clinical experience, we find inherent utility in cognitive and neuropsychological assessment for SLD identification and treatment. Therefore, the purposes of this chapter are to describe our operational definition of SLD and to highlight the importance and utility of gathering data from cognitive and neuropsychological tests (among other quantitative and qualitative data sources) within this framework.

A BRIEF PERSPECTIVE ON THE DEFINITION OF SLD

According to Kavale, Spaulding, and Beam (2009), the federal definition of SLD in IDEA 2004 and its regulations does not reflect the best thinking about the SLD construct because it has not changed in over 30 years. This fact is astonishing, as several decades of inquiry into the nature of SLD resulted in numerous proposals over the years to modify the definition. For example, the National Joint Committee on Learning Disabilities (NJCLD)—a group of organizations with a common concern about SLD—articulated several points of contention with the federal definition and, in 1981, put forth its own definition of SLD (Kavale et al., 2009). Although the NJCLD definition was well received (e.g., it was endorsed by the Interagency Committee on Learning Disabilities), it had little influence on the federal definition. As such, Kavale and Forness (2000) asserted that if the field of SLD is to recapture its status as a reliable entity in special education and psychology, then more attention must be paid to the federal definition. Accordingly, Kavale et al. (2009) have proposed a "richer" description of SLD that specifies the boundaries of the term and the class of things to which it belongs. In addition, their definition delineates what SLD is and what it is not. Although their description is not a radical departure from the federal definition, it provides a more comprehensive description of the nature of SLD. The Kavale et al. definition is as follows:

> Specific learning disability refers to heterogeneous clusters of disorders that significantly impede the normal progress of academic achievement . . . The lack of progress is exhibited in school performance that remains below expectation for chronological and mental ages, even when [the student is] provided with high-quality instruction. The primary manifestation of the failure to progress is significant underachievement in a basic skill area (i.e., reading, math, writing) that is not associated with insufficient educational, cultural/familial, and/or sociolinguistic experiences. The primary severe ability–achievement discrepancy is coincident with deficits in linguistic competence (receptive and/or expressive), cognitive functioning (e.g., problem solving, thinking abilities, maturation), neuropsychological processes (e.g., perception, attention, memory), or any combination of such contributing deficits that are presumed to originate from central nervous system dysfunction. The specific learning disability is a discrete condition differentiated from generalized learning failure by average or above (>90) cognitive ability and a learning skill profile exhibiting significant scatter indicating areas of strength and weakness. The major specific learning disability may be accompanied by secondary learning difficulties that also may be considered when [educators are] planning the more intensive, individualized special education instruction directed at the primary problem. (p. 46)

Kavale and colleagues state that their richer description of SLD "can be readily translated into an operational definition providing more confidence in the validity of a diagnosis of SLD" (p. 46). In the following section, we describe an operational definition of SLD that captures the nature of SLD as reflected in the federal definition and in Kavale and colleagues' definition. In addition, the reasons why operational definitions are important and necessary for SLD identification are highlighted.

THE NEED FOR AN OPERATIONAL DEFINITION OF SLD

An operational definition of SLD is needed to provide more confidence in the validity of the SLD diagnosis (Flanagan, Fiorello, & Ortiz, 2010; Kavale et al., 2009). For the purpose of this chapter, an *operational definition* is conceived of as one that provides a process for the identification and classification of concepts that have been defined formally (see Sotelo-Dynega, Flanagan, & Alfonso, 2011, for a summary). With no change in the federal definition of SLD, attention within the field has turned to articulating ways to operationalize SLD, with the intent of improving the clinical identification of this condition (Flanagan, Ortiz, Alfonso, & Mascolo, 2002, 2006; Kavale & Flanagan, 2007; Kavale & Forness, 2000; Kavale et al., 2009; Swanson, 1991).

For more than three decades, the main operational definition of SLD was the so-called "discrepancy criterion." Discrepancy was first introduced in Bateman's (1965) definition of learning disabilities (LD) and later was formalized in federal regulations as follows:

> (1) The child does not achieve commensurate with his or her age and ability when provided with appropriate educational experiences, and (2) the child has a *severe discrepancy between achievement and intellectual ability* in one or more areas relating to communication skills and mathematics abilities. (U.S. Office of Education, 1977, p. 65083; emphasis added)

Several problems with the traditional ability–achievement discrepancy approach to SLD identification have been discussed extensively in the literature and are highlighted elsewhere (e.g., Fiorello, Hale, & Wycoff, Chapter 20, this volume; Hale, Wycoff, & Fiorello, 2011); therefore, they are not repeated here.

With the reauthorization of IDEA in 2004, and the corresponding deemphasis on the traditional ability–achievement discrepancy criterion for SLD identification, there have been several attempts to operationalize the federal definition, many of which can be found in Flanagan and Alfonso (2011). Table 26.1 provides examples of how the 2004 federal definition of SLD has been operationalized.

Perhaps the most comprehensive operational definition of SLD was described over a decade ago by Kavale and Forness (2000). These researchers critically reviewed the available definitions of LD and methods for their operationalization, and found them to be largely inadequate. Therefore, they proposed a modest, hierarchical operational definition that reflected current research on the nature of LD. This operational definition is illustrated in Figure 26.1.

In their definition, Kavale and Forness (2000) attempted to incorporate the complex and multivariate nature of LD. Figure 26.1 shows that LD is determined through evaluation of performance at several "levels," each of which specifies particular diagnostic conditions. Furthermore, each level of the evaluation hierarchy depicted in Figure 26.1 represents a necessary, but not sufficient, condition for LD determination. Kavale and Forness contended that it is only when the specified criteria are met at all five levels of their operational definition that LD can be established as a "discrete and independent condition" (p. 251). Through their operational definition, Kavale and Forness provided a much more rational and defensible ap-

proach to the practice of LD identification than that which had been offered previously. In short, their operationalization of LD used "foundation principles in guiding the selection of elements that explicate the nature of LD" (p. 251); this represented both a departure from and an important new direction for current practice.

Flanagan and colleagues (2002) identified some aspects of Kavale and Forness's (2000) operational definition that they believed needed to be modified. For example, although Kavale and Forness's operational definition captured the complex and multivariate nature of LD, it was not predicated on any particular theoretical model, and it did not specify what methods might be used to satisfy criteria at each level. In addition, the hierarchical structure depicted in Figure 26.1 seems to imply somewhat of a linear approach to LD identification, whereas the process is typically more recursive and iterative. Consequently, Flanagan and colleagues proposed a similar operational definition of SLD, but based their definition primarily on the Cattell–Horn–Carroll (CHC) theory and its research base. In addition, these researchers provided greater specification of methods and criteria that may be used to identify SLD (Flanagan, Alfonso, & Mascolo, 2011; Flanagan et al., 2002; Flanagan, Ortiz, & Alfonso, 2007; Flanagan, Ortiz, Alfonso, & Mascolo, 2006).

Because operational definitions represent only temporary assumptions about a concept, they are subject to change (Kavale et al., 2009). Flanagan and colleagues have modified their operational definition over the last decade to ensure that it reflects the most current theory, research, and thinking with regard to (1) the nature of SLD; (2) the methods of evaluating various elements and concepts inherent in SLD definitions (viz., the federal definition); and (3) criteria for establishing SLD as a discrete condition separate from undifferentiated low achievement. The most recent iteration of Flanagan and colleagues' operational definition of SLD is presented in Figure 26.2. Because this definition is primarily grounded in CHC theory, it has been labeled "the CHC-based operational definition of SLD" (Flanagan, Alfonso, & Mascolo, 2011). However, it is important to note that we encourage a continuum of data-gathering methods, beginning with curriculum-based measurement (CBM) and progress monitoring, and culminating in norm-referenced tests of cognitive abilities and neuropsychological processes for students who demonstrate an inadequate response to interven-

TABLE 26.1. Examples of How the IDEA 2004 Federal Definition of SLD Has Been Operationally Defined

- Absolute low achievement (see Lichtenstein & Klotz, 2007, for a discussion)
- Ability–achievement discrepancy (see Zirkel & Thomas, 2010, for a discussion)
- Dual discrepancy (e.g., Fuchs & Fuchs, 1998)
- Failure to respond to scientifically based intervention (e.g., Fletcher, Barth, & Stuebing, 2011; Fletcher, Lyon, Fuchs, & Barnes, 2007)
- Pattern of academic and cognitive strengths and weaknesses (also called alternative research-based approaches or "third-method" approaches; e.g., Flanagan, Alfonso, & Mascolo, 2011; Hale, Flanagan, & Naglieri, 2008; Hale, Wycoff, & Fiorello, 2011; Naglieri, 2011)

Note. All examples in this table include a consideration of exclusionary factors as specified in the federal definition of SLD.

Level

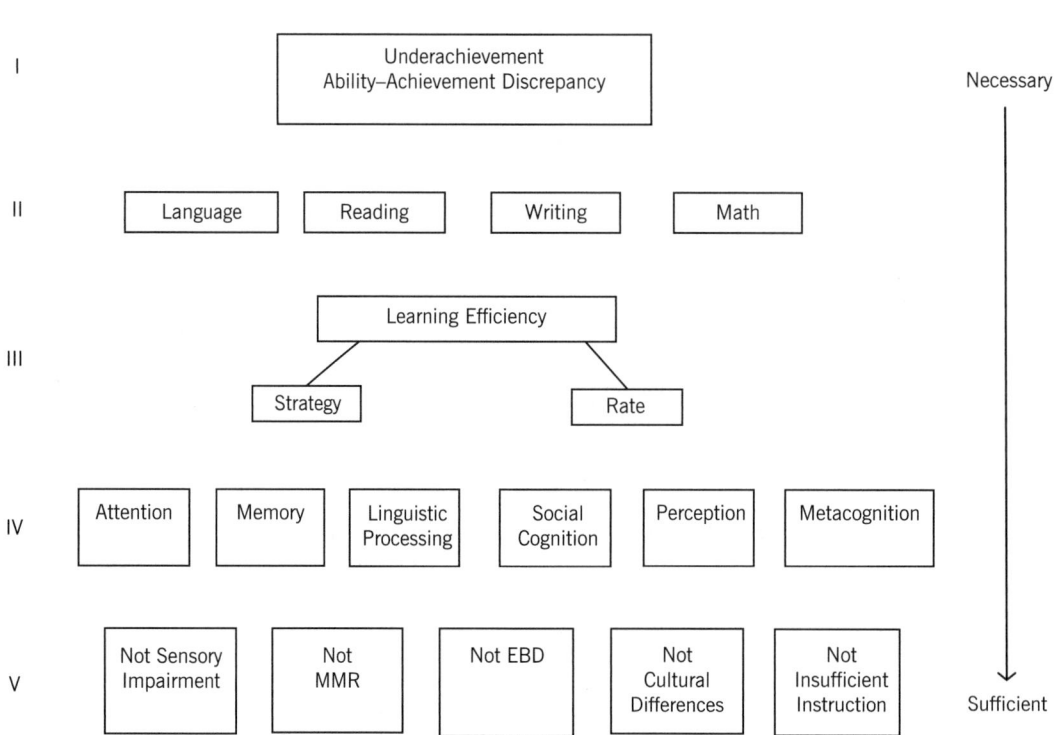

FIGURE 26.1. Kavale and Forness's operational definition of SLD. MMR, mild mental retardation (intellectual disability); EBD, emotional or behavioral disorder. From Kavale and Forness (2000). Copyright 2000 by the Hammill Institute on Disabilities. Reprinted by permission.

tion. This type of systematic approach to understanding learning difficulties can emanate from any similar and well-researched theory.

Figure 26.2 shows that the CHC-based operational definition of SLD is arranged according to levels, as Kavale and Forness's (2000) definition is. At each level, the definition includes (1) defining characteristics regarding the nature of SLD (e.g., a child has difficulties in one or more areas of academic achievement); (2) the focus of evaluation for each characteristic (e.g., academic achievement, cognitive abilities and neuropsychological processes, exclusionary factors); (3) examples of evaluation methods and relevant data sources (e.g., standardized, norm-referenced tests and educational records, respectively); and (4) the criteria that need to be met to establish that an individual possesses a particular characteristic of SLD (e.g., below-average performance in an academic area, such as basic reading skill). As may be seen in Figure 26.2, the "Nature of SLD" column includes a

description of what SLD is and what it is not. Overall, the levels represent adaptations and extensions of the recommendations offered by Kavale and colleagues (e.g., Kavale & Forness, 2000; Kavale et al., 2009), but they also include concepts from various other researchers (e.g., Berninger, 2011; Fletcher-Janzen & Reynolds, 2008; Geary, Hoard, & Bailey, 2011; Hale & Fiorello, 2004; Hale et al., 2010; Naglieri, 2011; Reynolds & Shaywitz, 2009a, 2009b; Siegel, 1999; Stanovich, 1999; Vellutino, Scanlon, & Lyon, 2000).

The CHC-based operational definition of SLD presented in Figure 26.2 differs from the one presented by Kavale and Forness (2000; see Figure 26.1) in four important ways. First, it is grounded in a well-validated contemporary theory on the structure of abilities (i.e., CHC theory). Second, in lieu of the traditional ability–achievement discrepancy method, a specific pattern of cognitive and academic ability and neuropsychological processing strengths and weaknesses is used as a defining characteristic or marker for SLD.[1] (It is important to understand that any pattern used for SLD determination should be supported by research on the relations among CHC abilities, processes, and academic outcomes—and, where possible, evidence on the neurobiological correlates of learning disorders in reading, math, and writing.) Third, the evaluation of exclusionary factors occurs earlier in the SLD identification process in our operational definition, to prevent individuals from having to undergo additional testing. Fourth, we emphasize that SLD assessment is a recursive process rather than a linear one, and that information generated and evaluated at one level may inform decisions made at other levels. The recursive nature of the SLD identification process is reflected by the circular arrows in Figure 26.2. Each level of the CHC-based operational definition of SLD is described in more detail in the next section.

THE CHC-BASED OPERATIONAL DEFINITION OF SLD

A diagnosis identifies the nature of a specific learning disability and has implications for its probable etiology, instructional requirements, and prognosis. Ironically, in an era when educational practitioners are encouraged to use evidence-based instructional practices, they are not encouraged to use evidence-based differential diagnoses of specific learning disabilities.

—BERNINGER (2011, p. 204)

The CHC-based operational definition of SLD described here is consistent with the alternative research-based "third option" for SLD identification specified in the U.S. Department of Education (2006) regulations. It is assumed that the levels of evaluation depicted in Figure 26.2 are undertaken after prereferral intervention activities (consistent with Tiers 1 and 2 of a response-to-intervention [RTI] approach) have been conducted with little or no success, and therefore a focused evaluation of specific abilities and processes through standardized testing is deemed necessary (see Brown-Chidsey & Andren, Chapter 35, this volume; Flanagan, Fiorello, et al., 2010). Moreover, before an SLD assessment is begun, other data from multiple sources may have (and probably should have) already been uncovered within the context of intervention implementation. These data may include results from informal testing, direct observation of behaviors, work samples, reports from people familiar with the child's difficulties

(e.g., teachers, parents), and information provided by the child him- or herself. In principle, level I assessment should begin only after the nature of a child's learning difficulties has been fully investigated and documented. It is beyond the scope of this chapter to provide a detailed discussion of assessment- and interpretation-related activities for each level of the operational definition. Therefore, only a brief summary of each level follows (see Flanagan, Alfonso, & Mascolo, 2011, for a more comprehensive description of the operational definition included in Figure 26.2).

Level I: Difficulties in One or More Areas of Academic Achievement

By definition, SLD is marked by dysfunction in learning. That is, learning is somehow disrupted from its normal course by some type of internal disorder or dysfunction. Although the specific mechanism that inhibits learning is not directly observable, one can proceed on the assumption that it manifests in observable phenomena, particularly academic achievement. Thus level I of the operational definition involves documenting that some type of *learning* deficit exists. Accordingly, the process at level I involves comprehensive measurement of the major areas of academic achievement (e.g., reading, writing, math, oral language). Noteworthy is the fact that a finding of low academic achievement is not sufficient for SLD identification because this condition alone may be present for a variety of reasons, only one of which is SLD.

The academic areas that are generally assessed at this level in the operational definition include the eight areas of achievement specified in the federal definition of SLD (IDEA 2004). These eight areas are math calculation, math problem solving, basic reading skill, reading fluency, reading comprehension, written expression, listening comprehension, and oral expression. Most of the skills and abilities measured at level I represent an individual's stores of acquired knowledge. These specific knowledge bases (e.g., quantitative knowledge [Gq], reading and writing ability [Grw], vocabulary knowledge [Gc]) develop largely as a function of formal instruction, schooling, and educationally related experiences (Carroll, 1993). Typically, the eight areas of academic achievement are measured via standardized, norm-referenced tests. In fact, many comprehensive achievement batteries, such as the Wechsler Individual Achievement Test—Third Edition (WIAT-III; Pearson, 2009; see Table 26.2),

Level	Nature of SLD[a]	Focus of Evaluation	Examples of Evaluation Methods and Data Sources	Criteria for SLD	SLD Classification and Eligibility
					Necessary →
I	Difficulties in one or more areas of academic achievement, including (but not limited to) basic reading skill, reading comprehension, reading fluency, oral expression, listening comprehension,[b] written expression, math calculation, math problem solving.	**Academic Achievement:** Performance in specific academic skills (e.g., Grw, Gq, Gc); may also include performance on measures of phonological and orthographic processing.	Response to high-quality instruction and intervention via progress monitoring; performance on norm-referenced, standardized achievement tests; evaluation of work samples; observations of academic performance; teacher/parent/child interview; history of academic performance; data from other members of multidisciplinary team (MDT) (e.g., speech–language pathologist, interventionist, reading specialist).	Performance in one or more academic areas is *weak or deficient[c]* (despite attempts at delivering high-quality instruction) as evidenced by converging data from multiple sources.	
II	SLD does not include learning problems that are the result of visual, hearing, or motor disabilities; of intellectual disability; of social or emotional disturbance; or of environmental, educational, cultural, or economic disadvantage.	**Exclusionary Factors:** Identification of potential primary causes of academic skill weaknesses or deficits, including intellectual disability, cultural or linguistic difference, sensory impairment, insufficient instruction or opportunity to learn, organic or physical health factors, social/ emotional or psychological disturbance.	Data from the methods and sources listed at levels I and III, as well as these: behavior rating scales; medical records; prior evaluations; interviews with current or past counselors, psychiatrists, etc.	Performance is not *primarily* attributed to these exclusionary factors, although one or more of them may contribute to learning difficulties.	
III	Disorders in one or more of the basic psychological/ neuropsychological processes involved in understanding or in using language, spoken or written; such disorders are presumed to originate from central nervous system dysfunction.	**Cognitive Abilities and Processes:** Performance in cognitive abilities (e.g., Gc, Gf, Gv, Ga, Glr, Gsm, Gs) and neuropsychological processes (e.g., attention, executive functioning).	Performance on norm-referenced tests, evaluation of work samples, observations of cognitive performance, task analysis/testing limits, teacher/parent/child interview, history of academic performance, and records review.	Performance in one or more cognitive abilities and/or neuropsychological processes (related to academic skill deficiency) is *weak or deficient[b]* as evidenced by converging data sources.	

			Sufficient for SLD Identification →
IV	Unexpected underachievement: An SLD is a discrete condition differentiated from generalized learning failure by average or better cognitive ability and a learning skill profile exhibiting significant variability indicating processing areas of strength and weakness.	**Data Integration—Analysis of a Pattern of Strengths and Weaknesses Consistent with SLD:** Determination of whether academic skill weaknesses or deficits are related to specific cognitive area(s) of weakness or deficit, as well as of whether pattern of data reflects a below-average aptitude–achievement *consistency* with otherwise average or better ability to think and reason.	Data gathered at all previous levels, as well as any additional data following a review of initial evaluation results (e.g., hypothesis testing, demand analysis).	No statistically significant or clinically meaningful difference between cognitive and academic deficits (e.g., circumscribed aptitude–achievement consistency); statistically significant or clinically meaningful difference between cognitive and academic deficits and cognitive and academic strengths (e.g., circumscribed ability–achievement discrepancy with cognitive areas of strength represented by standard scores ≥90); clinical judgment supports the impression that the child's overall ability to think and reason will enable him or her to benefit from tailored or specialized instruction/intervention, compensatory strategies, and accommodations, such that his or her performance rate and level will be likely to approximate those of more typically achieving, nondisabled peers.
V	An SLD has an adverse impact on educational performance.	**Special Education Eligibility:**[d] Determination of least restrictive environment for delivery of instruction and educational resources.	Data from all previous levels, MDT meeting, and parents.	Child demonstrates significant difficulties in daily academic activities that cannot be remediated, accommodated, or otherwise compensated for *without* the assistance of individualized special education services.
				Necessary for Special Education Eligibility

[a]This column includes concepts inherent in the federal definition (IDEA 2004) and in Kavale, Spaulding, and Beam's (2009) definition of SLD.

[b]Poor spelling with adequate ability to express ideas in writing is often typical of dyslexia and/or dysgraphia. Even though IDEA 2004 includes only the broad category of written expression, poor spelling and handwriting are often symptomatic of a specific writing disability and should not be ignored (Wending & Mather, 2009).

[c]Weak or deficient performance (also called *normative weakness*) is defined typically by standard score performances that are low average (i.e., ≤89) or significantly below average (i.e., ≤84), respectively, and that have ecological validity (e.g., standardized test performance is consistent with performance observed in the child's everyday classroom or educational environment).

[d]The primary SLD may be accompanied by secondary learning difficulties that also may be considered when educators are planning the more intensive, individualized special education instruction directed at the primary problem.

FIGURE 26.2. A CHC-based operational definition of specific learning disabilities (SLD).

649

TABLE 26.2. Correspondence between Eight Areas of SLD and WIAT-III Subtests and Composites

Areas in which SLD may be manifested (listed in IDEA 2004)	WIAT-III subtests	WIAT-III composites
Oral expression	Oral Expression	Oral Language
Listening comprehension	Listening Comprehension	Oral Language
Written expression	Alphabet Writing Fluency Sentence Composition Essay Composition Spelling	Written Expression
Basic reading skills	Early Reading Skills Word Reading Pseudoword Decoding	Basic Reading
Reading fluency skills	Oral Reading Fluency	Reading Comprehension and Fluency
Reading comprehension	Reading Comprehension	Reading Comprehension and Fluency
Mathematics calculation	Numerical Operations	Mathematics
Mathematics calculation	Math Fluency—Addition Math Fluency—Subtraction Math Fluency—Multiplication	Math Fluency
Mathematics problem solving	Math Problem Solving	Mathematics

Note. From Lichtenberger and Breaux (2010), Table 2.1, p. 21. Copyright 2010 by John Wiley & Sons. Adapted by permission.

measure all eight areas. It is important to realize that data on academic performance may (and should) come from multiple sources (see Figure 26.2, level I, column 4). Following the collection of data on academic performance, it is necessary to determine whether the child has a weakness or deficit in one or more specific academic skills.

A *weakness* is typically defined as performance on standardized, norm-referenced tests that falls below average (where *average* is defined as standard scores between 90 and 110 [inclusive], based on a scale having a mean of 100 and standard deviation of 15). A deficit is often defined as performance on norm-referenced tests that falls more than one standard deviations below the mean (i.e., standard scores <85). See Table 26.3 for an example of a classification system that may be used to describe performance on norm-referenced tests.

Determining whether a child has a weakness or deficit usually involves making normative-based comparisons of the child's performance against a representative sample of same-age or same-grade peers from the general population. If weaknesses

TABLE 26.3. System for Classifying Performance on Norm-Referenced Tests

Standard score range	Percentile range	Normative classification
<70	<2nd	Lower extreme
70–84	2nd–15th	Below average/normative weakness
85–89	16th–24th	Low average[a,b]
90–110	25th–75th	Average[a]
111–115	76th–84th	High average[a]
116–129	85th–97th	Above average/normative strength
>130	>97th	Upper extreme

[a]Within normal limits.
[b]Clinical judgment is likely necessary to determine if the construct underlying a score falling in this range is or is not functionally limiting for the individual.

or deficits in the child's academic achievement profile are not identified, then the issue of SLD may be moot because such weaknesses are a necessary component of the definition.

Nevertheless, some children who struggle academically may not demonstrate academic weaknesses or deficits on standardized, norm-referenced tests of achievement; this is particularly true of very bright students, for a variety of reasons. For example, some children may have figured out how to compensate for their processing deficits. Therefore, it is important not to assume that a child with a standard score of 90 on a "broad reading" composite is "OK," particularly when a parent, a teacher, or the student him- or herself expresses concern. Under these circumstances, a more focused assessment of the CHC and neuropsychological processes related to reading should be conducted.

The presence of a normative weakness or deficit established through standardized testing and corroborated by other data sources—such as CBM, clinical observations of academic performance, work samples, and so forth—is a necessary (but insufficient) condition for SLD determination. Therefore, when weaknesses or deficits in academic performance are found (irrespective of the particular methods by which they are identified), the process advances to level II.

Level II: Exclusionary Factors

Level II involves evaluating whether any documented weaknesses or deficits found through level I evaluation are or are not *primarily* the result of factors that may be, for example, largely external to the child, noncognitive in nature, or the result of a disorder other than SLD. Because there can be many reasons for weak or deficient academic performance, causal links to SLD should not be ascribed prematurely. Instead, reasonable hypotheses related to other potential causes should be developed. For example, cultural and linguistic differences are two common factors that can affect both test performance and academic skill acquisition adversely and can result in achievement data that appear to suggest SLD (see Ortiz, 2011, and Ortiz, Ochoa, & Dynda, Chapter 22, this volume). In addition, lack of motivation, social-emotional disturbance, performance anxiety, psychiatric disorders, sensory impairments, and medical conditions (e.g., hearing or vision problems) also need to be ruled out as potential explanatory correlates to any weaknesses or deficits identified at level I. Figure 26.3 is a form that may be used to document

systematically and thoroughly that the exclusionary factors listed in the federal definition of SLD (as well as other factors) were evaluated.

Note that because the process of SLD determination does not necessarily occur in a strict linear fashion, evaluations at levels I and II often take place concurrently, as data from level II are often necessary to understand performance at level I. The circular arrows between levels I and II in Figure 26.2 are meant to illustrate the fact that interpretations and decisions that are based on data gathered at level I may need to be informed by data gathered at level II. Ultimately, at level II, the practitioner must judge the extent to which any factors other than cognitive impairment can be considered the *primary* reason for the academic performance difficulties. The form in Figure 26.3 provides space for documenting this judgment. If performance cannot be attributed primarily to other factors, then the second criterion necessary for establishing SLD according to the operational definition is met, and assessment may continue to the next level.

It is important to recognize that although factors such as having English as a second language may be present and may affect performance adversely, SLD can also be present. Certainly, children who may have vision problems, chronic illnesses, limited English proficiency, and so forth may also have SLD. Therefore, when these or other factors at level II are present or even when they are determined to be *contributing* to poor performance, SLD should not be ruled out. Rather, only when such factors are determined to be *primarily* responsible for weaknesses in learning and academic performance—not merely contributing to them—should SLD be discounted as an explanation for dysfunction in performance. Examination of exclusionary factors is necessary to ensure fair and equitable interpretation of the data collected for SLD determination, and, as such, is not intended to *rule in* SLD. Rather, careful examination of exclusionary factors is intended to rule out other possible explanations for deficient academic performance.

One of the major reasons for placing evaluation of exclusionary factors at this (early) point in the SLD assessment process is to provide a mechanism that is efficient in both time and effort and that may prevent the unnecessary administration of additional tests. However, noteworthy is the fact that it may not be possible to rule out all of the numerous potential exclusionary factors completely and convincingly at this stage in the assessment

Evaluation and Consideration of Exclusionary Factors for SLD Identification

An evaluation for specific learning disabilities (SLD) requires consideration of factors other than a disorder in one or more basic psychological processes that may be the primary cause of a student's academic skill weaknesses and learning difficulties. These factors include (but are not limited to) vision/hearing[a] or motor disabilities, intellectual disability (ID), social-emotional or psychological disturbance, environmental or economic disadvantage, cultural and linguistic factors (e.g., limited English proficiency), insufficient instruction or opportunity to learn, and physical/health factors. These factors may be evaluated via behavior rating scales, parent and teacher interviews, classroom observations, attendance records, social/developmental history, family history, vision/hearing exams, medical records, prior evaluations, and interviews with current or past counselors, psychiatrists, and paraprofessionals who have worked with the student. Noteworthy is the fact that students with (and without) SLD often have one or more factors (listed below) that *contribute* to academic and learning difficulties. However, the practitioner must rule out any of these factors as being the *primary* cause of a student's academic and learning difficulties to maintain SLD as a viable classification/diagnosis.

Vision (check all that apply):

- ☐ Vision test recent (within 1 year)
- ☐ Vision test outdated (>1 year)
- ☐ Passed
- ☐ Failed
- ☐ Wears glasses

- ☐ History of visual disorder/disturbance
- ☐ Diagnosed visual disorder/disturbance

Name of disorder: ____________________

- ☐ Vision difficulties suspected or observed (e.g., difficulty with far- or near-point copying; misaligned numbers in written math work; squinting or rubbing eyes during visual tasks such as reading, computer use)

Notes: ____________________

____

____

Hearing (check all that apply):[b]

- ☐ Hearing tested (within 1 year)
- ☐ Hearing tested (>1 year)
- ☐ Passed
- ☐ Failed
- ☐ Uses hearing aids/devices

- ☐ History of auditory disorder/disturbance
- ☐ Diagnosed auditory disorder/disturbance
- ☐ Name of disorder: ____________________
- ☐ Hearing difficulties suspected or observed (e.g., frequent requests for repetition of auditory information; misarticulated words; attempts to self-accommodate by moving closer to sound source; obvious attempts to read speech)

Notes: ____________________

____

____

Motor functioning (check all that apply):

- ☐ Fine motor delay/difficulty
- ☐ Gross motor delay/difficulty
- ☐ Improper pencil grip (describe: ____________)
- ☐ Assistive devices/aids used (e.g., weighted pens, pencil grip, slant board)

- ☐ History of motor disorder
- ☐ Diagnosed motor disorder

Name of disorder: ____________________

- ☐ Motor difficulties suspected or observed (e.g., illegible writing; difficulty with letter or number formation, size, spacing; difficulty with fine motor tasks, such as using scissors, folding paper)

Notes: ____________________

____

____

(cont.)

FIGURE 26.3. Form for documenting evaluation of exclusionary factors in the SLD identification process.

Cognitive and adaptive functioning (check all that apply):
☐ Subaverage intellectual functioning (e.g., IQ of 70–75 or below)
☐ Pervasive cognitive deficits (e.g., weaknesses or deficits in many cognitive areas, including Gf *and* Gc)
☐ Deficits in adaptive functioning (e.g., social, communication, self-care)
  Areas of significant adaptive skill weaknesses (check all that apply):
  ☐ Motor skills   ☐ Communication   ☐ Socialization skills
  ☐ Daily living skills ☐ Behavioral/emotional skills ☐ Other
Notes: _____
_____
_____

Social-emotional/psychological factors (check all that apply):
☐ Diagnosed psychological disorder (specify: _____)
☐ Date of diagnosis: _____
☐ Specify current treatment modality (e.g., counseling, medication): _____
☐ Family history significant for psychological difficulties (specify: _____)
☐ Difficulties with social-emotional functioning (e.g., social phobia, anxiety, depression)
☐ Home–school adjustment difficulties
☐ Emotional stress
☐ Lack of motivation
☐ Autism
☐ Present medications (type, dosage, frequency, duration): _____
☐ Prior medication use (type, dosage, frequency, duration): _____
☐ Hospitalization(s) for psychological difficulties (date[s]: _____)
☐ Deficits in social, emotional, or behavioral (SEB) functioning (e.g., as assessed by standardized rating scales)
Notes: _____
_____
_____

Environmental/economic factors (check all that apply):
☐ Limited access to educational materials in the home   ☐ History of educational neglect
☐ Caregivers unable to provide instructional support   ☐ Frequent transitions (e.g., shared custody)
☐ Economic considerations precluded treatment   ☐ Environmental space factors (e.g., no space
  of identified issues (e.g., filling a prescription,   for studying; sleep disruptions due to shared
  replacing broken glasses, tutoring)   sleeping space)
☐ Temporary crisis
Notes: _____
_____
_____

Cultural/linguistic factors (check all that apply):[c]
☐ Limited number of years in U.S.: _____   ☐ Language(s) other than English spoken in home
☐ No history of early or developmental   ☐ Lack of or limited instruction in primary language
  problems in primary language   (# of years: _____)
☐ Current primary-language proficiency: ☐ Current English-language proficiency:
  (Dates: _____ Scores: _____)   (Date: _____ Scores: _____)
☐ Acculturative knowledge development   ☐ Parental educational and socioeconomic level
  (Circle one: High Moderate Low)   (Circle one: High Moderate Low)
Notes: _____
_____
_____

(cont.)

FIGURE 26.3. *(cont.)*

Physical/health factors (check all that apply):

☐ Limited access to health care

☐ Chronic health condition (specify: _____)

☐ Temporary health condition (date/duration: _____)

☐ History of medical condition (date diagnosed: _____)

☐ Medical treatments (specify: _____)

☐ Repeated visits to the school nurse/doctor

☐ Medication (type, dosage, frequency, duration: _____)

Notes: _____

_____

_____

Instructional factors (check all that apply):

☐ Interrupted schooling (e.g., midyear school move)　☐ Number of days absent/tardy: _____

☐ New teacher (past 6 months)　Specify why: _____

☐ Nontraditional curriculum (e.g., home-schooled)　☐ Retained or advanced a grade(s)

☐ Accelerated curriculum (e.g., advanced-placement classes)

Notes: _____

_____

_____

Determination of primary and contributory causes of academic weaknesses and learning difficulties (check one):

☐ From the available data, it is reasonable to conclude that one or more factors is *primarily* responsible for the student's observed learning difficulties. Specify: _____

☐ From the available data, it is reasonable to conclude that one or more factors *contributes* to the student's observed learning difficulties. Specify: _____

☐ *No* factors listed here appear to be the primary cause of the student's academic weaknesses and learning difficulties.

[a]For a vision or hearing disorder, it is important to understand the nature of the disorder, its expected impact on achievement, and the time of diagnosis. It is also important to understand what was happening instructionally at the time the disorder was suspected and/or diagnosed.

　　With regard to hearing, even mild loss can affect initial receptive and expressive language skills, as well as academic skill acquisition. When loss is suspected, the practitioner should consult professional literature to further understand the potential impact of a documented hearing issue (see American Speech–Language–Hearing Association guidelines at www.asha.org).

　　With regard to vision, refractive error (i.e., hyperopia and anisometropia), accommodative and vergence dysfunctions, and eye movement disorders are associated with learning difficulties, whereas other vision problems are not (e.g., constant strabismus and amblyopia). As such, when a vision disorder is documented or suspected, the practitioner should consult professional literature or websites to further understand the impact of the visual disorder (e.g., the American Optometric Association, www.aoa.org).

[b]When there is a history of hearing difficulties and an SLD diagnosis is being considered, hearing testing should be recent (i.e., conducted within the past 6 months).

[c]When evaluating the impact of language and cultural factors on a student's functioning, the practitioner should consider whether and to what extent other individuals with similar linguistic and cultural backgrounds as the referred student are progressing and responding to instruction in the present curriculum. For example, if a student with limited English proficiency is not demonstrating academic progress or is not performing as expected on a classwide or districtwide assessment when compared to peers who possess a similar level of English proficiency and acculturative knowledge, it is unlikely that cultural and linguistic differences are the sole or primary factors for the referred student's low performance. In addition, it is important to note that as the number of cultural and linguistic differences in a student's background increase, the greater the likelihood becomes that poor academic performance is attributable primarily to such differences rather than to a disability.

Note. All 50 U.S. states specify eight exclusionary criteria. Namely, learning difficulties cannot be primarily attributed to (1) visual impairment; (2) hearing impairment; (3) motor impairment; (4) ID; (5) emotional disturbance; (6) environmental disadvantage; (7) economic disadvantage; and (8) cultural difference. Noteworthy is the fact that certain states have adopted additional exclusionary criteria, including autism (CA, MI, VT, and WI), emotional stress (LA and VT), home or school adjustment difficulties (LA and VT), lack of motivation (LA and TN), and temporary crisis situation (LA, TN, and VT). We have integrated these additional criteria under "social-emotional/psychological factors" and "environmental/economic factors," and have added two additional categories—namely, "instructional factors" and "physical/health factors"—to this form.

FIGURE 26.3. (*cont.*)

process. For example, the data gathered at levels I and II may be insufficient to draw conclusions about such conditions as intellectual disability (ID; formerly called mental retardation; see Armstrong, Hangauer, & Nadeau, Chapter 30, this volume), which often requires more thorough and direct assessment (e.g., administration of an intelligence test and adaptive behavior scale). When exclusionary factors—at least those that can be evaluated at this level—have been evaluated carefully and eliminated as possible *primary* explanations for poor academic performance, the process may advance to the next level.

Level III: Deficits in Cognitive Abilities or Neuropsychological Processes

The criterion at level III is similar to the one specified in level I, except that it is evaluated with data from an assessment of cognitive abilities and neuropsychological processes. Analysis of data generated from the administration of standardized tests represents the most common method available by which cognitive and neuropsychological functioning in children is evaluated. However, other types of information and data are relevant to cognitive performance (see Figure 26.2, level III, column 4). Practitioners should seek out and gather data from other sources as a means of providing corroborating evidence for standardized test findings. For example, when test findings are found to be consistent with the child's performance in the classroom, a greater degree of confidence may be placed on test performance because interpretations of cognitive deficiency have ecological validity—an important condition for any diagnostic process (Hale & Fiorello, 2004). Table 26.4 provides an example of the cognitive abilities and neuropsychological processes measured by the Wechsler Intelligence Scale for Children—Fourth Edition (WISC-IV; Wechsler, 2003). For similar information on all major intelligence tests and selected neuropsychological instruments, see Flanagan, Ortiz, and Alfonso (in press) and Flanagan, Alfonso, Ortiz, and Dynda (2010).

A particularly salient aspect of the CHC-based operational definition of SLD is the concept that a weakness or deficit in a cognitive ability or process underlies difficulties in academic performance or skill development. Because research demonstrates that the relationship between the cognitive dysfunction and the manifest learning problems may be causal in nature (e.g., Fletcher, Taylor, Levin, & Satz, 1995; Hale & Fiorello, 2004; Hale et al.,

2010), data analysis at this level should seek to ensure that identified weaknesses or deficits on cognitive and neuropsychological tests bear an empirical relationship to those weaknesses or deficits in achievement identified previously. It is this very notion that makes it necessary to draw upon cognitive and neuropsychological theory and research to inform operational definitions of SLD and increase the reliability and validity of the SLD identification process. Theory and its related research base not only specify the relevant constructs that ought to be measured at levels I and III, but predict the manner in which they are related. Furthermore, application of current theory and research provides a substantive empirical foundation from which interpretations and conclusions may be drawn. Tables 26.5 and 26.6 provide a summary of the relations between CHC cognitive abilities and processes and reading and math achievement, respectively.

Tables 26.5 and 26.6 provide two sets of findings from two different literature reviews (i.e., Flanagan, Ortiz, Alfonso, & Mascolo, 2006; McGrew & Wendling, 2010). Because these literature reviews yielded some differences with regard to which abilities and processes are most relevant to academic achievement, each of these tables includes a "Comments" column that offers some possible explanations for the differences. A more extensive discussion of the implications of the findings reported in these tables may be found in McGrew and Wendling (2010) and Flanagan, Ortiz, and Alfonso (2012). Similarly, Table 26.7 provides a summary of the literature on the relations between CHC cognitive abilities and writing achievement (Flanagan, Ortiz, Alfonso, & Mascolo, 2006).

The information contained in Tables 26.5–26.7 may be used to guide how practitioners organize their assessments at this level. That is, prior to selecting cognitive and neuropsychological tests, a practitioner should have knowledge of those cognitive abilities and processes that are most important for understanding a child's academic performance in the area(s) in question (i.e., the area[s] identified as weak or deficient at level I). Evaluation of cognitive performance should be comprehensive in the areas of suspected dysfunction. Because evidence of a cognitive weakness or deficit is a necessary condition for SLD determination, if no weaknesses or deficits in cognitive abilities or processes are found, then an essential criterion for SLD determination is not met. When the criterion at level III is not met, an evaluation of whether or not the obtained cognitive data represent an eval-

TABLE 26.4. Cognitive Abilities and Neuropsychological Processes Measured by the Wechsler Intelligence Scale for Children—Fourth Edition (WISC-IV) Subtests

Subtest	CHC broad and narrow abilities					Neuropsychological domains							
	Gf	Gc	Gsm	Gv	Gs	Sensory–motor	Speed and efficiency	Attention	Visual-spatial (RH) and detail (LH)	Auditory-verbal	Memory and/or learning	Executive	Language[a]
Arithmetic[b]	✓ (RQ)		✓ (MW)					✓		✓	✓	✓	✓R
Block Design				✓ (SR,Vz)		✓			✓			✓	
Cancellation					✓ (P,R9)	✓	✓	✓	✓			✓	
Coding					✓ (R9)	✓	✓	✓	✓		✓	✓	
Comprehension		✓ (K0,LD)								✓	✓		✓E/R
Digit Span			✓ (MS,MW)					✓		✓	✓	✓	
Information		✓ (K0)								✓	✓		✓E
Letter–Number Sequencing			✓ (MW)					✓		✓	✓	✓	
Matrix Reasoning	✓ (I,RG)								✓			✓	
Picture Completion		✓ (K0)		✓ (CF)				✓	✓		✓		
Picture Concepts	✓ (I)	✓ (K0)								✓	✓	✓	
Similarities	✓ (I)	✓ (VL,LD)								✓	✓	✓	✓E
Symbol Search					✓ (P,R9)	✓	✓	✓	✓			✓	
Vocabulary		✓ (VL)								✓	✓		✓E
Word Reasoning	✓ (I)	✓ (VL)								✓	✓	✓	✓E/R

Note. Gf, fluid intelligence; Gc, crystallized intelligence; Gsm, short-term memory; Gv, visual processing; Gs, processing speed. RQ, quantitative reasoning; MW, working memory; SR, spatial relations; Vz, visualization; P, perceptual speed; R9, rate of test taking; K0, general (verbal) knowledge; LD, language development; MS, memory span; I, induction; RG, general sequential reasoning; CF, flexibility of closure; VL, lexical knowledge. The following Cattell–Horn–Carroll (CHC) broad abilities are omitted from this table because none is a primary ability measured by the WISC-IV: Glr (long-term storage and retrieval), Ga (auditory processing), Gt (decision/reaction time or speed), and Grw (reading and writing ability). Most CHC test classifications are from Flanagan, Ortiz, and Alfonso (2007). Classifications according to neuropsychological domains were based on our readings of neuropsychological texts (e.g., Fletcher-Janzen & Reynolds, 2008; Hale & Fiorello, 2004; Lezak, 1995; Miller, 2007, 2010) and are also found in Flanagan, Alfonso, Mascolo, and Hale (2011).
[a]E, expressive; R, receptive.
[b]Cognitive ability classifications for the Arithmetic subtest are based on the analyses conducted by Keith, Fine, Taub, Reynolds, and Kranzler (2006). It is important to note that the Keith et al. analyses did not include any other measures of math achievement; therefore, Gq was not represented adequately in their study. Arithmetic has been identified in many other studies as a measure of Gq, particularly math achievement (A3) (see Flanagan & Kaufman, 2009, for a discussion).

uation that was sufficient in breadth and depth vis à vis what is known about the relations between abilities, processes and academic skill acquisition and development is warranted. Furthermore, a more in-depth exploration of exclusionary factors evaluated at level II may be warranted.

Also, because new data are gathered at level III, it is now possible to evaluate the exclusionary factors that could not be evaluated earlier (e.g., ID). The circular arrows between levels II and III in Figure 26.2 are meant to illustrate the fact that interpretations and decisions that are based on data gathered at level III may need to be informed by data gathered at level II. Likewise, data gathered at level III are often necessary to rule out (or in) one or more factors listed at level II in Figure 26.2. Reliable and valid identification of SLD depends in part on being able to understand academic performance (level I), cognitive performance (level III), and the many factors that may facilitate or inhibit such performances (level II).

Level IV: Data Integration

The fourth level of evaluation involves an analysis of the individual's pattern of strengths and weaknesses. It revolves around a theory- and research-guided examination of performance across academic skills, cognitive abilities, and neuropsychological processes to determine whether the child's underachievement (as identified at level I) is indeed *unexpected*. When the process of SLD identification has reached this level, three necessary criteria for SLD identification have already been met: (1) One or more weaknesses or deficits have been found in academic performance; (2) one or more weaknesses or deficits have been found in cognitive abilities and/or neuropsychological processes; and (3) exclusionary factors have been determined not to be the primary causes of the academic and cognitive weaknesses or deficits. What has not been determined, however, is whether the pattern of results supports the notion of unexpected underachievement in a manner that suggests SLD. Within the context of the CHC-based operational definition, the nature of unexpected underachievement suggests that not only does a child possess specific, circumscribed, and related academic and cognitive weaknesses or deficits—referred to as a *below-average cognitive aptitude–achievement consistency*—but that these weaknesses exist along with generally average or better ability to think and reason (i.e., overall average intelligence).

The term *cognitive aptitude* within the context of the CHC-based operational definition of SLD represents the specific cognitive ability or neuropsychological processing deficits that are empirically related to the academic skill deficiency. For example, if a child's basic reading skill deficit is related to cognitive deficits in phonological processing (a Ga ability) and rapid automatic naming (a Glr ability), then the combination of below-average Ga and Glr performances represents his or her aptitude for basic reading. Moreover, the finding of below-average performance on measures of phonological processing, rapid automatic naming, and basic reading skill represents a below-average cognitive aptitude–achievement consistency (or, more specifically, a below-average *reading* cognitive aptitude–*reading* achievement consistency). The concept of cognitive aptitude–achievement consistency reflects the notion that there are documented relationships between specific cognitive abilities/processes and specific academic skills (see Tables 26.5–26.7; see also Hale et al., 2010). Therefore, the finding of below-average performance in related cognitive and academic areas is an important marker for SLD. Figure 26.4 depicts the relationships between cognitive and academic areas that are consistent with the operational definition of SLD presented here, as well as with alternative research-based methods of SLD identification (e.g., Fiorello et al., Chapter 20, this volume).

It is important to understand that discovery of consistencies among cognitive abilities and/or processes and academic skills in the below-average (or lower) range (depicted by the bottom two ovals in Figure 26.4) could result from ID or generally below-average cognitive ability. Therefore, identification of SLD cannot rest on below-average cognitive aptitude–achievement consistency alone. A child must also demonstrate evidence of average or better functioning (i.e., standard scores generally ≥ 90) in cognitive and neuropsychological domains that are not as highly correlated with the presenting problem. For example, in the case of a young child with reading decoding difficulties, it would be necessary to determine that performance in areas less related to this skill (e.g., Gf, math ability) are average or better. Such a finding would suggest that the related weaknesses in cognitive and academic domains are not due to a more pervasive form of cognitive dysfunction, thus supporting the notion of *unexpected underachievement*—that the child could in all likelihood perform within normal limits (e.g., at or close to grade level) in whatever achievement skill he or she was found

TABLE 26.5. Important Findings on Relations between CHC Abilities and Reading Achievement

CHC ability	Flanagan, Ortiz, Alfonso, and Mascolo (2006): General reading review[a] (116 independent studies)	McGrew and Wendling (2010): Basic reading skills and reading comprehension findings[b] (19 CHC/Woodcock–Johnson [WJ] studies)	Comments
Gf	Induction (I) and general sequential reasoning (RG) abilities play a moderate role in reading comprehension.	Quantitative reasoning (RQ) is tentative/speculative at ages 6–8 and 14–19 years for basic reading skills (BRS).[c] Broad Gf is tentative/speculative at ages 14–19 years for reading comprehension (RC).	The lack of a relationship between Gf abilities and reading in the McGrew and Wendling summary may be related to the nature of the dependent measures. For example, RC was represented by the WJ Passage Comprehension and Reading Vocabulary tests, both of which draw minimally on reasoning (e.g., they do not require an individual to draw inferences or make predictions).
Gc	**Language development (LD), lexical knowledge (VL), and listening abilities (LS) are important. These abilities become increasingly important with age.**	LS is moderately consistent at ages 6–8 years for BRS. LS is highly consistent at ages 6–19 years for RC. General fund of information (K0) is consistent at ages 6–8 years and moderately consistent at ages 9–19 years for BRS. K0 is highly consistent at ages 6–19 years for RC. Broad Gc is moderately consistent at ages 6–13 years and highly consistent at ages 14–19 years for BRS. Broad Gc is highly consistent at ages 6–19 years for RC.	The findings across the Flanagan et al., and McGrew and Wendling summaries are quite similar, given that broad Gc in the McGrew and Wendling summary is defined primarily by the narrow abilities of LD and VL. However, Flanagan et al. did not find a consistent relationship between the narrow ability of K0 and reading, as K0 was not well represented in the studies they reviewed.
Gsm	Memory span (MS) is important, **especially when evaluated within the context of working memory.**	Working memory (MW) is moderately consistent at ages 6–19 years for BRS and highly consistent at ages 6–19 years for RC. MS is tentative/speculative at ages 6–8 years and moderately consistent at ages 9–19 years for BRS. MS is consistent at ages 6–13 years and moderately consistent at ages 14–19 years for RC. Broad Gsm is consistent at ages 6–8 years and highly consistent at ages 9–19 years for BRS. Broad Gsm is consistent at ages 6–8 and 14–19 years for RC.	Both the Flanagan et al. and McGrew and Wendling summaries highlight the importance of Gsm for reading.
Gv	Orthographic processing	Visual memory (MV) is moderately consistent at ages 14–19 years for RC. Broad Gv is not consistently related to BRS or RC.	One possible explanation for the lack of a Gv relationship with BRS in the McGrew and Wendling summary is that the types of tasks used to measure visual processing in the studies they reviewed do not measure the visual aspects of reading (e.g., orthographic).

			Orthographic processing or awareness (the ability to rapidly map graphemes to phonemes) may be more related to the perceptual speed tasks found on cognitive tests (e.g., Symbol Search on the Wechsler scales).
Ga	**Phonetic coding (PC) or phonological awareness/processing is very important during the elementary school years.**	PC is moderately consistent at ages 6–13 years and consistent at ages 14–19 years for BRS. PC is consistent at ages 6–8 and 14–19 years, and tentative/speculative at ages 9–13 years, for RC. Speech sound discrimination and resistance to auditory stimulus distortion (US/UR) are consistent at ages 9–19 years for BRS. Broad Ga is not consistently related to BRS. Broad Ga is moderately related at ages 6–8 years to RC.	Interestingly, and in contrast to Flanagan et al.'s summary, McGrew and Wendling's summary does not show a strong relation between PC/phonological processing and reading at any age level. Given the wealth of research on the relations between PC/phonological processing and reading coupled with the neuroimaging research showing normalization of brain function in response to effective interventions for PC/phonological processing deficits, a reasonable assumption is that PC/phonological processing plays an important role in reading development during the early elementary school years. The relationship between PC/phonological processing and reading may be more prominent in students with reading difficulties (a population not included in the McGrew and Wendling samples).
Glr	**Naming facility (NA), or rapid automatic naming, is very important during the elementary school years.** Associative memory (MA) was also found to be related to reading at young ages.	MA is consistent at ages 6–8 years for BRS. Meaningful memory (MM) is highly consistent at ages 9–19 years for RC. NA is consistent at ages 14–19 years and moderately consistent at ages 9–13 years for RC. Broad Glr is consistent at ages 6–8 years for BRS. Broad Glr is consistent at ages 9–13 years for RC.	The lack of a significant relation between NA and BRS in the early elementary school years (ages 6–8 years) in the McGrew and Wendling summary is surprising, as rapid automatized naming or rate has always been implicated in young children who struggle with reading achievement, particularly reading fluency. However, the outcome measures in the studies reviewed by McGrew and Wendling may not have measured reading fluency well or at all.
Gs	**Perceptual speed (P) is important during all school years, particularly the elementary school years.**	P is consistent at ages 6–8 and 14–19 years, and moderately consistent at ages 9–13 years, for BRS. P is consistent at ages 14–19 years and moderately consistent at ages 6–13 years for RC.	Flanagan et al.'s summary shows a stronger relation between Gs and reading than McGrew and Wendling's summary. Nevertheless, the findings of both investigations show that Gs and P, in particular, are important for reading.

Note. For a discussion of the limitations of the findings reported in this table, see McGrew and Wendling (2010).

[a] Comments in bold represent the CHC abilities that demonstrated the strongest and most consistent relationships to reading achievement.

[b] Qualitative descriptors of consistency for the McGrew and Wendling (2010) analyses were coded as follows: The label "highly consistent" means that a significant finding was noted in 80% or more of the studies reviewed; "moderately consistent" means that a significant finding was noted in 50–79% of the studies reviewed; and "consistent" means that a significant finding was noted in 30–49% of the studies reviewed.

[c] "Tentative/speculative" results were those that were (1) between 20% and 29% in consistency; (2) based on a very small number of analyses (e.g., *n* = 2); and/or (3) based only on McGrew's exploratory multiple-regression analysis of manifest WJ III variables at the individual test level (see McGrew & Wendling, 2010).

TABLE 26.6. Important Findings on Relations between CHC Abilities and Mathematics Achievement

CHC ability	Flanagan, Ortiz, Alfonso, and Mascolo (2006): General math review[a] (32 independent studies)	McGrew and Wendling (2010): Basic math skills and math reasoning findings[b] (10 CHC/WJ studies)	Comments
Gf	**Induction (I) and general sequential reasoning (RG) abilities are consistently related to math achievement at all ages.**	Quantitative reasoning (RQ) is highly consistent at ages 6–19 years. RG is highly consistent at ages 14–19 years for math reasoning (MR) and consistent at ages 6–19 years for basic math skills (BMS).	Broad Gf is highly consistent at ages 6–13 years and moderately consistent at ages 14–19 years for MR, and moderately consistent at ages 6–19 years for BMS. In McGrew and Wendling's analyses, Induction was part of the RQ tasks and also was subsumed by Gf.
Gc	**Language development (LD), lexical knowledge (VL), and listening abilities (LS) are important. These abilities become increasingly important with age.**	LD and VL are consistent at ages 9–13 years and highly consistent at ages 14–19 years for BMS. LD and VL are consistent at ages 6–8 years, moderately consistent at ages 9–13 years, and highly consistent at ages 14–19 years for MR. LS is consistent at ages 6–8 years and highly consistent at ages 9–19 years for MR. LS is highly consistent for BMS at ages 6–19 years. KO is moderately consistent up to age 13 years and highly consistent at ages 14–19 years for MR only.	The lack of a relationship between LD/VL and BMS at ages 6–8 years in McGrew and Wendling is surprising, as elementary math contains several language concepts (e.g., *less than, greater than, sum, in all, together*). This finding is probably related to the nature of the math tasks used in the studies reviewed. General fund of information (KO) was either not represented or did not demonstrate a consistent relationship with math achievement in the Flanagan et al. review. Broad Gc is moderately consistent at ages 9–19 years for BMS. Broad Gc is consistent at ages 6–8 years, moderately consistent at ages 9–13 years, and highly consistent at ages 14–19 years for MR.
Gsm	**Memory span (MS) is important, especially when evaluated within the context of working memory.**	Working memory (MW) is highly consistent at ages 6–19 years. MS is consistent at ages 6–8 years for MR only.	Broad Gsm is consistent at ages 14–19 years for MR only.
Gv	May be important primarily for higher-level or advanced mathematics (e.g., geometry, calculus).	Spatial scanning (SS) is consistent at ages 6–8 years for BMS only.	Gv abilities related to math achievement are either not measured or not measured adequately by current intelligence batteries. Alternatively, the importance of an adequately measured Gv ability may be masked by the presence of other important variables (e.g., Gc, Gsm) included in the analyses (McGrew & Wendling).

Ga	Phonetic coding (PC) is consistent at ages 6–13 years for BMS. PC is moderately consistent at ages 6–8 years and consistent at ages 9–19 years for MR. Speech sound discrimination and resistance to auditory stimulus distortion (US/UR) are moderately consistent at ages 9–13 years for MR only.	The relationship in the McGrew and Wendling study between PC and BMS reflects the use of WJ Sound Blending as the PC indicator. Memory span is necessary for optimal performance on Sound Blending, which may account for the presence of the relationship.
Glr	Meaningful memory (MM) is moderately consistent at ages 14–19 years for MR. MM is moderately consistent at ages 9–13 years for BMS. Associative memory (MA) is consistent at ages 6–8 years. NA is consistent at ages 6–19 years for BMS only.	MM and MA either were not represented or did not demonstrate a consistent relationship with math achievement in the Flanagan et al. review. The relationship between naming facility (NA) and BMS would probably be more robust if the cognitive task stimuli involved the rapid naming of numbers rather than pictures.
Gs	**Speed of processing (Gs) and, more specifically, perceptual speed (P) are important during all school years, particularly during elementary school.**	In McGrew and Wendling's summary of the relations between Gs and math, P is also described as attention–concentration/executive functioning (AC/EF).
	Broad Gs is moderately consistent at ages 6–13 years and consistent at ages 14–19 years for BMS. Broad Gs is consistent at ages 6–8 years and moderately consistent at ages 9–13 years for MR. AC/EF is consistent at ages 6–8 years for BMS. AC/EF is highly consistent for ages 9–13 and consistent for ages 14–19 years for BMS. P is highly consistent at ages 6–19 years for BMS and moderately consistent at ages 6–19 years for MR.	

Note. For a discussion of the limitations of the findings reported in this table, see McGrew and Wendling (2010).

[a]The absence of comments for a particular CHC ability and achievement area (e.g., Ga and mathematics) in the Flanagan et al. review indicates that the research reviewed either did not report any significant relations between the respective CHC ability and the achievement area, or if significant findings were reported, they were only for a limited number of studies. Comments in bold represent the CHC abilities that demonstrated the strongest and most consistent relationships to mathematics achievement.

[b]Qualitative descriptors of consistency for McGrew & Wendling (2010) analyses were coded as follows: The label "highly consistent" denotes that a significant finding was noted in 80% or more of the studies reviewed; "moderately consistent" denotes that a significant finding was noted in 50–79% of the studies reviewed; and "consistent" denotes that a significant finding was noted in 30–49% of the studies reviewed.

TABLE 26.7. Summary of Findings on Relations between CHC Abilities and Writing Achievement

CHC ability	General writing achievement review
Gf	Induction (I) and general sequential reasoning (RG) abilities are related to basic writing skills primarily during the elementary school years (i.e., ages 6–13 years) and are consistently related to written expression at all ages.
Gc	**Language development (LD), lexical knowledge (VL), and general fund of information (K0) are important primarily after age 7. These abilities become increasingly important with age.**
Gsm	**Memory span (MS) is important to writing, especially spelling skills, whereas working memory has shown relations with advanced writing skills (e.g., written expression).**
Gv	Orthographic processing.
Ga	Phonetic coding (PC) or phonological awareness/processing is very important during the elementary school years for both basic writing skills and written expression (primarily before age 11).
Glr	Naming facility (NA) or rapid automatic naming has demonstrated relations with written expression, primarily the fluency aspect of writing.
Gs	**Perceptual speed (P) is important during all school years for basic writing and is related to written expression at all ages.**

Note. The limited comments for Gv indicates either that the research reviewed did not report any significant relations between that CHC ability and writing achievement, or that if significant findings were reported, they were for only a limited number of studies. Comments in bold represent the CHC abilities that showed the strongest and most consistent relationships to writing achievement. From Flanagan, Ortiz, Alfonso, and Mascolo (2006). Copyright 2006 by John Wiley and Sons. All rights reserved.

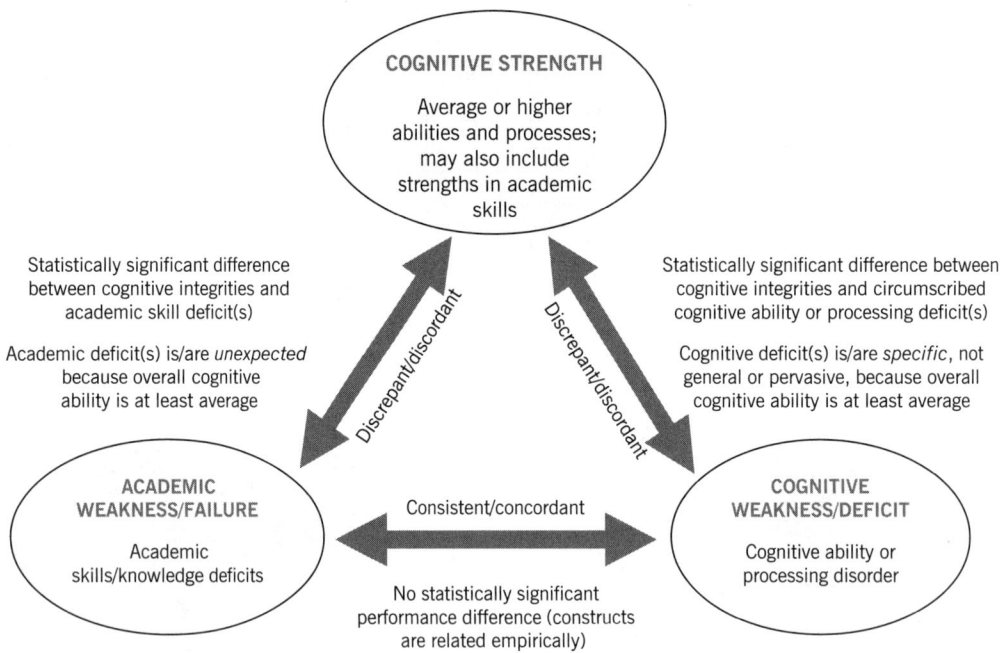

FIGURE 26.4. Common components of "third-method" approaches to SLD identification. Based on Flanagan, Fiorello, and Ortiz (2010) and Hale, Flanagan, and Naglieri (2008).

to be deficient, if not for *specific* cognitive ability or processing weaknesses or deficits. Moreover, because the child has generally average or better overall cognitive ability (depicted by the top oval in Figure 26.4), the academic skill deficiency is indeed unexpected. In sum, the finding of a pattern of circumscribed and related deficits (i.e., below-average cognitive aptitude–achievement consistency) within a generally average or better ability profile is convincing evidence of SLD, particularly when the student who demonstrates this pattern does not respond well to high-quality instruction and when exclusionary factors have been ruled out as the primary causes of the deficits.

Determining an otherwise average (or better) ability profile for a child who has a below-average cognitive aptitude–achievement consistency is not a straightforward task, and there is no agreed-upon method for determining this condition. Nevertheless, there is increasing agreement that a child who meets criteria for SLD has at least some cognitive capabilities that are indeed average or better, as represented in Figure 26.4 (e.g., Berninger, 2011; Fiorello et al., Chapter 20, this volume; Flanagan et al., 2008; Flanagan, Ortiz, & Alfonso, in press; Geary et al., 2011; Hale & Fiorello, 2004; Hale et al., 2010; Kaufman, 2008; Kavale & Flanagan, 2007; Kavale & Forness, 2000; Kavale et al., 2009; Naglieri, 2011). In fact, the earliest recorded definitions of LD were based on clinicians' observations of individuals who experienced considerable difficulties with the acquisition of basic academic skills, despite their average or above-average general intelligence (Kaufman, 2008). Indeed, "all historical approaches to SLD emphasize the spared or intact abilities that stand in stark contrast to the deficient abilities" (Kaufman, 2008, pp. 7–8). When SLD is not differentially diagnosed from other conditions that impede learning, such as ID and low average ability (e.g., slow learning [SL]), the SLD construct loses its meaning, and there is a tendency (albeit well intentioned) to accept anyone under the SLD rubric who has learning difficulties for reasons other than cognitive dysfunction.

When a student does not meet criteria specified in the CHC-based operational definition of SLD, it is possible that the student has SL (i.e., below-average cognitive ability). According to Kavale, Kauffman, Bachmeier, and LeFever (2008, p. 145), "About 14% of the school population may be deemed [to have] SL, but this group does not demonstrate unexpected learning failure, but rather an achievement level consonant with IQ level . . .

slow learn[ing] has never been a special education category, and 'What should not happen is that a designation of SLD be given to a [child with] slow learning' (Kavale, 2005, p. 555)." As such, it seems prudent for practitioners to adhere closely to an operational definition of SLD (or other alternative research-based model), so that SLD can be differentiated from other disorders that also manifest themselves in academic difficulty (Berninger, 2011; Della Toffalo, 2010).

Although it may be some time before consensus is reached on what constitutes "average or better ability" for the purpose of SLD identification, a child who has SLD, generally speaking, ought to be able to perform academically at a level approximating that of his or her more typically achieving peers *when provided with individualized instruction as well as appropriate accommodations, curricular modifications, and the like.* In addition, in order for a child with SLD to reach performances (in terms of both rate of learning and level of achievement) approximating those of his or her nondisabled peers, the child must possess the ability to learn compensatory strategies and apply them independently; this often requires higher-level thinking and reasoning, including intact executive functioning/processing (Maricle & Avirett, Chapter 34, this volume; McCloskey, Perkins, & Van Divner, 2009). Individuals with SLD can minimize or bypass their disabilities under certain circumstances. Special education provides the mechanism to assist a child with SLD in minimizing or bypassing his or her processing deficits through individualized instruction and intervention and through the provision of appropriate adaptations, accommodations, remediation, and compensatory strategies. However, to succeed in minimizing or bypassing the effects of an individual's SLD in the educational setting to the point of achieving at or close to grade level, overall average cognitive or intellectual ability is very likely requisite (see Fuchs & Young, 2006, for a discussion of the mediating effects of IQ on response to intervention). Of course, it is important to understand that while at least average overall cognitive ability is probably necessary for a child with SLD to be successful at minimizing or overcoming his or her cognitive processing deficits, many other factors may facilitate or inhibit academic performance, including motivation, determination, perseverance, familial support, quality of individualized instruction, student–teacher relationships, and existence of comorbid conditions (see Flanagan et al., 2012, for a discussion).

In an attempt to determine whether a child who demonstrates a below-average cognitive aptitude–achievement consistency also has average or better overall cognitive ability, Flanagan and colleagues have developed two programs: the SLD Assistant (Flanagan, Ortiz, & Alfonso, 2007) and the Ability, Aptitude, and RTI Estimator (Flanagan, Ortiz, & Alfonso, 2012). Each program provides a means of parceling out cognitive deficits from global functioning and judging the robustness of the spared abilities or cognitive strengths. These programs are not meant to replace clinical judgment, but rather to inform it. Others have also developed methods and suggested formulae for determining whether individuals have cognitive strengths that are in stark contrast to their cognitive weaknesses (see Fiorello et al., Chapter 20, this volume; Naglieri, 2011). Ultimately, the determination regarding whether or not a child with a below-average cognitive aptitude–achievement consistency has an SLD (and not SL or ID, for example), or exhibits unexpected (not expected) underachievement, must rely to some extent on clinical judgment.[2] Such judgment, however, is bolstered by converging data from multiple sources that were gathered via multiple methods and clinical tools (Flanagan & Alfonso, 2011).

Level V: SLD's Adverse Impact on Educational Performance

When a child meets criteria for an SLD diagnosis (i.e., when criteria for levels I through IV are met), it is typically obvious that the child has difficulties in daily academic activities that need to be addressed. The purpose of this final level of evaluation is to determine whether the identified condition (i.e., SLD) impairs academic functioning to such an extent that special education services are warranted.

Children with SLD require individualized instruction, accommodations, and curricular modifications to varying degrees, based on such factors as the nature of the academic setting, the severity of the SLD, the developmental level of each child, the extent to which each child is able to compensate for specific weaknesses, the manner in which instruction is delivered, the content being taught, and so forth. As such, some children with SLD may not require special education services, such as when their academic needs can be met through classroom-based accommodations (e.g., use of a word bank during writing tasks, extended time on tests) and/or differentiated instruction (e.g., allow-

ing a student with a writing deficit to record reflections on a reading passage and transcribe them outside the classroom prior to submitting a written product). Other children with SLD may require both classroom-based accommodations *and* special education services. And in a case where a child with SLD is substantially impaired in the general education setting, a self-contained special education classroom may be required to meet his or her academic needs adequately.

There are two possible questions at level V that must be answered by the multidisciplinary team (MDT). First, can the child's academic difficulties be remediated, accommodated, or otherwise compensated for without the assistance of individualized special education services? If the answer is yes, then services (e.g., accommodations, curricular modifications) may be provided, and their effectiveness monitored, in the general education setting. If the answer is no, then the MDT must answer the second question: What is the nature and extent of special education services that will be provided to the child? In answering this question, the MDT must ensure that individualized instruction and educational resources are tailored to the child in the least restrictive environment.

Summary of the CHC-Based Operational Definition of SLD

In the preceding paragraphs, we have provided a brief summary of the CHC-based operational definition of SLD. This definition provides a research-based framework for the practice of SLD identification and is likely to be most effective when it is informed continually by cognitive and neuropsychological theory and research that supports (1) the identification and measurement of constructs associated with SLD, (2) the relationships between academic skills and cognitive abilities and processes, and (3) a defensible method of interpreting results. Among the many important components of the definition, we have focused primarily on specifying criteria at the various levels of evaluation that should be met to establish the presence of SLD. These criteria include identification of empirically related academic and cognitive abilities and processes in the below-average range, compared to those of same-age peers from the general population; determination that exclusionary factors are not the primary cause of the identified academic and cognitive deficits; and identification of a pattern of performance consistent with unexpected underachievement, including identification of at least average overall cognitive ability.

When the criteria specified at each level of the operational definition are met, it may be concluded that the data gathered are sufficient to support a diagnosis of SLD in a manner consistent with IDEA 2004 and its attendant regulations, as well as with Kavale et al.'s (2009) definition of SLD. Because the conditions outlined in Figure 26.2 are based on current SLD research, the CHC-based operational definition presented here represents progress toward a more complete and defensible approach to the process of evaluating SLD than previous methods (see also Flanagan, Ortiz, Alfonso, & Dynda, 2006; Hale, Flanagan, & Naglieri, 2008; Kavale, Kaufman, Naglieri, & Hale, 2005; Kavale et al., 2008).

CONCLUSIONS AND FUTURE DIRECTIONS

The operational definition of SLD presented in this chapter is grounded in CHC theory and research, which assists in (1) determining whether specific cognitive ability and/or processing deficits are the probable cause of a student's academic difficulties; (2) distinguishing between SLD and other conditions and disorders (e.g., ID, SL), through both inclusionary and exclusionary criteria; and (3) identifying targets for remediation, compensation, accommodation, and/or curriculum modification (see also Flanagan, Fiorello, & Ortiz, 2010; Flanagan, Ortiz, & Alfonso, 2012). Because the operational definition is informed by the network of validity evidence in support of CHC theory in particular, it has the potential to increase the reliability and validity of SLD identification.

Like other alternative research-based methods to SLD identification, however, the CHC-based operational definition of SLD presented in this chapter must be studied further to determine its reliability and validity. Keogh (2005) has discussed criteria for determining the adequacy and utility of diagnostic systems, such as the ability–achievement discrepancy, RTI, and alternative research-based approaches. These criteria are included in Table 26.8.

Keogh (2005) declares that "LD is real and that it describes problems that are distinct from other conditions subsumed under the broad category of problems in learning and achievement" (p. 101). The question is how best to capture the distinctiveness of SLD. Therefore, we have offered the

TABLE 26.8. Keogh's (2005) Criteria for Determining the Adequacy and Utility of Diagnostic Systems

- Homogeneity (Do category members resemble one another?)[a]
- Reliability (Is there agreement about who should be included in the category?)
- Validity (Does category membership provide consistent information?)

[a]Because individuals with SLD are a *heterogeneous* group, it seems unreasonable to expect that this criterion of an SLD diagnostic system can be met. However, individuals with SLD share a particular set of features, as outlined in Figure 26.2 (i.e., academic skill deficit, cognitive ability or processing weaknesses, cognitive integrities or overall average intellectual ability, statistically significant differences between cognitive strengths and cognitive/academic weaknesses). Thus category members may possess a common set of characteristics (thereby meeting the homogeneity criterion), but may still be heterogeneous in nature (e.g., some have academic deficits in reading, others in math; some have cognitive deficits in phonological processing, others in memory).

CHC-based operational definition for SLD identification. Future directions in SLD identification should focus on evaluating this and other "third-method" approaches according to Keogh's criteria. Until such research is made available, the operational definition presented here remains a viable and inherently practical alternative to the traditional ability–achievement discrepancy method and the RTI-only approach, and it certainly rests on a substantial bed of evidence (derived primarily from the CHC, neuropsychology, assessment, and SLD literature). Indeed, when speaking about his own approach to identifying and intervening with students who have SLD, Della Toffalo (2010) has stated:

> Make no mistake . . . integrated models of identifying (and serving) students with LDs do not arrive prepackaged along with dozens of studies touting their "scientific validation." However, they are evidence-based because they emanate from the marriage of a collective body of knowledge that has been acquired through research in the fields of neuroscience, pedagogy, assessment, and intervention. (pp. 180–181)

Like most alternatives to the discrepancy and RTI-only approaches, the CHC-based operational definition *expands* the methods of assessment available to the practitioner, and culminates in a comprehensive understanding of the child that is clear and of value to all (Flanagan, Fiorello, & Ortiz, 2010). When commenting on their own operational definition as well as Flanagan and colleagues' (2002) definition, Kavale, Holdnack, and Mostert (2005) stated,

> Even if a student never enters the special education system, the general education teacher, the student's parents, and the student him- or herself would receive valuable information regarding *why* there was such a struggle in acquiring academic content, to the point of possibly needing special education. (p. 12; emphasis added)

Not surprisingly, understanding *why* often leads to determining *how*—how to remediate, compensate for, and accommodate weaknesses. As such, it makes practical and clinical sense to gather data from a variety of assessment tools, including cognitive and neuropsychological tests, when students demonstrate an inadequate response to intervention. The developers and supporters of such comprehensive assessment approaches agree on this point (see Hale et al., 2010).

In sum, SLD identification is complex and requires a great deal of empirical and clinical knowledge on the part of practitioners. Although many children's academic needs can be served well in the absence of information garnered from evaluations that include measurement of specific cognitive abilities and processes, there continue to be children whose difficulties warrant this type of comprehensive evaluation. According to Reynolds and Shaywitz (2009b),

> At the current stage of scientific knowledge, it is only through a comprehensive evaluation of a student's cognitive and psychological abilities and processes that insights into the underlying proximal and varied root causes of [academic] difficulties can be ascertained and then specific interventions be provided targeted to each student's individual needs, a process long advocated. (p. 140)

Because of its foundation in CHC theory and research, the operational definition presented here identifies specific targets for remediation, thereby significantly increasing the possibilities for truly individualized intervention (Kavale, Holdnack, & Mostert, 2005). Obscuring the differences between individuals with general cognitive deficiencies (e.g., ID, SL), and those with SLD by adopting simpler methods of identification (e.g., absolute low achievement, RTI-only) interferes with our ability to study these groups and intervene with them more effectively. A greater correspondence between diagnosis and treatment may be achieved

through a more discrete and operational definition of SLD.

ACKNOWLEDGMENT

This chapter is adapted from Flanagan, Alfonso, and Mascolo (2011). Copyright 2011 by John Wiley & Sons, Inc. Adapted by permission.

NOTES

1. Most individuals have statistically significant strengths and weaknesses in their cognitive ability and processing profiles. Intraindividual differences in cognitive abilities and processes are commonplace in the general population (McGrew & Knopik, 1996; Oakley, 2006). Therefore, statistically significant variation in cognitive and neuropsychological functioning in and of itself must not be used as de facto evidence of SLD. Instead, the pattern must reflect what is known about the nature of SLD (see Figure 26.2).

2. Overall average (or better) cognitive ability is difficult to determine in students with SLD because their specific cognitive deficits often attenuate total test scores (e.g., IQ). Therefore, such decisions should be based on multiple data sources and data-gathering methods. For example, a student with an SLD in mathematics may have a below-average WISC-IV Full Scale IQ due to deficits in processing speed and working memory (Geary et al., 2011). However, if the student has an average or better WISC-IV GAI and average or better reading and writing ability, for example, then it is reasonable to assume that this student has at least average cognitive ability. Of course, the more converging data sources that are available to support this conclusion, the more confidence one can place in such a judgment.

REFERENCES

Bateman, B. (1965). An educational view of a diagnostic approach to learning disorders. In J. Hellmuth (Ed.), *Learning disorders* (Vol. 1, pp. 219–239). Seattle, WA: Special Child.

Berninger, V. W. (2011). Evidence-based differential diagnosis and treatment of reading disabilities with and without comorbidities in oral language, writing, and math: Prevention, problem-solving consultation, and specialized instruction. In D. P. Flanagan & V. C. Alfonso (Eds.), *Essentials of specific learning disability identification* (pp. 203–232). Hoboken, NJ: Wiley.

Carroll, J. B. (1993). *Human cognitive abilities: A survey*

of factor-analytic studies. Cambridge, UK: Cambridge University Press.

Della Toffalo, D. A. (2010). Linking school neuropsychology with response-to-intervention models. In D. C. Miller (Ed.), *Best practices in school neuropsychology: Guidelines for effective practice, assessment, and evidence-based intervention* (pp. 159–183). New York: Wiley.

Flanagan, D. P., & Alfonso, V. C. (Eds.). (2011). *Essentials of specific learning disability identification.* Hoboken, NJ: Wiley.

Flanagan, D. P., Alfonso, V. C., & Mascolo, J. T. (2011). A CHC-based operational definition of SLD: Integrating multiple data sources and multiple data-gathering methods. In D. P. Flanagan & V. C. Alfonso (Eds.), *Essentials of specific learning disability identification* (pp. 233–298). Hoboken, NJ: Wiley.

Flanagan, D. P., Alfonso, V. C., Mascolo, J. T., & Hale, J. B. (2011). The Wechsler Intelligence Scale for Children—Fourth Edition in neuropsychological practice. In A. Davis (Ed.), *Handbook of pediatric neuropsychology* (pp. 397–414). New York: Springer.

Flanagan, D. P., Alfonso, V. C., Ortiz, S. O., & Dynda, A. (2010). Integrating cognitive assessment in school neuropsychological evaluations. In D. C. Miller (Ed.), *Best practices in school neuropsychology: Guidelines for effective practice, assessment, and evidence-based intervention* (pp. 101–140). Hoboken, NJ: Wiley.

Flanagan, D. P., Fiorello, C., & Ortiz, S. O. (2010). Enhancing practice through application of Cattell–Horn–Carroll theory and research: A "third method" approach to specific learning disability identification. *Psychology in the Schools, 47,* 739–760.

Flanagan, D. P., & Kaufman, A. S. (2009). *Essentials of WISC-IV assessment* (2nd ed.). Hoboken, NJ: Wiley.

Flanagan, D. P., Kaufman, A. S., Kaufman, N. L., & Lichtenberger, E. O. (2008). *Agora: The marketplace of ideas. Best practices: Applying response to intervention (RTI) and comprehensive assessment for the identification of specific learning disabilities* [6-hour training program/DVD]. Bloomington, MN: Pearson.

Flanagan, D. P., Ortiz, S. O., & Alfonso, V. C. (2007). *Essentials of cross-battery assessment* (2nd ed.). Hoboken, NJ: Wiley.

Flanagan, D. P., Ortiz, S. O., & Alfonso, V. C. (2012). *Essentials of cross-battery assessment* (3rd ed.). Hoboken, NJ: Wiley.

Flanagan, D. P., Ortiz, S. O., Alfonso, V. C., & Dynda, A. (2006). Integration of response-to-intervention and norm-referenced tests in learning disability identification: Learning from the Tower of Babel. *Psychology in the Schools, 43*(7), 807–825.

Flanagan, D. P., Ortiz, S. O., Alfonso, V. C., & Mascolo, J. (2002). *The achievement test desk reference (ATDR):*

Comprehensive assessment and learning disabilities. Boston: Allyn & Bacon.

Flanagan, D. P., Ortiz, S. O., Alfonso, V. C., & Mascolo, J. (2006). *The achievement test desk reference (ATDR): A guide to learning disability identification* (2nd ed.). Hoboken, NJ: Wiley.

Fletcher, J. M., Barth, A. E., & Stuebing, K. K. (2011). A response to intervention (RTI) approach to SLD identification. In D. P. Flanagan & V. C. Alfonso (Eds.), *Essentials of specific learning disability identification* (pp. 115–144). Hoboken, NJ: Wiley.

Fletcher, J. M., Lyon, G. R., Fuchs, L. S., & Barnes, M. A. (2007). *Learning disabilities: From identification to intervention.* New York: Guilford Press.

Fletcher, J. M., Taylor, H. G., Levin, H. S., & Satz, P. (1995). Neuropsychological and intellectual assessment of children. In H. Kaplan & B. Sadock (Eds.), *Comprehensive textbook of psychiatry* (6th ed., pp. 581–601). Baltimore: Williams & Wilkins.

Fletcher-Janzen, E., & Reynolds, C. R. (Eds.). (2008). *Neuropsychological perspectives on learning disabilities in the era of RTI: Recommendations for diagnosis and intervention.* Hoboken, NJ: Wiley.

Fuchs, D., & Young, C. L. (2006). On the irrelevance of intelligence in predicting responsiveness to reading instruction. *Exceptional Children, 73,* 8–30.

Fuchs, L. S., & Fuchs, D. (1998). Treatment validity: A unifying concept for reconceptualizing the identification of learning disabilities. *Learning Disabilities Research and Practice, 13,* 204–219.

Geary, D. C., Hoard, M. K., & Bailey, D. H. (2011). How SLD manifests in mathematics. In D. P. Flanagan & V. C. Alfonso (Eds.), *Essentials of specific learning disability identification* (pp. 43–64). Hoboken, NJ: Wiley.

Hale, J., Alfonso, V., Berninger, V., Bracken, B., Christo, C., Clark, E., et al. (2010). Critical issues in response-to-intervention, comprehensive evaluation, and specific learning disabilities identification and intervention: An expert white paper consensus. *Learning Disability Quarterly, 33,* 223–236.

Hale, J. B., Flanagan, D. P., & Naglieri, J. A. (2008). Alternative research-based methods for IDEA (2004) identification of children with specific learning disabilities. *Communiqué, 36*(8), 1, 14–15.

Hale, J. B., & Fiorello, C. A. (2004). *School neuropsychology: A practitioner's handbook.* New York: Guilford Press.

Hale, J. B., Wycoff, K. L., & Fiorello, C. A. (2011). RTI and cognitive hypothesis testing for identification and intervention of specific learning disabilities: The best of both worlds. In D. P. Flanagan & V. C. Alfonso (Eds.), *Essentials of specific learning disability identification* (pp. 173–201). Hoboken, NJ: Wiley.

Individuals with Disabilities Education Improvement Act of 2004 (IDEA 2004), Pub. L. No. 108-446, 118 Stat. 2647 (2004).

Kaufman, A. S. (2008). Neuropsychology and specific learning disabilities: Lessons from the past as a guide to present controversies and future clinical practice. In E. Fletcher-Janzen & C. Reynolds (Eds.), *Neuropsychological perspectives on learning disabilities in an era of RTI: Recommendations for diagnosis and intervention* (pp. 1–13). Hoboken, NJ: Wiley.

Kavale, K. A. (2005). Identifying specific learning disability: Is responsiveness to intervention the answer? *Journal of Learning Disabilities, 38,* 553–562.

Kavale, K. A., & Flanagan, D. P. (2007). Utility of RTI and assessment of cognitive abilities/processes in evaluation of specific learning disabilities. In S. Jimerson, M. Berns, & A. Van Der Heyden (Eds.), *Handbook of response to intervention: The science and practice of assessment and intervention* (pp. 130–147). New York: Springer.

Kavale, K. A., & Forness, S. R. (2000). What definitions of learning disability say and don't say: A critical analysis. *Journal of Learning Disabilities, 33,* 239–256.

Kavale, K. A., Holdnack, J. A., & Mostert, M. P. (2005). Responsiveness to Intervention and the identification of specific learning disability: A critique and alternative proposal. *Learning Disabilities Quarterly, 28,* 2–16.

Kavale, K. A., Kauffman, J. M., Bachmeier, R. J., & LeFever, G. B. (2008). Response-to-intervention: Separating the rhetoric of self-congratulation from the reality of specific learning disability identification. *Learning Disability Quarterly, 31,* 135–150.

Kavale, K. A., Kaufman, A. S., Naglieri, J. A., & Hale, J. B. (2005). Changing procedures for identifying learning disabilities: The danger of poorly supported ideas. *School Psychologist, 59,* 16–25.

Kavale, K. A., Spaulding, L. S., & Beam, A. P. (2009). A time to define: Making the specific learning disability definition prescribe specific learning disability. *Learning Disability Quarterly, 32,* 39–48.

Keith, T. Z., Fine, J. G., Taub, G. E., Reynolds, M. R., & Kranzler, J. H. (2006). Higher-order, multisample, confirmatory factor analysis of the Wechsler Intelligence Scale for Children—Fourth Edition: What does it measure? *School Psychology Review, 30,* 89–119.

Keogh, B. K. (2005). Revisiting classification and identification. *Learning Disability Quarterly, 28,* 100–102.

Lezak, M. (1995). *Neuropsychological assessment* (3rd ed.). New York: Oxford University Press.

Lichtenberger, E. O., & Breaux, K. C. (2010). *Essentials of WIAT III and KTEA-II assessment.* Hoboken, NJ: Wiley.

Lichtenstein, R., & Klotz, M. B. (2007). Deciphering the Federal Regulations on identifying children with specific learning disabilities. *Communique, 36*(3), 1, 13–16.

Mather, N., & Kaufman, N. (2006). Introduction to the special issue, part one: It's about the what, the how well, and the why. *Psychology in the Schools, 43,* 747–752.

McCloskey, G., Perkins, L. A., & Van Divner, B. (2009). *Assessment and intervention for executive function difficulties.* New York: Routledge.

McGrew, K. S., & Knopik, S. N. (1996). The relationship between intra-cognitive scatter on the Woodcock–Johnson Psycho-Educational Battery—Revised and school achievement. *Journal of School Psychology, 34,* 351–364.

McGrew, K. S., & Wendling, B. (2010). Cattell–Horn–Carroll cognitive–achievement relations: What we have learned from the past 20 years of research. *Psychology in the Schools, 47,* 651–675.

Miller, D. C. (2007). *Essentials of school neuropsychological assessment.* Hoboken, NJ: Wiley.

Miller, D. C. (Ed.). (2010). *Best practices in school neuropsychology: Guidelines for effective practice, assessment, and evidence-based intervention.* Hoboken, NJ: Wiley.

Naglieri, J. A. (2011). The discrepancy/consistency approach to SLD identification using the PASS theory. In D. P. Flanagan & V. C. Alfonso (Eds.), *Essentials of specific learning disability identification* (pp. 145–172). Hoboken, NJ: Wiley.

Oakley, D. (2006). Intra-cognitive scatter on the Woodcock–Johnson Tests of Cognitive Abilities—Third Edition and its relation to academic achievement. *Dissertation Abstracts International, 67,* 1199B.

Ortiz, S. O. (2011). Separating cultural and linguistic differences (CLD) from specific learning disability (SLD) in the evaluation of diverse students: Difference or disorder. In D. P. Flanagan & V. C. Alfonso (Eds.), *Essentials of specific learning disability identification* (pp. 299–325), Hoboken, NJ: Wiley.

Pearson. (2009). *Wechsler Individual Achievement Test—Third Edition (WIAT-III).* San Antonio, TX: Author.

Reynolds, C. R., & Shaywitz, S. A. (2009a). Response to intervention: Prevention and remediation, perhaps. Diagnosis, no. *Child Development Perspectives, 3,* 44–47.

Reynolds, C. R., & Shaywitz, S. A. (2009b). Response to intervention: Ready or not? Or, from wait-to-fail to watch-them-fail. *School Psychology Quarterly, 34,* 130–145.

Siegel, L. S. (1999). Issues in the definition and diagnosis of learning disabilities: A perspective on *Gu-*

ckenberger v. Boston University. Journal of Learning Disabilities, 32, 304–320.

Sotelo-Dynega, M., Flanagan, D. P., & Alfonso, V. C. (2011). Overview of specific learning disabilities. In D. P. Flanagan & V. C. Alfonso (Eds.), *Essentials of specific learning disability identification* (pp. 1–19). Hoboken, NJ: Wiley.

Stanovich, K. E. (1999). The sociopsychometrics of learning disabilities. *Journal of Learning Disabilities, 32,* 350–361.

Swanson, H. L. (1991). Operational definitions and learning disabilities: An overview. *Learning Disability Quarterly, 14*(4), 242–254.

U.S. Department of Education. (2006, August 14). 34 C.F.R. Parts 300 and 301: Assistance to states for the education of children with disabilities and preschool grants for children with disabilities: Final rule. *Federal Register, 71*(156), 46539–46845.

U.S. Office of Education. (1977). Assistance to states for education of handicapped children: Procedures for evaluating specific learning disabilities. *Federal Register, 42*(250), 65082–65085.

Vellutino, F. R., Scanlon, D. M., & Lyon, G. R. (2000). Differentiating between difficult-to-remediate and readily remediated poor readers: More evidence against the IQ–achievement discrepancy definition of reading disability. *Journal of Learning Disabilities, 33,* 223–238.

Wechsler, D. (2003). *Wechsler Intelligence Scale for Children—Fourth Edition.* San Antonio, TX: Psychological Corporation.

Wendling, B., & Mather, N. (2009). *Essentials of evidenced-based academic interventions.* Hoboken, NJ: Wiley.

Zirkel, P. A., & Thomas, L. B. (2010). State laws for RTI: An updated snapshot. *Teaching Exceptional Children, 42*(3), 56–63.

CHAPTER 27

Assessment of Intellectual Functioning in Autism Spectrum Disorder

Laura Grofer Klinger
Sarah E. O'Kelley
Joanna L. Mussey
Sam Goldstein
Melissa DeVries

Even though most of these children were at one time or another looked upon as feebleminded, they are all unquestionably endowed with good cognitive potentialities . . . The astounding vocabulary of the speaking children, the excellent rote memory for events of several years before, the phenomenal rote memory for poems and names, and the precise recollection of complex patterns and sequences, bespeak good intelligence . . .

—KANNER (1943, p. 217)

K anner's (1943) original description of the intellectual abilities of children with autism highlights the juxtaposition of cognitive delays and cognitive strengths that characterize this disorder. Although intellectual evaluations frequently suggest that children with autism are developmentally delayed, these children often have some peaks in their abilities. This combination of strengths and weaknesses creates an uneven profile of cognitive abilities, which presents a conundrum for psychologists trying to decide which IQ test to administer to individuals with autism.

The goal of this chapter is to provide a set of guidelines for deciding which intelligence test may be the most appropriate for evaluating a child with autism spectrum disorder (ASD). The term ASD is a relatively new term meant to convey the heterogeneity or "spectrum" of symptom presentation

and cognitive functioning in individuals with this diagnosis. The proposed *Diagnostic and Statistical Manual of Mental Disorders*, fifth edition (DSM-5; *www.dsm5.org*) uses the term ASD to replace the previous DSM-IV term of pervasive developmental disorder (PDD; American Psychiatric Association, 1994). This new concept of autism as a spectrum diagnosis emphasizes the importance of assessing severity as part of the diagnosis. Indeed, DSM-5 will require a severity specifier when making a diagnosis. The child's level of cognitive or intellectual functioning will be an important component of making this determination. However, there is no "best test" for measuring intellectual functioning in such children. Instead, the psychologist must consider the reasons why an intellectual evaluation is being requested for this particular individual; the literature on intellectual strengths and weaknesses in ASD; the unique social, communication, and behavioral symptoms of ASD that may interfere with intellectual testing; and the specific properties of the intellectual tests being considered.

OVERLAP BETWEEN ASD AND INTELLECTUAL DISABILITY

In his review of 36 epidemiological studies published between 1966 and 2003, Fombonne (2005) reported that the median rate of intellectual disability in individuals diagnosed with autism was 70.4% (range 40–100%). Across these studies, 29.3% of individuals were reported to have mild to moderate intellectual disability, and 38.5% were reported to have severe to profound intellectual disability. More recent studies, however, suggest that the rates of intellectual disability in persons with ASD are considerably lower, with rates ranging from 40% to 71% for individuals diagnosed with DSM-IV-defined autistic disorder and 6% to 49% for individuals diagnosed with pervasive developmental disorder not otherwise specified (PDD-NOS) or Asperger's disorder (see Fombonne, 2005, for a review). A population-based epidemiological study similarly showed lower rates of intellectual disability, with 55% of children with all ASDs receiving IQ scores within the range of intellectual disability (Baird et al., 2006). These lower rates could be a result of a broadening of the DSM diagnostic criteria to include diagnoses such as Asperger's disorder in the fourth edition (which, by definition, does not have a dual diagnosis of intellectual disability) and/or could be a result of more effective early intervention. Regardless of why the rates of comorbid diagnoses of ASD and intellectual disability are decreasing, there is a growing need for intellectual assessments that are appropriate for children with ASD across a wide range of ability.

Lower IQ scores have been associated with both gender and the presence of comorbid medical conditions. Females with autism tend to receive lower scores on both verbal and nonverbal measures of intelligence (Volkmar, Szatmari, & Sparrow, 1993). Volkmar and colleagues (1993) reported that proportionately more females with autism scored in the range of severe intellectual disability (IQ below 35) and that males with autism were 8.8 times more likely to receive scores indicating average intelligence. The prevalence rate of seizure disorders in persons with ASD ranges from 11% to 39% (see Ballaban-Gil & Tuchman, 2000, for a review). Individuals with ASD and a comorbid seizure disorder are more likely to have intellectual disability.

PROFILE OF COGNITIVE STRENGTHS AND WEAKNESSES IN ASD

Traditionally, it has been believed that individuals with ASD have a specific profile of intellectual ability characterized by a higher nonverbal IQ than verbal IQ (Lincoln, Allen, & Kilman, 1995; see Lincoln, Hansel, & Quirmbach, 2007, for a review). For example, individuals with ASD have frequently shown relative and absolute strengths on nonverbal visual–spatial tasks involving puzzles and arranging patterns or blocks into designs (e.g., Ghaziuddin & Mountain-Kimchi, 2004; Lincoln et al., 1995; Mayes & Calhoun, 2008; Ozonoff, South, & Miller, 2000). However, this profile has not received uniform support in the literature (Ehlers et al., 1997; Siegel, Minshew, & Goldstein, 1996; Venter, Lord, & Schopler, 1992). Mayes and Calhoun (2003) examined intellectual profiles of 164 children with autism across a wide chronological age range (3–15 years) and range of intellectual functioning (IQ scores of 14–143). In their sample, the profile of greater nonverbal than verbal IQ was present in preschool children, but gradually disappeared during the school-age years. Children with IQ scores above 80 displayed an even pattern of verbal and nonverbal abilities by 6–7 years of age. Children with IQ scores below 80 maintained a greater nonverbal than verbal IQ through the preschool years and did not show similar verbal and nonverbal scores until 9–10 years of age. Thus discrepancies between verbal and nonverbal IQ scores are related to both age and IQ and, contrary to prevailing beliefs, no single pattern is indicative of an ASD diagnosis. Instead, patterns may be present for specific IQ tests.

REFERRAL QUESTIONS FOR INTELLECTUAL TESTING IN ASD

There are several different reasons for evaluating developmental and intellectual abilities in individuals with ASD, including (1) as part of a diagnostic battery to determine whether an ASD is present; (2) as part of an educational battery to evaluate the strengths and weaknesses that should be targeted by a child's individualized education program; (3) as a measure of treatment effectiveness; and (4) as one means of estimating long-term prognosis.

Diagnostic Assessment

Intellectual testing is a recommended part of an interdisciplinary diagnostic evaluation for ASD (Filipek et al., 1999; Johnson, Myers, & the Council on Children with Disabilities, 2007). Klin, Saulnier, Tsatsanis, and Volkmar (2005) described developmental testing for infants and preschool-age children, and intellectual assessment for school-age children and older, as a "frame" for interpreting the results of diagnostic testing. This frame can be used to evaluate whether a child's social and communicative delays are greater than expected from the child's developmental level or whether they are equivalent to the child's developmental level. In order for a child to receive a diagnosis of ASD, social and communicative skills must be delayed below developmental level. For example, if a developmental evaluation indicates that a 4-year-old child has the cognitive development of a 2-year-old, then the child's social and communication skills (e.g., eye contact, pointing, symbolic play, reciprocal interactions, affect) should be compared to the skills expected of a 2-year-old. If a discrepancy between developmental level and social communication skills is not present, then diagnoses of developmental delay or language disorder should be considered.

Assessment of Current Strengths and Weaknesses

Intellectual testing is often helpful in clarifying the specific strengths and weaknesses present in an individual child and to highlight the areas that need to be addressed by intervention. Klin and colleagues (2005) recommended that intellectual assessment should

> describe patterns of both verbal and nonverbal functioning across several domains: (1) problem solving (e.g., can the child generate strategies and integrate information?), (2) concept formation (e.g., can the child abstract rules from specific instances or understand principles of categorization, order, time, number, and causation, and generalize knowledge from one context to another?), (3) reasoning (e.g., can the child transform information to solve visual-perceptual and verbal problems?), (4) style of learning (e.g., can the child learn from modeling, imitation, using visual cues, or verbal prompts?), and (5) memory skills (e.g., how many items of information

> can the child retain; . . . are the child's memory skills in one modality better than in another such as visual or verbal?). (Klin et al., 2005, p. 777)

This assessment of strengths and weaknesses is especially important, given the uneven profile of cognitive skills that typically characterizes a child with ASD.

Assessment of Intervention Effectiveness

Although IQ scores are commonly used as a measure of treatment effectiveness, there are many cautions involved in using IQ testing for this purpose. Importantly, the use of the same IQ test on multiple occasions raises concerns about possible practice effects and concerns about whether the testing is developmentally appropriate at both testing points. For example, a developmental test such as the Bayley Scales of Infant and Toddler Development, Third Edition (Bayley-III; Bayley, 2005) may be appropriate for a 2-year-old beginning intervention, but would no longer be appropriate for a 4-year-old at the conclusion of intervention. However, if different tests are administered at pre- and posttreatment, it is unclear whether gains are due to testing error or to the different social and communication requirements of the two tests, or whether a true increase in development or IQ has occurred. Even when the same test is administered at both time points, there are concerns that the items may measure different skills at different ages. For example, an instrument may include measures of social skills (playing peek-a-boo, reading a book with the examiner) for infants and toddlers that may not be a component of the same test at older ages. In this example, earlier low scores could partially be attributed to the child's social rather than intellectual delays.

Despite these cautions, changes in cognitive abilities are considered a hallmark of effective interventions; this is especially true of early intervention programs, where the goal is often to facilitate inclusion in regular education kindergarten classrooms (e.g., Eikeseth, Smith, Jahr, & Eldevik, 2007; Lovaas, 1987; Smith, Groen, & Wynn, 2000). The National Research Council (NRC) Committee on Educational Interventions for Children with Autism (2001) has stated that although intellectual testing provides useful information in measuring treatment effectiveness, this type of testing is not sufficient and should not be used as the sole measure of treatment outcome.

Predictions of Long-Term Outcome

IQ testing is often used as a prognostic indicator of long-term outcome for children and adolescents with ASD. Indeed, scores in children with ASD are considered to be as stable as IQ scores in children with other forms of developmental disabilities (NRC, 2001). However, this does not mean that IQ scores are stable across the lifespan. Mayes and Calhoun (2003) reported that in their sample of 164 children (ages 3–15) with ASD, the average IQ score increased from 53 for children 3 years of age to 91 for children 8 years of age or older. For children with IQ scores below 80, both verbal and nonverbal IQ scores increased. For children with IQ scores greater than or equal to 80, only verbal IQ increased significantly with age. After 8 years of age, both verbal IQ and nonverbal IQ were relatively stable. Because this was a cross-sectional study, it is possible that the increase in IQ can be attributed to the fact that lower-functioning children are evaluated at a younger age, whereas higher-functioning children are not seen until school age. However, longitudinal studies have also reported some significant improvement in IQ, particularly when comparing preschool performance to school-age performance (Sigman & McGovern, 2005) and when focusing on children with high-functioning autism (Freeman, Ritvo, Needleman, & Yokota, 1985). Less improvement has been observed in children with both autism and intellectual disability (Lord & Schopler, 1989). This significant change in IQ scores from early to middle childhood suggests that low IQ scores in early childhood do not necessarily predict later outcome.

However, more stability in IQ scores has been reported from middle childhood to adolescence and adulthood (Beadle-Brown, Murphy, & Wing, 2006; Howlin, Goode, Hutton, & Rutter, 2004; Seltzer, Shattuck, Abbeduto, & Greensberg, 2004; Sigman & McGovern, 2005). In Sigman and McGovern's (2005) longitudinal study of IQ in a sample of 48 individuals with autism, 74% of participants showed stable IQ between middle childhood and adolescence and early adulthood. Notably, 21% of their sample showed a significant decrease in IQ scores (i.e., a loss of 10 or more points). This decrease during adolescence may be due to a failure to make gains rather than a regression in skills. This stability in IQ scores from middle childhood to adolescence and early adulthood suggests that IQ scores may assist in predicting long-term cognitive ability and outcome.

Howlin and colleagues (2004) conducted a long-term follow-up study on 68 individuals seen initially at an average age of 7 years and followed until the average age of 29 years. All participants were required to have an initial IQ score of 50 or greater, to ensure that long-term outcome was not confounded with severe intellectual disability. Among the 45 children receiving IQ scores greater than or equal to 70 at the initial assessment, 78% remained in this range of intellectual functioning during adulthood. Furthermore, this higher-functioning group was more likely to live independently, although outcome varied considerably in this group. Those with initial IQ scores between 50 and 69 appeared to have a much poorer prognosis in terms of independent living, education attainment, employment, and friendships. Howlin et al. concluded that "only individuals with an IQ in the normal range (70+) have a real chance of living independently as they reach adulthood" (p. 225). Other follow-up studies from middle childhood to adulthood (Beadle-Brown et al., 2006; see Seltzer et al., 2004, for a review) have reported similar findings indicating that IQ is a good predictor of long-term educational attainment, communication skills, and independent living skills.

Taken together, these studies suggest that IQ scores may be an important predictor of long-term outcome in terms of cognitive functioning and independent living skills once a child reaches middle childhood. Thus an IQ test will be an important component of an assessment battery designed to estimate long-term prognosis in older children and adolescents with ASD.

DEVELOPMENTAL AND BEHAVIORAL ISSUES IN ASSESSING CHILDREN WITH ASD

Successful performance on an IQ test requires the ability to sit and attend to another person's instructions. However, children with ASD have difficulty with attention, social interaction, and language understanding. Thus the traditional standardized assessment paradigm is often a challenge for children with ASD (and for the examiner trying to administer the test). At a minimum, the examiner should have experience administering intellectual assessments to children and have some knowledge about how the symptoms of ASD may interfere with test administration and performance. Ideally, the examiner will have experience interacting with individuals with ASD. An understanding of the symptoms and treatment approaches for ASD will assist the examiner in choosing an appropriate test and structuring the testing session to ensure that the child's performance is representative of his or her true abilities.

Developmental Issues in IQ Assessment

It is important for an examiner to consider a child's chronological and mental age when choosing and administering an IQ test. This is particularly important when the child has significant developmental delays (i.e., there is a wide discrepancy between chronological and mental age). Such a child is likely to receive the lowest standard score provided by an assessment instrument. When this happens, it is difficult to translate the score into a meaningful description of the child's current ability. For example, if an IQ score of 50 is the lowest standard score provided by the assessment instrument, it is impossible to know whether the child's IQ is truly in this moderate range of intellectual disability, or whether a test with a wider range of standard scores would indicate severe or profound disability.

For an older child with significant developmental delays, it will be more appropriate to administer a test with a wider age range that will accommodate the child's level of delay. For example, a 12-year-old who is functioning at a 4-year-old level will probably be unable to complete any items on a test designed for elementary-school-age children, but may be able to perform some of the simpler tasks on a test designed for ages that span the preschool and elementary school years. For a young child, it may be more useful to consider the child's mental age (by calculating age equivalents) than to focus on a standard score (Akshoomoff, 2006). A focus on mental age equivalents in young children has several advantages. First, it highlights a focus on current developmental level rather than IQ. This is particularly important for young children with ASD, as the research discussed above on the stability of IQ in children with ASD suggests that such children can show large improvements in IQ scores from the preschool to elementary school years. Thus the use of a mental age score provides information about current ability without implying permanent intellectual disability. Second, the use of mental age equivalents may be more meaningful to caregivers or teachers, as they provide an estimate of developmentally appropriate academic, behavioral, and adaptive expectations. For example, it would be developmentally

inappropriate to expect a 3½-year-old child who is functioning at the 15-month level to learn to write his or her name, be toilet-trained, or understand the link between actions and time-out as a discipline technique.

Finally, when a child with significant developmental delays is tested, Akshoomoff (2006) recommends allowing caregivers to observe developmental testing and provide feedback about whether the child seemed to be performing to the best of his or her abilities. Allowing parents to observe and provide their opinions is helpful in preparing the parents for the feedback meeting. Parents who feel that their child showed his or her best skills during tests are more likely to accept estimates of developmental level or IQ as accurate representations of their child's current abilities.

Interference of ASD Symptoms

Children with ASD have more difficulty on tests involving the use of social and language skills, and less difficulty on nonverbal tasks that do not require speed or motor skills (NRC, 2001). More specifically, tests requiring skills that are specifically impaired in ASD—including attending to social information (Dawson et al., 2004), imitation (Rogers, Hepburn, Stackhouse, & Wehner, 2003), joint attention (Sigman, Mundy, Sherman, & Ungerer, 1986), and understanding of personal pronouns—are likely to produce lower scores than tests requiring skills that are often strengths in individuals with ASD (e.g., perception, rote memory). This is particularly evident when very young children with ASD (i.e., children ages 2–4 years) are tested. For example, young children with ASD may have difficulty completing tasks that assess the ability to play reciprocal social games (e.g., peek-a-boo), the ability to use an index finger to point to objects, the ability to imitate the examiner's actions, and the ability to understand directions that use the pronouns "I" and "you."

Akshoomoff (2006) reported that young children with ASD spent significantly less time attending to tasks as they were being presented and significantly more time in off-task behaviors, including leaving their seats or whining and crying. Furthermore, Askhoomoff found that scores on the Mullen Scales of Early Learning (Mullen, 1995) were positively correlated with engagement and negatively correlated with off-task behavior. Akshoomoff hypothesized that this relationship was a reflection both of poor cooperation and attention to the tasks (i.e., behavioral regulation problems) and of task demands that were related to the core symptoms of ASD. For example, she noted that both imitation and pointing skills are required for several of the Mullen subtests. Similarly, other tests designed for this age group (e.g., the Bayley-III and the Stanford–Binet Intelligence Scales, Fifth Edition [SB5]) include items that involve these types of skills. Although it may be impossible to find a test that does not involve these social and communication skills, the examiner should be aware of which tasks are likely to be particularly difficult for a child with ASD.

MEASURES OF INTELLECTUAL FUNCTIONING

Clinicians and researchers have a number of tools available for assessing the developmental level and intellectual ability of individuals with ASD. Some of these measures included children with ASD in the standardization sample, although inclusion criteria for each measure may have differed. Other measures did not specifically include children with ASD during standardization; however, children with ASD were not explicitly excluded, according to the norming criteria provided in the technical manuals.

Bayley Scales of Infant and Toddler Development, Third Edition

The Bayley-III (Bayley, 2005) measures the strengths and abilities of children from 1–42 months of age in the areas of Cognitive, Motor, Language, Social-Emotional, and Adaptive Behavior. Composite standard scores are available for each area assessed. Depending on a child's age, the Bayley-III can be administered in approximately 30–90 minutes. Administration time for the entire battery is approximately 50 minutes for children ages 12 months and younger, and approximately 90 minutes for children ages 13 months and older.

During standardization, data were collected on a group of 70 children between the ages of 16 and 42 months who met DSM-IV criteria for a pervasive developmental disorder (PDD), including autistic disorder, Asperger's disorder, Rett's disorder, childhood disintegrative disorder, and PDD-NOS. On the Bayley-III, the children with PDD obtained significantly lower scores on all subtest scales (Cognitive, Receptive Communication, Expressive Communication, Fine Motor, Gross Motor, and Social-Emotional) and composite measures (Language and Motor) than did children in the age-matched control group.

The Bayley-III is one of the few standardized instruments that are available to evaluate young children with significant developmental delays who would not meet basal requirements on most preschool instruments, resulting in an inability to calculate meaningful standard scores. The Bayley-III was extended upward to include 3½-year-old children; thus it is a good choice for testing a 2- or 3-year-old who is functioning below the 24-month level of development. However, a standard score of 50 is the lowest score provided by the Bayley-III, making it impossible to get a specific standard score for extremely delayed children and necessitating the use of age equivalent scores. The Bayley-III can also be administered to a child older than 42 months to estimate the child's developmental level (i.e., to obtain an age equivalent) if other measures are inappropriate due to a low mental age. However, these results must be interpreted cautiously, as a standard score cannot be computed.

Mullen Scales of Early Learning

The Mullen Scales of Early Learning (Mullen, 1995) battery is designed to measure cognitive functioning in children from birth through 68 months of age. This instrument assesses a child's Gross Motor, Fine Motor, Visual Reception, Receptive Language, and Expressive Language abilities. Each of the individual scales yields T scores (mean = 50) and age equivalents. The Mullen also provides an overall Early Learning Composite standard score, which is based on the standardized T scores from the four cognitive scales (Visual Reception Scale, Fine Motor Scale, Receptive Language Scale, and Expressive Language Scale). The amount of time necessary to administer the Mullen varies between approximately 15 and 60 minutes, depending on a child's age, with older children requiring more time. During standardization of the Mullen, children who had known physical or mental disabilities (including ASD) were not included in the sample.

Several recent studies have used the Mullen to test young children with ASD (Akshoomoff, 2006; Landa & Garrett-Mayer, 2006). The Mullen was used to examine the early development of children at high risk for ASD at 6, 14, and 24 months of age in a prospective study conducted by Landa and Garrett-Mayer (2006). They compared children showing clinical symptoms of ASD, language delay, and no impairment. By 14 months of age, children in the ASD symptom group were delayed in all areas except the Visual Reception domain, compared to children in the no impairment group. In addition, the children with ASD symptoms showed higher Visual Reception scores than Receptive Language scores. This is consistent with the intellectual profile research described earlier, indicating that preschool children with ASD show a strength in visual spatial processing and a weakness in verbal processing. Nearly half of the group with ASD symptoms showed decreasing composite scores between 14 and 24 months, suggesting that this is a particularly vulnerable developmental period for children with ASD. It is difficult to know whether this indicates a true decline, whether children were experiencing a plateau in skill development leading to lower standard scores, or whether task demands at 24 months involved skills that are more specifically impaired in children with ASD.

Akshoomoff (2006) compared Mullen scores in children with ASD (ages 16–43 months) and an age-matched group of children with typical development (Akshoomoff, 2006). Children with ASD had significantly lower standard scores on every scale. In addition, the children with ASD performed relatively better on the Fine Motor scale and relatively worse on the Receptive Language scale, again supporting a specific weakness in verbal processing in young children with ASD.

Like the Bayley-III, the Mullen is one of the few standardized instruments that are available to evaluate young children with significant developmental delays who would not meet basal requirements on most preschool assessment instruments. The Mullen is appropriate for children up to 5½ years of age, and thus is a good choice for testing preschool-age children with significant delays. Because the Mullen covers the entire preschool age range, it is also a good choice for early intervention studies examining change across the preschool years. However, even with this range, 73% of children with ASD in Akshoomoff's (2006) study received the lowest standard score (a T score of 20) provided by the Mullen on one or more scale. A T score of 20 is more than three standard deviations below average and represents an overall standard score of 55 or below. In this situation, age equivalents may be a more appropriate way to interpret test performance (Akshoomoff, 2006).

Differential Ability Scales—Second Edition

The Differential Ability Scales—Second Edition (DAS-II; Elliott, 2007, see Elliott, Chapter 13, this volume) is a brief but comprehensive measure of ability, which makes it attractive for use with individuals with ASD. The DAS-II is designed to measure cognitive strengths and weaknesses in individuals between the ages of 2 years, 6 months and 17 years, 11 months (2:6–17:11). The Early Years battery, which was labeled the Preschool level in the original DAS (Elliott, 1990), consists of a Lower Level (four subtests for ages 2:6–3:5 that take approximately 20 minutes to administer) and an Upper Level (six subtests for ages 3:6–6:11 that take approximately 30 minutes to administer). The School-Age battery consists of six subtests for individuals ages 7:0–17:11 that take approximately 40 minutes to administer. Testing at each level of the DAS-II yields a General Conceptual Ability (GCA) composite score. For the Early Years Lower Level battery, cluster scores for Verbal and Nonverbal ability are also calculated. For both the Early Years Upper Level and the School-Age batteries, cluster scores for Verbal, Nonverbal Reasoning, and Spatial ability are calculated. In addition, for children age 3:6 or older, a Special Nonverbal Composite (SNC) may be derived from the appropriate nonverbal core subtests from each battery, which may be a useful measure of cognitive ability for nonverbal individuals with ASD. For individuals between the ages of 5:0 and 8:11, examiners have the option of administering the Early Years battery "out of level" for children with significant intellectual disability. The DAS-II provides standard scores and age equivalents even for children tested within this extended age range for the Early Years battery. This is particularly useful for assessment of individuals with ASD, as it allows for more accurate assessment based on these individuals' mental age rather than their chronological age. Additional diagnostic subtests that measure working memory, processing speed, and school readiness are also available for individuals of different ages for the DAS-II.

Unlike most other cognitive assessment instruments, the DAS-II does not require a strict administration order for its subtests, which allows the testing session to be individualized for each examinee. For example, it may be of benefit to begin with a nonverbal task for individuals with ASD, to build rapport and familiarity with the testing environment. Examiners may also choose to begin with a subtest that overlaps both batteries, such as the Pattern Construction subtests, in order to observe and estimate informally an examinee's level of functioning (e.g., receptive and expressive language, cognitive flexibility) to guide in selection of the most appropriate test battery (i.e., choosing either the Early Years or School-Age level, or only administering tasks that yield the SNC).

Because individuals with ASD were not included in the standardization samples, no information is available regarding specific profiles of individuals with ASD. Furthermore, given the newness of the DAS-II, no research studies are available regarding its utility with individuals with ASD at this time. Joseph, Tager-Flusberg, and Lord (2002) administered the original DAS (Elliott, 1990) to 120 individuals with autism who were considered high-functioning (i.e., mean GCA was 76.7 and 84.5 for the Preschool and School-Age levels of the DAS, respectively) in an exploration of cognitive profiles and symptomatology in ASD. A profile of higher nonverbal than verbal abilities was observed in 48% of the preschool-age group and 34% of the school-age group of children; this is consistent with research discussed above showing nonverbal–verbal discrepancies in preschool children with ASD. In comparison, a profile of higher verbal than nonverbal abilities was observed in 8% of preschool-age children and 28% of school-age children.

Overall, the DAS-II offers the opportunity to identify a child's specific strengths and weaknesses; is appropriate across a wide chronological and mental age range; and has some flexibility in test administration, which is helpful when testing children with ASD. Because of the large age range, the DAS-II may be a good choice for intervention studies that will use IQ testing as one measure of outcome across an extended period of time. The DAS-II is particularly useful for testing children up to age 8:11 who have significant intellectual disability because of the option to administer the Early Years battery. It is less useful for children over 9 years of age who are functioning at the preschool level. The DAS-II is also less useful for testing young children with ASD who are performing below the 2½-year level, as they are unlikely to meet basal requirements on most subtests, resulting in an inability to calculate meaningful standard scores.

Stanford–Binet Intelligence Scales, Fifth Edition

The SB5 (Roid, 2003; see Roid & Pomplun, Chapter 10, this volume) assesses intelligence and cognitive abilities in individuals ages 2–85+ years. To obtain a Full Scale IQ (FSIQ), the SB5 requires an average 45–75 minutes of testing time. The SB5 also contains separate Nonverbal IQ (based on five

Nonverbal subtests) and Verbal IQ (based on five Verbal subtests) sections, which can be useful for testing individuals with ASD who are nonverbal or have limited language abilities. Each of these sections requires approximately 30 minutes. In addition, five factor scores can be computed (Fluid Reasoning, Knowledge, Quantitative Reasoning, Visual–Spatial Processing, and Working Memory), which can be used to identify a pattern of strengths and weaknesses in performance. Each factor score includes a Verbal and a Nonverbal subtest. Finally, an Abbreviated Battery IQ can be calculated from two subtests if necessary. This is often helpful when a child is displaying difficulty attending to task demands and the examiner is concerned about being able to complete the lengthier full battery of tests. The SB5 revision was designed to make the test more sensitive to assessing younger children with developmental delays than the previous version.

The SB5 standardization sample included 83 children and adolescents with diagnoses of autistic disorder between the ages of 2 and 17 years. This sample included 79% males and was predominantly European American. Individuals with autistic disorder performed similarly to those in the developmental delay group, but had slightly lower means on all subtest and composite scales. Although no studies to date have examined a specific pattern of subtest performance on the SB5 in children with ASD, several studies have examined the performance of children with ASD on the fourth edition of the Stanford–Binet (SB-IV; Carpentieri & Morgan, 1994; Harris, Handleman, & Burton, 1990; Mayes & Calhoun, 2003). Overall, children with ASD were found to be more impaired on SB-IV verbal reasoning tasks (especially the Absurdities task, which requires social comprehension and reasoning) than on nonverbal reasoning tasks (such as Pattern Analysis, Bead Memory, and Quantitative Reasoning, which involve visual perception skills). Children with autism demonstrated delays in verbal reasoning that were significantly greater than those of chronological-age-matched children with intellectual disability (Carpentieri & Morgan, 1994).

Because of its wide age range, the SB5 may be an appropriate measure for testing a child with significant developmental delays (e.g., a 10-year-old child with the mental age of a preschool child) who might not meet basal requirements on tests that are solely developed for school-age children. In addition, the SB5 may be a good choice for intervention studies that will use IQ testing as one measure of outcome across an extended period of time. Although the SB5's Nonverbal IQ score may be appropriate for children with limited language, some of the Nonverbal tasks require imitation and receptive language skills, which are both areas of weakness in children with ASD. For example, the Nonverbal Working Memory task requires the child to imitate the examiner's motor movements by tapping a series of blocks. At a more sophisticated level, the child is asked to imitate the examiner's movements in reverse order; this requires that the child understand the verbal directions to do so. Thus the Nonverbal measures on the SB5 are not completely independent of language understanding and can be negatively affected by symptoms of ASD.

Kaufman Assessment Battery for Children—Second Edition

The Kaufman Assessment Battery for Children—Second Edition (KABC-II; Kaufman & Kaufman, 2004; see also Kaufman Singer et al., Chapter 11, this volume) is a measure of intelligence and achievement for use with individuals ages 3–18 years. It was developed to be a culturally fair assessment to evaluate minority groups and children with learning disabilities, and is used in educational planning and placement decisions, neuropsychological assessment, and research. Administration of the KABC-II takes between 35 and 85 minutes. Global test scores include a Mental Processing Index (if the Luria model, which measures mental processing in the absence of verbal ability, for test interpretation, which includes measures of verbal ability, is chosen) or a Fluid–Crystallized Index (if the Cattell–Horn–Carroll model is chosen). A supplemental Nonverbal Index is also provided.

The utility of the KABC-II as a measure of intellectual function in children with ASD has not yet been formally evaluated. However, the original version, the K-ABC (Kaufman & Kaufman, 1983), has been examined in children with ASD. Freeman, Lucas, Forness, and Ritvo (1985) used the K-ABC to evaluate 6- to 12-year-old children with autism. Similar to performance on other IQ tests, children with autism demonstrated a distinct and uneven pattern of cognitive development. In contrast, however, Stavrou and French (1992) proclaimed support for the usefulness of the K-ABC as a measure of general intelligence in children (ages 5–12 years) with autism because their performance was not significantly different from that of their peers with typical development. Because of its large age range, the KABC-II may be particularly

useful for elementary-age children and adolescents with ASD who have significant intellectual disabilities.

Wechsler Preschool and Primary Scale of Intelligence—Third Edition

The Wechsler Preschool and Primary Scale of Intelligence—Third Edition (WPPSI-III; Wechsler, 2002; see also Wahlstrom, Breaux, Zhu, & Weiss, Chapter 9, this volume;) is designed to assess intelligence in children ages 2:6 through 7:3. For younger children (ages 2:6–3:11), the WPPSI-III yields a Verbal IQ, a nonverbal Performance IQ, an overall FS IQ, and an optional supplemental General Language Composite. The core subtests can be completed in 25–35 minutes for this age group. For older children (ages 4:0–7:3), the WPPSI-III yields a Verbal IQ, a Performance IQ, an FSIQ, and an optional supplemental Processing Speed Quotient. For older children, the core subtests can be completed in approximately 40–50 minutes.

To determine the clinical utility of the WPPSI-III, a group of 21 children between the ages of 3:0 and 6:11 who met DSM-IV criteria for autistic disorder were included in the standardization sample. This group of children contained more males than females, to reflect the higher prevalence rate of autistic disorder in males. Children were excluded from this group if they had existing overall cognitive ability scores more than 2.67 standard deviations below the mean. On all composites, children in the autistic disorder group scored significantly lower than the matched control group. The children with autistic disorder obtained higher mean Performance IQ scores than Verbal IQ scores. Scaled scores on all subtests, except for the Block Design and Object Assembly subtests, were lower for the children in the autistic disorder group than the control group.

Because the WPPSI-III provides both Verbal and Performance IQ scores, it offers an opportunity to identify a pattern of strengths and weaknesses in children with ASD. However, some of the Performance IQ tasks require language understanding, and thus the Performance IQ score is not completely independent of a child's language delays. The WPPSI-III was extended to include both younger preschool-age children and older children entering elementary school, making it appropriate for beginning school-age children who have significant developmental delays. However, the WPPSI-III is less useful for testing 2- and 3-year-old children with ASD who are performing below the 2½-year level as they are unlikely to meet basal requirements on most subtests, resulting in an inability to calculate meaningful standard scores.

Wechsler Intelligence Scale for Children—Fourth Edition

The Wechsler Intelligence Scale for Children—Fourth Edition (WISC-IV; Wechsler, 2003; see also Wahlstrom et al., Chapter 9, this volume) is designed to assess intelligence in children ages 6:0–16:11. It assesses intelligence in the cognitive domains of Verbal Comprehension, Perceptual Reasoning, Working Memory, and Processing Speed, as well as providing a composite FSIQ score of general intellectual ability. The amount of time required to administer the WISC-IV varies, depending on the number of subtests administered to a child, but administration of the 10 core subtests can be completed within approximately 65–80 minutes. During standardization testing, 182 children ages 6–7 were given both the WISC-IV and the WPPSI-III. There was less than a 1-point difference between the two tests on the corresponding index and FSIQ scores (Wechsler, 2003). Thus the WISC-IV may be a good choice for reevaluating a child who has previously been given the WPPSI-III.

A sample of 19 children between the ages of 7 and 16 years who met DSM-IV criteria for autistic disorder were included in the standardization sample. This sample included 89% males, and all children had an IQ score above 60. Compared to a matched control group of children, the children in the autistic disorder group scored significantly lower on all composites. There were significant group differences at the subtest level on all subtests except Block Design and Arithmetic. There was some support for a higher Perceptual Reasoning Index (PRI) score than a Verbal Comprehension Index (VCI) score, although the difference was relatively small (5.5 points).

Lincoln and colleagues (2007) administered the WISC-IV to a sample of 41 children between the ages of 6 and 14 years who met DSM-IV criteria for autistic disorder. These children showed the strongest performance on the Block Design subtest and the weakest performance on the Comprehension subtest. In comparison to the standardization sample, children in Lincoln and colleagues' younger sample showed a much larger discrepancy (18.5 points) between the PRI and VCI scores. When children with IQ scores below 60 were excluded, the large discrepancy remained (16.7 points). More

research is needed to confirm whether the profile of scores on the WISC-IV will parallel research on the WISC-III suggesting that visual–verbal processing differences are most pronounced in younger and more intellectually delayed individuals with ASD (Lincoln et al., 1995; Manjiviona & Prior, 1999; Mayes & Calhoun, 2003).

Preliminary data are available on WISC-IV profiles in children with high-functioning ASD. In the standardization testing, an additional group of 27 children between the ages of 9 and 15 years who met DSM-IV criteria for Asperger's disorder were administered the WISC-IV. This group consisted of 93% males, and children were excluded if they had existing overall cognitive ability scores below 70. In this sample, the individuals in the Asperger's disorder group exhibited significantly lower performance on the Processing Speed Index (PSI), Working Memory Index (WMI), and FSIQ than that of a matched control group. Mayes and Calhoun (2008) conducted a profile analysis on 54 children with high-functioning ASD (e.g., IQ of 70 or higher) on the WISC-IV. They also reported that children with ASD scored significantly lower on the PSI (average score of 85) and the WMI (average score of 89) compared to their performance on the VCI (average of 107) and the PRI (average score of 115). Additionally, although children with ASD showed VCI scores within the average range these scores were lower than their PRI. On average, the lowest verbal scores were obtained on the Comprehension subtest presumably because of the social understanding required on this task. Taken together, the WISC-IV may identify specific weaknesses in attention, graphomotor skills, processing speed, and social comprehension that have the potential to impact daily life even in individuals with average or higher intelligence.

Because the WISC-IV provides separate measures of verbal and nonverbal reasoning, working memory, and processing speed, it provides an opportunity to identify a pattern of strengths and weaknesses in children with ASD. The addition of the WMI and PSI to the WISC-IV provides a measurement of the poor motor skills and attention difficulties experienced by individuals with ASD. However, the General Abilities Index (GAI) based on VCI and PRI alone may represent the best global measure of intelligence on the WISC-IV for individuals with high-functioning ASD. Indeed, the GAI was an average of 12 points higher than the FSIQ for children in the Mayes and Calhoun (2008) study. Despite the significant strength of the WISC-IV in its ability to separate the impact of working memory and processing speed on the GAI, however, the use of timed tests, and the need for verbal understanding even on measures of perceptual reasoning, may lead to underestimates of the nonverbal abilities of some children and adolescents with ASD (Klin et al., 2005). Furthermore, younger school-age children with significant delays are unlikely to meet basal requirements on most subtests, resulting in an inability to calculate meaningful standard scores.

Leiter International Performance Scale—Revised

The Leiter International Performance Scale—Revised (Leiter-R; Roid & Miller, 1997) is designed to assess nonverbal intellectual ability, memory, and attention in children and adolescents between the ages of 2:0 and 20:11. Administration requires no verbal instructions from the examiner or verbal responses from the child. This instrument contains 20 subtests, which are equally divided between a Visualization and Reasoning Battery and an Attention and Memory Battery. Although the number of subtests administered varies according to a child's age, the Visual Reasoning and Attention and Memory batteries combined can generally be completed within 90 minutes. In addition to an FSIQ score, a Brief IQ screener can be computed based on four subtests. The Brief IQ screener can be completed in approximately 25 minutes, whereas the FSIQ measure requires approximately 40 minutes to administer. In a comparison of the Leiter-R Brief IQ and FSIQ scores in a group of children with autism and language limitations, Tsatsanis and colleagues (2003) found a very strong relationship ($r = .97$) between these two measures of intelligence. Thus the Leiter-R Brief IQ is particularly useful when a child is unable to complete the full battery of tests due to poor motivation, attention, or autism symptoms.

Although ASD was not one of the special groups included in the Leiter-R standardization sample, the test was administered to 701 individuals with developmental, language, sensory, or learning difficulties. When investigating the profile of scores obtained on the Leiter-R in a group of children with autism who had limited language abilities and low nonverbal IQ (average Leiter-R Brief IQ of 68), Tsatsanis and colleagues (2003) found that in three out of four cases, these children performed significantly better on the Fundamental Visualization composite than on Fluid Reasoning. These findings are consistent with research findings of

higher perceptual and visual–spatial reasoning skills in children with ASD. Kuschner, Bennetto, and Yost (2007) used the Leiter-R Brief IQ to examine the cognitive profile of preschool-age children with high-functioning ASD (average Leiter-R Brief IQ of 80). They found that, compared to children of similar chronological and nonverbal mental age with developmental delays, children with ASD showed specific strengths in tasks measuring the ability to focus on specific visual details (Figure Ground subtest) and to mentally manipulate and synthesize visual information (Form Completion subtest). The children with ASD were specifically impaired on a subtest measuring abstract reasoning and concept formation (Repeated Patterns subtest). These results suggest that children with ASD do not have overall strengths in nonverbal processing, and instead have strengths in visual perception. This is consistent with cognitive theories of ASD, including weak central coherence (Happé & Frith, 2006) and enhanced perceptual processing (Mottron, Dawson, Soulières, Hubert, & Barack, 2006).

The Leiter-R is an excellent choice for testing either a nonverbal child with ASD or a child with significantly impaired receptive and expressive language. This is one of the few tests that would be appropriate for an older child with very few words in his or her vocabulary (e.g., a 15-year-old who is able to speak in single words only). An additional strength of the Leiter-R is the presence of teaching trials, including examiner demonstrations and the ability to take the child's hand to teach task demands. However, many instructions are provided via gestures and facial expressions—both social stimuli that are very difficult for children with ASD to understand. Furthermore, this test is not appropriate for young, delayed children. Like other tests that begin at the 2½-year range, preschool children with ASD who have developmental delays are unlikely to understand task demands and achieve a basal score.

Raven's Standard Progressive Matrices Test

The Raven's Standard Progressive Matrices (Raven, Court, & Raven, 1992) test measures a person's ability to form perceptual relations and to reason by analogy. Variations of the Standard Matrices are the Coloured and Advanced Matrices. Each test is considered to be a measure of Spearman's g, which is independent of language and formal schooling; thus they are often used as measures of nonverbal intelligence. The Raven's Standard is normed for use with persons ranging in age from 6 years to adult. An overall percentile score is available. Administration time for the Raven's Standard is approximately 45 minutes.

A number of studies have been conducted in an attempt to establish the utility of the Raven's Standard as a measure of intellectual function in individuals with ASD, with mixed results. Hayashi, Kato, Igarashi, and Kashima (2008) used the Raven's Standard to examine the fluid reasoning abilities of youth ages 6–12 years with Asperger's disorder, relative to those of typically developing children matched on age, gender, and FSIQ. Their results indicated that the participants with Asperger's disorder, on average, received raw scores significantly higher than those of their peers with typical development.

Another study examining performance of a group of children with autism and a group of typical peers on the Raven's Standard demonstrated that significant differences were not present with regard to accuracy scores, but that the children with autism did demonstrate faster response time in completing the test than their typical peers did (Soulières et al., 2009).

Bolte, Dziobek, and Poustka (2009) used the Raven's Standard to measure intelligence in 48 individuals with autism, 28 individuals with other psychiatric diagnoses, and 25 peers with typical development. Individuals with autism functioning in the lower ranges of intelligence according to German versions of the Wechsler intelligence scales (Tewes, 1991; Tewes, Roßmann, & Schallberger, 1999) demonstrated a larger discrepancy between their Raven's Standard score and Wechsler score, with better performance on the Raven's. No other participant group showed this magnitude of score discrepancy, suggesting that the Raven's Standard may provide an appropriate measure of nonverbal intelligence for lower-functioning individuals with autism.

Dawson, Soulières, Gerusbacher, and Mottron (2007) demonstrated the utility of the Raven's Standard as a measure of intelligence for individuals with autism. Their sample included 38 children with autism, ages 7–16 years, and 24 peers with typical development of similar ages. The performance of these participants on the Raven's Standard was compared with their performance on the WISC-III. The children with autism performed significantly better on the Raven's than on the Verbal IQ, Performance IQ, and FSIQ of the WISC-III; this difference was not observed in the comparison group of typically developing individuals. Furthermore, in contrast to the findings of Bolte and colleagues (2009), these discrepancies in performance were observed for individuals with autism regardless of their intellectual level.

Chen, Planche, and Lemonnier (2010) administered the Coloured Raven's to 14 males with high-functioning autism and 26 age-matched peers with typical development, and found that participants with autism who had WISC-III FSIQ scores greater than or equal to 90 received Raven's scores statistically higher than their FSIQ scores. These results suggest that versions of the Raven's may be excellent measures of nonverbal reasoning skills in children with ASD, and that traditional language-based measures may underestimate reasoning skills in children with ASD. Thus the Raven's Standard or one of its variations may be an excellent addition to an assessment battery to highlight a child's strengths. However, it may not be a good "stand-alone" measure, as it may fail to capture the language difficulties that affect day-to-day functioning in children with ASD.

Test of Nonverbal Intelligence—Fourth Edition

The Test of Nonverbal Intelligence—Fourth Edition (TONI-4; Brown, Sherbenou, & Johnsen, 2010) is a nonverbal, motor-free measure of intelligence, aptitude, abstract reasoning, and problem solving for use with individuals ages 6:0–89:11. Administration time is 5–20 minutes. Two equivalent forms are available for repeated administrations. Items contain one or more of eight salient characteristics: (1) shape, (2) position, (3) direction, (4) rotation, (5) contiguity, (6) shading, (7) size, and (8) movement. Although the standardization sample of this measure did not include a group with ASD, it is purportedly useful with individuals who are difficult to assess because of its language-free format.

Although no studies have examined the utility of the TONI-4 for use with individuals having ASD, two such studies have been conducted with earlier versions of the test. Edelson, Schubert, and Edelson (1998) examined the TONI-2 (Brown, Sherbenou, & Johnsen, 1990) performance of 258 individuals with autism who were between the ages of 4 and 41 years. They found that 66% of their sample was "testable" with the TONI-2; ability to sustain attention was a determining factor in testability. Edelson (2005) later measured intellectual functioning in 35 individuals with autism, ages 4–18 years. Individuals were assessed with the TONI-3 (Brown, Sherbenou, & Johnsen, 1997) and the Universal Nonverbal Intelligence Test (UNIT; Bracken & McCallum, 1998; see also McCallum & Bracken, Chapter 14, this volume). Edelson suggested that the TONI-3 may be a more culturally fair measure of intelligence for individuals with autism, given the absence of any real-world knowledge requirement (as in the Analogic Reasoning tasks of the UNIT). These results support other findings in research using the TONI that symptoms and associated features of autism, such as language deficits and deficits in social and "real-world" knowledge, can adversely affect the performance of an individual with autism on a more traditional measure of intelligence. Thus the TONI-4 may be an excellent choice for testing either a nonverbal child with ASD or a child with significantly impaired receptive and expressive language. Furthermore, for verbal children with ASD, the TONI-4 may be a good additional measure to provide information regarding nonverbal strengths. The TONI-4 is less useful for children with mental ages below 6 years because of floor effects. Like the other nonverbal IQ tests, the TONI-4 may not be a good stand-alone measure if it is important to document a child's language abilities.

GUIDELINES FOR CHOOSING A MEASURE OF INTELLECTUAL FUNCTIONING

As is clear from this review, there are multiple options for assessment of cognitive functioning in individuals with ASD. There is no clear "gold standard" for assessing intelligence in children and adolescents with ASD. Instead, the flexibility of available instruments allows researchers and clinicians to adopt an individualized assessment approach rather than a static ASD cognitive battery. From our review of existing measures and assessment issues, we encourage examiners to take the following considerations into account when choosing the appropriate tools for a cognitive assessment.

Language Ability

Perhaps one of the most limiting factors in cognitive assessment of individuals with ASD is the verbal ability of the examinees. Some of the available measures allow for separate assessment of nonverbal and verbal ability in producing qualitatively

and quantitatively useful scores. However, some assessments, including the Wechsler intelligence tests and the SB5, require examinees to have a certain level of receptive language to understand nonverbal task directions. As a result, determining both an individual's level of language use and his or her level of understanding of verbal directions is essential in choosing an appropriate measure. Even when the nonverbal tasks are appropriate, individuals with limited language may not receive any credit on the language measures, resulting in an invalid assessment. Given research showing discrepancies in verbal and nonverbal functioning in individuals with ASD, evaluators are encouraged to consider whether administration of both a traditional test and a nonverbal test would provide the most comprehensive view of a child's abilities. Although it is important to assess language functioning to capture the extent of language delay and its impact on daily life, a nonverbal measure may provide a measure of a child's strengths and suggest intervention techniques that utilize these strengths.

Chronological Age and Developmental Level

With available measures spanning the age range from birth to 90 years, there is no age level at which an individual's ability may not be assessed. In measuring cognitive skills, it is best to choose a measure for which standard scores based on population norms are available for the individual's chronological age. Choosing an age-appropriate measure will add to the reliability and validity of the scores yielded by a cognitive measure and will aid in greater communication regarding the individual's abilities. When several measures are appropriate, the examiner should consider choosing an instrument that is appropriate for children several years younger than the examinee. For example, when deciding which developmental test to administer to a 3-year-old with ASD, the examiner has a wide range of tests that are appropriate for the child's chronological age, including the Bayley-III, Mullen, DAS-II, SB5, and WPPSI-III. However, a child who is delayed may have difficulty completing tests that are designed for children 2½ years of age or older, and floor effects are likely. Thus the examiner might consider a developmental test that is appropriate for younger children, such as the Bayley-III or the Mullen. If the age-appropriate measure is too difficult (e.g., requires too much receptive or expressive language) and no other instruments are available, it is reasonable to choose an alternative measure that may provide age equivalents rather than standard scores. For example, if an individual has a chronological age of 5½ years or above, but a mental age below 2½ years, there is no appropriate instrument. In this case, either the Bayley-III or Mullen may be administered and age equivalents calculated.

Behavioral Severity

Some examinees may exhibit behavioral difficulties that make it difficult to complete a lengthy evaluation or that raise concerns about the validity of the results. The examiner is encouraged to use behavioral strategies (e.g., use of a structure schedule of activities, a reward system, frequent breaks) to increase the chance of obtaining an accurate score. (See Klinger, O'Kelley, & Mussey, 2009, for a discussion of behavioral strategies.) Furthermore, behavioral difficulties are often signs of frustration and fatigue in individuals with ASD. When individuals have short attention spans or low tolerance of seated, formalized testing, examiners are encouraged to choose the most succinct measure that will yield informative data for the purposes of assessment. This approach will prove much more satisfying for both the examiners and examinees than engaging in a standard test choice for every individual. The DAS-II was designed to be a relatively brief assessment instrument and is a good choice when time is a concern. In addition, several measures (the DAS-I, Leiter-R, SB5) have a brief IQ measure that may be more appropriate than an entire battery.

The Purpose of the Assessment

Determining the need for assessment and the value of the obtained results for the individual is of ultimate importance in choosing a measure of cognitive ability for a child or adolescent with ASD. The underlying need is typically for a comprehensive measure of a range of cognitive abilities, but in other situations a screener of cognitive ability will suffice. Examiners should keep in mind what will happen to the scores after the assessment is complete as well. For example, certain agencies (e.g., school systems) may only accept comprehensive measures and full-scale or composite scores when making eligibility decisions. If an assessment is intended to be part of a series of administrations to track an individual's development over time, one of the instruments that covers a wider age range

may be of preference (e.g., the SB5 for the entire lifespan, the Mullen for measurements across the preschool years, or the Leiter-R or DAS-II for multiple assessments throughout childhood and adolescence).

Because of the uneven profile of strengths and weaknesses characterizing individuals with ASD, examiners are often faced with the decision to choose an instrument that highlights an examinee's strengths or weaknesses. For example, a child with limited language but good nonverbal perception abilities may receive higher scores on a nonverbal IQ test such as the Leiter-R, but may perform much more poorly on a test with receptive and expressive language demands such as the WISC-IV. This choice between these measures depends on the purpose of the evaluation. If the goal of the evaluation is to highlight the fact that the child is not developmentally delayed in all areas and in fact has some age-level skills, the Leiter-R may be a good choice. However, if the purpose of the assessment is to identify strengths and weaknesses that may affect school performance, a test that includes verbal ability will be important for providing a good predictor of the child's performance in a classroom that requires verbal comprehension and expression in order to be successful. Identifying the child's verbal weaknesses will be likely to lead to additional school accommodations that may not be offered if a nonverbal IQ test is administered.

SUMMARY

In this chapter, we have asserted that there is no "best test" for measuring intellectual functioning in persons with ASD. Because of the uneven profiles that characterize individuals with ASD and the behavioral difficulties that often occur during standardized testing, the examiner needs to have not only experience in administering standardized assessments, but an understanding of how the symptoms of ASD may interfere with test performance. The examiner is encouraged to provide additional structure to increase the examinee's attention and motivation to complete the assessment while maintaining a standardized test administration. In addition, it is important to choose the right instrument in order to ensure that an accurate estimate of developmental ability is obtained. The examiner is encouraged to consider the following sequence of questions when deciding which test is most appropriate:

1. Which instruments are appropriate for the examinee's chronological age?
2. Is the child nonverbal, necessitating the need for a nonverbal IQ test?
3. Given the examinee's estimated mental age, is it appropriate to choose a test that extends several years below the examinee's chronological age?
4. If there are no appropriate measures that include both the examinee's chronological age and expected mental age, is a test that provides age equivalents available?
5. Is a full battery or a brief IQ score more appropriate? The answer to this question depends on whether the referral agency would prefer one type of measure and whether behavioral difficulties may interfere with testing success.
6. If the assessment is being conducted to measure whether the examinee is showing an increase or decrease in skills across time, which measure is most appropriate, given the proposed range of assessments? For example, if the child was previously evaluated with a Wechsler scale, it may be most appropriate to administer another Wechsler scale. If the child is participating in a longitudinal research project, which measure is most appropriate, given the proposed age range of the study?
7. Is the assessment being conducted to highlight the individual's strengths or to highlight areas of weakness that may need additional intervention? This is particularly important if the examinee has discrepant verbal and nonverbal abilities or if the examiner wants to highlight difficulties with attention, processing speed, and/or working memory that impact everyday functioning.

ACKNOWLEDGMENT

This chapter is adapted in part from Klinger, O'Kelley, and Mussey (2009). Copyright 2009 by The Guilford Press. Adapted by permission.

REFERENCES

Akshoomoff, N. (2006). Use of the Mullen Scales of Early Learning for the assessment of young children with autism spectrum disorders. *Child Neuropsychology*, 12, 269–277.

American Psychiatric Association. (1994). *Diagnostic and statistical manual of mental disorders* (4th ed.). Washington, DC: Author.

Baird, G., Simonoff, E., Pickles, A., Chandler, S., Loucas, T., Meldrum, D., et al. (2006). Prevalence of disorders of the autism spectrum in a population cohort of children in South Thames: The Special Needs and Autism Project (SNAP). *Lancet*, 368, 210–215.

Ballaban-Gil, K., & Tuchman, R. (2000). Epilepsy and epileptiform EEG: Association with autism and language disorders. *Mental Retardation and Developmental Disabilities Research Reviews*, 6, 300–308.

Bayley, N. (2005). *Manual for the Bayley Scales of Infant and Toddler Development, Third Edition* (Bayley-III). San Antonio, TX: Harcourt Assessment.

Beadle-Brown, J., Murphy, G., & Wing, L. (2006). The Camberwell cohort 25 years on: Characteristics and changes in skills over time. *Journal of Applied Research in Intellectual Disabilities*, 19, 317–329.

Bolte, S., Dziobek, I., & Poustka, F. (2009). Brief report: The level and nature of autistic intelligence revisited. *Journal of Autism and Developmental Disorders*, 39, 678–682.

Bracken, B. A., & McCallum, R. S. (1998). *Universal Nonverbal Intelligence Test: Examiner's manual*. Itasca, IL: Riverside.

Brown, L., Sherbenou, R. J., & Johnsen, S. K. (1990). *Manual for the Test of Nonverbal Intelligence—Second Edition*. Austin, TX: PRO-ED.

Brown, L., Sherbenou, R. J., & Johnsen, S. K. (1997). *Manual for the Test of Nonverbal Intelligence—Third Edition*. Austin, TX: PRO-ED.

Brown, L., Sherbenou, R. J., & Johnsen, S. K. (2010). *Manual for the Test of Nonverbal Intelligence—Fourth Edition*. Austin, TX: PRO-ED.

Carpentieri, S. C., & Morgan, S. B. (1994). Brief report: A comparison of patterns of cognitive functioning of autistic and nonautistic retarded children on the Stanford–Binet—Fourth Edition. *Journal of Autism and Developmental Disorders*, 24, 215–223.

Chen, F., Planche, P., & Lemonnier, E. (2010). Superior nonverbal intelligence in children with high-functioning autism or Asperger's disorder. *Research in Autism Spectrum Disorders*, 4, 457–460.

Dawson, M., Soulières, I., Gerusbacher, M. A., & Mottron, L. (2007). The level and nature of autistic intelligence. *Psychological Science*, 18, 657–662.

Dawson, G., Toth, K., Abbott, R., Osterling, J., Munson, J., Estes, A., et al. (2004). Early social attention impairments in autism: Social orienting, joint attention, and attention to distress. *Developmental Psychology*, 40, 271–283.

Edelson, M. G. (2005). A car goes in the garage like a can of peas goes in the refrigerator: Do deficits in real world knowledge affect the assessment of intelligence in individuals with autism. *Focus on Autism and Other Developmental Disabilities*, 20, 2–9.

Edelson, M. G., Schubert, D. T., & Edelson, S. M. (1998). Factors predicting intelligence scores on the TONI in individuals with autism. *Focus on Autism and Other Developmental Disabilities, 13,* 17–26.

Ehlers, S., Nyden, A., Gillberg, C., Sandberg, A. D., Dahlgren, S., Hjelmquist, E., et al. (1997). Asperger syndrome, autism, and attention disorders: A comparative study of the cognitive profiles of 120 children. *Journal of Child Psychology and Psychiatry, 38,* 207–217.

Eikeseth, S., Smith, T., Jahr, E., & Eldevik, S. (2007). Outcomes for children with autism who began intensive behavioral treatment between ages 4 and 7: A comparison controlled study. *Behavior Modification, 31,* 264–278.

Elliott, C. D. (1990). *Differential Ability Scales.* San Antonio, TX: Psychological Corporation.

Elliott, C. D. (2007). *Differential Ability Scales—Second edition.* San Antonio, TX: Harcourt Assessment.

Filipek, P. A., Accardo, P. J., Baranek, G. T., Cook, E. H., Jr., Dawson, G., et al. (1999). The screening and diagnosis of autistic spectrum disorders. *Journal of Autism and Developmental Disorders, 29,* 439–484.

Fombonne, E. (2005). Epidemiological studies of pervasive developmental disorders. In F. R. Volkmar, R. Paul, A. Klin, & D. Cohen (Eds.), *Handbook of autism and pervasive developmental disorders: Vol. 1. Diagnosis, development, neurobiology, and behavior* (3rd ed., pp. 42–69). Hoboken, NJ: Wiley.

Freeman, B. J., Lucas, J. C., Forness, S. R., & Ritvo, E. R. (1985). Cognitive processing of high-functioning autistic children: Comparing the K-ABC and the WISC-R. *Journal of Psychoeducational Assessment, 3,* 357–362.

Freeman, B. J., Ritvo, E. R., Needleman, R., & Yokota, A. (1985). The stability of cognitive and linguistic parameters in autism: A five-year prospective study. *Journal of the American Academy of Child Psychiatry, 24,* 459–464.

Ghaziuddin, M., & Mountain-Kimchi, K. (2004). Defining the intellectual profile of Asperger syndrome: Comparison with high-functioning autism. *Journal of Autism and Developmental Disorders, 34,* 279–284.

Happé, F., & Frith, U. (2006). The weak coherence account: Detail-focused cognitive style in autism spectrum disorders. *Journal of Autism and Developmental Disorders, 36,* 5–25.

Harris, S. L., Handleman, J. S., & Burton, J. L. (1990). The Stanford–Binet profiles of young children with autism. *Special Services in the Schools, 6,* 135–143.

Hayashi, M., Kato, M., Igarashi, K., & Kashima, H. (2008). Superior fluid intelligence in children with Asperger's disorder. *Brain and Cognition, 66,* 306–310.

Howlin, P., Goode, S., Hutton, J., & Rutter, M. (2004). Adult outcomes for children with autism. *Journal of Child Psychology and Psychiatry, 45,* 212–229.

Johnson, C. P., Myers, S. M., & the Council on Children with Disabilities. (2007). Identification of and evaluation of children with autism spectrum disorders. *Pediatrics, 120,* 1183–1215.

Joseph, R. M., Tager-Flusberg, H., & Lord, C. (2002). Cognitive profiles and social-communicative functioning in children with autism spectrum disorder. *Journal of Child Psychology and Psychiatry, 43,* 807–821.

Kanner, L. (1943). Autistic disturbances of affective contact. *Nervous Child, 2,* 217–250.

Kaufman, A. S., & Kaufman, N. L. (1983). *Kaufman Assessment Battery for Children (K-ABC): Administration and scoring manual.* Circle Pines, MN: American Guidance Service.

Kaufman, A. S., & Kaufman, N. L. (2004). *Kaufman Assessment Battery for Children—Second Edition: Manual.* Circle Pines, MN: American Guidance Service.

Klin, A., Saulnier, C., Tsatsanis, K., & Volkmar, F. R. (2005). Clinical evaluation in autism spectrum disorders: Psychological assessment within a transdisciplinary framework. In F. R. Volkmar, R. Paul, A. Klin, & D. J. Cohen (Eds.), *Handbook of autism and pervasive developmental disorders: Vol. 2. Assessment, interventions, and policy* (3rd ed., pp. 772–798). Hoboken, NJ: Wiley.

Klinger, L. G., O'Kelley, S. E., & Mussey, J. L. (2009). Assessment of intellectual functioning in autism spectrum disorders. In S. Goldstein, J. Naglieri, & S. Ozonoff (Eds.), *Assessment of autism spectrum disorders* (pp. 209–252). New York: Guilford Press.

Kuschner, E. S., Bennetto, L., & Yost, K. (2007). Patterns of nonverbal cognitive functioning in young children with autism spectrum disorders. *Journal of Autism and Developmental Disorders, 37,* 795–807.

Landa, R., & Garrett-Mayer, E. (2006). Development in infants with autism spectrum disorders: A prospective study. *Journal of Child Psychology and Psychiatry, 47,* 629–638.

Lincoln, A. J., Allen, M. H., & Kilman, A. (1995). The assessment and interpretation of intellectual abilities in people with autism. In E. Schopler & G. B. Mesibov (Eds.), *Learning and cognition in autism* (pp. 89–117). New York: Plenum Press.

Lincoln, A. J., Hansel, E., & Quirmbach, L. (2007). Assessing intellectual abilities of children and adolescents with autism and related disorders. In S. R. Smith & L. Handler (Eds.), *The clinical assessment of children and adolescents: A practitioner's handbook* (pp. 527–544). Mahwah, NJ: Erlbaum.

Lord, C., & Schopler, E. (1989). The role of age at assessment, developmental level, and test in the stability of intelligence scores in young autistic children. *Journal of Autism and Developmental Disorders, 19*, 483–499.

Lovaas, I. (1987). Behavioral treatment and normal educational and intellectual functioning in young autistic children. *Journal of Consulting and Clinical Psychology, 55*, 3–9.

Manjiviona, J., & Prior, M. (1999). Neuropsychological profiles of children with Asperger syndrome and autism. *Autism, 3*, 327–356.

Mayes, S. D., & Calhoun, S. L. (2003). Analysis of the WISC-III, Stanford–Binet: IV, and academic achievement test scores in children with autism. *Journal of Autism and Developmental Disorders, 33*, 329–341.

Mayes, S. D., & Calhoun, S. L. (2008). WISC-IV and WIAT-III profiles in children with high functioning autism. *Journal of Autism and Developmental Disorders, 38*, 428–439.

Mottron, L., Dawson, M., Soulières, I., Hubert, B., & Burack, J. (2006). Enhanced perceptual functioning in autism: An update, and eight principles of autistic perceptions. *Journal of Autism and Developmental Disorders, 36*, 27–43.

Mullen, E. M. (1995). *Mullen Scales of Early Learning.* Circle Pines, MN: American Guidance Service.

National Research Council (NRC). (2001). Committee on Educational Interventions for Children with Autism, Division of Behavioral and Social Sciences and Education. *Educating children with autism.* Washington, DC: National Academy Press.

Ozonoff, S., South, M., & Miller, J. N. (2000). DSM-IV defined Asperger syndrome: Cognitive, behavioral and early history differentiation from high-functioning autism. *Autism, 4*, 29–46.

Raven, J. C., Court, J. H., & Raven, J. (1992). *Raven manual: Section 3. The standard progressive matrices.* Oxford: Oxford Psychologists Press.

Rogers, S. J., Hepburn, S., Stackhouse, T., & Wehner, E. (2003). Imitation performance in toddlers with autism and those with other developmental disorders. *Journal of Child Psychology and Psychiatry, 44*, 763–781.

Roid, G. H. (2003). *Stanford–Binet Intelligence Scales, Fifth Edition.* Itasca, IL: Riverside.

Roid, G. H., & Miller, L. J. (1997). *Leiter International Performance Scale—Revised: Examiner's Manual.* Wood Dale, IL: Stoelting.

Seltzer, M. M., Shattuck, P., Abbeduto, L., & Greenberg, J. (2004). Trajectory of development in adolescents and adults with autism. *Mental Retardation*

and *Developmental Disabilities Research Reviews, 10*, 234–247.

Siegel, D. J., Minshew, N. J., & Goldstein, G. (1996). Wechsler IQ profiles in diagnosis of high-functioning autism. *Journal of Autism and Developmental Disorders, 26*, 389–406.

Sigman, M., & McGovern, C. W. (2005). Improvement in cognitive and language skills from preschool to adolescence in autism. *Journal of Autism and Developmental Disorders, 35*, 15–23.

Sigman, M., Mundy, P., Sherman, T., & Ungerer, J. (1986). Social interactions of autistic, mentally retarded, and normal children with their caregivers. *Journal of Child Psychology and Psychiatry, 27*, 647–656.

Smith, T., Groen, A. D., & Wynn, J. W. (2000). A randomized trial of intensive early intervention for children with pervasive developmental disorder. *American Journal on Mental Retardation, 5*, 269–285.

Soulières, I., Dawson, M., Samson, F., Barbeau, E. B., Sahyoun, C. P., Strangman, G. E., et al. (2009). Enhanced visual processing contributes to matrix reasoning in autism. *Human Brain Mapping, 30*, 4082–4107.

Stavrou, E., & French, J. L. (1992). The K-ABC and cognitive processing styles in autistic children. *Journal of School Psychology, 30*, 259–267.

Tewes, U. (1991). *Hamburg–Wechsler-Intelligenztest für Erwachsene—Revision.* Göttingen, Germany: Hogrefe.

Tewes, U., Roßmann, P., & Schallberger, U. (1999). *Hamburg–Wechsler-Intelligenztest für Kinder—III (HAWIK-III).* Bern, Switzerland: Hogrefe.

Tsatsanis, K. D., Dartnall, N., Cicchetti, D., Sparrow, S. S., Klin, A., & Volkmar, F. R. (2003). Concurrent validity and classification accuracy of the Leiter and Leiter-R in low-functioning children with autism. *Journal of Autism and Developmental Disorders, 33*, 23–30.

Venter, A., Lord, C., & Schopler, E. (1992). A follow-up study of high-functioning autistic children. *Journal of Child Psychology and Psychiatry, 33*, 489–507.

Volkmar, F. R., Szatmari, P., & Sparrow, S. S. (1993). Sex difference in pervasive developmental disorders. *Journal of Autism and Developmental Disorders, 23*, 579–591.

Wechsler, D. (2002). *Wechsler Preschool and Primary Scale of Intelligence—Third Edition (WPPSI-III).* San Antonio, TX: Psychological Corporation.

Wechsler, D. (2003). *Wechsler Intelligence Scale for Children, Fourth Edition (WISC-IV).* San Antonio, TX: Psychological Corporation.

Cognitive and Neuropsychological Assessment of Attention-Deficit/Hyperactivity Disorder
Redefining a Disruptive Behavior Disorder

James B. Hale
Megan Yim
Andrea N. Schneider
Gabrielle Wilcox
Julie N. Henzel
Shauna G. Dixon

BEHAVIORAL DEFINITIONS OF ADHD: THE SOURCE OF THE PROBLEM

Attention-deficit/hyperactivity disorder (ADHD) is one of the most commonly diagnosed psychiatric problems in children, affecting approximately 5% of children worldwide (Polanczyk, Silva de Lima, Lessa Horta, Biederman, & Rohde, 2007). Although typically defined as a disruptive behavior disorder, ADHD also interferes with cognitive, neuropsychological, academic, and social functioning (Hale, Reddy, et al., 2010). Behavioral ADHD criteria based on informant report have been used to identify three interrelated symptom clusters as subtypes in the *Diagnostic and Statistical Manual of Mental Disorders*, fourth edition, text revision (DSM-IV-TR; American Psychiatric Association, 2000): the predominantly inattentive, predominantly hyperactive–impulsive, and combined subtypes, with 80% of cases displaying symptoms of all three (Barkley, 1997). Although behavioral manifestations of the disorder are typically considered for diagnostic and intervention purposes, ADHD is clearly a neurobiological disorder (Dickstein, Bannon, Castellanos, & Milham, 2006). Accordingly, researchers and practitioners alike could benefit from examining children with attention problems from a cognitive and neuropsychological perspective.

A neuropsychological perspective may be advantageous because attention difficulties are ubiquitous in clinical practice and have many different causes. There are many disorders that exhibit ADHD-like symptom profiles, making it difficult for behavioral criteria to have diagnostic specificity for ADHD (Hale, Reddy, et al., 2010). In addition, ADHD frequently occurs comorbidly with other learning disorders (e.g., specific learning disabilities [SLD]) and psychiatric diagnoses (e.g., oppositional defiant disorder, anxiety disorders), further complicating diagnostic and treatment practices (Friedman et al., 2007). As a result, practitioners conducting cognitive and intellectual assessments of children with attention problems can expect mixed findings, depending on whether children have "true ADHD," which ADHD subtype they have, or whether some other disorder is affecting attention (Hale et al., 2009). Redefining ADHD as a neuropsychological disorder, in which patterns of intellectual, cognitive, and neuropsychological test performance help differentiate the various causes of attention problems, could lead to clearer diagnostic decisions that have both ecological and treatment validity.

IS ADHD A BEHAVIOR DISORDER OR A NEUROLOGICAL DISORDER?

Despite the behavioral focus in both defining ADHD and determining the presence of the disorder, it has been clear for some time that ADHD is in fact an inherited neurological disorder in most cases, related to catecholamine (e.g., dopamine and/or norepinephrine) neurotransmitter dysregulation (Arnsten, 2001; Faraone, 2008; Kieling, Goncalves, Tannock, & Castellanos, 2008; Pliszka, 2005). This dysregulation affects optimal frontal–subcortical circuit function (Castellanos et al., 2002), with prefrontal, basal ganglia (e.g., striatum), and cerebellar regions most frequently found to be dysmorphic and/or dysfunctional in ADHD (Casey, Nigg, & Durston, 2007; Dickstein et al., 2006). Children with ADHD may also be predisposed to atypical development of white matter tracts in frontal–subcortical circuits (Casey et al., 2007). These circuits can be depicted in a "top-down" or "anterior–posterior" axis for clinical interpretation of test findings (see Figure 28.1), and their dysfunction is the source of most brain-based psychopathologies, such as ADHD, obsessive–compulsive disorder, other anxiety disorders, and depression (Hale, Reddy, et al., 2010).

These executive circuits serve to manage and control other brain functions. Acting as the brain's "boss," they are responsible for planning, organizing, strategizing, problem solving, monitoring, evaluating, and changing behavior (Hale & Fiorello, 2004). In addition, it is clear that "true ADHD" is not a deficiency of primary attention, but rather one of attention control, making it a disorder of *intention* (Denckla, 1996; Hale, Reddy, et al., 2010). Other structures affected include the anterior cingulate (e.g., Rubia, Smith, Brammer, Toone, & Taylor, 2005; Schulz et al., 2004) and the corpus callosum (e.g., Giedd et al., 1994; Semrud-Clikeman et al., 1994), which effectuate information transfer and control (Liotta et al., 2007; Moll et al., 2000). These combined deficits can not only affect behavior during cognitive and intellectual testing, but also affect scores on subtests that either directly or indirectly require executive functions for optimal task performance. As a result, a child with ADHD may perform adequately on many cognitive and intellectual tasks, but may show subtest variability leading to small decrements in performance as a result of his or her executive dysfunction.

Although circuit dysfunction likely explains the cognitive and behavioral manifestations of ADHD (Dickstein et al., 2006; Hale, Reddy, et al., 2010; Voeller, 2001), other neuropsychiatric disorders show impairment in these frontal–subcortical circuits, with attention regulation problems a common finding (Miller & Cummings, 2007). Children with depression, anxiety disorders, tic disorders, pervasive developmental disorders, posttraumatic stress disorder, sleep disorders, thought disorders, seizure disorders, and learning disorders can all show significant attention problems. Because the core symptoms of ADHD are not specific to the disorder, using behavioral criteria to differentiate ADHD from other disorders is remarkably difficult and leads to considerable population heterogeneity (Wahlstedt, Eninger, Thorell, & Bohlin, 2008); this limits the sensitivity and specificity of our di-

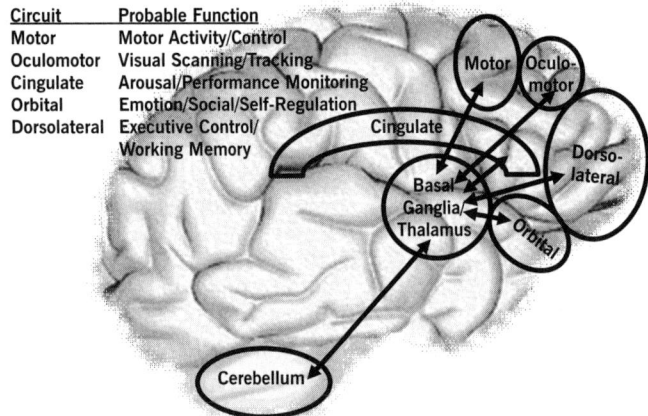

Circuit	Probable Function
Motor	Motor Activity/Control
Oculomotor	Visual Scanning/Tracking
Cingulate	Arousal/Performance Monitoring
Orbital	Emotion/Social/Self-Regulation
Dorsolateral	Executive Control/Working Memory

FIGURE 28.1. Brain circuits most often found to be dysmorphic and/or dysfunctional in ADHD, and their probable functions.

agnostic tools, and attenuates treatment effects (Hale et al., 2011). Is it because there are so many causes of "ADHD" that only behavioral criteria are relevant for diagnosis (e.g., Brown & LaRosa, 2002), or is it that using behavioral definitions of ADHD results in heterogeneous samples, with different putative neurological causes?

SPECIFYING NEUROPSYCHOLOGICAL ADHD SUBTYPES

The heterogeneity of the population currently diagnosed with ADHD has led to several theories and debates regarding putative causes for the disorder, with several authors positing multiple ADHD endophenotypes or subtypes that may differ in etiology and symptom expression (Doyle et al., 2005). Several leading explanations for ADHD symptom variability include Sonuga-Barke's (2005) delay aversion theory; Sergeant's (2000) cognitive-energetic model; Sagvolden, Aase, Johansen, and Russell's (2005) reinforcement/motivation theory; Nigg and Casey's (2005) theory of cognitive and affective control; and Barkley's (1997) response inhibition theory. Although further review of these theories is beyond the scope of this chapter, there are probably children with these various causes of attention problems, and as a result, they are likely to show different cognitive and neuropsychological profiles.

Despite inconsistent evidence across samples, some empirical support can be found for each of the theoretical models described above. However, the majority of evidence supports Barkley's (1997) theory that children with "true ADHD," at least those children who have the combined type and who respond to stimulant medication, have a deficit in response inhibition (Hale, Reddy, et al., 2010; Hale et al., 2011). In fact, of the neuropsychological measures most likely to be impaired, response inhibition is the most common finding in meta-analyses, with vigilance, working memory, and planning measures also likely to be impaired (Willcutt, Doyle, Nigg, Faraone, & Pennington, 2005). These findings suggest differential executive deficits in ADHD; that is, ADHD may be accounted for by "cool" (e.g., working memory, mental flexibility, sustained attention) and "hot" (e.g., behavioral regulation, inhibition) executive deficits (Castellanos, Sonuga-Barke, Milham, & Tannock, 2006; Hale, Reddy, et al., 2010). Although evidence suggests that response inhibition is the primary deficit in ADHD combined type,

some have suggested that the inattentive type of ADHD may be a neuropsychologically and behaviorally distinct disorder (Diamond, 2005). It is also possible that some inattentive children may have ADHD but do not meet the behavioral threshold for hyperactive–impulsive symptoms; others may have other psychiatric or learning disorders (Hale, Reddy, et al., 2010), even though they would all behaviourally be considered to have ADHD inattentive type.

Given that there is clearly a neurobiological basis for ADHD (Castellanos et al., 2002), exploration of endophenotypes can help elucidate why cognitive profile variability is common in this heterogeneous disorder. One child may respond to test stimuli impulsively and not check the final answers before saying "done"; another may carefully look at all stimuli and responses, proceeding slowly and methodically through a task, which would also lead to a lower score. Although both children may be considered to have "ADHD" according to DSM-IV-TR criteria, it is clear that these children have different symptoms and presentations, and may require different intervention strategies as a result.

Delineation of the genetic, neuropsychological, cognitive, psychosocial, behavioral, and environmental determinants of ADHD endophenotypes may translate into scientific advances in ADHD practice (Coghill, Nigg, Rothenberger, Sonuga-Barke, & Tannock, 2005). Until scientific clarification is achieved, many will continue to advocate adherence to behavioral criteria in defining ADHD, arguing that these have more diagnostic utility than neuropsychological measures (Brown & LaRosa, 2002). Unfortunately, advocates of this behavioral diagnostic approach to understanding ADHD fail to recognize the circularity of their research design and conclusions. If behavioral criteria are used to define (e.g., informant report) and then test for the disorder (e.g., informant ratings), it is not surprising that these ratings have more discriminant validity (Hale et al., 2009).

Given that ADHD is a disorder characterized by both neurostructural abnormalities and neurochemical dysregulation, it seems that attention should be shifted from behavioral to neuropsychological definitions of the disorder. Until the shift is made from using behavioral criteria to neuropsychological criteria in diagnosing ADHD (e.g., Nigg, Blaskey, Stawicki, & Sachek, 2004), cognitive and neuropsychological tests are likely to have limited sensitivity and specificity; treatment effects will also remain attenuated for large samples because some will respond while others will not (e.g., Hale, Fiorello, & Brown, 2005; Hale, Kaufman, Naglieri, & Kavale, 2006; Hale et al., 2008, 2009; Hale, Reddy, et al., 2010; Hale et al., 2011). Given that ADHD is a neurobiological disorder, it makes sense that it should be diagnosed on the basis of cognitive and neuropsychological functioning. Once ADHD definitions are based on such functioning, researchers can begin to examine the discriminant and treatment validity of behavior ratings. We propose here that this paradigm shift in diagnostic practice may ultimately lead to greater understanding of "true ADHD" versus "pseudo-ADHD" (Hale et al., 2009), and to more specifically targeted interventions that have both ecological and treatment validity.

COGNITIVE AND INTELLECTUAL FUNCTIONING IN ADHD

Given that behavioral definitions of ADHD undermine our understanding of cognitive and neuropsychological functioning in this heterogeneous population, it should not be surprising that previous research on cognitive and intellectual functioning in ADHD has been mixed. Part of the problem is that cognitive and intellectual tests seldom measure executive functions directly. In addition, since these tests are multifactorial and tap perceptual and memory systems as well, the executive deficits seen in ADHD may only limit optimal performance and may not lead to specific subtest or factor deficit patterns (Chow & Cummings, 2007). The multiplicity of ADHD cognitive symptoms makes differential diagnosis via cognitive and neuropsychological tests both challenging and controversial. Given the current state of ADHD behavioral diagnosis, Table 28.1 is presented to reflect this heterogeneity in cognitive and neuropsychological functions found for children with ADHD (see Hale, Reddy, et al., 2010). Of particular interest in Table 28.1 is that our position—namely, that ADHD is a problem with attention control, not with primary attention—suggests problems in "true ADHD" with executive attention and vigilance, not a primary attention deficit.

Given the questionable utility of global intelligence in populations with ADHD (Fiorello et al.,

TABLE 28.1. Cognitive/Neuropsychological Characteristics of Children with ADHD

Construct	Probable impairment level	Reliability
Inhibitory control	Moderate to severe	Consistent
Basic attention	None to mild	Consistent
Executive attention/vigilance	Moderate to severe	Consistent
Motor activity (hyperactivity)	Mild (old) to severe (young)	Consistent
Fine motor/praxis	Mild to moderate	Inconsistent
Motor timing/cerebellar motor	Mild to moderate	Inconsistent
Tactile, auditory, visual sensory	None to mild	Inconsistent
Executive functioning/fluid reasoning	Mild to severe[a]	Inconsistent
Working memory	Mild to severe[b]	Inconsistent
Long-term memory encoding	None to mild	Consistent
Long-term memory storage	None to mild	Consistent
Long-term memory retrieval	Moderate to severe	Inconsistent
Processing speed	Mild to severe	Inconsistent
Visual–spatial–holistic ability	None to moderate	Inconsistent
Auditory–verbal–crystallized ability	None to mild	Inconsistent
Global intelligence	None to mild	Consistent

[a]Depends on cortical–subcortical circuit examined.
[b]Verbal impairment < visual impairment.

2007), the following review of the neuropsychological and cognitive characteristics of children with this disorder is based on the premise that idiographic interpretation of intellectual, cognitive, and neuropsychological patterns of performance is preferred over nomothetic score interpretation. This position is supported by cognitive and neuropsychological research showing that cognitive and neuropsychological processes, not stimulus input or response output, are critical for understanding ADHD and other high-prevalence disorders (Hale, Reddy, et al., 2010; Hale, Wycoff, & Fiorello, 2010). As a result, we emphasize the cognitive and neuropsychological processes that could affect cognitive and intelligence test performance, and deemphasize global intelligence score interpretation because of its questionable validity (e.g., Hale, Fiorello, Kavanagh, Holdnack, & Aloe, 2007). Thus global intelligence is addressed at the end of this section.

Inhibitory Control

Inhibitory control is the ability to suppress responses to irrelevant stimuli. Impulsivity is a common problem with inhibitory control, often leading to problematic behaviors such as sensation seeking, risk taking, carelessness, indulgence, and fearlessness (Hollander & Evers, 2001). As previously discussed, the dorsolateral, orbital, and anterior cingulate prefrontal regions regulate stimulus judgment, goal setting, and goal maintenance, as well as the adaptive response patterns needed to control impulsive behaviors (D'Amato, Fletcher-Janzen, & Reynolds, 2005). Neuroimaging data have suggested that disruption in the white matter tract of the orbitofrontal circuit is correlated with impulsivity in ADHD (Konrad, Gauggel, Manz, & Scholl, 2000). In addition, the right inferior or ventrolateral prefrontal cortices are most often associated with motor inhibition and emotion regulation (Congdon & Canli, 2005). However, it is important to recognize that multiple cortical and subcortical regions are typically involved in impulsivity (Barkley, 1997), including the dorsolateral circuit (Hale, Reddy, et al., 2010), where prefrontal structures are involved in "top-down" executive-mediated inhibitory control as opposed to the "bottom-up" subcortical influence related to reinforcement and punishment in situations requiring inhibition (Nigg, 2000).

Inhibitory control is central to the successful execution of higher-order behaviors such as working memory (for avoiding extraneous informa-

tion), goal-directed behavior (for delayed gratification), and emotional self-control (for minimizing emotionally laden reactions) (Quay, 1977). Working memory is clearly tapped on several cognitive measures, such as Differential Ability Scales—Second Edition (DAS-II) Recall of Digits—Backward; Stanford–Binet Intelligence Scales, Fifth Edition (SB5) Nonverbal Working Memory; and Wechsler Intelligence Scale for Children—Fourth Edition (WISC-IV) Arithmetic. And goal-directed behavior is important for persistence during difficult cognitive tests or items, such as Woodcock–Johnson III (WJ III) Concept Formation, Kaufman Assessment Battery for Children—Second Edition (KABC-II) Rebus, and Cognitive Assessment System (CAS) Planning. However, difficulties with executive self-control may be seen in variable motivation following response failure, or in poor frustration tolerance. Children with ADHD may also start responding before all the instructions are provided, become distracted by the testing environment or extraneous stimuli, or respond without considering the consequences of their actions (Solanto et al., 2001)—all of which can interfere with optimal cognitive and intellectual test performance.

Attention Deficit or Sustained-Attention (Vigilance) Deficit?

Attention affects so many areas of cognitive, academic, and behavioral functioning that children with attention problems are at considerable risk for school failure and social problems (Biederman et al., 2004; Clark, Prior, & Kinsella, 2002; Lawrence et al., 2004). As noted earlier, attention problems are ubiquitous in clinical practice (Reddy & Hale, 2007) and can be due to dysfunction in posterior (e.g., parietal) and/or anterior (e.g., frontal–subcortical circuits) regions (Hale, Reddy, et al., 2010). Thus recognizing the different causes of attention problems is critical for both assessment and intervention (e.g., academic remediation, behavioral treatments, and/or medication).

Attention is critical for successful performance on any cognitive or intellectual task, so attention problems can lead to inconsistent and often poor test performance. Attention demands may vary from minimal to substantial on these measures, so an individual with ADHD or other attention problems may have lower intellectual/cognitive scores on some measures but not others. Interpretation is further complicated by the fact that there are multiple attention systems in the brain (e.g., orienting, sustained, divided; Mirsky, 1996; Posner & Petersen, 1990). In addition, Brieber and colleagues (2007) found frontal gray matter correlates with attention, and volume reductions in gray and white matter have been reported in several frontal areas in ADHD (Mostofsky, Cooper, Kates, Denckla, & Kaufmann, 2002), which may affect multiple interrelated aspects of attention (Hale, Reddy, et al., 2010). Furthermore, atypical development of frontal–striatal white matter tracts has been associated with poor cognitive control of attention (Casey et al., 2007). As suggested earlier, frontal–striatal circuit dysfunction is related to the attention control problems seen in ADHD (Brieber et al., 2007; Castellanos et al., 2006; Williams, Stott, Goodyer, & Sahakian, 2007), but the posterior parietal attention network, implicated in some children's attention problems (e.g., Hale et al., 2006), is not likely to be the cause of "true ADHD" (Huang-Pollock & Nigg, 2003). As a result, a useful distinction in understanding ADHD is attempting to evaluate whether the problem with a posterior attention activation or allocation (Sergeant, 2000), which may be common in ADHD inattentive type, or with the executive control of attentional resources required for sustained attention or vigilance (Huang-Pollock, Nigg, & Halperin, 2006), which may be more common in the ADHD combined type. Children with "true ADHD" may then have difficulty maintaining attention, while those with "pseudo-ADHD" may have difficulty allocating attention. However, this clinical distinction is not an easy one, as modulation of attention could be due to dysfunctional interconnectivity between frontal and posterior attention systems (Gazzaley, Cooney, McEvoy, Knight, & D'Esposito, 2005).

Consistent with Barkley's (1997) theory, Hale and colleagues (Hale et al., 2005, 2011; Hale, Blaine-Halperin, & Beakley, 2007) found that DSM-IV-TR inattention symptoms did not correlate with executive and self-regulation neuropsychological factors, but that hyperactive–impulsive symptoms were correlated with these neuropsychological factors. They found that children with impaired executive function were more likely to have ADHD combined type and respond to stimulants, whereas children with low impairment were more likely to have ADHD inattentive type and not respond to medication. However, others have suggested that there are few neuropsychological differences between ADHD subtypes, and have questioned the primacy of executive deficits in ADHD (Geurts, Verte, Oosterlaan, Roeyers, & Sergeant, 2004). The mixed findings again may be related to behavioral definitions of ADHD, which lead to population heterogeneity and limit the sensitivity and specificity of our neuropsychological measures (Hale et al., 2009, 2011; Hale, Reddy, et al., 2010).

Although response inhibition may be the primary deficit in the behaviorally defined combined type of ADHD, the inattentive type is probably quite heterogeneous: Some children with this type may not meet the behavioral threshold for hyperactive–impulsive symptoms and thus may have a milder form of ADHD, while others in this group may have multiple other causes for their attention problems (Hale et al., 2009; Reddy & Hale, 2007). Since multiple disorders and brain areas can lead to attention problems, heterogeneity among children referred for attention problems must be carefully considered by examining the types of attention problems displayed on cognitive and neuropsychological measures to determine whether children have "true ADHD" or "pseudo-ADHD" due to some other cause (Hale, Reddy, et al., 2010). For instance, arousal or attention activation is necessary for quick, efficient performance or processing speed, and may be more common in children identified with the inattentive type; those with the combined type may have more difficulty with sustained attention or persistence, which interferes with processing efficiency (Lockwood, Marcotte, & Stern, 2001).

Activity Level and Sensory–Motor Functioning

Given the frontal–subcortical nature of "true ADHD," it is not surprising that these children have difficulty with motor activity and control, as the frontal lobes are also responsible for motor activity. Research has confirmed that children with ADHD have hypoactivity in the dopamine neurotransmitter system, which in turn leads to overt motor hyperactivity (Jucaite, Fernell, Halldin, Forssberg, & Farde, 2005), at least for ADHD combined type. However, children with the inattentive type of ADHD are often characterized as being slow-moving, sluggish, and *hypoactive* (i.e., as having "slow cognitive tempo"), which again suggests a different etiology and course (Barkley, 1997; Diamond, 2005; Milich, Balentine, & Lynam, 2001). Although hyperactivity or hypoactivity is not directly tapped by cognitive or intellectual tasks, it can be observed during test administration. A child who is hyperactive displays fidgeting behavior or moves around excessively in his or her seat, whereas a child who is hypoactive may present as preoccupied, sluggish, lethargic, and listless or may show poor processing or decision speed.

Even more likely to affect cognitive and intellectual task performance is the difficulty children with ADHD experience with motor precision and consistency (Rommelse et al., 2008), which can lead to a comorbid diagnosis of developmental coordination disorder (Sergeant, Piek, & Oosterlaan, 2006; Watemberg, Waiserberg, Zuk, & Lerman-Sagie, 2007). The motor circuit dysfunction found in ADHD affects not only self-directed motor skills, but motor control while performing external tasks (Mostofsky et al., 2002; Suskauer et al., 2008), with the basal ganglia being especially important for maintaining executive control of motor functions (Castellanos et al., 2006; Halperin & Schultz, 2006). Although this is likely to affect graphomotor skills during testing (e.g., copying shapes, handwriting), it is important to consider whether the problem is due to frontal (e.g., premotor cortex) or subcortical (e.g., basal ganglia, cerebellar) motor dysfunction, or both (e.g., Castellanos et al., 2006). In addition, some children with ADHD have difficulties with motor timing or sequencing (Mostofsky, Newschaffer, & Denckla, 2003; Rommelse et al., 2008), which may influence other psychomotor tasks, such as processing speed tasks.

Do children with ADHD have sensory or perceptual processing problems? The executive problems experienced by children with ADHD are more likely to affect what the children do (i.e., output) than what they perceive (i.e., input), so sensory problems should be secondary to problems with executive control. However, children with ADHD do have more sensory problems than controls (e.g., Mangeot et al., 2001; Yochman, Parush, & Ornoy, 2004). These problems are logical, since executive control requires frontal–striatal–*thalamic* circuit functioning. The thalamus is an important sensory relay station (it can be thought of as the "Grand Central Station" of sensory processing), so impaired circuit function could lead to thalamic problems in ADHD (Rowe et al., 2005) and sensory processing difficulties. In addition, problems with anterior–posterior and left–right connectivity (e.g., corpus callosum, cingulate, other white matter tracts) could lead to difficulty with sensory–motor integration and bimanual coordination during motor performance (e.g., Klimkeit, Sheppard, Lee, & Bradshaw, 2004; Liotti et al., 2007; Moll, Heinrich, Trott, Wirth, & Rothenberger, 2000).

Executive Functioning, Fluid Reasoning, Working Memory, and Processing Speed

Difficulties with executive function, fluid reasoning, working memory, and processing speed are probably the most consistent, albeit still controversial, neuropsychological findings in children with ADHD (Castellanos et al., 2006; Hale, Reddy, et al., 2010). As these cognitive and neuropsychological constructs are related to planning, organizing, strategizing, monitoring, evaluating, and shifting/changing behaviors (Hale & Fiorello, 2004), and to dorsolateral and inferior prefrontal–subcortical circuit function (Dickstein et al., 2006), it should not be surprising that they are most likely to be impaired in children with ADHD.

Several meta-analyses have examined measures of these interrelated executive functions (e.g., Homack & Riccio, 2004; Romine et al., 2004; Sergeant, Guerts, & Oosterlaan, 2002; Willcutt et al., 2005). Willcutt and colleagues (2005) found that deficits in response inhibition, vigilance, working memory, and planning were most indicative of ADHD, and that these deficits could not be caused by intelligence, achievement, or comorbidity problems. Meta-analyses for measures of executive decision making, online performance monitoring, and interference control (the Stroop Color–Word Test); sustained attention and inhibitory control (a continuous-performance test [CPT]); and problem solving, mental flexibility, cognitive set shifting, and response to feedback (i.e., the Wisconsin Card Sorting Test) also found these measures to be sensitive to ADHD deficits, but poor performances on these measures are not specific to the disorder (Homack & Riccio, 2004; Riccio, Reynolds, Lowe, & Moore, 2002; Romine et al., 2004). However, CPT deficits may be specific to the combined type of ADHD (Collings, 2003; Henzel, 2010), consistent with the notion that "true ADHD" is a disorder of response inhibition and that the inattentive type may have a different etiology and course (e.g., Barkley, 1997; Castellanos et al., 2006; Hale, Reddy, et al., 2010). Importantly, while executive measures may be sensitive to ADHD deficits, other childhood disorders are linked to impairments on these measures (Sergeant et al., 2002; Sonuga-Barke, Sergeant, Nigg, & Willcutt, 2008); this suggests that clinicians must not only attend to the level of performance (e.g., average, below average, impaired), but also examine the *pattern* among these measures of executive performance for differential diagnosis of ADHD (Hale, Reddy, et al., 2010).

Of the intelligence and cognitive tests available, several tap working memory (e.g., the WJ III, WISC-IV, SB5, DAS-II, KABC-II) and processing speed (e.g., the WJ III, WISC-IV, DAS-II), both of which have been found to be deficient in children with ADHD (Mayes & Calhoun, 2006). Children with ADHD have both verbal and nonverbal working memory impairments, with meta-analyses revealing moderate and large effect sizes, respectively; these findings suggest that visual–spatial working memory is more impaired than verbal working memory (Martinussen, Hayden, Hogg-Johnson, & Tannock, 2005; Willcutt et al., 2005). Although Hale and colleagues (2011) found executive factors that included working memory to be related to DSM-IV-reported hyperactive–impulsive symptoms (Hale et al., 2005), consistent with the assumption that visual–spatial working memory and inhibition deficits were both being related to right frontal dysfunction (Clarke et al., 2007), executive functions have been found to be related to inattentive symptoms in other studies (Chhabildas, Pennington, & Willcutt, 2001; Martinussen & Tannock, 2006). These differences may in part be explained by divided (left) and sustained (right) prefrontal attention influences on verbal and nonverbal working memory, respectively (e.g., Pasini, Paloscia, Allesandrelli, Porfirio, & Curatolo, 2007; Smith & Jonides, 1997), or it may be that working memory deficits are secondary to response inhibition problems (Barkley, 1997; Dennis et al., 2009; Nigg, 2005). However, these types of working memory may be differentially impaired by ADHD subtype: Deficits in verbal working memory may be more indicative of the inattentive type, whereas nonverbal working memory may be more impaired in the combined type (e.g., Henzel, 2010; Martinussen et al., 2005).

Children with ADHD also exhibit deficits in processing speed and efficiency (Mayes & Calhoun, 2006). Consistent with Sergeant's (2000) cognitive-energetic model, slow and variable performance on information processing and rapid CPTs could result from poor connectivity or energy supply (Russell et al., 2006), which may be more related to the inattentive type's slow cognitive tempo (Hartman, Willcutt, Rhee, & Pennington, 2004; Weiler, Holmes Bernstein, Bellinger, & Waber, 2000) than to the combined type. However, deficits have been reported in both subtypes (Chhabildas et al., 2001; Nigg, Blaskey, Huang-Pollock, & Rappley, 2002). Processing speed measures typically require visual–motor skills and sustained attention/vigilance. Since motor timing,

organization, and control deficits are common in ADHD (Mostofsky et al., 2003; Piek, Dyck, Francis, & Conwell, 2007; Rommelse et al., 2008), and sustained attention or persistence is also deficient in ADHD (Huang-Pollock et al., 2008; Willcutt et al., 2005), it may be that different patterns of processing speed deficits can be found in different subtypes (i.e., arousal problems leading to slow processing in the inattentive type, poor motor timing and control or limited persistence in the combined type) (Lockwood et al., 2001). Consistent with these differences, Rucklidge and Tannock (2002) found that children with the inattentive type had reaction time deficits due to performance variability, while those with the combined type had problems with reaction time due to interference control.

Fluid reasoning abilities are not traditionally thought of as executive functions, but they are clearly related to executive measures (Decker, Hill, & Dean, 2007), suggesting that they could be impaired in children with ADHD (Miller & Hale, 2008). Several fluid reasoning measures can be found on the WJ III, WISC-IV, DAS-II, SB5, and KABC-II, and the executive deficits experienced by children with ADHD can influence performance on these measures and reduce subtest scores as a result. Other tests (e.g., the CAS, WJ III) have measures that in part tap other executive constructs like attention and planning, and more direct impairments are observed on these measures (e.g., Goldstein & Naglieri, 2008). There may be subtype differences, at least on the CAS Planning and Attention measures: Children with the combined type are more likely to have deficits on the former, suggesting self-regulation deficits, while those with the inattentive type are more likely to have primary attention deficits (Goldstein & Naglieri, 2008).

Learning and Memory

Given that children with ADHD have executive or output problems, one might conclude that they do not have difficulty with learning and memory—especially with storage of information in long-term memory, which appears to be intact (Kaplan, Dewey, Crawford, & Fisher, 1998). However, academic deficits are perhaps the most consistent findings for children with ADHD (Shaywitz & Shaywitz, 1988), so the impact on learning and memory is clearly evident, and this may be apparent on intellectual measures of crystallized abilities (see below). New learning requires executive functions for governing a gradiential shift from new information processing to long-term storage; this suggests that executive functions are necessary to take information from right frontal to left posterior regions (Goldberg, 2001; Hale & Fiorello, 2004), consistent with the executive–fluid abilities relationship discussed above (Decker et al., 2007; Kane & Engle, 2002).

Working memory is clearly important for both long-term memory encoding and retrieval, which appear to be related to left and right frontal functions, respectively (Tulving & Markowitsch, 1997). It should not be surprising that children with ADHD have more difficulty with working memory for retrieval, given the preponderance of evidence pointing, to right frontal impairment in the disorder (e.g., Clarke et al., 2007; Martinussen et al., 2005; Willcutt et al., 2005). As a result, long-term memory as tapped by crystallized measures may be intact in ADHD, but difficulty with long-term retrieval may lead to lower performance on crystallized/knowledge measures, such as those found on the DAS-II, KABC-II, SB5, WISC-IV, and WJ III. Interestingly, those with depression and attention problems may show the opposite pattern, with right prefrontal hyperactivity and left prefrontal hypoactivity (e.g., Hecht, 2010), which could lead to more problems with long-term memory encoding than with retrieval.

Finally, the basal ganglia structures are important for associative, procedural, and habit learning (Myers et al., 2003; Packard & Knowlton, 2002), and nucleus accumbens deficiencies may lead to deficient motivation or reinforcement during new learning situations (Sonuga-Barke, 2005). Learning problems are sometimes associated with cerebellar deficits in ADHD (Castellanos et al., 2006). Although the cerebellum was once thought to serve only motor functions, we now know that it is important for executive coordination of cognitive functions, including learning, memory, timing, and automaticity (Doya, 2000; Ivry, 1993; Rapoport, van Reekum, & Mayberg, 2000). ADHD deficits due to these subortical structures could in part result in lower performance on processing speed measures, especially those requiring associative learning (e.g., the WISC-IV Coding subtest).

Visual–Spatial–Holistic and Auditory–Verbal–Crystallized Functioning

Visual–spatial–holistic and auditory verbal–crystallized psychological processes are typically not as impaired as executive processes (e.g., work-

ing memory, processing speed) in children with ADHD, and are often in the average range (Mayes & Calhoun, 2006). However, since frontally mediated executive functions govern all other aspects of cognition (Luria, 1973), measures of these high-g-loading processes may be negatively affected. In addition, since anterior–posterior and left–right hemisphere functions are in part related to the integrity of white matter "roads and highways" tracts (e.g., the corpus callosum and other fasciculi)— pathways negatively affected in ADHD (e.g., Castellanos et al., 2002; Durston, 2003; Hale & Fiorello, 2004; Rubia et al., 1999; Vaidya et al., 1998; Valera, Faraone, Murray, & Seidman, 2007)—children with ADHD may show subtle decrements in performance on these measures.

There is some debate whether the visual–spatial–holistic deficits seen in children with ADHD are directly related to executive dysfunction or whether these deficits are in fact due to comorbid processing problems. Visual–spatial–holistic processes are often associated with the posterior regions of the right hemisphere (Hale & Fiorello, 2004), so they should not be significantly impaired in "true ADHD." However, the right hemisphere is dominant for attention in general, and there is a strong relationship between executive and visual–spatial performance measures (Denckla, 1996). Posterior right-hemisphere regions seem to be important for attention orienting, and the anterior regions to be responsible for sustained attention and inhibition (Aman, Roberts, & Pennington, 1998; Berger & Posner, 2000; Casey et al., 1997; Mirsky, 1996; Pliszka, Liotti, & Woldorff, 2000). Right frontal impairment seems likely in ADHD (e.g., Aron, Robbins, & Poldrack, 2004; Carter, Krener, Chaderjian, & Northcutt, 1995; Castellanos, 2001; Congdon & Canli, 2005; Durston, 2003; Rubia, 2002; Sandson, Bachna, & Morin, 2000; Vaidya et al., 2005), and meta-analyses suggest that these children have few problems with visual orienting, which would suggest more right posterior attention problems (e.g., Huang-Pollock & Nigg, 2003). As a result, behaviorally defined ADHD may be largely a right-hemisphere disorder. The combined type may be more a right frontal problem (due to frontal–subcortical circuit dysfunction), and the inattentive type may be more a right posterior problem, directly affecting visual–spatial–holistic processes (Hale et al., 2006, 2009). Attention orienting and attentional neglect can occur with right posterior dysfunction (Gross-Tsur, Shalev, Manor, & Amir, 1995; Posner & Petersen, 1990; Reddy & Hale, 2007), so it is important for differential diagnosis to determine whether visual–spatial–holistic processing deficits are primary—as would be the case in "nonverbal" learning disabilities (Hain, Hale, & Glass-Kendorski, 2008; Hale et al., 2006)—or whether they are secondary to executive dysfunction and "true ADHD" (Hale, Reddy, et al., 2010).

Visual–spatial–holistic processes are more likely to be impaired than auditory–verbal–crystallized ones in ADHD (Martinussen et al., 2005; Sandson et al., 2000), but attention deficits are also found in children with auditory processing and language disorders (McGrath et al., 2008; Moss & Sheiffele, 1994). In early studies, many children with speech–language disorders (Love & Thompson, 1988) and central auditory processing disorders (Riccio, Hynd, Cohen, Hall, & Molt, 1994) met criteria for ADHD. Barkley (1997) argues that poor internalization of language in ADHD is in part responsible for poor behavior regulation and impulse control, consistent with findings that ventrolateral frontal regions responsible for expressive language are also response inhibition tasks (Liddle, Kiehl, & Smith, 2001).

These early reports of auditory–verbal–crystallized deficits in ADHD have not been substantiated in recent years, leading some to question the language–ADHD relationship (Ors et al., 2005; Williams et al., 2000). Children who do not process language well will certainly appear inattentive in the classroom (Buttross, 2000), and could meet criteria for "comorbid" ADHD according to the DSM-IV-TR criteria, but their ADHD symptoms may be secondary to their learning/language problems. These early studies did not screen for comorbid SLD, and more recent studies have shown that auditory processing and language deficits are more often associated with SLD than with ADHD (Gomez & Condon, 1999; Pisecco, Baker, Silva, & Brooke, 2001; Purvis & Tannock, 1997). ADHD executive deficits appear to be independent of SLD (Klorman et al., 1999; McInnes, Humphries, Hogg-Johnson, & Tannock, 2003), and the language deficits these children experience may be more related to the executive/expressive aspects of language (Goodyer, 2000)—such as working memory required during verbal retrieval, language organization/formulation, and pragmatic language—which are known to be impaired in ADHD and affected by frontal/executive dysfunction (e.g., Hale et al., 2005; Hurks et al., 2004; Kim & Kaiser, 2000; Kourakis, Katachanakis, Vlahonikolis, & Paritsis, 2004; Purvis & Tannock, 1997; Tannock & Schachar, 1996; Thorell, 2007; Westby & Cutler, 1994).

Intellectual "Ability" in ADHD

Children with ADHD have been shown to score lower on IQ tests than nondisordered controls, but this disparity ranges from approximately 2 points (Jepsen, Fagerlund, & Mortensen, 2009) to 9 points (Kuntsi, Wood, Van Der Meere, & Asherson, 2009), suggesting that most children with ADHD fall within the average range of global intelligence. Approximately 9% of the variance was shared between IQ and ADHD symptoms in one twin study (Kuntsi et al., 2004), with an 86% association between ADHD symptom scores and IQ; to the authors of several studies, such findings suggest a strong genetic relationship. When examining genetic links between dopaminergic polymorphisms and intelligence in ADHD (recall that dopamine dysregulation is the most likely cause of ADHD), Mill et al. (2006) found a relationship, but this was not confirmed in other larger-sample studies (Genro et al., 2006; Sonuga-Barke et al., 2008). In their longitudinal study, Polderman and colleagues (2006) found high heritability for IQ (80%), executive function (50%), and attention (60%) at age 12, but executive functions were weakly correlated with IQ, and attention ratings were only moderately correlated with IQ at this age. In another twin study, inattentive symptoms were negatively correlated with intelligence and positively correlated with depression, but this was not the case for hyperactive–impulsive symptoms (Willcutt, Pennington, Chhabildas, Friedman, & Alexander, 1999).

Although overall general intelligence scores have been found to be significantly lower for children with ADHD, and some have even suggested that ADHD is largely a deficit in intellectual functioning (Frazier, Demaree, & Youngstrom, 2004), this variation may be in part due to lower performance on subtests sensitive to executive deficits, as has been suggested throughout this chapter. It has been argued that global IQ interpretation is not warranted for children with ADHD because global IQ is characterized by large amounts of unique factor variance (49.7%) and significant amounts of shared variance among two or three factor scores (38.6%), but little shared variance among all four factor scores on the WISC-IV (2.4%) (Fiorello et al., 2007). If global IQ interpretation is limited for children with ADHD, what is the influence of ADHD symptoms on intelligence test performance? For a potential answer to this question, let us examine Polderman and colleagues' (2009) findings for the relationship between executive measures of inhibitory control and intelligence ($r = -.24$, $r^2 = .058$) and attention problems and intelligence ($r = -.34$, $r^2 = .116$) for 12-year-olds, with a correlation between attention problems and response inhibition of .18 ($r^2 = .032$). This would suggest that approximately 14% of intelligence and cognitive ability test scores are influenced by inattentive and hyperactive–impulsive ADHD symptoms, while 3% of these scores are influenced by the combined effects of inattention, hyperactivity, and impulsivity. This suggests that the executive influences on IQ are separable, and that lower IQ scores are not only due to lower overall ability.

Although of course these correlational data do not suggest that ADHD symptoms cause decrements in intelligence, they are clearly related, and the effects are difficult for practitioners to disentangle. With ADHD symptoms potentially affecting a large portion of subcomponent subtest and/or factor scores, the question remains as to which measures are most affected. Subtests found to contribute to the IQ disparity include Wechsler Digit Span subtests (Assesmany, McIntosh, Phelps, & Rizza, 2001; Reddy, Braunstein, & Dumont, 2008), particularly Digits Backward versions (Hale, Hoeppner, & Fiorello, 2002; Hale et al., 2005); WJ III auditory and verbal working memory tasks (Ford, Keith, Floyd, Fields, & Schrank, 2003); and SB5 Nonverbal Working Memory subtests (Marusiak & Janzen, 2005)—all of which are often part of working memory factor scores found to be deficient in ADHD (Dennis et al., 2009; Mayes & Calhoun, 2006). However, these working memory deficits are inconsistent in meta-analyses (Willcutt et al., 2005) and may be differentially affected for ADHD subtypes (Henzel, 2010; Martinussen et al., 2005). Processing speed measures are also frequently impaired in ADHD, as noted earlier, particularly associative learning/processing speed tasks (e.g., WISC-IV Coding) (Mayes & Calhoun, 2006). However, slow processing speed may be more prevalent in ADHD inattentive type (Mayes, Calhoun, Chase, Mink, & Stagg, 2009; Weiler et al., 2000), consistent with the finding that slow cognitive tempo is associated with inattentive symptoms (Hartman et al., 2004).

Other measures found to be deficient in children with ADHD include crystallized measures that tap executive-mediated functions like language organization/formulation and retrieval from long-term memory, as well as visual–spatial measures that require attention to visual detail and retrieval from long-term visual memory (Assesmany et al., 2001). In fact, the "ACID" profile (Arithmetic, Coding, Information, and Digit Span), which includes working memory, processing speed, and long-term memory retrieval demands, was found to be deficient for children with ADHD in WISC-III studies (Ek et al., 2007; Snow & Sapp, 2000). As noted earlier, Planning and Attention as measured by the CAS also seem to be impaired in children with ADHD (Naglieri, Salter, & Edwards, 2004; Van Luit, Kroesbergen, & Naglieri, 2005), and given the relationship between executive function and fluid reasoning (Blair, 2006; Decker et al., 2007), we can expect that children with ADHD will struggle on fluid reasoning tests like the WJ III Concept Formation subtest (Harrier & DeOrnellas, 2005) or the DAS-II Sequential and Quantitative Reasoning subtest (e.g., Gibney, McIntosh, Dean, & Dunham, 2002). Executive dysfunction may in part mediate deficits in crystallized and fluid abilities found for children with ADHD, but the relationship for fluid abilities, intelligence, and ADHD is complex, with fluid decrements reflecting executive attention deficits (Tillman, Bohlin, Sorensen, & Lundervold, 2009).

This pattern of poor intellectual/cognitive subtest performance has led to considerable debate regarding the nature of intelligence tests, especially since IQ is characterized by little shared variance among the factors that contribute to the global score (Fiorello et al., 2007), as noted earlier. It remains plausible that executive deficits lead to variable performance and lower scores on particular intelligence subtests, indirectly lowering overall intelligence scores as a result. Given the relatively small difference in average overall intelligence scores of children with ADHD and controls, it is quite plausible that this discrepancy can be attributed to attention and response inhibition problems, in addition to other executive impairments found in ADHD (e.g., Willcutt et al., 2005). Interestingly, when children with ADHD are treated with methylphenidate, which has been shown to improve cognitive and academic function in children with ADHD (see Hale et al., 2005; Hale, Reddy, et al., 2010), the executive impairments associated with ADHD and cognitive performance appear to be ameliorated (Gimpel et al., 2005; Pearson et al., 2003). In addition, children with high IQ and ADHD show cognitive, psychiatric, and behavioral features similar to those of children with ADHD and lower IQs (Antshel et al., 2007). Together, these findings suggest that lower IQ scores among individuals with ADHD may reflect deficits in executive and attention control processes, rather than deficiencies in general intelligence.

CONCLUSIONS AND FUTURE DIRECTIONS

Despite convincing evidence that children with ADHD have significant cognitive, neuropsychological, academic, and behavioral problems (Barkley, 2006) due to frontal–subcortical circuit and executive dysfunction (Dickstein et al., 2006), it is common practice to focus largely on behavioral criteria for determining ADHD diagnosis and evaluating treatment effects. This leads to heterogeneous ADHD groups, which limit the sensitivity and specificity of cognitive and neuropsychological tests in determining ADHD diagnosis; they also attenuate treatment results because children with "true ADHD" will respond, while those with "pseudo-ADHD" will not (Hale et al., 2005, 2006, 2011; Hale, Reddy, et al., 2010). Although some suggest that behavior ratings are more important than neuropsychological measures in determining ADHD diagnosis (e.g., Brown & LaRosa, 2002), these conclusions are inherently circular because the indirect summative judgments of informants are used to diagnose (i.e., define) the disorder, and then the same judgments are used to determine whether it exists (Hale et al., 2009).

Redefining ADHD as a neurobiological disorder for which cognitive and neuropsychological tests can be used to provide a direct evaluation of the attention, working memory, and executive deficits displayed by children will be a critical step in advancing ADHD diagnostic and treatment practices in the years to come. With this change, researchers and practitioners can begin to differentiate neuropsychiatric disorders on the basis of frontal–subcortical circuit function, and then examine how performance measures can differentiate these disorders. Until then, judging ADHD on the basis of summative judgments provided by indirect informant reports will limit our understanding of ADHD, and of how intellectual, cognitive, and neuropsychological measures can be used to judge the presence of the disorder and evaluate treatment effects (Hale, Reddy, et al., 2010). This behavioral approach to ADHD limits our understanding of which children have "true ADHD" due to frontal–striatal hypoactivity affecting response inhibition and other executive functions, and which have "pseudo-ADHD" due to numerous other causes (e.g., Barkley, 1997; Diamond, 2005; Dickstein et al., 2006; Hale et al., 2009; Willcutt et al., 2005).

With the limitations of the behavioral definition of ADHD in mind, assessment of intellectual, cognitive, neuropsychological, and academic functioning in children with ADHD and other disorders affecting attention remains a critical function of practicing psychologists. The issues raised in this chapter are especially critical for practitioners when one considers the ubiquity of attention problems found in clinical practice (Reddy & Hale, 2007) and the legal requirements for thorough comprehensive evaluations for disability identification (Dixon, Eusebio, Turton, Wright, & Hale, 2011). In this chapter we have not only provided readers with the scientific impetus to reconceptualize ADHD as a neurobiological disorder, but have also provided a detailed review of the cognitive and neuropsychological patterns of performance seen in this heterogeneous population, which can help practitioners differentiate ADHD from other disorders affecting attention. We argue that comprehensive evaluations that take historical, cognitive, neuropsychologial, academic, and behavioral data into account can help practitioners discern the nature of children's attention problems for diagnostic purposes, and can aid in the development of targeted intervention programs that may ultimately establish the ecological and treatment validity of assessment findings.

Making Assessment Meaningful for Intervention: Cognitive Hypothesis Testing

Given that intellectual, cognitive, and neuropsychological assessment of ADHD is currently limited by the behavioral definition of the disorder, we feel it is important to conduct comprehensive evaluations that address the concurrent, ecological, and treatment validity of these measures. Careful, comprehensive evaluations are critical, given the neurobiological basis of ADHD and the ubiquity of attention problems in clinical practice (Hale, Reddy, et al., 2010; Reddy & Hale, 2007). To overcome the problems associated with traditional profile analysis of intellectual and cognitive tests, Hale and Fiorello (2004) have developed *cognitive hypothesis testing* (CHT), a model in which assessment results are examined within the context of multiple data sources to ensure the utility of results for identifying childhood disorders and providing instructional and behavioral supports (see Figure 20.1 in Fiorello, Hale, & Wycoff, Chapter 20, this volume). CHT helps clarify the nature of the attention deficits observed, as well as whether subtle or direct effects of executive impairments are influencing a child's behavior and performance. In CHT, assessment data are not only considered for differential diagnosis, but also used to develop interventions that are subsequently monitored via single-subject designs to ensure treatment efficacy (Hale & Fiorello, 2004).

The CHT identification and intervention model is based on four premises (Fiorello, Hale, Decker, & Coleman, 2009; Hale & Fiorello, 2004). The first premise is that complex cognitive and neuropsychological processes are related to real-world outcomes such as academic achievement and psychosocial functioning. The second premise is that children with disabilities have significant cognitive strengths and weaknesses that interact with the environmental determinants of behavior to lead to adaptive or problem learning and behavior. The third premise is that direct assessment of cognitive and neuropsychological processes, and examination of ecological and treatment validity, can lead to more effective interventions for children with disabilities. The final premise is that weaknesses or deficits must be remediated or compensated for, based on the underlying cognitive strengths and weaknesses.

The CHT model uses a scientist-practitioner approach for integrating cognitive and neuropsychological assessment and intervention for children who do not respond to standard interventions (Fiorello et al., 2009; Hale & Fiorello, 2004). The CHT approach requires ongoing data-based decision making over time, using the scientific method (e.g., theory, hypothesis, data collection, data interpretation) not only to establish the concurrent and ecological validity of results, but also to link this information to subsequent intervention to establish treatment efficacy. Although empirical profile analysis (see Elliott, Hale, Fiorello, Dorvil, & Moldovan, 2010; Fiorello et al., 2009; Hale et al., 2006) is encouraged when subcomponent scores are significantly different within factors, the CHT model overcomes the limitations of traditional profile analyses by using the intellectual/cognitive tests only as *screening* tools. Any hypotheses derived from these cognitive/intellectual screening tools and other data sources (e.g., prior intervention data, history, ratings) must be tested by using other cognitive or neuropsychological measures with greater sensitivity and specificity, and then subsequently evaluated to ensure that they have concurrent, ecological, and ultimately treatment

validity. The methods of CHT are thus not unlike the methods described by Flanagan and colleagues for cross-battery assessment (Flanagan, Ortiz, & Alfonso, 2007). Only when children are provided with comprehensive evaluations in all areas of suspected disability can we be confident in our diagnostic decisions, and this cannot be accomplished with intelligence tests alone (Dixon et al., 2011). Once the CHT evaluation is completed, problem-solving consultation is undertaken to develop, implement, monitor, and evaluate interventions designed to help children overcome their difficulties.

CHT is designed to help practitioners address the valid criticism that cognitive and neuropsychological assessment is not related to intervention (e.g., Reschly, 2005), by helping practitioners use the problem-solving approach to develop, implement, monitor, evaluate, and recycle interventions until treatment efficacy is achieved (Hale & Fiorello, 2004). The CHT approach has been used to document brain–behavior–intervention relationships in children with reading (Fiorello, Hale, & Snyder, 2006), math (Hale et al., 2006), and attention (Reddy & Hale, 2007) disorders, and has been advocated for use in both educational (Elliott et al., 2010; Fiorello et al., 2009; Hale et al., 2008) and neuropsychological (Fletcher-Janzen, 2005; Miller, Getz, & Leffard, 2006) settings.

Given the problems with global intelligence or IQ interpretation for children with ADHD and other high-prevalence disorders (Elliott et al., 2010; Fiorello et al., 2007; Hale, Fiorello, et al., 2007), and the significant limitations of traditional profile analysis (Hale, Wycoff, & Fiorello, 2010), a scientific approach to understanding psychological processes and interpreting cognitive and neuropsychological tests is critical for understanding and helping children with ADHD and other disabilities (e.g., Dixon et al., 2011; Fiorello et al., 2009; Hale & Fiorello, 2004). Using CHT methodology, practitioners can use cognitive and neuropsychological assessment data in an informed, scientific, and responsible manner to better understand children who present with ADHD and other attention problems for both diagnostic and treatment purposes. Not only will this approach help pinpoint the exact nature of a child's attention problems, and help differentiate "true ADHD" from "pseudo-ADHD" (Hale, Reddy, et al., 2010); it can also lead to effective interventions that include all available diagnostic information, not just behavioral criteria that undermine our efforts to serve children with ADHD and other disorders affecting attention.

REFERENCES

Aman, C. J., Roberts, R. J., Jr., & Pennington, B. F. (1998). A neuropsychological examination of the underlying deficit in attention deficit hyperactivity disorder: Frontal lobe versus right parietal lobe theories. *Developmental Psychology, 34,* 956–969.

American Psychiatric Association. (2000). *Diagnostic and statistical manual of mental disorders* (4th ed., text rev.). Washington, DC: Author.

Antshel, K. M., Faraone, S. V., Stallone, K., Nave, A., Kaufmann, F. A., Doyle, A., et al. (2007). Is attention deficit hyperactivity disorder a valid diagnosis in the presence of high IQ?: Results from the MGH Longitudinal Family Studies of ADHD. *Journal of Child Psychology and Psychiatry, 48,* 687–694.

Arnsten, A. (2001). Neurobiology of executive functions: Catecholamine influences on prefrontal cortical functions. *Biological Psychiatry, 57,* 1377–1384.

Aron, A. R., Robbins, T. W., & Poldrack, R. A. (2004). Inhibition and the right inferior prefrontal cortex. *Trends in Cognitive Sciences, 8,* 170–177.

Assemany, A., McIntosh, D. E., Phelps, L., & Rizza, M. G. (2001). Discriminant validity of the WISC-III with children classified with ADHD. *Journal of Psychoeducational Assessment, 19,* 137–147.

Barkley, R. A. (1997). *ADHD and the nature of self-control.* New York: Guilford Press.

Barkley, R. A. (2006). *Attention-deficit hyperactivity disorder* (3rd ed.). New York: Guilford Press.

Berger, A., & Posner, M. I. (2000). Pathologies of brain attentional networks. *Neuroscience and Biobehavioral Reviews, 24,* 3–5.

Biederman, J., Monuteaux, M. C., Doyle, A. E., Seidman, L. J., Wilens, T. E., Ferrero, F., et al. (2004). Impact of executive function deficits and attention-deficit/hyperactivity disorder (ADHD) on academic outcomes in children. *Journal of Consulting and Clinical Psychology, 72,* 757–766.

Blair, C. (2006). How similar are fluid cognition and general intelligence?: A developmental neuroscience perspective on fluid cognition as an aspect of human cognitive ability. *Behavioral and Brain Sciences, 29,* 109–125.

Brieber, S., Neufang, S., Bruning, N., Kamp-Becker, I., Remschmidt, H., Herpertz-Dahlmann, B., et al. (2007). Structural brain abnormalities in adolescents with autism spectrum disorder and patients with attention deficit/hyperactivity disorder. *Journal of Child Psychology and Psychiatry, 48*(12), 1251–1258.

Brown, R. T., & LaRosa, A. L. (2002). Recent developments in the pharmacotherapy of attention deficit/hyperactivity disorder (ADHD). *Professional Psychology: Research and Practice, 33,* 591–595.

Buttross, S. (2000). Attention deficit-hyperactivity disorder and its deceivers. *Current Problems in Pediatrics, 30,* 41–50.

Carter, C. S., Krener, P., Chaderjian, M., & Northcutt, C. (1995). Asymmetrical visual–spatial attentional performance in ADHD: Evidence for a right hemispheric deficit. *Biological Psychiatry, 37,* 789–797.

Casey, B. J., Castellanos, F. X., Giedd, J. N., Marsh, W. L., Hamburger, S. D., Schubert, A. B., et al. (1997). Implications of right frontostriatal circuitry in response inhibition and attention-deficit/hyperactivity disorder. *Journal of the American Academy of Child and Adolescent Psychiatry, 36*(3), 374–383.

Casey, B. J., Nigg, J. T., & Durston, S. (2007). New potential leads in the biology and treatment of attention deficit-hyperactivity disorder. *Current Opinion in Neurology, 20,* 119–124.

Castellanos, F. X. (2001). Neuroimaging studies of attention-deficit/hyperactivity disorder. In M. Solanto, A. Arnsten, & F. X. Castellanos (Eds.), *Attention-deficit/hyperactivity disorder and stimulants: Basic and clinical neuroscience* (pp. 243–258). New York: Oxford University Press.

Castellanos, F. X., Lee, P. P., Sharp, W., Jeffries, N. O., Greenstein, D. K., Clasen, L. S., et al. (2002). Developmental trajectories of brain volume abnormalities in children with attention-deficit/hyperactivity disorder. *Journal of the American Medical Association, 288,* 1740–1748.

Castellanos, F. X., Sonuga-Barke, E. J., Milham, M. P., & Tannock, R. (2006). Characterizing cognition in ADHD: Beyond executive dysfunction. *Trends in Cognitive Sciences, 10*(3), 117–123.

Chhabildas, N., Pennington, B. F., & Willcutt, E. G. (2001). A comparison of the neuropsychological profiles of the DSM-IV subtypes of ADHD. *Journal of Abnormal Child Psychology, 29,* 529–540.

Chow, T. W., & Cummings, J. L. (2007). Frontal–subcortical circuits. In B. L. Miller & J. L. Cummings (Eds.), *The human frontal lobes: Functions and disorders* (2nd ed., pp. 25–43). New York: Guilford Press.

Clark, C., Prior, M., & Kinsella, G. (2002). The relationship between executive function abilities, adaptive behaviour, and academic achievement in children with externalising behaviour problems. *Journal of Child Psychology and Psychiatry, 43,* 785–796.

Clarke, S. D., Kohn, M. R., Hermens, D. F., Rabbinge, M., Clark, C. R., Gordon, E., et al. (2007). Distinguishing symptom profiles in adolescent ADHD using an objective cognitive test battery. *International Journal of Adolescent Medicine and Health, 19,* 355–367.

Coghill, D., Nigg, J., Rothenberger, A., Sonuga-Barke, E., & Tannock, R. (2005). Whither causal models in the neuroscience of ADHD? *Developmental Science*, 8, 105–114.

Collings, R. D. (2003). Differences between ADHD inattentive and combined types on the CPT. *Journal of Psychopathology and Behavioral Assessment, 25*, 177–189.

Congdon, E., & Canli, T. (2005). The endophenotype of impulsivity: Reaching consilience through behavioral, genetic, and neuroimaging approaches. *Behavioral and Cognitive Neuroscience Reviews, 4*, 262–281.

D'Amato, R. C., Fletcher-Janzen, E., & Reynolds, C. R. (Eds.). (2005). *Handbook of school neuropsychology.* Hoboken, NJ: Wiley

Decker, S. L., Hill, S. K., & Dean, R. S. (2007). Evidence of construct similarity in executive functions and fluid reasoning ability. *International Journal of Neuroscience, 117*, 735–748.

Denckla, M. B. (1996). Biological correlates of learning and attention: What is relevant to learning disability and attention-deficit hyperactivity disorder? *Journal of Developmental and Behavioral Pediatrics, 17*, 114–119.

Dennis, M., Francis, D. J., Cirino, P. T., Schachar, R., Barnes, M. A., & Fletcher, J. M. (2009). Why IQ is not a covariate in cognitive studies of neurodevelopmental disorders. *Journal of the International Neuropsychological Society, 15*, 331–343.

Diamond, A. (2005). Attention-deficit disorder (attention-deficit/hyperactivity disorder without hyperactivity): A neurobiologically and behaviourally distinct disorder from attention-deficit/hyperactivity disorder (with hyperactivity). *Development and Psychopathology, 17*(3), 807–825.

Dickstein, S. G., Bannon, K., Castellanos, F. X., & Milham, M. P. (2006). The neural correlates of attention deficit hyperactivity disorder: An ALE meta-analysis. *Journal of Child Psychology and Psychiatry, 47*(10), 1051–1062.

Dixon, S. G., Eusebio, E. C., Turton, W. J., Wright, P. W. D., & Hale, J. B. (2011). *Forest Grove School District v. T.A.* Supreme Court case: Implications for school psychology practice. *Journal of Psychoeducational Assessment, 29*(2), 103–113.

Doya, K. (2000). Complementary roles of basal ganglia and cerebellum in learning and motor control. *Current Opinion in Neurobiology, 10*, 732–739.

Doyle, A. E., Willcutt, E. G., Seidman, L. J., Biederman, J., Chouinard, V. A., Silva, J., et al. (2005). Attention-deficit/hyperactivity disorder endophenotypes. *Biological Psychiatry, 57*, 1324–1335.

Durston, S. A. (2003). A review of the biological bases of ADHD: What have we learned from imaging studies? *Mental Retardation and Developmental Disabilities Research Reviews, 9*, 184–195.

Ek, U., Fernell, E., Westerlund, J., Holmberg, K., Olsson, P., & Gillberg, C. (2007). Cognitive strengths and deficits in schoolchildren with ADHD. *Acta Paediatrica, 96*, 756–761.

Elliott, C., Hale, J. B., Fiorello, C. A., Dorvil, C., & Moldovan, J. (2010). Differential Ability Scales–II prediction of reading performance: Global scores are not enough. *Psychology in the Schools, 47*, 698–720.

Faraone, S. V. (2008). Statistical and molecular genetic approaches to developmental psychopathology: The pathway forward. In J. J. Hudziak (Ed.), *Developmental psychopathology and wellness: Genetic and environmental influences* (pp. 245–265). Arlington, VA: American Psychiatric Publishing.

Fiorello, C. A., Hale, J. B., Decker, S. L., & Coleman, S. (2009). Neuropsychology in school psychology. In E. Garcia-Vazquez, T. D. Crespi, & C. A. Riccio (Eds.), *Handbook of education, training and supervision of school psychologists in school and community* (Vol. 1, pp. 213–232). New York: Taylor & Francis.

Fiorello, C. A., Hale, J. B., Holdnack, J. A., Kavanagh, J. A., Terrell, J., & Long, L. (2007). Interpreting intelligence test results for children with disabilities: Is global intelligence relevant? *Applied Neuropsychology, 14*, 2–12.

Fiorello, C. A., Hale, J. B., & Snyder, L. E. (2006). Cognitive hypothesis testing and response to intervention for children with reading disabilities. *Psychology in the Schools, 43*, 835–854.

Flanagan, D. P., Ortiz, S. O., & Alfonso, V. C. (2007). *Essentials of cross-battery assessment* (2nd ed.). Hoboken, NJ: Wiley.

Fletcher-Janzen, E. (2005). The school neuropsychological examination. In R. C. D'Amato, E. Fletcher-Janzen, & C. R. Reynolds (Eds.), *Handbook of school neuropsychology* (pp. 172–212). Hoboken, NJ: Wiley.

Ford, L., Keith, T. Z., Floyd, R. G., Fields, C., & Schrank, F. A. (2003). Using the Woodcock–Johnson III Tests of Cognitive Abilities with students with attention-deficit/hyperactivity disorder. In F. A. Schrank & D. P. Flanagan (Eds.), *WJ III clinical use and interpretation: Scientist-practitioner perspectives* (pp. 320–344). San Diego, CA: Academic Press.

Frazier, T. W., Demaree, H. A., & Youngstrom, E. (2004). Meta-analysis of intellectual and neuropsychological test performance of children with attention-deficit/hyperactivity disorder. *Neuropsychology, 18*, 543–555.

Friedman, N. P., Haberstruck, B. C., Willcutt, E. G., Miyake, A., Young, S. E., Corle, R. P., et al. (2007). Greater attention problems during childhood predict poorer executive functioning in late adolescence. *Psychological Science, 18*, 893–900.

Gazzaley, A., Cooney, J. W., McEvoy, K., Knight, R. T., & D'Esposito, M. (2005). Top-down enhancement and suppression of the magnitude and speed of neural activity. *Journal of Cognitive Neuroscience, 17,* 507–517.

Genro, J. P., Roman, T., Zeni, C. P., Grevet, E. H., Schmitz, M. P., Abreu, B. P., et al. (2006). No association between dopaminergic polymorphisms and intelligence variability in attention-deficit/hyperactivity disorder. *Molecular Psychiatry, 11,* 1066–1067.

Geurts, H. M., Verte, S., Oosterlaan, J., Roeyers, H., & Sergeant, J. A. (2004). ADHD subtypes: Do they differ in their executive functioning profile? *Archives of Clinical Neuropsychology, 20,* 457–477.

Gibney, L., McIntosh, D. E., Dean, R., & Dunham, M. (2002). Diagnosing attention disorders with measures of neurocognitive functioning. *International Journal of Neuroscience, 112,* 539–564.

Giedd, J. N., Castellanos, F. X., Casey, B. J., Kozuch, P., King, A. C., Hamburger, S. D., et al. (1994). Quantitative morphology of the corpus callosum in attention deficit hyperactivity disorder. *American Journal of Psychiatry, 151,* 665–669.

Gimpel, G., Collett, B., Veeder, M., Gifford, J., Sneddon, P., Bushman, B., et al. (2005). Effects of stimulant medication on cognitive performance of children with ADHD. *Clinical Pediatrics, 44,* 405–411.

Goldberg, E. (2001). *The executive brain: Frontal lobes and the civilized mind.* New York: Oxford University Press.

Goldstein, S., & Naglieri, J. A. (2008). The school neuropsychology of ADHD: Theory, assessment, and intervention. *Psychology in the Schools, 45,* 859–874.

Gomez, R., & Condon, M. (1999). Central auditory processing ability in children with ADHD with and without learning disabilities. *Journal of Learning Disabilities, 32,* 150–158.

Goodyer, I. M. (2000). Language difficulties and psychopathology. In D. V. M. Bishop & L. B. Leonard (Eds.), *Speech and language impairments in children: Causes, characteristics, intervention and outcome* (pp. 227–244). New York: Psychology Press.

Gross-Tsur, V., Shalev, R. S., Manor, O., & Amir, N. (1995). Developmental right-hemisphere syndrome: Clinical spectrum of the nonverbal learning disability. *Journal of Learning Disabilities, 28,* 80–86.

Hain, L. A., Hale, J. B., & Glass-Kendorski, J. (2008). The enigmatic population of specific learning disabilities: Comorbidity of psychopathology in cognitive and academic subtypes. In S. G. Feifer & G. Rattan (Eds.), *Emotional disorders: A neuropsychological, psychopharmacological, and educational perspective* (pp. 199–226). Middletown, MD: School Neuropsych Press.

Hale, J. B., Blaine-Halperin, D., & Beakley, K. (2007, February). *Executive impairment determines ADHD*

response to methylphenidate treatment. Paper presented at the 35th annual meeting of the International Neuropsychological Society, Portland, OR.

Hale, J. B., & Fiorello, C. A. (2004). *School neuropsychology: A practitioner's handbook.* New York: Guilford Press.

Hale, J. B., Fiorello, C. A., & Brown, L. (2005). Determining medication treatment effects using teacher ratings and classroom observations of children with ADHD: Does neuropsychological impairment matter? *Educational and Child Psychology, 22,* 39–61.

Hale, J. B., Fiorello, C. A., Kavanagh, J. A., Holdnack, J. A., & Aloe, A. M. (2007). Is the demise of IQ interpretation justified?: A response to special issue authors. *Applied Neuropsychology, 14,* 37–51.

Hale, J. B., Fiorello, C. A., Miller, J. A., Wenrich, K., Teodori, A. M., & Henzel, J. (2008). WISC-IV assessment and intervention strategies for children with specific learning disabilities. In A. Prifitera, D. H. Saklofske, & L. G. Weiss (Eds.), *WISC-IV clinical assessment and intervention* (2nd ed., pp. 109–171). Amsterdam: Elsevier.

Hale, J. B., Hoeppner, J. B., & Fiorello, C. A. (2002). Analyzing Digit Span components for assessment of attention processes. *Journal of Psychoeducational Assessment, 20,* 128–143.

Hale, J. B., Kaufman, A., Naglieri, J. A., & Kavale, K. A. (2006). Implementation of IDEA: Integrating response to intervention and cognitive assessment methods. *Psychology in the Schools, 43,* 753–770.

Hale, J. B., Reddy, L. A., Decker, S. L., Thompson, R., Henzel, J., Teodori, A., et al. (2009). Development and validation of an executive function and behavior rating screening battery sensitive to ADHD. *Journal of Clinical and Experimental Neuropsychology, 31,* 897–912.

Hale, J. B., Reddy, L. A., Semrud-Clikeman, M., Hain, L., Whitaker, J., Morley, J., et al. (2011). Executive impairment determines ADHD medication response: Implications for academic achievement. *Journal of Learning Disabilities, 44*(2), 196–212.

Hale, J. B., Reddy, L. A., Wilcox, G., McLaughlin, A., Hain, L., Stern, A., et al. (2010). Assessment and intervention for children with ADHD and other frontal–striatal circuit disorders. In D. C. Miller (Ed.), *Best practices in school neuropsychology: Guidelines for effective practice, assessment, and evidence-based intervention* (pp. 225–279). Hoboken, NJ: Wiley.

Hale, J. B., Wycoff, K. L., & Fiorello, C. A. (2010). RTI and cognitive hypothesis testing for specific learning disabilities identification and intervention: The best of both worlds. In D. P. Flanagan & V. C. Alfonso (Eds.), *Essentials of specific learning disability identification* (pp. 173–202). Hoboken, NJ: Wiley.

Halperin, J. M., & Schultz, K. P. (2006). Revisiting the

role of the prefrontal cortex in the pathophysiology of attention-deficit/hyperactivity disorder. *Psychological Bulletin, 132*(4), 560–581.

Harrier, L. K., & DeOrnellas, K. (2005). Performance of children diagnosed with ADHD on selected planning and reconstitution tests. *Applied Neuropsychology, 12,* 106–119.

Hartman, C. A., Willcutt, A. G., Rhee, S. H., & Pennington, B. F. (2004). The relation between sluggish cognitive tempo and DSM-IV ADHD. *Journal of Abnormal Child Psychology, 32,* 491–503.

Hecht, D. (2010). Depression and the hyperactive right hemisphere. *Neuroscience Research, 68,* 77–87.

Henzel, J. (2010). *Neuropsychological processes in children with ADHD and comorbid conditions.* Unpublished doctoral dissertation, Philadelphia College of Osteopathic Medicine.

Hollander, E., & Evers, M. (2001). New developments in impulsivity. *Lancet, 358,* 949–950.

Homack, S., & Riccio, C. A. (2004). A meta-analysis of the sensitivity and specificity of the Stroop Color and Word Test with children. *Archives of Clinical Neuropsychology, 19,* 725–743.

Huang-Pollock, C. L., & Nigg, J. T. (2003). Searching for the attention deficit in attention deficit hyperactivity disorder: The case of visuospatial orienting. *Clinical Psychology Review, 23,* 801–830.

Huang-Pollock, C. L., Nigg, J. T., & Halperin, J. M. (2006). Single dissociation findings of ADHD deficits in vigilance but not anterior or posterior attention systems. *Neuropsychology, 20,* 420–429.

Hurks, P. P., Hendriksen, J. G., Vles, J. S., Kalff, A. C, Feron, F. J., Kroes, M., et al. (2004). Verbal fluency over time as a measure of automatic and controlled processing in children with ADHD. *Brain and Cognition, 55,* 535–544

Ivry, R. B. (1993). Cerebellar involvement in the explicit representation of temporal information. *Annals of the New York Academy of Sciences, 682,* 214–230.

Jepsen, J. R. M., Fagerlund, B., & Mortensen, E. L. (2009). Do attention deficits influence IQ assessment in children and adolescents with ADHD? *Journal of Attention Disorders, 12,* 551–562.

Jucaite, A., Fernell, E., Halldin, C., Forssberg, H., & Farde, L. (2005). Reduced midbrain dopamine transporter binding in male adolescents with attention-deficit/hyperactivity disorder: Association between striatal dopamine markers and motor hyperactivity. *Biological Psychiatry, 57,* 229–238.

Kane, M. J., & Engle, R. W. (2002). The role of the prefrontal cortex in working memory capacity, executive attention, and fluid intelligence: An individual differences perspective. *Psychonomic Bulletin and Review, 9,* 637–671.

Kaplan, B. J., Dewey, D. M., Crawford, S. G., & Fisher, G. C. (1998). Deficits in long-term memory are not characteristic of ADHD. *Journal of Clinical and Experimental Neuropsychology, 20,* 518–528.

Kieling, C., Goncalves, R. R., Tannock, R., & Castellanos, F. X. (2008). Neurobiology of attention-deficit/hyperactivity disorder. *Child and Adolescent Clinics of North America, 17,* 285–307.

Kim, O. H., & Kaiser, A. P. (2000). Language characteristics of children with ADHD. *Communication Disorders Quarterly, 21,* 154–165.

Klimkeit, E. I., Sheppard, D. M., Lee, P., & Bradshaw, J. L. (2004). Bimanual coordination deficits in attention deficit/hyperactivity disorder (ADHD). *Journal of Clinical and Experimental Neuropsychology, 26,* 999–1010.

Klorman, R., Hazel-Fernandez, L. A., Shaywitz, S. E., Fletcher, J. M., Marchione, K. E., Holohan, J., et al. (1999). Executive functioning deficits in attention-deficit/hyperactivity disorder are independent of oppositional defiant or reading disorder. *Journal of the American Academy of Child and Adolescent Psychiatry, 38,* 1148–1155.

Konrad, K., Gauggel, S., Manz, A., & Scholl, M. (2000). Inhibitory control in children with traumatic brain injury (TB1) and children with attention deficit/hyperactivity disorder (ADHD). *Brain Injury, 14,* 859–875.

Kourakis, L. E., Katachanakis, C. N., Vlahonikolis, L. G., & Paritsis, N. K. (2004). Examination of verbal memory and recall time in children with attention deficit hyperactivity disorder. *Developmental Neuropsychology, 26,* 565–570.

Kuntsi, J., Wood, A. C., Van Der Meere, J., & Asherson, P. (2009). Why cognitive performance in ADHD may not reveal true potential: Findings from a large population-based sample. *Journal of the International Neuropsychological Society, 15,* 570–579.

Lawrence, V., Houghton, S., Douglas, G., Durkin, K., Whiting, K., & Tannock, R. (2004). Executive function and ADHD: A comparison of children's performance during neuropsychological testing and real-world activities. *Journal of Attention Disorders, 7,* 137–149.

Liddle, P. F., Kiehl, K. A., & Smith, A. M. (2001). Event-related fMRI study of response inhibition. *Human Brain Mapping, 12,* 100–109.

Liotti, M., Pliszka, S. R., Perez, R., Luus, B., Glahn, D., & Semrud-Clikeman, M. (2007). Electrophysiological correlates of response inhibition in children and adolescents with ADHD: Influence of gender, age, and previous treatment history. *Psychophysiology, 44,* 936–948.

Lockwood, K. A., Marcotte, A. C., & Stern, C. (2001).

Differentiation of attention-deficit/hyperactivity disorder subtypes: Application of a neuropsychological model of attention. *Journal of Clinical and Experimental Neuropsychology, 23,* 317–330.

Love, A. J., & Thompson, M. G. (1988). Language disorders and attention deficit disorders in young children referred for psychiatric services: Analysis of prevalence and a conceptual synthesis. *American Journal of Orthopsychiatry, 58,* 52–64.

Luria, A. R. (1973). *The working brain.* New York: Basic Books.

Mangeot, S. D., Miller, L. J., McIntosh, D. N., McGrath-Clarke, J., Simon, J., Hagerman, et al. (2001). Sensory modulation dysfunction in children with attention-deficit-hyperactivity disorder. *Developmental Medicine and Child Neurology, 43,* 399–406.

Martinussen, R., Hayden, J., Hogg-Johnson, S., & Tannock, R. (2005). A meta-analysis of working memory impairments in children with attention-deficit/hyperactivity disorder. *Journal of the American Academy of Child and Adolescent Psychiatry, 44,* 377–384.

Martinussen, R., & Tannock, R. (2006). Working memory impairments in children with attention-deficit hyperactivity disorder with and without comorbid language learning disorders. *Journal of Clinical and Experimental Neuropsychology, 28,* 1073–1094.

Marusiak, C. W., & Janzen, H. L. (2005). Assessing the working memory abilities of ADHD children using the Stanford–Binet Intelligence Scales, Fifth Edition. *Canadian Journal of School Psychology, 20,* 84–97.

Mayes, S. D., & Calhoun, S. L. (2006). WISC-IV and WISC-III profiles in children with ADHD. *Journal of Attention Disorders, 9,* 486–493.

Mayes, S. D., Calhoun, S. L., Chase, G. A., Mink, D. M., & Stagg, R. E. (2009). ADHD subtypes and co-occurring anxiety, depression, and oppositional-defiant disorder. *Journal of Attention Disorders, 12,* 540–550.

McGrath, L. M., Hutaff-Lee, C., Scott, A., Boada, R., Shriberg, L. D., & Pennington, B. F. (2008). Children with comorbid speech sound disorder and specific language impairment are at increased risk for attention-deficit/hyperactivity disorder. *Journal of Abnormal Child Psychology, 36,* 151–163.

McInnes, A., Humphries, T., Hogg-Johnson, S., & Tannock, R. (2003). Listening comprehension and working memory are impaired in attention-deficit hyperactivity disorder irrespective of language impairment. *Journal of Abnormal Child Psychology, 31,* 427–443.

Milich, R., Balentine, A. C., & Lynam, D. R. (2001). ADHD combined type and ADHD predominantly inattentive type are distinct and unrelated disorders. *Clinical Psychology: Science and Practice, 8,* 463–488.

Mill, J., Caspi, A., Williams, B. S., Craig, I., Taylor, A.,

Polo-Tomas, M., et al. (2006). Prediction of heterogeneity in intelligence and adult prognosis by genetic polymorphisms in the dopamine system among children with attention-deficit/hyperactivity disorder. *Archives of General Psychiatry, 63,* 462–469.

Miller, B. L., & Cummings, J. L. (Eds.). (2007). *The human frontal lobes: Functions and disorders* (2nd ed.). New York: Guilford Press.

Miller, D. C., & Hale, J. B. (2008). Neuropsychological applications of the WISC-IV and WISC-IV Integrated. In A. Prifitera, D. H. Saklofske, & L. G. Weiss (Eds.), *WISC-IV clinical assessment and intervention* (2nd ed., pp. 445–495). Amsterdam: Elsevier.

Miller, J. A., Getz, G., & Leffard, S. A. (2006). *Neuropsychology and the diagnosis of learning disabilities under IDEA 2004.* Poster presented at the 34th annual meeting of the International Neuropsychological Society, Boston.

Mirsky, A. F. (1996). Disorders of attention: A neuropsychological perspective. In G. R. Lyon & N. A. Krasnegor (Eds.), *Attention, memory, and executive function* (pp. 71–95). Baltimore: Brookes.

Moll, G. H., Heinrich, H., Trott, G., Wirth, S., & Rothenberger, A. (2000). Deficient intracortical inhibition in drug-naive children with attention-deficit hyperactivity disorder is enhanced by methylphenidate. *Neuroscience Letters, 284,* 121–125.

Moss, W. L., & Sheiffele, W. A. (1994). Can we differentially diagnose an attention deficit disorder without hyperactivity from a central auditory processing problem? *Child Psychiatry and Human Development, 25,* 85–96.

Mostofsky, S. H., Cooper, K. L., Kates, W. R., Denckla, M. B., & Kaufmann, W. E. (2002). Smaller prefrontal and premotor volumes in boys with attention-deficit/hyperactivity disorder. *Biological Psychiatry, 52,* 785–794.

Mostofsky, S. H., Newschaffer, C. J., & Denckla, M. B. (2003). Overflow movements predict impaired response inhibition in children with ADHD. *Perceptual and Motor Skills, 97,* 1315–1331.

Myers, C. E., Shohamy, D., Gluck, M. A., Grossman, S., Kluger, A., Ferris, S., et al. (2003). Dissociating hippocampal versus basal ganglia contributions to learning and transfer. *Journal of Cognitive Neuroscience, 15,* 185–193.

Naglieri, J. A., Salter, C. J., & Edwards, G. H. (2004). Assessment of ADHD and reading disabilities using the PASS theory and Cognitive Assessment System. *Journal of Psychoeducational Assessment, 22,* 93–105.

Nigg, J. T. (2000). On inhibition/disinhibition in developmental psychopathology: Views from cognitive and personality psychology and a working inhibition taxonomy. *Psychological Bulletin, 126,* 220–246.

Nigg, J. T. (2005). Neuropsychologic theory and findings in attention-deficit/hyperactivity disorder: The state of the field and salient challenges for the coming decade. *Biological Psychiatry, 57,* 1424–1435.

Nigg, J. T., Blaskey, L. G., Huang-Pollock, C. L., & Rappley, M. D. (2002). Neuropsychological Executive functions and DSM-IV ADHD subtypes. *Journal of the American Academy of Child and Adolescent Psychiatry, 41,* 59–66.

Nigg, J. T., Blaskey, L. G., Stawicki, J. A., & Sachek, J. (2004). Evaluating the endophenotype model of ADHD neuropsychological deficit: Results for parents and siblings of children with ADHD combined and inattentive subtypes. *Journal of Abnormal Psychology, 113,* 614–625.

Nigg, J. T., & Casey, B. J. (2005). An integrative theory of attention-deficit/hyperactivity disorder based on cognitive and affective neurosciences. *Development and Psychopathology, 17,* 785–806.

Ors, M., Ryding, E., Lindgren, M., Gustafsson, P., Blennow, G., & Rosen, I. (2005). SPECT findings in children with specific language impairment. *Cortex, 41,* 316–326.

Packard, M. G., & Knowlton, B. J. (2002). Learning and memory functions of the basal ganglia. *Annual Review of Neuroscience, 25,* 563–593.

Pasini, A., Paloscia, C., Allessandrelli, R., Porfirio, M. C., & Curatolo, P. (2007). Attention and executive functions profile in drug naïve ADHD subtypes. *Brain and Development, 29,* 400–408.

Pearson, D. A., Santos, C., Roache, J., Casat, C., Loveland, K. A., Lachar, D., et al. (2003). Treatment effects of methylphenidate on behavioral adjustment in children with mental retardation and ADHD. *Journal of the American Academy of Child and Adolescent Psychiatry, 42,* 209–216.

Piek, J. P., Dyck, M. J., Francis, M., & Conwell, A. (2007). Working memory, processing speed, and set-shifting in children with developmental coordination disorder and attention-deficit-hyperactivity disorder. *Developmental Medicine and Child Neurology, 49,* 678–683.

Pisecco, S., Baker, D. B., Silva, P. A., & Brooke, M. (2001). Boys with reading disabilities and/or ADHD: Distinctions in early childhood. *Journal of Learning Disabilities, 34,* 98–106.

Pliszka, S. R. (2005). The neuropsychopharmacology of attention-deficit/hyperactivity disorder. *Biological Psychiatry, 57,* 1385–1390.

Pliszka, S. R., Liotti, M., & Woldorff, M. G. (2000). Inhibitory control in children with attention-deficit/hyperactivity disorder: Event related potentials identify the processing component and timing of an impaired right-frontal response-inhibition mechanism. *Biological Psychiatry, 48,* 238–246.

Polanczyk, G., Silva de Lima, M., Lessa Horta, B., Biederman, J., & Rohde, L. A. (2007). The worldwide prevalence of ADHD: A systematic review and metaregression analysis. *American Journal of Psychiatry, 164,* 942–948.

Polderman, T. J. C., de Geus, E. J. C., Hoekstra, R. A., Bartels, M., van Leeuwen, M., Verhulst, F. C., et al. (2009). Attention problems, inhibitory control, and intelligence index overlapping genetic factors: A study in 9-, 12-, and 18-year-old twins. *Neuropsychology, 23,* 381–391.

Polderman, T. J. C., Gosso, M. F., Posthuma, D., van Beijsterveldt, T. C., Heutink, P., Verhulst, F. C., et al. (2006). A longitudinal twin study on IQ, executive functioning, and attention problems during childhood and early adolescence. *Acta Neurologica Belgica, 106,* 191–207.

Posner, M. I., & Petersen, S. E. (1990). The attention system of the human brain. *Annual Review of Neuroscience, 13,* 25–42.

Purvis, K., & Tannock, R. (1997). Language abilities in children with attention deficit hyperactivity disorder, reading disabilities, and normal controls. *Journal of Abnormal Child Psychology, 25,* 133–144.

Quay, H. C. (1977). Measuring dimensions of deviant behavior: The Behavior Problem Checklist. *Journal of Abnormal Child Psychology, 5,* 277–287.

Rapoport, M., van Reekum, R., & Mayberg, H. (2000). The role of the cerebellum in cognition and behavior: A selective review. *Journal of Neuropsychiatry and Clinical Neurosciences, 12,* 193–198.

Reddy, L. A., Braunstein, D. J., & Dumont, R. (2008). Use of the Differential Ability Scales for children with attention-deficit/hyperactivity disorder. *School Psychology Quarterly, 23,* 39–48.

Reddy, L. A., & Hale, J. B. (2007). Inattentiveness. In A. R. Eisen (Ed.), *Clinical handbook of childhood behavior problems: Case formulation and step-by-step treatment programs* (pp. 156–211). New York: Guilford Press.

Reschly, D. J. (2005). Learning disabilities identification: Primary intervention, secondary intervention, and then what? *Journal of Learning Disabilities, 38,* 510–515.

Riccio, C. A., Hynd, G. W., Cohen, M. J., Hall, J., & Molt, L. (1994). Comorbidity of central auditory processing disorder and attention-deficit hyperactivity disorder. *Journal of the American Academy of Child and Adolescent Psychiatry, 33,* 849–857.

Riccio, C. A., Reynolds, C. R., Lowe, P., & Moore, J. J. (2002). The continuous performance test: A window on the neural substrates for attention? *Archives of Clinical Neuropsychology, 17,* 235–272.

Romine, C. B., Lee, D., Wolfe, M. E., Homack, S., George, C., & Riccio, C. A. (2004). Wisconsin Card

Sorting Test with children: A meta-analytic study of sensitivity and specificity. *Archives of Clinical Neuropsychology, 19,* 1027–1041.

Rommelse, N. N. J., Altink, M. E., Oosterlaan, J., Beem, L., Buschgens, C. J. M., Buitelaar, J., et al. (2008). Speed, variability, and timing of motor output in ADHD: Which measures are useful for endophenotypic research? *Behavior Genetics, 38,* 121–132.

Rowe, D. L., Robinson, P. A., Lazzaro, I. L., Powles, R. C., Gordon, E., & Williams, L. M. (2005). Biophysical modeling of tonic cortical electrical activity in attention deficit hyperactivity disorder. *International Journal of Neuroscience, 115,* 1273–1305.

Rubia, K. (2002). The dynamic approach to neurodevelopmental psychiatric disorders: Use of fMRI combined with neuropsychology to elucidate the dynamics of psychiatric disorders, exemplified in ADHD and schizophrenia. *Behavioural Brain Research, 130,* 47–56.

Rubia, K., Overmeyer, S. O., Taylor, E., Brammer, M., Williams, S. C. R., Simmons, A., et al. (1999). Hypofrontality in attention deficit hyperactivity disorder during higher order motor control: A study with functional MRI. *American Journal of Psychiatry, 156,* 891–896.

Rubia, K., Smith, A. B., Brammer, M. J., Toone, B., & Taylor, E. (2005). Abnormal brain activation during inhibition and error detection in medication-naive adolescents with ADHD. *American Journal of Psychiatry, 162,* 1067–1075.

Rucklidge, J. J., & Tannock, R. (2002). Neuropsychological profiles of adolescents with ADHD: Effects of reading difficulties and gender. *Journal of Child Psychology and Psychiatry, 43,* 988–1003.

Russell, V. A., Oades, R. D., Tannock, R., Killeen, P. R., Auerback, J. G., Johansen, E. B., et al. (2006). Response variability in attention-deficit/hyperactivity disorder: A neuronal and glial energetic hypothesis. *Behavioral and Brain Functions, 2*(30), 1–25.

Sagvolden, T., Aase, H., Johansen, E. B., & Russell, V. A. (2005). A dynamic developmental theory of attention-deficit/hyperactivity disorder (ADHD) predominantly hyperactive/impulsive and combined subtypes. *Behavioral and Brain Sciences, 28,* 397–468.

Sandson, T. A., Bachna, K. J., & Morin, M. D. (2000). Right hemisphere dysfunction in ADHD: Visual hemispatial inattention and clinical subtype. *Journal of Learning Disabilities, 33,* 83–90.

Schulz, K. P., Fan, J., Tang, C. Y., Newcorn, J. H., Buchsbaum, M. S., Cheung, A. M., et al. (2004). Response inhibition in adolescents diagnosed with attention deficit hyperactivity disorder during childhood: An event-related fMRI study. *American Journal of Psychiatry, 161,* 1650–1657.

Semrud-Clikeman, M., Filipek, P. A., Biederman, J., Steingard, R., Kennedy, D., Renshaw, M., et al. (1994). Attention-deficit hyperactivity disorder: Magnetic resonance imaging morphometric analysis of the corpus callosum. *Journal of the American Academy of Child and Adolescent Psychiatry, 33,* 875–881.

Sergeant, J. A. (2000). The cognitive-energetic model: An empirical approach to attention-deficit hyperactivity disorder. *Neuroscience and Biobehavioral Reviews, 24,* 7–12.

Sergeant, J. A., Geurts, H., & Oosterlaan, J. (2002). How specific is a deficit in executive functioning for attention-deficit/hyperactivity disorder? *Behavioural Brain Research, 130,* 3–28.

Sergeant, J. A., Piek, J. P., & Oosterlaan, J. (2006). ADHD and DCD: A relationship in need of research. *Human Movement Science, 25,* 76–89.

Shaywitz, S. E., & Shaywitz, B. A. (1988). Increased medication use in attention-deficit hyperactivity disorder: Regressive or appropriate? *Journal of the American Medical Association, 260,* 2270–2272.

Smith, E. E., & Jonides, J. (1997). Working memory: A view from neuroimaging. *Cognitive Psychology, 33,* 5–42.

Snow, J. B., & Sapp, G. L. (2000). WISC-III subtest patterns of ADHD and normal samples. *Psychological Reports, 87,* 759–765.

Solanto, M. V., Abikoff, H., Sonuga-Barke, E., Schachar, R., Logan, G. D., Wigal, T., et al. (2001). The ecological validity of delay aversion and response inhibition as measures of impulsivity in AD/HD: A supplement to the NIMH Multimodal Treatment Study of AD/HD. *Journal of Abnormal Child Psychology, 29,* 215–228.

Sonuga-Barke, E. J. S. (2005). Causal models of attention-deficit/hyperactivity disorder: From common simple deficits to multiple developmental pathways. *Biological Psychiatry, 57,* 1231–1238.

Sonuga-Barke, E. J. S., Sergeant, J. A., Nigg, J., & Willcutt, E. (2008). Executive dysfunction and delay aversion in attention deficit hyperactivity disorder: Nosologic and diagnostic implications. *Child and Adolescent Psychiatric Clinics of North America, 17,* 367–384.

Suskauer, S., Simmonds, D., Caffo, B. S., Denckla, M. B., Pekar, J., & Mostofsky, S. (2008). fMRI of intrasubject variability in ADHD: Anomalous premotor activity with prefrontal compensation. *Journal of the American Academy of Child and Adolescent Psychiatry, 10,* 1141–1150.

Tannock, R., & Schachar, R. (1996). Executive dysfunction as an underlying mechanism of behavior and language problems in attention deficit hyperactivity disorder. In J. H. Beitchman, N. J. Cohen, M.

M. Konstantareas, & R. Tannock (Eds.), *Language, learning, and behavior disorders: Developmental, biological, and clinical perspectives* (pp. 128–155). New York: Cambridge University Press.

Thorell, L. B. (2007). Do delay aversion and executive function deficits make distinct contributions to the functional impact of ADHD symptoms?: A study of early academic skill deficits. *Journal of Child Psychology and Psychiatry, 48,* 1061–1070.

Tillman, C. M., Bohlin, G., Sorensen, L., & Lundervold, A. J. (2009). Intellectual deficits in children with ADHD beyond central executive and nonexecutive functions. *Archives of Clinical Neuropsychology, 24,* 769–782.

Tulving, E., & Markowitsch, H. J. (1997). Memory beyond the hippocampus. *Current Opinion in Neurobiology, 7,* 209–216.

Vaidya, C. J., Austin, G., Kirkorian, G., Ridlehuber, H. W., Desmond, J. E., Glover, G. H., et al. (1998). Selective effects of methylphenidate in attention deficit hyperactivity disorder: A functional magnetic resonance study. *Proceedings of the National Academy of Sciences USA, 95,* 14494–14499.

Vaidya, C. J., Bunge, S. A., Dudukovic, N. M., Zalecki, C. A., Elliott, G. R., & Gabrieli, J. D. E. (2005). Altered neural substrates of cognitive control in childhood ADHD: Evidence from functional magnetic resonance imaging. *American Journal of Psychiatry, 162,* 1605–1613

Valera, E. M., Faraone, S. V., Murray, K. E., & Seidman, L. J. (2007). Meta-analysis of structural imaging findings in attention-deficit/hyperactivity disorder. *Biological Psychiatry, 61,* 1361–1369.

Van Luit, J. E. H., Kroesbergen, E. H., & Naglieri, J. A. (2005). Utility of the PASS theory and Cognitive Assessment System for Dutch children with and without ADHD. *Journal of Learning Disabilities, 38,* 434–439.

Voeller, K. K. S. (2001). Attention-deficit/hyperactivity disorder as a frontal–subcortical disorder. In D. G. Lichter & J. L. Cummings (Eds.), *Frontal–subcortical circuits in psychiatric and neurological disorders* (pp. 334–371). New York: Guilford Press.

Wahlstedt, K. C., Eninger, L., Thorell, L. B., & Bohlin, G. (2008). Interrelations between executive function and symptoms of hyperactivity/impulsivity and inattention in preschoolers: A two year longitudinal study. *Journal of Abnormal Child Psychology, 38,* 163–171.

Watemberg, N., Waiserberg, N., Zuk, L., & Lerman-Sagie, T. (2007). Developmental coordination disorder in children with attention-deficit-hyperactivity disorder and physical therapy intervention. *Developmental Medicine and Child Neurology, 49,* 920–925.

Weiler, M. D., Holmes Bernstein, J., Bellinger, D. C., & Waber, D. P. (2000). Processing speed in children with attention deficit/hyperactivity disorder, inattentive type. *Child Neuropsychology, 6,* 218–234.

Westby, C. E., & Cutler, S. K. (1994). Language and ADHD: Understanding the bases and treatment of self-regulatory deficits. *Topics in Language Disorders, 14,* 58–76.

Willcutt, E. G., Doyle, A. E., Nigg, J. T., Faraone, S. V., & Pennington, B. F. (2005). Validity of the executive function theory of attention-deficit/hyperactivity disorder: A meta-analytic review. *Biological Psychiatry, 57,* 1336–1346.

Willcutt, E. G., Pennington, B. F., Chhabildas, N. A., Friedman, M. C., & Alexander, J. (1999). Psychiatric comorbidity associated with DSM-IV ADHD in a nonreferred sample of twins. *Journal of the American Academy of Child and Adolescent Psychiatry, 38,* 1355–1362.

Williams, D., Stott, C. M., Goodyer, I. M., & Sahakian, B. J. (2000). Specific language impairment with or without hyperactivity: Neuropsychological evidence for frontostriatal dysfunction. *Developmental Medicine and Child Neurology, 42,* 368–375.

Yochman, A., Parush, S., & Ornoy, A. (2004). Responses of preschool children with and without ADHD to sensory events in daily life. *American Journal of Occupational Therapy, 58,* 294–302.

Intellectual and Neuropsychological Assessment of Individuals with Sensory and Physical Disabilities and Traumatic Brain Injury

Scott L. Decker
Julia A. Englund
Alycia M. Roberts

Neuropsychology differs from traditional forms of cognitive assessment in that it is based on a theoretical understanding of the underlying biological mechanisms that cause or influence cognition and behavior. This chapter outlines the neuropsychological basis and assessment of physical and sensory deficits, as well as traumatic brain injury (TBI), in children. These disabilities are discussed together and addressed within a neuropsychological framework because behavioral deficits resulting from these disabilities clearly originate in biological function. Understanding the clinical manifestations of these disabilities will enhance interventions and services for children with such conditions.

Assessments of physical and sensory functioning have long been part of standard neuropsychological evaluations (Finger, 1994). Interestingly, sensory measures have been correlated not only with academic measures (Decker, 2004), but also with measures of intellectual functioning (Decker, 2002; Roberts, Pallier, & Goff, 1999; Stankov, Seizova-Cajic, & Roberts, 2001). Although the mechanistic connection is debatable, both sensory and physical abilities are prerequisites for input and output mechanisms of cognitive faculties and provide indicators of the cognitive system's integrity.

There are shared areas of the brain that participate in sensory–motor behaviors as well as higher cognitive abilities. For example, lesions in the left frontal area of the brain may result in contralateral motor impairment (right-side hemiplegia) as well as language deficits (expressive aphasia), due to localized proximity of both functions in a spatially similar area of the brain (Kolb & Whishaw, 2003). Although deficits in either function may be obvious to the trained clinician, it is only neuropsychological theory—informed by the understanding of brain–behavior correspondence—that can explain the connections between sensory deficits and intellectual deficits, as well as between sensory functions and higher cognitive faculties like language.

In the sections that follow, we focus specifically on sensory, physical, and TBI-caused disabilities. Each section provides both practical and legal definitions for each type of disability. In addition, assessment and intervention issues are addressed. Both individual child factors and test-related factors important to consider when clinicians are selecting, administering, and interpreting neuropsychological and cognitive tests are included.

SENSORY DISABILITIES

According to the U.S. Census Bureau (2000), 9.3 million people in the United States, or about 3.6% of the general population, are estimated to suffer from sensory disabilities (limitations in sight or hearing). The *Standards for Educational and Psychological Testing* volume (American Educational Research Association [AERA], American Psychological Association [APA], & National Council on Measurement in Education [NCME], 1999) emphasizes fairness in testing for individuals with such disabilities and suggests common accommodations for these individuals, including modifying presentation or response format, timing, or setting; using only portions of a test; or substituting assessment instruments/using alternative tests. Individual factors may affect which tests are given and what modifications are made, as well as how accurately the resultant test scores reflect a child's cognitive and neuropsychological functioning. It is therefore the clinician's responsibility to ensure selection of appropriate instruments, nonbiased test administration and interpretation of results, and application and consideration of necessary modifications for each child.

In a school setting, children with visual impairment or blindness (VI/B) are served mainly under the Individuals with Disabilities Education Improvement Act of 2004 (IDEA 2004) category of *visual impairment*, defined in federal regulations (U.S. Department of Education, 2006) as follows:

> *Visual impairment including blindness* means an impairment in vision that, even with correction, adversely affects a child's educational performance. The term includes both partial sight and blindness. (p. 46757)

According to the IDEA Data Accountability Center (DAC) (n.d.), in fall 2008 U.S. public schools in the 50 states served 3,420 children ages 3–5 (of 708,481 total preschool students served under all categories) and 25,790 children and youth ages 6–21 (of 5,884,739 total) under the IDEA 2004 category of visual impairment. Slightly more children and youth (8,416 ages 3–5 and 70,682 ages 6–21 in fall 2008) were served under the combined *deafness* and *hearing impairment* IDEA categories, defined, respectively, as follows:

> *Deafness* means a hearing impairment that is so severe that the child is impaired in processing linguistic information through hearing, with or without amplification that adversely affects a child's educational performance. . . . *Hearing impairment* means an impairment in hearing, whether permanent or fluctuating, that adversely affects a child's educational performance but that is not included under the definition of deafness in this section. (p. 46756)

And, lastly, in fall 2008, 207 children ages 3–5 and 1,735 children and youth ages 6–21 were served under the IDEA *deaf-blindness* definition:

> *Deaf-blindness* means concomitant hearing and visual impairments, the combination of which causes such severe communication and other developmental and educational needs that [the children] cannot be accommodated in special education programs solely for children with deafness or children with blindness. (p. 46756)

Few studies focus specifically on the cognitive and neuropsychological assessment of children with deaf-blindness, which involves multiple disabilities that may or may not be interrelated, and so the populations with VI/B and deafness/hearing impairment (D/HI) are our main focus in this portion of the chapter. Briefly, however, in a recent review of individual variables for examiners to consider when evaluating children and individuals with deaf-blindness, Dalby and colleagues (2009) specified etiology as a major factor. According to Dalby and colleagues, individuals with congenital deaf-blindness are more likely to experience cognitive, adaptive, and social impairments than those whose deaf-blindness is acquired. Those with acquired deaf-blindness are more likely to use speech as their primary mode of communication. The American Association of the Deaf-Blind's website (*www.aadb.org*) offers educational resources to address the needs of these multiply disabled children, such as listings of state organizations, service providers, and support groups; frequently asked questions and fact sheets; newsletters and magazines; and information about assistive technology. *Best Practices in School Psychology V* (Thomas & Grimes, 2008) offers broad-based information helpful for designing instruction and intervention for individuals with multiple disabilities like deaf-blindness. In particular, Powell-Smith, Stoner, Bilter, and Sansosti (2008) emphasize the importance of systemic collaboration, considering each child's optimal learning environment and mode of communication, and encouraging family involvement.

Etiologies: A Brief Overview

In a typically developing child, vision begins with the eye detecting light in the environment and transducing the stimulus energy into neurological impulses. These impulses are sent from the eye (retina) to the occipital lobes of the brain via the optic nerve, which travels through the lateral geniculate nucleus in the midbrain before transferring information to the primary visual cortex for basic visual processing; then information such as orientation, contrast, color, location in space, and identity is saved for higher-level processing in either the occipitoparietal dorsal visual stream or the temporoparietal ventral visual stream, depending on information type. In some children with VI/B, abnormal pigment production in the eye (albinism, a congenital condition; Bradley-Johnson & Morgan, 2008) disrupts this process early in the stream. Other congenital causes include retinitis pigmentosa, which involves degeneration of light-sensitive retinal cells, or various forms of prenatal damage to the visual system. If the damage occurs during or after birth, the vision loss is considered acquired. Bradley-Johnson and Morgan (2008) list the following possible diseases and accidents that may result in acquired vision loss: head injury, anoxia at birth, central nervous system infections (e.g., meningitis), and medication reactions. Damage to any part of the visual pathway can lead to observable difficulties with visual tasks, but most children's vision loss can be traced to the eye or optic nerve early on in the pathway. One exception is cortical visual impairment, sometimes called cortical blindness, which occurs with damage to the brain's visual system from head injuries, infections, and other accidents or diseases. Children with this condition experience problems not only with basic visual processing, but also with attention and other cognitive functions (Bradley-Johnson & Morgan, 2008). Understanding the etiology of a particular child's vision loss can aid in individualized and sensitive psychoeducational assessment and planning.

Children without hearing impairments first receive sound information as sound waves, or vibrations, entering the outer, middle, and then inner ear. The vibrations travel from the eardrum to three tiny bones in the middle ear, and then one of those bones, called the stirrup, sends the vibrations along the coiled cochlea in the inner ear. When the cochlea vibrates, tiny hairs called cilia move, and the sound information passes through the auditory nerve to the auditory cortex in the temporal lobes of the brain for processing. The auditory cortex organizes information from different sound frequencies in higher cortical areas, which individuals "hear" as different sounds.

According to the American Speech–Language–Hearing Association (ASHA, 2010), sensorineural hearing loss—which occurs when the cochlea or auditory nerve is damaged, is permanent, and cannot be corrected with surgery or other medical procedures—can result from disease (e.g., viruses or tumors); exposure to toxins (e.g., drugs) or high noise levels; head injuries; inherited genetic syndromes; or perinatal injury. These children not only have trouble hearing low-level sound, but also experience difficulty understanding speech and hearing sounds clearly (ASHA, 2010). Conductive hearing loss, on the other hand, results primarily in an inability to hear faint sounds or a reduction in sound level that is often surgically correctable. Conductive hearing loss can be caused by middle ear pathology (e.g., otitis media or ear infection), impacted earwax, ear canal infection, irritation from a foreign body in the ear, or malformation or absence of any physical part of the outer or middle ear (ASHA, 2010). If there is damage to or malfunction of both the outer or middle ear and the inner ear or auditory nerve, mixed (sensorineural and conductive) hearing loss can occur. In addition, hearing loss can be unilateral (occurring only in one ear) or bilateral. According to ASHA (2010), about 1 in 1,000 children is born with unilateral hearing loss, and approximately 3% of all school-age children suffer from it. Children with both unilateral and bilateral hearing loss are at risk for academic, speech–language, and social-emotional difficulties (ASHA, 2010).

Special Considerations for Assessment: Child Factors

A variety of individual factors can influence the test performance of children with sensory disabilities and can affect the interpretation of results. Selected chapters in the Thomas and Grimes (2008) volume offer helpful educational programming information for students with VI/B (Bradley-Johnson & Morgan, 2008) and students with D/HI (Lukomski, 2008), highlighting the diversity of these populations and the lack of a "one-size-fits-all" solution for their psychoeducational planning. For both populations, early intervention and family collaboration, as well as a multidisciplinary approach to assessment, placement, and intervention, are imperative for appropriate data-based decision making in the schools. The school psychologist must cooperate with a team of specialists and other professionals—such as speech–hearing therapists and educators, medical personnel, and VI/B educators—to develop a comprehensive, interdisciplinary educational plan for each child that addresses child-environment fit, considers preferred modes of communication, and includes objectives and strategies for improving social interaction and communication skills. For a child with D/HI, Lukomski (2008) stresses including the following specific elements in the child's plan: strategies for handling communication breakdowns, handling the child's fatigue, school staff training in communication strategies, and American Sign Language (ASL) parent training. In addition, decision-making and planning teams must keep in mind that most children with hearing problems have average IQs but exhibit lags in literacy and academic achievement because of developmental differences in the acquisition and internalization of language. For children with VI/B, having a basic understanding of the variety and availability of adaptive technologies and materials, such as raised-line paper, computer programs with speech or Braille output, and closed-circuit television that electronically magnifies text for children with low vision, is crucial (Bradley-Johnson & Morgan, 2008). Since many visual cues in the environment are unavailable to these children, the school psychologist must also include strategies targeted at improving organizational skills and social communication. For children with either D/HI or VI/B, evaluation should include systematic observation of the children in a variety of settings, since social interactions, communication modes, and behavior may vary among contexts.

Next, we consider specific areas of heterogeneity in the populations with VI/B and D/HI that may affect test selection, administration, and interpretation, including the following: age at onset; quantitative and qualitative nature of the vision or hearing loss; etiology; comorbidity; and (for children with D/HI) reading and language ability, preferred mode of communication, and parental hearing status.

Individual Factors to Consider in Assessment of Children with VI/B

One major individual factor to consider in the assessment of children with VI/B is age at onset of the sensory impairment, which contributes to the heterogeneity of this population. For example, in the standardization sample for the Comprehensive Vocational Evaluation System (CVES; Dial, Chan, Mezger, et al., 1991)—an empirically developed, VI/B-specific neuropsychological battery—56% of cases were considered "congenital," with onset of vision impairment occurring from birth to 1 year of age; 8% were "early blind" (2 years to 5 years, 11 months); 9% were "school age" (6 years to 17

years, 11 months); and the rest were adult-onset cases (Hill-Briggs, Dial, Morere, & Joyce, 2007). Joyce, Isom, Dial, and Sandel (2004) found that adults with early-onset VI outperformed those with adult-onset VI in shape and texture discrimination on tests from the Haptic Sensory Discrimination Test (HSDT) and McCarron Assessment of Neuromuscular Development, VI/B Version (MAND-VI), providing evidence that age at onset of VI substantially impacts neuropsychological test results. Conversely, adult-onset participants excelled at persistent motor control, and the school-onset group performed significantly better than early-onset individuals in bimanual dexterity (Joyce et al., 2004). On the other hand, MacCluskie, Tunick, Dial, and Paul (1998) compared Wechsler Adult Intelligence Scale—Revised (WAIS-R) and Cognitive Test for the Blind (CTB) performance for groups of adults ($N = 60$) with early-onset (before age 2) versus late-onset (after age 5) VI and found no significant differences. However, years of education significantly contributed to variance in cognitive ability scores. The authors tested a small sample of adults and did not control for degree of residual vision, so these results should be interpreted with caution. Notwithstanding, one implication for professionals assessing persons with VI/B is that while age of onset itself may not contribute to variability in cognitive test scores, number of years of education seems to matter. Thus, it is important to consider how the examinee's current age and grade level may influence scores in individuals with both congenital and late-onset VI/B.

Another variable that can affect test performance and interpretation of results is level of blindness or amount of vision loss. The Texas School for the Blind and Visually Impaired (2010) reminds clinicians that an individual with congenital (onset prior to 18 months of age) blindness and no vision—a Braille or tactile learner—is at the most severe end of the spectrum, and will require the most modifications both to testing and to educational content and delivery methods; a print learner with low vision will require fewer testing and educational modifications. Consider the illustrative case of the CVES standardization sample, in which 71% of cases were considered "legally blind," 18% "visually impaired," and 11% "totally blind." It is also worth noting that even two individuals with the same optical refraction score (e.g., 20/100) may have different functional levels of vision (Hill-Briggs et al., 2007). In the Joyce and colleagues (2004) study, participants who had some residual functional vision performed significantly better on various subtests of the HSDT and MAND-VI (included in the CVES battery) than those who were "totally blind"; again, this demonstrates the importance of considering level of vision loss in assessing individuals with VI/B.

Clinicians should keep in mind that VI/B has different etiologies in different people, and that multiple etiologies may even be present within the same individual. Studies have found differences in cognitive and neuropsychological performance based on these different etiologies. For example, participants whose blindness was caused by early birth (retinopathy of prematurity, or ROP) performed significantly worse on spatial and auditory analysis (verbal–spatial cognitive abilities) and hand strength (perceptual–motor functions) tests from the CVES battery than participants with either retinitis pigmentosa or congenital cataracts as etiologies (Nelson, O'Brien, Dial, & Joyce, 2001). It was concluded that ROP caused more cognitive impairment than other common etiologies of VI/B. Similarly, McGee (1994) found that those with diabetes-related blindness performed worse on tasks measuring left-lateralized perceptual–motor functions, as well as on nonverbal cognitive tasks.

Many individuals with VI/B suffer from comorbid disabilities or conditions that may or may not be related to their vision loss, including neuropsychological conditions (such as head injuries, cerebral palsy, and tumors) and other disabilities commonly seen in school settings (e.g., learning, hearing, or physical disabilities). In fact, throughout the CVES standardization process, only 25% of the individuals who presented with vision loss did *not* have profiles consistent with another such disorder (Hill-Briggs et al., 2007), and standardization was based only on this 25%. However, since the majority of individuals with VI/B seem to suffer from comorbid disorders, it is debatable whether or not a group without comorbidity is truly representative of the population with VI/B in the United States. In fact, according to Miller (2007), almost all children with sensory impairments have additional impairments in academic, social, cognitive, adaptive, and/or behavioral domains. It is vital for the evaluator to keep in mind that the cognitive and neuropsychological profile observed during evaluation of an individual with VI/B and a comorbid condition may be the effect of the VI/B, of the other neuropsychological disorder, of the additive combination of both independent conditions, or of the multiplicative effects of both conditions acting together.

Individual Factors to Consider in Assessment of Children with D/HI

Age at onset should also be considered in assessing children with D/HI. Because hearing, verbal communication, and language development are linked, children with early-onset (prior to 18 months old) hearing loss and those whose hearing loss occurred after significant language development exhibit significantly different profiles of linguistic and communicative functioning (Braden, 1994; Marschark & Clark, 1993; Meadow, 1980). Although severe and profound hearing loss will have the most significant impact on test administration, any level of hearing loss can have some effect on standardized test performance (Braden, 1994). In addition, examiners should consider whether or not the hearing loss is progressive, as an examinee's current level of hearing loss may not be the same as it was earlier in development or will be later in life (Hill-Briggs et al., 2007). Finally, as in the evaluation of children with VI/B, clinicians must also consider the additive and interactive influences of any comorbid disability or medical condition. A learning disability, for example, may be overlooked if diagnostic overshadowing causes the examiner to erroneously attribute all verbal reasoning deficits to hearing loss.

One relatively unique factor in assessing individuals with D/HI is their level of reading and language ability. According to the Gallaudet Research Institute (2005), 18-year-olds with severe hearing loss usually perform on tests of reading comprehension at a grade 4.5 level, and those with profound hearing loss at a grade 3.8 level. Competency with reading and writing tasks may also be negatively affected by the different grammatical structures of traditional spoken English and many signing systems, such as ASL. Therefore, asking children with D/HI to read the directions for a test is not an appropriate modification. Variability in reading and language levels should also be taken into account when examiners are selecting tests that include high verbal loadings or rely substantially on reading instructions and/or stimuli.

A further consideration for evaluators in testing an individual with D/HI is the examinee's primary or preferred mode of communication—both current and during development. Current communication mode has implications for communication methods during testing; for example, this affects the decision of whether to use an interpreter, to seek an examiner fluent in ASL or another visual communication system, or to modify the test administration in some other way so as to accommodate the individual child's hearing loss level and preferred communication style. Several studies have also shown that mode of communication during development—for example, cued speech, oral communication, combined methods, or sign language (ASL or another signing system)—affects cognitive functioning and performance, and even lateralization of neuropsychological tasks (e.g., Bosworth & Dobkins, 1999; Cattani & Clibbens, 2005; Charlier & Leybaert, 2000; LaSasso, Crain, & Leybaert, 2003).

Parental hearing status (i.e., whether or not the parents also have D/HI) can also affect a child's development of language and communication (Anderson, 2006), achievement and psychosocial adjustment (Polat, 2003), as well as cultural and identity development as the child decides whether to identify primarily with deaf culture or to assimilate him- or herself into the hearing world (Leigh, Marcus, Dobosh, & Allen, 1998). Clinicians should not only be sensitive to these cultural issues, but remember that the hearing status of a child's parents will affect the child's cognitive functioning (Braden, 1994; Vernon, 2005) and his or her preferred or primary communication mode in adolescence and adulthood. Although debates continue on this issue, it has been shown that deaf children born to hearing parents function at a lower cognitive level than those born to deaf parents (Braden, 1994; Vernon, 2005).

Special Considerations for Assessment: Test Factors

In addition to addressing individual child factors, clinicians should consider the inadequacies of the assessment instruments themselves—from instructions, to stimuli, to norms and norming samples—for use with special populations, as such inadequacies have historically plagued both research and application of evaluation methods for individuals with VI/B and D/HI.

For individuals with VI/B, some tests can be administered without vision requirements, such as subtests from the Halstead–Reitan Battery (HRB), including the Tactual Performance Test, Grip Strength, and Finger Oscillation, as well as the haptic version of Raven's Progressive Matrices (Rich & Anderson, 1965). However, tests for general cognition and memory that lack vision requirements are more difficult to find. Furthermore, the appropriateness of these tests for the population with VI/B is debatable, considering

inadequate norms for special populations and the need to control for examinees' varying levels of residual vision (Hill-Briggs et al., 2007). Although traditional IQ tests (e.g., the Stanford–Binet and Wechsler scales) have been adapted for individuals with VI/B, the norming samples for this group have historically been very small and included children with comorbid disabilities (Gutterman, Ward, & Genshaft, 1985). For example, in the original norming sample for the CVES battery created specifically for examinees with VI/B, 44% of those tested displayed profiles indicative of some kind of neuropsychological disorder (Dial, Chan, Tunick, Gray, & Marme, 1991). As noted earlier, the CVES norms were ultimately based on the final 25% of tested cases that had no other disability or medical condition besides VI/B (Hill-Briggs et al., 2007); therefore, practitioners should be wary of the inherent problems faced by test creators in finding and selecting appropriate norming samples. If much of the normative sample already exhibits the very class of disorders the test is designed to detect, sensitivity for doing so is severely limited.

Examiners testing children with D/HI must consider that these individuals' need for basic communication accommodations during the test automatically breaks standard administration. Oral administration without a sign language interpreter, therefore, is often impossible and is always inappropriate with individuals who do not primarily use oral communication outside the testing situation (Hill-Briggs et al., 2007). For example, individuals who typically use sign language or other visual communication strategies may seem to have adequate oral expression abilities but may have difficulty processing incoming auditory information. Informal communication abilities can be similarly deceiving, but the testing situation is a formal communication context with different demands and a higher imperative to ensure that each individual sound and word is being expressed and received precisely as it is intended. These individuals need to spend extra time processing auditory information, and when interpreters are used, time delays and inconsistencies in wording and meaning can have a negative impact on test performance. Use of interpreters also makes it difficult to adhere closely to standardized administration. This is because ASL and spoken English have different syntactical rules and grammatical structure, which render verbatim or direct translation impossible. Because of these difficulties, test instructions should be given in the examinee's preferred communication mode—such as ASL, if possible—and the examiner should allow extra practice trials and modeling when necessary (Hill-Briggs et al., 2007). If the examiner is not fluent in the examinee's primary communication mode, an experienced interpreter who is familiar with the examinee's particular dialect or signing approaches, as well as with mental health interpreting idiosyncrasies (Miller & Vernon, 2001), should be sought. Moreover, sensory distractions—both visual and auditory—should be carefully minimized. Hill-Briggs and colleagues (2007) also caution against asking examinees with D/HI to cover their eyes or wear a blindfold during perceptual and motor tasks (since this eliminates their sole mode of communication), and recommend using visual barriers instead.

The question of which tests to use in assessing individuals with D/HI is as important as deciding how to modify them, and is further discussed below. Although the Wechsler scales have been used with such individuals in the past (Braden, 1994), "adapting" a Wechsler test by only considering the nonverbal half of the test (Performance IQ, in older editions) is problematic, as excluding the other half of the test may lead to under- or overestimation of overall cognitive ability. Furthermore, as a general rule, tests with high verbal loading should be avoided. Testing considerations for individuals with D/HI may seem complex, but with appropriate evaluation of materials and methods employed, accurate measures of functioning are possible. As we discuss in the next section, selecting testing instruments for individuals with D/HI is similarly complex.

Instruments for Assessing Individuals with VI/B

Clinicians might consider using a cognitive measure developed specifically for individuals with VI/B, such as the Cognitive Test for the Blind (CTB), which was standardized on and designed for such individuals. The CTB is one of several tests included in the CVES for assessing individuals with VI/B (Hill-Briggs et al., 2007), and it covers three primary neuropsychological factors: verbal–spatial cognitive abilities, perceptual–motor functions, and emotional–coping concerns. Although the CTB has acceptable reliability and validity (Nelson, Dial, & Joyce, 2002), it can only be used with individuals age 14 and older. Despite the positive results from test development of the CVES showing its utility for populations with VI/B (Chan, Lynch, Dial, Wong, & Kates, 1993;

Dial, Chan, Mezger, et al., 1991; Kaskel, Dial, Chan, & Roldan, 1991), the test was developed for adults; although some measures suggested in the battery (e.g., the Wechsler Intelligence Scale for Children—Fourth Edition [WISC-IV]) are well suited for children, the battery as a whole is not.

Although there have been attempts to create and disseminate child-friendly cognitive tests specifically for individuals with VI/B, most of these tests are no longer commercially available due to problems with test reliability and validity, as well as inadequately made comparisons between samples of children with VI/B and typically developing children. Creators of the Bielefeld Developmental Test for Blind Infants and Preschoolers, for example, attempted to create "blind-neutral" items for young children but were not successful, and the test was removed from circulation (Brambring & Tröster, 1994). The best option remaining for practitioners working with children who have VI/B, then, is to try to select from the available children's standardized cognitive and neuropsychological tests, those that most easily lend themselves to modification. Tests such as the WISC-IV, for example, are appropriate for a pediatric population and can be used with these children if interpreted with caution. The Texas School for the Blind and Visually Impaired (2010) suggests using only the verbal subtests from the various Wechsler scales or the Woodcock–Johnson III Tests of Cognitive Abilities (WJ III COG), but they stress that clinical judgment is needed for interpreting results from only half of the entire test. Because the WJ III COG, however, includes tests that are designed to be used selectively, interpretation of only verbal subtests on this measure may be preferable to using those from the Wechsler scales, in which subtests are designed to contribute to an interpretable composite. Also, minimizing the inclusion of subtests that are heavily nonverbally loaded or that comprise several tasks dependent on visual–spatial information is essential. Examiners' manuals for several popular tests like the WJ III COG provide tables listing appropriate subtests for populations with VI/B and suggested accommodations specifically for these examinees (Mather & Woodcock, 2001). According to a test manual search we conducted, however, neither the WISC-IV nor the WJ III COG manual offers VI/B norms. Table 29.1 displays commonly used cognitive tests that provide suggested accommodations and/or lists of appropriate subtests for individuals with VI/B (and other disabilities).

Flanagan, Ortiz, and Alfonso (2007) have revised their recommendations for the cross-battery

TABLE 29.1. Availability of Special Testing Consideration Information in Cognitive Test Manuals

Test	Suggested accommodations provided				Norms/clinical sample scores provided				Chart of appropriate subtests provided			
	VI/B	D/HI	PI	TBI	VI/B	D/HI	PI	TBI	VI/B	D/HI	PI	TBI
WISC-IV		✓	✓			✓	✓			✓		
WJ III COG	✓	✓	✓						✓	✓		
SB5	✓	✓	✓				✓			✓		
KABC-II						✓						
NEPSY-II						✓	✓					
DAS-II	✓	✓	✓			✓				✓		

Note. VI/B, visual impairment/blindness; D/HI, deafness/hearing impairment; PI, physical impairment; WISC-IV, Wechsler Intelligence Scale for Children—Fourth Edition; WJ III COG, Woodcock–Johnson III Tests of Cognitive Abilities; SB5, Stanford–Binet Intelligence Scales, Fifth Edition; KABC-II, Kaufman Assessment Battery for Children—Second Edition; NEPSY-II, NEPSY—Second Edition; DAS-II, Differential Ability Scales—Second Edition.

assessment (XBA) approach to cognitive evaluation of children. This approach is based on the Cattell–Horn–Carroll (CHC) model of intelligence (Carroll, 1993 and Appendix, this volume; Horn & Noll, 1997), which purports that general intelligence, or *g*, comprises a number of broad-stratum abilities, such as fluid reasoning (Gf), crystallized knowledge (Gc), quantitative reasoning (Gq), visual–spatial processing (Gv), and short-term memory (Gsm). Instead of administering only one cognitive test battery to children, examiners using this approach systematically select tests from more than one battery, to ensure that the abilities and processes most germane to the referral are assessed comprehensively. The XBA approach often results in a more psychometrically stable and complete picture of cognitive abilities than that which can be obtained by a single battery. This approach may aid examiners of children with VI/B in selecting test instruments, as subtests from different batteries can be administered according to both their contributions to the CHC broad abilities and their level of appropriateness for these children. If one Gf subtest, as an illustration, involves visual stimulus material—as does the WJ III COG Analysis–Synthesis test—then Gf tests that are less dependent on visual information can be selected. Evaluators applying the XBA approach, however, must note that some broad-ability cluster scores (such as Gv) may be difficult or impossible to obtain or interpret, depending on the individual child and his or her level of vision loss.

Various tests from the HRB or Luria–Nebraska Battery (LNB) can be used for individuals with VI/B, according to the Texas School for the Blind and Visually Impaired (2010), if careful attention is paid to the examinee's need for modifications and if these modifications are considered in interpreting results. The NEPSY-II, which may be more appropriate for school-age children, does not offer VI/B norms or suggested accommodations, but includes subtests similar to those found in the HRB and LNB and may be administered with similar accommodations. Ultimately, test selection should be a collaborative decision between a clinician and a specialist or vision teacher knowledgeable about and experienced in working with children who have VI/B. In addition, formal evaluation methods should be supplemented by informal, often more subjective methods (e.g., student work samples, personal interactions with the child, and interviews with parents and teachers), in order to gain a more complete picture of the child's neuropsychological strengths and weaknesses than may not be obtainable from test scores alone.

Instruments for Assessing Individuals with D/HI

Although the earlier-discussed issues of mode of communication, use of interpreters, and other standardized test problems still make cognitive and neuropsychological assessment of individuals with D/HI complex, there is considerably more research on this topic (for overviews, see Braden, 2001; Maller, 2003) than is available for the population with VI/B. Braden (1994) reviewed over 300 studies on IQ and deafness and found that IQ distributions for deaf people without comorbid conditions and for hearing people are nearly identical, which has also helped to raise awareness of the intellectual potential of students with D/HI. Again, test selection and interpretation should include awareness of individual variables, and, as noted above for individuals with VI/B, should be a multi-disciplinary team effort involving hearing teachers and other special professionals.

For cognitive assessment, clinicians can use the Comprehensive Test of Nonverbal Intelligence, the WJ III COG, or the Universal Nonverbal Intelligence Test (UNIT), with the understanding that the verbal subtests of the WJ III COG should only be administered and interpreted when the clinician has specific experience using these scales for individuals with D/HI (Hill-Briggs et al., 2007). Nonverbal tests such as the UNIT can provide accurate estimates of overall cognitive functioning, since the tasks minimize verbal requirements and stimulus material. When examiners are assessing fluid reasoning skills, Hill-Briggs and colleagues (2007) suggest emphasizing spatial reasoning tasks, keeping in mind that language differences and cognitive processing delays or use of an interpreter may affect the delivery of instructions. On Digit Span working memory tasks, they also remind clinicians that the average forward span for deaf signers is approximately five digits, and that the backward span is usually equivalent. Differences between signing system and English grammatical structure or syntax must be taken into account in using subtests such as the WJ III COG Visual–Auditory Learning test and other sentence or story recall tasks.

Notably, the Stanford–Binet Intelligence Scales, Fifth Edition (SB5) test manual includes an entire appendix titled "Use of the Stanford–Binet Intelligence Scales, Fifth Edition, with Deaf and Hard of Hearing Individuals: General Considerations and Tailored Administration" (Roid, 2003, Appendix E). The appendix divides individuals with D/HI into four categories: those who use sign language, simultaneous communication, cued speech, or auditory verbal–oral communication. The categories are based on the SB5 standardization administration to a special sample of individuals with D/HI, and suggestions for the appropriateness of administering each SB5 subtest to each of these groups are provided. In addition, the WJ III COG manual provides suggested accommodations specifically for individuals with D/HI, as well as a table of appropriate subtests for use with such children by primary mode of communication (see Table 29.1).

Miller (2007) suggests including the SB5 in CHC-based cognitive assessment of children with D/HI, as the SB5 provides scores for the five broad abilities Gf, Gc, Gq, Gsm, and Gv, and has adequate information in Appendix E of the test manual (Roid, 2003). In the Kaufman Assessment Battery for Children—Second Edition (KABC-II; Kaufman & Kaufman, 2004) manual, the authors report no significant differences between a subgroup ($n = 18$) of students with D/HI and the hearing standardization group. Therefore, the KABC-II can also be used as part of a CHC-based cognitive assessment for children with D/HI. The KABC-II manual (Kaufman & Kaufman, 2004) reports that hearing and D/HI norms for the following factors were not significantly different, suggesting that the KABC-II is a stable measure of these abilities in children with D/HI: long-term retrieval (Glr), Gf, and Gv. Lastly, the Differential Ability Scale—Second Edition (DAS-II; Elliott, 2007) manual reports equivalent performances for children with D/HI and a matched hearing control group on subtests composing the test's Gf and Gv cluster scores. The DAS-II manual (Elliott, 2007) also includes tables of suggestions for administration to children with D/HI by subtest and communication mode, as well as a sign language CD and norming information from a clinical sample with D/HI. Instead of using one of these batteries alone to assess cognitive functioning in a child with D/HI, clinicians should consider employing the XBA approach (Flanagan et al., 2007) based on Miller's suggestions for this special population. It is worth noting, however, that subtests contributing to cluster scores for broad-stratum abilities such as auditory processing (Ga) may be inappropriate to administer to these children or may have problematic interpretations.

With perceptual–motor tests, clinicians can usually use standard tasks from neuropsychological batteries such as the HRB and LNB, with careful attention to how directions are given and processed by the examinee. Again, the NEPSY-II is perhaps more appropriate for use with school-age children but not yet empirically validated for individuals with D/HI, although it offers D/HI norms from a special D/HI clinical sample. As mentioned previously, examiners should provide an alternative to blindfolding or to asking individuals with D/HI to close their eyes during some neuropsychological tasks (e.g., balance tasks), as these modifications restrict their use of vision, an important mode of communication for individuals with D/HI. Hill-Briggs and colleagues (2007) note that standard visual–motor tasks in neuropsychological batteries are suitable for individuals with D/HI, but that caution should be exercised in interpreting the Rey Complex Figure task because children with D/HI may have different organizational strategies from those of typically developing children.

PHYSICAL DISABILITIES

According to the U.S. Census Bureau (2000), an estimated 8.2% of the general population had a physical disability (i.e., some limitation in basic physical activities), amounting to 21.2 million people in the United States. Difficulties surrounding the assessment of individuals with physical disabilities have recently become more prevalent—due in part to an increase in the number of individuals with such disabilities, but also in part to the proliferation of health services for these individuals (O'Keefe, 1994). Many of these difficulties stem from an inability to measure abilities adequately or to interpret test scores on various assessments when an individual's disability inhibits him or her in some way. The difficulties specific to assessing individuals with physical disabilities, as well as the potential testing accommodations, are dependent on the type and severity of the disabilities.

Typically, children with some sort of physical impairment (PI) are served under the IDEA 2004 category of *orthopedic impairment*. Federal guidelines (U.S. Department of Education, 2006) define this as follows:

> *Orthopedic impairment* means a severe orthopedic impairment that adversely affects a child's educational performance. The term includes impairments caused by a congenital anomaly, impairments caused by disease (e.g., poliomyelitis, bone tuberculosis), and impairments from other causes (e.g., cerebral palsy, amputations, and fractures or burns that cause contractures). (pp. 46756–46757)

According to the IDEA DAC (n.d.), approximately 7,680 children ages 3–5 and an additional 62,332 children and youth ages 6–21 in the United States were served under this category in the fall of 2008. Occasionally, children with a PI may qualify for special education services under the category of *other health impaired* (OHI). According to IDEA, OHI is defined as

> having limited strength, vitality, or alertness, including a heightened alertness to environmental stimuli, that results in limited alertness with respect to the educational environment, that—
>
> (i) Is due to chronic or acute health problems such as asthma, attention deficit disorder or attention deficit hyperactivity disorder, diabetes, epilepsy,

> a heart condition, hemophilia, lead poisoning, leukemia, nephritis, rheumatic fever, sickle cell anemia, and Tourette syndrome; and
>
> (ii) Adversely affects a child's educational performance. (p. 46757)

According to the IDEA DAC (n.d.), 18,080 children ages 3–5 and 648,112 children and youth ages 6–21 in the United States were served under this category in the fall of 2008. However, OHI covers more than just students with PI, so these figures are overestimates. Nevertheless, each individual with PI, whether qualifying for school services under orthopedic impairment or OHI, or in the workforce under a federal Section 504 plan, requires some unique testing considerations at both the individual and test level.

Etiologies: A Brief Overview

Motor skills development occurs in stages, preceded and accompanied by the growth and development of the endocrine and nervous systems. The typically developing child passes through a sequence of milestones, such as holding his or her own head up at about 2 months of age, crawling at about 6 months, and walking at about 1 year of age (Sigelman & Rider, 2009). It is during this time of rapid development that some types of PI become apparent. Specifically, delayed walking is often indicative of a motor impairment. PI can be either acquired (e.g., spinal cord injury [SCI] and amputation) or congenital. Congenital disabilities become apparent either at birth or during infancy and toddlerhood when a child fails to reach one or more typical milestones. Cerebral palsy (CP), for example—the third-ranked childhood disability as of 1999, occurring 1.4–2.4 times in every 1,000 live births (Cummings, Nelson, Grether, & Velie, 1993; Hagberg, Hagberg, & Olow, 1993; Stanley, Blair, Hockey, Petterson, & Watson, 1993)—has many potential causes, including genetic abnormality, intrauterine infection, complications during labor or birth, or experiencing a TBI before the age of 5. CP generally causes problems associated with movement and posture, although comorbid disorders (e.g., intellectual disabilities, sensory disorders, seizures, and growth abnormalities) often occur (Pellegrino, 1997).

Special Considerations for Assessment: Child Factors

There is little literature on the neuropsychological testing of children with PI, and much of what exists is very specific to one disorder or another. Two of the most researched conditions are CP and SCI. Another variable contributing to the heterogeneity of this population is a child's age at onset of a disability. Many physical disabilities are the result of congenital defects or diseases (e.g., CP, muscular dystrophy [MD], and multiple sclerosis). The age of onset can significantly affect one's ability to compensate for mild to severe PI. Individuals with congenital disabilities learn to cope with their limitations from birth. Those who acquire impairments at a relatively young age are less likely to have multiple deficits as adults. Li and Moore (1998) found that both younger participants and those with congenital disabilities had higher levels of disability acceptance. Those with PI acquired as the result of disease, amputation, or accidents have the added difficulty of relearning many tasks without the full use of a particular body part. Research conducted on motor recovery following stroke, SCI, and CP has indicated that motor recovery, if it occurs, can be incomplete or deficient (Krishnan, 2006).

To qualify for services under federal programs (IDEA or Section 504), an individual's disability must be severe. The type and severity of disability will greatly affect test selection and interpretation. For individuals who fatigue easily as a result of their disability, for example, it may be appropriate to extend the time to allow for additional breaks (AERA et al., 1999). Individuals with PI may also suffer from comorbid conditions. For example, in assessing individuals with CP, associated difficulties—such as learning difficulties, attention-deficit/hyperactivity disorder, intellectual disability, and sensory impairment—warrant consideration. It is these problems that put students at the greatest disadvantage when contrasted with their peers (Pellegrino, 1997). In the case of students with chronic disease or those with PI, distinguishing gaps in achievement resulting from the illness or impairment from indirect effects, such as those caused by school absence, pain or fatigue, depression, and low self-efficacy, is imperative (Donnelly, 2005). Comorbidity is also a possible source of construct-irrelevant variance,[1] which should be considered in interpreting the results of assessments conducted on individuals with PI.

Special Considerations for Assessment: Test Factors

Historically, accommodations for PI have been considered less salient than those for sensory disabilities, such as VI/B or D/HI (Lezak, Howieson,

& Loring, 2004). In the past, clinical judgment and prior experience alone were considered acceptable standards for modifying test administration (Pratt & Moreland, 1998). Currently, many assessments suggest accommodations in the administration or technical manuals in an attempt to retain standardization, even in working with special populations (see Table 29.1). Common test accommodations include modifications in presentation, response format, or timing, as well as in test selection (AERA et al., 1999). Test setting and environment can also be modified for accessibility and physical comfort due to problems associated with a disability (AERA et al., 1999; Pratt & Moreland, 1998). A few test manuals provide normative information for clinical populations such as those with PI (see Table 29.1), but those that do are typically based on small samples that are not necessarily representative of the greater population with PI.

Motor functioning is a primary consideration for those assessing individuals with PI to bear in mind (Hill-Briggs et al., 2007), as motor functioning dictates the use of various response options. Specifically, impairment or loss of motor function in the upper extremities is of utmost concern, as it can affect fine motor control and/or dexterity. Impairments in this area will significantly reduce response format options because such individuals will not be able to complete tasks such as those requiring the manipulation of stimuli, or holding or utilizing a writing utensil (e.g., writing, drawing, or copying a figure). If standardized test administration requires such motor skills, then test accommodations for these individuals are a necessity (Nester, 1994). The only exception would be when the goal of testing is to determine the extent of limitation caused by the PI.

Awareness of the individual's level of discomfort is another important variable for consideration and may require continual evaluation throughout the duration of testing. Individuals with PI may require repositioning or additional breaks to combat discomfort or fatigue, and some individuals (e.g., those with CP or MD) may additionally experience pain or cramping. Studies conducted on secondary pain (often the result of treatment) in adults with CP illustrated the immense impact of pain. From 67% to 84% of participants across three studies reported chronic pain (Engel, Jensen, Hoffman, & Kartin, 2003; Schwartz, Engel, & Jensen, 1999; Turk, Geremski, Rosenbaum, & Weber, 1997), and 18–56% reported daily incidents of pain (Andersson & Mattsson, 2001; Engel et al., 2003; Schwartz et al., 1999). Similarly, Zebracki and Drotar (2008) found that 54% of those with Duchenne MD and 80% of those with Becker MD reported experiencing pain associated with their disease. Also, according to the Child Activity Limitations Interview (CALI; Palermo, Witherspoon, Valenzuela, & Drotar, 2004), sitting was endorsed most frequently as causing discomfort in daily life, further justifying the need to monitor discomfort during an assessment (Zebracki & Drotar, 2008). Accessibility is also a concern. For example, if an individual uses a wheelchair, the testing location needs to be wheelchair-accessible.

Instruments for Assessing Individuals with PI

Since specialized cognitive tests do not exist for persons with PI in the same way that they do for individuals with VI/B or D/HI, great care must be taken to accommodate varying degrees of impairment within the framework of existing measures such as the WISC-IV, WJ III COG, or SB5. Many popular tests like these provide recommended test modifications and norming information (see Table 29.1). Although the norms exist, they are unlikely to be representative. Resultant scores should therefore be interpreted with caution.

Within SCI research, certain measures have been noted as being particularly useful in cases of paraplegia and quadriplegia. Others should be avoided; for example, the Trail Making Tests would not be an ideal selection for someone with a fine motor impairment because of construct-irrelevant variance. The following are some of the most commonly used measures within a motor-free neuropsychological assessment battery: the Wechsler Memory Scale, minus visual reproduction; the verbal subtests of the WAIS; the Symbol Digit Modalities Test; the Stroop Test; the Rey Auditory Verbal Learning Test; the Hooper Visual Organization Test; the Halstead Category Test; and the California Oral Word Association Test (Davidoff, Roth, & Richards, 1992; Dowler et al., 1997; Richards, Bown, Hagglund, Bua, & Reeder, 1988; Roth et al., 1989). Using various tests in this way is reminiscent of the XBA cognitive assessment approach (Flanagan et al., 2007), in which subtests from a variety of batteries can be combined in order to provide a comprehensive assessment of an individual's cognitive abilities. A mixed approach, like XBA, can provide the opportunity to more fully assess individuals with PI. Using such an approach could allow for subtest substitutions, which could assess an individual's skills in a different way, independent of his or her PI.

TRAUMATIC BRAIN INJURY

Approximately 1.4 million individuals suffer from a TBI every year, and children and youth between the ages of 0–4 and 15–19 are in the highest risk categories for sustaining a TBI (Brain Injury Association of America, 2010). Approximately 24% of children with severe head injuries do not survive (White et al., 2001). Comprehensive evaluations that include neuropsychological assessment are critical in assisting neurologists, determining the degree and severity of functional impairment resulting from the injury, and documenting changes in impairment over time (American Academy of Neurology, 1996). Schools and educational institutions are obligated under federal law to identify and provide special educational assistance to children with TBI. TBI is specified in IDEA 2004 as one of 13 categories under which students may receive special education services. IDEA 2004 defines TBI as:

> an acquired injury to the brain caused by an external physical force, resulting in total or partial functional disability or psychosocial impairment, or both, that adversely affects a child's educational performance. The term applies to open or closed head injuries resulting in impairments in one or more areas, such as cognition; language; memory; attention; reasoning; abstract thinking; judgment; problem-solving; sensory, perceptual, and motor abilities; psychosocial behavior; physical functions; information processing; and speech. [The term] does not apply to brain injuries that are congenital or degenerative, or to brain injuries induced by birth trauma. (p. 46757)

The federal definition explicitly excludes children whose brains may be affected by congenital problems or injury at birth; however, these children may still be eligible for special education under Section 504.

TBI may result from penetrating or nonpenetrating wounds. Impairment may range from none to severe, and injuries to the brain may result from direct damage to the brain or from indirect damage caused by brain swelling or bruising. Because falls and motor vehicle accidents are the most common causes of TBI and usually result in diffuse injury, the deficits and symptoms associated with TBI vary widely. Early research on the developmental sequelae of brain injuries in childhood suggested that most children fully recover from the injury by adulthood due to brain plasticity. However, more contemporary research has suggested that TBI sustained during childhood—even a mild brain injury—may in fact have lasting deficits in adulthood that include not only cognitive but psychiatric problems (Pirozzolo & Papanicolaou, 1986).

The specific location of injury also influences long-term outcomes. Counterintuitively, right-hemispheric injuries have been shown to result in more long-term impairments than left-hemispheric injuries, even though the left hemisphere is typically the dominant hemisphere and highly involved in language functions. However, the right hemisphere seems to deal with new learning experiences (novelty) more proficiently than the left hemisphere—and, for children, almost all experiences are new learning experiences.

Neuropsychological Assessment

No specific cognitive profile or cluster of symptoms has been considered diagnostic of TBI; this is not surprising, considering that injuries may be focal (one specific area) or diffuse (general). Focal neurological damage results in more specific behavioral dysfunction than does diffuse damage (Berninger & Richards, 2002; Halstead, 1947; Kolb & Whishaw, 2003; Luria, 1980). Clinical hypothesis testing within an individualized assessment plan is important to match the clinical symptoms and measured neuropsychological deficits to the type and location of the injury. This requires a basic understanding of neuropsychology. Two common cognitive deficits of children with TBI are slowed processing speed and attention problems (Rutter, 1981). These and other cognitive deficits resulting from TBI invariably result in academic and educational problems, which require specialized attention from educational professionals (Blosser & DePompei, 1991; D'Amato & Rothlisberg, 1996).

Although processing speed deficits in TBI have been known for some time, only recently have the neurological mechanisms been understood through the use of new technologies. Thatcher, Walker, Gerson, and Geislerm (1989) used quantitative electroencephalography to compare 264 patients with mild head injuries to a control group and found differences in the frontal and frontotemporal regions of the brain, such that the data could distinguish patients from controls with 93% accuracy. Using functional magnetic resonance imaging, Kraus and colleagues (2007) found that TBI resulted in white matter disruption, and that the degree of disruption was correlated with neuropsychological impairment, particularly with measures of executive functions and attention. In another study, children with TBI who had persistent motor control deficits as a result of white matter disruption were shown to exhibit different cortical acti-

vation patterns during movement tasks. Compared to controls, these children showed greater brain activation in the parietal and cerebellum areas (Caeyenberghs, Wenderoth, Smits-Engelsman, Sunaert, & Swinnen, 2009). The authors interpreted these results as reflecting the greater attentional resources needed by the children with TBI to carry out motor acts in comparison to the control group, in which such acts were automatized. Together, these studies suggest that TBI causes white matter disruption of the brain, which interferes with automatized behaviors. Compensation with effortful behaviors ultimately results in slowed performance, detected as slowed processing speed and attentional problems on standardized tests.

Neuropsychological consultation has been recommended as a core educational service to be provided by school psychologists (D'Amato, 1990; Decker, 2008; Hale & Fiorello, 2004; Miller, 2007). School psychologists who serve children with TBI, but who lack neuropsychological training, may consider referring the children to or directly consulting with a neuropsychologist. Neuropsychological consultation involves not only direct service delivery, but also an understanding of recovery patterns, rehabilitation and effective interventions, and school reentry assistance. Critically, families commonly experience an often overlooked emotional reaction to loss of a "normal" child. Consultation with families is necessary to help set appropriate expectations for academic and behavioral performance.

Special Considerations for Assessment: Child and Test Factors

One primary function of the school psychologist is to conduct a comprehensive, broad-based assessment of a child with TBI to ensure that a valid picture of the child can be communicated to parents and teachers and incorporated into intervention (Havey, 2002). Test accommodations are most needed for children with TBI when sensory impairments or PI are evident. When such impairments are not evident, most measures frequently used by school psychologists are appropriate for assessing the underlying impairment that has resulted from the TBI. However, it is important for clinicians to be aware of how core deficits caused by a TBI may inadvertently affect a variety of test constructs, thereby creating construct irrelevant variance. For example, attention problems and slowed processing speed may have an impact on any variety of cognitive measures, not just those subtests explicitly targeting attention and processing speed. To minimize construct-irrelevant factors, it may be necessary to administer directions at a slower pace to children with TBI to ensure comprehension. In addition, children with TBI may need examiners to repeat directions to ensure proper encoding. When engaging in longer tasks, children with TBI may require more frequent prompting to prevent lapses in attention. More frequent breaks may be necessary, too, as children with TBI may become fatigued more quickly than other children of a similar developmental age but without a TBI. Most adaptations needed for assessment of children with mild TBI should not seriously jeopardize test validity.

As previously mentioned, age is an important variable for several reasons. First, age is a risk factor in two ways: Younger children (ages 0–4) are at higher risk for TBI due to falls, and older adolescents (ages 17–20) are at higher risk for TBI due to automobile accidents. Age also moderates the sequelae of behavioral impairment: TBI in younger children may interfere with the later development of skills, whereas TBI in adolescents may result in the loss of learned skills.

Estimating preinjury functional status is important to determine the degree to which cognition has changed as a result of the injury. Premorbid intelligence is typically estimated by a qualitative review of historical records (past educational achievement) and quantitative performance on cognitive measures typically resistant to neurological injury. Measures of crystallized intelligence (e.g., vocabulary) are used to measure abilities most resistant to neurological injury (Lezak et al., 2004; Russell, 1980).

Instruments for Assessing Individuals with TBI

As with standard school psychology assessment procedures, no one test or test battery can comprehensively assess the emotional, cognitive, and behavioral status of a child with TBI. Thus various measures from different domains are required. The Glasgow Coma Scale is widely used in making the initial determination of injury severity (mild, moderate, or severe). This is a short rating scale of eye, verbal, and motor responses that is used at or near the time of injury. Scores range from 3 to 15, with 3 representing no eye, verbal, or motor response and 15 representing a fully awake and functioning person. Similarly, a structured interview specifically tailored to important factors related to neurological injury is recommended (Dean, Woodcock, Decker, & Schrank, 2003). Sensory–motor

measures are useful adjuncts to intellectual assessment, to rule out basic input–output deficits as a source of impairment on cognitive measures and to validate clinical hypotheses of cortical injury. Residual sensory–motor impairment from a brain injury has been demonstrated in children several weeks after release from the hospital (Gagnon, Forget, Sullivan, & Friedman, 1998).

Telzrow (1991) recommends assessing a variety of domains of intellectual functioning in children with TBI. Although a variety of assessment models may work for this purpose (Hale & Fiorello, 2004; Miller, 2007), a cross-battery model (e.g., the XBA approach) provides ample coverage to comprehensively assess different domains of cognitive functioning. A cross-battery model not only provides a close correspondence between cognitive functions of interest to neuropsychologists, but also enjoys wide familiarity among school psychologists (Decker, 2008). The cognitive domains incorporated in the XBA approach (Flanagan et al., 2007) include processing speed, a crucial area of assessment for children with TBI. Attention is not an explicit cognitive domain within the model, and so clinicians should be familiar with test-specific attentional demands and how attention may influence underlying test performance.

SUMMARY

This chapter has discussed issues related to sensory and physical disabilities as well as TBI within a neuropsychological framework. This framework is necessary because the causes of VI/B, D/HI, PI, and TBI all have some basis in the physiological disruption of typical sensory, motor, and cognitive pathways in the brain and body. In a school setting, individuals with all of these impairments may be eligible for services under IDEA 2004. We have reviewed the ways in which individual child factors—such as age at onset, nature and severity of the disability, etiology, comorbidity, primary modes of communication, and reading and language ability—can affect test selection, administration, and interpretation. We have also offered examples of the ways in which individual differences within each disability category may manifest themselves during academic and testing situations. Some important considerations noted for all disability categories include attention to within-category heterogeneity; the child's communicative style and linguistic skill level; the fit between educational environment and child; and the necessity of collaborating with both families and a multidisciplinary team to achieve systematic data-based decision making on a case-by-case basis.

In addition, we have reviewed the availability of cognitive and neuropsychological test batteries with special sections for these categories of children, including standardized test manuals with suggested accommodations, appropriate subtests, and clinical sample and normative information. We have also explained particular precautions that must be taken and modifications that must be made when examiners are using several widely used standardized tests. These cautions include the prerequisite skills and training needs for test interpretation, limitations in tests and test availability, and inadequate normative information. Specific issues for each population have been described, such as the use of nonvisual subtest materials for students with VI/B, interpreters for individuals with D/HI, modifications to motor tests for children with PI, and extra attention to pacing and frequent breaks for children with TBI. With careful attention to both child and test factors, and the help of a multidisciplinary team, many currently available cognitive and neuropsychological test batteries can be used effectively for the assessment of children with VI/B, D/HI, PI, and TBI. Cautious interpretation of the results, along with multisource information from systematic observations and from professional colleagues and specialists, can be integrated to provide a sound psychoeducational plan for every child, regardless of sensory or physical disability.

NOTE

1. The term *construct-irrelevant variance* is used to describe instances in which variability in responses is affected by something unrelated to the interpreted construct (Messick, 1995). This can occur as a result of changes in methodology, and as such, is especially important to keep in mind when testing individuals who require modifications to standardized procedures.

REFERENCES

American Academy of Neurology. (1996). Assessment: Neuropsychological testing in adults: Considerations for neurologists. *Neurology, 47,* 592–599.

American Educational Research Association (AERA), American Psychological Association (APA), National Council on Measurement in Education (NCME).

(1999). *Standards for educational and psychological testing.* Washington, DC: AER.

American Speech–Language–Hearing Association (ASHA). (2010). Type, degree, and configuration of hearing loss. Retrieved from *www.asha.org/public/hearing/disorders/types.htm*.

Anderson, D. (2006). Lexical development of deaf children acquiring signed languages. In B. Schick, M. Marschark, & P. Spencer (Eds.), *Advances in the sign language development of deaf children* (pp. 135–160). New York: Oxford University Press.

Andersson, C., & Mattsson, F. (2001). Adults with cerebral palsy: A survey describing problems, needs, and resources with special emphasis on locomotion. *Developmental Medicine and Child Neurology, 43*(2), 76–82.

Berninger, V. W., & Richards, T. L. (2002). *Brain literacy for educators and psychologists.* San Diego, CA: Academic Press.

Blosser, J. L., & DePompei, R. (1991). Preparing education professionals for meeting the needs of students with traumatic brain injury. *Journal of Head Trauma Rehabilitation 6*(1), 73–82.

Bosworth, R. G., & Dobkins, K. R. (1999). Left-hemisphere dominance for motion processing in deaf signers. *Psychological Science, 10*(3), 256–262.

Braden, J. P. (1994). *Deafness, deprivation, and IQ.* New York: Plenum Press.

Braden, J. P. (2001). The clinical assessment of deaf people's cognitive abilities. In M. D. Clark, M. Marschark, & M. Karchmer (Eds.), *Context, cognition, and deafness* (pp. 14–37). Washington, DC: Gallaudet University Press.

Bradley-Johnson, S., & Morgan, S. K. (2008). Best practices for instructing students who are visually impaired or blind. In A. Thomas & T. Grimes (Eds.), *Best practices in school psychology V* (pp. 1833–1846). Bethesda, MD: National Association of School Psychologists.

Brain Injury Association of America. (2010). Facts about traumatic brain injury. Washington, DC: Author. Retrieved from *www.biausa.org/Default.aspx?SiteSearchID=1192&ID=/search-results.htm*.

Brambring, M., & Tröster, H. (1994). The assessment of cognitive development in blind infants and preschoolers. *Journal of Visual Impairment and Blindness, 88*(1), 9–18.

Caeyenberghs, K., Wenderoth, N., Smits-Engelsman, B. C. M., Sunaert, S., & Swinnen, S. P. (2009). Neural correlates of motor dysfunction in children with traumatic brain injury: Exploration of compensatory recruitment patterns. *Brain, 132,* 684–694.

Carroll, J. B. (1993). *Human cognitive abilities: A survey of factor analytic studies.* New York: Cambridge University Press.

Cattani, A., & Clibbens, J. (2005). Atypical lateralization of memory for location: Effects of deafness and sign language use. *Brain and Cognition, 58*(2), 226–239.

Chan, F., Lynch, R. T., Dial, J. G., Wong, D. W., & Kates, D. (1993). Applications of the McCarron–Dial System in vocational evaluation: An overview of its operational framework and empirical findings. *Vocational Evaluation and Work Adjustment Bulletin, 26*(2), 57–65.

Charlier, B. L., & Leybaert, J. (2000). The rhyming skills of deaf children educated with phonetically augmented speechreading. *Quarterly Journal of Experimental Psychology, 53a,* 349–375.

Cummings, S. K., Nelson, K. B., Grether, J. K., & Velie, E. M. (1993). Cerebral palsy in four northern California counties, births 1983 through 1985. *Journal of Pediatrics, 123*(2), 230–237.

Dalby, D., Hirdes, J., Stolee, P., Strong, J., Poss, J., Tjam, E., et al. (2009). Characteristics of individuals with congenital and acquired deaf-blindness. *Journal of Visual Impairment and Blindness, 103*(2), 93–102.

D'Amato, R. C. (1990). A neuropsychological approach to school psychology. *School Psychology Quarterly, 5,* 141–160.

D'Amato, R. C., & Rothlisberg, B. A. (1996). How education should respond to students with traumatic brain injury. *Journal of Learning Disabilities, 29,* 670–683.

Davidoff, G. N., Roth, E. J., & Richards, J. S. (1992). Cognitive deficits in spinal cord injury: Epidemiology and outcome. *Archives of Physical Medicine and Rehabilitation, 73,* 275–284.

Dean, R. S., Woodcock, R. W., Decker, S. L., & Schrank, F. A. (2003). A cognitive neuropsychological assessment system. In F. L. Schrank & D. P. Flanagan (Eds.), *WJ III clinical use and interpretation* (pp. 345–375). Amsterdam: Elsevier.

Decker, S. L. (2002). Confirmatory models of sensory/motor and cognitive constructs. *Dissertation Abstracts International, 63,* 1083B.

Decker, S. L. (2004). Incremental validity of tactile measures in predicting letter–word identification skills. *Archives of Clinical Neuropsychology, 19*(7), 907–908.

Decker, S. L. (2008). School neuropsychology consultation in neurodevelopmental disorders. *Psychology in the Schools, 45*(9), 799–811.

Dial, J. G., Chan, F., Mezger, C., Parker, H. J., Zangla, K., Wong, D. W., et al. (1991). Comprehensive Vocational Education System for visually impaired and blind persons. *Journal of Visual Impairment and Blindness, 85,* 153–157.

Dial, J. G., Chan, F., Tunick, R., Gray, S. G., & Marme, M. (1991). Neuropsychological evaluation: A functional and behavioral approach. In B. T. McMahon & L. R. Shaw (Eds.), *Work worth doing: Advances in brain injury rehabilitation* (pp. 47–76). Orlando, FL: Paul M. Deutsch.

Donnelly, J. P. (2005). Providing neuropsychological services to learners with chronic illnesses. In R. C. D'Amato, E. Fletcher-Jensen, & C. R. Reynolds (Eds.), *Handbook of school neuropsychology* (pp. 511–532). Hoboken, NJ: Wiley.

Dowler, R. N., Harrington, D. L., Haaland, K. Y., Swanda, R. M., Fee, F., & Fiedler, K. (1997). Profiles of cognitive functioning in chronic spinal cord injury and the role of moderating variables. *Journal of the International Neuropsychological Society, 3,* 464–472.

Elliott, C. D. (2007). *Differential Ability Scales—Second Edition.* San Antonio, TX: Harcourt Assessment.

Engel, J. M., Jensen, M. P., Hoffman, A. J., & Kartin, D. (2003). Pain in persons with cerebral palsy: Extension and cross validation. *Archives of Physical Medicine and Rehabilitation, 84,* 1125–1128.

Finger, S. (1994). *Origins of neuroscience: A history of explorations into brain functions.* New York: Oxford University Press.

Flanagan, D. P., Ortiz, S. O., & Alfonso, V. C. (2007). *Essentials of cross-battery assessment* (2nd ed.). Hoboken, NJ: Wiley.

Gagnon, I., Forget, R., Sullivan, S. J., & Friedman, D. (1998). Motor performances following a mild traumatic brain injury in children: An exploratory study. *Brain Injury, 12,* 843–853.

Gallaudet Research Institute. (2005). Stanford Achievement Test—8th Edition for deaf and hard of hearing students: Reading comprehension subgroup results. Retrieved from *gri.gallaudet.edu/Assessment/sat-read. html.*

Gutterman, J., Ward, M., & Genshaft, J. (1985). Correlations of scores of low vision children on the Perkins–Binet tests of intelligence for the blind, the WISC-R, and the WRAT. *Journal of Visual Impairment and Blindness, 55*–58.

Hagberg, B., Hagberg, G., & Olow, I. (1993). The changing panorama of cerebral palsy in Sweden: VI. Prevalence and origin during the birth year period 1983–1986. *Acta Paediatrica, 82,* 387–393.

Hale, J. B., & Fiorello, C. A. (2004). *School neuropsychology: A practitioner's handbook.* New York: Guilford Press.

Halstead, W. C. (1947). *Brain and intelligence: A quantitative study of the frontal lobes.* Chicago: University of Chicago Press.

Havey, J. M. (2002). Working with students with traumatic brain injury. In A. Thomas & J. Grimes (Eds.), *Best practices in school psychology IV* (pp. 1433–1446). Bethesda, MD: National Association of School Psychology.

Hill-Briggs, F., Dial, J., Morere, D., & Joyce, A. (2007).

Neuropsychological assessment of persons with physical disability, visual impairment or blindness, and hearing impairment or deafness. *Archives of Clinical Neuropsychology, 22*(3), 389–404.

Horn, J. L., & Noll, J. (1997). Human cognitive capabilities: Gf-Gc theory. In D. P. Flanagan, J. L. Genshaft, & P. L. Harrison (Eds.), *Contemporary intellectual assessment: Theories, tests, and issues* (pp. 53–91). New York: Guilford Press.

Individuals with Disabilities Education Act (IDEA) Data Accountability Center (DAC). (n.d.) Data tables for OSEP state reported data. Retrieved from *www.ideadata.org/arc_toc10.asp#partbCC.*

Individuals with Disabilities Education Improvement Act of 2004 (IDEA 2004), Pub. L. No., 108-446, 118 Stat. 2647 (2004).

Joyce, A., Isom, R., Dial, J. G., & Sandel, M. G. (2004). Implications of perceptual–motor differences within blind populations. *Journal of Applied Rehabilitation Counseling, 35*(3), 3–7.

Kaskel, L. M., Dial, J. G., Chan, F., & Roldan, G. (1991). Evaluating work potential of persons with visual impairments: The Comprehensive Vocational Evaluation System (CVES) approach. In R. Fry (Ed.), *The issue papers: Fifth national forum on issues in vocational assessment* (pp. 167–173). Menomonie: University of Wisconsin–Stout, Materials Development Center.

Kaufman, A. S., & Kaufman, N. L. (2004). *Kaufman Assessment Battery for Children–Second Edition.* Circle Pines, MN: American Guidance Service.

Kolb, B., & Whishaw, I. Q. (2003). *Fundamentals of human neuropsychology.* New York: Worth.

Kraus, M. F., Susmaras, T., Caughlin, B. P., Walker, C. J., Sweeney, J. A., & Little, D. M. (2007). White matter integrity and cognition in chronic traumatic brain injury: A diffusion tensor imaging study. *Brain, 130*(10), 2508–2519.

Krishnan, R. V. (2006). Relearning toward motor recovery in stroke, spinal cord injury, and cerebral palsy: A cognitive neural systems perspective. *International Journal of Neuroscience, 116,* 127–140.

LaSasso, C., Crain, K., & Leybaert, J. (2003). Rhyme generation in deaf students: The effect of exposure to cued speech. *Journal of Deaf Studies and Deaf Education, 8,* 250–270.

Leigh, I. W., Marcus, A. L., Dobosh, P. K., & Allen, T. E. (1998). Deaf/hearing cultural identity paradigms: Modification of the Deaf Identity Development Scale. *Journal of Deaf Studies and Deaf Education, 3*(4), 329–338.

Lezak, M., Howieson, D. B., & Loring, D. W. (2004). *Neuropsychological assessment* (4th ed.). New York: Oxford University Press.

Li, L., & Moore, D. (1998). Acceptance of disability and its correlates. *Journal of Social Psychology, 138*(1), 13–25.

Lukomski, J. (2008). Best practices in planning effective instruction for children who are deaf/hard of hearing. In A. Thomas & T. Grimes (Eds.), *Best practices in school psychology V* (pp. 1819–1832). Bethesda, MD: National Association of School Psychologists.

Luria, A. R. (1980). *Higher cortical functions in man.* New York: Basic Books.

MacCluskie, K., Tunick, R., Dial, J., & Paul, D. (1998). The role of vision in the development of abstraction. *Journal of Visual Impairment and Blindness, 92*(3), 189.

Maller, S. (2003). Intellectual assessment of deaf people: A critical review of core concepts and issues. In M. Marschark & P. E. Spencer (Eds.), *Oxford handbook of deaf studies, language, and education* (pp. 451–463). New York: Oxford University Press.

Marschark, M., & Clark, M. D. (Eds.). (1993). *Psychological perspectives on deafness.* Hillsdale, NJ: Erlbaum.

Mather, N., & Woodcock, R. W. (2001). *Examiner's manual: Woodcock–Johnson III Tests of Cognitive Abilities.* Itasca, IL: Riverside.

McGee, J. M. (1994). *Neuropsychological functioning of adult subjects with diabetic retinopathy compared to a normal blind population.* Unpublished doctoral dissertation, University of North Texas, Denton.

Meadow, K. P. (1980). *Deafness and child development.* Berkeley: University of California Press.

Messick, S. (1995). Validity of psychological assessment: Validation of inferences from persons' responses and performances as scientific inquiry into score meaning. *American Psychologist, 50*(9), 741–749.

Miller, D. C. (2007). *Essentials of school neuropsychological assessment.* Hoboken, NJ: Wiley.

Miller, K. R., & Vernon, M. (2001). Linguistic diversity in deaf defendants and due process rights. *Journal of Deaf Studies and Deaf Education, 6*(3), 226–234.

Nelson, P. A., Dial, J. G., & Joyce, A. (2002).Validation of the Cognitive Test for the Blind as an assessment of intellectual functioning. *Rehabilitation Psychology, 47*(2), 184–193.

Nelson, P. A., O'Brien, E. P., Dial, J. G., & Joyce, A. (2001). Neuropsychological correlates of retinopathy of prematurity (ROP) compares to other causes of blindness [Abstract]. *Archives of Clinical Neuropsychology, 16,* 766–767.

Nester, M. A. (1994). Psychometric testing and reasonable accommodation for persons with disabilities. In S. M. Bruyere & J. O'Keefe (Eds.), *Implications of the Americans with Disabilities Act for psychology* (pp. 25–36). New York: Springer/American Psychological Association.

O'Keefe, J. (1994). Disability, discrimination, and the Americans with Disabilities Act. In S. M. Bruyere &

J. O'Keefe (Eds.), *Implications of the Americans with Disabilities Act for psychology* (pp. 1–14). New York: Springer/American Psychological Association.

Palermo, T. M., Witherspoon, D., Valenzuela, D., & Drotar, D. (2004). Development and validation of the Child Activity Limitations Interview: A measure of pain-related functional impairment in school-age children and adolescents. *Pain, 109,* 461–464.

Pellegrino, L. (1997). Cerebral palsy. In M. Batshaw (Ed.), *Children with disabilities* (4th ed., pp. 499–528). Baltimore: Brookes.

Pirozzolo, F. J., & Papanicolaou, A. C. (1986). Plasticity and recovery of function in the central nervous system. In J. E. Obrzut & G. W. Hynd (Eds.), *Child neuropsychology: Vol. 1. Theory and research* (pp. 141–154). Orlando, FL: Academic Press.

Polat, F. (2003). Factors affecting psychosocial adjustment of deaf students. *Journal of Deaf Studies and Deaf Education, 8*(3), 325–339.

Powell-Smith, K. A., Stoner, G., Bilter, K. J., & Sansosti, F. J. (2008). Best practices in supporting the education of students with severe and low-incidence disabilities. In A. Thomas & T. Grimes (Eds.), *Best practices in school psychology V* (pp. 1233–1248). Bethesda, MD: National Association of School Psychologists.

Pratt, S. I., & Moreland, K. L. (1998). Individuals with other characteristics. In J. Sandoval, C. L. Frisby, K. F. Geisinger, J. D. Scheuneman, & J. R. Grenier (Eds.), *Test interpretation and diversity* (pp. 349–371). Washington, DC: American Psychological Association.

Rich, C. C., & Anderson, R. P. (1965). A tactual form of the Progressive Matrices for use with blind children. *Personnel and Guidance Journal, 43*(9), 912–919.

Richards, J. S., Brown, L., Hagglund, K., Bua, G., & Reeder, K. (1988). Spinal cord injury and concomitant traumatic brain injury: Results of a longitudinal investigation. *American Journal of Physical Medicine and Rehabilitation, 67,* 211–216.

Roberts, R. D., Pallier, G., & Goff, G. N. (1999). Sensory processes within the structure of human cognitive abilities. In P. L. Ackerman, P. C. Kyllonen, & R. D. Roberts (Eds.), *Learning and individual differences: Process, trait, and content determinants* (pp. 339–370). Washington, DC: American Psychological Association.

Roid, G. H. (2003). *Stanford–Binet Intelligence Scales, Fifth Edition.* Itasca, IL: Riverside.

Roth, E., Davidoff, G., Thomas, P., Doljanac, R., Dijkers, M., Berent, S., et al. (1989). A controlled study of neuropsychological deficits in acute spinal cord injury patients. *Paraplegia, 27,* 480–489.

Russell, E. W. (1980). Fluid and crystallized intelligence: Effects of diffuse brain damage on the WAIS. *Perceptual and Motor Skills, 51,* 121–122.

Rutter, M. (1981). Psychological sequelae of brain damage in children. *American Journal of Psychiatry, 138*(12), 1533–1544.

Schwartz, L. S., Engel, J. M., & Jensen, M. P. (1999). Pain in persons with cerebral palsy. *Archives of Physical Medicine and Rehabilitation, 80,* 1243–1246.

Sigelman, C. K., & Rider, E. A. (2009). *Life-span human development* (6th ed.). Belmont, CA: Wadsworth Cengage Learning.

Stankov, L., Seizova-Cajic, T., & Roberts, R. D. (2001). Tactile and kinesthetic perceptual processes within the taxonomy of human cognitive abilities. *Intelligence 29,* 1–29.

Stanley, F. J., Blair, E., Hockey, A., Petterson, B., & Watson, L. (2003). Spastic quadriplegia in Western Australia: A genetic epidemiological study: I. Case population and perinatal risk factors. *Developmental Medicine and Child Neurology, 35*(3), 191–201.

Telzrow, C. F. (1991). The school psychologist's perspective on testing students with traumatic brain injury. *Journal of Head Trauma Rehabilitation, 6,* 23–34.

Texas School for the Blind and Visually Impaired. (2010). Resources. Retrieved from *www.tsbvi.edu/resources.*

Thatcher, R. W., Walker, R. A., Gerson, I., & Geislerm, F. H. (1989). EEG discriminant analyses of mild head trauma. *Electroencephalography and Clinical Neurophysiology, 73,* 94–106.

Thomas, A., & Grimes, T. (Eds.). (2008). *Best practices in school psychology V.* Bethesda, MD: National Association of School Psychologists.

Turk, M. A., Geremski, C. A., Rosenbaum, P. F., & Weber, R. J., (1997). The health status of women with cerebral palsy. *Archives of Physical Medicine and Rehabilitation, 78,* 810–817.

U.S. Census Bureau. (2000). Disability status: 2000. Retrieved from *www.census.gov/hhes/www/disability/disabstat2k.html.*

U.S. Department of Education. (2006, August 14). 34 C.F.R. Parts 300 and 301: Assistance to states for the education of children with disabilities and preschool grants for children with disabilities: Final rule. *Federal Register, 71*(156), 46539–46845.

Vernon, M. (2005). Fifty years of research on intelligence of deaf and hard-of-hearing children: A review of literature and discussion of implications. *Journal of Deaf Studies and Deaf Education, 10*(3), 225–231.

White, J. R., Farukhi, Z., Bull, C., Christensen, J., Gordon, T., Paidas, C., et al. (2001). Predictors of outcome in severely head-injured children. *Critical Care Medicine, 29*(3), 534–540.

Zebracki, K., & Drotar, D. (2008). Pain and activity in children with Duchenne or Becker muscular dystrophy. *Developmental Medicine and Child Neurology, 50,* 546–552.

CHAPTER 30

Use of Intelligence Tests in the Identification of Children with Intellectual and Developmental Disabilities

Kathleen Armstrong
Jason Hangauer
Joshua Nadeau

BRIEF OVERVIEW OF INTELLECTUAL AND DEVELOPMENTAL DISABILITIES

The term *intellectual and developmental disabilities* (IDD) is used to describe a group of chronic and clinically distinct disorders affecting developmental progress in one or more domains as compared with established norms. Formerly referred to as *mental retardation*, IDD is one of the more common groups of developmental disabilities, affecting nearly 3 out of 100 individuals in the United States (American Association on Intellectual and Developmental Disabilities [AAIDD], 2010). The *Diagnostic and Statistical Manual of Mental Disorders,* fourth edition, text revision (DSM-IV-TR), using the term *mental retardation,* defines IDD as a disorder with an onset before age 18, in which an individual shows "significantly subaverage intellectual functioning: an IQ of approximately 70 or below on an individually administered IQ test," along with delays in adaptive behavior performance (American Psychiatric Association [APA], 2000, p. 49). The AAIDD (2010) defines the upper limit of subaverage intelligence as an IQ score of 75, when there are also concerns related to adaptive functioning. This association stresses that factors including linguistic diversity, culture differences, and the environment must be taken into account in assessing for IDD. A comparable definition, also using the term *mental retardation,* is found in the Individuals with Disabilities Education Improvement Act of 2004 (IDEA 2004).

IDD has traditionally been defined by levels (mild, moderate, severe, profound), reflecting IQ ranges. These ranges are most often used for purposes of diagnosis, determining eligibility for services, allocating resources, and stratifying individuals for research and legal purposes (Shevell, 2008; Walker & Johnson, 2006). The overall prevalence rate for IDD is 2–3% of the overall population, with 85% of those individuals classified as functioning within the mild range, 10% within the moderate range, 3–4% within in the severe range, and 1–2% within the profound range (Walker & Johnson, 2006). The majority of children with mild IDD are not identified until school entry or later, particularly when there is no history of medical or physical problems or significant delays in milestones. Furthermore, many adults with mild IDD become indistinguishable from other members of the community because they no longer have academic demands, and their adaptive strengths make them successfully integrated in vocational and community settings (Hamilton, 2006). IDD disproportionately affects males and those from lower socioeconomic populations; thus both nature and nurture are thought to play important roles in cognitive development (Oakland, Mpofu, Glasgow, & Junel, 2003).

At least 50% of the variance in IQ scores is gene-related, while the remaining causes have been linked to prenatal causes such as brain malformations and maternal substance abuse, and postnatal causes including seizures, infections, malnutrition, and traumatic brain injury (Walker & Johnson, 2006). The three most common known medical and physical causes of IDD are fragile X syndrome (FXS) and Down syndrome (DS) (both genetic disorders), and fetal alcohol syndrome (FAS), which results from prenatal exposure to alcohol (Walker & Johnson, 2006). In children with FAS, IQ scores range from 20 to 120, with a mean score of 65; in comparison, IQ scores for children with FXS range from 25 to 65, while those for children with DS range from 40 to 60 (Walker & Johnson, 2006). In general, the more severe the disability, the greater the likelihood of an underlying genetic cause (Zeanah, 2009). Lastly, IDD may also be associated with other developmental disabilities, neurological disorders, or behavior disorders, including autism spectrum disorder (ASD), in which about 50% of affected individuals score below 50 and 20% score between 50 and 70 on IQ tests (National Institute of Mental Health, 2008).

COMPARISON OF IDD AND DEVELOPMENTAL DELAY

Developmental delay (DD) is a descriptive term used in both medicine and education to describe lags in the skill development of infants and young children across one or more developmental domains (e.g., communication, motor, adaptive, cognitive, and social-emotional); it is presumed to be transitory or temporary, and thus amenable to intervention (Nickel & Desch, 2000). For example, certain conditions in infancy and early childhood may mimic IDD, such as communication disorders or cerebral palsy, or may reduce adaptive functioning, such as the sequelae of child abuse or neglect. However, functioning may improve when the conditions are altered. Use of the term DD is thought to prevent unjustified diagnostic conclusions of IDD, based on assessments that are less reliable and valid for young children (Nickel & Desch, 2000).

Global developmental delay (GDD) refers to delays across a variety of developmental domains, and is defined operationally as scoring two or more standard deviations from the mean on objective, norm-referenced testing in two or more developmental domains (Shevell, 2008). GDD is more likely to be associated with an underlying, presumably causative pathology, and portends a worse prognosis than DD. In some definitions, GDD is considered equivalent to IDD; however, studies have shown that the initial diagnosis of GDD is not necessarily associated with objective measures of cognitive impairment after age 5 (Riou, Ghosh, Francoeur, & Shevell, 2009). These authors recommend that along with intellectual and developmental evaluation, functional performance of young children has important implications related to diagnosis and prognosis, and should therefore be taken into account.

Both the 1997 reauthorization of the original IDEA and IDEA 2004 include a definition for DD, which may be used to provide special education services to children under age 5 (Danaher, 2005). Eligibility policies related to children with DD vary across the United States. The majority of states (43) use a norm-referenced criterion of two or more standard deviations below the mean in one developmental area, or 1.5 standard deviations below the mean in two or more developmental domains (Danaher, 2005), to define a significant delay.

Although there is a need for standardized assessment activities in very young children, there are also concerns about these activities. The concerns are related to the rapid developmental changes that occur in young children, the desirability of avoiding premature labeling and stigma, and the limitations of assessment tools available for this population. Predictive validity studies for norm-referenced tests for children under age 2 generally show that tests are not good at predicting later intellectual performance (Fagan & Singer, 1983; Sternberg, Grigorenko, & Bundy, 2001). No predictive validity data are available for infant and toddler assessment tools with contemporary norms, including such well-known tools as the Bayley Scales of Infant and Toddler Development, Third Edition (Bayley-III; Bayley, 2005); the Merrill–Palmer—Revised Scales of Development (M-P-R; Roid & Sampers, 2004); and the Battelle Developmental Inventory, Second Edition (BDI-2; Newborg, 2004). Furthermore, the adequacy of floors and item gradients in these tools is weak (e.g., the standard scores do not go below 55, thus limiting their use with significantly delayed or very young children; Bradley-Johnson & Johnson, 2007). In particular with measures of cognitive abilities, test scores are most appropriately inter-preted as reflecting current developmental lev-els rather than IQ (Flanagan & Alfonso, 1995). Using repeated developmental assessments over time, and documenting changes in rates of devel-opment and function, will lead to a more accurate diagnosis of IDD.

LIMITATIONS OF INTELLIGENCE TESTS FOR ASSESSING CHILDREN WITH IDD OR DD

Administration and Scoring Procedures

Standardized tests are of limited use for children with IDD because of numerous factors: inflexibili-ty in administrative procedures; limited number of items at extreme ranges of ability; insensitivity to small increments of change; and children's sensory or physical limitations, short attention span, and communication delays. Several intelligence tests used in preschool populations have been identi-fied as having inadequate test floors (Flanagan & Alfonso, 1995). Specifically, in order to differen-tiate between subgroups (e.g., children with DD who are lower-functioning), the test must have an adequate number of beginning items that can allow an examiner to establish a sufficient basal level. That is, the examiner interested in deter-mining what a child *can* do may find that the test does not have enough items to realistically assess skills or changes in functioning. This limitation prevents establishing an accurate range of func-tioning (mild, moderate, or severe range) and can be problematic for educational planning purposes. Later in this chapter, we discuss another approach to the identification of children with IDD, which may yield more useful information for educational planning.

Culture and Language Differences

Differences among individual cultures, languages, and dialects are crucial for any examiner to con-sider in assessment. For instance, children who are bilingual and are in the earlier stages of learning English may not understand test questions and therefore may earn a lower score. If a child is a dual-language learner (mastering his or her native as well as a new language), great care must be taken in selecting and administering standardized tests (Padilla & Borsato, 2008). Best practice in assess-ment of a dual-language learner involves observing

the child in multiple contexts—among other chil-dren and with parents, as well as during informal interactions with the child (e.g., playing a game). This process will help the examiner gauge whether the child truly has a language disorder needing in-tervention or is in the process of mastering both languages (Espinosa, 2005). These issues are also important to consider when an examiner sees chil-dren with different dialects and accents.

INSTRUMENTS FREQUENTLY USED TO MEASURE COGNITION

Table 30.1 briefly reviews two commonly used standardized assessment instruments for infants and toddlers. As in the assessment of any child, multiple pieces of information should be gathered and integrated to formulate diagnostic or eligibil-ity decisions and assist in intervention planning. Table 30.1 discusses the strengths and weaknesses of these two developmental tests, each of which derives a standard score for each of five develop-mental areas (adaptive, personal–social, commu-nication, motor, and cognitive) and an overall composite score.

Table 30.2 summarizes assessment tools for chil-dren over 2 years of age and focuses only on cogni-tive scales. The strengths and weaknesses of each measure as they relate to assessing young children as well as school-age children are discussed. The tests are highlighted because of their particular at-tention to assessing young children and attempts to provide adequate floors (e.g., easier questions) to assess lower-functioning children.

IQ TESTING AND ADAPTIVE BEHAVIOR FUNCTIONING

Adaptive behavior is a critical component to con-sider in evaluating a child for concerns related to IDD. *Adaptive behavior* is defined by the Ameri-can Association on Mental Retardation (AAMR; 2002) as a collection of conceptual, social, and practical skills learned by individuals in order to function in daily life. Adaptive behavior is consid-ered an integral component of diagnosis for IDD by DSM-IV-TR (APA, 2000). In addition, both IDEA 2004 and the AAMR (2002) define IDD as a disability in which an individual has significant limitations in adaptive behavior coexisting with limitations in intelligence. It is critical for profes-sionals assessing children for IDD to consider the

TABLE 30.1. Assessment Tools Frequently Used to Measure Development and Cognition in Infants and Toddlers

Instrument name	Age range, areas assessed, and materials	Strengths	Weaknesses
Battelle Developmental Inventory, Second Edition (BDI-2; Newborg, 2004)	**Age range:** Birth–7 years **Areas assessed:** Adaptive, Social–Emotional, Language, Motor, and Cognitive **Materials:** Administration manual, manipulatives box, scoring protocol, stimulus book	Large representative norm sample of U.S. children Engaging materials Internal consistency for Cognitive domain is adequate Format of BDI-2 is especially suitable for a multidisciplinary approach Computer-assisted scoring available	Norm sample did not include children at risk for developmental delays Poor portability of test materials No test–retest reliability data provided for children under the age of 2 Item gradients for children 23 months old versus 24 months old can change substantially (i.e., children can earn significantly different scores between 23 and 24 months of age) Standard scores do not go below 55, thus limiting use with children who are very low-functioning
Bayley Scales of Infant and Toddler Development, Third Edition (Bayley-III; Bayley, 2005)	**Age range:** 1–42 months **Areas assessed:** Adaptive, Social-Emotional, Language, Motor, and Cognitive **Materials:** Administration manual, technical manual, stimulus manipulative, scoring protocol	Large representative norm sample of U.S. children Children with atypical development included in overall sample Engaging materials Adequate floor (beginning at 16 days of age) as well as item gradients (e.g., change is not dramatic when child's age changes by 1 day)	Portion of children in overall norm sample with atypical development were not described by category or diagnosis (e.g., cognitive, behavioral delays) Concerns regarding educational relevance of some cognitive items (Bradley-Johnson & Johnson, 2007) Numerous cognitive items are timed and can be problematic in assessing young children (Chandlee et al., 2002)

extent to which the children can take care of their own needs and interact socially with other children and adults. In fact, the inclusion of adaptive behavior functioning in assessment for IDD has resulted from significant legislative efforts (Reschly, Myers, & Hartel, 2002). Specifically, in the past individuals were said to have met diagnostic criteria for IDD if they earned a score more than two standard deviations below the mean on an intelligence test alone. Excluding the consideration of adaptive behavior functioning led to wrongly identifying many individuals as having IDD.

Numerous methods exist for objectively assessing adaptive behavior functioning. The majority of standardized scales used to measure adaptive behavior assess the following core areas: (1) communication, (2) social interaction, (3) daily living skills, (4) community living skills, and (5) motor skills. A person familiar with the individual being assessed can typically provide accurate information regarding the aforementioned skills. It is best practice to have multiple sources of information (e.g., parent, teacher, community member), in order to ascertain the extent to which a child has a deficit in adaptive functioning compared to same-age peers.

Adaptive behavior functioning along with cognitive performance must be considered in the diagnosis of IDD or in determining eligibility for services. The assessment of adaptive behavior functioning is one way that functional skills in an individual may be identified and linked to intervention strategies. The next section summarizes the use of *response to intervention* (RTI) within a

TABLE 30.2. Assessment Tools Used to Measure Cognitive Development in Children 2+ Years of Age

Instrument name	Age range and areas assessed	Strengths	Weaknesses
Differential Ability Scales—Second Edition (DAS-II; Elliott, 2007)	**Age range:** 2:6–17:11 **Areas assessed:** Divided into two age levels, which overlap: Early Years battery for ages 2:6–8:11 (typical age administered, 2:6–6:11) and School-Age battery for ages 5:0–17:11 (typical age administered, 7:0–17:11) Consists of Verbal, Nonverbal Reasoning, Spatial, and diagnostic subtests	Good internal-consistency reliability as well as test–retest stability over time Flexibility to administer a battery at a lower level of the test if a sufficient basal level has not been achieved Includes 12 groupings of exceptional children (both with disabilities and with intellectual giftedness) in norm sample Separate test batteries for younger and older children, reflecting brisk progression of intellectual development in young children, and providing unique flexibility to move from one battery to another if necessary (see above)	Some subtests may not be appropriate for children with severe sensory or motor disabilities, as it may unfairly disadvantage them The array of subtests and choice of which diagnostic tests to use beyond the core battery can be confusing for some examiners
Kaufman Assessment Battery for Children—Second Edition (KABC-II; Kaufman & Kaufman, 2004)	**Age range:** Two separate batteries: 3-year-old (yielding one global measure of ability) and 3- to 18-year-old (yielding two measures of ability, to reflect dual theoretical orientation of the instrument) **Areas assessed:** Two theoretical models: Luria (Learning ability, Planning and knowledge, Sequential processing, Simultaneous processing) and CHC[a] (Long-Term Storage and Retrieval, Short-Term Memory, Fluid Reasoning and Crystallized Ability, Visual Processing)	Special attention paid by test developers to addressing adequate floor issues (scales yield standard scores more than three standard deviations from the mean) Allows examiners to accept correct responses via a variety of communication modalities (e.g., signing, another language, writing)	Test kit is cumbersome to carry Record forms are long and complex Bonus points given across numerous subtests Certain subtests may be difficult for lower-functioning children to understand (e.g., Rebus)
Stanford–Binet Intelligence Scales, Fifth Edition (SB5; Roid, 2003)	**Age range:** 2–85+ years **Areas assessed:** Consists of 10 subtests (five Nonverbal and five Verbal); each subtest is organized into five separate CHC factors (Fluid Reasoning, Knowledge, Quantitative Reasoning, Visual–Spatial Processing, and Working Memory)	Includes numerous features making it useful for preschool populations (e.g., multiple types of toys, engaging activities) Better floors, leading to the ability to discriminate among subgroups of preschool children (i.e., delayed and/or low-functioning) Includes reliable and valid method to calculate Full Scale IQ from 10 to 225	Some subtests have limited floors and ceilings (particularly problematic for children who are very low-functioning) Numerous subtests have a steep item gradient; specifically, the difficulty of items moves upward very quickly, which can be problematic in assessing children for IDD

(cont.)

TABLE 30.2. *(cont.)*

Instrument name	Age range and areas assessed	Strengths	Weaknesses
Stanford–Binet Intelligence Scales, Fifth Edition *(cont.)*		Change-sensitive scores assist in determining whether a young child has made progress despite stagnant standard scores Better ability to discern (by using Nonverbal and Verbal quotients) whether English-language proficiency has adversely affected performance (Roid, 2003)	
Wechsler Preschool and Primary Scale of Intelligence—Third Edition (WPPSI-III; Wechsler, 2002)	**Age range:** 2:6–7:3 years of age **Areas assessed:** Close alliance with CHC theory	Excellent standardization sample Good subtest floors compared to other measures, enabling distinction among average, below-average, and lower-extreme-range abilities Examiner's manual provides subtest and profiles for 16 different disorders (e.g., learning disabilities, IDD)	Latest edition reduced the number of interesting manipulatives that keep young children and lower-functioning individuals engaged User manual can be cumbersome; specifically, interpretive steps and tables are not in sequential order Examiner's manual provides limited guidance on interpretation of scores; examiners must consult outside resources for this information
Wechsler Intelligence Scale for Children—Fourth Edition (WISC-IV; Wechsler, 2003)	**Age range:** 6–16:11 years **Areas assessed:** Verbal Comprehension, Perceptual Reasoning, Working Memory, Processing Speed; 10 additional subtests can be administered beyond the core battery as well	Excellent standardization sample Increased attention to developmental appropriateness (e.g., specific teaching items), which may be beneficial in assessing children for IDD Four-factor structure across all age ranges of the test	WISC-IV has fewer manipulatives than previous editions, which may decrease engagement in children being assessed for IDD One subtest, Matrix Reasoning, may be unfairly biased to children with visual deficits
Wechsler Adult Intelligence Scale—Fourth Edition (WAIS-IV; Wechsler, 2008)	**Age range:** 16:0–90:11 years **Areas assessed:** Verbal Comprehension, Perceptual Reasoning, Working Memory, Processing Speed	Excellent standardization sample Closely matches WISC-IV in domains assessed	Some evidence exists that the WAIS-IV may overestimate intellectual ability in some cases when compared to other measures, such as the SB5 (Silverman et al., 2010)

[a]CHC, Cattell–Horn–Carroll.

tiered service delivery model that may be of assistance in assessment and intervention planning in educational setting for children with IDD or DD.

INTELLIGENCE TESTING AND THE RTI FRAMEWORK

Response to Intervention

RTI is a decision-making framework that relies solely upon collected data to drive instructional, intervention, and placement decision, and has gained considerable attention in special education legislation (IDEA 2004). Although RTI models vary, Batsche and colleagues (2005) provide a commonly accepted conceptualization of assessment within RTI as having two purposes: to facilitate the development and implementation of evidence-based interventions (EBIs) within the general education classroom; and to provide a reliable means of determining the extent to which students respond to EBIs—a method typically referred to as *progress monitoring.*

Similar to the practice of evidence-based medicine, RTI requires that interventions must be evidence-based; that is, there must be empirical data showing that a planned intervention has been effective for the population which the target child belongs. An EBI must be implemented *within the general education classroom.* The reasoning behind this requirement is twofold: An intervention is clearly of no use to the general education teacher if it does not help the child succeed in their classroom. In addition, if interventions are being planned and implemented within a more restrictive environment such as a self-contained special education classroom, then an implicit decision has been made that the student does not belong in the general education classroom. This presumption of student deficit heightens the chance of confirmatory bias against the student.

The third concern—and the origin of the term *response to intervention*—is that there must be a means in place that reliably indicates whether or not, and to what extent, the student responds to the chosen intervention. The idea here should be clear: If the intervention doesn't improve the student's performance, then its continuation is a waste of time and resources. And, if the intervention is not effective, then further consideration is warranted as to what is causing the deficit in student performance and how to address those concerns.

Problem Solving and RTI

RTI is commonly considered to provide a decision-making framework across three educational arenas: student assessment, school and/or district resource management, and eligibility for special education services. Addition of a problem-solving component to the RTI model provides an efficient manner of driving actions taken during the RTI process. To wit, in a problem-solving/RTI (PS/RTI) model, assessment is focused upon identifying a problem, analyzing its possible cause(s), finding and implementing an appropriate intervention to address the identified problem, and monitoring the effectiveness of the implemented intervention with respect to the originally identified problem. An in-depth examination of the PS/RTI model is beyond the scope of the current discussion. However, to set the context for the topic at hand, a brief overview of the assessment, resource management, and eligibility methodology is necessary.

PS/RTI and Student Assessment

Assessment within a PS/RTI model is very different from traditional assessment methodologies. Bergan and Kratochwill (1990) describe a typical PS/RTI model as a four-stage cycle, with multiple actions occurring within each stage. The four stages are problem identification, problem analysis, plan development/implementation, and program evaluation/RTI.

The problem identification stage generally consists of operationally defining a replacement behavior or skill in terms that are recognizable and (perhaps more important) measurable. Once the behavior is defined, authentic in-class assessments are conducted to determine the student's current level of performance, that of his or her peers, and that expected by the teacher (or by benchmark). From these data, a gap analysis is used to determine whether or not a problem exists (i.e., the presence of a significant discrepancy between actual and expected performance), as well as the appropriate intervention and analysis point (the entire class, small groups of students, or an individual).

Within the problem analysis stage, hypotheses are generated across six contextual domains in an attempt to determine which area(s) are contributing to the identified problem. The areas include quality of instruction, level and quality of curricular materials, the classroom environment, the target student, the classroom peers, and the home and family environment. An important idea to keep in mind is that from this point on in the problem-solving process, data collection is focused solely upon validating or refuting the generated hypotheses. In addition, the only interventions selected for implementation will be those addressing hypotheses that have been validated by further data collection.

At this point, a replacement behavior has been defined, a problem identified, and hypotheses generated to explain the problem. Within the plan development/implementation stage, one or more EBIs are designed and put in place to address the hypothesized barriers to the student's learning. Although the gap analysis conducted during problem identification will determine the level at which to intervene (e.g., whole-class, small-group, individual), any potential intervention must be directly tied to a valid hypothesis, as well as empirically supported for use in the given situation.

During program evaluation/RTI, the effectiveness of the selected intervention is tracked and analyzed via the student's measured response—with respect to both the gap analysis and the student's rate of growth. Quite simply, any intervention that serves to narrow the gap is maintained or increased in intensity, while any intervention resulting in low, no, or negative growth is either modified or discontinued. Note that this stage serves as a continuous planning tool, as well as a backup to the generated hypotheses.

PS/RTI and Resource Management

A secondary, though important, use of the PS/RTI model is to enhance school/district resource management via a tiered delivery system of academic and behavioral interventions. Although various models exist, with differing numbers of tiers, the overarching concept is unchanged: organizing school resource usage to match the needs of all students. The least complex model (three-tiered) is optimal for explaining the impact on resource management.

A basic academic PS/RTI model consists of three tiers, with tier 1 (T1) representing the entire population in question—a classroom, a grade level, a school, or a district. At this tier, assessment is characterized by the use of periodic academic screeners, which are used to determine the impact of schoolwide instruction, as well as to identify those students who display a poor response to intervention. Note that in T1, the "intervention" is core instruction.

When students show poor RTI, two hypotheses are addressed: Core instruction is inadequate (i.e., fewer than 80% of students are achieving the targeted benchmarks), and/or exposure to instruction is inadequate (i.e., nonresponding students display an excessive number of absences). If either of these hypotheses reveals a problem, intervention at T1 is indicated. These interventions consist of curricular modifications to improve the quality of instruction, and/or increasing parental involvement to address student absenteeism. If neither hypothesis is valid (i.e., at least 80% of students are achieving benchmarks, and nonresponding students do not display excessive absences), intervention at the second tier (T2) is indicated.

At the second tier, supplemental interventions—that is, interventions *in addition to core instruction*—are implemented to increase both the *exposure* to instruction (small groups in multiple settings) and the *intensity* of instruction (focus on smaller number of skills). At this point, if the students display a positive RTI (the gap narrows), they will either continue to receive T2 interventions or be faded to T1 intervention (core instruction only). However, if the students display zero or negative RTI, then intervention at the third tier (T3) is indicated.

The third tier consists of individualized, intensive interventions implemented in addition to core *and* supplementary interventions. Again, note that T3 interventions must be based upon all data collected to date. These interventions are characterized by increased instruction time (core instruction, supplementary instruction, and intensive instruction), individualized materials, and additional instructional personnel as necessary. If a student displays a positive response to T3 interventions, maintenance or fading to the supplementary (T2) level occurs. If the student displays a zero or negative RTI, a key decision point is reached: Will T3 resources continue to be used to target the replacement behavior, or instead be used to address lower-priority (though still important) academic skills?

PS/RTI and Student Eligibility

Eligibility determination for specialized education services, though one of the most hotly debated topics between proponents and detractors of RTI (Hale, Kaufman, Naglieri, & Kavale, 2006), is a tertiary purpose of the PS/RTI model. As opposed to discrepancy models, eligibility within the PS/

RTI model relies upon two separate though related questions at the T3 level. First, do the amount and nature of resources equating to positive student RTI exceed those typically found within the general education classroom? Second, are observed gains in student growth maintained when these augmenting resources are removed? Thus, in the PS/RTI model, if such surplus resources are required to *achieve and maintain* positive RTI, then a student is eligible for specialized education services.

To summarize, the conceptualization of RTI within a problem-solving framework addresses three critical needs in using available funds to meet the requirements of the No Child Left Behind Act of 2001 and IDEA 2004. The model provides an algorithm to drive service delivery decisions, using EBIs linked directly to skill or behavioral deficits. The model maximizes effective prioritization of funds via a tiered service delivery framework. Finally, the model bases determination of specialized education services eligibility solely upon the continuing necessity of resources beyond those available within the general education classroom.

INTEGRATING RTI WITH INTELLIGENCE TESTING FOR CHILDREN WITH IDD OR DD

Norm-referenced tests, including intelligence tests, have often been deemphasized by proponents of "RTI-only" models (e.g., Espin & Wallace, 2004; Thurlow & Ysseldyke, 1980). However, in certain facets of assessment, norm-referenced tests and the PS/RTI model have something in common: They both seek to identify and/or rule out problems.

The PS/RTI model is one driven entirely through the collection of data: Data are collected to identify existing problems, to drive hypotheses and design EBIs, to monitor intervention effectiveness, and to determine student eligibility for specialized education services. With this in mind, it stands to reason that any source of reliable data about a student is important to the effectiveness of a data-driven process. When educators maintain an awareness of these similar goals, tests of cognitive ability and adaptive behavior can be integrated into a tiered problem-solving model. RTI is a framework for improving student outcomes through systemic change. In this respect, such a model relies upon inter- and intrasystem relationships to define expectations and assess performance. Although it is fair to state that an IQ test

cannot judge the effectiveness of core instruction, it must also be considered that such tests were not designed to do so. Similarly, a PS/RTI model cannot diagnose a disability or student-centered condition; however, such a model was never meant to do so. Worth mentioning is the notion that best practice does not involve a question as to whether or not norm-referenced tests are appropriate; rather, it is knowing at what point—and for which questions—such tests should be used within the PS/RTI model.

When T1 intervention is not indicated, this finding implies that the identified problem is related to curricular materials, the classroom environment, peer relationships, sociocultural issues, or a student-centered deficiency. Although materials and the environment are not subject to norm-referenced assessment, the remaining issues (relationships with peers, issues and behaviors related to home and/or culture, and cognitive abilities) are well within the purview of adaptive behavior and cognitive measures.

These measures have the potential to contribute much-needed data about a student's cognitive abilities and processes, as well as his or her adaptive behavior, to hypothesis generation and intervention planning. As such, IQ testing within the PS/RTI model becomes appropriate once the information such tests can contribute becomes germane to the hypotheses being generated to address the problem at hand. When educators are designing and implementing interventions at the small-group and individual level, IQ tests provide a reliable, unique, and empirically justified source of information for intervention selection and implementation planning.

SUMMARY AND CONCLUSIONS

This chapter has provided an overview of the traditional use of intelligence tests and adaptive behavior measures in the identification of children with IDD; our particular focus has been on integrating this process within the more contemporary PS/RTI model for determining instructional goals and placement decisions. For many years, standardized assessments of IQ and adaptive behavior constituted the gold standard for diagnosis of IDD, and these scores led to the placement of children in special education programs or opened eligibility for other services. Limitations of standardized IQ testing for individuals with IDD have been widely publicized, and include issues such as limited floors, steep item gradients, language or sensory deficits, and attention problems, which may interfere with performance and bias results. As a result, some children have been overrepresented in special education settings and have had less opportunity to participate in more inclusive settings. The inclusion of adaptive behavior measures in the assessment process is intended to provide a less biased and more comprehensive understanding of an individual's daily functioning across his or her daily routines. The results can then be used to develop interventions and tailor supports that help these individuals live more independently.

Similarly, the PS/RTI model has been developed to improve students' performance and help make educational decisions, including special education placement. Especially in the case of children with mild IDD, this model may prove to be a superior method to determine need and eligibility for special education services.

However, it must be kept in mind that the PS/RTI model was never meant to diagnose a disability, and has not yet demonstrated clinical or research utility; for those reasons, the more traditional psychological assessments may be necessary. Examiners must stay abreast of a wide variety of well-standardized assessment tools with the potential to answer referral questions and address the specific needs of individuals with IDD. The relationship between assessment and intervention is likely to be emphasized in the future, and the role that IQ testing may play in the identification of IDD will depend upon the advances of the science.

REFERENCES

American Association on Intellectual and Developmental Disabilities (AAIDD). (2010). *Intellectual disability: Definition, classification, and systems of support* (11th ed.). Washington, DC: Author.

American Association on Mental Retardation (AAMR). (2002). *Mental retardation: Definition, classification, and systems of support* (10th ed.). Washington, DC: Author.

American Psychiatric Association (APA). (2000). *Diagnostic and statistical manual of mental disorders* (4th ed., text rev.). Washington, DC: Author.

Batsche, G., Elliott, J., Graden, J. L., Grimes, J., Kovaleski, J. F., Prasse, D., et al. (2005). *Response to intervention: Policy considerations and implementation.* Alexandria, VA: National Association of State Directors of Special Education.

Bayley, N. (2005). *Bayley Scales of Infant and Toddler Development, Third Edition.* San Antonio, TX: Harcourt Assessment.

Bergan, J. R., & Kratochwill, T. R. (1990). *Behavioral consultation and therapy.* New York: Plenum Press.

Bradley-Johnson, S., & Johnson, M. (2007). Infant and toddler cognitive assessment. In B. A. Bracken & R. J. Nagle (Eds.), *Psychoeducational assessment of preschool children* (pp. 325–358). Mahwah, NJ: Erlbaum.

Chandlee, J., Heathfield, I., Sclganik, M., Damokosh, A., & Radcliffe, J. (2002). Are we consistent in administering and scoring the Bayley Scales of Infant Development-II? *Journal of Psychoeducational Assessment, 20,* 183–200.

Danaher, J. (2005). *Eligibility policies and practices for young children under Part B of IDEA* (NECTAC Notes No. 15). Chapel Hill: University of North Carolina, FPG Child Development Institute, National Early Childhood Technical Assistance Center.

Elliott, C. D. (2007). *Differential Ability Scales—Second Edition.* San Antonio, TX: Harcourt Assessment.

Espin, C., & Wallace, T. (2004). *Research Institute for Progress Monitoring.* Minneapolis: University of Minnesota.

Espinosa, L. (2005). Supporting learners with diverse educational needs in general education settings. *Psychology in the Schools, 42,* 837–853.

Fagan, J. F., & Singer, L. T. (1983). Infant recognition memory as a measure of intelligence. In L. Lipsitt & C. Rovee-Collier (Eds.), *Advances in infancy research* (Vol. 2, pp. 31–78). Norwood, NJ: Ablex.

Flanagan, D., & Alfonso, V. (1995). A critical review of the technical characteristics of new and recently revised intelligence tests for preschool children. *Journal of Psychoeducational Assessment, 13,* 66–90.

Hale, J., Kaufman, A., Naglieri, J., & Kavale, K. (2006). Implementation of IDEA: Integrating response to intervention and cognitive assessment methods. *Psychology in the Schools, 43,* 753–770.

Hamilton, S. (2006). Screening for developmental delay: Reliable, easy to use tools. *Journal of Family Practice, 55(5),* 2–9.

Individuals with Disabilities Education Improvement Act of 2004 (IDEA 2004), Pub. L. No. 108-446, 118 Stat. 2647 (2004).

Kaufman, A. S., & Kaufman, N. L. (2004). *Kaufman Assessment Battery for Children—Second Edition.* Circle Pines, MN: American Guidance Service.

National Institute of Mental Health. (2008). *Autism spectrum disorders.* Bethesda, MD: Author.

Newborg, J. (2004). *Battelle Developmental Inventory, Second Edition.* Itasca, IL: Riverside.

Nickel, R., & Desch, L. (2000). *Caring for children with disabilities and chronic conditions.* Baltimore: Brookes.

Oakland, T., Mpofu, E., Glasgow, K., & Junel, B. (2003). Diagnosis and administration of assessments for students with mental retardation in Australia, France, United States, and Zimbabwe 98 years after Binet's first intelligence test. *International Journal of Testing, 3,* 59–75.

Padillo, A., & Borsato, G. (2008). Issues in culturally appropriate psychoeducational assessment. In L. Suzuki, J. Ponterotto, & P. Meller (Eds.), *Handbook of multicultural assessment: Clinical, psychological, and educational applications* (3rd ed., pp. 5–21). San Francisco: Jossey-Bass.

Reschly, D., Myers, T., & Hartel, C. (Eds.). (2002). *Disability determination for mental retardation.* Washington, DC: National Academy Press.

Riou, E., Ghosh, S., Francoeur, E., & Shevell, M. (2009). Global developmental delay and its relationship to cognitive skills. *Developmental Medicine and Child Neurology, 51*(8), 600–606.

Roid, G. H. (2003). *Stanford–Binet Intelligence Scales, Fifth Edition, Technical manual.* Itasca, IL: Riverside.

Roid, G. H., & Sampers, J. L. (2004). *Merrill–Palmer—Revised Scales of Development.* Wood Dale, IL: Stoelting.

Shevell, M. (2008). Global delay and mental retardation or intellectual disability: Conceptualization, evalua-

tion, and etiology. *Pediatric Clinics of North America, 55,* 1–6.

Silverman, W., Miezejeski, C., Ryan, R., Zigman, W., Krinsky-McHale, S., & Urv, T. (2010). Stanford–Binet and WAIS-IV IQ differences and their implications for adults with intellectual disability. *Intelligence, 38,* 242–248.

Sternberg, R. J., Grigorenko, E. L., & Bundy, D. A. (2001). The predictive value of IQ. *Merrill–Palmer Quarterly, 47,* 1–41.

Thurlow, M., & Ysseldyke, J. E. (1980). Instructional planning: Information collected by school psychologists vs. information considered useful by teachers. *Journal of School Psychology, 20*(1), 3–10.

Walker, W., & Johnson, C. (2006). Mental retardation: Overview and diagnosis. *Pediatrics Review, 27,* 204–212.

Wechsler, D. (2002). *WPPSI-III technical and interpretive manual.* San Antonio, TX: Psychological Corporation.

Wechsler, D. (2003). *Wechsler Intelligence Scale for Children—Fourth Edition.* San Antonio, TX: Psychological Corporation.

Wechsler, D. (2008). *Wechsler Adult Intelligence Scale—Fourth Edition.* San Antonio, TX: Pearson.

Zeanah, C. H. (Ed.). (2009). *The handbook of infant mental health* (3rd ed.). New York: Guilford Press.

PART VI

CONTEMPORARY AND EMERGING ISSUES IN INTELLECTUAL ASSESSMENT

Using the Joint Test Standards to Evaluate the Validity Evidence for Intelligence Tests

Jeffery P. Braden
Bradley C. Niebling

The current edition of the *Standards for Educational and Psychological Testing* (American Educational Research Association [AERA], American Psychological Association [APA], & National Council on Measurement in Education [NCME], 1999) provides a framework for evaluating contemporary tests of intelligence. The *Standards* help test publishers and test users decide how to present, use, and evaluate tests, and help users to select and interpret tests as well. However, we believe that many users of intelligence tests may not be familiar with the *Standards*, and may be uncertain how to apply them to such tests. Although we appreciate that the *Standards* are undergoing revision as this chapter goes to press, we begin our chapter with a brief description of the 1999 *Standards* to proceed with our argument. In the next section of the chapter, we articulate a framework for judging the validity evidence provided by test developers. We then use the framework to evaluate the validity evidence presented for selected contemporary tests of intelligence at their time of publication, and include the emerging assessment paradigm of response to intervention (RTI). We conclude our discussion by assessing common strengths, weaknesses, and challenges confronting test developers and users in understanding the validity of intelligence tests.

DEVELOPMENT AND CONTENT OF THE *STANDARDS*

The *Standards* first appeared as a joint publication in 1974 (APA, AERA, & NCME, 1974). The joint publication combined three distinct sets of standards promulgated by different groups interested in educational and psychological tests (i.e., APA, 1954, 1966; AERA, 1955). The *Standards* were revised in 1985 (AERA, APA, & NCME, 1985) and again in 1999. The goal is to revise the *Standards* approximately every 10 years; therefore, another revision is underway, and is planned to culminate in a new (fourth) edition by 2012.

Each edition of the *Standards* has attempted to reflect professional consensus regarding expectations for the development and use of educational and psychological tests. As stated in the 1999 version, "the purpose of publishing the *Standards* is to provide criteria for the evaluation of tests, testing practices, and the effects of test use" (AERA et al., 1999, p. 2). That is, the *Standards* are intended to apply both to those who produce tests (developers) and to those who use tests (examiners). Additional standards apply to test users (e.g., APA, 2002) and to test takers (e.g., APA, 1998), but the *Standards* are intended to reflect the contemporary and common consensus for the use of educational and psychological tests.

The 1999 edition of the *Standards* contains three sections, covering the following topics: (1) test construction, evaluation, and documentation; (2) fairness in testing; and (3) testing applications. Although specific standards in all three sections apply to test publishers and users, the standards applying to test developers appear primarily in the first section.

The 1999 edition differs from previous editions in a number of important ways. First, specific standards are no longer identified as either primary or secondary. Instead, the salience of any given standard is determined by its relevance for the intended uses of the test. Second, the 1999 *Standards* volume specifies that standards cannot be applied in a literal or rote checklist. Rather, professional judgment, the degree to which the test developer and user satisfy each standard, the availability of alternatives, and research must influence the degree to which a test is deemed acceptable.

Third, the *Standards* employ an important shift in the use of the term *construct*. Rather than meaning unobservable characteristics, this term is broadened to mean "the concept or characteristic that a test is designed to measure" (AERA et al., 1999, p. 5). This redefinition alters the understanding of *validity* from that of previous versions. Instead of describing three distinct types of validity (*content*, *construct*, and *criterion*), the 1999 *Standards* regard validity as being "the degree to which evidence and theory support the interpretations of test scores entailed by proposed uses of tests" (p. 9). In other words, validity is the degree to which evidence supports the assumption that a test score reflects the construct the test aims to assess. Therefore, the distinctions among content, construct, and criterion validity in previous versions are replaced by the notion that multiple sources of evidence must support the claim that the test measures the construct.

The *Standards* identify five sources of evidence: (1) *test content*, (2) *response processes*, (3) *internal structure*, (4) *relations to other variables*, and (5) *consequences of testing*. Three of these sources appeared in previous editions: test content (content validity), internal structure (construct validity), and relations to other variables (criterion validity). However, the other two sources of evidence are new. Response process evidence supports the contention that test takers use the intended psychological processes when responding to items

(e.g., a reasoning test elicits reasoning rather than recall). Test consequence evidence should support the case that testing and test outcomes actually fulfill the claims made for test use (e.g., a test demonstrates that results are useful for designing psychoeducational interventions).

In this chapter, we focus on the intersection of the 1999 *Standards* and intelligence tests. We attempt to identify those standards that are more or less relevant to particular intelligence tests, based on the claims of those tests. Our primary focus is on validity claims and evidence, mainly because of the importance of these standards for intellectual assessment. Intelligence tests are more often criticized for failing to assess their intended construct (intelligence) than for lacking reliability, norms, and other attributes found in other parts of the *Standards*; also, it is no accident that validity is covered in the first chapter of the *Standards* because ultimately the meaning of a test result determines its value to the test developer, test user, and test taker.

Although we appreciate that appropriate use of intelligence tests is a joint responsibility shared by test developers and test users, our primary focus is on evaluating the validity evidence provided by test developers at the time of publication to support tests of intelligence. Standard 11.1 states: "Prior to the adoption and use of a published test, the test user should study and evaluate the materials provided by the test developer" (AERA et al., 1999, p. 113). Although Standard 11.1 goes on to specify four areas of particular importance for test users to consider, our review focuses on two: (1) the purposes of the test, and (2) the validity data available to support score interpretations consistent with those purposes. We suggest a framework for evaluating the materials and information provided by a test developer to help test users fulfill their obligation to meet Standard 11.1, although we also appreciate that users should obtain and consider evidence from other sources as well (e.g., professional publications, test reviews). We focus primarily on those standards dealing with validity, which are found in Chapter 1 of the *Standards*.

VALIDITY EVIDENCE FRAMEWORK

We developed an organizational and conceptual framework for evaluating the importance and quality of validity evidence presented by test developers shortly after the publication of the 1999

Standards. The original draft of this framework was used to evaluate the validity evidence presented by the test developers of a wide variety of assessment instruments commonly used by school psychologists (Braden et al., 2001, 2002). Although the content of the new *Standards* was written to represent a shift in philosophy for establishing validity, no explicit guidance was provided for applying the new *Standards.* Therefore, we developed a framework for evaluating validity claims and evidence (Braden & Niebling, 2005), and we have updated and extended the application of that framework to include RTI assessment approaches in this chapter.

Application to Published Intelligence Tests

Our original framework assigned each of the 24 validity standards (AERA et al., 1999, Ch. 1) to one of the five evidence domain areas: content, response processes, internal structure, relation to other variables, and consequences. To increase the functionality and objectivity of these standards, and to help users meet the spirit of Standard 11.1, we created two Likert-type scales. The first Likert-type scale rates the *importance* of the validity evidence presented in each of the five domain areas for the claims made by the test developer. For example, evidence of test content is more important for tests claiming to measure specific content (e.g., tests of mathematics abilities that employ a state's math standards) than for tests not making such claims (e.g., projective tests). Ratings on this scale range from 1 = "not important" to 5 = "critical/very important." The second Likert-type scale asks test users to rate the *quality* of the validity evidence presented in each of the five domain areas by the test developer. Ratings on this scale range from 1 = "weak" to 5 = "strong," with a 0 rating for "no evidence present."

As we applied our framework to these psychological tests, we invited test developers and other experts to provide feedback to us about our efforts (see Braden et al., 2001, 2002). On the basis of that feedback, we realized that our framework was inadequate. Consequently, we altered the framework in two ways. First, we created an additional domain area called the *cross-cutting* domain. This domain was created for the standards dealing with validity issues that cut across, or serve as a type of umbrella for, the other five domain areas. For example, Standard 1.1 directs test developers to

justify and support recommended interpretations, and does not clearly fall into a specified domain of evidence. Second, we decided that some standards fit into more than one of the five evidence domain areas. Third, we felt that standards in multiple domains serve either a **primary** (in bold) or *secondary* (in italics) role within each domain. For example, the primary emphasis of Standard 1.14 relates to a test's relations to other variables, but it is also related to internal test structure when test evidence includes factor-analytic evidence, such as the kind of evidence presented to support cross-battery analyses of cognitive processes. Figure 31.1 graphically presents the allocation of standards to the six categories. Table 31.1 presents an organizational framework for jointly considering the importance of a body of evidence or standards, and the quality of available evidence to respond to the domain.

We then developed a set of coding procedures (Niebling & Braden, 2003) to evaluate validity claims and the evidence test developers provide to support those claims. The materials accompanying each assessment instrument (e.g., technical manuals, administration manuals, test publisher bulletins) formed the foundations for evaluating test claims and validity. The first step was to identify each of the claims listed by the test developer for use of the test. These claims guided the collection of validity evidence and determined the relative importance of evidence. For example, a test claiming to assess cognitive processes has a greater obligation to provide evidence of response processes than a test that does not make such a claim. Next, the validity evidence was identified and evaluated within each evidence domain area; the standards in those domain areas were used as the lens through which to examine that evidence. The next step was to rate the importance of the gathered evidence for the domain. We repeated the process for each of the six domain areas to provide a structured, but subjective, evaluation of evidence supporting the claims made for the test.

Application to the RTI Paradigm

Subsequent to our revision of our framework and development of coding procedures was the codification of a set of practices collectively known as *response to intervention* (RTI) in the Individuals with Disabilities Education Improvement Act of 2004 (IDIEA 2004). RTI is "an integrated approach to service delivery that encompasses general and spe-

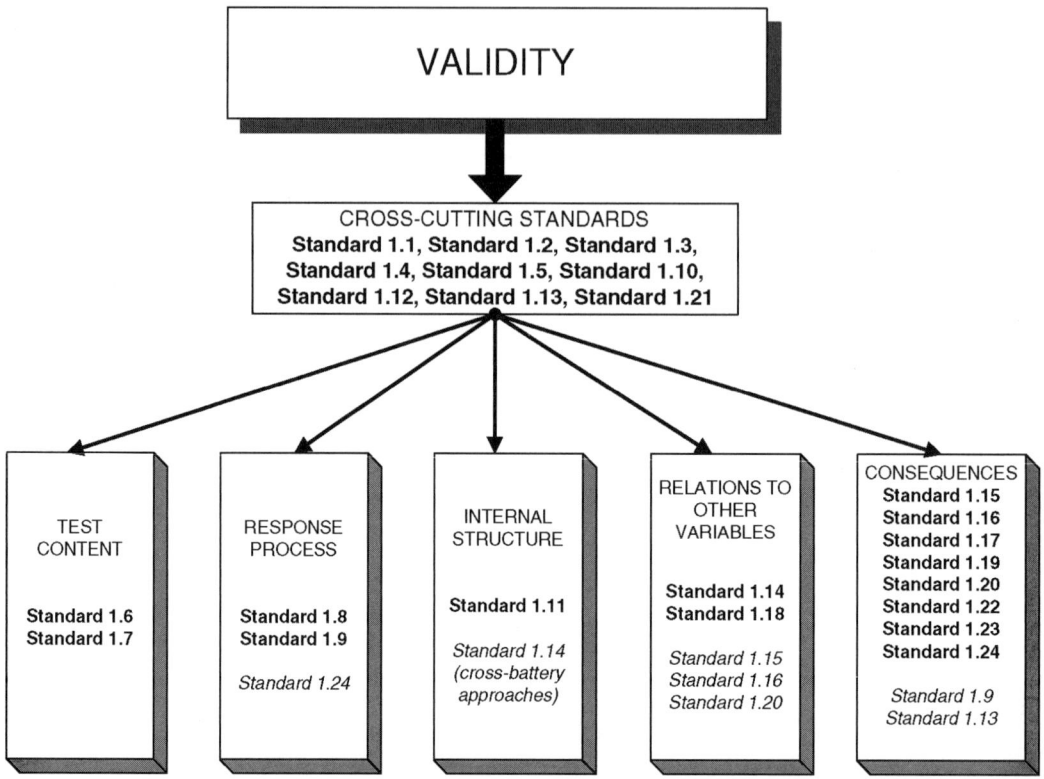

FIGURE 31.1. Conceptual framework for understanding and applying validity standards.

cial education" that includes "the practice of (1) providing high-quality instruction/intervention matched to student needs and (2) using learning rate over time and level of performance to (3) make important educational decisions" (Batsche et al., 2005, p. 6). This is a broad definition that encompasses several issues and sets of practices, including assessment as a process as opposed to a singular "test."

When we applied the validity framework to the assessment process in an RTI framework, we distinguished between dynamic assessment and the

determination of a student's eligibility and need for special education services. *Dynamic assessment* (Grigorenko & Sternberg, 1998; Schulte & Grigorenko, 2004) has a long history in intellectual assessment as a mechanism to distinguish an individual's low levels of performance (i.e., a history or pattern of not learning) from the individual's potential to learn by measuring levels of performance before and after intervention. Large improvements in performance imply greater potential (and therefore intellectual abilities) relative to small improvements or no changes. We distinguish this tradition

TABLE 31.1. Validity Evidence Rating Grid

Standard domain	Importance of Evidence					Quality of Evidence					
Cross-cutting	1	2	3	4	5	0	1	2	3	4	5
Test content	1	2	3	4	5	0	1	2	3	4	5
Response processes	1	2	3	4	5	0	1	2	3	4	5
Internal structure	1	2	3	4	5	0	1	2	3	4	5
Relation to other variables	1	2	3	4	5	0	1	2	3	4	5
Consequences	1	2	3	4	5	0	1	2	3	4	5

from the RTI framework, which is focused not on whether an individual has potential to learn (all students are assumed to have potential); instead, RTI focuses on whether a given intervention can result in sufficient improvement in a student's performance to render special education unnecessary. Although there are many overlaps between dynamic assessment in the intellectual tradition and RTI as an eligibility assessment mechanism (Grigorenko, 2009), we see their foci as distinct. Dynamic assessment seeks to draw inferences about an individual's potential to learn (e.g., intelligence), whereas RTI collects information about a student's performance discrepancy, rate of learning progress, and educational needs to determine whether the student is entitled to and in need of special education services.

Using this broad definition of RTI and assessment as being process-oriented challenged us to apply the *Standards* and our validity framework. The *Standards* and our framework are better suited for individual assessment instruments or tests. Nevertheless, we contend that our framework can be usefully applied to the assessment aspects of RTI. Furthermore, any test authors or users who claim that the results of intelligence tests can be used for any type of decision making within an RTI framework should use the *Standards* to guide their provision or examination of validity evidence for those claims.

The framework described here was designed to increase the functionality and objectivity of the *Standards* for evaluating validity evidence presented by test developers. We note, however, that this framework is not intended to remove the importance of professional judgment in using the *Standards* to examine validity evidence. Furthermore, our framework is not a checklist or test; rather, the framework describes the *process* of collecting and evaluating validity evidence. Ratings represent the importance and quality of evidence presented relative to *test claims*, and are not a rote application of the *Standards*. Our ratings should be viewed in this context.

ANALYSIS OF VALIDITY EVIDENCE FOR SELECTED TESTS OF INTELLIGENCE

In this section, we describe how we applied the framework we developed to tests of intelligence. We used three criteria to select tests for review: (1) The tests are described in other chapters of the present book; (2) the test was published after the

publication of the 1999 *Standards* (so test developers had the opportunity to use this edition of the *Standards*); and (3) publication data were available to us in time for inclusion in our chapter. These criteria identified the following tests for review: (1) the Wechsler Intelligence Scale for Children—Fourth Edition (WISC-IV; Wechsler, 2003); (2) the Stanford–Binet Intelligence Scales, Fifth Edition (SB5; Roid, 2003a); (3) the Woodcock–Johnson III Tests of Cognitive Abilities (WJ III COG; Woodcock, McGrew, & Mather, 2001); (4) the Reynolds Intellectual Assessment Scales (RIAS; Reynolds & Kamphaus, 2003); and (5) Kaufman Assessment Battery, Second Edition (KABC-II; Kaufman & Kaufman, 2004). Exclusion of other tests is in no way intended to convey judgments about those tests; our review is not exhaustive. Rather, our review is intended to illustrate one way that test users might respond to Standard 11.1 regarding review of test developer information, particularly as it applies to the purposes and validity of contemporary tests of intelligence.

Review of the WISC-IV

We reviewed the administration (Wechsler, 2003) and technical (Psychological Corporation, 2003) manuals for claims regarding the WISC-IV. The claims we identified are presented in Table 31.2. We then consulted these sources, as well as three technical bulletins provided by the test developers (Williams, Weiss, & Rolfhus, 2003a, 2003b, 2003c), for evidence to support test claims. Our ratings of importance for various domains, and the quality of evidence within those domains, are presented in Figure 31.2.

Review of the SB5

We reviewed the administrative (Roid, 2003a), interpretive (Roid, 2003b), and technical (Roid, 2003c) manuals for the SB5 to identify test claims and evidence. These three sources substantially overlap, and in some cases replicate some sections in their entirety. In addition, we included three Assessment Services Bulletins distributed by the test developer (i.e., Becker, 2003; Braden & Elliott, 2003; Ruf, 2003) for additional evidence in support of test claims. The claims we identified for the test are presented in Table 31.3. Our ratings of importance for various domains, and the quality of evidence within those domains, are presented in Figure 31.3.

TABLE 31.2. Claims Made for the WISC-IV by the Test Developer

Administration manual (Wechsler, 2003, pp. 7–8)

- The WISC-IV is for use with examinees 6 years, 0 months to 16 years, 11 months of age.
- It provides comprehensive assessment of general intellectual functioning.
- It identifies giftedness, intellectual disability, and cognitive strengths and weaknesses.
- Specific suggestions for use with adaptive behavior, memory, and achievement measures are provided.
- Results can guide treatment planning and placement decisions.
- The WISC-IV provides invaluable clinical information for neuropsychological evaluation.
- It is also useful in research.

Technical manual (Psychological Corporation, 2003)

- The WISC-IV measures four major cognitive clusters loosely aligned with Cattell–Horn–Carroll (CHC) theory (Ch. 1, pp. 7–8):
  - Fluid Reasoning
  - Verbal Comprehension
  - Working Memory
  - Processing Speed
- Subtests measure specific cognitive processes (pp. 16–20).

Technical Bulletin No. 2 and other sources (in parentheses)

- Use for clients with the following special conditions is implied by directions and data:
  - Deafness and hearing impairments (Wechsler, 2003, pp. 12–18)
  - Physical/motor disabilities (Wechsler, 2003, p. 11; Psychological Corporation, 2003, pp. 100–101)
  - Language or speech disabilities (Wechsler, 2003, p. 11; Psychological Corporation, 2003, pp. 91–93)
  - Sensory disabilities (Wechsler, 2003, p. 11)
  - English-language learner status (Wechsler, 2003, p. 12)
  - Non-English-speaking status (Wechsler, 2003, p. 12)
  - Intellectual giftedness (Psychological Corporation, 2003, pp. 79–80)
  - Mild to moderate intellectual disability (Psychological Corporation, 2003, pp. 80–84)
  - Learning disorders (Psychological Corporation, 2003, pp. 84–88)
  - Attention-deficit/hyperactivity disorder (Psychological Corporation, 2003, pp. 89–91)
  - Traumatic brain injury (Psychological Corporation, 2003, pp. 93–97)
  - Autistic disorder (Psychological Corporation, 2003, pp. 98–100)

Cross-cutting standards	Importance	4
Standards **1.1, 1.2, 1.3, 1.4, 1.5, 1.10, 1.12, 1.13, 1.21**	Quality	3

- Clear statements are made regarding test user qualifications and responsibilities.
- Theoretical descriptions/rationales for claims regarding general intelligence are extensive and well documented.
- Little to no direct evidence is provided for specific claims regarding treatment planning or links to neuropsychological foundations.
- Clear statements help users distinguish between statistically reliable differences and unusual (base rate) differences among test scores.
- The norming sample is described in detail, including information regarding age, grade level, census region, community size, gender, race, type of school attended, and status of parents. The sample matches the target population very well.
- Collection procedures of the norming data are described in detail, as are procedures for test administration.
- Extensive discussion of how to identify intraindividual strengths and weaknesses by using Index, subtest, and within-subtest responses does not include discussion of contradictory findings available in the literature.

Test content	Importance	4
Standards **1.6, 1.7**	Quality	3

- Test content is described extensively, and inferences about the psychological processes they elicit are based in part on test content. Research findings on previous versions of the Wechsler scales are also cited to support the contention that subtests elicit specific processes.

(continued)

FIGURE 31.2. Summary of validity evidence for the WISC-IV.

- Test items were developed and reviewed by expert panels to ensure that they reflect their intended constructs. However, details regarding the selection and composition of the panels are lacking.

Response processes	Importance	5
Standards **1.8, 1.9**, *1.24*	Quality	3

- Research on previous versions of the Wechsler scales is cited as evidence that subtests and Index scores elicit specific processes; however, most of the cited evidence is inferential, because it relies on subjective identification of common item content and infers the psychological processes that would explain the correlation between the items. For example, factor loadings are explained by invoking common psychological processes, without direct evidence that examinees used those processes.
- Multiple-choice item errors were analyzed for common patterns that might suggest measurement of unintended processes.
- Interview evidence from examinees was obtained and analyzed for two new subtests, but not for other subtests.
- The use of the term *process score* implies scores reflect neuropsychological processes, although no direct evidence is provided to support this implication.

Internal structure	Importance	5
Standards **1.11**, *1.14*	Quality	5

- Ample evidence of correlations among items and subtests provides convergent and divergent validity evidence.
- Confirmatory and exploratory factor analyses concur in strongly supporting the four-factor model claimed by the test developers.
- Stability and reliability indices also provide evidence of internal consistency and the stability of the constructs measured within the battery.

Relationship to other variables	Importance	5
Standards **1.14, 1.18**, *1.15, 1.16, 1.20*	Quality	4

- Correlations among a variety of measures are provided; these generally support the notion that the test measures general intelligence, predicts academic achievement, is related to clinical diagnostic categories, and is consistent with previous versions of the test.
- Corrected correlations are provided; uncorrected correlations are not.
- A rationale for including unusual or unexpected measures is provided; although a rationale for expected measures (e.g., other tests of intelligence, achievement) is not provided, it is not needed. References to other measures allow test users to find and evaluate the quality of external measures.
- Extensive data are provided for a variety of clinical samples, supporting test performance across a range of relevant conditions.
- An extensive narrative review of research on previous editions, coupled with evidence that the new edition is highly related to older editions, provides unusually broad evidence linking the test to many attributes. However, the narrative review is selective, and could have been more powerful if it used contemporary methods to summarize research findings (e.g., meta-analysis).

Test consequences	Importance	5
Standards **1.15, 1.16, 1.17, 1.19, 1.20, 1.22, 1.23, 1.24**, *1.9, 1.13*	Quality	1

- The technical manual (p. 101) addresses this issue in a single paragraph, arguing that it is the sole responsibility of the test user to supply evidence regarding test consequences.
- Extensive data from clinical groups imply support for claims of diagnostic utility; however, these data are not provided at the individual level, and therefore are difficult to evaluate.
- The omission of research on previous test editions that addresses test consequences stands in stark contrast to the extensive use of research on previous editions to support other claims.
- The extensive description of how users may use test results to identify cognitive strengths and weaknesses in the technical manual (Ch. 6) implies value for meeting claims regarding clinical and educational interventions; however, no evidence is cited or provided in direct support of these claims.
- Item bias indices were used to identify and eliminate or modify items indicating evidence of bias. However, no summary evidence is provided regarding means, variances, or item bias influence for groups.
- Unintended consequences (particularly as they relate to score differences between groups defined by ethnic, gender, and socioeconomic status) are not mentioned. This omission is puzzling, given the extensive research and debate that previous editions of the same test have sparked on this topic, as well as the substantial (but unreported) differences in means between some ethnic groups on this test.

FIGURE 31.2. (*cont.*)

TABLE 31.3. Claims Made for the SB5 by the Test Developer

Administration manual (Roid, 2003a)

- The SB5 is appropriate for examinees 2–85 years of age (p. 1).
- It is useful for clients with the following special conditions (pp. 1–2):
  o Deafness and hearing impairments
  o Communication disorders
  o Autism
  o Specific learning disabilities
  o Limited English-language background
  o Traumatic brain injury
  o Other conditions affecting language ability (e.g., aphasia, stroke)
  o Limited vision
  o Orthopedic impairment
  o Highest level of gifted performance
  o Low intellectual functioning or mental retardation
  o Various neuropsychological difficulties
- Appropriate uses include the following (pp. 4–5):
  o Diagnosis of developmental disabilities and exceptionalities, including intellectual disability, learning disabilities, developmental cognitive delays, and intellectual giftedness
  o Clinical and neuropsychological assessment
  o Research on abilities
  o Early childhood assessment
  o Psychoeducational evaluations for special education placements
  o Adult Social Security and workers' compensation evaluations
  o Provide information for interventions such as individualized family service plans, individualized education programs, career assessment, employee selection and classification, and adult neuropsychological treatment
  o Must be used with additional measures for diagnostic purposes (e.g., adaptive behavior for intellectual disability diagnosis)
- The SB5 measures intelligence and five broad cognitive abilities or factors (Ch. 2):
  o Fluid Reasoning
  o Knowledge
  o Quantitative Reasoning
  o Visual–Spatial Processing
  o Working Memory
- Subtests measure unique, narrow cognitive abilities (pp. 138–143).
- Cognitive strengths and weaknesses are identified via score contrasts (pp. 147–150).
  o Abbreviated Battery IQ is useful for neuropsychological examinations when used with additional tests (p. 1).

Interpretive and technical manuals (Roid, 2003b, 2003c)

- Claims made in the administration manual are reiterated.

Cross-cutting standards	Importance	4
Standards **1.1, 1.2, 1.3, 1.4, 1.5, 1.10, 1.12, 1.13, 1.21**	Quality	5

- Clear statements are made regarding test user qualifications and responsibilities.
- Theoretical descriptions/rationales for claims regarding general intelligence are extensive and well documented.
- Little to no direct evidence is provided for specific claims regarding value for treatment planning.
- Clear statements help users distinguish between statistically reliable differences and unusual (base rate) differences among test scores.
- The norm sample is described in detail, including information regarding age, grade level, census region, gender, race, and education level. The sample matches the target population very well.
- Collection procedures for norms data are described in detail, as are procedures for test administration.
- Extensive discussion of how to identify intraindividual strengths and weaknesses by using index, subtest, and within-subtest responses includes some discussion of contradictory findings available in the literature, but no justification is provided for subtest-specific interpretations beyond content analyses.
- Extended discussion is provided of administration and interpretation issues for special populations, including detailed guides for test accommodations.

(continued)

FIGURE 31.3. Summary of validity evidence for the SB5.

Test content	Importance	4
Standards **1.6, 1.7**	Quality	5

- Test content is described extensively, and inferences about the psychological processes they elicit are made in part based on test content. Research findings on previous versions of the SB are also cited to support the contention that subtests measure general intelligence.
- Test items were developed and reviewed by expert panels to ensure that they reflect their intended constructs. Explicit details about the processes, and names of expert consultants and review committee members, are provided.

Response processes	Importance	4
Standards **1.8, 1.9**, *1.24*	Quality	1

- Research on previous versions of the SB is cited as evidence to justify the realignment of factor structures and processes to CHC theory.
- Claims that subtests and index scores elicit specific processes rest exclusively on subjective identification of common item content and inferences about psychological processes that would explain correlations among items and scores. For example, factor loadings are explained by invoking common psychological processes, without direct evidence that examinees used those processes.
- Although the *Standards* volume is cited frequently in all manuals, the chapter on validity evidence (Roid, 2003c) omits response processes.
- Change-sensitive scores (i.e., Rasch item scores) are described and provide general evidence that the test measures processes that increase and change across the developmental spectrum.

Internal structure	Importance	5
Standards **1.11**, *1.14*	Quality	5

- Exploratory and confirmatory factor-analytic data strongly support test claims, and were replicated by dividing the norm sample in half. Comparisons of factor models support five-factor claim; internal fit statistics are strong, although residual mean squares are slightly higher than desired.
- Cross-battery factor analysis (with WJ III) statistics strongly support factor structure claims within and between tests.
- Stability and reliability indices also provide evidence of internal consistency and the stability of the constructs measured within the battery.
- Correlation tables reporting relationships among subtests are not provided.

Relationship to other variables	Importance	5
Standards **1.14, 1.18**, *1.15*, *1.16*, *1.20*	Quality	4

- Overall, correlations among a variety of measures are provided; these generally support the notion that the test measures general intelligence, predicts academic achievement, is related to clinical diagnostic categories, and is consistent with previous versions of the test.
- A rationale for expected measures (e.g., other tests of intelligence, achievement) is not provided, but it is not needed. References to other measures allow test users to find and evaluate the quality of external measures.
- Data are provided for a variety of clinical samples, supporting test performance across a range of relevant conditions.
- An extensive narrative review of research on previous editions, coupled with evidence that the new edition is highly related to older editions, provides unusually broad evidence linking the test to many attributes. However, the narrative review is selective; could have been more powerful if it used contemporary methods to summarize research findings (e.g., meta-analysis); and notes that research on previous versions of the test does not generalize well beyond broad measures of general intelligence (i.e., research on factor structures and processes in previous editions does not generalize to the new version).
- Relationships between test scores, abilities, and performance in important social contexts are theoretically justified (Roid, 2003b, Ch. 5), but no direct evidence is provided to support the rationale.
- Correlations with other intelligence tests (previous versions of the SB, two other contemporary intelligence tests) are inexplicably characterized as criterion validity. However, correlations are moderate and appropriate, with a few anomalies (e.g., the correlation between Visual–Spatial Processing scores and WISC-III Performance IQ are lower than the correlation with Verbal IQ).
- Correlations with two achievement batteries (the WJ-III Tests of Achievement [WJ III ACH] and the Wechsler Individual Achievement Test—Second Edition [WIAT-II]) are described as predictive, but are concurrent. Correlations are moderate and appropriate, with a few anomalies (e.g., the SB5 Knowledge score is more highly correlated with WJ III ACH Reading Comprehension than with Mathematics Reasoning, but the opposite pattern occurs on the WIAT-II).

(continued)

FIGURE 31.3. *(cont.)*

Test consequences	Importance	5
Standards **1.15, 1.16, 1.17, 1.19, 1.20, 1.22, 1.23, 1.24**, *1.9*, *1.13*	Quality	2

- Extensive data from clinical groups imply support for claims of diagnostic utility. Although the administration manual does not provide data at the individual level, the interpretive manual does so, and includes recommended cutoff scores.
- The extensive description of how users may use test results to identify cognitive strengths and weaknesses in all three manuals implies value for meeting claims regarding clinical and educational interventions; however, no direct evidence is cited nor provided in direct support of these claims.
- Case studies elaborate the recommended seven-step interpretive procedure. It is noteworthy that the first three steps intend to establish the validity of scores for the examinee; the last four steps are similar to profile interpretation recommended for other tests, and are not explicitly justified via treatment response studies or other direct evidence.
- Item bias indices were used to identify and eliminate or modify items indicating evidence of bias. Summary evidence of item bias statistics, correlations, and internal consistency for various groups are provided, but no summary evidence is provided regarding means and variances for groups.
- Unintended consequences and concerns with diagnosis (particularly as they relate to score differences between groups defined by ethnic, gender, disability, and socioeconomic status) are discussed often, and include references to critical research and appropriate ethical guidelines and cautions.
- Although the chapter on validity in the technical manual does not include a section on consequential validity (despite citing the *Standards*), the interpretive manual includes a chapter addressing consequential validity in the context of test bias and fairness for groups.
- Explicit directions to examiners to include data from other sources are provided for some diagnostic decisions (e.g., intellectual disability, learning disability).

FIGURE 31.3. *(cont.)*

Review of the WJ III COG

We reviewed the examiner's (Woodcock et al., 2001) and technical (McGrew & Woodcock, 2001) manuals for the WJ III COG to identify test claims. We also consulted three technical bulletins provided by the test developers (Flanagan, 2001; Mather & Schrank, 2001; Schrank, McGrew, & Woodcock, 2001) for test claims and evidence to support test claims. The claims we identified are presented in Table 31.4. Our ratings of importance

for various domains, and the quality of evidence within those domains, are presented in Figure 31.4.

Review of the RIAS

We reviewed the professional manual (Reynolds & Kamphaus, 2003) for the RIAS to identify test claims. The claims we identified are presented in Table 31.5. We then consulted this source, and information on the test publisher's webpage (Psycho-

TABLE 31.4. Claims Made for the WJ III COG by the Test Developers

Examiner's manual (Woodcock, McGrew, & Mather, 2001)

- The WJ III COG is for use with preschool through geriatric levels.
- It measures intelligence according to the domains set forth in CHC theory.
- Appropriate uses include the following:
  - Diagnosis (p. 5)
  - Determination of intraindividual ability discrepancies (in conjunction with WJ III ACH; p. 5):
    - Understanding strengths and weaknesses
    - Diagnosing and documenting specific disabilities (however, multiple sources of information in addition to a discrepancy are needed for a learning disability diagnosis)
    - Acquiring *most* relevant information for educational and vocational planning
  - Educational and vocational programming
  - Planning individual programs
  - Guidance
  - Assessing growth
  - Research and evaluation
  - Psychometric training

Cross-cutting standards	Importance	4
Standards **1.1, 1.2, 1.3, 1.4, 1.5, 1.10, 1.12, 1.13, 1.21**	Quality	3

- The test user is encouraged to integrate other, "nontest" information when making diagnostic and classification decisions.
- The test developers strongly discourage making interpretations based on subtests only, but rather when each score is interpreted within the context of all other scores and assessment data.
- Discussion of "strengths" and "weaknesses," and of using test and cluster scores to examine them, is ambiguous. Although warnings against the practice are provided, ample directions and case examples illustrate the practice. Little to no empirical support is provided for how these analyses are beneficial, despite abundant evidence regarding intraindividual differences.
- Several of the tests can be interpreted according to the executive functions required and the corresponding processes used to perform the tasks (e.g., attention, working memory, planning, and cognitive flexibility).
- The norming sample is described in detail, including information regarding age, grade level, census region, community size, gender, race, type of school/college attended, education of adults, employment status, and occupation.
- Collection procedures of the norming data are described in detail. Based on this information, test users should be able to judge the relevance of statistical findings in the technical manual to local conditions.
- The examiner's manual provides detailed and accessible information about administration, scoring, qualifications, and training suggestions.

Test content	Importance	4
Standards **1.6, 1.7**	Quality	4

- A detailed description is provided of the CHC theory of cognitive abilities, around which content was crafted.
- Multiple tests cover each domain of the CHC theory.
- The Rasch model was employed to ensure that all items in each test measure the same narrow ability or trait. This process of item selection also helped the test developers to avoid selecting items that measured processes extraneous to the intended construct.
- Cognitive items range from lower-level processing to high-level thinking and reasoning.
- An expert panel was utilized in decisions about test content, but no details are given regarding panel selection or membership.
- Nine reviewers examined all WJ III COG items to identify potentially sensitive issues for women, individuals with disabilities, and cultural or linguistic minorities. Again, details about panel selection and composition are lacking.

Response processes	Importance	4
Standards **1.8, 1.9**, *1.24*	Quality	1

- Again, an extensive description is provided of the CHC theory of cognitive abilities, and of the theoretical response processes associated with each test within this framework.
- Descriptions are given of the WJ III cognitive performance model and the WJ III information-processing model. These models provide additional information regarding the processes theorized to be necessary for answering the test items.
- The CHC broad and narrow abilities measured by each of the WJ III COG tests are outlined. Also, a brief description is given of the test content by defining the nature of the stimuli, test requirements, and response modalities.
- A description of each test with its relationship to the CHC theory is included in the examiner's manual. This description includes the type of responses required from the test taker and the theorized psychological processes necessary to answer the items.
- Evidence is primarily theoretical, not empirical.
- No evidence is provided to guide examiners how to select among the three different characterizations of response processes (i.e., the CHC, cognitive performance, and information-processing models); all three frameworks are implied to be potentially valid for understanding clients' cognitive processes, but no guidance or evidence is provided to help users decide which model is appropriate for a given client.

Internal structure	Importance	5
Standards **1.11**, *1.14*	Quality	5

- Fit statistics for all five age levels are lower for WJ III than for competing intelligence models; evidence supporting the WJ III CHC model of intelligence from age 6 to late adulthood is provided.
- Confirmatory factor analyses are provided at five different age levels; the CHC interpretation is generally stable across age levels, providing evidence for structural integrity of the measure across the lifespan.

(continued)

FIGURE 31.4. Summary of validity evidence for the WJ III COG.

- Items were selected to reflect an average difference in difficulty of 3–4 *W* scale points between items.
- Extensive statistical evidence is provided for developmental patterns of cognitive performance on the tests and for the CHC-based structure of the tests.
- Internal-structure data are provided in Appendices D and E, the technical manual, and technical bulletins.

Relationship to other variables	Importance	4
Standards **1.14, 1.18**, *1.15*, *1.16*, *1.20*	Quality	4

- Special study samples were employed to provide evidence for diagnostic utility and for use with a range of populations.
- The test developers provide convergent and divergent validity evidence in the form of correlations between the WJ III COG and other measures of cognitive abilities and achievement. They reference the measures they use, so that readers will be able to find additional information about those instruments. However, they do not provide a rationale for selecting the other measures.
- All evidence presented in the technical manual and technical bulletins is concurrent, with no predictive evidence presented.

Test consequences	Importance	5
Standards **1.15, 1.16, 1.17, 1.19, 1.20, 1.22, 1.23, 1.24**, *1.9*, *1.13*	Quality	1

- Evidence for diagnosis of common learning and attention difficulties is provided for groups, but not for individuals.
- Theoretical and conceptual evidence to support claims that the test measures intelligence is provided, but no direct evidence to support claims of value for planning educational or psychological interventions is provided.

FIGURE 31.4. (*cont.*)

logical Assessment Resources, 2003), for evidence to support test claims. Our ratings of importance for various domains, and the quality of evidence within those domains, are presented in Figure 31.5.

Review of the KABC-II

We reviewed the examiner's manual (Kaufman & Kaufman, 2004) of the KABC-II to identify test claims. The claims we identified are presented in Table 31.6. We also reviewed information available on Pearson's website (*www.pearsonassessments.com/haiweb/cultures/en-us/productdetail.htm?pid=PAa21000&Community=CA_Ed_AI_Ability*) for supporting evidence. Our ratings of importance for various domains, and the utility of evidence within those domains, are presented in Figure 31.6.

TABLE 31.5. Claims Made for the RIAS by the Test Developers

Professional manual (Reynolds & Kamphaus, 2003)

- The RIAS is for use with examinees ages 3–94 years.
- It is a measure of verbal and nonverbal intelligence (p. 12).
- It can be used for diagnosis and educational placement of individuals with these conditions (pp. 11–13):
  - Learning disability
  - Intellectual disability
  - Giftedness
  - Memory impairment/central nervous system disturbances
  - Various forms of childhood psychopathology where intellectual functioning is an issue
- It can also be used for individuals with these conditions (p. 13):
  - Visual impairment (verbal subtests only)
  - Hearing deficiency (professional judgment on case-by-case basis)
  - Physical/orthopedic impairment
  - Neuropsychological impairments (other than those noted above)
  - Emotional/psychotic disturbances (due to brevity of measure)
- Other uses include the following:
  - Informing evaluation recommendations and remediation strategies (p. 14)
  - Research (p. 14)
  - Predicting specific outcomes (e.g., academic success) (Table 1.5, p. 12)

Cross-cutting standards	Importance	4
Standards **1.1, 1.2, 1.3, 1.4, 1.5, 1.10, 1.12, 1.13, 1.21**	Quality	4

- Theoretical descriptions/rationales for test developers' usage claims are clear.
- Little to no empirical evidence is provided to suggest treatment utility of assessment results.
- Theoretical and empirical evidence warning against profile analysis is provided.
- The norming sample is described in detail, including information regarding age, grade level, census region, community size, gender, race, type of school/college attended, education of adults, employment status, and occupation.
- Collection procedures for the norming data are described in detail. An appropriate description is given of statistical correction procedures used to account for regional overrepresentation.
- The examiner's manual provides detailed and accessible information about administration, scoring, qualifications, and training suggestions.

Test content	Importance	4
Standards **1.6, 1.7**	Quality	4

- A brief description is given of the qualifications of expert panel members, but details are omitted.
- Content evidence is primarily in the form of historical reference, theory, and logical argument.
- Final items were chosen based on the basis of item statistics derived from true-score theory.
- Carroll's three-stratum theory was the primary foundational theory for the content of this instrument.

Response processes	Importance	4
Standards **1.8, 1.9**, *1.24*	Quality	1

- The test developers place primary responsibility for gathering this evidence on the test user during test administration.
- The developers provide little to no direct evidence for this domain.
- Primary evidence is based on theory and logical argument, and this is limited.
- The developers spend some time describing the hypothesized types of response processes that should be invoked for each subtest, but do not provide evidence to support their hypotheses.

Internal structure	Importance	5
Standards **1.11**, *1.14*	Quality	5

- All items are correlated at least .40 with subtest total scores, with most at least .50.
- Extensive empirical evidence that individual subtest internal-consistency measures are high and significant is provided.
- Internal consistency of subtests across different age and other subgroups is above .90.
- Exploratory and confirmatory factor analyses support test structure.

Relationship to other variables	Importance	5
Standards **1.14, 1.18**, *1.15, 1.16, 1.20*	Quality	4

- The test developers provide convergent and divergent validity evidence via correlations between the RIAS and other measures of cognitive abilities and achievement. They reference the measures they use, so that readers will be able to find additional information about those instruments.
- The developers provide a rationale for selecting the other measures.
- A rationale and good validity evidence are provided for relations to variables besides other IQ tests, such as developmental trends and clinical status.
- A detailed description is given of clinical group performance relative to other groups.
- No evidence is presented on the individual level, only group-level data.

Test consequences	Importance	5
Standards **1.15, 1.16, 1.17, 1.19, 1.20, 1.22, 1.23, 1.24**, *1.9, 1.13*	Quality	1

- Group-level evidence of accurate diagnoses made with the RIAS is provided, but no individual-level data are given, and there is no differential comparison over other measures used for diagnosis.
- The test developers provide evidence indicating a minimization of item and cultural bias.
- No direct evidence is presented relating stated test purposes to test consequences.

FIGURE 31.5. Summary of validity evidence for the RIAS.

TABLE 31.6. Claims Made for the KABC-II by the Test Developers

Examiner's manual (Kaufman & Kaufman, 2004)

- The KABC-II is for use with preschool through young adult (3–18 years) levels.
- It measures cognitive abilities according to two models: one based on CHC theory, and one based on Luria's neuropsychological processing approach.
- Appropriate uses include the following:
  - Measures range of abilities (p. 1)
  - Identifies cognitive strengths and weaknesses (multiple citations)
  - Informs how processing strengths and weaknesses affect academic skills (pp. 2, 9)
  - Measures two distinct cognitive models (CHC and Luria) (pp. 2–5)
  - Measures ability with less cultural and linguistic influences (p. 5)
  - Measures abilities especially well/more fairly for minority and non–English language examinees (p. 2, 5)
  - Facilitates clinical and educational diagnoses, educational planning, treatment planning, and placement decisions (p. 9)
  - Improves understanding of brain–behavior relationships (p. 9)

Cross-cutting standards	Importance	4
Standards **1.1, 1.2, 1.3, 1.4, 1.5, 1.10, 1.12, 1.13, 1.21**	Quality	4

- Theoretical descriptions/rationales for test developers' usage claims are clear.
- Little to no empirical evidence is provided to suggest treatment utility of assessment results.
- Theoretical and empirical evidence describing practices for profile analysis is provided.
- The norming sample is described in detail, including information regarding age, grade level, census region, community size, gender, race, schooling, and parental status.
- Collection procedures for the norming data are described adequately. An appropriate description is given of statistical correction procedures used to account for regional overrepresentation.
- The examiner's manual provides detailed and accessible information about administration, scoring, qualifications, and training suggestions.

Test content	Importance	4
Standards **1.6, 1.7**	Quality	2

- The description largely refers to the original K-ABC development, which appeals primarily to historical reference, theory, and logical argument.
- Changes were described to newer subtests, but a clear rationale was not provided for why those changes were made.
- No reference to or description of item review processes (e.g., expert panel) is mentioned in manual.

Response processes	Importance	5
Standards **1.8, 1.9**, *1.24*	Quality	1

- The manual makes strong claims that the test measures cognitive processes but not content.
- However, the developers provide little to no direct evidence for this claim.
- Primary evidence is based on theory and logical argument, and this is limited to indirect evidence (e.g., item response data) which is not specifically invoked in support of response processes.
- No brain-related data (e.g., fMRI, glucose uptake, TBI studies) to support claims of Luria's model or brain–behavior links.
- Also, no direct evidence provided to show test "more fairly" assesses cognitive processes in minority children (e.g., differential structures for majority vs. minority groups, differential relationships of Gc to other tests for minority groups).
- The developers spend considerable space describing the hypothesized types of response processes that should be invoked for each subtest, but do not provide evidence to support their hypotheses.

(cont.)

FIGURE 31.6. Summary of validity evidence for the KABC-II.

Internal structure	Importance	5
Standards **1.11**, *1.14*	Quality	4

- Extensive empirical evidence that individual subtest internal-consistency measures are high and significant is provided.
- Internal consistency of subtests across different ages and other subgroups is generally above .90.
- Exploratory and confirmatory factor analyses support CHC test structure.
- However, no data provided to support claims that Luria's model is better for nonstandard language or background children (e.g., differential factor structures, changes in conclusions when Gc included).

Relationship to other variables	Importance	5
Standards **1.14, 1.18**, *1.15, 1.16, 1.20*	Quality	3

- The test developers provide convergent validity evidence via correlations between the KABC-II and other measures of cognitive abilities and achievement.
- Patterns of relationship support meaning of general index and Gc index; however, correlation patterns suggest other indexes less consistent (e.g., correlations are too high with measures of different abilities or too low with measures expected to be similar).
- The developers provide a rationale for selecting the other measures.
- Special group studies support claims of smaller differences in means between groups, but do not address claims of "more fair" assessment for special groups (i.e., no evidence of differential validity is provided).
- No evidence is shown to link test to measures representing Luria's model (i.e., all comparisons are to instruments using CHC model or to measures of achievement).
- A detailed description is given of clinical group performance relative to other groups.
- No evidence is presented on the individual level (e.g., diagnostic sensitivity); only group-level data are reported.

Test consequences	Importance	5
Standards **1.15, 1.16, 1.17, 1.19, 1.20, 1.22, 1.23, 1.24**, *1.9, 1.13*	Quality	1

- Group-level evidence of accurate diagnoses made with the KABC-II is provided, but no individual-level data are given, and there is no differential comparison over other measures used for diagnosis.
- The test developers provide evidence indicating a minimization of item and cultural bias, and smaller differences on cognitive measures than is commonly found on other tests—but no supporting data to show that these smaller differences lead to better placement or intervention are provided.
- No direct evidence is presented relating stated test purposes (e.g., diagnosing strengths and weaknesses for clinical and educational treatment planning; illuminating brain–behavior links that influence achievement).

FIGURE 31.6. *(cont.)*

CONCEPTS FOR VALIDATING RTI

The codification and increasing emphasis on RTI for making instructional and entitlement decisions warrant discussion, as one of the frequently mentioned purposes of intellectual assessment is to help make similar decisions. That is, disability is often defined at least partly in terms of intelligence, either as an inclusionary characteristic (e.g., mental retardation—now, in fact, increasingly referred to as intellectual disability—has historically been defined in large part by unusually low IQ), or as an exclusionary characteristic (e.g., definitions of learning disability typically exclude low IQ as a cause of poor academic performance). Therefore,

the question arises whether RTI processes produce valid data for identifying disabilities, particularly those that have been historically defined with reference to intelligence.

As we have noted earlier, dynamic assessment has typically compared an individual's performance on a cognitive task under standardized conditions to performance under other (sometimes standardized) conditions, and it has been argued that improvements in performance between different conditions reveal cognitive potential not evident under standardized conditions. Presumably, improvement in performance within an RTI framework demonstrates the potential for an individual to learn, and would therefore imply that intellectual (dis)abilities are not responsible for impeding learning. In other words, if learning occurs, by definition the individual's intellectual abilities must be sufficient to allow learning.

However, the obverse is not necessarily true. That is, if no learning occurs, it is not logical to assume that the individual's intellectual abilities are insufficient to allow for learning. Just as the failure of efforts to produce heavier-than-air flight over many centuries did not prove it impossible, likewise a student's failure to respond to instruction does not mean that the student lacks the capacity to respond; it only means that the interventions that have been tried are not sufficient to induce improvement. We note a disturbing, and illogical, leap in assuming that RTI is sufficient for determining eligibility and entitlement. That is, although a failure to induce a response cannot be interpreted to mean that a child lacks the intellectual abilities to respond, this is the inference that is implicitly or explicitly supported by RTI (viz., that a child who fails to respond after reasonable attempts has a disability of unspecified origin).

There is little to no evidence for the validity of intellectual assessments we reviewed for use within an RTI decision-making process. This is not surprising because those advocating the use of intellectual assessments within an RTI framework are often trying to retrofit intelligence tests to an application that the tests were not created to accomplish (i.e., assisting RTI processes).

Yet others argue that intellectual assessment should be part of a comprehensive assessment process *in addition* to RTI (e.g., Willis & Dumont, 2006). This argument rests on the assumption that the data generated by RTI processes are insufficient for making entitlement decisions. Advocates for using RTI processes without the use of intellectual assessment to make entitlement decisions need to answer the question "Is there sufficient validity evidence to support the use of an RTI process to make entitlement decisions?" The short answer is "Yes" in places where eligibility criteria have been modified to specify that such data are sufficient. Whether such changes to policy are appropriate is beyond the scope of this chapter. Those advocating for the use of intellectual assessment in addition to RTI because such data would lead to better intervention selection or adaptation (and therefore would maximize student outcomes), need data to show the incremental utility of intellectual assessment in an RTI framework. Given that there is essentially no evidence for the utility of intellectual assessment for treatment selection or

maximization in isolation, we would contend that the argument that intellectual assessment adds incremental value to RTI is unsupported—and, given the current state of research, unlikely. The primary value of intellectual assessment in eligibility determination is diagnosis, and if diagnostic criteria are modified to eliminate intelligence as a criterion, then there is no current evidential basis for supporting intellectual assessment within an RTI framework.

CONCLUSIONS

In our reviews of the four test batteries, we have attempted to illustrate how test users might evaluate validity claims and evidence for tests claiming to measure intelligence. The degree to which tests make additional claims (e.g., value for selecting psychoeducational or psychological interventions, diagnosis) places greater burdens on the test developers to provide evidence showing that those claims are met. Not all forms of evidence are equal in supporting test claims, nor does an abundance of some forms of evidence compensate for a lack of other forms. Despite the differences in claims and evidence in the tests we reviewed, we note two clear strengths shared by most tests.

First, contemporary tests of intelligence provide a substantial amount of evidence to support their validity. Contemporary intelligence tests compare favorably to most other instruments used in psychology and education; for example, most of the tests we have reviewed devote one or more volumes, such as a technical manual, to supporting evidence. This is also a substantial improvement over earlier versions of intelligence tests, which often failed to provide any meaningful validity evidence.

Second, test developers tend to provide an abundance of evidence in two primary forms: the internal structure of the test, and relationships to other variables. Extensive evidence regarding items (e.g., bias), scales or subtests (e.g., reliability, stability), and relationships among scales (e.g., correlations, exploratory and confirmatory factor analyses) help test users understand the internal structure of the test. Also, test developers provide a strong array of relationships between test scores and other variables. This evidence is primarily in the form of correlations with other tests, and secondarily in the form of relating test scores to diagnoses in clinical samples.

However, we have also noted some weaknesses in the validity evidence provided by test developers. We appreciate at the outset that test users are somewhat analogous to prosecuting attorneys, whose primary guiding principle is "One can never have too much evidence." Test developers are constrained by economic, ethical, and practical issues, and cannot be expected to provide all the evidence that test users might want. Therefore, we limit our criticisms to those forms of validity evidence that are absent but are highly relevant, or absent but could be made available at little additional cost.

None of the tests we have reviewed provides much direct evidence of response processes, and none provides much evidence for test consequences. In our first version of this chapter, we were not surprised because these domains were new to the *Standards*. However, tests developed and published since the *Standards* were released could be reasonably expected to meet evidential standards. Furthermore, intelligence tests claim to measure cognitive processes (e.g., rather than past learning or "test-wiseness"), and psychology's capacity for identifying such response processes provides ample opportunities to measure response processes.

Likewise, none of the tests we have reviewed provides much evidence of testing consequences—although all tests claim beneficial test consequences as a purpose for using the test. We appreciate that test developers cannot be held accountable for all possible consequences of test scores; nor can they be responsible for the quality of educational, medical, or social programs to which examinees are often assigned in part on the basis of test scores. Instead, we believe that test developers should be held accountable to a standard similar to the one applied to drug companies. That is, test developers should provide some evidence that when the test is used as specified, some real benefit is conferred on the test taker that would not be conferred in the absence of testing (e.g., random assignment to a treatment or program vs. assignment guided by test results). This is particularly pertinent for claims that tests are helpful in selecting and planning psychoeducational interventions (a claim common to all the tests we have reviewed). If a test developer claims that test results are valuable for this purpose, then we believe the test developer should demonstrate that test scores are more valuable than the psychological equivalent of a placebo or other tests currently available for similar purposes via response to treatment studies. This standard is even more important in an era of RTI, where alternative methods of assessment introduce interventions and assess outcomes as a critical feature of the diagnostic process. If intellectual assessment will continue to contribute to the K–12 arena, proponents must show that intellectual assessment is relevant to intervention selection and outcome.

Test development and use constitute an evolving and symbiotic enterprise, with shared responsibilities for obtaining, providing, and using validity evidence. Clearly, test developers provide much more evidence for contemporary tests than was available for previous tests, and the evidence available generally supports the claims that contemporary intelligence tests are well aligned with the theoretical constructs that define intelligence. Evidence relating to the clinical application of tests to improve client welfare is more limited, or altogether absent. We appreciate that theory typically develops more rapidly than practical application, and we hope that by examining the strengths and weaknesses in the evidence regarding intelligence test validity through the lens of the 1999 *Standards*, we will encourage test users and developers to continue the progress in developing validity evidence to support tests of intelligence.

ACKNOWLEDGMENTS

We would like to acknowledge the efforts of our colleagues Lori Bruno, Latrice Green, Ryan Kettler, Patricia Aleman, and Elisa Steele-Shernoff, for their assistance in developing and applying the original validity standards framework. We also acknowledge feedback on our efforts from test developers James DiPerna, Stephen Elliott, Randy Kamphaus, Nancy Mather, Cecil Reynolds, Larry Weiss, and Richard Woodcock. We further thank David Goh for his assistance, which was instrumental in helping us conceptualize how to apply the *Standards*.

We also note that Jeffrey P. Braden received funds from Riverside Publishing, Inc., for preparing a guide to test accommodations for the SB5, and that he has accepted grants providing test materials to support test training from The Psychological Corporation, Riverside Publishing, and the Woodcock–Muñoz Foundation.

REFERENCES

American Educational Research Association (AERA) Committee on Test Standards. (1955). *Technical recommendations for achievement tests*. Washington, DC: Author.

American Educational Research Association (AERA), American Psychological Association (APA), & National Council on Measurement in Education (NCME). (1985). *Standards for educational and psychological testing* (2nd ed.). Washington, DC: APA.

American Educational Research Association (AERA), American Psychological Association (APA), & National Council on Measurement in Education (NCME). (1999). *Standards for educational and psychological testing* (3rd ed.). Washington, DC: AERA.

American Psychological Association (APA). (1954). *Technical recommendations for psychological tests and diagnostic techniques.* Washington, DC: Author.

American Psychological Association (APA). (1966). *Standards for educational and psychological tests and manuals.* Washington, DC: Author.

American Psychological Association (APA). (1998). *The rights and responsibilities of test takers: Guidelines and expectations.* Retrieved from *www.apa.org/science/ttrr.html.*

American Psychological Association (APA), American Educational Research Association (AERA), & National Council on Measurement in Education (NCME). (1974). *Standards for educational and psychological tests.* Washington, DC: APA.

Batsche, G., Elliott, J., Graden, J., Grimes, J., Kovaleski, J., Prasse, D., et al. (2005). *Response to intervention: Policy considerations and implementation.* Alexandria, VA: National Association of State Directors of Special Education.

Becker, K. A. (2003). *History of the Stanford–Binet Intelligence Scales: Content and psychometrics* (Stanford–Binet Intelligence Scales, Fifth Edition, Assessment Services Bulletin No. 1). Itasca, IL: Riverside.

Braden, J. P., & Elliott, S. N. (2003). *Accommodations on the Stanford–Binet Intelligence Scales, Fifth Edition* (Stanford–Binet Intelligence Scales, Fifth Edition, Assessment Services Bulletin No. 2). Itasca, IL: Riverside.

Braden, J. P., & Niebling, B. C. (2005). Using the Joint Test Standards to evaluate the validity evidence for intelligence tests. In D. P. Flanagan & P. L. Harrison (Eds.), *Contemporary intellectual assessment: Theories, tests and issues* (2nd ed., pp. 615–630). New York: Guilford Press.

Braden, J. P., Niebling, B. C., Bruno, L., Green, L. Y., Kettler, R. J., Aleman, P., et al. (2001, August). *New validity standards for educational and psychological tests: An overview and application.* Symposium conducted at the annual meeting of the American Psychological Association, San Francisco.

Braden, J. P., Niebling, B. C., Bruno, L., Green, L. Y., Kettler, R. J., Aleman, P., et al. (2002, April). *New validity standards for educational and psychological tests: An overview and application.* Symposium conducted at the annual meeting of the National Association of School Psychologists, Washington, DC.

Flanagan, D. P. (2001). *Comparative features of the WJ III Tests of Cognitive Abilities* (Woodcock–Johnson III Assessment Service Bulletin No. 1). Itasca, IL: Riverside.

Grigorenko, E. L. (2009). Dynamic assessment and response to intervention: Two sides of one coin. *Journal of Learning Disabilities, 42*(2), 111–132.

Grigorenko, E. L., & Sternberg, R. J. (1998). Dynamic testing. *Psychological Bulletin, 124*(1), 75–111.

Individuals with Disabilities Education Improvement Act of 2004, Publ L. No. 108-446, 20 U.S.C. §1400 et seq. (2004).

Kaufman, A. S., & Kaufman, N. L. (2004). *Kaufman Assessment Battery for Children Second Edition manual.* Circle Pines, MN: AGS Publishing.

Mather, N., & Schrank, F. A. (2001). *Use of the WJ III discrepancy procedures for learning disabilities identification and diagnosis* (Woodcock–Johnson III Assessment Service Bulletin No. 3). Itasca, IL: Riverside.

McGrew, K. S., & Woodcock, R. W. (2001). *Woodcock–Johnson III technical manual.* Itasca, IL: Riverside.

Niebling, B. C., & Braden, J. P. (2003). *Coding procedures: Evaluating the validity of test instrument interpretation.* Unpublished manuscript.

Psychological Assessment Resources. (2003). Reynolds Intellectual Assessment Scales. Retrieved from *www.parinc.com/RIAS.cfm.*

Psychological Corporation. (2003). *Wechsler Intelligence Scale for Children—Fourth Edition: Technical manual.* San Antonio, TX: Author.

Reynolds, C. R., & Kamphaus, R. W. (2003). *Reynolds Intellectual Assessment Scales and the Reynolds Intellectual Screening Test: Professional manual.* Lutz, FL: Psychological Assessment Resources.

Roid, G. H. (2003a). *Stanford–Binet Intelligence Scales, Fifth Edition: Examiner's manual.* Itasca, IL: Riverside.

Roid, G. H. (2003b). *Stanford–Binet Intelligence Scales, Fifth Edition: Interpretive manual.* Itasca, IL: Riverside.

Roid, G. H. (2003c). *Stanford–Binet Intelligence Scales, Fifth Edition: Technical manual.* Itasca, IL: Riverside.

Ruf, D. L. (2003). *Use of the SB5 in the assessment of high abilities* (Stanford–Binet Intelligence Scales, Fifth Edition, Assessment Services Bulletin No. 3). Itasca, IL: Riverside.

Schrank, F. A., McGrew, K. S., & Woodcock, R. W. (2001). *Technical abstract* (Woodcock–Johnson III Assessment Service Bulletin No. 2). Itasca, IL: Riverside.

Schulte, A. C., & Grigorenko, E. L. (2004). Dynamic testing: The nature and measurement of learning potential. *School Psychology Quarterly, 19*(1), 88–92.

Wechsler, D. (2003). *Wechsler Intelligence Scale for Children—Fourth Edition.* San Antonio, TX: Psychological Corporation.

Williams, P. E., Weiss, L. G., & Rolfhus, E. L. (2003a).

Wechsler Intelligence Scale for Children—Fourth Edition: Clinical validity (Technical Report No. 3). Retrieved from *www.wisc-iv.com*.

Williams, P. E., Weiss, L. G., & Rolfhus, E. L. (2003b). *Wechsler Intelligence Scale for Children—Fourth Edition: Psychometric properties* (Technical Report No. 2). Retrieved from *www.wisc-iv.com*.

Williams, P. E., Weiss, L. G., & Rolfhus, E. L. (2003c). *Wechsler Intelligence Scale for Children—Fourth Edition: Theoretical model and test blueprint* (Technical Report No. 1). Retrieved from *www.wisc-iv.com*.

Willis, J. O., & Dumont, R. (2006). And never the twain shall meet: Can response to intervention and cognitive assessment be reconciled? *Psychology in the Schools, 43*(8), 901–908.

Woodcock, R. W., McGrew, K. S., & Mather, N. (2001). *Woodcock–Johnson III Tests of Cognitive Abilities.* Itasca, IL: Riverside.

CHAPTER 32

Using Confirmatory Factor Analysis to Aid in Understanding the Constructs Measured by Intelligence Tests

Timothy Z. Keith
Matthew R. Reynolds

Factor analysis is inexorably linked with the development of intelligence theory and intelligence tests. Early intelligence theories and factor-analytic methods were developed in tandem, and the connection continues to this day. Carroll's (1993) three-stratum theory of intelligence was developed, in part, through the use of *exploratory factor analysis* (EFA).

For much of its history, the term *factor analysis* meant what is now called EFA. In its simplest form, EFA involves making a series of decisions about the method of factor extraction to use, the number of factors to retain, and the method of rotation to use. For researchers who do not wish to make these decisions, most computer programs will default to a common method if none is specified (not always a wise choice). The output from the analysis consists of factor loadings of each variable on each factor and, if an oblique rotation was used, correlations among the factors. The researcher then assigns names to the factors based on the loadings of the variables on the factors, along with relevant theory and previous research.

In the hands of an expert, EFA can be much more complex and elegant than the simple approach just described. A variety of extraction methods can be used, depending on the questions of interest; complex decision rules and expert judgment can be used to determine how many factors should be extracted; and a variety of graphical and mathematical methods can be used to rotate the extracted factors to simple structure. For example, Carroll (1993, Ch. 3) outlined an approach to EFA that was an elegant combination of consistency and judgment (see also McDonald, 1999, p. 187). Whether simple or complex, EFA involves judgment on the part of the researcher: judgment concerning the decisions required, and judgment concerning the meaning of the extracted factors. It is this aspect of EFA that can be disconcerting to those wanting yes–no answers to questions, but it is also this requirement for thought that makes the approach so alluring and so powerful.

In its simplest form, *confirmatory factor analysis* (CFA) requires the researcher to decide, in advance, the nature of the factor structure underlying the data. He or she must specify the number of factors and the variables that load on each factor. So, for example, the researcher may specify that variable 1 loads on factor 1, but not on factor 2. The researcher may specify that factors are correlated, or may specify that they are uncorrelated. The results of the analysis provide *fit statistics*, which provide feedback as to the adequacy of the specified factor structure, or the degree to which the *model* (factor structure) *fits* the data (reproduces the covari ances among the data). In CFA, in other words, the researcher tests the adequacy of a particular factor structure by restricting the factor solution (thus the method is sometimes called *restricted factor analysis*; Allen & Thorndike, 1995) and seeing whether that restricted solution is consistent with the data. In contrast, in EFA (sometimes called *unrestricted factor analysis*), the researcher examines and imparts meaning to the best factor structure (given the decision rules used).

CFA is often described as a more theory-driven approach than EFA. This assertion probably involves some overstatement. It is possible, for example, to use EFA in a theory-driven, hypothesis-testing manner (cf., Thorndike, 1990; Thurstone, 1947), just as it is possible to use CFA in an exploratory, theory-absent manner. Indeed, Jöreskog and Sörbom (1993, p. 115) have argued that a combination exploratory–confirmatory "model-generating" approach is probably the most common approach to *structural equation modeling* (SEM) and CFA. Nevertheless, the simple fact that CFA requires the specification of a model—and thus knowledge about the probable structure of the characteristic being measured—means that some sort of theory (formal or informal, strong or weak) is required. EFA can easily be conducted in the absence of theory, although theoretically driven analyses are almost invariably more complete and informative than atheoretical ones. EFA can be a valuable tool for *developing* theory, whereas CFA may be better suited for *testing* existing theory.

This chapter demonstrates the use of CFA, with particular attention to using CFA to understand the constructs measured by modern intelligence tests. It begins with a "simple" CFA model, and gradually moves to CFA methods that provide a more complete evaluation of the theories underlying tests (e.g., hierarchical analysis, the comparison of alternative models, multisample analyses). It demonstrates how the method can be used to test formal theories as well. The emphasis is on the use of CFA to *test hypotheses* about *theories*.

There are several computer programs available that conduct CFA. These programs are designed to conduct latent-variable SEM; SEM includes and subsumes CFA (the *measurement model*, in the jargon of SEM), and thus SEM programs also conduct CFA. The oldest program is LISREL (LInear Structural RELations; Jöreskog & Sörbom, 1996); extensive information about the program is available at *www.ssicentral.com*. Other common programs include EQS (Bentler, 1995; *www.mvsoft. com*) and Mplus (Muthén & Muthén, 1998–2010;

www.statmodel.com), perhaps the most powerful and flexible SEM program. The analyses presented in this chapter were conducted using Amos (Analysis of MOment Structures; Arbuckle, 1995–2010; *www.spss.com/amos*), probably the easiest-to-use such program. Amos uses a drawing program to provide pictorial input and output of models. The figures in this chapter were drawn with Amos, and the graphic output shown was produced by the Amos program.

A SAMPLE CFA

The Kaufman Adult and Adolescent Intelligence Test (KAIT) is an older measure of cognitive abilities for individuals ages 11 through adulthood (Kaufman & Kaufman, 1993). According to the manual, the KAIT was designed to measure intelligence according to the Cattell–Horn theory of intelligence, although only two of the Cattell–Horn factors are included in the KAIT model (*fluid intelligence*, also known as *novel reasoning*, and *crystallized intelligence*, also known as *comprehension–knowledge*). In addition, the KAIT was designed to measure *delayed recall*, or a person's memory for material learned earlier in the test. Thus the KAIT includes 10 subtests designed to measure three abilities: fluid intelligence (Gf), crystallized intelligence (Gc), and delayed recall.

Figure 32.1 shows this "theory" of the KAIT in figural form. The 10 subtests are shown in rectangles, and the abilities they are designed to measure are enclosed in ovals. Directed arrows or paths point from the abilities to the subtests in recognition of the implicit assumption that the abilities residing within the person are what cause him or her to score a certain way on a subtest. So, for example, examinees' levels of fluid intelligence are the primary determinant of their scores on the Mystery Codes subtest.

Figure 32.1 is also the beginning of a CFA model; a more complete CFA model is shown in Figure 32.2.[1] In the jargon of CFA, the variables enclosed in rectangles (the subtests) are the *measured* variables, whereas the variables enclosed in ovals (e.g., the KAIT abilities) are *unmeasured* variables, also known as *latent* variables, or *factors*. The paths from latent to measured variables represent the factor loadings. Notice that not all possible paths are drawn. Theoretically, the lack of a path from, say, Gf to Double Meanings means that the test authors believe Double Meanings does not measure fluid intelligence, or that variation in fluid

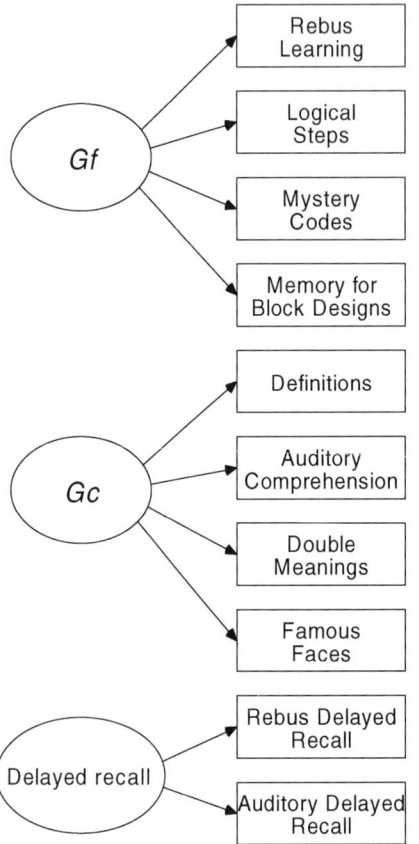

FIGURE 32.1. Theoretical structure of the KAIT.

underlying the tests maintains that the factors are independent). The figure also includes small ovals, labeled u1 through u10, with paths drawn to each of the subtests. The factors are not the only cause of a person's scores on the subtest; each subtest is also partially the result of other influences that are unique to each subtest, generally called *unique* or *specific variances* (see Keith, 2006). In addition, each subtest is also affected by errors of measurement (*error variance*). These unique and error variances, combined, are represented by u1 through u10; they are enclosed in ovals because they are unmeasured. These unique and error variances are hereafter termed *unique variances*, although they are referred to by a variety of names here and in the literature, including *errors* and *residuals*.

Several of the paths in Figure 32.2 have the value 1 beside them. The measured variables in the model have a defined scale, and that scale is whatever scale was used for each subtest (e.g., a scaled score from 1 to 19). But none of the latent variables (neither the factors nor the unique variances) have a predetermined scale. The 1's beside paths serve the purpose of setting the scales of the latent variables by setting the path to 1.0. The path of 1.0 from Gf to Rebus Learning, for exam-

intelligence does not produce variation in scores on the Double Meanings subtest. Rather, scores on Double Meanings are a reflection of crystallized intelligence, as indicated by the path drawn from Gc to Double Meanings. At a practical level, the path from Gc to Double Meanings means that the factor loading will be estimated in the analysis, and the lack of a path from Gf to Double Meanings means that the factor loading of Double Meanings on Gf will be constrained to 0.

Figure 32.2 includes information beyond that included in Figure 32.1. The curved, two-headed arrows between factors represent covariances (or, in the standardized output, correlations). Although the KAIT manual does not say so explicitly, it is reasonable to expect that the abilities measured by the KAIT are not independent of (uncorrelated with) one another. Modern intelligence theories recognize this relation among factors (e.g., Carroll, 1993, Chs. 2–3), and CFAs of intelligence tests should specify correlated factors (unless the theory

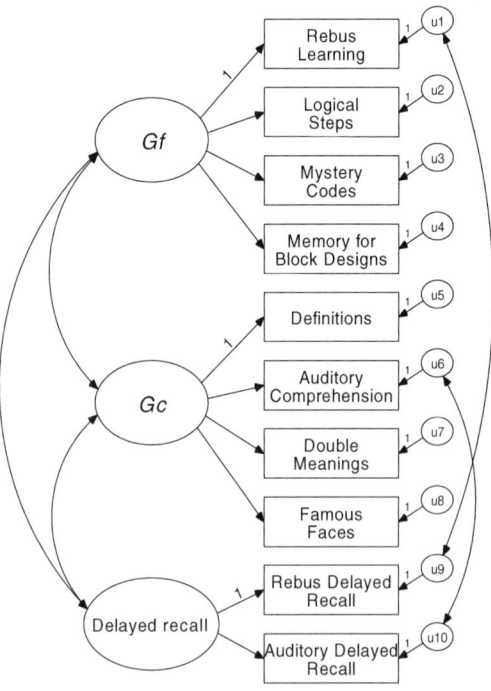

FIGURE 32.2. A CFA model of the structure of the KAIT.

ple, sets the scale of the Gf factor to be the same as the scale for Rebus Learning. Thus each factor includes one path of 1.0, and the paths from each of the unique variances to the measured variables are set to 1.0 (to set the scale to be the same as the corresponding measured variable). The use of 1.0 is arbitrary—any value could be used—and once all of the parameters of the model are estimated with these constraints (called the *unstandardized* or *metric solution*), all values are restandardized (the *standardized solution*).

Finally, the model in Figure 32.2 includes a less common characteristic: correlations among the unique variances, as represented by the curved lines connecting several of the unique variances (e.g., u1 and u9). The Rebus Delayed Recall test on the KAIT requires examinees to remember rebuses learned earlier in the test for the Rebus Learning subtest. Since Rebus Delayed Recall builds on Rebus Learning, it seems likely that the unique variances affecting Rebus Delayed Recall will be related to those affecting Rebus Learning. Similarly, the *error* variances affecting Rebus Delayed Recall may well be related to those affecting Rebus Learning. These possibilities (i.e., specific factors) may be built into the CFA model by specifying that the unique variances of these two subtests are allowed to correlate (there are other ways of doing so as well).

The KAIT standardization data were used to estimate the model. The KAIT manual includes correlation matrices of subtests for the KAIT at each age level, along with an average correlation matrix for the entire sample (Kaufman & Kaufman, 1993, p. 136). The matrix and standard deviations for the entire standardization sample were used as input for the Amos computer program (Arbuckle, 1995–2010). The average sample size (*N* = 143) for the different age groups was used as the sample size.

The results of the analysis are shown in Figure 32.3. First, notice the fit indices for the model in the lower left of the figure. The model is *overidentified*, meaning that we could have estimated many more parameters in the model than we actually did (e.g., the path from Gf to Definitions was constrained to 0, as were many other possible paths). In an overidentified model, the number of parameters estimated is less than the number of covariances among the measured variables. As a result, the model has *degrees of freedom*. Degrees of freedom are an index of the degree of overidentification of a model; they are not, as in most other statistical analyses, related to the sample size. It is

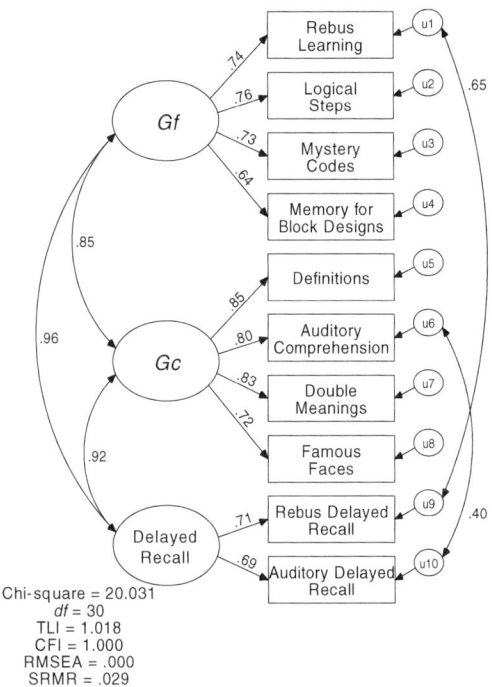

FIGURE 32.3. Results of a CFA of the structure of the KAIT. The results are for the standardized solution.

also possible to conduct the analysis in reverse: to estimate the correlation or covariance matrix from the solved model. But because the model is overidentified, the estimates of the covariances will not be identical to the covariance matrix used to estimate the model in the first place (see Keith, 2006, Ch. 12, or Kline, 2011, Ch. 6, for a discussion of overidentification). The fit indices shown in the figure are all measures of the degree to which the matrix *implied* by the model differs from the *actual* matrix used to estimate the model.

Five fit indices are shown in the figure, although there are dozens to choose from. Chi-squared (χ^2) is the most commonly reported fit statistic. It has the advantage of allowing a statistical test of the fit of the model; it can be used with the degrees of freedom to determine the probability that the model is, in some sense, "correct." Thus a large χ^2 in comparison to the *df* (and a small probability—e.g., $p < .05$) suggests that the actual and implied covariance matrices are statistically significantly different, that the model provides a poor fit to the data, or that the model could not have produced the data. The model therefore is not a good representation of the "true" factor structure. In contrast, a small χ^2 in comparison to the *df* is statistically insignificant ($p > .05$), and suggests that the model does provide a reasonable explanation of the data.

Although χ^2 fits well within the tradition of significance testing in psychology, it also has well-known problems (as does the tradition of either–or significance testing itself; cf. Cohen, 1994; Thompson, 2006): In particular, it is directly related to sample size, so that with large samples, virtually all χ^2's will be significant, even when the model is only trivially incorrect (see Tanaka, 1993, among others, for further discussion). With small samples, even inadequate models may have a good fit, as judged by χ^2. For this and other reasons, other fit statistics have been developed; the ones listed for this analysis were chosen because they highlight different dimensions of fit, and have shown promise in simulation studies (Fan, Thompson, & Wang, 1999; Hu & Bentler, 1998, 1999). Methodologists generally recommend using a combination of criteria.

One criticism of χ^2 is that it is a measure of the exact fit of the model to the data, whereas, at best, models are designed to *approximate* reality. The *root mean square error of approximation* (RMSEA) is therefore a measure of approximate fit. Smaller values suggest a better fit, with values of .06 or smaller suggesting a good fit (Hu & Bentler, 1999), and those of approximately .08 suggesting an adequate fit (Browne & Cudeck, 1993). The RMSEA is sometimes reported along with its 90% confidence interval. The *standardized root mean square residual* (SRMR) may be one of the more intuitively appealing measures of fit. Recall that fit indices are derived from the similarity or dissimilarity between the actual covariance matrix used to estimate the model and the matrix implied by the model. The *root mean square residual* (RMR) represents the average of these differences, and the SRMR is the *standardized* average of these differences. Because a standardized covariance is a correlation, the SRMR therefore represents the average difference in the actual *correlations* among the measured variables and those implied by the model. Values of .08 or less suggest little difference in the two matrices (Hu & Bentler, 1999).

The *Tucker–Lewis index* (TLI) and the *comparative fit index* (CFI) both compare the fit of the model with that of a "null" model, one in which the measured variables are assumed to be unrelated. The TLI appears to be relatively unaffected by sample size; the CFI is designed to estimate the fit in the population. For both, values of .95 or greater suggest a "good fit" of the model to the data (Hu

& Bentler, 1999), with values above .90 suggesting an adequate fit. We sometimes report one of these indices (because they often are fairly similar in magnitude), sometimes both.

Briefly, all of the fit indices suggest that the KAIT model provides an excellent fit to the standardization data. χ^2 is small and statistically nonsignificant ($p = .668$); the TLI and CFI are large; and both the RMSEA and the SRMR are quite small. Thus the "theory" underlying the KAIT appears to fit the KAIT standardization data; the test appears to measure what the authors designed it to measure; and the structure of the KAIT appears valid. The next step, then, is to interpret the substantive results.

The paths from latent to measured variables show the factor loadings. They are all large, and examination of their standard errors and *t* values (shown in the detailed printout, but not included here or in the figure) shows that they are all statistically significant. Likewise, the factor correlations are large and statistically significant, ranging from .96 for the correlation between the latent delayed-recall and Gf factors to .85 between Gf and Gc. Finally, the correlations among unique variances suggest that there is a substantial correlation between the variance of the Rebus Learning test that is not accounted for by the Gf factor and the variance of the Rebus Delayed Recall subtest that is not accounted for by the delayed-recall factor ($r = .65$). Similarly, the unique variances of Auditory Comprehension and Auditory Delayed Recall are substantially correlated.

These findings generally support the validity of the KAIT. One curious finding, however, is that the correlations between the delayed-recall and the Gf and Gc factors (.96 and .92, respectively) are higher than the correlations between the two presumably more intellectual factors, Gf and Gc (.85). Such a finding could be investigated by comparing this model with alternative models, as shown below.

An Alternative Method of Specifying Factor Models

Before we illustrate the comparison of competing alternative models, it is worth illustrating an alternative method of specifying factor models. The previous model set the scale of the latent factors by fixing a single factor loading from each factor to 1.0 (what Kline, 2011, refers to as *unit loading identification*). An alternative is to fix the *factor variances* to 1.0 (*unit variance identification*), and then estimate all factor loadings; a KAIT model using this method is shown in Figure 32.4. This procedure has advantages over the method of fixing a factor loading. When the factor variances are set to 1, the factor covariances in the unstandardized solution are in fact correlations. Because constraints to models are made in the unstandardized metric, this method makes it possible to set factor correlations to 1, or 0, or some other value to see what this constraint does to the fit of the model (this procedure is used in several subsequent examples). With hierarchical models (to be discussed below), however, only the highest factor level can use this alternative method.

The results of the analysis of the model shown in Figure 32.4 are identical to those shown in Figure 32.3 and are not repeated here. It is worth noting, however, that this method can occasionally produce slightly different estimates than unit loading identification does (Millsap, 2001).

COMPARING ALTERNATIVE MODELS

The previous section has presented the basics of CFA, but has also presented a fairly sterile approach: the simple rejection of or support for a single model. Such an approach is problematic. The simple fact that a model does or does not fit the data provides only partial support for the validity of a test or theory. A model may fit the data well, but there may be other, competing models that fit the data as well or better. Or a given model may provide an inadequate fit to the data, but may be the best model among the alternatives. Formal or informal theory may suggest several possible models to explain the test scores we observe; if all fit the data well, how is one to decide which is the *best* model? What is needed is the ability to compare competing models, or to compare a target model with one or several alternative models. "At best, a given model represents a tentative explanation of the data. The confidence with which one accepts such an explanation depends, in part, on whether other, rival explanations have been tested and found wanting" (Loehlin, 2004, p. 61).

Fortunately, fit statistics can be used to compare competing models as well. If two models are *nested*—that is, if one model can be derived from another by placing additional constraints on the model—then the χ^2 for the two models can be compared. The χ^2 for the less constrained model (the model with smaller df and smaller χ^2) can be subtracted from the χ^2 for the more constrained model. The χ^2 difference, or *likelihood ratio test* ($\Delta\chi^2$), can then be compared to the change in degrees of freedom (Δdf) to determine whether the relaxation in the model results in a statistically significant decrease in χ^2. If the $\Delta\chi^2$ is not statistically significant—if one model is not significantly better than another—then, as scientists, we generally prefer the more *parsimonious* (more constrained) model. If the $\Delta\chi^2$ is statistically significant, then the less parsimonious model is preferred. Parsimony is reflected in CFA models by df; the larger the df, the more constraints in the model, and therefore the more parsimonious the model.

The *Akaike information criterion* (AIC; Akaike, 1987) is another useful measure for comparing competing models, and does not require that the models be nested. The AIC is not interpreted in isolation; rather, the AICs for two or more competing models are compared, with the smaller AIC suggesting the better model. Other, related fit indices include the *Bayes information criterion* (BIC; Schwarz, 1978) and the sample-size-adjusted BIC (aBIC; Sclove, 1987). Likewise, the other fit statistics already discussed may be compared across models, although such comparison is generally a subjective one rather than a test of significance. Finally, a highly constrained "baseline" model may be used instead of a null model in the calculation

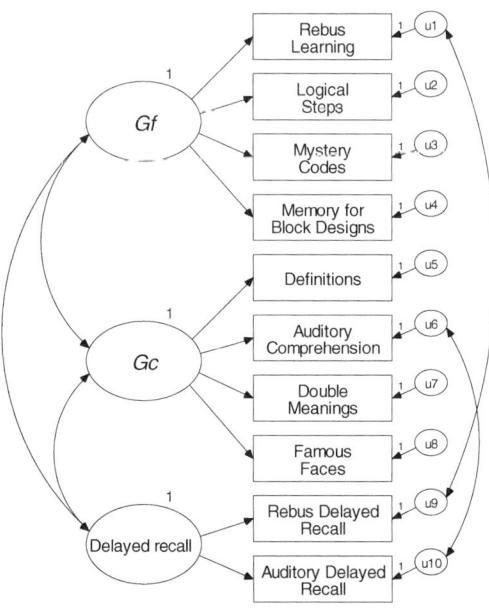

FIGURE 32.4. An alternative method of specifying factor models. Factor variances rather than factor loadings are set to 1 to set the scale of the factors.

of fit indexes such as TLI and CFI. For example, a one-factor *g* model may provide a useful baseline model in CFAs of intelligence tests (Humphreys, 1990). Of course, with these alternative baseline models, the resulting values will generally not approach the .95 cutoff recommended for these fit statistics when null models are used.

Comparing Alternative Models for the KAIT

Figure 32.3 has displayed the results of an initial CFA of the KAIT. The model fits the data well, and thus the model seems a good explanation of the KAIT standardization data. Nevertheless, questions concerning the structure, as displayed, are also reasonable. Since, for example, Rebus Delayed Recall asks examinees to recall material first learned in the Rebus Learning test, isn't RDR also a measure of Gf? Similarly, is Auditory Delayed Recall also a measure of Gc in addition to delayed recall? And why does the delayed-recall factor correlate so highly with Gf and Gc? If it is indeed a measure of delayed recall, shouldn't it correlate at a lower level with these highly intellectual factors than they do with each other?

Figure 32.5 shows a model that tests the first two of these questions: whether the Rebus and Auditory Delayed Recall subtests also measure Gf and Gc abilities. In addition to allowing RDR to load on the delayed-recall factor, it was also allowed to load on the Gf factor; Auditory Delayed Recall loaded on both the delayed-recall and Gc factors. Otherwise, the model shown in Figure 32.5 is the same as that shown in Figure 32.4, with one exception: For the model to be properly identified, some sort of additional constraint was required for the Rebus and Auditory Delayed Recall subtests. To allow estimation, the factor loadings for these two subtests on the delayed-recall factor were constrained to be equal.[2]

The results of this analysis are also shown in the figure. Like the earlier model, this variation provides an excellent fit to the averaged standardization data. But does the model provide any better fit than the structure as intended by the test authors? The χ^2 for the model is 15.779 for Figure 32.5 versus 20.031 for Figure 32.3. As shown in Table 32.1, the change in χ^2 is 4.232, which, given the change in *df* ($\Delta df = 1$), is statistically significant ($p < .05$) (the table does not include RMSEA values, which do not vary from model to model). Thus specifying that the Rebus and Auditory Delayed Recall subtests measure Gf and Gc in addition to delayed re-

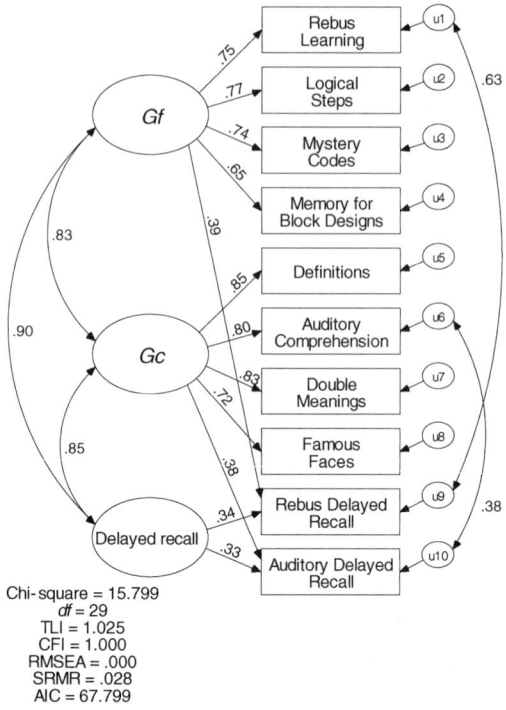

Chi-square = 15.799
df = 29
TLI = 1.025
CFI = 1.000
RMSEA = .000
SRMR = .028
AIC = 67.799

FIGURE 32.5. An alternative model of the structure of the KAIT. Rebus Delayed Recall and Auditory Delayed Recall are assumed to measure Gf and Gc, respectively, in addition to delayed-recall ability.

call leads to a statistically significant improvement in fit; Figure 32.5 may be a better explanation of the structure of the KAIT than Figures 32.3 and 32.4. The AIC shown in Figure 32.5 (67.799) is also smaller than the AIC for the models shown in Figures 32.3 and 32.4 (70.031), also suggesting that the model shown in Figure 32.5 is a better explanation of the structure of the KAIT than are the earlier models.

But what about substantive interpretation? With the changes in the model, it appears that Rebus Delayed Recall is a slightly better measure of Gf than it is of delayed recall, although it provides a strong measure of neither ability. Likewise, Auditory Delayed Recall appears as good, or slightly better, as a measure of Gc as it does of delayed recall, but appears a strong measure of neither ability. As in Figure 32.3, the delayed-recall factor correlates with the Gf and Gc factors as highly as or more highly than they correlate with each other, suggesting that a more intellectually laden name might be more appropriate (e.g., Glr, or *long-term storage and retrieval*).

TABLE 32.1. Comparison of Various CFA Models of the KAIT

Model (Figure no.)	χ^2 (df)	$\Delta\chi^2$ (Δdf)[a]	p	TLI	CFI	SRMR	AIC
Actual structure (Figure 32.3)	20.031 (30)			1.018	1.000	.029	70.031
Delayed recall and Gf-Gc (Figure 32.5)	15.799 (29)	4.232 (1)	.0397	1.025	1.000	.028	67.799
Gf-Gc (Figure 32.6)	19.158 (32)	3.359 (3)	.3395	1.022	1.000	.032	65.158
Subtests affect delayed recall (Figure 32.7)	15.833 (30)			1.026	1.000	.028	65.833

[a]All comparisons are with the preceding model.

Given the small paths from delayed recall to the Rebus and Auditory Delayed Recall subtests in Figure 32.5, it is reasonable to ask whether these two subtests should be considered measures of fluid and crystallized ability only, and not measures of delayed recall. The results of the test of such a model are shown in Figure 32.6. This model is more constrained than the model shown in Figure 32.5, so the question of interest now becomes whether these constraints on the model result in a statistically significantly *worse* fit to the data over the model in Figure 32.5.[3]

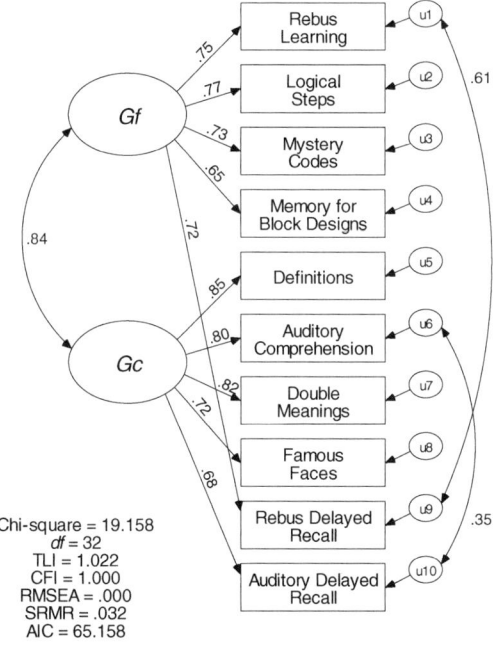

Chi-square = 19.158
df = 32
TLI = 1.022
CFI = 1.000
RMSEA = .000
SRMR = .032
AIC = 65.158

FIGURE 32.6. Another alternative model of the structure of the KAIT. The two Delayed Recall subtests (Rebus and Auditory) are assumed to measure Gf and Gc only, not a separate delayed-recall ability.

The fit statistics suggest that the model in Figure 32.6 provides as good a fit to the data as does that in Figure 32.5: The change in χ^2 is not statistically significant (see Table 32.1). The model in Figure 32.6 is more parsimonious, but with an equivalent fit to Figure 32.5; we prefer the more parsimonious model. Likewise, the AIC suggests a better fit for the model in Figure 32.6.

The substantive interpretation of the model in Figure 32.6 is straightforward. The Rebus and Auditory Delayed Recall subtests provide measures of Gf and Gc abilities, respectively, that are almost as strong as the tests intended to measure those abilities.

The model shown in Figure 32.6 can also be compared to the one in Figure 32.3. Although the two models appear to fit the data equally well, the model in Figure 32.6 is a more parsimonious explanation of the data. Taken together, these comparisons of models are not definitive, but do suggest that the Rebus and Auditory Delayed Recall subtests of the KAIT should be considered additional measures of the abilities measured by the two primary KAIT scales (fluid and crystallized) more than measures of learning or delayed recall.

One final model is discussed before another topic is raised because it illustrates an important point about CFA and SEM. In the models shown so far, the presumed overlap between the delayed-recall tests and the nondelayed versions of the tests (i.e., Rebus Learning and Auditory Comprehension) has been modeled by using correlated error terms. This is a common method of dealing with such overlap, but it is not the only way of doing so. It is not simply the case that performances on the Rebus and Auditory Delayed Recall tests *share* unique and error variance with the tests from which they were derived. Rather, performances on these two tests should depend, in part, on how well the material was learned when first presented. Thus, in addition to being affected by delayed recall, Gf, and Gc, these two tests should also be *affected* by their original versions. Figure 32.7 shows a model that embodies this reasoning, by having Rebus Learning affect Rebus Delayed Recall and having Auditory Comprehension affect Auditory Delayed Recall. As shown in this figure and in Table 32.1, this model fits the data quite well. The model is not nested with the other models, and thus the $\Delta\chi^2$ test is not appropriate (and is not shown). Judging by the AIC, this model fits better than most of the other models shown (and better than the model in Figure 32.3, with which it is most directly comparable). Note the strong effect of Rebus Learning on Rebus Delayed Recall, and the moderate effect of Auditory Comprehension on Auditory Delayed Recall. We believe that this example illustrates the power and the flexibility of CFA and, more generally, SEM, and their ability to model our conceptions of the way the world works. If we can think through the way we believe that intelligence works on various outcomes (including the subtests we use to measure it), then we can

probably model that notion and test it against our data.

The only model that fits better than that shown in Figure 32.7 is the model in Figure 32.6. Although not shown, a version of Figure 32.7 in which Rebus and Auditory Delayed Recall load on Gf and Gc (with no delayed-recall factor) has a fit and *df* identical to those in Figure 32.6. These, then, are *equivalent models*—models that cannot be evaluated on the basis of fit. It is always worth considering alternative models to one's preferred model; Keith (2006) and Kline (2011) have demonstrated rules for generating equivalent, alternative models (see also Lee & Hershberger, 1990). (Interestingly, although these two models are equivalent, the models shown in Figures 32.3 and 32.7 are not. The rules for equivalent models explain why.) Before turning to the next topic, we simply note that these models are not an exhaustive examination of the structure of the KAIT; there are other plausible models from other perspectives (see, e.g., Cole & Randall, 2003; Flanagan & McGrew, 1998).

HIERARCHICAL CFA

Many modern theories of intelligence recognize a factor that is more general and broader than the specific abilities tested in first-order CFA. This *general factor* is often considered to subsume, affect, or partially cause the more narrow abilities, and is often symbolized as *g*. For example, Carroll's (1993) three-stratum theory of intelligence includes *g* as the most general, highest-order factor. Although it is conceptually similar to Spearman's *g*, most modern theories assume that *g* is a higher-order factor (cf. Burt, 1949; Vernon, 1950). Most modern intelligence tests also tacitly recognize such a general, overall factor by summing subtests or subscales into an overall score. Although this general score may go by a variety of names—Full Scale IQ, General Cognitive Ability, or General Intellectual Ability—it generally represents an overall, general, summative ability.

If *g* is recognized in formal theory (as a latent variable that explains, in part, the positive correlations among all tests of mental ability) and through the informal theory of the scoring of intelligence tests, it would also be valuable to test such a construct through CFA. One common approach has been to specify a single-factor model, such as the one shown in Figure 32.8 (a *g*-model version of the Wechsler Intelligence Scale for Children—Fourth Edition [WISC-IV]). Such a model suggests that

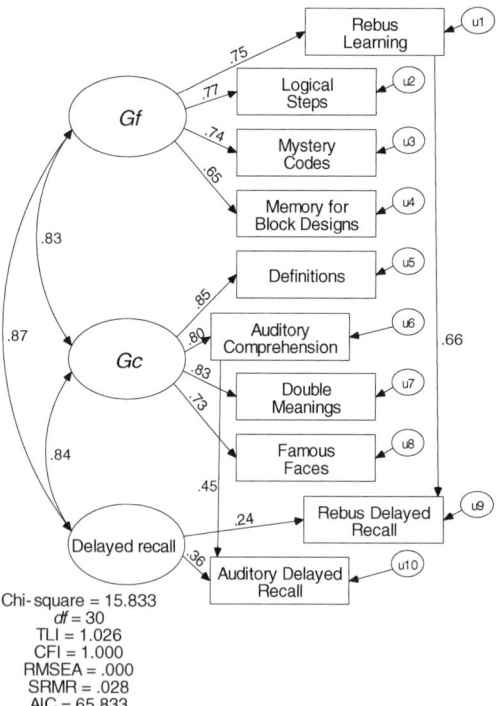

FIGURE 32.7. Yet another alternative model of the structure of the KAIT. The Rebus Learning and Auditory Comprehension tests are assumed to *affect* performance on the subsequent Rebus Delayed Recall and Auditory Delayed Recall tests.

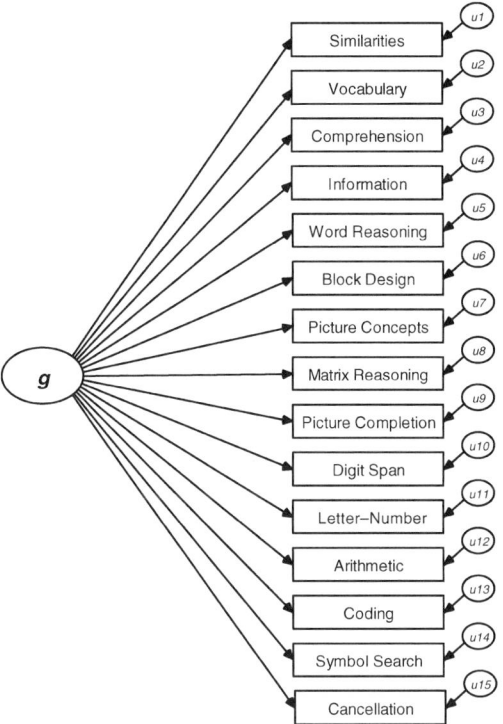

FIGURE 32.8. A general intelligence, or *g*, model of the structure of cognitive abilities as assessed by the WISC-IV. The model assumes that the WISC-IV tests are reflections of general intelligence only, rather than more specific, shared abilities, such as verbal or perceptual abilities.

scores on the individual subtests are a product of a general factor and of unique and error variances. Such an approach is fairly common (see Psychological Corporation, 2003), and it mirrors, to some degree, the common practice of isolating a *g* factor in EFA by examining the unrotated first factor in principal-components analysis. However, it is also an unsatisfying solution for several reasons. First, *g* is generally recognized as a *hierarchical* factor; a more realistic structure for the tests from Figure 32.8 is shown in Figure 32.9, in which the subtests are explained (in part) by first-order factors, and the first-order factors are in turn explained (in part) by a second-order *g* factor. Second, if Figure 32.9 represents the *true* structure of the abilities measured by the 15 WISC-IV tests, then Figure 32.8 represents an inadequate test of the second-order *g* factor. The presence of first-order factors means that the Verbal Comprehension tests measure something in common other than general intelligence; the Perceptual Reasoning tests measure something in common other than *g*; and so on. These first-order factors may be identified by characteristics shared among groups of subtests, whereas *g* cannot. To reiterate, Figure 32.8 represents an inadequate test of a higher-order *g* factor.

Figure 32.10 shows a CFA model to test the higher-order structure of the Differential Ability Scales—Second Edition (Elliott, 2007). In scoring the School-Age version of the DAS-II, the "core" subtests are added together to form Verbal, Nonverbal Reasoning, and Spatial scores, and these three scores are added together to form a General Cognitive Ability score. Thus the core subtests are designed to measure both a *general* ability and more specific abilities (Gc, Gf, Gv). The informal theory underlying the test is clearly hierarchical in nature. There are three memory subtests included as well, two of which are added together to form a Working Memory composite. Here we have used all three as measures of Gsm, which is also affected by a second-order *g* factor. To simplify presentation, these analyses do not include the subtests measuring long-term retrieval or processing speed.

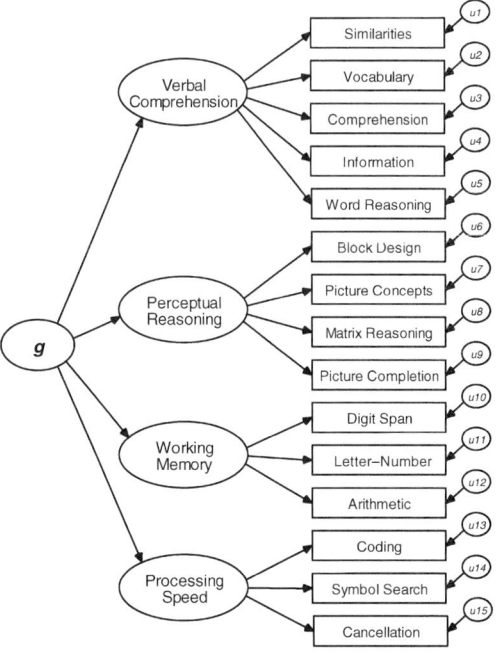

FIGURE 32.9. A higher-order model of the structure of the WISC-IV. The model assumes that each test is a reflection of narrow, shared abilities (e.g., Verbal Comprehension), and that these narrow abilities are in turn partially explained by *g*.

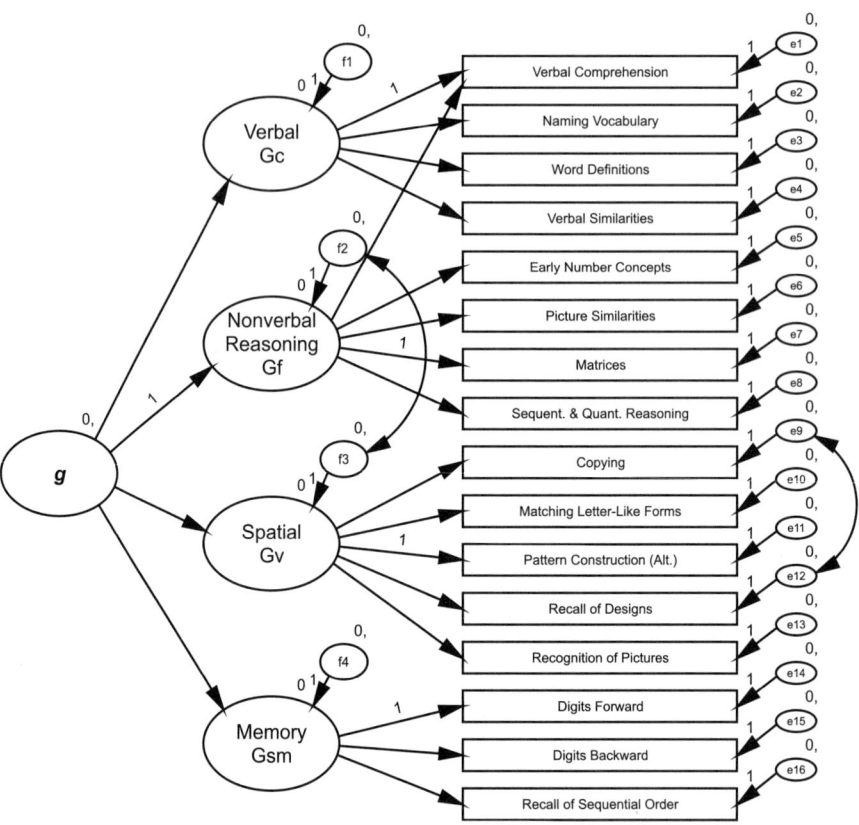

FIGURE 32.10. A hierarchical, higher-order model of the structure of the DAS-II.

One interesting feature of the DAS-II is that although the composition and structure of the test change in going from the Early Years to the School-Age version, all tests were given to children ages 5–8 in the standardization sample; these age levels, with multiple indicators of each construct, are the ones used here. The structure shown (including the correlated errors and cross-loading) is based on findings presented in Keith, Low, Reynolds, Patel, and Ridley (2010); see this article for more complete analyses of the structure of the DAS-II, including cross-age tests of measurement invariance.

Figure 32.10 is quite similar to the general hierarchical model in Figure 32.9, except for the presence of small ovals (f1 through f4) pointing to the first-order factors. These represent the *unique* variances of each of the first-order factors. Just as the first-order factors are not the only causes of the scores on the subtests, g is not the only cause of a child's Verbal or Spatial ability; there is also something unique about Verbal ability as opposed

to Spatial ability. This *unique factor* variance, with the test specific and general factor variance removed, is recognized in the model through the presence of the latent variables f1 through f4.[4] As in earlier models, each latent variable (including g and the unique factor variances) have their scales set by fixing one loading to 1.0. As noted above, the model has been estimated by using the standardization data for ages 5–8.

The results of the higher-order CFA of the DAS-II are shown in Figure 32.11. The fit statistics suggest that the model provides an excellent fit to the data, and thus support the scoring structure of the DAS-II. The first-order factor loadings suggest that the core subtests are generally good measures of their corresponding factors, although Verbal Comprehension appears to require both Verbal Ability (or Gc) and Nonverbal Reasoning (or Gf) for successful completion.

The second-order factor loadings are perhaps even more interesting. In scoring the DAS-II, the Verbal, Nonverbal Reasoning, and Spatial ability

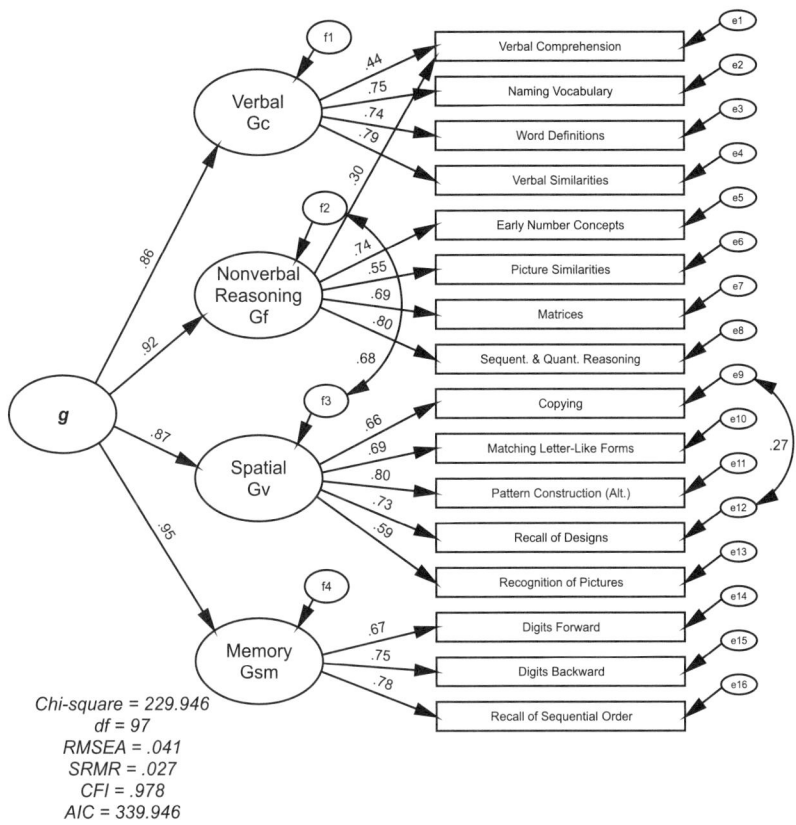

FIGURE 32.11. Standardized solution for a higher-order model of the structure of the DAS-II.

scores are combined to create an overall score. The figure shows that the three corresponding latent factors are indeed strongly affected by *g*, thus supporting the hierarchical structure of the scale. Also of interest, the Nonverbal Reasoning factor has a very high loading, .92, on the second-order *g* factor. Although the factors are statistically distinguishable (based on $\Delta\chi^2$), the loading is quite high. This finding lends support to the claim that the Nonverbal Reasoning scale of the DAS-II should be considered a measure of Gf (Elliott, 2007; Keith et al., 2010), given evidence that Gf is often quite similar to, and sometimes indistinguishable from, *g* (e.g., Carroll, 1993, Ch. 15; Gustafsson, 1984). The high loading by Gsm is less common, and may suggest that this factor is more cognitively complex (e.g., working memory) than the label Gsm would suggest.

Researchers and clinicians are often interested in the loading of the subtests on *g*, or the relative strength or weakness of tests as measures of *g*. It is not necessary to resort to *g*-only models (Figure 32.8) or nested-factors models (discussed below) to get such estimates, however. In higher-order models, the loadings of the subtests on higher-order factors are calculated as the indirect (and total) effects of the hierarchical factors on the subtests, through the intermediate factors. So, for example, in Figure 32.11, the loading of Sequential and Quantitative Reasoning on *g* is .736 (.92 × .80). SEM (and CFA) programs will easily calculate these indirect effects. The *g* loadings of the DAS-II are shown in Table 32.2 (arranged from largest to smallest). Note that these *g* loadings are model-specific; the estimates shown in Table 32.2 apply to the model shown in Figure 32.11. If the model is correct, then the *g* loadings will be accurate.

Nested-Factors Models

An alternative method of testing hierarchical models is through what is called a *nested-factors model*, not to be confused with nested, competing models. In a nested-factors model, all subtests are

TABLE 32.2. Loadings of DAS Subtests on a Higher-Order g Factor

Subtest	g
Recall of Sequential order	.740
Sequent. and Quant. Reasoning	.736
Digits Backward	.717
Pattern Construction (Alt.)	.695
Verbal Similarities	.682
Early Number Concepts	.680
Verbal Comprehension	.651
Naming Vocabulary	.649
Matrices	.641
Word Definitions	.636
Recall of Designs	.635
Digits Forward	.634
Matching Letter-Like Forms	.597
Copying	.576
Recognition of Pictures	.512
Picture Similarities	.507

loaded directly both on a G factor and on narrow factors, with the factors generally orthogonal or uncorrelated (cf. Carroll, 1995; Gignac, 2008; Gustafsson & Balke, 1993).

A nested-factors version of the DAS-II model is shown in Figure 32.12. (The ovals representing the unique variances of the subtests are not shown in the figure to help simplify it, but were included in the analysis.) This initial version of the model did not estimate well and required modification. (The residual variance of the Sequential and Quantitative Reasoning test was negative, an impossibility, and was set to 0. None of the Gf factor loadings were statistically significant, and the correlated error was not significant; these nonsignificant parameters were deleted. These changes allowed the Sequential and Quantitative Reasoning residual variance to be unconstrained again.) A working, solved version of the nested-factors model is shown in Figure 32.13. This model also fit the data well, although not quite as well as the higher-order model (the models are not nested, so this comparison is based on the AIC).

We first focus on the findings of this model and then discuss how this model relates to the previous higher-order model. First, the loadings of the subtests on the (first-order) G factor are similar, but not identical, to those shown as indirect effects in Table 32.2 (we refer to such first-order general factors as G, rather than g, to make the distinction

between first- and second-order general factors explicit). In contrast, the loadings of the subtests on the Gc, Gv, and Gsm factors are much smaller than in the previous model. The practical and conceptual differences in the two models lead to these differences.

How do the models differ, and in what ways are they similar? Some researchers treat nested-factors models as equivalent to higher-order models, but clearly they are not (indeed, we question whether the nested-factors model should be considered hierarchical, but it generally is). Although both models suggest that the subtests are affected both by general intelligence and one or more less broad abilities, the nature of that influence differs. The higher-order model assumes that g, general intelligence, influences individual tests through the broad abilities, or less general abilities, or multiple intelligences. The nested-factors model seemingly makes no assumptions about the relation between g and the broad (first-order) factors, instead only specifying that the subtests measure both g and broad abilities. Strictly speaking, however, the model asserts that G is *unrelated* to the broad abilities. The upshot of this difference is that the higher-order model places constraints on the possible loadings of the subtests on the second-order g factor, as the effect of g on the first-order factors are the same for each subtests that loads on a particular broad factor (in the higher-order model). Said differently, the nested-factors model assumes only direct effects for G on the measured variables, whereas the higher-order model asserts indirect effects. For those approaching CFA from a regression orientation, the nested-factors model is analogous to a simultaneous regression, whereas the higher-order model is more like a path model.

Because of these constraints, the higher-order model is a more constrained model than is the nested-factors model. In fact, it is possible to go from one model to another in several ways (Yung, Thissen, & McLeod, 1999). Most simply, both models may be considered subsets of a model in which g influences both first-order factors and subtests (a model that would be underidentified without additional constraints), but the higher-order model influences subtests indirectly, and the nested-factors model affects them directly.

One seeming advantage of the nested-factors approach is that by including all factors at the same level the paths may be considered *partialed* effects. That is, the loadings of the Gc, Gf, and Gsm factors are the effects of these factors on the subtests, *with G statistically removed, or partialed* out. As a result (and if the factors are uncorrelat-

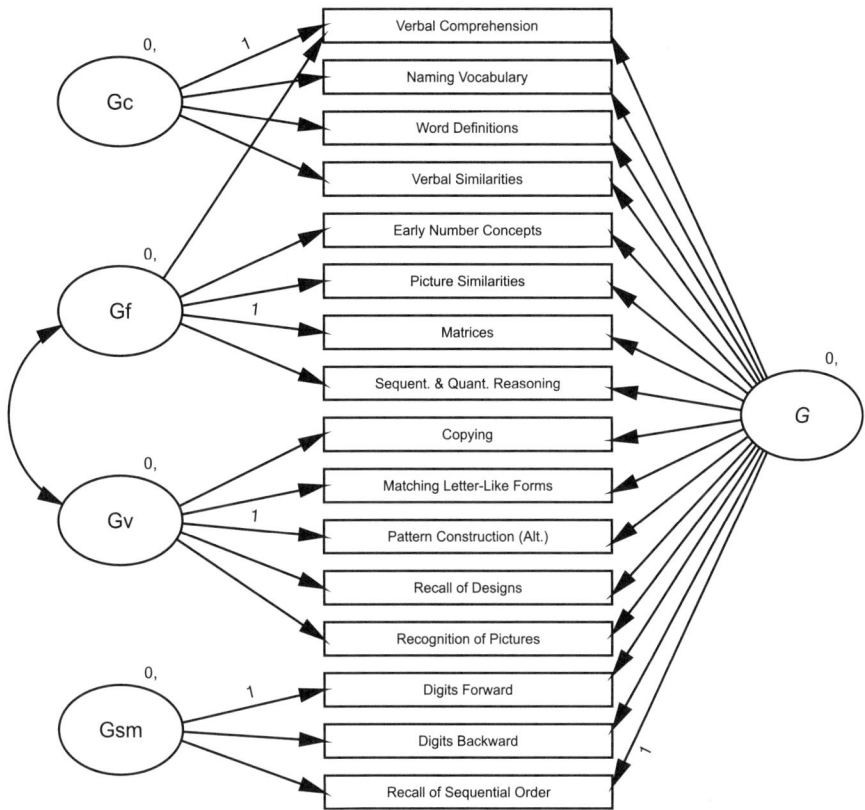

FIGURE 32.12. A nested-factors model of the structure of the DAS-II. Although such a model may be considered an alternative to the higher-order model, in that each test is assumed to be a product of both narrow, shared abilities and G, the model assumes that the narrow abilities are unrelated to G beyond this shared influence.

ed), the findings from such models are analogous to a Schmid–Leiman transformation (Schmid & Leiman, 1957), in which first-order and higher-order loadings are orthogonalized to aid in interpretation. This would seem to be an important practical advantage for the nested-factors approach. But it is also very simple to obtain such orthogonalized results in a higher-order model (see Reynolds & Keith, in press, for an illustration; that chapter also compares these models in more detail). A nested-factors approach requires a partialed approach; in fact, that is the only interpretation allowed. A higher-order approach allows for interpretation of both simple effects of first-order factors and (with a little more work) partialed effects, with g removed.

Another potential advantage of the nested-factors approach is that it appears agnostic as to the relation between the g factor and the other factors. Said differently, this approach may be somewhat more exploratory than a higher-order approach. But this advantage does not come without a cost. All CFA models (and, indeed, all EFA models) make assumptions about the nature of intelligence. The models shown in Figures 32.10 and 32.12 make very different assumptions about the nature of intelligence. The higher-order model says that g is a superordinate ability. Moreover, in a higher-order model g is further removed from the subtests, indicating a higher level of abstraction. There are no direct effects from g to the subtests, which seems consistent with the inability to define g based on surface characteristics of specific tests (see Jensen, 1998, Ch. 4); g is more abstract than the broad abilities.[5]

The nested-factors approach, in contrast, says that G is no more important than other abilities. That is, it does not affect those abilities; rather, it affects more test scores, and it is a breadth factor rather than a superordinate factor (Gignac,

2008). The nested-factors approach is a top-down approach, with G taken into account first, whereas the higher-order approach is more of a bottom-up approach. In sum, models imply theories, and we should know what theory our models are implying. Given the intertwined nature of measurement and theory, it is important to choose a model on theoretical grounds as well as well as practical ones.

A practical disadvantage of the nested-factors approach is that the model is often difficult to estimate. Factors must include more than two indicators, or empirical underidentification will result. To avoid this, additional indicators, or meaningful factor intercorrelations (cf. Keith, Reynolds, Patel, & Ridley, 2008), are required; or we must make additional constraints, which may result in a worse

fit and which require justification. Even with three or more tests per factor, nested-factors model can be touchy. In our own experience, it often helps to specify start values for many parameters.

Model choice should reflect a guiding theory. Theoretically, the model analyzed should, at a minimum, reflect the theory underlying the test, or an alternative theoretical specification. The higher-order model would seem to have a clear advantage in this regard, given that most theories including a general factor suggest that this is a higher-order, hierarchical factor (Jensen, 1998). Tests are not always scored this way (e.g., subtests, rather than scales, are often added together to form IQ composites), but most test manuals reference a higher-order type structure if theoretical justifica-

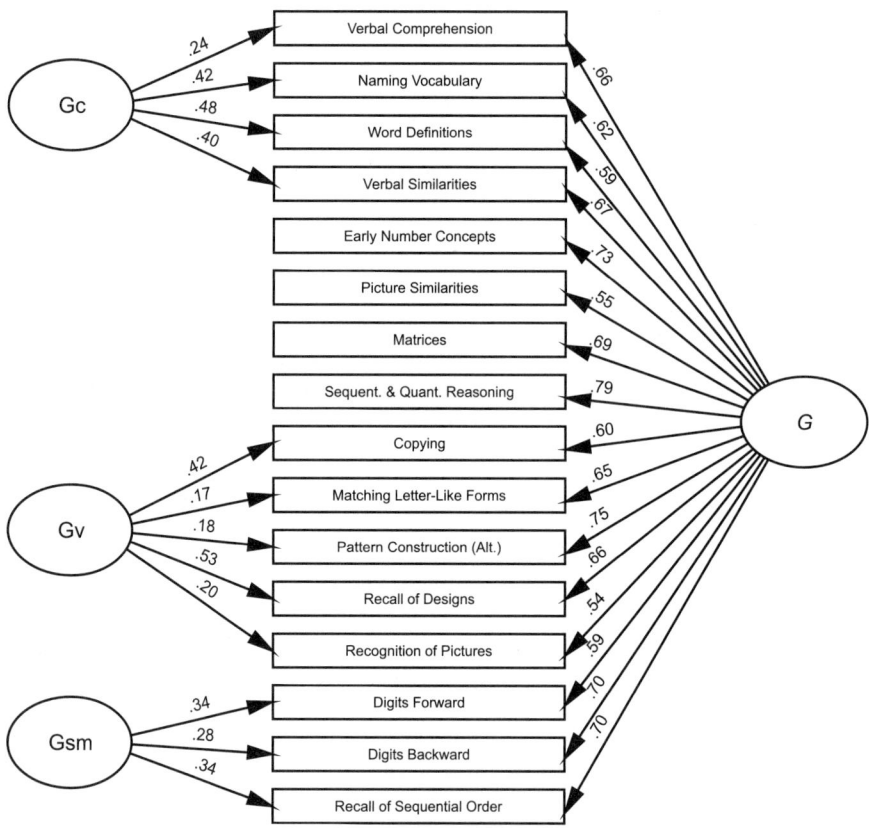

Chi-square = 237.183
df = 92
RMSEA = .044
SRMR = .029
CFI = .977
AIC = 057.183

FIGURE 32.13. DAS-II nested-factors model standardized solution.

tion for the test structure is presented. In contrast, the nested-factors model is not consistent with most modern theoretical orientations with which we are familiar. Indeed, even the Schmid–Leiman transformation was originally developed to transform, for interpretive purposes, results of *higher-order* EFAs. For these reasons, we would argue that a higher-order hierarchical model should generally be preferred. See Gustafsson and Aberg-Bengtsson (2010) and Reynolds and Keith (in press) for further discussion.

Before we change topics again, it is worth revisiting nomenclature. We have noted that calling the model in Figures 32.12 and 32.13 a *nested-factors model* could lead to confusion because we also speak of models' being *nested* with each other. Prepare to be more confused. Both types of models are generally considered types of hierarchical models (thus the title of this section), although, strictly speaking, the nested-factors model is not hierarchical in nature. But the nested-factors model is often referred to as simply the *hierarchical model* (Reynolds & Keith, in press), as opposed to a higher-order model. Gignac (2008) refers to it as the *direct hierarchical model*, which is perhaps a more useful name. It is also sometimes referred to as the *bifactor model*, presumably because all (or most) tests are assumed to measure two common factors. It is sometimes difficult to know what is meant, given such confusing nomenclature.

TESTING HYPOTHESES ABOUT THE SIMILARITY OF FACTORS

CFA is also a useful method for testing hypotheses about how factors or tests should be interpreted. Such research often involves testing the similarity of factors within a test or between two tests. CFA can be used to test whether two tests designed to measure the same factors (e.g., the Gf factors from the Woodcock–Johnson III [WJ III] and the KAIT) do, in fact, measure statistically indistinguishable factors. By the same token, the method can be used to test whether two tests designed to measure *different* abilities do, in fact, measure distinguishable factors.

What Types of Abilities Does the Cognitive Assessment System Measure?

The Cognitive Assessment System (CAS; Naglieri & Das, 1997) is a nonstandard measure of cognitive abilities based on the *planning, attention, si-*

multaneous, and successive (PASS) theory of intelligence. The PASS model is a neuropsychological and information-processing theory of cognition, and the CAS is the only test based entirely on this theory (see Naglieri, Das, & Goldstein, Chapter 7, this volume, and Das, Naglieri, & Kirby, 1994, for more information).

Cattell–Horn–Carroll (CHC) theory is a combination of Carroll's three-stratum theory and Cattell and Horn's Gf-Gc theory, theories that already overlapped considerably. (For more information about CHC theory, see Schneider & McGrew, Chapter 4, this volume.) Although the CAS was designed to measure the PASS abilities, several authors have questioned whether the CAS in fact measures those abilities or whether it measures several abilities from CHC theory (Carroll, 1995; Kranzler & Keith, 1999). In particular, Kranzler and Keith (1999; see also Keith & Kranzler, 1999; Kranzler, Keith, & Flanagan, 2000) have argued that the Planning and Attention tests of the CAS measure components of processing speed (Gs); that the Simultaneous tests measure a mixture of visual processing and fluid reasoning (Gv and Gf); and that the Successive tests measure components of short-term memory (Gsm).

CFA across tests can be used to help settle this debate. The WJ III Tests of Cognitive Abilities (WJ III COG) are closely tied to and appear to provide strong measures of the CHC abilities (McGrew & Woodcock, 2001; Taub & McGrew, 2004). If so, then joint CFA of the WJ III COG and the CAS can be used to test the similarity of the CAS factors and those from the WJ III COG.

Keith, Kranzler, and Flanagan (2001) reported a series of joint CFAs of these two instruments; a few of these are described briefly here to illustrate the CFA methodology. Figure 32.14 shows one of the initial models tested in this research. The model shows a CFA of the WJ III tests on the left, and a CFA of the CAS tests on the right. The CAS factors have been labeled with both the CHC theory-derived names and those from the PASS/CAS orientation.

If the CAS tests in fact measure the PASS abilities, the correlations of the CAS factors with the WJ III factors Gs, Gv, Gf, and Gsm should be of moderate magnitude, presumably close to the average correlation among the WJ III factors (average $r = .490$). In contrast, if the CAS tests measure CHC abilities, the corresponding correlations should be considerably higher. Figure 32.15 shows the results of a joint CFA in which the correlations among factors have been unconstrained and freely estimated. To simplify the display, only the

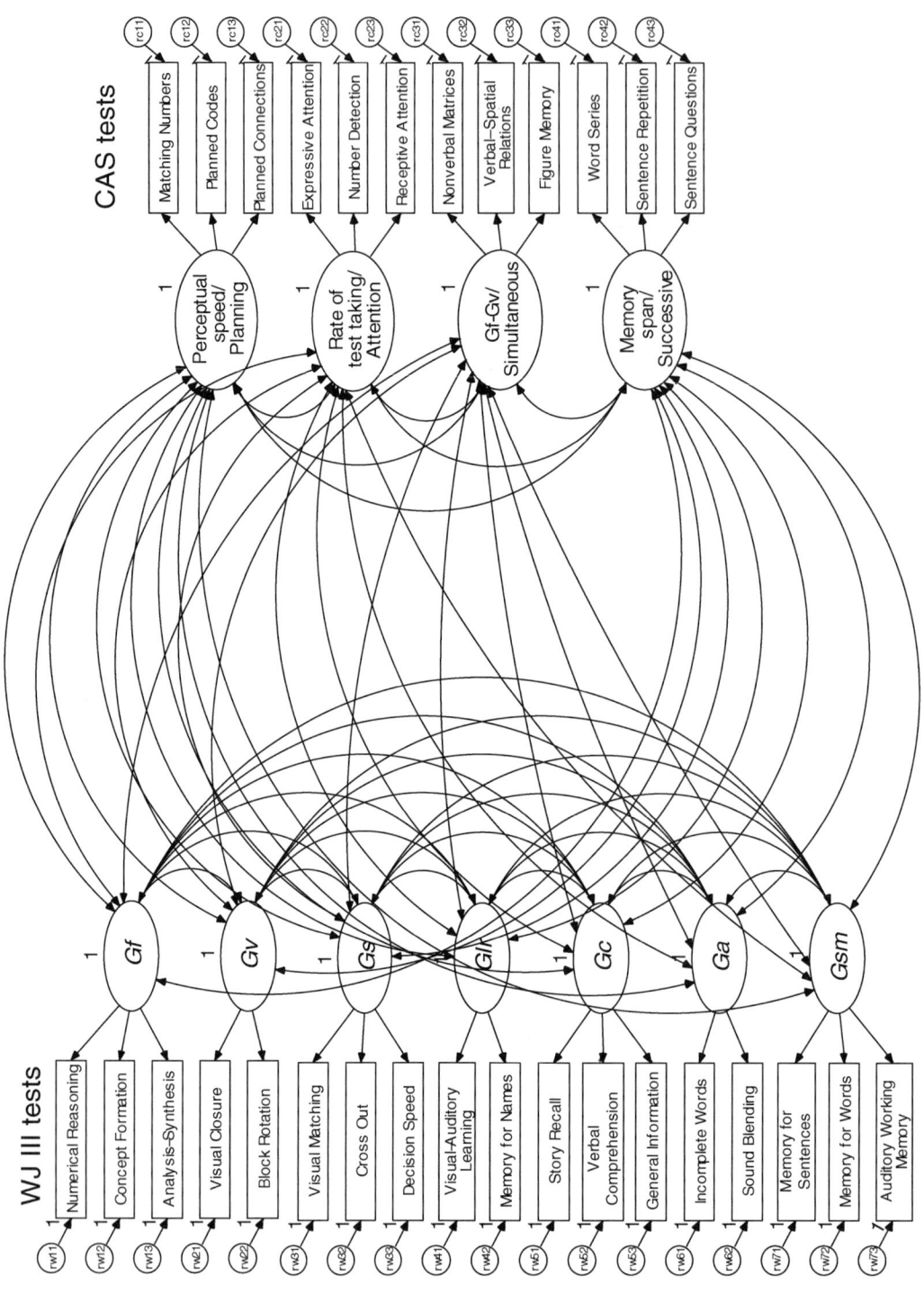

FIGURE 32.14. A cross-battery CFA model designed to test the similarity or dissimilarity of the constructs measured by the CAS and the WJ III COG. From Keith, Kranzler, and Flanagan (2001). Copyright 2001 by the National Association of School Psychologists. Adapted by permission.

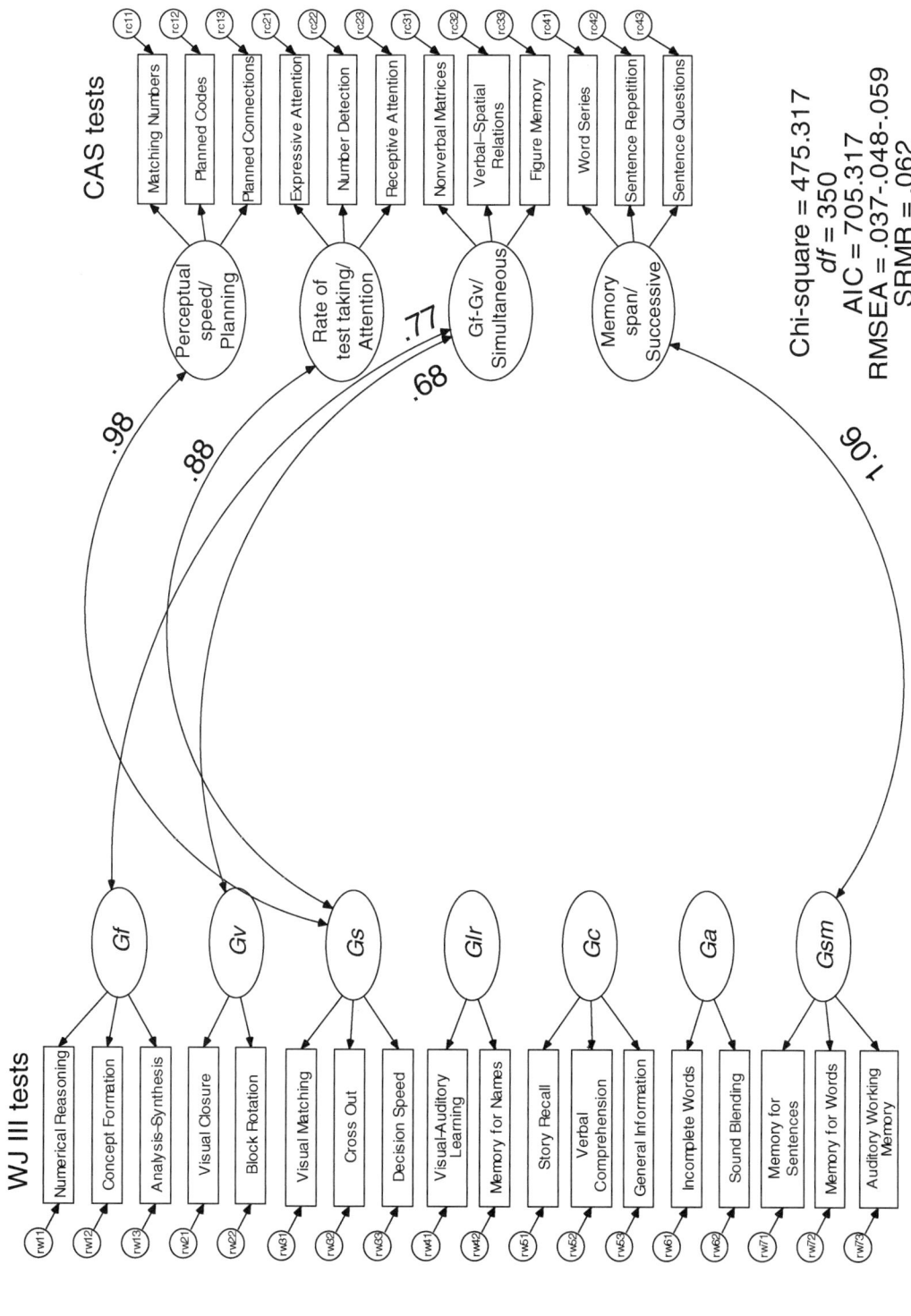

FIGURE 32.15. Correlations between selected factors from the WJ III COG and the CAS. The factor correlations suggest that the CAS tests overlap considerably with the WJ III COG CHC abilities.

relevant correlations are shown, but all have been estimated (for the complete factor correlation matrix, see Keith et al., 2001).

As shown in Figure 32.15, all of the relevant correlations are higher than the average factor correlation. The Simultaneous–Gf and Simultaneous–Gv correlations are .77 and .68, respectively; the Planning–Gs and Attention–Gs correlations are .98 and .88, respectively; and the correlation between Successive and Gsm is greater than 1 (1.06; this value is not statistically significantly different from 1.0, however). The overall fit of the model is adequate to good. These initial, unconstrained analyses support a CHC interpretation of the CAS abilities rather than a PASS interpretation.

It is possible to conduct a stronger test of the convergence or divergence of factors by constraining correlations among factors and comparing the fit of those models. Note that the initial model has been specified by setting factor variances to 1.0 (rather than factor loadings), so that constraints to factor covariances are in fact made to factor correlations (because correlations are standardized covariances). Figure 32.16 shows the second step in these analyses, in which the correlations between the WJ Gs factor and the CAS Planning and Attention factors have been constrained to .49, the average correlation among WJ factors. (All other factor correlations have been allowed to vary, but are not shown so as to simplify the figure.) A comparison of the fit of this model with the initial model tests whether the correlations between Gs and Planning and Attention are no higher than would be expected for mental factors measuring distinct abilities. As shown in Table 32.3, these constraints to the model result in a statistically significant increase in $\Delta\chi^2$, however, suggesting the rejection of this hypothesis. In step 3, these same factor correlations have been constrained to a value of 1.0, to test whether the Planning and Attention factors are instead statistically indistinguishable from processing speed (Gs). As shown in the table, these constraints result in a statistically insignificant increase in $\Delta\chi^2$, thus supporting the contention that the Planning and Attention tests of the CAS measure processing speed.

Keith and colleagues (2001) conducted numerous additional analyses to test whether the CAS measures PASS or CHC abilities. In addition to testing the similarity of factors, the authors tested a series of joint hierarchical, integrated, and PASS-derived models; for additional information, see the original article. The article is a good illustration of the use of CFA to test competing hypotheses

about the nature of constructs measured by intelligence tests.

TESTING THE SIMILARITY OF FACTOR STRUCTURE ACROSS GROUPS: INVARIANCE

An important subset of questions about the constructs measured by intelligence tests involves questions about whether the test measures the same constructs across groups. Does a multiage battery, for example, measure the same set of constructs for 8-year-olds as it does for 18-year-olds? Does a new intelligence test measure Gf and Gc abilities for white students, but merely test-taking skills for minority students? Does a verbal comprehension composite score have the same meaning for boys as it does for girls? These questions ask, in essence, whether the factor structure and corresponding factor loadings of the tests vary across groups. These are questions of factorial invariance.

The method of *multigroup* CFA (MG-CFA) provides an excellent method for answering such questions. In MG-CFA, any of the parameters that are estimated or fixed in a model can be specified as being invariant across two or more groups. For example, suppose we wish to determine whether a set of tests measures the same constructs for boys and girls. We could specify that the factor loadings of that series of tests are the same for boys and girls. We could also specify that the factor covariances, the factor variances, and the unique and error variances are identical across groups.

In one of the earliest examples of using CFA to test for invariance (Jöreskog, 1971), MG-CFA was used to test for invariance of covariance structures. Meredith (1993) extended and formalized the testing of factorial invariance under the more general scope of measurement invariance. Evidence of measurement invariance indicates that a person's observed test score (e.g., WISC Block Design test score) depends on the person's latent Gv ability, and not other variables such as group membership (e.g., sex, ethnicity, or socioeconomic status). All of the models tested thus far in this chapter have focused on structuring covariances (solving for CFA models by using variances and covariances), and have not involved structuring the means. Meredith demonstrated the use of MG-CFA with mean structures, often referred to as *multigroup mean and covariance structure analysis* (MG-MACS), to test various aspects of measurement invariance. This

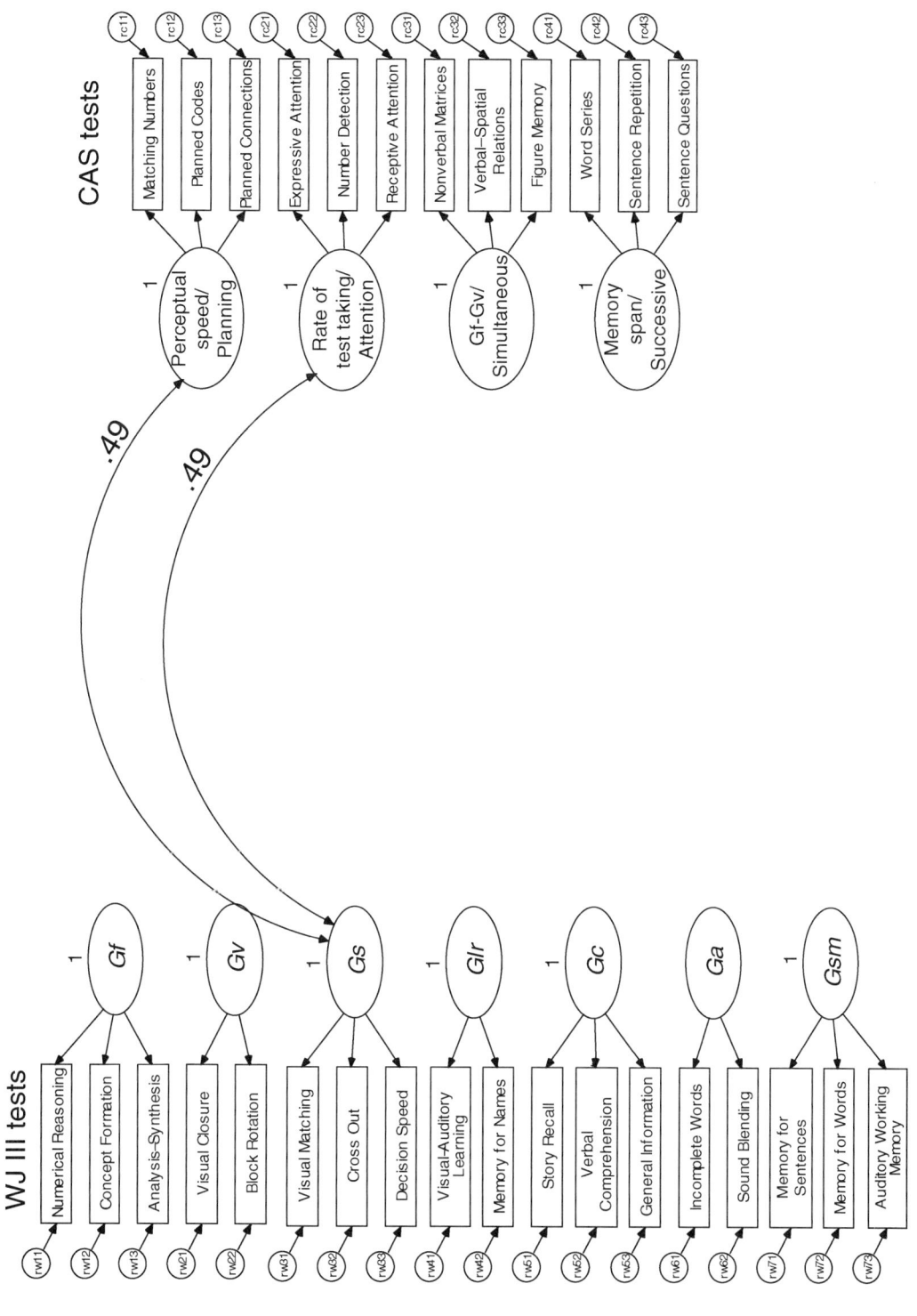

FIGURE 32.16. Testing hypotheses using the CAS/WJ III COG model. The correlations between WJ III Processing Speed and the CAS Planning and Attention factors are set to the average value for factor correlations. The fit is degraded as a result of these model constraints.

777

TABLE 32.3. Comparison of the Competing Hypotheses about the Nature of the CAS Planning and Attention Tests

Model	$\Delta\chi^2$ (df)	p	AIC
Unconstrained conjoint model	475.317 (350)[a]		705.317
Factors are distinct; correlation of Planning, Attention with Gs = .49	43.259 (2)	<.001	744.576
Factors are indistinguishable; correlation of Planning, Attention with Gs = 1.00	4.902 (2)	.086	706.219

[a]χ^2 value for the unconstrained model is the χ^2 rather than the $\Delta\chi^2$.
Note. Each model is compared to the unconstrained model. The $\Delta\chi^2$ value reported for the unconstrained model is the χ^2. From Keith, Kranzler, and Flanagan (2001). Copyright 2001 by the National Association of School Psychologists. Adapted by permission.

model-based framework compares various models specifying different degrees of invariance in a structured approach using MG-CFA. The following is an example of this approach.

This example uses test score data from 128 girls and 122 boys who were a part of the Kaufman Assessment Battery for Children—Second Edition (KABC-II; Kaufman & Kaufman, 2004) norming sample to test for measurement invariance across the sexes. The example tests whether the KABC-II subtests measure the CHC abilities in the same way for 4-year-old boys as they do

for 4-year-old girls. For children who are 4 years of age, the KABC-II provides four index scores designed to reflect four CHC abilities: Gsm, Glr, Gv, and Gc. These composite scores are generated from scores obtained from two or three subtests. The factor model is shown in Figure 32.17. This factor model is consistent with the CHC scoring structure of the KABC-II. Note that the KABC-II also includes a global composite score, but in this example we focus on testing for measurement bias in the broad-ability composites only and not the global composite (see Reynolds, Keith, Ridley,

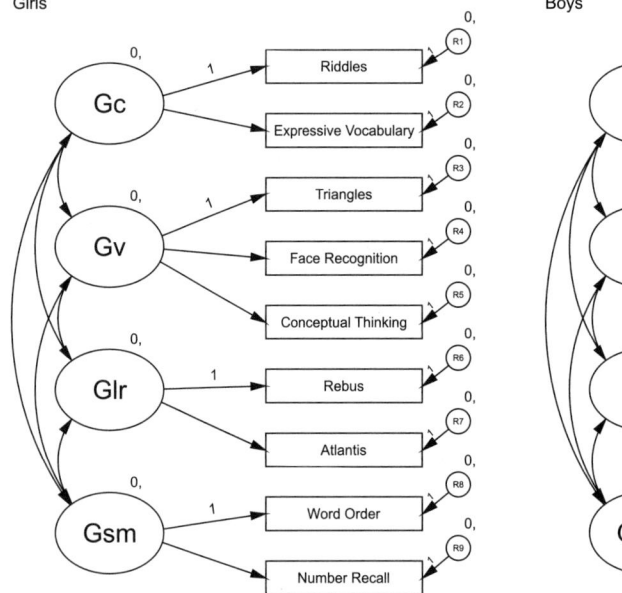
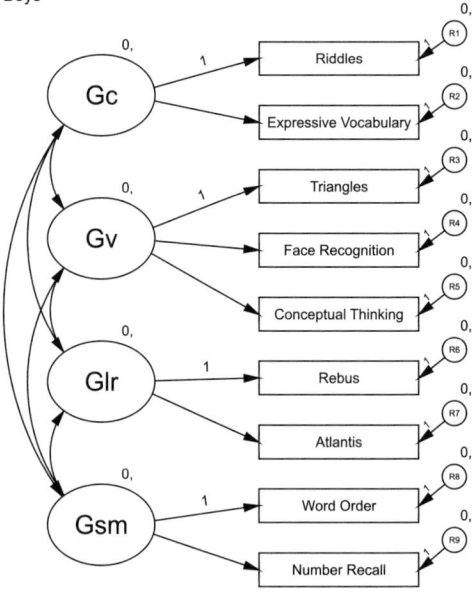

FIGURE 32.17 MG-CFA set-up for testing configural invariance across sexes for the KABC-II for 4-year-olds. The same configuration of factors is specified for girls (left) and boys (right).

& Patel, 2008, for higher-order models and the KABC-II).

The model shown is slightly different from previous models. Note the values of 0 next to all of the latent variables ("0," in the figure). These are the means of the latent variables. This model also estimates the intercepts for the subtests, although these are not shown in the figure. What are the *intercepts*? The intercepts are the same things as in a regression model: The intercept for the Riddles subtest, for example, is the expected Riddles score for someone with a value of 0 on the latent Gc factor. Alternatively, the intercepts may be considered as the average score on Riddles for the group, after level of Gc is controlled for. In previous models we have not been concerned with means or intercepts (they have, in essence, been set to 0 for latent variables and freely estimated for intercepts of measured variables). As will be seen, it is necessary to consider, and explicitly model, means and intercepts in testing for measurement invariance. All SEM programs can explicitly model means and intercepts (i.e., mean structures).

Steps in Invariance Testing

Testing for measurement invariance via MG-CFA typically involves the application of increasingly restrictive sets of equality constraints. Different researchers use different terms to describe the different facets of invariance; we generally use the hierarchy discussed by Meredith (1993). In the first step, the same factor structure is imposed on each group. This initial step is often referred to as *configural invariance* (cf. Thurstone's [1947] *configurational invariance*). This type of invariance requires the same CFA model to be configured across groups. This step may be performed with multigroup analysis; alternatively, models can be estimated separately for each group. After that step, steps for testing for *metric invariance* (also known as *weak factorial* or *factor-loading invariance*), *strong factorial* (*scalar* or *intercept*) *invariance*, and *strict factorial* (*residual*) *invariance* are followed. Greater detail about the meaning of invariance at each step is provided as the example is worked through. This particular order is not strictly required. For example, some might first test for invariance of the covariance structure (factor loadings and residuals) and then introduce the means (intercepts). There are some important considerations, however. For example, factor loadings should be invariant if the intercepts associated with those loadings are to be constrained.

Configural Invariance

Configural invariance simply entails establishing the same configuration of factors across the groups. In this example, the model shown in Figure 32.17 has been estimated for both boys and girls by using MG-CFA (the model for girls is on the left, the model for boys on the right). The factors and patterns of free and fixed loadings within groups are the same across the groups. Factor loadings have been fixed to 1 to scale the factors. This is an important consideration because the factor variances (and covariances) should vary freely across groups; thus unit loading identification should be used.

The fit of this MG-CFA model is excellent (Table 32.4). The parameter estimates within each group are reasonable. The fit within each group is excellent as well. The factor model thus appears to be a good fit to the data for boys and girls. Note that if these models were run separately, the sum of the χ^2 and df for boys ($\chi^2 = 17.5$, $df = 21$) and girls ($\chi^2 = 23.3$, $df = 21$) would be equal to the results from the MG-CFA. Configural invariance is typically thought of as a baseline model, one that future models may be tested against. If modifications are needed to the factor model, this step is the best place to make those modifications.

Metric Invariance

The configuration of the factor structure has been established in each group in the configural invariance model. The next step is to restrict corresponding factor loadings to be equal across groups, and is referred to as a test of *metric* (or *weak factorial*) *invariance*. Each factor has one loading already fixed to 1, and those remain.[6] The factor loadings estimated freely within each group in the configural model are now constrained so that corresponding factor loadings are set to be equal across groups. These constraints are made to the unstandardized

TABLE 32.4. Tests of Factorial Invariance for the KABC-II Data for 4-Year-Olds

Model	χ^2	df	$\Delta\chi^2$	Δdf	p
Configural	40.8	42			
Metric (factor loadings)	44.0	47	3.2	5	.67
Strong (intercepts)	49.5	52	5.5	5	.36
Strict (residuals)	63.0	61	13.5	9	.14

Note. Each model is compared to the previous model.

loadings. So for example, the (unstandardized) loading of Expressive Vocabulary on Gc is fixed to be equal across the sexes. Such a constraint, if supported, means that a one-unit increase in Gc should result in the same unit increase in Expressive Vocabulary for boys as for girls. In all, five constraints have been added: one loading on each Gc, Glr, and Gsm factor, and two loadings on the Gv factor. Figure 32.18 shows the models for boys and girls with these constraints. In Amos, these are accomplished by giving the parameters the same labels in the two groups (*a* for the factor loading of Expressive Vocabulary, etc.). Other programs use other methods, but such constraints are possible in all SEM programs. These constraints resulted in a change of 5 degrees of freedom. Because this model is nested within the configural model, $\Delta\chi^2$ may be used to test for degradation in model fit (other criteria are also possible). The inclusion of these five additional constraints does not result in degradation of model fit ($\Delta\chi^2 = 3.18[5]$, $p = .67$). Metric invariance is tenable. This finding means that the relations between the factors and the subtests are the same across groups, or that the factors are the "same" (in some sense of the word) for both groups. Group comparisons of *factor* variances and covariances are now considered acceptable. Such a test does not indicate that observed subtest variances may be compared (Gregorich, 2006). Moreover, even though metric invariance is tenable, there is not enough evidence yet for us to say that boys and girls with the same latent levels of the CHC factors will indeed have the same observed scores. Such a statement requires further tests, tests that specifically include the intercepts.

Strong Factorial Invariance

Strong factorial invariance needs to be established before group comparisons may be made with regard to the common factor means (or composite score means). Strong invariance requires that covariances *and* means are analyzed and modeled. In the metric invariance model, the corresponding unstandardized factor loadings have been fixed to be equal across groups. As in previous models, the means have not been modeled. Or, more exactly, the factor means have been fixed to 0, and subtest intercepts have been allowed to vary across group. Specification of strong invariance requires that the subtest intercepts (means) are modeled. Specifically, factor mean differences are allowed, while all corresponding subtest intercepts are constrained to be equal across groups. This specification imposes the restriction that all subtest mean differences *are the result of the common factors* (un-

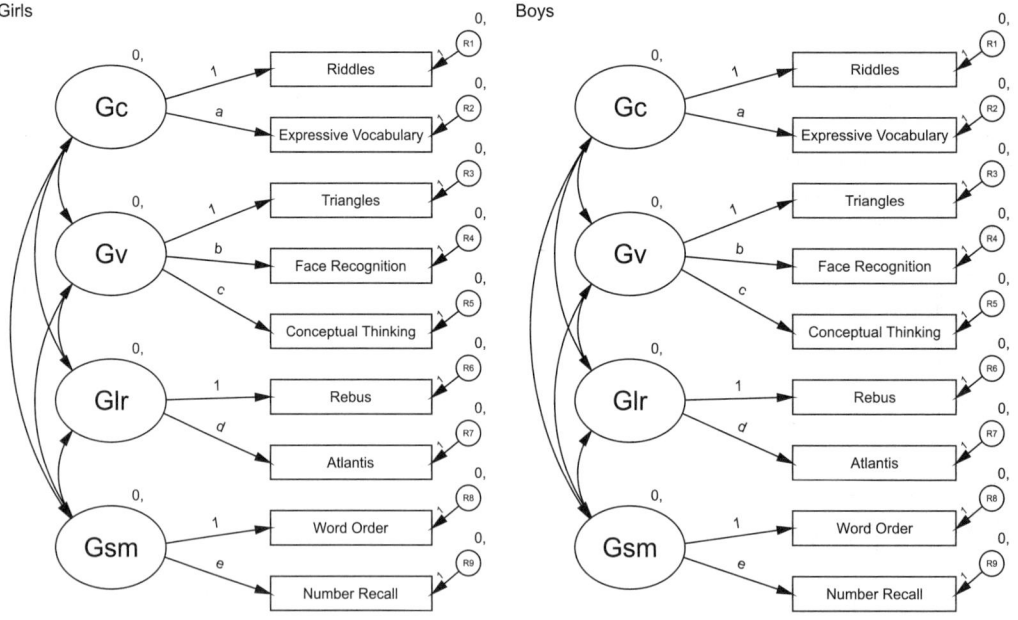

FIGURE 32.18. Testing for metric invariance. Factor loadings are constrained to be equal for girls (left) and boys (right).

standardized results are shown in Figure 32.19). Nine equality constraints, one per subtest, have been added to the corresponding subtest intercepts (e.g., the Expressive Vocabulary intercepts have been constrained to be equal across boys and girls). Note that in previous models the latent factor means have been fixed to be 0 (this is the default). To allow differences in the common factors across groups, the latent means of one group have been freed, while the other "reference" group means have remained fixed to 0. Here we denote girls as the reference group and keep their latent means fixed to 0. Boys are the comparison group, and their latent factor means are freed (note that the 0's have been removed from the boys' factors). Technically speaking, the latent means are not estimated; rather, the boys' latent mean estimate represents the difference from the female mean because the constraints on corresponding intercepts essentially forces mean differences "up" through the factor means. Freeing these four factor means results in 4 fewer degrees of freedom. Therefore, the Δ*df* for this model compared to the

metric invariance model should equal 5 (i.e., 9 subtest intercept constraints minus 4 latent mean differences allowed).

Given that girls are the reference group, positive latent mean values for boys indicate that boys have higher latent means, and negative values indicate that girls have higher latent means (because the female latent mean will be 0). Before those latent means may be interpreted, however, strong invariance must be tenable. That is, those differences in latent means should account for the differences across the sexes in the observed test scores. If these constraints are added and model fit is degraded, then the researcher should investigate the reasons for this misfit, and the latent mean differences at this point will be misleading. Similarly, the composite scores from the test should not be compared across the sexes.

Because the metric invariance model is tenable, all prior constraints are maintained, nine additional intercept constraints are applied, and the boys' Gc, Gv, Gsm, and Glr factor means are freed. The addition of these constraints does not

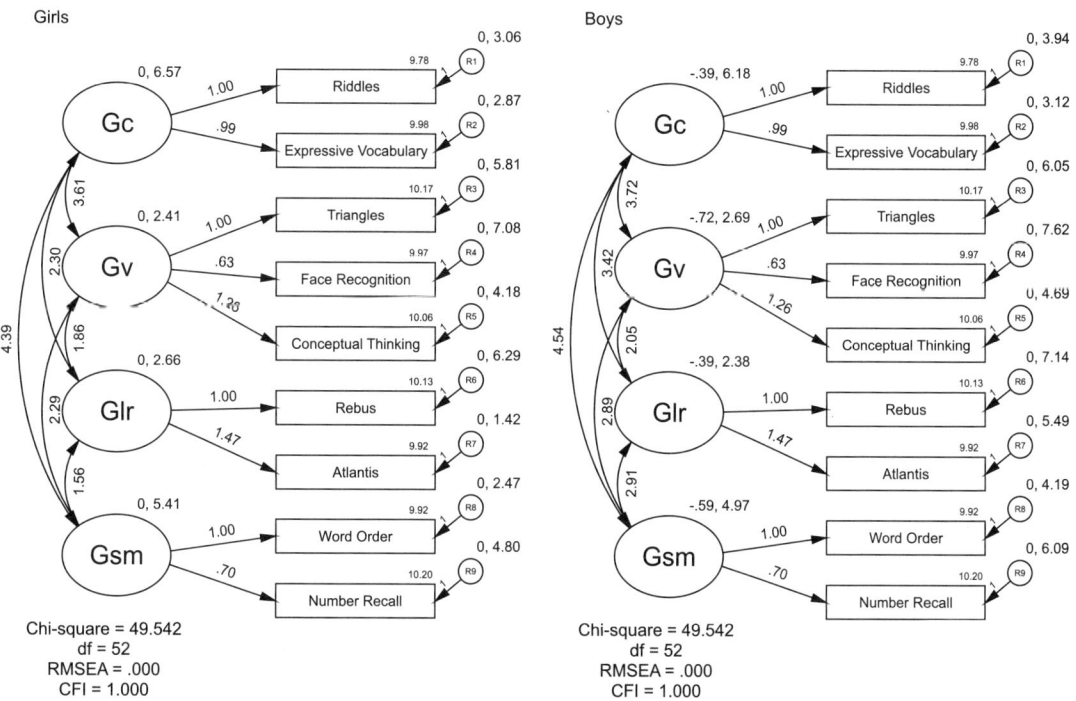

FIGURE 32.19. Unstandardized results for a test of strong (intercept) invariance. Note the numbers above each measured variable. These are the intercepts, which are constrained to be equal across the sexes in this step. The numbers above the latent variables are the means and variances. The latent means for the broad abilities are allowed to vary for boys, and the numbers shown are the latent mean differences for boys as compared to girls.

result in a statistically significant degradation in model fit ($\Delta\chi^2 = 5.5[5]$, $p = .36$). Strong invariance is tenable. That is, differences in subtest means across the sexes are explained by differences in the latent factor means between boys and girls. Stated differently, boys and girls with the same level of Gc (or Gv, etc.) will earn the same score on the subtests. It is thus acceptable for a researcher to compare boys and girls in their latent factor or observed composite means. However, before discussing differences in factor means, we first test for strict invariance.

Strict Factorial Invariance

The last step in testing for measurement invariance is referred to as *strict factorial invariance*. In tests of strict invariance, additional equality constraints are imposed on the variances of the residuals (error + specific variance, R1 through R9 in the figures). Strict invariance allows for group comparisons of observed subtest means and variances. There is disagreement about the necessity of strict invariance (cf. Little, 1997; Lubke & Dolan, 2003). Some of it boils down to the purpose of the research. Strictly speaking, however, strict factorial invariance is consistent with measurement invariance (Meredith & Teresi, 2006).

The application of these nine additional constraints on the residuals does not result in a degradation of model fit (Table 32.4). All sex differences in observed (subtest) score means and variances are due to differences in the common factor means and variances/covariances. The CHC composites from the KABC-II are completely unbiased with respect to sex (for 4-year-olds). Observed scores on the KABC-II depend on the latent factors, not on sex.

In this example, measurement invariance has been established with relative ease. In many other situations, the findings may be more complicated, and partial measurement invariance may be investigated. Such a topic is beyond the scope of this chapter (Byrne, Shavelson, & Muthén, 1989).

Substantive Questions

We have thus far focused on tests of measurement invariance, which may subsume many interesting research questions. Researchers are often interested in testing for construct bias for a test across two or more groups (e.g., Keith, Quirk, Schartzer, & Elliott, 1999). Such questions may be modeled by using tests of factorial invariance. Metric

invariance is often seen as the most important step in such testing. Intercept invariance is also increasingly recognized as important because it is important that tests have the same zero point (intercepts) for a given level of a latent ability. Otherwise, a score of, say, 110 would have a different meaning for one group versus the other.

Other interesting research questions may also be answered. For example, we have mentioned that differences in latent means are estimated and can be compared because strong invariance is tenable (and even better, strict invariance is). Girls' latent means for each factor are 0, while the boys' are estimated. Negative latent mean values thus indicate that boys' levels of abilities are lower. Each latent mean is negative (Gc = −.39, Gv = −.72, Glr = −.39, Gsm = −.59), though only Gv is statistically significant at the $p < .05$ level (see Figure 32.19). To be clear, a mean difference on this latent factor does *not* indicate that the test is biased; rather, it indicates that there is a true mean difference between boys and girls in these latent constructs. That mean difference in the latent factor accounts for the differences in the observed scores, so at age 4, boys on average score lower on Gv (it may also be of interest to include a g factor and test for differences by using higher-order models; see Chen, Keith, Weiss, Zhu, & Li, 2010; Keith et al., 2008; Reynolds et al., 2008). Latent mean differences can also be tested with model-fitting procedures by constraining the factor mean to be equal (i.e., by fixing the boys' factor means back to 0) for boys and girls and checking for degradation in model fit.

Other questions may also be of interest. Are the factor variances equal across groups? Or are the latent factors equally differentiated across groups? To answer those questions, a researcher may want to test for equality of the variances and covariances/correlations (see Little, 1997). It is once again important to note that these are substantive questions, and measurement invariance must be established before these comparisons are made. These questions may follow tests of measurement invariance, but *during* testing for measurement invariance, it is imperative to allow for group differences in factor variances and covariances, and (when the means are modeled) for differences in the factor means.

Intercepts and Means

As already noted, means are often not modeled in factor analysis, so it may be worth describing intercept (strong factorial) invariance in a bit more detail. Meredith (1993) described intercept invariance as a test of equality in specific factor means (controlling for the factor). If there is a *difference* in specific factor means (at equal levels of the latent trait), a constant score is added to the mean of the latent trait that is specific, and not related to the common factor.

Say, for example, there is an interest in comparing boys and girls on a composite score from a test battery designed to measure visual–spatial ability (Gv). The composite score includes four subtests that are supposed to measure four aspects of visual–spatial ability (e.g., closure speed, visual memory, spatial scanning, and spatial visualization). Measurement invariance is investigated. Metric invariance is demonstrated. Strong factorial (intercept) invariance, however, is not tenable. Specifically, the intercept associated with spatial visualization differs across groups, such that boys score higher on this test when boys and girls have the same level of Gv. When the constraint on this test is removed, strong invariance is tenable, and boys and girls do not demonstrate a latent Gv mean difference (note that there still could be a mean difference in Gv and strong invariance would hold). If mean scores are compared on a Gv composite score (or latent mean) without the spatial visualization test included, the composite means will probably not show a statistically significant difference. If spatial visualization tests are included in the calculation of that mean, however, boys will show higher scores on that Gv composite than girls, even though they do not differ in true level of Gv. Thus the apparent advantage is not due to the latent Gv ability; rather, it is due to a difference in the specific factor mean of spatial visualization (this is one hypothesis). That difference in the specific factor mean is thus a source of constant or additive bias.

Here is another way of putting it. If the linear factor model is considered in terms of a linear equation, then the expected score for a person equals the intercept plus the product of the factor loading times the true latent ability. Imagine a boy and girl with exactly the same latent Gv mean (e.g., 10). Metric invariance is established so that the factor loading (.5) is equivalent across groups. Say that intercept invariance is found for all of the tests, except for spatial visualization. Now say that the intercept values for spatial visualization are 15 for boys and 10 for girls. The expected score for boys is $15 + (.5 \times 10) = 20$. The expected score for girls is $10 + (.5 \times 10) = 15$. The expected score for boys is

higher, even though the latent Gv ability is identical. The composite scores are then confounded with a difference in a specific mean (referred to as *uniform bias*). The Gv composite score for boys will be overestimated because of an advantage in spatial visualization, not Gv. Note that in contrast, if the intercept is invariant, the expected scores are the same for boys and girls (see Gregorich, 2006, for more examples).

Finding intercept differences (or other differences) may be discouraging for a researcher. But from a substantive point of view, as well as from that of research and understanding what intelligence tests measure, the finding may be quite informative. In this Gv example, *partial* strong factorial invariance is demonstrated and it is found that there are no sex differences in the broad Gv factor, but only specific factors. Such knowledge will be interesting substantively, and may lead to a better understanding of sex differences and a better understanding of the measurement of Gv. For example, it may be that there are indeed sex differences, but only in specific aspects of Gv (e.g., spatial visualization). It will be important, however, to consider other possible reasons for this difference. Item content is only one of many possible reasons why such bias may occur. For example, perhaps a time limit is imposed on girls when they performed this task, while for boys there is no such limit. That is, there are many potential sources for uniform bias, but thinking critically about the potential reasons for these differences may also lead to interesting hypotheses for future research. What should be obvious, however, is that the application of a model-based framework allows for more specificity and sophistication in investigating such measurement and substantive questions.

REFERENCE VARIABLES: COMBINING SAMPLES

A major difficulty in conducting CFA-guided intelligence test research is the time commitment involved for both researchers and participants. An individually administered test of intelligence will generally take 90 minutes to administer, and substantial sample sizes are needed (150 or more are useful, although see Keith, 2006, or Kline, 2011, for more detail on power analysis and sample size). As some of the examples in this chapter have shown, research using tests from multiple batteries allows for powerful tests of competing theories (for a further discussion, see Keith & Reynolds, 2010).

Data collection for such research also requires a considerable increase in time commitment. It is also likely to reduce participation rates; how many participants (or their parents) are willing to spend 3–4 hours taking tests to aid in a research project? Even if they are willing, examinee fatigue is likely to be an issue, so data collection for one examinee is likely to require multiple sessions. On the other hand, imagine how useful the inclusion of additional batteries or parts of batteries would be, allowing for more comprehensive tests of specific questions and even underlying theories. Needless to say, despite the appeal, such studies are quite rare.

One possible solution is the use of a reference variable approach (McArdle, 1994) as a way of combining data from different samples, if those samples share a subset of subtests given to all participants. McArdle (1994) outlined the approach as a method of reducing data collection requirements by instituting "planned missingness." That is, a large number of measures could be administered to participants, but no one would take all measures. Instead, each participant might take one, two, or a few tests per factor measured, or subsets of participants would take a different subset of measures. The methodology builds on several topics already discussed, especially multisample analysis and invariance testing, and it requires expanding our thinking about what "latent" variables are. Cheung and Chan (2005) have advocated the method as a way of combining correlation matrices for meta-analysis. Keith and colleagues (2010) have illustrated the use of the method to conduct cross-age invariance testing when the structure of a test changes across age groups. Here, we illustrate the method as a way of combining overlapping batteries from multiple samples.

Stone (1992) conducted a cross-battery CFA of the original Differential Ability Scales (DAS) and the second edition of the WISC, the Wechsler Intelligence Scale for Children—Revised (WISC-R). His primary purpose was to compare models similar in structure to that guiding the WISC-R to those guiding the DAS (the DAS-type structure was more strongly supported). The data presented by Stone, however, can also be used to test specific hypotheses about the abilities measured by either measure. As a huge help to those who might want to investigate further, he reported the correlation matrix among the tests in these two batteries, thus allowing us (or anyone else) to further analyze those data. We used those data in previous versions of this chapter to illustrate cross-

battery analysis and its utility in answering questions about the constructs measured by tests (viz., whether the Block Design subtest of the WISC-R measures visual processing [Gv] or fluid intelligence [Gf]).

As noted earlier, one enduring question concerning the Wechsler scales is what exactly is being measured by the Arithmetic test. In previous versions of the WISC, Arithmetic was a component of the Verbal scale, but it was often combined with Digit Span and Coding into a (probably misnamed) Freedom from Distractibility factor in EFA. In the WISC-IV and the WAIS-IV, there is evidence that Arithmetic measures Gf (Benson, Hulac, & Kranzler, 2010; Keith, Fine, Taub, Reynolds, & Kranzler, 2006), but that it may also measure short-term memory (Gsm) and crystallized intelligence. A cross-battery CFA of the WISC-III with the WJ III COG has suggested that Arithmetic is best considered a measure of Gq, or mathematics achievement (Phelps, McGrew, Knopik, & Ford, 2005). Thus, although the Stone data do not focus on the most recent versions of the WISC and the DAS, they may still be useful for helping understand the construct measured by previous (and probably current) versions of the Arithmetic test.

The DAS includes two good measures of Gf, one of which (Sequential and Quantitative Reasoning) appears to measure quantitative reasoning (RQ). Thus a joint CFA of the WISC-R and the DAS could determine whether the Arithmetic test "fits" on the same factor with Sequential and Quantitative Reasoning. But what about alternative competing hypotheses? The original DAS also included three short measures of achievement (Basic Number Skills, Spelling, and Word Reading), so with a cross-battery CFA of the WISC-R, the DAS, and the DAS achievement scale, it would be possible to test whether WISC-R Arithmetic measures Gf, achievement, neither, or both. Because the two measures also include other measures of Gsm (each includes a digit span measure), it would also be possible to test whether Arithmetic measures short-term memory skills.

The second sample in this research was a portion of the DAS standardization sample, ages 8–15 (the age range of the Stone DAS/WISC-R data), using the DAS cognitive and achievement tests. These data are accessible as age-related matrices in the DAS technical handbook (Elliott, 1990). There are thus two samples used in this example. The first sample includes 115 children ages 8–15 who were administered both the DAS and the

WISC-R. The second sample includes children ages 8–15 in the standardization sample who were administered the DAS cognitive battery and the three DAS achievement tests. For both samples, the correlation matrix of tests and standard deviations were used as input for the analysis.[7]

Figure 32.20 shows the model developed and tested for the DAS/WISC-R data, and Figure 32.21 shows the model developed and tested for the DAS/achievement data (the Recall of Digits residual has been constrained based on the results of the DAS/WISC-R data). As shown in the figures, both models fit the data well, and we are likely to accept them as reasonable. Figure 32.22 shows the setup for the reference variable analysis, with the DAS/WISC-R sample on the top and the DAS/achievement sample on the bottom. This is a basic multisample analysis, but with different models across samples. What is unusual in these are that some variables that are normally measured variables appear as latent variables in one sample (e.g., the subtests of the WISC-R in the lower figure). This may seem strange, but consider some alternative ways of thinking about latent variables: They are unmeasured, or even imaginary variables, and an imaginary variable is also a *missing variable*. The latent variables Gc, or u13, do not appear anywhere in either dataset; they are missing. Likewise, in the DAS/WISC-R sample, there is no Basic Arithmetic variable, and thus it is missing or latent.

Both models will be underidentified (and therefore impossible to estimate) if analyzed separately, but they can be analyzed in tandem, with certain parameter constraints. These are also shown in the figure. Thus the path from achievement to Basic Arithmetic in the DAS/WISC-R sample is constrained to the value estimated in the DAS/achievement sample, and the path from Gc to Information in the DAS/achievement sample is constrained to the value estimated in the DAS/WISC-R sample, and so on. In fact, every parameter that has the same label across the two figures is constrained to be equal across the groups. These include some of the factor loadings, factor variances, variances of residuals, and covariances among factors and residuals. The constrained parameters are those related to measured variables that do not exist in one sample versus the other.

These constraints are *required* for estimation, but are they reasonable? What if the DAS/WISC-R sample were very different from the DAS/achievement sample? In that case, assumptions concerning the equivalence of these parameters would not

be justified. It is possible, however, to get an idea of the reasonableness of these assumptions by testing for invariance for the parts of the model that exist in *both* groups. The DAS cognitive battery was administered to both samples (these are the *reference* variables), and thus it is possible to go through the invariance testing steps for these portions of the models. Table 32.5 shows the results of such testing. The configural model is the model shown in Figure 32.22, with no cross-sample constraints beyond those required for identification and estimation. For the metric invariance model, the paths from the factors to the DAS cognitive tests are constrained to be equal across groups. As shown in the table, these constraints do not result in a statistically significant decrement in model fit, and thus we are likely to accept these loadings as equal across groups. The table shows that the results of each level of invariance testing are plausible.[8] If the common structure is equivalent across groups, it makes sense to assume that the unmeasured/missing portions of that structure are equivalent also. As a result, we can now proceed confidently to using these combined data to test hypotheses of interest. If we were using raw data (and if intercept invariance were also tested and established), it would now also be reasonable to combine the two datasets and let the SEM program deal with the missing data. (Given that most SEM programs, by default, use maximum-likelihood methods for dealing with missing data, the results should be the same as in the reference variable approach, with structures estimated via maximum-likelihood estimation.)

The model shown in Figure 32.22, and those discussed so far in Table 32.5, have assumed that the WISC-R Arithmetic test is a measure of quantitative reasoning, and thus of Gf, fluid intelligence. With the Test Arithmetic 1 model, a cross-loading has also been allowed for Arithmetic on the achievement factor. As shown in the table, this model relaxation results in an improvement in χ^2, but that improvement is not statistically significant. We are likely to accept the stricter model, the one specifying that Arithmetic is a measure of RQ/Gf, over the one that specifies that Arithmetic measures both Gf and achievement. Interestingly, in the model in which both loadings are allowed, neither is statistically significant (probably due to the smallish sample size), but they are of similar magnitude (.41 for Gf, .39 for achievement). If we stopped our model testing here, we would be likely to conclude that Arithmetic is better considered a measure of RQ and Gf than of achievement.

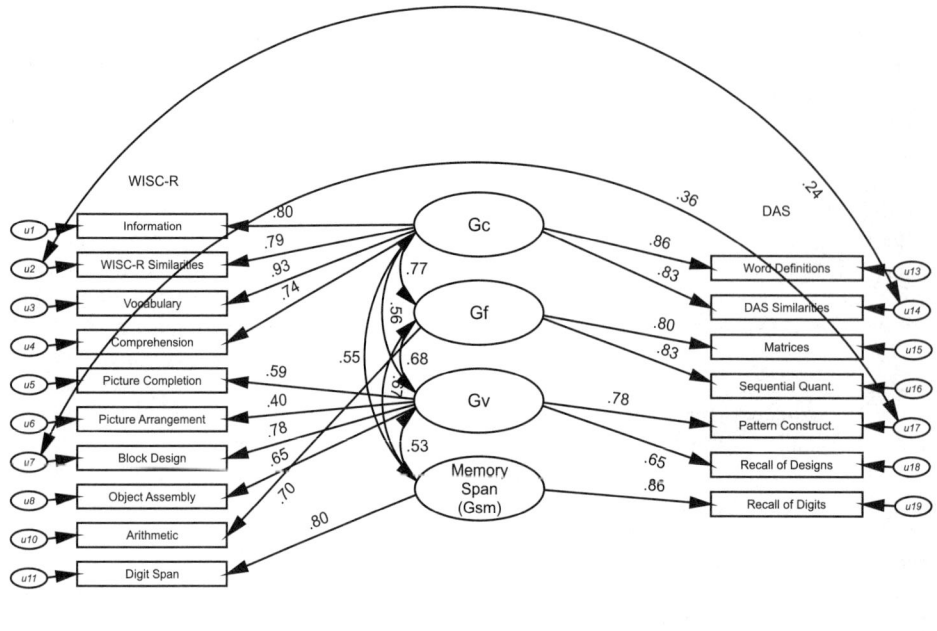

Chi-square = 107.130
df = 111
TLI = 1.004
CFI = 1.000
RMSEA = .000
SRMR = .044
AIC = 191.130

FIGURE 32.20. Cross-battery CFA of the DAS and the WISC-R.

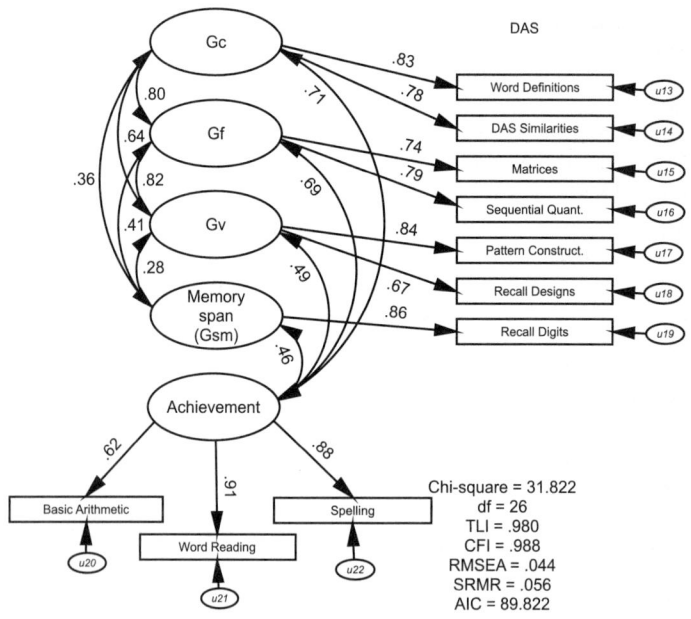

Chi-square = 31.822
df = 26
TLI = .980
CFI = .988
RMSEA = .044
SRMR = .056
AIC = 89.822

FIGURE 32.21. CFA of the DAS and the DAS achievement tests.

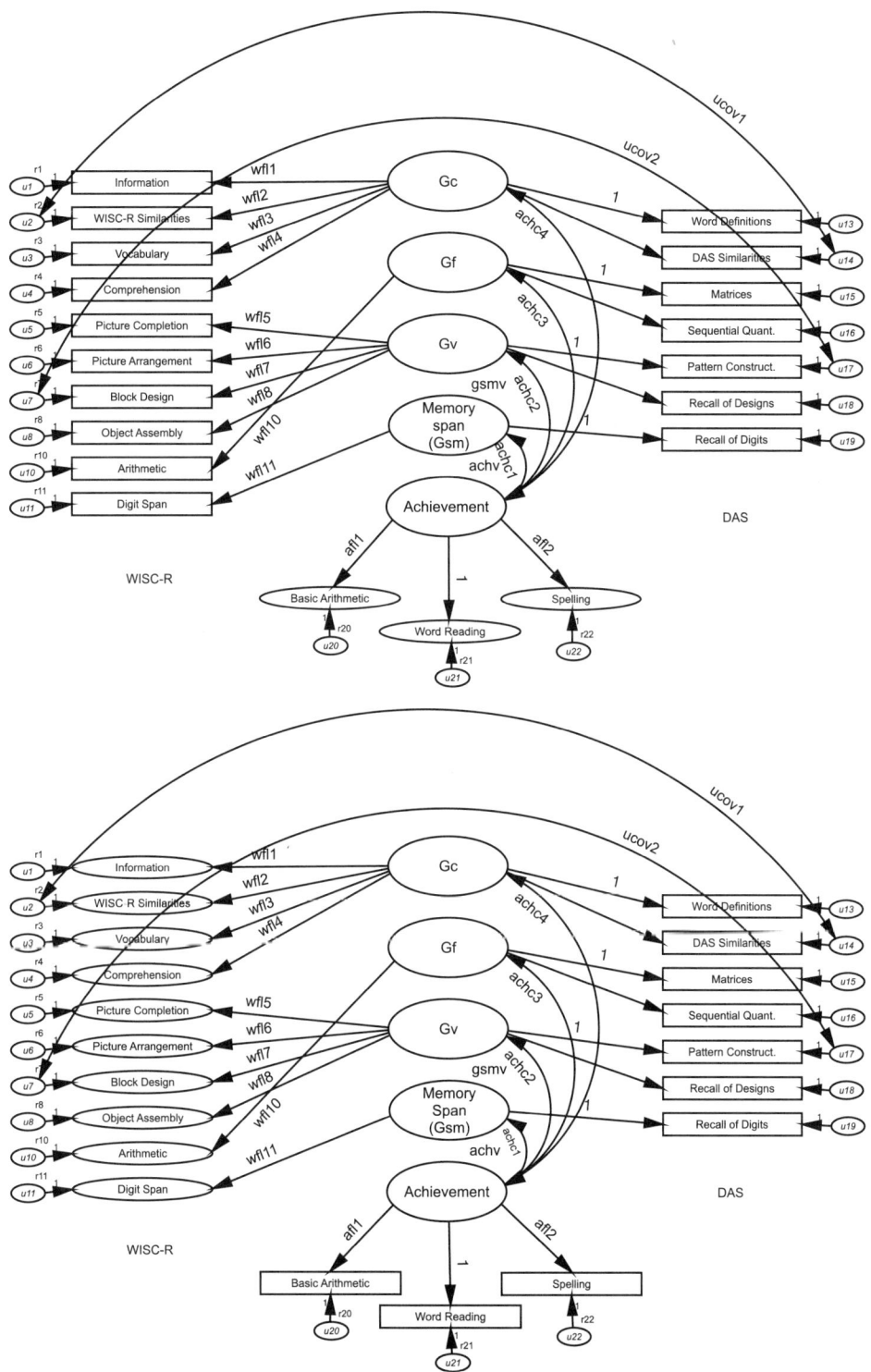

FIGURE 32.22. Reference variable set-up for a multigroup, cross-battery analysis of the DAS/WISC-R and the DAS/DAS achievement. Some variables are measured in one sample and latent (missing) in the other.

TABLE 32.5. Comparisons of Reference Variable Models: Invariance and Hypothesis Testing

Model	χ^2	df	$\Delta\chi^2$	Δdf	p	RMSEA	SRMR	AIC
Configural	138.952	137				.008	.044	280.952
Metric	139.029	140	0.077[a]	3	.994	.000	.044	275.029
Subtest residual	143.471	147	4.442[a]	7	.728	.000	.045	265.471
Factor variances	143.675	150	0.204[a]	3	.977	.000	.046	259.675
Factor covariances	152.271	156	8.596[a]	6	.198	.000	.054	256.271
Test Arithmetic 1	150.431	155	1.840[a]	1	.175	.000	.052	256.431
Test Arithmetic 2	152.198	156	1.767[a]	1	.184	.000	.052	256.198
Test Gsm 1	151.351	155	0.920[b]	1	.337	.000	.053	257.351
Test Gsm 2	178.475	156	28.044[a]	1	<.001	.025	.074	282.475

[a]Compared to the previous model.
[b]Compared to the factor covariances model.

The Test Arithmetic 2 model specifies that Arithmetic loads only on the achievement factor. This model can also be compared to the Test Arithmetic 1 model. The difference is not statistically significant, suggesting that a model with Arithmetic loading only on the achievement factor is better than a model allowing it to load on both Arithmetic and Gf. The model comparisons are not definitive in this case (e.g., AIC of 256.271 vs. 256.198), so it is still not clear whether Arithmetic is better considered a measure of Gf or of achievement. Larger sample sizes, additional measures of RQ, and additional measures of arithmetic achievement would help in making this determination.

The most recent version of the WISC (the WISC-IV) includes the Arithmetic test on the Working Memory Index, suggesting that it is a measure of the narrow ability working memory and the broad ability short-term memory (Gsm). Table 32.5 also shows two models testing this possibility. The results of these comparisons are more definitive. Allowing Arithmetic to cross-load on a Gsm factor does not improve model fit, and with a model allowing such cross-loading, the Gf-to-Arithmetic path is statistically significant, whereas the Gsm-to-Arithmetic path is not. In addition, a model allowing Arithmetic to load only on the Gsm factor fits statistically significantly worse than does a model allowing cross-loadings, and worse (based on the AIC) than does a model allowing it to load only on a Gf factor. The models suggest that Arithmetic (at least the version of Arithmetic on the WISC-R) probably measures Gf more than it measures Gsm. Of course, additional measures of

Gsm and additional measures of working memory abilities on the Gsm factor would improve these comparisons as well.

Figure 32.23 shows another way to specify this model (this is the configural invariance model). With this specification, variables that are measured in one sample but missing in the other simply are not included in that second sample. Note that the latent variable referencing achievement does appear in both, with its variance and covariances constrained to be equal across groups. Note that the fit statistics for this version of the model match those for the original configural invariance specification shown in Table 32.5.

Although these results and speculation are interesting, the main purpose of this example has been to illustrate the reference variable approach. Clearly, this is a useful approach for increasing the number of tests and broadening the factor representation in CFA. It can be useful for combining extant datasets, as we have done here, but a more useful approach would be to use this to plan data collection so that the breadth of measurement is increased without increasing the time commitment per participant. And the approach is not limited to two samples. Elsewhere (Reynolds, Keith, Flanagan, & Alfonso, 2010), for example, we combined data from four samples in a comprehensive test of CHC theory. This research also tested for measurement invariance in many of the major tests used (e.g., the WISC-IV, the WJ III, and the reference test, the KABC-II) against their standardization data to ensure that the smaller cross-battery samples were representative of the underlying factor structures.

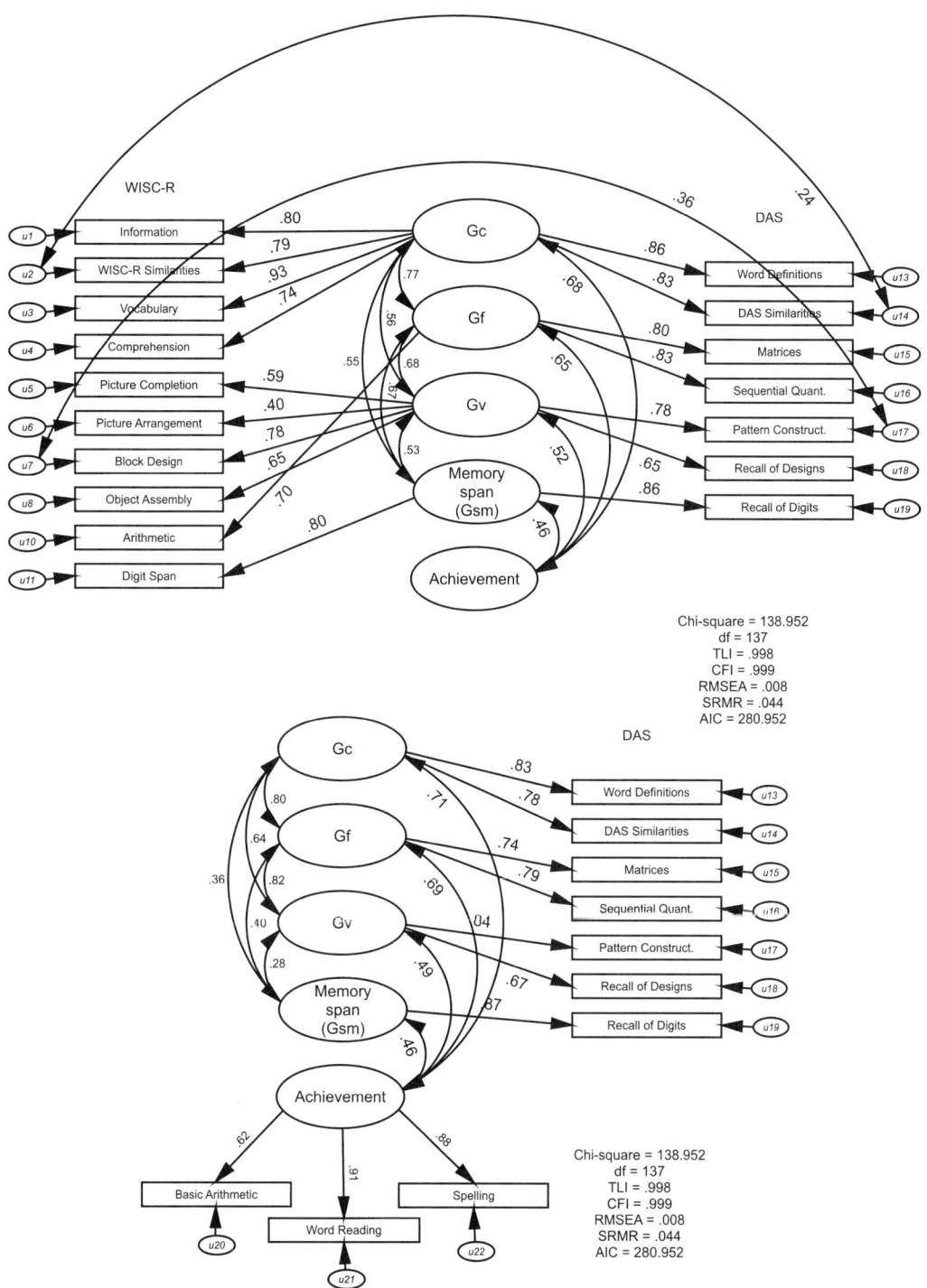

FIGURE 32.23. An alternative model specification for the reference variable approach.

TESTING THEORIES OF INTELLIGENCE

Most of the examples used in this chapter are examples of CFA used to understand the constructs measured by specific tests. The method is equally applicable, however, for asking and answering questions about *theories* of intelligence. Some analyses serve both functions; the joint CFA of the WJ III and CAS discussed earlier has implications for CHC and PASS theory, in addition to the tests derived from these theories. That is, the fact that the hypotheses derived from CHC theory are supported provides support for that theory.

CHC and Three-Stratum Theory

CHC theory is based, in part, on Carroll's three-stratum theory of cognitive abilities. Both theories posit a higher-order model of intelligence with narrow-order abilities at the bottom and the most general ability, g, at the apex. The theory is described in detail in Carroll (1993) and in Schneider and McGrew (Chapter 4, this volume).

Carroll speculated that there might well be *intermediate* factors between his second-stratum (e.g., Gf, Gc, Gv) and third-stratum abilities, but he left the task of describing this intermediate structure up to other researchers. Bickley, Keith, and Wolfle (1995) addressed the possibility of intermediate factors and tested one such model, and Keith (1997) explored several such possible models, but neither pursued the matter in depth. One difference between three-stratum theory and Gf-Gc theory (the other component of CHC theory) is the nature of quantitative reasoning and quantitative knowledge. Gf-Gc theory has traditionally treated quantitative skills as a separate achievement-related construct, Gq, whereas Carroll focused on quantitative reasoning (RQ) and found it to be a part of fluid or novel reasoning (Gf). To demonstrate CFA's applicability to testing theory, one model with intermediate factors is explored here, and several models exploring the nature of quantitative reasoning are tested.

The WJ III COG is based on CHC theory, and research suggests that it provides valid measures of CHC constructs (McGrew & Woodcock, 2001; Taub & McGrew, 2004), so it is a good tool for testing basic questions about CHC theory. A basic CHC model is shown in Figure 32.24 (cf. Floyd, Keith, Taub, & McGrew, 2007). The data used were the matrices of correlations and standard deviations for children ages 9–13 from the WJ III standardization data (McGrew & Woodcock,

2001). Not all WJ III COG tests were used; the model includes three good measures of each factor. The sample sizes for tests in this matrix varied, so an overall sample size of 1,000 was used in these analyses (the EM [expectation maximization] algorithm was used to deal with incomplete data in the calculation of the matrices).

Figure 32.24 also shows the results of the analysis of this initial model for 9- to 13-year-olds in the WJ III standardization sample. As shown in the figure, the initial model provides a good fit to the WJ III data; the SRMR, RMSEA, TLI, and CFI all suggest an excellent fit to the data. The RMSEA information in the figure is a little different from that presented previously; the figure shows the point value of the RMSEA (.043) surrounded by the 90% confidence interval of the RMSEA (.039–.047).

The model shown in Figure 32.25 presents one possible set of intermediate factors between the second and third stratum from CHC/three-stratum theory (in the model, these intermediate factors are second-order factors, and g is a third-order factor). Woodcock (1993) proposed a *cognitive performance model* (CPM) of abilities as a method of explaining how abilities work in concert to affect a person's overall functioning, and this model has been refined and built into the scoring of the WJ III COG. The CPM includes three intermediate factors between the broad abilities (Gf, Gc, etc.) and g: *verbal ability*, *thinking ability*, and *cognitive efficiency*. Two of these intermediate factors are included in the model; verbal ability and Gc are the same, so there was no need to build a verbal ability intermediate factor into the model (an intermediate factor could have been built into the model, but the fit would be the same as the more simple model shown).

As shown in the figure and in Table 32.6, this categorization of second-stratum abilities into thinking abilities and cognitive efficiency leads to an improvement in the fit of the model. In particular, the intermediate CPM factors produce a statistically significant decrease in χ^2, thus suggesting the division of some of the second-stratum abilities into thinking and cognitive efficiency as a worthwhile addition to the three-stratum theory.

One interesting aspect of this model is the essential equivalence of g and thinking abilities. (The path from g to thinking ability is actually 1.02, but is not statistically significantly different from 1.) A common fix would be to constrain the disturbance of the thinking ability factor to 0, which would fix the standardized loading to 1.0. Shown in Figure

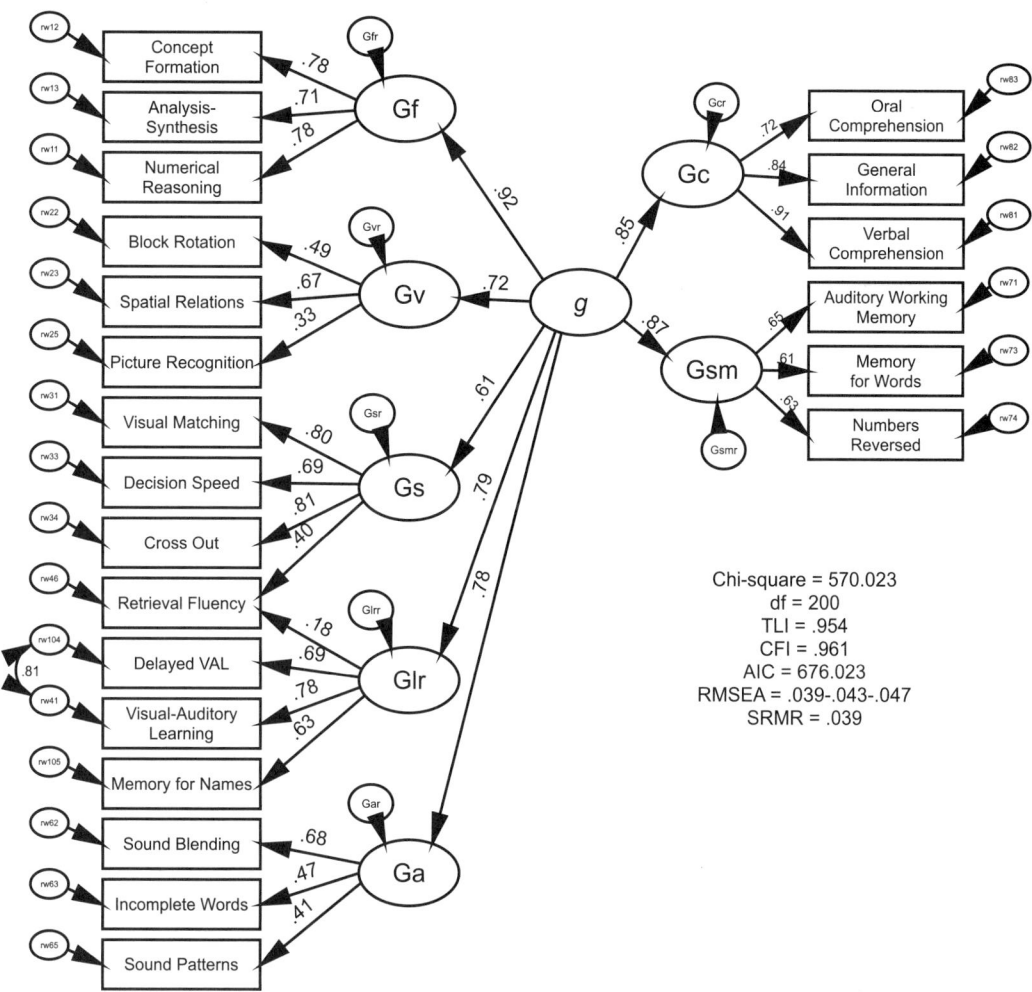

FIGURE 32.24. A three-stratum-theory-derived model of the WJ III COG. The model fits the data well.

32.26 is a model in which the g and thinking ability factors are combined; this model is equivalent to one in which the thinking disturbance is set to 0. As shown in the table, this model does not result in a statistically significant increase in χ^2, and thus is preferred as a more parsimonious version of the CPM. This modified model supports the combination of the Gs and Gsm factors into a hierarchical cognitive efficiency factor, but suggests that g and thinking ability are statistically indistinguishable.

One final variation of this model is mentioned briefly. One could argue that the path from cognitive efficiency to g should be reversed, so that efficiency affects g rather than the reverse. This modification could be based on the assumption

that processing speed and short-term memory (and cognitive efficiency) are fundamental mental skills that influence one's level of general intelligence—essentially, gatekeepers of general cognitive ability (see Schneider & McGrew, Chapter 4, this volume). Unfortunately, without further modification, this model is statistically equivalent to the modified CPM model, and the two cannot be distinguished on the basis of fit statistics. The rules for generating equivalent and nonequivalent models mentioned earlier (e.g., Keith, 2006, Ch. 12) could be used to develop some nonequivalent versions of these two alternative models, thus allowing a test of whether g should be considered an influence on cognitive efficiency, or an effect.

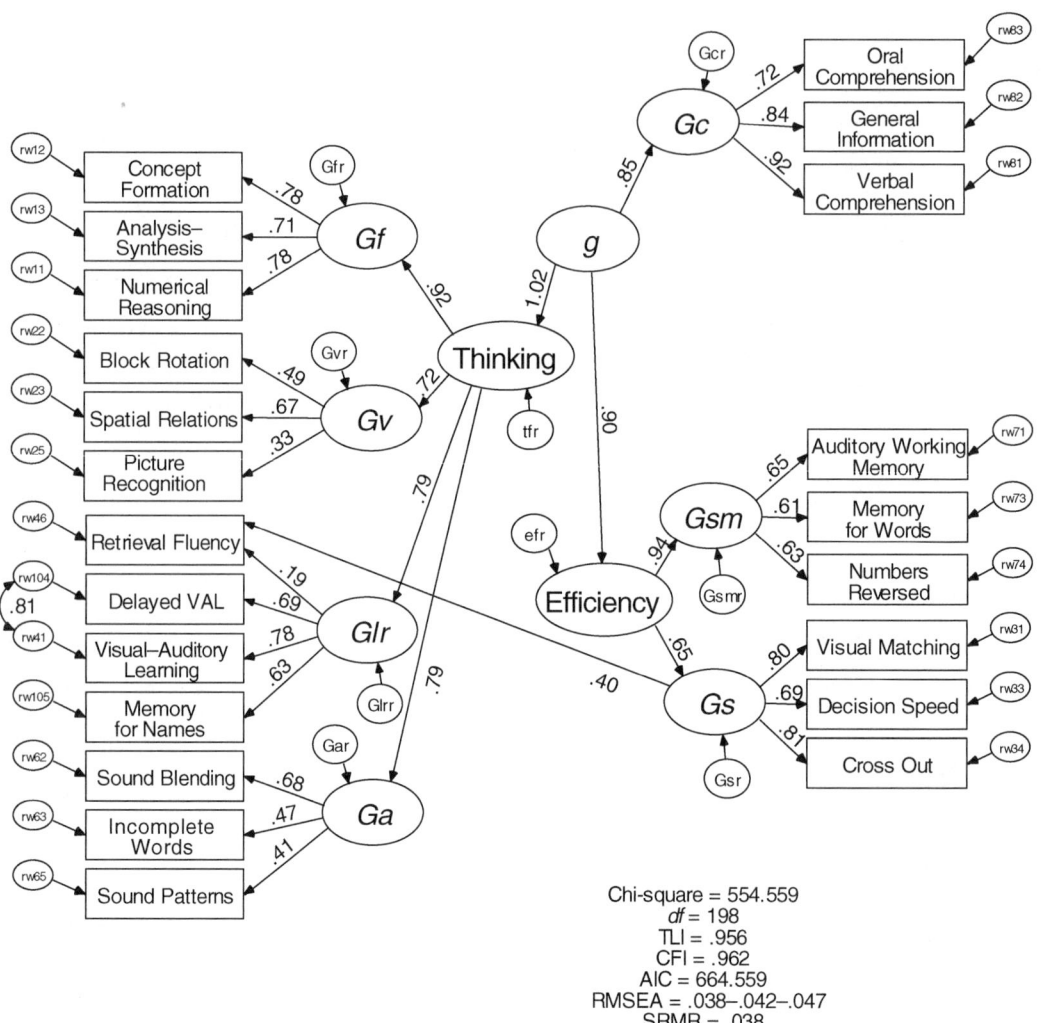

FIGURE 32.25. A test of possible intermediate factors between Carroll's stratum II and stratum III abilities. The model is based on Woodcock's cognitive performance model (CPM).

TABLE 32.6. Comparison of the Fit of Models Testing Different Intermediate-Level Factors in the Three-Stratum Theory, and the Relation of Gf and RQ factors

Model description	χ^2 (df)	$\Delta\chi^2$ (df)	p	AIC
1. Initial model: No intermediate factors	570.023 (200)			676.023
2. Cognitive performance model (CPM)	554.559 (198)	15.464 (2)[a]	<.001	664.559
3. Cognitive performance model 2	556.827 (199)	2.268 (1)[a]	.132	664.827
4. Initial Gf-RQ model: Separate factors	1914.426 (198)			2068.426
5. Gf subsumes Gf (narrow) and RQ	1873.621 (197)	40.805 (1)[a]	<.001	2029.621

[a]Compared to the previous model.

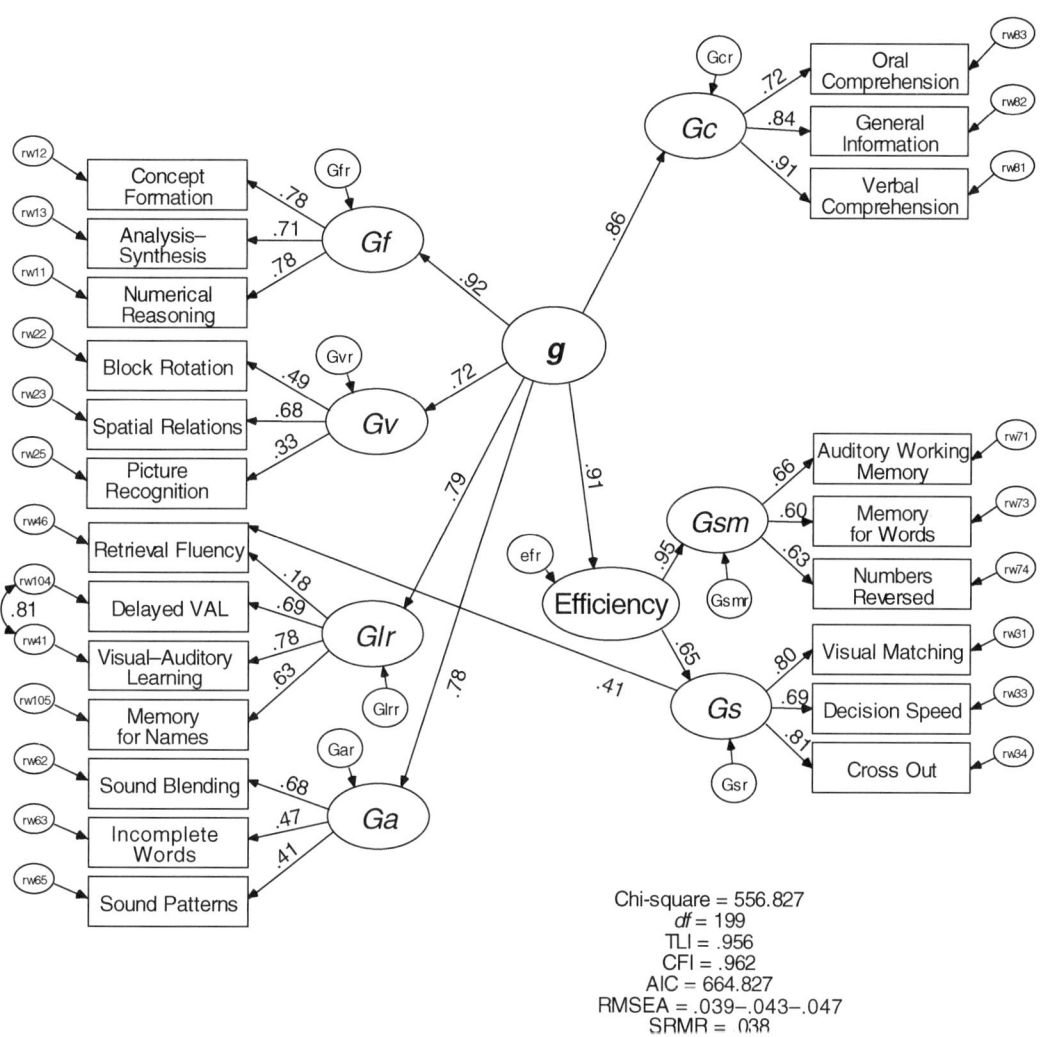

Chi-square = 556.827
df = 199
TLI = .956
CFI = .962
AIC = 664.827
RMSEA = .039–.043–.047
SRMR = .038

FIGURE 32.26. A simplified version of the CPM in Figure 32.25.

The final two models in this chapter (Figures 32.27 and 32.28) test Carroll's contention that quantitative reasoning (RQ) is a part of Gf rather than a separate second-stratum factor. The models do not address the existence or nature of a Gq (quantitative knowledge) factor. These analyses have been conducted on over 5,000 participants from the WJ III standardization sample. The advantage of these data are that they include two clear measures of quantitative reasoning: number series and number matrices (these two tests were combined into a Numerical Reasoning test when the WJ III COG was first released). The sample is

described in more detail in Keith and colleagues (2008).

The initial quantitative reasoning model set-up with separate Gf and RQ factors (in the upper right of the figure) is shown in Figure 32.27, and the fit statistics for comparing models are shown in the figure and in Table 32.6. As shown in the figure, the initial quantitative reasoning model provides a good fit to the data using common criteria. There are missing cases in the data, and Amos does not produce SRMR when there are missing data (some other programs, such as Mplus, do); thus SRMR is not reported.

There are several possible ways to test whether

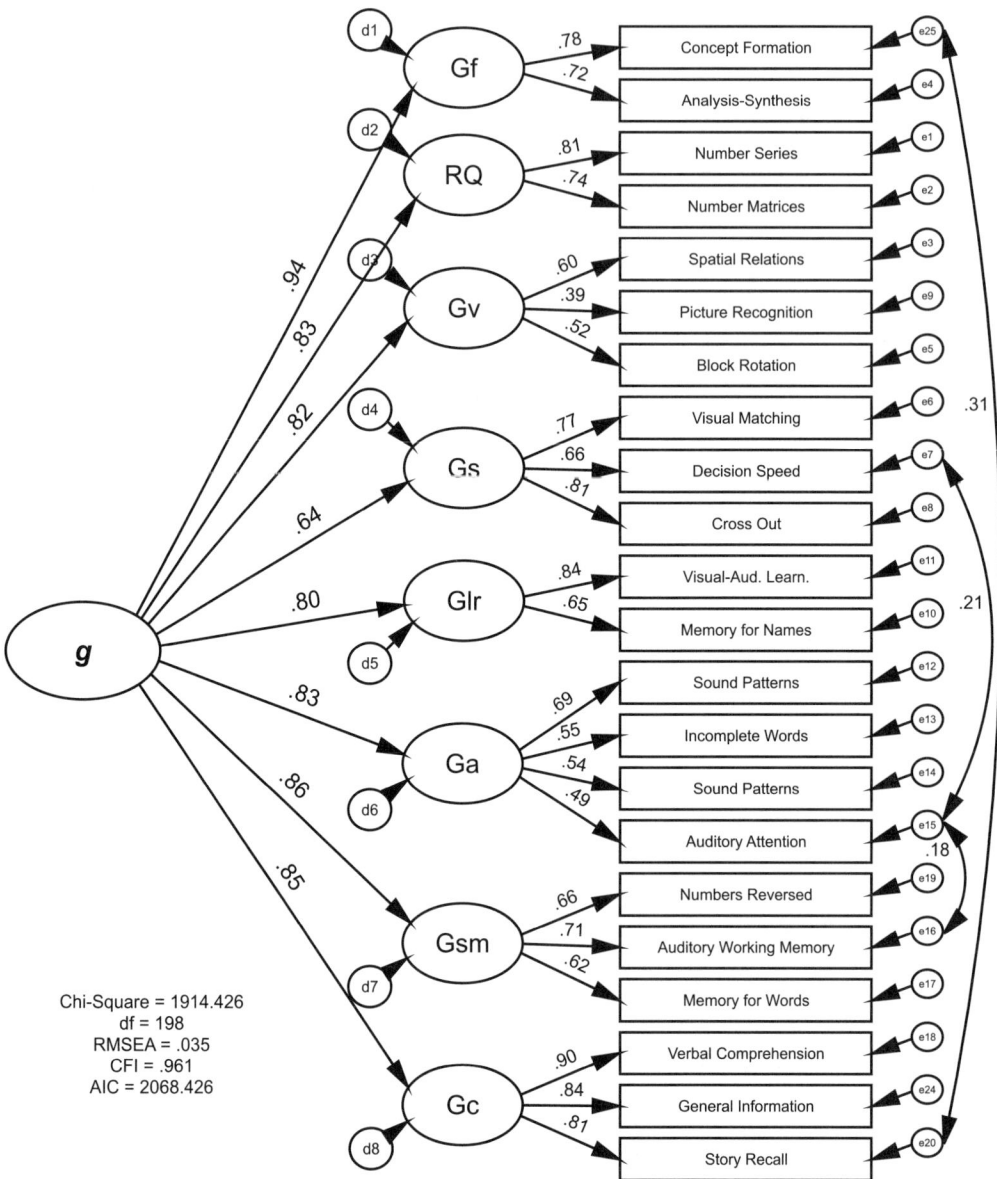

FIGURE 32.27. A model designed to probe the nature of the relation between Gf and RQ.

the RQ factor should be subsumed under a broader Gf factor. One common method—the most agnostic approach—would be to specify correlated errors for the disturbances of the Gf and RQ factors. Such a model suggests that these two factors measure something in common besides general intelligence. Figure 32.28 shows a model in which the narrow Gf (symbolized as "Gf narrow") and RQ factors are subsumed under a broader Gf factor.

This model is, in fact, statistically equivalent to the correlated disturbance model, but better symbolizes the hypothesis of interest. A third method would be to delete the path from g to RQ and include one from Gf to RQ (this model is neither shown nor tested here). As shown in Table 32.6, the loading of the original Gf and RQ factors onto a broader Gf factor results in a considerable improvement in model fit over the initial quantita-

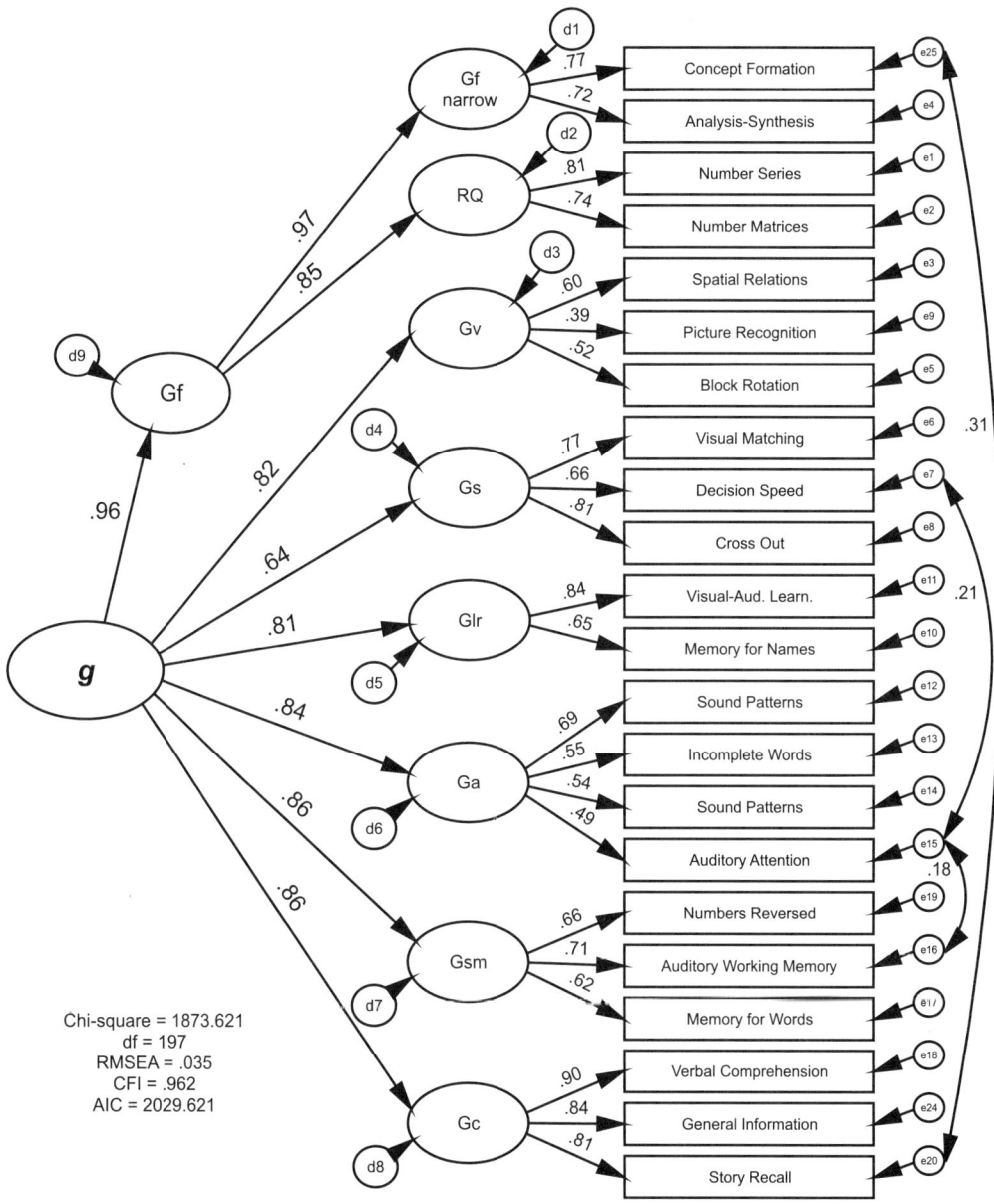

FIGURE 32.28. In this model, Gf subsumes RQ and a narrow Gf factor. The model shows an improvement in fit over the previous model.

tive reasoning model. Said differently, the broad Gf factor may be considered an intermediate factor between the narrow Gf and RQ factors and g. This preliminary investigation supports the contention that quantitative reasoning is a part of fluid/novel reasoning (Gf).

SUMMARY

This chapter has provided an overview of and introduction to the method of CFA, with particular attention to the use of the method as an aid in understanding the constructs measured by modern tests of intelligence. The chapter has covered "simple" CFA—in other words, first-order CFA, a method that is fairly common in the factor-analytic/intelligence literature.

We believe, however, that additional uses of CFA are needed if we are really interested in understanding the constructs we are measuring. Thus we encourage the comparison of *meaningful* alternative explanations to a researcher's pet theory through the testing and comparison of alternative factor models. This practice, too, is becoming more common, although alternative models are not always meaningful. For example, we argue that a single-factor model is generally not a meaningful alternative and does not represent modern thinking about the nature of *g* as a construct.

Many modern theories of intelligence are hierarchical in nature, with the most prominent example being the three-stratum theory, a "metatheory" developed and tested by John Carroll (and incorporated into CHC theory). Most tests of intelligence tacitly recognize a hierarchical nature of intelligence as well (Keith & Reynolds, 2010). We strongly believe that our research should therefore test these hierarchical notions of intelligence if we are to fully understand the constructs we are measuring. Put another way, a test of a first-order version of a hierarchical theory/test is an incomplete test of that theory. Furthermore, higher-order hierarchical analysis provides a more thorough understanding of the first-order abilities (Carroll, 1993, Ch. 3). This chapter has demonstrated several variations of hierarchical CFA, using second- and even third-order factors.

This chapter has demonstrated several other important uses of CFA: to compare the constructs measured across different tests, and to compare the constructs measured by one test across different groups. Many of the most vexing problems in the intelligence field revolve around these issues, and CFA is an excellent method for answering these important questions. Cross-battery CFA can be a powerful method for answering questions about the nature of constructs measured by specific tests, and for understanding the nature of intelligence. Use of a reference variable approach can enable larger and more comprehensive tests of such theories. Multisample CFA provides an organized, effective method for testing for the equivalence of structures across groups, and for testing for construct bias across groups. Finally, CFA provides a powerful method for testing theory, and especially for testing competing theories of intelligence.

We have not covered or tried to cover all possible uses of CFA; those uses are limited primarily by the imagination of the researcher. In addition, CFA is a subset of a more general approach—SEM—and this broader approach is also useful for understanding the nature of the constructs measured by tests of intelligence. To mention only two examples, SEM provides an excellent method for testing the stability over time of the *constructs* we measure, independent of the method of measurement, and multigroup SEM provides an excellent method for evaluating the presence of *predictive* bias in our measurements (cf. Borsboom, Romeijn, & Wicherts, 2008; McArdle, 1994). Nevertheless, we hope that this chapter has provided enough of an overview to stimulate thought and further study, and to fire the imaginations of future CFA readers and researchers. For those interested in additional study, there are numerous resources available (e.g., Keith, 2006; Kline, 2011; Loehlin, 2004; Reynolds & Keith, in press).

NOTES

1. The factor model tested is one that matches the intended structure of the KAIT. Other models (e.g., Flanagan & McGrew, 1998) are certainly plausible, but are not evaluated here.
2. Without this constraint, this portion of the model would have been underidentified.
3. More generally, if $\Delta\chi^2$ is statistically significant, the less constrained model (the model with the smaller *df*) is selected; if $\Delta\chi^2$ is not statistically significant, the more parsimonious model (the model with the larger *df*) is selected. It may not be immediately obvious why the model in Figure 32.6 is a constrained version of that in Figure 32.5. Figure 32.6 is statistically identical to Figure 32.5 with the paths from delayed recall to the Rebus and Auditory Delayed Recall subtests set to 0, and the correlations between delayed recall and the other two factors set to 0.
4. In SEM, these are known as *disturbances* and represent all other causes not included in the model. Thus, for the DAS example, f1 represents all causes of Verbal ability/Gc other than *g*.
5. Anyone who has had to explain IQ test scores to parents will probably note that it is much easier to talk about broad-ability scores than about the global composite because those tests are grouped together according to explainable, surface characteristics of tests. This is a reflection of the abstractness of *g* versus the broad abilities.
6. See Widaman and Reise (1997) for alternative specifications.
7. The DAS standardization sample included approximately 1,600 children, but the sample size was set to 115 in the multisample analyses so as not to overwhelm the findings for the other group. The matrix

reported in Stone (1992) did not include standard deviations, which are needed to test for later levels of invariance. For purposes of illustration, we set these to the average *SD* for each test (10 for the DAS and 3 for the WISC-R). Information presented in the DAS manual (Elliott, 1990), from where these data originated, suggests that these values are likely reasonable.

8. The variance steps may be plausible, in part, because we have guessed at values for the subtest variances in the DAS/WISC-R sample. If our purpose were to rigorously test hypotheses instead of to illustrate the method, this would be an important limitation. In this example, we are interested in the covariance structure more than the mean structure; thus we have not tested for intercept invariance or the equality of latent means. If questions of latent means were important, it would also be important to include these steps in the invariance testing.

REFERENCES

Akaike, H. A. (1987). Factor analysis and AIC. *Psychometrika*, *52*, 317–332.

Allen, S. R., & Thorndike, R. M. (1995). Stability of the WPPSI-R and WISC-III factor structure using cross-validation of covariance structure models. *Journal of Psychoeducational Assessment*, *13*, 3–20.

Arbuckle, J. L. (1995–2010). *Amos 19.0 user's guide.* Crawfordville, FL: Amos Development.

Benson, N., Hulac, D. M., & Kranzler, J. H. (2010). Independent examination of the Wechsler Adult Intelligence Scale—Fourth Edition (WAIS-IV): What does the WAIS-IV measure? *Psychological Assessment*, *22*, 121–130.

Bentler, P. M. (1995). *EQS structural equations program manual.* Encino, CA: Multivariate Software.

Bickley, P. G., Keith, T. Z., & Wolfle, L. M. (1995). The three-stratum theory of cognitive abilities: Test of the structure of intelligence across the life span. *Intelligence*, *20*, 309–328.

Borsboom, D., Romeijn, J. W., & Wicherts, J. M. (2008). Measurement invariance versus selection invariance: Is fair selection possible? *Psychological Methods*, *13*(2), 75–98.

Browne, M. W., & Cudeck, R. (1993). Alternative ways of assessing model fit. In K. A. Bollen & J. S. Long (Eds.), *Testing structural equation models* (pp. 136–162). Newbury Park, CA: Sage.

Burt, C. L. (1949). The structure of the mind: A review of the results of factor analysis. *British Journal of Educational Psychology*, *19*, 100–111, 176–199.

Byrne, B. M., Shavelson, R. J., & Muthén, B. O. (1989). Testing for equivalence of factor covariance and means structures: The issue of partial measurement invariance. *Psychological Bulletin*, *105*, 456–466.

Carroll, J. B. (1993). *Human cognitive abilities: A survey of factor-analytic studies.* New York: Cambridge University Press.

Carroll, J. B. (1995). [Review of the book *Assessment of cognitive processes: The PASS theory of intelligence*]. *Journal of Psychoeducational Assessment*, *13*, 397–409.

Chen, H., Keith, T. Z., Weiss, L., Zhu, J., & Li, Y. (2010). Testing for multigroup invariance of second-order WISC-IV structure across China, Hong Kong, Macau, Taiwan. *Personality and Individual Differences*, *49*, 677–682.

Cheung, M. W.-L., & Chan, W. (2005). Meta-analytic structural equation modeling: A two-stage process. *Psychological Methods*, *10*, 40–64.

Cohen, J. (1994). The earth is round (*p* < .05). *American Psychologist*, *49*, 997–1003.

Cole, J. C., & Randall, M. K. (2003). Comparing cognitive ability models of Spearman, Horn and Cattell, and Carroll. *Journal of Psychoeducational Assessment*, *21*, 160–179.

Das, J. P., Naglieri, J. A., & Kirby, J. R. (1994). *Assessment of cognitive processes: The PASS theory of intelligence.* Boston: Allyn & Bacon.

Elliott, C. D. (1990). *Differential Ability Scales: Introductory and technical manual.* San Antonio, TX: Psychological Corporation.

Elliott, C. D. (2007). *Differential Ability Scales—Second Edition: Introductory and technical manual.* San Antonio, TX: Harcourt Assessment.

Fan, X., Thompson, B., & Wang, L. (1999). Effects of sample size, estimation methods, and model specification on structural equation modeling fit indexes. *Structural Equation Modeling*, *6*, 56–83.

Flanagan, D. P., & McGrew, K. S. (1998). Interpreting intelligence tests from modern Gf-Gc theory: Joint confirmatory factor analysis of the WJ-R and Kaufman Adolescent and Adult Intelligence Test (KAIT). *Journal of School Psychology*, *36*, 151–182.

Floyd, R. G., Keith, T. Z., Taub, G. E., & McGrew, K. S. (2007). Cattell–Horn–Carroll cognitive abilities and their effects on reading decoding skills: *g* has indirect effects, more specific abilities have direct effects. *School Psychology Quarterly*, *22*(2), 200–233.

Gignac, G. E. (2008). Higher-order models versus direct hierarchical models: *g* as superordinate or breadth factor. *Psychological Science Quarterly*, *50*(1), 21–43.

Gregorich, S. E. (2006). Do self-report instruments allow meaningful comparisons across diverse population groups?: Testing measurement invariance using the confirmatory factor analysis framework. *Medical Care*, *44*, S78–S94.

Gustafsson, J.-E. (1984). A unifying model for the

structure of intellectual abilities. *Intelligence, 8,* 179–203.

Gustafsson, J.-E., & Aberg-Bengtsson, L. (2010). Unidimensionality and interpretability of psychological instruments. In S. Embretson (Ed.), *Measuring psychological constructs: Advances in model-based approaches* (pp. 97–121). Washington, DC: American Psychological Association.

Gustafsson, J.-E., & Balke, G. (1993). General and specific abilities as predictors of school achievement. *Multivariate Behavioral Research, 28,* 407–434.

Hu, L., & Bentler, P. M. (1998). Fit indices in covariance structure modeling: Sensitivity to underparameterized model misspecification. *Psychological Methods, 3,* 424–453.

Hu, L., & Bentler, P. M. (1999). Cutoff criteria for fit indexes in covariance structure analysis: Conventional criteria versus new alternatives. *Structural Equation Modeling, 6,* 1–55.

Humphreys, L. G. (1990). View of a supportive empiricist. *Psychological Inquiry, 1,* 153–155.

Jensen, A. R. (1998). *The g factor: The science of mental ability.* Westport, CT: Praeger.

Jöreskog, K. G. (1971). Simultaneous factor analysis in several populations. *Psychometrika, 36,* 409–426.

Jöreskog, K. G., & Sörbom, D. (1993). *LISREL 8: Structural equation modeling with the SIMPLIS command language.* Hillsdale, NJ: Erlbaum.

Jöreskog, K. G., & Sörbom, D. (1996). *LISREL 8 user's reference guide.* Lincolnwood, IL: Scientific Software.

Kaufman, A. S., & Kaufman, N. L. (1993). *Kaufman Adolescent and Adult Intelligence Test: Manual.* Circle Pines, MN: American Guidance Service.

Kaufman, A. S., & Kaufman, N. L. (2004). *Kaufman Assessment Battery for Children—Second Edition: Technical manual.* Circle Pines, MN: American Guidance Service.

Keith, T. Z. (1997). Using confirmatory factor analysis to aid in understanding the constructs measured by intelligence tests. In D. P. Flanagan, J. L. Genshaft, & P. L. Harrison (Eds.), *Contemporary intellectual assessment: Theories, tests, and issues* (pp. 373–402). New York: Guilford Press.

Keith, T. Z. (2006). *Multiple regression and beyond.* Boston: Allyn & Bacon.

Keith, T. Z., Fine, J. G., Taub, G. E., Reynolds, M. R., & Kranzler, J. H. (2006). Higher-order, multi-sample, confirmatory factor analysis of the Wechsler Intelligence Scale for Children—Fourth Edition: What does it measure? *School Psychology Review, 35,* 108–127.

Keith, T. Z., & Kranzler, J. H. (1999). The absence of structural fidelity precludes construct validity. Rejoinder to Naglieri on what the Cognitive Assessment System does and does not measure. *School Psychology Review, 28,* 303–321.

Keith, T. Z., Kranzler, J. H., & Flanagan, D. P. (2001). What does the Cognitive Assessment (CAS) measure?: Joint confirmatory factor analysis of the CAS and the Woodcock–Johnson Tests of Cognitive Ability (3rd Edition). *School Psychology Review, 30,* 89–119.

Keith, T. Z., Low, J. A., Reynolds, M. R., Patel, P. G., & Ridley, K. P. (2010). Higher-order factor structure of the Differential Ability Scales—II: Consistency across ages 4 to 17. *Psychology in the Schools, 47,* 676–697.

Keith, T. Z., Quirk, K. J., Schartzer, C., & Elliott, C. D. (1999). Construct bias in the Differential Ability Scales?: Confirmatory and hierarchical factor structure across three ethnic groups. *Journal of Psychoeducational Assessment, 17,* 249–268.

Keith, T. Z., & Reynolds, M. R. (2010). CHC and cognitive abilities: What we've learned from 20 years of research. *Psychology in the Schools, 47,* 635–650.

Keith, T. Z., Reynolds, M. R., Patel, P. G., & Ridley, K. P. (2008). Sex differences in latent cognitive abilities ages 6 to 59: Evidence from the Woodcock Johnson III Tests of Cognitive Abilities. *Intelligence, 36,* 502–525.

Kline, R. B. (2011). *Principles and practices of structural equation modeling* (3rd ed.). New York: Guilford Press.

Kranzler, J. H., & Keith, T. Z. (1999). Independent confirmatory factor analysis of the Cognitive Assessment System (CAS): What does the CAS measure? *School Psychology Review, 28,* 117–144.

Kranzler, J. H., Keith, T. Z., & Flanagan, D. P. (2000). Independent examination of the factor structure of the Cognitive Assessment System (CAS): Further evidence challenging the construct validity of the CAS. *Journal of Psychoeducational Assessment, 18,* 143–159.

Lee, S., & Hershberger, S. (1990). A simple rule for generating equivalent models in covariance structure modeling. *Multivariate Behavioral Research, 25,* 313–334.

Little, T. (1997). Mean and covariance structures (MACS) analyses of cross-cultural data: Practical and theoretical issues. *Multivariate Behavioral Research, 32,* 53–76.

Loehlin, J. C. (2004). *Latent variable models: An introduction to factor, path, and structural analysis* (4th ed.). Mahwah, NJ: Erlbaum.

Lubke, G. H., & Dolan, C. V. (2003). Can unequal residual variances across groups mask differences in residual means in the common factor model? *Structural Equation Modeling, 10,* 175–192.

McArdle, J. J. (1994). Structural factor analysis experiments with incomplete data. *Multivariate Behavioral Research, 29,* 409–454.

McArdle, J. J. (1998). Contemporary statistical models for examining test bias. In J. J. McArdle & R. W. Woodcock (Eds.), *Human cognitive abilities in theory and practice* (pp. 157–196). Mahwah, NJ: Erlbaum.

McDonald, R. P. (1999). *Test theory: A unified treatment.* Mahwah, NJ: Erlbaum.

McGrew, K. S., & Woodcock, R. W. (2001). *Technical manual: Woodcock–Johnson III.* Itasca, IL: Riverside.

Meredith, W. (1993). Measurement invariance, factor analysis, and factorial invariance. *Psychometrika, 58,* 525–543.

Meredith, W., & Teresi, J. A. (2006). An essay on measurement and factorial invariance. *Medical Care, 44*(11, Suppl. 3), S69–S77.

Millsap, R. E. (2001). When trivial constraints are not trivial: The choice of uniqueness constraints in confirmatory factor analysis. *Structural Equation Modeling, 8,* 1–17.

Muthén, L. K., & Muthén, B. O. (1998–2010). *Mplus user's guide* (6th ed.). Los Angeles: Authors.

Naglieri, J. A., & Das, J. P. (1997). *Cognitive Assessment System: Interpretive handbook.* Itasca, IL: Riverside.

Phelps, L., McGrew, K. S., Knopik, S. N., & Ford, L. (2005). The general (*g*), broad, and narrow CHC stratum characteristics of the WJ III and WISC-III tests: A confirmatory cross-battery investigation. *School Psychology Quarterly, 20,* 66–88.

Psychological Corporation. (2003). *Wechsler Intelligence Scale for Children—Fourth Edition: Technical manual.* San Antonio, TX: Author.

Reynolds, M. R., & Keith, T. Z. (in press). Measurement and statistical issues in child assessment research. In C. R. Reynolds (Ed.), *Oxford handbook of child and adolescent assessment.* New York: Oxford University Press.

Reynolds, M. R., Keith, T. Z., Flanagan, D. P., & Alfonso, V. C. (2010, December). *Utility of CHC taxonomy in identifying the factorial composition of intelligence subtests: A joint CFA.* Paper presented at the meeting of the International Society for Intelligence Research, Washington, DC.

Reynolds, M. R., Keith, T. Z., Ridley, K. P., & Patel, P. G. (2008). Sex differences in latent general and broad cognitive abilities for children and youth: Evidence

from higher-order MG-MACS and MIMIC models. *Intelligence, 36,* 236–260.

Schmid, J., & Leiman, J. M. (1957). The development of hierarchical factor solutions. *Psychometrika, 22,* 53–61.

Schwarz, G. (1978). Estimating the dimensions of a model. *Annals of Statistics, 6,* 461–464.

Sclove, S. L. (1987). Applications of some model-selection criteria to some problems in multivariate analysis. *Psychometrika, 52,* 333–343.

Stone, B. J. (1992). Joint confirmatory factor analyses of the DAS and WISC-R. *Journal of School Psychology, 30,* 185–195.

Tanaka, J. S. (1993). Multifaceted conceptions of fit in structural equation models. In K. S. Bollen & J. S. Long (Eds.), *Testing structural equation models* (pp. 10–39). Newbury Park, CA: Sage.

Taub, G. E., & McGrew, K. S. (2004). A confirmatory factor analysis of CHC theory and cross-age invariance of the Woodcock–Johnson Tests of Cognitive Abilities III. *School Psychology Quarterly, 19,* 72–87.

Thompson, B. (2006). *Foundations of behavioral statistics.* New York: Guilford Press.

Thorndike, R. M. (1990). Would the real factors of the Stanford–Binet Fourth Edition please come forward? *Journal of Psychoeducational Assessment, 8,* 412–435.

Thurstone, L. L. (1947). *Multiple-factor analysis: A development and expansion of The vectors of the mind.* Chicago: University of Chicago Press.

Vernon, P. E. (1950). *The structure of human abilities.* New York: Wiley.

Widaman, K., F., & Reise, S. F. (1997). Exploring the measurement invariance of psychological instruments: Applications in the substance use domain. In K. J. Bryant, M. Windle, & S. G. West (Eds.), *The science of prevention: Methodological advances from alcohol and substance abuse research* (pp. 281–324). Washington, DC: American Psychological Association.

Woodcock, R. W. (1993). An information processing view of Gf-Gc theory. *Journal of Psychoeducational Assessment, Monograph Series: Woodcock–Johnson Psycho-Educational Battery—Revised,* 80–102.

Yung, Y. F., Thissen, D., & McLeod, L. D. (1999). On the relationship between the higher-order factor model and the hierarchical factor model. *Psychometrika, 64,* 113–128.

CHAPTER 33

The Emergence of Neuropsychological Constructs into Tests of Intelligence and Cognitive Abilities

Daniel C. Miller
Denise E. Maricle

PERSPECTIVES ON NEUROCOGNITIVE ASSESSMENT

Baron (2004) has pointed out that "intelligence tests are not neuropsychological instruments" (p. 114). Historically, tests of intelligence were designed empirically to be predictive of academic achievement, and the lens through which they were viewed was very narrow. In the last 20 years, however, there has been a rapid advance in theoretically driven intelligence tests, with the Lurian and Cattell–Horn–Carroll (CHC) theories being the primary approaches used in intelligence test development, construction, and interpretation. Consequently, intelligence tests today are being used differently, with a broader lens; less attention is being given to the concept of g (general intellectual ability) as a predictor of academic achievement, and more emphasis is being placed on combinations of cognitive constructs as predictors of academic achievement.

The Lurian and CHC theories provide unique perspectives on the assessment of cognitive abilities. The Lurian perspective is grounded in clinical neuropsychology with extensive empirical evidence stemming from strong brain–behavior research. Currently, Lurian theory provides the foundation for the Cognitive Assessment System (CAS; Naglieri & Das, 1997) and can be used as an alternative interpretive approach for the Kaufman Assessment Battery for Children—Second Edition (KABC-II; Kaufman & Kaufman, 2004a). In contrast to Lurian theory, CHC theory is largely based on a factor-analytic cross-battery approach. The Woodcock–Johnson Tests of Cognitive Abilities Normative Update (WJ III COG NU; Woodcock, McGrew, & Mather, 2001b, 2007b) serves as the preeminent instrument that operationalizes CHC theory. CHC theory has since been applied to the Stanford–Binet Intelligence Scales, Fifth Edition (SB5; Roid, 2003), and the Differential Ability Scales—Second Edition (DAS-II: Elliott, 2007), as well as being the preferred interpretive model for the KABC-II (Kaufman & Kaufman, 2004a). CHC theory has thus become the "default" theoretical perspective in the majority of tests of cognitive ability.

Although there is significant psychometric research supporting CHC theory, one of its weaknesses is that there is no empirical evidence for the direct linkage between neuroanatomical functions and the cognitive constructs posited by the theory. As Baron (2004) has correctly pointed out, current intelligence tests have typically not been validated with respect to brain function. We agree with Baron that intelligence tests are not neuropsychological instruments. Presently, neuroimaging studies linking brain function to concurrent measures of commonly used tests of cognitive abilities are not available. Perhaps it is best to view intelligence tests as packaged samples of behavior that (1) may be a starting point for generating hypotheses about possible deficits in neuropsychological processing, and (2) may also be interpreted from a neuropsychological perspective.

Miller (2007, 2010) has introduced the school neuropsychological conceptual model (SNP model; see Figure 33.1) as a way of organizing cross-battery assessment data on school-age children. The purposes of the SNP model are (1) to facilitate clinical interpretation by providing an organizational framework for the assessment data; (2) to strengthen the linkage between assessment and evidence-based interventions; and (3) to provide a common frame of reference for evaluating the effects of neurodevelopmental disorders on neuropsychological processes. The complete SNP model includes the integration of academic achievement and social-emotional functioning with the major neuropsychological assessment components (see Miller, 2007, 2010, for reviews); however, we focus in this chapter only on the neurocognitive portions.

More recently, Flanagan, Alfonso, Ortiz, and Dynda (2010) have discussed the possible integration of the Lurian, CHC, and SNP models as a means of providing a common lens through which to examine neurocognitive constructs. For example, they have shown how neuropsychological constructs such as concept formation or working memory can be classified according to the three perspectives. Thus Flanagan and colleagues provide a much-needed framework for translating and integrating the concepts, principles, and nomenclature of the three models.

Historically, clinical neuropsychological assessment has attempted to link the cognitive and behavioral manifestations of neuropsychological processing with known brain structures or functions; it has relied on both quantitative and qualitative aspects of performance. Traditional neuropsychological tests consist of specifically designed tasks used to measure a psychological function known to be linked to a particular brain structure or pathway. The tests are typically used to assess impairment after an injury or illness known to affect neurocognitive functioning, or are used in research to compare neuropsychological abilities across experimental groups. In contrast, tests of cognitive abilities have traditionally focused

almost exclusively on quantitative measures of cognitive performance, while ignoring qualitative behaviors. Baron (2004) has stated that this limitation prevents the clinical detection of meaningful performance patterns, such as strategy selection, analysis of error patterns, and response latency.

In response to such limitations, test publishers have begun to gather the prevalence rates of observable qualitative behaviors and to provide practitioners with useful base rate data. Starting with the CAS (Naglieri & Das, 1997), followed by the Wechsler Intelligence Scale for Children—Third Edition as a Process Instrument (Kaplan, Fein, Kramer, Delis, & Morris, 1999) and the Wechsler Intelligence Scale for Children—Fourth Edition Integrated (WISC-IV: Integrated; Wechsler, 2004; Wechsler et al., 2004), test authors and publishers have provided a bridge between the fields of cognitive and neuropsychological assessment by including qualitative behaviors in tests of cognitive functions.

THE SCHOOL/PEDIATRIC NEUROPSYCHOLOGICAL CONCEPTUAL MODEL

The emerging subspecialization of school neuropsychology bridges the gap between traditional psychoeducational approaches and clinical neuropsychological approaches, allowing for both quantitative and qualitative assessment of performance. Miller's (2007, 2010) SNP model provides a framework for school psychologists to integrate quantitative and qualitative performance from commonly used tests of cognitive abilities and to interpret performance from a neuropsychological perspective. The bulk of this chapter is structured to provide information about how neuropsychological constructs are measured in traditional neuropsychological tests and current tests of cognitive ability. Within the SNP model, tasks from the various instruments are classified on the basis of their underlying neurocognitive demands, the theoretical perspectives from which they originate, and psychometric data from cross-battery research.

One of the limitations of this chapter is that we are only looking at the conceptual overlap between traditional neuropsychological instruments and tests of cognitive functions. In order to fully assess all of the neuropsychological constructs within the SNP model, practitioners would have to administer a broader array of instruments, such as specialized or targeted tests of learning

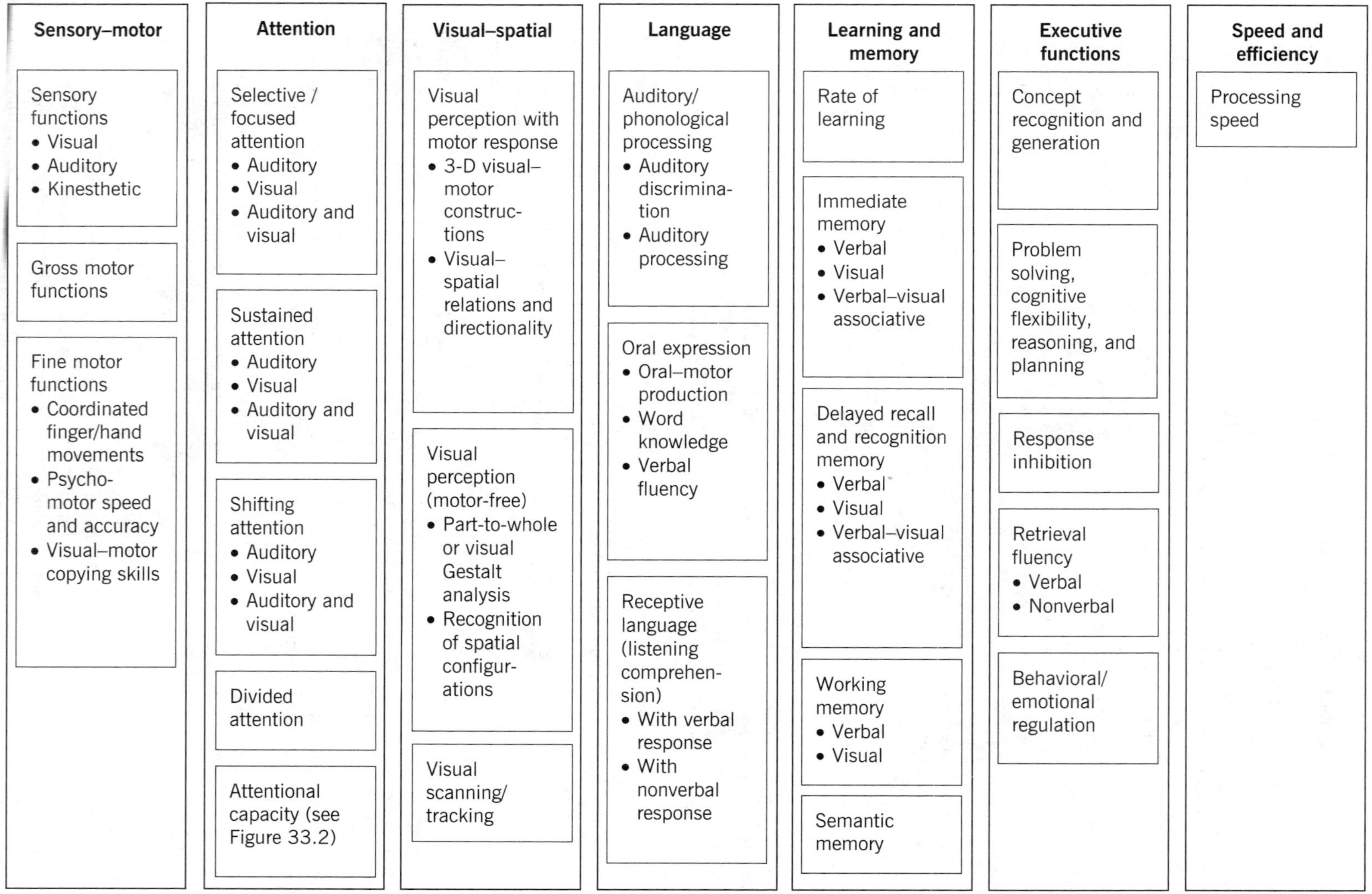

Sensory–motor	Attention	Visual–spatial	Language	Learning and memory	Executive functions	Speed and efficiency
Sensory functions • Visual • Auditory • Kinesthetic	Selective / focused attention • Auditory • Visual • Auditory and visual	Visual perception with motor response • 3-D visual–motor constructions • Visual–spatial relations and directionality	Auditory/phonological processing • Auditory discrimination • Auditory processing	Rate of learning	Concept recognition and generation	Processing speed
Gross motor functions	Sustained attention • Auditory • Visual • Auditory and visual	Visual perception (motor-free) • Part-to-whole or visual Gestalt analysis • Recognition of spatial configurations	Oral expression • Oral–motor production • Word knowledge • Verbal fluency	Immediate memory • Verbal • Visual • Verbal–visual associative	Problem solving, cognitive flexibility, reasoning, and planning	
Fine motor functions • Coordinated finger/hand movements • Psychomotor speed and accuracy • Visual–motor copying skills	Shifting attention • Auditory • Visual • Auditory and visual	Visual scanning/tracking	Receptive language (listening comprehension) • With verbal response • With nonverbal response	Delayed recall and recognition memory • Verbal • Visual • Verbal–visual associative	Response inhibition	
	Divided attention			Working memory • Verbal • Visual	Retrieval fluency • Verbal • Nonverbal	
	Attentional capacity (see Figure 33.2)			Semantic memory	Behavioral/emotional regulation	

FIGURE 33.1. Miller's school/pediatric neuropsychological assessment model.

and memory or of sensory–motor functions. The following constructs covered in common by traditional neuropsychological instruments and tests of cognitive abilities are discussed: sensory–motor and visual–motor functions; attentional processes; visual-perceptual, visual–spatial, and visual-constructional functions; language functions; learning and memory; and executive functions.

Sensory–Motor and Visual–Motor Functions

One of the major contrasts between intelligence testing and neuropsychological assessment is related to the assessment of sensory–motor functions. Neuropsychological evaluations typically assess for sensory functions of vision, hearing, and the sense of touch, as well as fine and gross motor functions, whereas the major tests of cognitive abilities have traditionally not included these neuropsychological functions as part of their core batteries. There are only two neuropsychological constructs within the sensory–motor domain that have been integrated into current tests of cognitive abilities: motor sequencing and visual–motor integration (see Table 33.1).

Traditional neuropsychological assessment has multiple examples of tests designed to measure motor sequencing actions with both the dominant and nondominant hands. These measures stem from Alexander Luria's original investigations of motor functions (Christensen, 1975), and all require the placement of the hand in three or more successive positions after either a verbal command or visual modeling from the examiner. Traditional neuropsychological measures of motor sequencing include the Finger Sequencing Test (Welsh, Pen-

nington, & Groisser, 1991), the Fist–Edge–Palm Test (Christensen, 1975), and the Oseretskii Test of Reciprocal Coordination (Buchanan & Heinrichs, 1989) (see Baron, 2004, for a review).

Various sensory–motor tasks (e.g., Fingertip Tapping, Imitating Hand Positions, and Manual Motor Sequences) have also been included in the NEPSY-II (Korkman, Kirk, & Kemp, 2007), which is a comprehensive neuropsychological battery designed for school-age children. The Test of Memory and Learning—Second Edition (TOMAL-2: Reynolds & Voress, 2007) also includes a Manual Imitations test. Among tests of cognitive abilities, only the KABC-II (Kaufman & Kaufman, 2004a) includes a motor sequencing task called Hand Movements.

One of the classic neuropsychological measures of visual–motor integration is the Rey–Osterrieth Complex Figure Test (ROCF), developed in the 1940s by Rey (1941) and Osterrieth (1944). The test has been revised and restandardized multiple times (e.g., a current version is the Rey Complex Figure Test and Recognition Trial; Meyers & Meyers, 1995), but the purpose of the test remains the same: to assess for visual–spatial constructional ability. The ROCF requires copying a complex figure drawing with an added delayed-recall component. Other two-dimensional copying tasks that may be used to supplement tests of cognitive abilities are the Beery–Buktenica Developmental Test of Visual–Motor Integration (VMI; Beery, Buktenica, & Beery, 2010) and the Design Copying test from the NEPSY-II (Korkman et al., 2007).

Only two current tests of cognitive abilities include a direct measure of visual–motor integration: the Copying test from the DAS-II (Elliott, 2007) and the Coding Copy test from the WISC-IV In-

TABLE 33.1. Sensory–Motor and Visual–Motor Functions Measured on Traditional Neuropsychological Tests and Current Tests of Cognitive Abilities

Neuropsychological construct(s)	Traditional neuropsychological measures	Examples of neuropsychological measures in tests of cognitive abilities
Motor sequencing	Finger Sequencing Test Fist–Edge–Palm Test NEPSY-II: Fingertip Tapping (dominant and nondominant hand combined), Imitating Hand Positions, and Manual Motor Sequences Oseretskii Test of Reciprocal Coordination TOMAL-2: Manual Imitations	KABC-II: Hand Movements
Visual–motor integration	VMI NEPSY-II: Design Copying Rey Complex Figure Test and Recognition Trial	DAS-II: Copying WISC-IV Integrated: Coding Copy

tegrated (Wechsler et al., 2004). Although other current tests of cognitive abilities do not include measures of visual–motor integration, it is common practice in psychoeducational assessment to include an additional test like the Beery VMI, to rule out the presence of any sensory–motor deficit that could explain a learning difficulty. For example, before a specific learning disability can be diagnosed, federal law (the Individual with Disabilities Education Improvement Act of 2004) requires that any sensory–motor impairment be ruled out as a primary causal factor.

Since many childhood disorders are known to have associated sensory–motor deficits (see Decker & Davis, 2010, for a review; see also Decker, Englund, & Roberts, Chapter 29, this volume), clinicians must not rely on using tests of cognitive abilities alone. Tests of cognitive abilities do not include other important sensory–motor constructs that should be measured, such as speed and accuracy of motor output, both of which have a direct impact upon a learner's achievement (Miller, 2007, 2010). When the referral questions raise serious concerns about sensory–motor functions, an appropriately trained clinician is encouraged to include the sensory–motor subtests from the NEPSY-II (Korkman et al., 2007) or to administer portions of the Dean–Woodcock Sensory–Motor Battery (DWSMB; Dean & Woodcock, 2003). The DWSMB consists of eight measures of sensory functioning, nine measures of motor functioning, and one measure of lateral dominance or preference. A valuable aspect of the DWSMB is that it is co-normed with a major test of cognitive abilities, the WJ III COG NU (Woodcock et al., 2001b, 2007b); this allows for direct comparisons between sensory–motor functions and cognitive processes.

Attentional Processes

Attentional processes and executive functions are often intertwined, and some neuropsychological tests such as the NEPSY-II (Korkman et al., 2007) combine these processes into a single domain for interpretation. In Miller's SNP model (2007, 2010), attentional processes are interpreted separately from executive functions. Consistent with prevailing neuropsychological theories of attention (see Riccio, Reynolds, & Lowe, 2001, for a review), the SNP model views attention as multidimensional, with five subcomponents: (1) selective/focused attention, (2) sustained attention, (3) shifting attention, (4) divided attention, and (5) attentional capacity. Miller has stated, "While attention is most probably multidimensional, many of the tests

that are designed to measure attention . . . do not isolate the subcomponents of attention very well. Many of the common tasks of attention measure, as one unit, multiple subcomponents of attention such as selective and sustained attention" (2010, pp. 95–96).

It is understood that some aspect of attentional processing is a basic requirement to perform almost any cognitive task. As an example, it is difficult to perform well on a memory task if attention is lacking during the encoding process. However, several current tests of cognitive abilities are specifically designed to measure one or more of the attentional subcomponents (see Table 33.2).

Selective and/or Sustained Attention

Traditional neuropsychological measures of selective and sustained attention include the d2 Test of Attention (Brickenkamp & Zilmer, 1998) and the Ruff 2 & 7 Selective Attention Test (Ruff & Allen, 1996). Both of these tests require the examinee to choose target stimuli quickly from a visual array. The NEPSY-II (Korkman et al., 2007) Auditory Attention and Response Set Test measures aspects of selective, sustained, and shifting attention. Continuous-performance tests (CPTs) measure sustained attention and are used by both neuropsychologists and school psychologists in the diagnosis of attention-deficit/hyperactivity disorder (ADHD). Examples of CPTs include the Conners' Continuous Performance Test II (Conners & Multi-Health Systems Staff, 2004) and the Integrated Visual and Auditory Continuous Performance Test (Sandford & Turner, 1993–2006).

Several tests of cognitive abilities have included measures of selective and sustained attention. The CAS (Naglieri & Das, 1997) has two tests: Number Detection and Receptive Attention; the WISC-IV (Wechsler, 2003) also has two tests: Cancellation and Coding. Each of these tests requires quickly finding a stimulus target within a larger visual array full of distracters. The WJ III COG NU (Woodcock et al., 2001b, 2007b) likewise includes two tests that require selective and/or sustained attention: Auditory Attention and Pair Cancellation.

Divided Attention

The Trail Making Test (TMT) from the Halstead–Reitan Neuropsychological Test Battery (Reitan & Wolfson, 1985) is one of the most widely used neuropsychological tests. The test has been adapted

TABLE 33.2. Attentional Processes Measured on Traditional Neuropsychological Tests and Current Tests of Cognitive Abilities

Neuropsychological construct(s)	Traditional neuropsychological measures	Examples of neuropsychological measures in tests of cognitive abilities
Selective and sustained attention	d2 Test of Attention Ruff 2 & 7 Selective Attention Test Continuous-performance tests NEPSY-II: Auditory Attention and Response Set	CAS: Number Detection and Receptive Attention WISC-IV: Cancellation and Coding WJ III COG NU: Auditory Attention and Pair Cancellation
Divided attention	Halstead–Reitan Trail Making Test D-KEFS: Trail Making	CAS: Planned Connections
Attentional capacity	CMS: Stories Immediate Corsi Block Span Knox Cube Test NEPSY-II: Narrative Memory and Sentence Repetition TOMAL-2: Digits Forward, Letters Forward, and Memory for Stories WRAML2: Finger Windows, Number/Letter, Sentence Memory, and Story Memory	CAS: Word Series DAS-II: Recall of Digits—Forward KABC-II: Number Recall and Word Order (without interference) WISC-IV: Digit Span WISC-IV Integrated: Letter Span, Spatial Span—Forward, and Visual Digit Span WJ III COG NU: Memory for Words

into many forms, including the Trail Making test on the Delis–Kaplan Executive Function System (D-KEFS; Delis, Kaplan, & Kramer, 2001). The traditional TMT has two parts: Part A requires the examinee to draw a line in sequence between numbered circles on a page, and Part B requires the examinee to draw a line between circles that contain alternating sequential numbers or letters of the alphabet. The D-KEFS version of the TMT contains multiple trials that parse out the neurocognitive demands of the task and aid in the interpretation of test performance. The CAS (Naglieri & Das, 1997) is the only test of cognitive ability that incorporates a measure of divided attention, which is called Planned Connections.

Attentional Capacity

Attentional capacity has a direct relationship with the cognitive capacity or load required on memory tasks. As the stimuli to be recalled increase in length (e.g., in number of digits or letters), and as the semantic loading increases from words to sentences to stories, there are concurrent changes in the attentional demands of the tasks. Figure 33.2 illustrates the relationship of attentional capacity to memory tasks. Attentional capacity, or immediate short-term memory for numbers, letters, or visual sequences, is measured on common tasks in both neuropsychological tests and tests of cognitive functions. Digit span tests are routinely included

in tests of cognitive abilities, such as the Recall of Digits—Forward test on the DAS-II (Elliott, 2007), the Number Recall test on the KABC-II (Kaufman & Kaufman, 2004a), the Digit Span—Forward test on the WISC-IV (Wechsler, 2003), and the Letter Span and Visual Digit Span tests on the WISC-IV Integrated (Wechsler et al., 2004). The WISC-IV Integrated also includes a visual form of digit span tests, Spatial Span—Forward, which is similar to two classic neuropsychological visual span tests: the Corsi Block Span test (Milner, 1971) and the Knox Cube Test (Arthur, 1947; Knox, 1914). Two targeted tests of memory and learning for children include measures of digit or visual sequence spans: the Digits Forward test on the TOMAL-2 (Reynolds & Voress, 2007) and the Finger Windows and Number/Letter tests on the Wide Range Assessment of Memory and Learning, Second Edition (WRAML2; Sheslow & Adams, 2003).

Attentional capacity and contextual cues increase with memory for words and sentences. Among neuropsychological assessment tasks, the NEPSY-II and the WRAML2 both have sentence memory tests. There are similar memory-for-words tasks on three tests of cognitive abilities: Word Series on the CAS (Naglieri & Das, 1997), Word Order (without interference) on the KABC-II (Kaufman & Kaufman, 2004a), and Memory for Words on the WJ III COG NU (Woodcock et al., 2001b, 2007b).

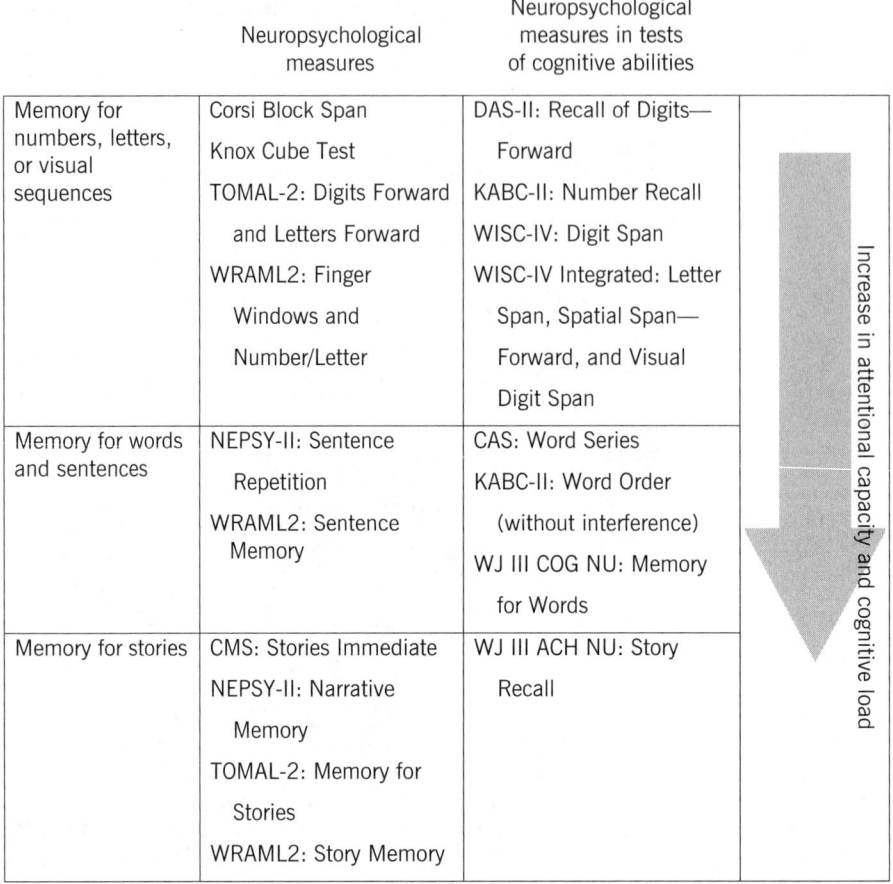

	Neuropsychological measures	Neuropsychological measures in tests of cognitive abilities	
Memory for numbers, letters, or visual sequences	Corsi Block Span Knox Cube Test TOMAL-2: Digits Forward and Letters Forward WRAML2: Finger Windows and Number/Letter	DAS-II: Recall of Digits—Forward KABC-II: Number Recall WISC-IV: Digit Span WISC-IV Integrated: Letter Span, Spatial Span—Forward, and Visual Digit Span	Increase in attentional capacity and cognitive load
Memory for words and sentences	NEPSY-II: Sentence Repetition WRAML2: Sentence Memory	CAS: Word Series KABC-II: Word Order (without interference) WJ III COG NU: Memory for Words	
Memory for stories	CMS: Stories Immediate NEPSY-II: Narrative Memory TOMAL-2: Memory for Stories WRAML2: Story Memory	WJ III ACH NU: Story Recall	

FIGURE 33.2. Relationship of attentional capacity to memory tasks.

Finally, attentional capacity is maximized with increased cognitive load and semantic content with memory for stories. The three major stand-alone tests of memory and learning—the Children's Memory Scale (Cohen, 1997), the TOMAL-2, and the WRAML2—all contain tests that assess memory for stories. Although the Woodcock–Johnson Tests of Achievement Normative Update (WJ III ACH NU: Woodcock, McGrew, & Mather, 2001a, 2007a), the companion instrument to the WJ III COG NU, has a Story Recall test, no test of cognitive ability directly measures story recall.

Visual-Perceptual, Visual–Spatial, and Visual–Constructional Functions

In the SNP model (Miller, 2007, 2010), tests of visual–spatial processing are conceptually divided into three categories: (1) tests that require visual

perception with a motoric response, (2) tests that require visual perception but are motor-free, and (3) tests that require visual scanning or tracking (see Table 33.3).

Visual Perception with Motor Response

Three-dimensional, visual–motor constructions and visual planning and organization are two neurocognitive constructs shared between neuropsychological measures and tests of cognitive abilities (see Table 33.3). The Block Construction test on the NEPSY-II (Korkman et al., 2007) is an example of a neuropsychological measure that requires three-dimensional construction of blocks. Similar visual–motor, constructional tasks on tests of cognitive abilities include Pattern Construction on the DAS-II (Elliott, 2007), Triangles on the KABC-II (Kaufman & Kaufman, 2004a), Block Design and

TABLE 33.3. Visual-Perceptual, Visual–Spatial, and Visual–Constructional Processes Measured on Traditional Neuropsychological Tests and Current Tests of Cognitive Abilities

Neuropsychological construct(s)	Traditional, europsychological measures	Examples of neuropsychological measures in tests of cognitive abilities
	Visual perception with motor response	
Visual–motor three-dimensional constructions	NEPSY-II: Block Construction (total)	DAS-II: Pattern Construction KABC-II: Triangles WISC-IV: Block Design and Block Design—No Time Bonus WISC-IV Integrated: Block Design Process Approach
Visual planning and organization	NEPSY-II: Route Finding Porteus Maze Test	WISC-IV Integrated: Elithorn Mazes
	Visual perception (motor-free)	
Part-to-whole analysis–synthesis and visual Gestalt closure	Hooper Visual Organization Test	KABC-II: Gestalt Closure RIAS: What's Missing WISC-IV: Picture Completion WISC-IV Integrated: Block Design Multiple Choice and Block Design Multiple Choice—No Time Bonus WJ III DS: Visual Closure
Recognizing spatial configurations	NEPSY-II: Arrows Total, Geometric Puzzles, and Picture Puzzles	DAS-II: Matching Letter-Like Forms KABC-II: Block Counting WJ III COG NU: Spatial Relations WJ III DS: Block Rotation
	Visual scanning/tracking	
Visual scanning/ tracking	D-KEFS: Trail Making—Condition 1 NEPSY-II: Picture Puzzles	WISC-IV: Cancellation, Coding, and Symbol Search

Block Design—No Time Bonus on the WISC-IV (Wechsler, 2003), and Block Design Process Approach on the WISC-IV Integrated (Wechsler et al., 2004).

The Porteus Maze Test (Porteus, 1965) is a classic neuropsychological test designed to assess visual planning, route finding, and visual–motor control. A more contemporary neuropsychological measure of visual planning and organization is the Route Finding test from the NEPSY-II (Korkman et al., 2007). Only one test of cognitive abilities, the WISC-IV Integrated (Wechsler et al., 2004) has a task, the Elithorn Mazes, that requires visual planning and organization.

Visual Perception (Motor-Free)

For the purposes of this discussion, motor-free visual-perceptual tasks are divided into two groups based on the neurocognitive demands of the task: (1) tasks requiring part-to-whole analysis–synthesis or visual Gestalt closure, and (2) tasks requiring recognition of spatial configurations (see Table 33.3). These two sets of neurocognitive constructs are shared between neuropsychological measures and tests of cognitive abilities.

The Hooper Visual Organization Test (HVOT; Hooper, 1958) is a classic neuropsychological test designed to measure visual analysis and synthesis, conceptual reorganization, and mental rotation. The HVOT consists of a set of line drawings of familiar objects that have been divided into fragments. The examinee is asked to reassemble the fragments mentally and then name the object. Tests of cognitive abilities designed to measure similar neurocognitive constructs include Gestalt Closure from the KABC-II (Kaufman & Kaufman, 2004); What's Missing from the Reynolds

Intellectual Assessment Scale (RIAS; Reynolds & Kamphaus, 2003); Picture Completion from the WISC-IV (Wechsler, 2003); the Block Design Multiple Choice and Block Design Multiple Choice—No Time Bonus from the WISC-IV Integrated (Wechsler et al., 2004); and Visual Closure from the WJ III Diagnostic Supplement (WJ III DS; Woodcock, McGrew, Mather, & Schrank, 2003, 2007).

The second neurocognitive construct shared between neuropsychological measures and tests of cognitive abilities is the recognition of spatial configurations. An example of a neuropsychological test that measures the recognition of spatial configurations is the Arrows test from the NEPSY-II (Korkman et al., 2007). Tests of cognitive abilities that measure this same construct include Matching Letter-Like Forms from the DAS-II (Elliott, 2007); Block Counting from the KABC-II (Kaufman & Kaufman, 2004a); Spatial Relations from the WJ III COG NU (Woodcock et al., 2001b, 2007b); and Block Rotation from the WJ III DS (Woodcock et al., 2003, 2007).

Visual Scanning/Tracking

There are few tests that directly measure visual scanning or tracking (see Table 33.3). The first condition of the D-KEFS Trail Making test requires the examinee to visually scan and identify as many numeral 3's on a page as quickly as possible. Other tests require visual scanning or tracking, which is a secondary neurocognitive construct rather than what the test is principally designed to measure. For example, the Picture Puzzles test on the NEPSY-II (Korkman et al., 2007) requires visual scanning, but is principally measuring visual discrimination and spatial localization. Likewise, tests of cognitive abilities such as Cancellation, Coding, and Symbol Search on the WISC-IV (Wechsler, 2003) and Visual Matching, Decision Speed, Pair Cancellation, and Cross Out from the WJ III batteries (Woodcock et al., 2001b, 2007b; 2003, 2007), which are designed principally to measure processing speed, also secondarily require visual scanning for successful performance.

Language Functions

The SNP model (Miller, 2007, 2010) classifies language functions assessed on neuropsychological and cognitive abilities measures into three broad categories: (1) auditory/phonological processing, (2) expressive language or oral expression, and (3) receptive language or listening comprehension (see Table 33.4). It is recognized that other language functions, such as pragmatics, semantics, and prosody of speech, are typically included in test batteries administered by speech–language pathologists.

Auditory/Phonological Processing

Within the auditory/phonological processing category, there are two traditional neuropsychological tests designed to measure basic auditory discrimination skills: the Seashore Rhythm Test from the Halstead–Reitan Neuropsychological Test Battery (Reitan & Wolfson, 1985) and the Wepman's Auditory Discrimination Test (Wepman & Reynolds, 1986) (see Table 33.4). The Sounds Patterns—Voice and Sound Patterns—Music tests on the WJ III DS (Woodcock et al., 2003, 2007) are also designed to measure basic auditory discrimination skills. The WJ III ACH NU battery (Woodcock et al., 2001a, 2007a), the companion instrument to the WJ III COG NU, also has a Sound Awareness test that measures auditory discrimination skills.

The Phonological Processing test on the NEPSY-II (Korkman et al., 2007) is a contemporary neuropsychological measure of both higher-order phonemic awareness and phonemic manipulation (e.g., blending or deleted sounds). Tests of cognitive abilities that measure this same auditory processing construct include Phonological Processing on the DAS-II (Elliott, 2007) and Incomplete Words and Sound Blending on the WJ III COG NU (Woodcock et al., 2001b, 2007b).

Oral Expression

The oral expression skills assessed on neuropsychological and cognitive abilities measures can be subdivided into three types of tasks: those requiring (1) oral–motor production, (2) word knowledge, or (3) verbal fluency. Oral–motor production is typically assessed by having an examinee repeat "tongue-twister" sentences or nonsense words rapidly (see Table 33.4). Two contemporary neuropsychological measures of oral–motor production are found on the NEPSY-II (Korkman et al., 2007): Oral Motor Sequences and Repetition of Nonsense Words. The Sentence Repetition and Speech Rate tests on the CAS (Naglieri & Das, 1997) are the only two tests within the major batteries of cognitive abilities that measure oral–motor production.

TABLE 33.4. Language Functions Measured on Traditional Neuropsychological Tests and Current Tests of Cognitive Abilities

Neuropsychological construct(s)	Traditional neuropsychological measures	Examples of neuropsychological measures in tests of cognitive abilities
	Auditory/phonological processing	
Auditory discrimination	Seashore Rhythm Test Wepman's Auditory Discrimination Test	WJ III ACH NU: Sound Awareness WJ III DS: Sound Patterns—Voice and Sound Patterns—Music
Auditory processing	NEPSY-II: Phonological Processing	DAS-II: Phonological Processing WJ III COG NU: Incomplete Words and Sound Blending
	Oral expression	
Oral–motor production	NEPSY-II: Oral Motor Sequences and Repetition of Nonsense Words	CAS: Sentence Repetition and Speech Rate
Word knowledge	NEPSY-II: Body Part Naming Test of Word Knowledge	DAS-II: Naming Vocabulary and Word Definitions KABC-II: Expressive Vocabulary WISC-IV: Vocabulary WISC-IV Integrated: Vocabulary Multiple Choice and Picture Vocabulary Multiple Choice
Verbal fluency	Boston Naming Test—Second Edition D-KEFS: Color–Word Interference—Condition 1 (Color Naming) and Condition 2 (Word Naming) NEPSY-II: Inhibition (Naming Condition) and Speeded Naming Rapid Automatized Naming and Rapid Alternating Stimulus	DAS-II: Rapid Naming KTEA-II: Naming Facility (RAN) WJ III COG NU: Rapid Picture Naming
	Receptive language (listening comprehension)	
Receptive language	NEPSY-II: Body Part Identification and Comprehension of Instructions Peabody Picture Vocabulary Test—Fourth Edition Receptive One-Word Picture Vocabulary Test Revised Token Test Token Test for Children—Second Edition	CAS: Verbal–Spatial Relations and Sentence Questions DAS-II: Verbal Comprehension

The Body Part Naming test on the NEPSY-II (Korkman et al., 2007) and the Test of Word Knowledge (Wiig & Secord, 1992) are neuropsychological tests designed to measure the construct of word knowledge, or the ability to know the meaning of words. Counterparts on tests of cognitive functioning include Naming Vocabulary and Word Definitions on the DAS-II (Elliott, 2007), Expressive Vocabulary on the KABC-II (Kaufman & Kaufman, 2004), Vocabulary on the WISC-IV (Wechsler, 2003), and Vocabulary Multiple Choice

and Picture Vocabulary Multiple Choice on the WISC-IV Integrated (Wechsler et al., 2004).

Verbal fluency is a neurocognitive construct that is included in both neuropsychological tests and tests of cognitive abilities. Neuropsychological measures of verbal fluency include the Boston Naming Test—Second Edition (Kaplan, Goodglass, & Weintraub, 1983), the Rapid Automatized Naming and Rapid Alternating Stimulus tests (Wolf & Denckla, 2005), the Color–Word Interference tests (Color Naming and Word Naming) on the D-KEFS (Delis et al., 2001), and the Inhibition (Naming Condition) and Speeded Naming tests on the NEPSY-II (Korkman et al., 2007). Tests of cognitive abilities that are designed to measure verbal fluency include Rapid Naming on the DAS-II (Elliott, 2007), Naming Facility (RAN) on the KTEA II (Kaufman & Kaufman, 2004b), and Rapid Picture Naming on the WJ III COG NU (Woodcock et al., 2001b, 2007b).

Receptive Language

Receptive language tests may also be referred to as tests of listening comprehension. A list of receptive language tests found on both neuropsychological tests and tests of cognitive abilities is presented in Table 33.4. The classic neuropsychological test designed to measure receptive language skills is the Token Test (DeRenzi & Vignolo, 1978; McGhee, Ehrler, & DiSimoni, 2007). The Token Test requires the examinee to listen to increasingly long and complex verbal directions that request specific interaction with the colored tokens (e.g., "Point to the blue one to the right of the first yellow one in the top row"). A contemporary neuropsychological measure of receptive language skills, modeled after the Token Test, is the Comprehension of Instructions test on the NEPSY-II (Korkman et al., 2007). Two additional receptive language tests that were developed in educational practice, but are used by both neuropsychologists and assessment specialists in the schools, are the Peabody Picture Vocabulary Test—Fourth Edition (Dunn & Dunn, 2006) and the Receptive One-Word Picture Vocabulary Test (Brownell, 2000). The major tests of cognitive abilities that include measures of receptive language are the Verbal–Spatial Relations and Sentence Questions tests on the CAS (Naglieri & Das, 1997) and the Verbal Comprehension test on the DAS-II (Elliott, 2007). Most frequently, measures of receptive and expressive language are found on tests of achievement or speech and language batteries.

Learning and Memory

Learning and memory tasks have been classified in many ways. Conceptualizations of memory and learning have recently been shifting away from traditional information-processing models to models based on neuroscience. The SNP model (Miller, 2007, 2010) classifies tests of memory and learning from neuropsychological tests and cognitive measures into five broad categories: (1) rate

of learning, (2) immediate memory, (3) delayed recall and recognition, (4) working memory, and (5) semantic memory (see Figure 33.1). The first four memory and learning constructs are shared between neuropsychological tests and tests of cognitive abilities. The fifth classification of memory and learning, semantic memory, is defined as the wealth of encyclopedic knowledge readily available for recall. However, since semantic memory relates more to areas of academic achievement, it is not commonly measured on neuropsychological tests; rather, it is uniquely measured on tests of cognitive abilities and tests of achievement.

Rate of Learning

Rate of learning is measured by the change in the number of correctly recalled words from a fixed list of words repeated over multiple trials. The major tests of cognitive abilities do not include tests that are designed to measure rate of learning. However, several neuropsychological batteries or comprehensive tests of memory and learning provide assessments of rate of learning. Examples include the Word Pairs—Learning and Word Lists—Learning scores from the CMS (Cohen, 1997), the List Memory Learning Effect score from the NEPSY-II (Korkman et al., 2007), and the Word Selective Reminding score from the TOMAL-2 (Reynolds & Voress, 2007). The California Verbal Learning Test—Children's Version (Delis, Kramer, Kaplan, & Ober, 1994) is a targeted rate-of-learning measure that is often administered by both neuropsychologists and school psychologists.

Immediate Memory

Immediate memory can be further subdivided according to the neurocognitive demands of a particular task. The first subdivision of immediate memory tasks takes into consideration the sensory input modality required to complete the task. As a result, immediate memory tasks can be subdivided into verbal immediate memory, visual immediate memory, and verbal–visual associative memory categories. In addition, the verbal and visual immediate memory tasks can be further subdivided according to the use of contextual cues (see Figure 33.3). For example, a simple memory-for-digits task is a verbal immediate memory task without contextual cues, whereas a memory-for-stories task is a verbal immediate memory task with contextual cues.

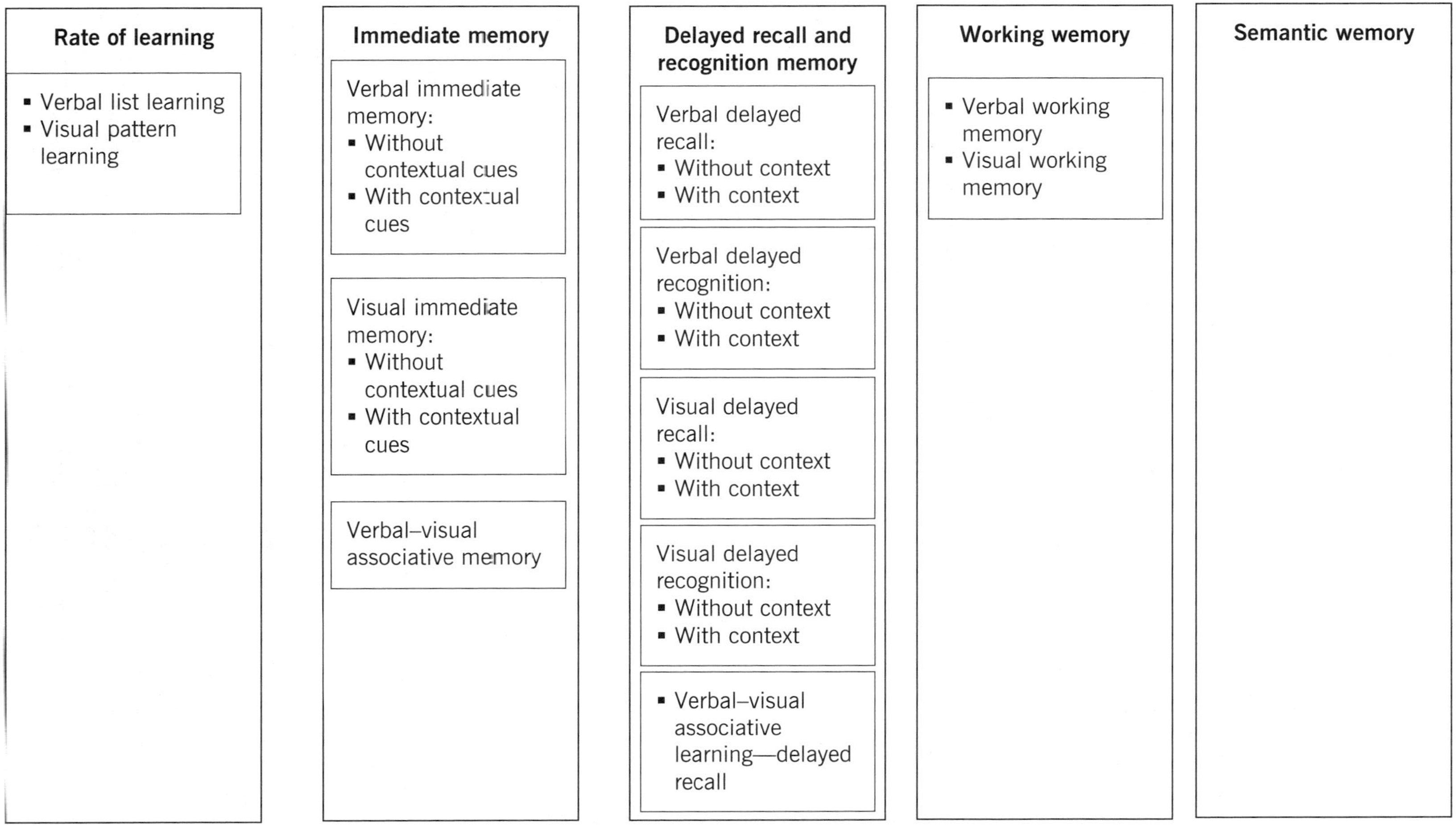

Rate of learning

- Verbal list learning
- Visual pattern learning

Immediate memory

Verbal immediate memory:
- Without contextual cues
- With contextual cues

Visual immediate memory:
- Without contextual cues
- With contextual cues

Verbal–visual associative memory

Delayed recall and recognition memory

Verbal delayed recall:
- Without context
- With context

Verbal delayed recognition:
- Without context
- With context

Visual delayed recall:
- Without context
- With context

Visual delayed recognition:
- Without context
- With context

Verbal–visual associative learning—delayed recall

Working memory

- Verbal working memory
- Visual working memory

Semantic memory

FIGURE 33.3. Subcomponents of learning and memory.

Verbal Immediate Memory with No Contextual Cues

Verbal immediate memory tasks with no contextual cues are common to both neuropsychological tests and tests of cognitive abilities (see Table 33.5). Strings of numbers, letters, or unrelated words are often used as stimuli in these types of tasks, and the examinee is asked to recall increasingly long spans of stimuli. Neuropsychological measures of verbal immediate memory that do not include contextual cues include Word Lists—Immediate Recall and Word Pairs—Immediate Recall on the CMS (Cohen, 1997); Word List Interference—Repetition on the NEPSY-II (Korkman et al., 2007); and Digits Forward, Letters Forward, and Word Selective Reminding on the TOMAL-2 (Reynolds & Voress, 2007).

The major tests of cognitive abilities that include measures of verbal immediate memory tasks without contextual cues are Word Series on the CAS (Naglieri & Das, 1997); Recall of Digits—Forward on the DAS-II (Elliott, 2007); Number Recall, Word Order, and Word Order (without color interference) on the KABC-II (Kaufman & Kaufman, 2004a); Digit Span—Forward on the WISC-IV (Wechsler, 2003); and Letter Span on the WISC-IV Integrated (Wechsler et al., 2004).

Verbal Immediate Memory with Contextual Cues

Verbal immediate memory tasks with contextual cues are also found on neuropsychological tests and tests of cognitive abilities, but to a lesser degree than the verbal immediate memory tasks without contextual cues (see Table 33.5). Sentences of increasing length and stories with increasing complexity are used as stimuli in these types of tasks. Neuropsychological measures of verbal immediate memory tests that include contextual cues are Stories—Immediate Recall on the CMS (Cohen, 1997), Narrative Memory and Sentence Repetition on the NEPSY-II (Korkman et al., 2007), Memory for Stories on the TOMAL-2 (Reynolds & Voress, 2007), and Sentence Memory and Story Memory on the WRAML2 (Sheslow & Adams, 2003).

Two major tests of cognitive abilities that include a measure of verbal immediate memory with added contextual cues are the Verbal Memory test on the RIAS (Reynolds & Kamphaus, 2003) and the Memory for Sentences test on the WJ III DS (Woodcock et al., 2003, 2007). The WJ III ACH NU (Woodcock et al., 2001a, 2007a), the compan-

ion instrument to the WJ III COG NU, also has a Story Recall test that measures verbal immediate memory with added contextual cues.

Visual Immediate Memory with No Contextual Cues

The types of stimuli used for visual immediate memory tasks with no contextual cues vary, but can include abstract designs, faces, objects, or pictures (see Table 33.5). Examinees are typically shown visual stimuli for a brief exposure and then asked to motorically reproduce the details of what was seen, or are asked to match, nonverbally or verbally, a newly presented visual stimulus with what was previously seen.

Neuropsychological tests that require visual immediate memory for abstract designs include Memory for Designs on the NEPSY-II (Korkman et al., 2007), Abstract Visual Memory and Visual Sequential Memory on the TOMAL-2 (Reynolds & Voress, 2007), and Design Memory on the WRAML2 (Sheslow & Adams, 2003). Tests of cognitive abilities that measure a comparable construct include Figure Memory on the CAS (Naglieri & Das, 1997) and Recall of Designs on the DAS-II (Elliott, 2007).

Neuropsychological tests requiring visual immediate memory for numbers, faces, objects, or pictures (see Table 33.5) include Faces—Immediate Recall on the CMS (Cohen, 1997), Memory for Faces—Immediate Recall on the NEPSY-II (Korkman et al., 2007), and Facial Memory on the TOMAL-2 (Reynolds & Voress, 2007). The major tests of cognitive abilities that include visual immediate memory for numbers, faces, objects, or pictures are Recognition of Pictures on the DAS-II (Elliott, 2007), Face Recognition on the KABC-II (Kaufman & Kaufman, 2004a), Nonverbal Memory on the RIAS (Reynolds & Kamphaus, 2003), Object Memory on the Universal Nonverbal Intelligence Test (UNIT; Bracken & McCallum, 1998), Coding Recall and Visual Digit Span on the WISC-IV Integrated (Wechsler et al., 2004), and Picture Recognition on the WJ III COG NU (Woodcock et al., 2001b, 2007b).

Neuropsychological tests requiring visual immediate memory for spatial locations (see Table 33.5) include Dot Location—Immediate Recall on the CMS (Cohen, 1997) and the Memory for Locations and Visual Selective Reminding tests on the TOMAL-2 (Reynolds & Voress, 2007). The major tests of cognitive abilities that include visual immediate memory for spatial locations are Spatial

TABLE 33.5. Learning and Memory Functions Measured on Traditional Neuropsychological Tests and Current Tests of Cognitive Abilities

Neuropsychological construct(s)	Traditional neuropsychological measures	Examples of neuropsychological measures in tests of cognitive abilities
	Immediate memory	
Verbal immediate memory for numbers, letters, or words (no contextual cues)	CMS: Word Lists—Immediate Recall and Word Pairs—Immediate Recall NEPSY-II: Word List—Interference Repetition TOMAL-2: Digits Forward, Letters Forward, and Word Selective Reminding	CAS: Word Series DAS-II: Recall of Digits—Forward KABC-II: Number Recall, Word Order, and Word Order (without color interference) WISC-IV: Digit Span—Forward WISC-IV Integrated: Letter Span WJ III COG NU: Memory for Words
Verbal immediate memory for sentences or stories	CMS: Stories—Immediate Recall NEPSY-II: Narrative Memory and Sentence Repetition TOMAL-2: Memory for Stories WRAML2: Sentence Memory and Story Memory	RIAS: Verbal Memory WJ III ACH NU: Story Recall WJ III DS: Memory for Sentences
Visual immediate memory for abstract designs	NEPSY-II: Memory for Designs TOMAL-2: Abstract Visual Memory and Visual Sequential Memory WRAML2: Design Memory	CAS: Figure Memory DAS-II: Recall of Designs
Visual immediate memory for numbers, faces, objects, or pictures	CMS: Faces—Immediate Recall NEPSY-II: Memory for Faces—Immediate Recall TOMAL-2: Facial Memory	DAS-II: Recognition of Pictures KABC-II: Face Recognition RIAS: Nonverbal Memory UNIT: Object Memory WISC-IV Integrated: Coding Recall and Visual Digit Span WJ III COG NU: Picture Recognition
Visual immediate memory for spatial locations	CMS: Dot Locations—Immediate Recall TOMAL-2: Memory for Locations and Visual Selective Reminding	UNIT: Spatial Memory WISC-IV Integrated: Spatial Span—Forward
Visual immediate memory with contextual cues	CMS: Family Pictures—Immediate Recall WRAML2: Picture Memory	UNIT: Symbolic Memory
Verbal–visual associative learning	NEPSY-II: Memory for Names—Immediate Recall TOMAL-2: Object Recall and Paired Recall WRAML2: Sound–Symbol	DAS-II: Recall of Objects—Immediate KABC-II: Atlantis and Rebus WJ III COG NU: Visual–Auditory Learning WJ III DS: Memory for Names
	Delayed recall and recognition	
Verbal–visual associative delayed recall	NEPSY-II: Memory for Names—Delayed Recall WRAML2: Sound–Symbol—Delayed	DAS-II: Recall of Object—Delayed KABC-II: Atlantis—Delayed and Rebus—Delayed WJ III COG NU: Visual–Auditory Learning—Delayed WJ III DS: Memory for Names—Delayed

(cont.)

TABLE 33.5. *(cont.)*

Neuropsychological construct(s)	Traditional neuropsychological measures	Examples of neuropsychological measures in tests of cognitive abilities
	<u>Working memory</u>	
Verbal working memory	CMS: Numbers Backwards and Sequences NEPSY-II: Word List Interference—Recall TOMAL-2: Digits Backwards and Letters Backwards WRAML2: Verbal Working Memory	DAS-II: Recall of Digits—Backward and Recall of Sequential Order KABC-II: Word Order (with color interference effect) SB5: Verbal Working Memory WISC-IV: Arithmetic, Digit Span—Backward, and Letter–Number Sequencing WISC-IV Integrated: Letter–Number Sequencing Process Approach WJ III COG NU: Auditory Working Memory and Numbers Reversed
Visual working memory	WRAML2: Symbolic Working Memory	SB5: Nonverbal Working Memory WISC-IV Integrated: Spatial Span—Backward

Memory on the UNIT (Bracken & McCallum, 1998) and Spatial Span—Forward on the WISC-IV Integrated (Wechsler et al., 2004).

Visual Immediate Memory with Contextual Cues

There are only a few neuropsychological and cognitive tests designed to measure visual immediate memory with added contextual cues. Neuropsychological measures requiring visual immediate memory with added contextual cues include Family Pictures—Immediate Recall on the CMS (Cohen, 1997) and Picture Memory on the WRAML2 (Sheslow & Adams, 2003). The Symbolic Memory test on the UNIT (Bracken & McCallum, 1998) is the only test on a major cognitive test battery to measure visual immediate memory with added contextual cues.

Verbal–Visual Associative Learning

Verbal–visual associative learning tasks have been included on both neuropsychological and cognitive abilities tests in the past decade. Each of the tasks requires the examinee to learn to associate a verbal label with either a picture, object, symbol, or face, often with corrective feedback. Neuropsychological tests requiring verbal–visual associative learning (see Table 33.5) include Memory for Names—Immediate Recall on the NEPSY-II (Korkman et al., 2007), Object Recall and Paired

Recall on the TOMAL-2 (Reynolds & Voress, 2007), and Sound–Symbol on the WRAML2 (Sheslow & Adams, 2003). The major tests of cognitive abilities designed to measure verbal–visual associative learning include Recall of Objects—Immediate on the DAS-II (Elliott, 2007), Atlantis and Rebus on the KABC-II (Kaufman & Kaufman, 2004), Visual–Auditory Learning on the WJ III COG NU (Woodcock et al., 2001b, 2007b), and Memory for Names on the WJ III DS (Woodcock et al., 2003, 2007).

Delayed Recall and Recognition

Tests of cognitive abilities do not typically include measures of delayed recall or recognition. A clinician who needs to assess delayed recall or recognition will need to use stand-alone tests of memory and learning (e.g., the WRAML2, TOMAL-2, or CMS) or the Memory and Learning tests from the NEPSY-II (Korkman et al., 2007).

Verbal–Visual Associative Delayed Recall

All of the verbal–visual associative learning tests mentioned in the section on verbal–visual associative learning, except for the Object Recall and Paired Recall tests on the TOMAL-2 (Reynolds & Voress, 2007), have a delayed-recall portion of their tests (see Table 33.5). The purpose of these tests is to assess long-term memory, or the degree of consolidation, for paired verbal–visual stimuli.

Working Memory

Working memory can be assessed according to the input modality, verbal or visual. Table 33.5 presents examples of tests designed to measure verbal working memory included in neuropsychological batteries (e.g., the NEPSY-II) or tests of memory and learning (e.g., the CMS, TOMAL-2, or WRAML2). All of these measures have in common the neurocognitive processing demand of active manipulation of information in immediate memory, which is the core requirement of a working memory task. An example of a working memory task is recalling a string of numbers or letters in reverse order after hearing them presented sequentially.

The major tests of cognitive abilities that include verbal working memory tests are Recall of Digits—Backward and Recall of Sequential Order on the DAS-II (Elliott, 2007); Word Order (with color interference effect) on the KABC-II (Kaufman & Kaufman, 2004a); Verbal Working Memory on the SB5 (Roid, 2003); Arithmetic, Digit Span—Backward, and Letter–Number Sequencing on the WISC-IV (Wechsler, 2003); Letter–Number Sequencing Process Approach on the WISC-IV Integrated (Wechsler et al., 2004); and Auditory Working Memory and Numbers Reversed on the WJ III COG NU (Woodcock et al., 2001b, 2007b).

There are very few tests designed to measure visual working memory. The WRAML2 provides a measure of visual working memory with its Symbolic Working Memory subtest (Sheslow & Adams, 2003). Two tests of cognitive abilities that include tasks designed to measure visual working memory are the Nonverbal Working Memory test on the SB5 (Roid, 2003) and the Spatial Span—Backward test on the WISC-IV Integrated (Wechsler et al., 2004).

Executive Functions

Among all neurocognitive constructs, the construct of executive functions has generated the most attention, interest, and research. Practitioners and researchers often equate executive functions with intelligence (Blair, 2006; Friedman et al., 2006). As a result, test publishers have included a broad array of executive function tasks on the major tests of cognitive abilities.

However, Maricle, Johnson, and Avirett (2010) point out that there is not "a mutually agreed upon list of cognitive components which comprise executive functions" (pp. 599–600). The SNP model (Miller, 2007, 2010) classifies tests of executive functions from neuropsychological and cognitive measures into four broad categories: (1) concept recognition and generation; (2) problem solving, cognitive flexibility, reasoning, and planning; (3) retrieval fluency; and (4) response inhibition (see Figure 33.1).

Concept Recognition and Generation

Concept recognition or generation tasks typically require the examinee to classify objects or pictures into groups that share a common attribute (e.g., same color or shape). The goal of these tasks is to identify as many classifications as possible; this requires divergent thinking and concept formation. Neuropsychological tests requiring concept recognition or generation (see Table 33.6) include Sorting and Twenty Questions on the D-KEFS (Delis et al., 2001) and Animal Sorting on the NEPSY-II (Korkman et al., 2007). Tests of cognitive abilities that include measures of concept recognition or generation are Picture Similarities and Verbal Similarities on the DAS-II (Elliott, 2007), Similarities on the WISC-IV (Wechsler, 2003), and Similarities Multiple Choice on the WISC-IV Integrated (Wechsler et al., 2004).

Problem Solving, Cognitive Flexibility, Reasoning, and Planning

Despite the multiple classification schemas developed for executive functions, most researchers and theorists agree that executive functions include measures of problem solving, cognitive flexibility, reasoning, and planning. Classic neuropsychological tests requiring the executive functions of cognitive flexibility or set shifting (see Table 33.6) include the Halstead–Reitan Category Test (Reitan & Davidson, 1974) and the Wisconsin Card Sorting Test (Grant & Berg, 1993). More recent neuropsychological tests measuring cognitive flexibility, set shifting, or response inhibition include Tower, Color Word Interference—Condition 4 (Switching), Proverbs, Verbal Fluency—Condition 3 (Switching), and Word Context on the D-KEFS (Delis et al., 2001), and Clocks and Inhibition (Switching Condition) on the NEPSY-II (Korkman et al., 2007).

TABLE 33.6. Executive Functions Measured on Traditional Neuropsychological Tests and Current Tests of Cognitive Abilities

Neuropsychological construct(s)	Traditional neuropsychological measures	Examples of neuropsychological measures in tests of cognitive abilities
Concept recognition and generation	D-KEFS: Sorting and Twenty Questions NEPSY-II: Animal Sorting	DAS-II: Picture Similarities and Verbal Similarities WISC-IV: Similarities WISC-IV Integrated: Similarities Multiple Choice
Problem solving, cognitive flexibility, reasoning, and planning	D-KEFS: Tower, Color Word Interference— Condition 4, Proverbs, Verbal Fluency— Condition 3, and Word Context Halstead–Reitan Category Test NEPSY-II: Clocks and Inhibition (Switching Condition) Wisconsin Card Sorting Test	CAS: Matching Numbers, Nonverbal Matrices, Planned Codes, and Planned Connections DAS-II: Matrices, and Sequential and Quantitative Reasoning KABC-II: Pattern Reasoning, Rover, and Story Completion RIAS: Guess What, Odd-Item Out, and Verbal Reasoning UNIT: Analogic Reasoning, Cube Design, and Mazes WJ III COG NU: Concept Formation and Analysis–Synthesis WISC-IV: Matrix Reasoning and Picture Concepts WISC-IV Integrated: Elithorn Mazes
Retrieval fluency	D-KEFS: Verbal Fluency and Design Fluency NEPSY-II: Design Fluency and Word Generation	WJ III COG NU: Retrieval Fluency
Response inhibition	D-KEFS: Color-Word Test—Condition 3 (Inhibition) NEPSY-II: Inhibition—Condition 2 and Statue Stroop Color–Word Test	CAS: Expressive Attention

Tests of cognitive abilities that are designed to measure similar executive function constructs are Matching Numbers, Nonverbal Matrices, Planned Codes, and Planned Connections on the CAS (Naglieri & Das, 1997); Matrices, and Sequential and Quantitative Reasoning, on the DAS-II (Elliott, 2007); Pattern Reasoning, Rover, and Story Completion on the KABC-II (Kaufman & Kaufman, 2004a); Guess What, Odd-Item Out, and Verbal Reasoning on the RIAS (Reynolds & Kamphaus, 2003); Analogic Reasoning, Cube Design, and Mazes on the UNIT (Bracken & McCallum, 1998); Concept Formation and Analysis–Synthesis on the WJ III COG NU (Woodcock et al., 2001b, 2007b); Matrix Reasoning and Picture Concepts on the WISC-IV (Wechsler, 2003); and Similarities Multiple Choice on the WISC-IV Integrated (Wechsler et al., 2004).

Retrieval Fluency

Retrieval fluency is the ability to recall information quickly and accurately from long-term memory. Miller (2007, 2010) has stated that the efficiency of the retrieval strategies is what makes retrieval fluency an executive function, rather than just a measure of long-term memory. On neuropsychological tests, retrieval fluency is measured by using either verbal or nonverbal stimuli. Typically, verbal retrieval fluency tasks require the examinee to recall words that start with a particular letter or fit within a specific semantic category (e.g., food, pieces of furniture); nonverbal fluency tests usually require the examinee to quickly generate unique designs or patterns, using structured or unstructured visual arrays.

The neuropsychological tests that measure verbal retrieval fluency are Verbal Fluency on the D-

KEFS (Delis et al., 2001) and Word Generation on the NEPSY-II (Korkman et al., 2007) (see Table 33.6). Nonverbal retrieval fluency measures include a Design Fluency test on both the D-KEFS and the NEPSY-II. The only test of cognitive abilities with a measure of retrieval fluency is the WJ III COG NU (Woodcock et al., 2001b, 2007b).

Response Inhibition

Response inhibition is "the ability to not respond to distracter stimuli while focusing on target stimuli" (Miller, 2007, p. 245). Response inhibition tasks typically involve the ability to inhibit a response after a particular response set has been established. For example, in the classic Stroop test, the examinee is asked to name the color of the ink a color word (e.g., *red*, *green*, or *blue*) is printed in, rather than reading the word itself.

The neuropsychological tests designed to measure response inhibition are Color Word Test—Condition 3 (Inhibition) on the D-KEFS (Delis et al., 2001); the Inhibition—Condition 2 (Inhibition) and Statue tests on the NEPSY-II (Korkman et al., 2007); and the numerous versions of the Stroop Color–Word Test (e.g., Golden & Freshwater, 2002). The only measure of cognitive abilities that includes a response inhibition task is Expressive Attention on the CAS (Naglieri & Das, 1997), which is modeled after the Stroop test.

CONCLUSIONS AND FUTURE DIRECTIONS

The major premise of this chapter—that the integration of neurocognitive constructs into tests of cognitive ability is somehow new or emerging—is actually false. In fact, many of these neurocognitive constructs have been found all along in tests of cognitive abilities. Early researchers in cognitive assessment (e.g., Binet, Norsworthy, Terman, and Wechsler) were interested in measuring such cognitive constructs as processing speed, memory, or executive functions, but advances in psychometrics and test development led to an emphasis on empirical measurement within the field of cognitive assessment. As a result, there was an interpretive overemphasis on a singular global score as the best measure of intellectual functioning or the best predictor of academic achievement. Other developments within the field of psychology were also influential in the evolution of cognitive assessment. For example, as psychology moved away

from the medical model, training programs in school, counseling, and clinical psychology gave less emphasis to the biological bases of behavior. For the most part, training programs in neuropsychology were the exceptions in this particular trend. In addition, as a result of the natural expansion in the knowledge base within the field (as well as a certain amount of territorialism/protectionism), psychology became more specialized or fractured, and the transfer of knowledge between related disciplines became less common. In cognitive assessment, this led to a narrow lens through which cognitive abilities were viewed and interpreted.

In actuality, there is far more integration between the disciplines of neuropsychology and cognitive assessment than many professionals realize. For example, many current tests of cognitive abilities are composed of tasks that measure commonly identified neurocognitive constructs. In addition, current trends in interpretation of intellectual abilities are more theoretically driven than in the past and are being influenced by research on cognitive constructs of intelligence, which lends itself to a common nomenclature with the field of neuropsychology. Finally, the surge of interest in the neurosciences resulting from remarkable findings in brain science has generated a corresponding surge of research in the applicability of neuropsychology to cognitive assessment, bringing the field back to its historical origins.

In order to progress as a discipline, the next major advance in the integration of neuroscience and cognitive assessment has to be the use of neuroimaging techniques to validate associations between cognitive constructs and neurological functioning or brain structure, and then to validate the applicability of the various tasks or subtests being used to measure these neurocognitive constructs. This research should lead to more definitive conclusions about the connection between theoretical cognitive constructs and actual brain functioning, as well as to better identification of neurocognitive deficits with more targeted and applicable measures. Assessing neurocognitive functioning more accurately and parsimoniously should ideally lead to greater applicability for recommendations and interventions to address the manifestation of neurocognitive deficits in real-world settings.

In the meantime, best practice in assessment would suggest that individuals conducting cognitive and neurocognitive assessments need to (1) realize that current cognitive instruments are limited in their comprehensiveness, measuring only limited aspects of cognitive or neurocognitive constructs, and interpret them with this in mind; (2) understand that current cognitive instruments are best used as screeners for neurocognitive functioning, and that further assessment with more targeted measures (in the use of which they must be trained) may be required in the presence of suspected neurocognitive deficits; (3) recognize that a strong foundation or knowledge base in the neurosciences is necessary to use and interpret cognitive measures correctly from a neuropsychological perspective; and (4) appreciate the need for a theoretically based interpretive framework (Luria's theory, CHC theory, SNP model, Flanagan et al.'s integrative interpretive model) within which to draw their conclusions.

The disciplines of cognitive assessment and neuropsychology have been, are, and will continue to be intertwined. Cognition, by definition, is brain-based; therefore, the assessment of cognition needs to be a brain-based endeavor. As the 21st century progresses, these two fields will evolve together, and perhaps psychologists in the future will express surprise that they were ever considered separate fields of study.

REFERENCES

Arthur, G. (1947). *A point scale of performance tests (Rev. Form II)*. New York: Psychological Corporation.

Baron, I. S. (2004). *Neuropsychological evaluation of the child*. New York: Oxford University Press.

Beery, K. E., Buktenica, N. A., & Beery, N. A. (2010). *Beery–Buktenica Developmental Test of Visual–Motor Integration, 6th Edition* Minneapolis, MN: Pearson Assessments.

Blair, C. (2006). Towards a revised theory of general intelligence: Further examination of fluid cognitive abilities as a unique aspect of human cognition. *Behavioral and Brain Sciences, 29*, 145–153.

Bracken, B. A., & McCallum, R. S. (1998). *Universal Nonverbal Intelligence Test*. Itasca, IL: Riverside.

Brickenkamp, R., & Zilmer, E. (1998). *d2—Test of Attention*. Ashland, OH: Hogrefe & Huber.

Brownell, R. (2000). *Receptive One-Word Picture Vocabulary Test*. Novato, CA: Academic Therapy.

Buchanan, R. W., & Heinrichs, D. W. (1989). The Neurological Evaluation Scale (NES): A structured instrument for the assessment of neurological signs in schizophrenia. *Psychiatry Research, 27*, 335–350.

Christensen, A.-L. (1975). *Luria's neuropsychological investigation: Text*. New York: Spectrum.

Cohen, M. J. (1997). *Children's Memory Scale*. San Antonio, TX: Psychological Corporation.

Conners, C. K., & Multi-Health Systems Staff. (2004). *Conners' Continuous Performance Test II Version 5 for Windows (CPT II V.5)*. North Tonawanda, NY: Multi-Health Systems.

Dean, R. S., & Woodcock, R. W. (2003). *Dean–Woodcock Neuropsychological Battery*. Itasca, IL: Riverside.

Decker, S., & Davis, A. (2010). Assessing and intervening with children with sensory–motor impairments. In D. C. Miller (Ed.), *Best practices in school neuropsychology: Guidelines for effective practice, assessment, and evidence-based intervention* (pp. 673–692). Hoboken, NJ: Wiley.

Delis, D., Kaplan, E., & Kramer, J. H. (2001). *Delis–Kaplan Executive Function System: Examiner's manual*. San Antonio, TX: Psychological Corporation.

Delis, D. C., Kramer, J. H., Kaplan, E., & Ober, B. A. (1994). *California Verbal Learning Test: Children's Version*. San Antonio, TX: Psychological Corporation.

DeRenzi, E., & Vignolo, L. (1978). *Revised Token Test*. Shreveport, LA: Dysphagia Plus.

Dunn, L. M., & Dunn, L. M. (2006). *Peabody Picture Vocabulary Test—Fourth Edition*. Minneapolis, MN: Pearson Assessments.

Elliott, C. D. (2007). *Differential Ability Scales—Second Edition*. San Antonio, TX: Harcourt Assessment.

Flanagan, D. P., Alfonso, V. C., Ortiz, S. O., & Dynda, A. M. (2010). Integrating cognitive assessment in school neuropsychological evaluations. In D. C. Miller (Ed.), *Best practices in school neuropsychology: Guidelines for effective practice, assessment, and evidence-based intervention* (pp. 101–140). Hoboken, NJ: Wiley.

Friedman, N. P., Miyake, A., Corley, R. P., Young, S. E., DeFries, J. C., & Hewitt, J. K. (2006). Not all executive functions are related to intelligence. *Psychological Science, 17*, 172–179.

Golden, C. J., & Freshwater, S. M. (2002). *Stroop Color–Word Test*. Odessa, FL: Psychological Assessment Resources.

Grant, D. A., & Berg, E. A. (1993). *Wisconsin Card Sorting Test: Manual*. Odessa, FL: Psychological Assessment Resources.

Hooper, H. E. (1958). *Hooper Visual Organization Test: Manual*. Los Angeles: Western Psychological Services.

Individuals with Disabilities Education Improvement Act of 2004 (IDEA 2004), Pub. L. No. 108-446, 20 U.S.C. §1400 et seq. (2004).

Kaplan, E., Fein, D., Kramer, J., Delis, D., & Morris, R. (1999). *WISC-III PI: Manual*. San Antonio, TX: Psychological Corporation.

Kaplan, E. F., Goodglass, H., & Weintraub, S. (2001).

The Boston Naming Test—Second Edition. Philadelphia: Lippincott Williams & Wilkins.

Kaufman, A. S., & Kaufman, N. L. (2004a). *Kaufman Assessment Battery for Children—Second Edition.* Circle Pines, MN: American Guidance Service.

Kaufman, A. S., & Kaufman, N. L. (2004b). *Kaufman Test of Educational Achievement—Second Edition.* Circle Pines, MN: American Guidance Service.

Knox, H. A. (1914). Mental defectives. *New York Medical Journal, 99,* 215–222.

Korkman, M., Kirk, U., & Kemp, S. (2007). *NEPSY-II: A developmental neuropsychological assessmentt.* San Antonio, TX: Harcourt Assessment.

Maricle, D. E., Johnson, W., & Avirett, E. (2010). Assessing and intervening in children with executive function disorders. In D. C. Miller (Ed.), *Best practices in school neuropsychology: Guidelines for effective practice, assessment, and evidence-based intervention* (pp. 599–640). Hoboken, NJ: Wiley.

McGhee, R. L., Ehrler, D. J., & DiSimoni, F. (2007). *Token Test for Children—Second Edition.* Austin, TX: PRO-ED.

Meyers, J. E., & Meyers, K. R. (1995). *Rey Complex Figure Test and Recognition Trial.* Odessa, FL: Psychological Assessment Resources.

Miller, D. C. (2007). *Essentials of school neuropsychological assessment.* Hoboken, NJ: Wiley.

Miller, D. C. (2010). School neuropsychological assessment and intervention. In D. C. Miller (Ed.), *Best practices in school neuropsychology: Guidelines for effective practice, assessment, and evidence-based intervention* (pp. 81–100). Hoboken, NJ: Wiley.

Milner, B. (1971). Interhemispheric differences in localization of psychological processes in man. *British Medical Bulletin, 27,* 272–277.

Naglieri, J. A., & Das, J. P. (1997). *Das–Naglieri Cognitive Assessment System.* Itasca, IL: Riverside.

Osterrieth, P. A. (1944). Le test de copie d'une figure complex: Contribution a l'étude de la perception et de la mémoire. *Archives de Psychologie, 30,* 286–356.

Porteus, S. D. (1965). *Porteus Maze Test: Fifty years' application.* New York: Psychological Corporation.

Reitan, R. M., & Davidson, L. A. (Eds.). (1974). *Clinical neuropsychology: Current status and applications.* Washington, DC: Winston.

Reitan, R. M., & Wolfson, D. (1985). *The Halstead–Reitan Neuropsychological Test Battery: Theory and clinical interpretation.* Tuscon, AZ: Neuropsychological Press.

Rey, A. (1941). L'examen psychologique data les can d'eencephalopathie traumatique. *Archives de Psychologie, 28,* 286–340.

Reynolds, C. R., & Kamphaus, R. W. (2003). *Reynolds Intellectual Assessment Scales.* Lutz. FL: Psychological Assessment Resources.

Reynolds, C. R., & Voress, J. K. (2007). *Test of Memory and Learning—Second Edition.* Austin, TX: PRO-ED.

Riccio, C. A., Reynolds, C. R., & Lowe, P. A. (2001). *Clinical applications of continuous performance tests: Measuring attention and impulsive responding in children and adolescents.* New York: Wiley.

Roid, G. H. (2003). *Stanford–Binet Intelligence Scales, Fifth Edition.* Itasca, IL: Riverside.

Ruff, R. M., & Allen, C. C. (1996). *Ruff 2 & 7 Selective Attention Test.* Odessa, FL: Psychological Assessment Resources.

Sandford, J. A., & Turner, A. (1993–2006). *Integrated Visual and Auditory Continuous Performance Test.* Richmond, VA: BrainTrain.

Sheslow, D., & Adams, W. (2003). *Wide Range Assessment of Memory and Learning—Second Edition.* Wilmington, DE: Wide Range.

Wechsler, D. (2003). *Wechsler Intelligence Scale for Children—Fourth Edition.* San Antonio, TX: Psychological Corporation.

Wechsler, D., Kaplan, E., Fein, D., Morris, E., Kramer, J. H., Maerlender, A., et al. (2004). *The Wechsler Intelligence Scale for Children—Fourth Edition Integrated: Technical and interpretative manual.* San Antonio, TX: Harcourt Assessment.

Welsh, M. C., Pennington, B. F., & Groisser, D. B. (1991). A normative-developmental study of executive function: A window on prefrontal function in children. *Developmental Neuropsychology, 7,* 131–149.

Wepman, J. M., & Reynolds, W. M. (1986). *Wepman's Auditory Discrimination Test—Second Edition.* Los Angeles: Western Psychological Services.

Wiig, E. H., & Secord, W. (1992). *Test of Word Knowledge.* San Antonio, TX: Psychological Corporation.

Wolf, M., & Denckla, M. B. (2005). *Rapid Automatized Naming and Rapid Alternating Stimulus Tests.* Austin, TX: PRO-ED.

Woodcock, R. W., McGrew, K. S., & Mather, N. (2001a, 2007a). *Woodcock–Johnson III Tests of Achievement Normative Update.* Rolling Meadows, IL: Riverside.

Woodcock, R. W., McGrew, K. S., & Mather, N. (2001b, 2007b). *Woodcock–Johnson III Tests of Cognitive Abilities Normative Update.* Rolling Meadows, IL: Riverside.

Woodcock, R. W., McGrew, K. S., Mather, N., & Schrank, F. A. (2003, 2007). *Woodcock–Johnson III Diagnostic Supplement to the Tests of Cognitive Abilities.* Rolling Meadows, IL: Riverside.

CHAPTER 34

The Role of Cognitive and Intelligence Tests in the Assessment of Executive Functions

Denise E. Maricle
Erin Avirett

The study of executive functions is a relatively new, but popular, area of research in the field of neuroscience (Ardilla, 2008). In the last 10 years there has been a proliferation of articles, books, and research about executive functions. Psychologists and other professionals have referred to "executive functions" or "executive functioning" as if it is a known, singular cognitive construct that is well understood and easily measured. In fact, despite the wealth of available information, we still know very little about executive functions.

The purpose of this chapter is to provide a review of how the major measures of intellectual functioning can be used in the assessment of executive functions. However, assessment of executive functioning involves more than just the choice of tools. In order to evaluate executive functions effectively, an understanding of how such functions are defined and conceptualized, knowledge about the neuroanatomical correlates and developmental trajectories of executive functioning, and familiarity with how executive functions are operationalized and measured is required. Therefore, a brief discussion of definitional issues, theoretical conceptualizations, and neuropsychological underpinnings is provided to assist the reader in understanding the complexity of the topic. Then each of the major instruments of broad cognitive functioning is reviewed for how it can be used in

the evaluation of executive functions. Within this chapter, the terms *executive functions*, *executive function*, and *executive functioning* are used interchangeably.

DEFINITIONAL ISSUES

The terminology for executive functions is frequently used inconsistently and interchangeably, with little understanding of, or even mutual agreement as to, what the terms actually imply. The complex reciprocal nature of executive functions makes developing a cohesive definition challenging (Maricle, Johnson, & Avirett, 2010). Researchers cannot even agree on whether executive functions are a single process, or a descriptive term for a collection of cognitive processes. In the fields of school psychology, neuropsychology, school neuropsychology, and cognitive psychology, the prevailing perspective is that executive functions consist of separate but related cognitive processes. Despite this consensus, researchers have not agreed upon the components of executive functioning, although several domains are generally accepted. These domains include self-monitoring and regulation of cognition, emotion, and behavior; initiating, planning, and completing complex tasks; working memory; attentional control (in hibition, sustained attention, shifting attention); and cognitive flexibility (Alvarez & Emory, 2006; Anderson, Levine, & Jacobs, 2002; Baron, 2004; Chan, Shum, Toulopoulou, & Chen, 2008; Cheung, Mitsis, & Halperin, 2004; Hughes & Graham, 2002; Lezak, Howieson, & Loring, 2004; Stuss & Alexander, 2000). Overall, the concept of executive functioning includes the ideas of mental flexibility, the ability to filter out interference or distractions, the ability to engage in goal-directed behavior, and the ability to anticipate the consequences of one's actions (Ardilla, 2008; Ardilla & Surlof, 2007; Knight & Stuss, 2002).

This definitional debate is not an esoteric one. How executive functions are defined is critical to the assessment process because how test authors define the construct determines how it is operationalized and thus measured in a particular instrument. It is also necessary for the examiner to define what elements or components of executive function they are interested in, since executive functioning in and of itself has not been proven conclusively to really exist. In addition, no one measure or instrument is able to evaluate all of the proposed executive functions in their entirety. Thus examiners need to know what aspects of executive functions should be measured and how the instruments or tools they have chosen actually measure these specific aspects. Finally, understanding the limitations posed by definitional differences is important when researchers and clinicians alike are reading and filtering through the wealth of literature being presented on this important topic.

THEORETICAL MODELS

The variety of current models and theories reflects diverse and disparate perspectives on the nature, structure, and role of the executive functions; however, the literature is cluttered with competing claims and datasets that are inadequate for leveraging support for any one theory or model over another. Although the structure and role of executive functions have been debated and conceptualized in a multitude of ways by numerous researchers, no clear consensus has emerged regarding a specific theory or model of executive functioning. Executive function models can be categorized according to the way they conceptualize those functions (Zelazo, Muller, Frye, & Marcovitch, 2003). Two primary perspectives dominate the literature at this time. Executive functions are considered to be either a unitary and hierarchical system with control and monitoring processes, or a set of distinct but interlocking cognitive processes.

In the hierarchical perspective, executive functions are considered a unitary construct. In this view, executive functioning is regarded as metacognitive and is frequently seen as analogous to overall intelligence (Anderson, 2008; Blair, 2006; Friedman et al., 2006; Grafman, 2006; Kane & Engle, 2002). This view depicts executive functions as the supervisor of other subordinate and narrower cognitive processes. Accordingly, executive functioning is more difficult to operationalize, define, and assess in this perspective, due to the complexity of identifying and measuring the managerial metacognitive aspect in conjunction with the varied associated cognitive processes. Within this viewpoint, executive functions constitute a nebulous, overarching entity similar to *g*: We all know it when we see it, but no one can really "define" it. Examples of this perspective can be seen in Luria's theory of cognitive functioning (the theory that underlies the NEPSY-II, the Cognitive Assessment System [CAS], and one interpretive framework for the Kaufman Assessment Battery for Children—Second Edition [KABC-II]) and in Cattell–Horn–Carroll (CHC) theory (the primary theory underlying the Woodcock–Johnson III Tests of Cognitive Abilities [WJ III COG], the Stanford–Binet Intelligence Scales, Fifth Edition [SB5], the Differential Ability Scales—Second Edition [DAS-II], the other interpretive framework for the KABC-II, and other modern measures of cognitive functioning).

Luria described human cognitive processes within the framework of three functional units. In Luria's theory, the first functional unit (block I) is arousal and attention; the second unit (block II) codes information using simultaneous and successive processes; and the third functional unit (block III) is involved in the regulation of executive functioning (planning, strategizing, regulating performance, and solving problems). Luria identified the prefrontal lobes of the brain as primarily responsible for the third functional unit. Luria's work served as one impetus for the study of executive functions and has been used as a blueprint for defining components of human intellectual competence.

CHC theory describes human cognitive processes within the framework of three strata: a general overarching factor, broad cognitive factors, and multiple narrow abilities. CHC theory does not describe a specific and separate element of executive functioning; rather, components of executive functions are integrated primarily into the Gf (fluid reasoning) broad-ability factor (Kane & Engle, 2002; McGrew & Woodcock, 2001) and the narrow-ability factors of induction, general sequential reasoning, and attention and concentration. Drawing from more recent research, Flanagan, Alfonso, Ortiz, and Dynda (2010) present an integrated interpretive framework based on psychometric, neuropsychological, and Lurian perspectives, and provide a neurocognitive demand task analysis of the major test batteries using this framework. Defining executive functioning as a global neuropsychological domain represented by metacognition, planning, learning, memory, and cognitive efficiency, Flanagan et al. (2010) posit that the neuropsychological domain of executive functions corresponds well with eight broad CHC abilities: fluid reasoning (Gf), comprehension–knowledge (Gc), processing speed (Gs), short-term memory (Gsm), long-term storage and retrieval (Glr), quantitative knowledge (Gq), reading and writing ability (Grw), and general knowledge ability (Gkn).

Proponents of a unitary conceptualization of executive functions argue that their perspective is the most parsimonious view of executive functions, and that nonunitary models or perspectives are reductionistic and not helpful, given their fractionation of executive functions (Sugarman, 2002). In contrast, researchers from the second major viewpoint see executive functions as a label for a collection of distinct, yet associated, cognitively complex higher-order processes (Anderson, 2001; Ardilla, Pineda, & Rosselli, 2000; Baron, 2004; Elliott, 2003; McCabe, Roediger, McDaniel, Balota, & Hambrick, 2010). Proponents of this perspective would argue that the factorial evidence clearly supports distinct cognitive processes that correlate moderately with each other. However, as previously stated, researchers cannot reach a consensus as to what cognitive processes constitute these executive functions. Salthouse (2005) has suggested that reasoning and perceptual speed represent the underlying features of executive functions, whereas others have proposed working memory (Baddeley, 1996, 2000), verbal working memory (Sugarman, 2002), or inhibition (Barkley, 2000) as the clear foundation of executive functioning. Miyake, Friedman, Emerson, Witzki, and Howerter (2000) propose an intermediate position. They see executive functions as separate but moderately correlated constructs, and suggest that the executive system is composed of both unitary and nonunitary components. Other researchers have elaborated

on this idea and proposed two types of executive functions: metacognitive and behavioral (Fuster, 2001, 2002; Happaney, Zelazo, & Stuss, 2004). According to this perspective, the metacognitive type consists of the usual executive functions and is mediated by the dorsolateral prefrontal cortex (PFC), whereas the behavioral type is responsible for the coordination of cognition and emotion, with inhibition as its primary expression, and is mediated by the ventromedial PFC.

Miller's (2007) recently proposed school neuropsychology model also provides an intermediate perspective on neuropsychological constructs such as executive functions; he views them as independent but moderately correlated constructs. Miller's model is unique in that it uses neuropsychological, neuroanatomical, and neuroassessment research to conceptualize the model's components. It is specifically intended to be applied to the neuropsychological development of children and adolescents, and it can be utilized in conjunction with interpretive approaches specific to children, such as Hale and Fiorello's (2004) cognitive hypothesis-testing model. In Miller's conceptual model, tasks are classified as either primary or secondary. If a task is labeled as *primary*, it suggests that the primary neurocognitive construct being measured accounts for the majority of the test variance, whereas the label of *secondary* indicates that the neurocognitive construct contributes to performance on the task but to a lesser degree.

Miller categorizes executive functions as concept generation, inhibition, motor programming and planning, reasoning, and problem solving. He views these executive functions as being strongly related to fluid reasoning abilities or tasks that require novel problem-solving skills. In contrast to other researchers, Miller views other common aspects of executive functioning, such as working memory and attention, as separate neurocognitive constructs. For example, attentional processes in Miller's model are comprehensively addressed (i.e., the proposed category includes selective/focused attention, sustained attention, shifting attention, attentional capacity, and divided attention), but are considered to be distinct from executive functions. Memory is also considered a separate cognitive construct (consisting of visual and verbal immediate memory, working memory, and long-term memory) and is not viewed as a subset of executive functions.

Understanding these different theoretical perspectives is important because they shape the research being conducted on executive functions and influence the interpretation of the obtained data. Some theories have exerted considerable influence on the field even when there is no supporting evidence. It is also important to note that the primary theoretical models of executive functioning were developed from an adult perspective, and have been applied to children and adolescents on a post hoc basis. Children often display differential performance, which does not fit many of the models currently available.

THE NEUROPSYCHOLOGY OF EXECUTIVE FUNCTIONS

Understanding the neuropsychological underpinnings of executive functioning is also critical to the assessment of executive functions. Despite amazing progress in neuroimaging, the neuroanatomy and neurophysiology of executive functions continue to be debated in the literature. Historically, executive functions have been associated with the PFC, and more specifically with the anterior portions of the PFC. Exactly how the PFC supports executive functions is largely unknown and somewhat controversial (Alvarez & Emory, 2006; Hughes & Graham, 2008; Wood & Grafman, 2003). Attempts to localize executive functions to discrete areas in the PFC with neuroimaging techniques have been inconclusive (Roberts, Robbins, & Weiskrantz, 2002). A one-to-one correspondence between executive functions and the PFC has not yet been documented in the research, and many claims are speculative at best (Alvarez & Emory, 2006). Moreover, some neuroimaging results have implicated posterior, cortical, and subcortical regions in executive functioning, and it has been posited that executive functioning may be a more flexible distributed network than previously thought (Roberts et al., 2002).

The PFC comprises approximately one-third of the brain; maintains intricate connections to the rest of the brain; and continues to mature through synaptogenesis, myelination, and pruning well into early adulthood. Three systems—the dorsolateral PFC, the anterior cingulate circuit, and the orbitofrontal cortex—are thought to be involved in executive functions. The dorsolateral PFC is associated with most of the "typical" executive functions, including cognitive flexibility and behavioral spontaneity; maintaining and shifting cognitive attention; organization and planning; goal setting; performing dual-task activities; short-term memory; focusing and sustaining attention;

inhibition; and fluency (Alvarez & Emory, 2006; Hale & Fiorello, 2004; Romine & Reynolds, 2005). Deficits within the dorsolateral PFC are often associated with attention problems, poor problem solving, and difficulties with self-monitoring and control. The anterior cingulate circuit appears to control the behavioral processes associated with initiation, inhibition, motivation, selective or divided attention, response monitoring, and error detection (van Vreen & Carter, 2002; Zilmer, Spiers, & Culbertson, 2008). Damage to the anterior cingulate circuit often results in difficulties with response inhibition (Miller, 2007), slow completion time or decision speed, lack of persistence, and difficulty with self-monitoring (Hale & Fiorello, 2004). The orbitofrontal cortex is involved with emotional and social behaviors such as tact, sensitivity, impulsivity, and emotional inhibition (Bradshaw, 2001; Knight & Stuss, 2002). Deficits in the orbitofrontal cortex are associated with emotional dysregulation, aggression, sexual promiscuity, disinhibition, impulsivity and poor decision making. These three systems together create, support, and coordinate the complex cognitive functions involved in problem solving and decision making, which are the hallmarks of the construct being defined as *executive functions*.

Despite our neuroanatomical understanding of executive functioning, it is important to remember that our knowledge and understanding of how the brain functions when it is processing and performing executive function tasks is still very limited (P. Anderson, 2002). The PFC does not act in isolation; therefore, it is challenging to identify which brain regions contribute to which outcomes on specific measures of executive functions. In other words, a deficit in one area can lead to multiple behaviors or, conversely, one behavior may be the result of multiple underlying impairments. It is also important to remember that although a variety of neural correlates have been identified in adults for various components of executive functioning, no research to date has confirmed these findings with children.

DEVELOPMENTAL TRAJECTORIES OF EXECUTIVE FUNCTIONING IN CHILDREN

Until recently, executive functions were thought to emerge in adolescence and early adulthood. The belief was that they played little or no role in typical brain development during infancy and childhood. However, recent research has debunked this early perception and demonstrated the critical role executive functions play in typical brain development across the lifespan (V. Anderson, 2002; Reynolds, 2007). According to numerous researchers (Carlson, 2004; Hughes & Graham, 2008; Lidz, 2003), higher-order cognitive skills are present before they are observable, functional, or testable. In addition, research has demonstrated an interaction between developmental processes and the manifestation of executive functions (Blair, Zelazo, & Greenberg, 2005; Brocki & Bohlin, 2004; Zelazo et al., 2003). Executive functions appear to emerge, develop rapidly, and reach adult levels of performance differentially; therefore, research would suggest that developmental profiles or trajectories will depend on the executive skill(s) being examined (Archibald & Kerns, 1999; Romine & Reynolds, 2005). As a result, it is important for psychologists working with children in any capacity to be aware of and understand the developmental trajectories of the executive functions they seek to measure.

ASSESSMENT OF EXECUTIVE FUNCTIONS

Operationalizing definitions of executive functions in order to assess them is even more difficult and fraught with challenges than developing theoretical definitions. One of the challenges is obtaining valid, accurate, and reliable measures (Hughes & Graham, 2008), given the perspective that executive functions are not unitary but composed of multiple complex functions. Since there is no universal definition of what constitutes executive functions, or which domains are critical for successful executive functioning, there is no agreement as to what executive function domains should be measured or how these domains should be assessed. A second challenge is that by definition executive function tasks are complex, so task impurity becomes an issue, in that a task may require (and thus be influenced by) multiple cognitive processes. Thus it is difficult to distinguish executive function tasks from other tasks because the integrative simultaneous nature of frontal lobe functioning makes it difficult to parse out the specific cognitive functions being utilized in each type of task in order to create a pure measure of executive functioning (Hughes & Graham, 2002; Maricle et al., 2010; Romine & Reynolds, 2005).

Even when a task can be identified as a relatively valid, reliable, and somewhat pure measure of a particular executive function, the task or the individual's performance on the task is often misinterpreted. A common mistake is to equate deficient performance on an identified task of executive function with frontal lobe or neurological dysfunction. A second common mistake is to assume that each task taps an underlying cognitive process that is universal to all executive function tasks, or that all tasks of executive function are measuring the same aspects of the construct. Such presumptions lead to overly simplified, narrow, or inaccurate interpretations. Interpreting results from executive function tasks depends on precise specification of task demands; this necessitates a systematic understanding of the components of executive function, as well as an understanding that most executive function tasks require several cognitive skills for successful performance (Flanagan et al., 2010; Hughes & Graham, 2008; Miller, 2007). Research demonstrates that successful performance on most complex cognitive tasks requires a combination of cognitive skills, such as working memory, attention, concept formation, inhibition, and/or cognitive flexibility. The breakdown in an individual's performance can occur at any stage of cognitive processing, from lower-level skills such as attention to the higher-order skills such as planning (Delis, Kaplan, & Kramer, 2001). Accurate interpretation then requires determining the neurocognitive constructs that contribute to successful or poor performance on a specific task, and then considering those results within the context of a specific individual's assessment.

The broad range of skills implicated in executive functions has led to the use of many different assessment tools; however, no instrument has yet been developed to measure executive functioning in its entirety. Rather, there are tools available to measure specific components of executive functions. Assessment can be divided into broad overall measures of multiple cognitive constructs, or targeted measures of a specific cognitive construct. Executive functions can be more or less effectively evaluated by using both types of measures. Miller and Hale (2008) note that standardized intellectual measures are psychometrically some of the best tools available to practitioners, and that incorporating these tools into neuropsychological assessment is an essential practice. Thus a discussion of the major norm-referenced comprehensive batteries of intelligence and how they relate to the measurement of executive functions is warranted.

EVALUATION OF EXECUTIVE FUNCTIONS WITH THE MAJOR COGNITIVE BATTERIES

Woodcock–Johnson III Tests of Cognitive Abilities Normative Update

The WJ III COG Normative Update (Woodcock, McGrew, & Mather, 2001, 2007; we continue to refer to it here as the WJ III COG) is a compilation of tasks factorially designed to operationalize the CHC theory of cognitive functioning. CHC theory regards cognitive abilities as multidimensional and dynamic rather than as static domains of function. CHC theory, and by extension the WJ III COG, do not view executive functioning as a specific independent cognitive domain; rather, it is seen as a cognitive process and is represented as multiple independent narrow abilities involved in fluid reasoning (Gf), short-term memory (Gsm), and processing/decision speed (Gs).

Very little research involving the WJ III COG has focused exclusively on the cognitive construct of executive functions; the majority of the research has focused on the broad CHC factors and the underlying narrow abilities. One exception is a study by Floyd and colleagues (2006) that examined the relationship of the WJ III COG clinical clusters with the Delis–Kaplan Executive Function System (D-KEFS; Delis et al., 2001). Their results suggested that the clinical clusters correlated moderately with the D-KEFS tasks, and that both measures appeared to be assessing a general construct—most likely general intellectual ability because of the strong correlation with the General Intellectual Ability score.

On the WJ III COG, two clinical clusters, the Executive Processes cluster and the Broad Attention cluster, have been identified as measuring executive functions. The Broad Attention cluster appears to measure aspects of cognitive attention (Floyd, Shaver, & McGrew, 2003), including attentional capacity (Numbers Reversed), divided attention (Auditory Working Memory), selective attention (Auditory Attention), and sustained attention (Pair Cancellation). Subtests such as Numbers Reversed and Auditory Working Memory also contribute to the short-term memory factor as measures of working memory and short-term memory capacity. The Executive Processes cluster was designed to measure cognitive processes associated with executive functioning and consists of three subtests: Concept Formation, Planning, and Pair Cancellation. According to Floyd and colleagues (2003), these three subtests provide mea-

sures of inhibition or interference control, cognitive or mental flexibility, and strategic planning. Ford, Keith, Floyd, Fields, and Schrank (2003) describe Concept Formation as a controlled learning task that measures fluid reasoning and requires rule formation, categorical reasoning, inductive thinking, and logical deduction. Pair Cancellation is described as a complex measure that requires the examinee to identify a specific repeating pattern and successful performance requires attention, vigilance, speed of visual scanning, and interference control. The Planning subtest requires the examinee to trace a stimulus without removing the pencil from the paper or retracing any lines. As an executive function measure, it evaluates the examinee's ability to determine, select, and apply solutions involved in future planning, along with visual–spatial scanning and sequential reasoning (Read & Schrank, 2003). The complexity involved in scoring the Planning subtest keeps many examiners from administering the task regularly. Gregg and Coleman (2003) note that besides being indicative of executive function deficits, an individual's performance is also vulnerable to difficulties in attention and working memory.

Flanagan and colleagues' (2010) integrated interpretive framework would incorporate additional subtests besides those discussed above, including Analysis–Synthesis, Visual–Auditory Learning, Visual–Auditory Learning—Delayed, Retrieval Fluency, Decision Speed, and Visual Matching. These subtests are primarily measures of the Glr (long-term retrieval and storage), Gf (fluid reasoning), and Gs (processing speed) cognitive domains, which within the integrated interpretive framework would fall into the broader domain of executive functions.

Stanford–Binet Intelligence Scales, Fifth Edition

The SB5 (Roid, 2003b), the most recent revision of the popular Stanford–Binet series, was constructed on a five-factor hierarchical cognitive model consistent with current CHC theory (Roid & Barram, 2004). Using nonverbal and verbal tasks, the SB5 evaluates Fluid Reasoning (Gf), Knowledge (Gc), Quantitative Reasoning (Gq), Visual–Spatial Processing (Gv), and Working Memory (Gsm). Each subtest in the Verbal domain has a counterpart in the Nonverbal domain. Roid (2003a) indicates that the Nonverbal domain measures the general ability to reason, to solve problems, to visualize, and to recall information presented in pictorial, figural and symbolic formats; the Verbal domain measures the general ability to reason, solve problems, visualize, and recall information using spoken or written words or sentences.

Studies reported in the technical manual support the presence of a general factor, two group factors and five specific factors; however, research conducted by other investigators calls these results into question. Sattler, Dumont, Salerno, and Roberts-Pittman (2008), Canivez (2008), and DiStefano and Dombrowski (2006) found either no support or limited support for the group (i.e., two-factor) model or for the specific (i.e., five-factor) model. Canivez also noted issues of subtest migration or cross-loading, wherein subtests theoretically associated with one factor were in fact associated with multiple dimensions/factors. For example, some of the SB5 Nonverbal subtests actually accounted for more variance on the Verbal factor than the Nonverbal factor. Another issue of concern with the SB5 is that the subtests in each domain change as the individual progresses through the levels. Each subtest has one to three unique activities or variations of the task. For example, Verbal Fluid Reasoning is composed of Early Reasoning, Verbal Absurdities, and Verbal Analogies, and each variation taps verbal fluid reasoning differentially and utilizes other cognitive skills to a greater or lesser degree. This is problematic, in that it is difficult to determine that what is being measured at one level is the same thing being measured at another level within the same subtest. Given the massive task impurity issues, an examiner must have a good understanding of each task within each subtest, how and when the task changes form, what skills are being measured with each form of the task, and finally how the individual's performance and score may be affected as a result.

No research is currently available that addresses the specific use of the SB5 for assessing executive functions. The current literature indicates that interpretation of the SB5 should be primarily at the level of g or overall general intelligence. However, task analyses can suggest how various tasks within the SB5 may be measuring different aspects of executive functioning. If executive functions are conceptualized from a cognitive construct perspective, then tasks within the SB5 could be parsed into likely measures of different aspects of executive functioning. For example, the Nonverbal Fluid Reasoning task (Object Series/Matrices) requires sequential reasoning and deductive thinking for successful completion of items at the early levels, and then incorporates a classic matrix or

pattern reasoning task using inductive thinking at the more advanced levels. Matrix tasks have consistently been found to be good measures of Gf or fluid reasoning, one hypothesized executive functioning skill (Tranel, Manzel, & Anderson, 2008). In contrast, only the Verbal Analogies items of the Verbal Fluid Reasoning task would constitute true fluid reasoning or abstract thinking skills, and thus the Verbal Fluid Reasoning task should not be considered an adequate measure of verbal executive functioning. Roid (2003a) would take exception to this characterization, as he believes that the Verbal Fluid Reasoning task measures the ability to solve novel verbal problems, to identify cause-and-effect relationships, to classify according to form and function, and to use inductive reasoning with analogies. Another example can be found in the Nonverbal Working Memory subtest and its Verbal Working Memory counterpart. The Nonverbal Working Memory task measures visual short-term memory capacity and visual working memory capacity through a "shell game" at early levels and a block-tapping task at the more advanced levels. Its Verbal Working Memory counterpart uses memory for sentences and memory for a word in the presence of interference to assess verbal short-term memory and working memory capacity.

Differential Ability Scale— Second Edition

The DAS-II is a revision of the Differential Ability Scales (DAS; Elliott, 1990), which originated from the British Ability Scales (BAS; Elliott, 1983). According to Dumont, Willis, and Elliott (2009) the DAS-II is based on current knowledge of neuroscience and was designed to reflect cognitive processes that contribute to learning difficulties in children; it was not developed to reflect a unitary model of g or general intelligence. The selection of abilities to be assessed by the DAS-II was intended to be consistent with CHC theory.

The technical manual reports varying factor structures for the DAS-II at different age levels. At the earliest ages (2–3), a two-factor model (Verbal and Nonverbal) emerges; at ages 4–5, a five-factor model emerges (Verbal, Nonverbal Reasoning, Spatial, Visual–Verbal Memory, and Verbal Short-Term Memory); at ages 6–12, a seven-factor model emerges (Verbal, Nonverbal Reasoning, Spatial, Verbal Memory, Verbal–Visual Memory, Cognitive Speed, and Auditory Processing); and for ages 6–17, a six-factor model emerges (Verbal, Nonverbal Reasoning, Spatial, Verbal Short-Term

Memory, Visual–Verbal Memory, and Cognitive Speed). Sattler, Dumont, Willis, and Salerno (2008) conducted a principal-components factor analysis using data from the technical manual and identified for the Early Years Lower Level battery a three-factor solution that they found difficult to define, but that did not support the factor solutions cited in the technical manual. Sattler and colleagues identified a seven-factor solution for the Early Years Upper Level battery and felt that five were clearly identifiable as Verbal, Nonverbal, Spatial, Working Memory, and Processing Speed. For the School-Age battery, a six-factor solution was determined with five identifiable factors (Verbal, Nonverbal, Reasoning/Spatial, Working Memory, Processing Speed, and Visual Memory). Examiners using the DAS-II need to be cognizant of these varying factor structures and what they purportedly measure at different age levels when interpreting results.

No research is available that directly addresses the DAS-II's relationship to executive functions. According to Dumont and colleagues (2009), the DAS-II assesses seven broad abilities: verbal ability (Gc), spatial ability (Gv), nonverbal reasoning ability (Gf), retrieval (Glr), memory (Gsm), processing speed (Gs), and auditory processing (Ga). The Verbal and Spatial ability clusters are intended to reflect the major information-processing systems used to receive, perceive, remember, and process information using both auditory and visual modalities. Verbal ability as measured by the DAS-II essentially consists of language development and lexical knowledge. Spatial ability primarily consists of tasks requiring spatial relations and visualization, although one task, Recall of Designs, measures visual memory. The tasks of the Nonverbal Reasoning ability cluster (Matrices, Sequential and Quantitative Reasoning, and Picture Similarities) provide adequate to strong measures of inductive thinking and reasoning. The Matrices task assesses the ability to formulate and test hypotheses, inductive reasoning, verbal mediation, and visual perception. The Picture Similarities subtest evaluates the ability to formulate and test hypotheses about relationships and to solve nonverbal problems by attaching representation or conceptual meaning to a pictured object. The Sequential and Quantitative Reasoning task assesses the ability to perceive relationships, draw conclusions, reason inductively, formulate and test hypotheses, use analytic reasoning, and retrieve long-term information. The DAS-II also provides strong measures of another executive functioning

construct, that of memory (free recall, span, and working memory), through the broad Retrieval and Memory clusters. The subtests Recall of Designs, Recall of Digits (Forward and Backward), Recall of Objects (Immediate and Delayed), Recall of Sequential Order, and Recognition of Pictures allow for a comprehensive assessment of visual and auditory short-term memory capacity, working memory capacity, and long-term retrieval.

Wechsler Intelligence Scale for Children—Fourth Edition

The Wechsler scales are believed to be the most widely used measures of intelligence throughout the world (Flanagan & Kaufman, 2009). The Wechsler Intelligence Scale for Children—Fourth Edition (WISC-IV; Wechsler, 2003) embodies a fundamental shift from previous editions of the WISC, since it was redesigned to more adequately reflect the current CHC theoretical perspective on cognition. As such, the WISC-IV combines the traditionally derived Wechsler approach and CHC theory (Strauss, Sherman, & Spreen, 2006). Four factors have been identified in the WISC-IV technical manual to describe the cognitive constructs being measured: the Verbal Comprehension Index (VCI), the Perceptual Reasoning Index (PRI), the Working Memory Index (WMI), and the Processing Speed Index (PSI). In contrast, a study by Keith, Fine, Taub, Reynolds, and Kranzler (2006) identified five CHC factors: Gc, Gv, Gf, Gsm, and Gs. Flanagan and Kaufman (2009) resolve this structural debate by suggesting that both factor structures represent the cognitive constructs of the WISC-IV and that interpretation needs to include consideration of both perspectives, with CHC constructs taking the form of "clinical clusters." Sattler and Dumont (2008) also criticize the factor structure, noting that the factor structure does not hold true for all age groups, with the weakest factor being the WMI.

Given the dissension regarding the factor structure of the WISC-IV, a brief review is provided. The VCI is composed of tasks that measure verbal abilities utilizing reasoning, comprehension, and conceptualization. The index involves tasks that require comprehension–knowledge, verbal fluid reasoning, and long-term memory (Weiss, Beal, Saklofske, Packiam-Alloway, & Prifitera, 2008). Within the CHC perspective, the VCI comprises a measure of Gc or comprehension–knowledge (Keith et al., 2006), although Flanagan and Kaufman (2009) note that the two subtests of Similarities and Word Reasoning may share a verbal fluid reasoning construct. The PRI consists of tasks that measure perceptual fluid reasoning with some visual–spatial organization (Weiss et al., 2008). However, within the CHC perspective, the PRI is not a unitary factor; it appears to measure visual processing (Gv) and fluid reasoning (Gf) (Flanagan & Kaufman, 2009; Keith et al., 2006). The WMI is defined by the developers of the WISC-IV as a measure of the ability to concentrate, sustain attention, and exert mental control. Flanagan and Kaufman have classified the WMI as a narrowband ability factor (the narrow ability of working memory within the broad Gsm factor) within the CHC model. Weiss and colleagues (2008) take exception to this characterization and believe that the WMI tasks are strong measures of verbal short-term and working memory. Keith and colleagues (2006) determined that the WMI appears to be a mixture of Gsm and Gf. Finally, the PSI provides a measure of the speed of mental and graphomotor processing. Within CHC theory, the PSI tasks are seen as visual scanning and speed-of-processing tasks falling under the Gs factor.

None of the subtests on the WISC-IV are thought to measure executive functioning unequivocally, and no research could be found that specifically assesses the contribution of executive functioning to WISC-IV tasks. The Elithorn Mazes task, which is found only on the WISC-IV Integrated (Wechsler et al., 2004), is deemed a measure of executive function in that it focuses on immediate planning, self-monitoring, and the ability to inhibit impulsive responding. According to Weiss and colleagues (2008), the Elithorn Mazes task provides a preliminary estimate of the skills that constitute executive functions and correlates with other measures of executive functioning, although it certainly does not provide a comprehensive measure of the domain of executive functioning. Holdnack and Weiss (2006) clearly state that the Elithorn Mazes task assesses only some of the skills related to executive functioning, and that adequate performance on the task should not be construed as evidence that an individual's executive functioning is intact. Holdnack, Weiss, and Entwistle (2006) have proposed an Executive Functioning Index that could be used to provide initial evidence that an examinee may have difficulties with executive functioning. Holdnack and colleagues suggest using the Comprehension Multiple Choice, Elithorn Mazes, Spatial Span—Forward, and Cancellation—Random subtests from the WISC-IV Integrated for this purpose.

Miller (2007; see also Miller & Hale, 2008) conceptually groups the WISC-IV and WISC-IV Integrated subtests according to his school neuropsychology model. Miller labels Matrix Reasoning, Picture Concepts, and Elithorn Mazes as primary executive function measures. According to Miller and Hale (2008), Matrix Reasoning is principally a nonverbal reasoning or problem-solving task within the executive functions domain and is more of a fluid reasoning task (as per CHC theory) than a perceptual reasoning task (as identified by the developers of the WISC-IV). Another core perceptual reasoning subtest that Miller deems primarily a measure of executive functioning is Picture Concepts. Picture Concepts measures abstract categorical reasoning ability, and within CHC theory is a clear measure of fluid reasoning. Elithorn Mazes is included as a primary measure of executive functioning in the school neuropsychology model because, as previously stated, it is regarded as a measure of planning, organization, motor execution, and response inhibition. The Block Design subtest (and its variations within the WISC-IV Integrated), Similarities, Vocabulary, Comprehension, Arithmetic, and Word Reasoning are all considered secondary measures of executive functioning in the school neuropsychology model.

Flanagan and colleagues' (2010) integrated interpretive framework incorporates additional subtests besides those discussed in Miller's model, including Cancellation, Coding, Digit Span, Letter–Number Sequencing, Spatial Span—Forward and Backward, Symbol Search, and Visual Digit Span. These subtests are primarily seen as measures of Gsm (short-term and working memory) and Gs (processing speed), but within the integrated interpretive framework they fall into the broader domain of executive functions.

Kaufman Assessment Battery for Children—Second Edition

Kaufman and Kaufman (2004) deliberately designed the KABC-II to incorporate two distinct theoretical models: the CHC and Lurian models. However, the authors recommend using the CHC model interpretively for most purposes. The KABC-II is composed of 18 subtests grouped into four or five scales, depending on the child's age and the interpretive model chosen. The Lurian model organizes the subtests into four scales: Sequential, Simultaneous, Learning, and Planning. The CHC model organizes the same subtests into short-term memory (Gsm), visual processing (Gv), long-term storage and retrieval (Glr), fluid reasoning (Gf), and crystallized ability (Gc). The KABC-II may be a promising tool for assessing intelligence and cognitive impairments, but current research on its applicability within a neuropsychological framework for neuropsychological assessment is limited (Mays, Kamphaus, & Reynolds, 2009).

On the KABC-II, learning ability and planning ability from the Lurian perspective are the domains most applicable to executive functioning. Within the CHC perspective, these equate to the cognitive factors of Glr (long-term storage and retrieval) and Gf (fluid reasoning), respectively. Kaufman, Kaufman, Kaufman-Singer, and Kaufman (2005) consider Planning/Gf to be the domain most closely associated with executive functioning. On the KABC-II, Planning/Gf tasks are designed to require a variety of mental operations to solve novel problems, including cognitive flexibility, inductive and deductive reasoning, hypothesis generation, and impulse control. Tasks that encompass the domain of Learning/Glr also require the integration of several executive functions. Kaufman and colleagues note that Learning/Glr on the KABC-II emphasizes efficiency of the storage and retrieval, not the specific information being stored. They further emphasize that effective paired-associate learning requires considerable attention and planning skills, as well as storage and retrieval skills.

Kaufman and colleagues (2005) delineate narrow cognitive abilities underlying the KABC-II subtests, identifying induction, general sequential reasoning, and associative learning/memory as the primary narrow abilities representative of executive functioning. Three KABC-II subtests are considered measures of induction: Conceptual Thinking, Pattern Reasoning, and Story Completion. The Conceptual Thinking task is only administered to children ages 3 years, 0 months to 6 years, 11 months (3:0–6:11), and involves determining conceptual relationships by identifying the concept that does not fit the relationship parameters. The Pattern Reasoning subtest requires the examinee to complete a logical linear pattern (i.e., the examinee must identify what part of the pattern is missing and complete the missing section with the appropriate choice from among a series of choices). The Story Completion task is similar, in that the examinee completes the missing elements of a pictured story by deducing from the remaining story line what aspects of the story are missing. Two subtests, Rover and Riddles, assess general se-

quential reasoning. Rover requires the examinee to determine the quickest and shortest path from one point to another by using rules, strategy selection, and visual–spatial thinking. The Riddles task involves solving a verbal puzzle/riddle by using characteristics of concrete or abstract verbal concepts. Associative memory is assessed by two subtests, Atlantis and Rebus, both of which are controlled learning tasks associating a word with a picture/symbol/concept.

Flanagan and colleagues' (2010) integrated interpretive framework would add two subtests, Triangles and Word Order, to those discussed above. However, whereas the Gsm tasks on other instruments are also considered within this framework as being representative of executive functioning, these tasks on the KABC-II are not thus considered. Gsm tasks on the KABC-II are measures of short-term memory span or capacity only, and not of working memory.

The NEPSY-II

Conceptualized from Luria's perspective, the NEPSY-II (Korkman, Kirk, & Kemp, 2007) is an assessment that focuses specifically on the neuropsychological development of children. The original NEPSY was traditionally under the purview of child clinical psychologists and pediatric neuropsychologists. However, the NEPSY-II has recently become popular with school psychologists, who tend to use it more as a measure of cognitive functioning in the tradition of intelligence tests than for its intended neuropsychological purpose, and thus it is included in this discussion. The Lurian tradition requires that assessments identify and distinguish between primary and secondary deficits of cognitive functions. From this perspective, examining simple and complex components of specific domains, and the additional use of qualitative information, provide a more thorough assessment of possible deficits.

The NEPSY-II is purported to measure six domains of cognitive functioning (Attention and Executive Functioning; Language; Sensorimotor; Visuospatial Processing; Memory and Learning; and Social Perception). Korkman and her colleagues (2007) acknowledge that not all cognitive functions constituting a specific domain are assessed. They believe that these cognitive functions do not develop in isolation, but work in concert together, and that broad conclusions based on individual subtests measuring only limited aspects of particular domains should not be drawn.

The Attention and Executive Functioning domain is the most germane to this discussion. Titley and D'Amato (2008) describe the tasks in this domain as a continuum of skills ranging from simple attention to complex self-monitoring. Animal Sorting, Auditory Attention and Response Set, Clocks, Statue, Design Fluency, and Inhibition compose the Attention and Executive Functioning domain of the NEPSY-II. Of these six subtests, four span the widest age range (7–16 years), one is limited to preschoolers (3–6 years), and one is limited to children ages 5–12 years.

Research on the NEPSY-II is currently quite limited; therefore, users must rely on information provided in the technical manual by the test authors. Animal Sorting is a classic card-sorting task similar to the Wisconsin Card Sorting Test. Card-sorting tasks demonstrate good construct validity as measures of concept generation, which is thought to be a fundamental executive function. Animal Sorting was designed to measure the ability to form basic concepts, categorize, and shift fluently from one concept to another. The Auditory Attention and Response Set subtest consists of two discrete tasks. Auditory Attention requires sustained and selective auditory attention, whereas Response Set adds the element of shifting attention and the ability to maintain set while inhibiting previously learned responses. The Clocks task uses analog clocks to assess planning, organization, visual-perceptual, and visual–spatial skills. Similar tasks have been frequently used for adults with brain injuries, who often exhibit impaired performance. Cohen, Riccio, Kibby, and Edmonds (2000) evaluated the use of a clocks task with children and found that performance improvements were associated with age. Children at age 6 can draw the basic elements of a clock, and by ages 10–12 most children can generate an accurate picture of a clock but may make positioning errors. Adult levels of performance are reached in early adolescence. However, no research appears to have looked at the validity of clocks tasks as measures of either executive function or attention. The Design Fluency task was designed to assess the ability to generate as many unique designs as possible by connecting dots presented in either a structured or random array. It provides a measure of the efficiency and speed of cognitive visual processing. The Inhibition task is a variation of the classic Stroop task; it was designed to assess the ability to inhibit an automatic response in favor of a novel response and to shift or switch response types. The task requires the individual to view a series of shapes or arrows and then to name either the shape, the direction, or an alternative response.

To date, there are no published independent research studies examining the Attention and Executive Functioning domain of the NEPSY-II; the available research focuses on the original NEPSY. Since the NEPSY-II replaced three of the original six subtests in this domain with new tasks, conclusions from previous research cannot be brought to bear on the validity of the current domain as a measure of attention, executive function, or a mixture of both. Kemp (2007) has stated that the subtests in the Attention and Executive Functioning domain measure the core components of executive functioning (including strategic planning, cognitive flexibility, and self-regulation), as well as subcomponents such as initiation, fluency, inhibition, and working memory. However, Kemp notes that the domain does not measure all aspects of executive functioning or attention. A major limitation of the Attention and Executive Functioning domain is the lack of empirical research on the validity of the domain. More specifically, the merging of the cognitive constructs of attention and executive function, and the validity of the tasks chosen to measure these cognitive constructs, have received limited attention in the literature.

TARGETED EVALUATION OF EXECUTIVE FUNCTIONS: A BRIEF DISCUSSION

Friedman and colleagues (2006) suggest that current measures of intelligence do not capture the breadth and depth of executive functioning, and are best considered as screening tools for executive dysfunction. Evidence of executive function deficits would then warrant a more targeted evaluation of identified areas of dysfunction. There are numerous instruments that target the assessment of executive functions and related neurocognitive constructs. A complete overview of such assessment instruments is beyond the purview and scope of this chapter; the reader is referred to Maricle and colleagues (2010) for a more comprehensive review.

Targeted assessment instruments measure neurocognitive constructs such as executive functioning, attention, or working memory more specifically and narrowly. As such, they often require more specialized knowledge and training for proper use. However, several targeted instruments of executive functions are commonly used by school psychologists and other child clinicians, including the D-KEFS; the Behavior Rating Inventory of Executive Function (BRIEF); and various versions of category, trail-making, tower, and Stroop-like tasks. In addition, numerous measures are used to evaluate related neurocognitive constructs such as memory (Test of Memory and Learning—Second Edition; Wide Range Assessment of Memory and Learning, Second Edition; Children's Memory Scale) or attention (Test of Everyday Attention for Children; Conners' Continuous Performance Test II). Two targeted assessment instruments thought to measure executive functions, The BRIEF and the D-KEFS, are briefly discussed here because they are the most commonly used in psychoeducational, psychological, and neuropsychological evaluations.

Behavior Rating Inventory of Executive Functions

The BRIEF (Gioia, Isquith, Guy, & Kenworthy, 2000) is frequently used by school psychologists and other professionals to measure executive functions in children and adolescents. Unfortunately, the BRIEF is often the *only* measure used to assess executive functions. The BRIEF defines executive functioning as the ability to self-regulate cognitive and social problem solving, and was designed to assess impairment of these behaviors in the home and school environments (Gioia et al., 2000). It is an 86-item questionnaire for teachers and/or parents that utilizes a 3-point Likert scale ("never," "sometimes," "often") to determine how often a child performs a behavior that is thought to be a manifestation of executive dysfunction. The BRIEF provides *T* scores (higher scores are indicative of dysfunction) and yields a global measure of executive functioning (Global Executive Composite) and two indexes, Behavioral Regulation and Metacognition. Three subtests (Inhibition, Shift, Emotional Control) constitute the Behavioral Regulation Index, and five subtests make up the Metacognition Index (Initiate, Working Memory, Plan/Organize, Organization of Materials, and Monitor).

A significant limitation of the BRIEF is the adequacy and representativeness of its normative sample, which was obtained from one state (Maryland) and limited in size (1,419 parents and 720 teachers). Another important limitation for clinicians using the BRIEF to be aware of is its poor interrater reliability (<.50), in that parents have consistently been found to rate their children as having significantly greater difficulties than teachers rate the children as having. Professionals who choose to use the BRIEF need to realize that it is an indirect measure, and that what is being measured is an adult's perception of a child's behavioral manifestations of executive dysfunction, not the child's cognitive executive functions themselves. In fact, the research suggests that the BRIEF does not correlate with direct measures of executive functions (Anderson, Anderson, Northam, Jacobs, & Mikiewicz, 2002; Benjamin, 2004; Mangeot, Armstrong, Colvin, Yeates, & Taylor, 2002; Vriezen & Pigott, 2002). Instead, it should be considered more of a measure of attention or behavior, similar to measures such as the Behavior Assessment System for Children, Second Edition; the Achenbach System of Empirically Based Assessment; or the Conner's Behavior Rating Comprehensive Scales (CBRS). The consensus of most researchers is that the BRIEF should never be used as the sole measure of executive functions.

Delis–Kaplan Executive Function System

An instrument that is gaining in popularity among school psychologists is the D-KEFS (Delis et al., 2001). The D-KEFS consists of an assortment of standardized individual measures of executive functioning which Delis and colleagues combined into a comprehensive battery. There are nine tests, which may be administered in combination or separately: the Word Context Test, Sorting Test, Twenty Questions Test, Tower Test, Color Word Interference Test, Verbal Fluency Test, Design Fluency Test, Trail Making Test, and Proverbs Test. The tests are thought to measure mental flexibility, inhibition, problem solving, planning, impulse control, concept formation, abstract thinking, and verbal or spatial creativity (Homack, Lee, & Ricco, 2005). The D-KEFS does not yield an overall composite score representing executive functioning; rather, each test is scored and interpreted individually. Each test yields an aggregate score (scaled score and percentile) and relevant process scores (response accuracy, error rate, and response latency).

A primary limitation of the D-KEFS is that its clinical usefulness with children and adolescents is largely unknown, since the majority of its tasks were developed and standardized on adults. Research using the D-KEFS is scarce, with the majority of research having occurred previously on the individual measures incorporated into the D-KEFS rather than on the battery as a whole. Research using the battery, or even the individual tests, with children is very limited. This limitation is a critical one, as the D-KEFS is subject to strong age effects: Children at the youngest ages generally exhibit the lowest scores, and performance on most of the measures is highly influenced by speed of processing until early adolescence (Strauss et al., 2006). A second limitation of the D-KEFS is that it is a challenging instrument to learn to administer, score, and interpret. Clinicians wishing to use the battery should have appropriate training, practice, and supervision with the instrument, as well as an adequate background in neuropsychological assessment, in order to interpret the obtained results appropriately.

Currently, the research would indicate that the most defensible way to evaluate executive functioning is to assess executive function components separately, using targeted measures specifically developed for this purpose. This brings the clinician full circle, back to the dilemma of which executive functions should be measured. As previously stated, researchers disagree about this, and there are varying recommendations in the literature. The school neuropsychology model (Miller, 2007) would suggest the following: concept generation, inhibition, motor programming and planning, reasoning, and problem solving. Stuss (2009) would propose measuring initiation, planning, sequencing, inhibition, flexibility (shifting), and self-monitoring. Maricle and colleagues (2010) recommend evaluating the components of cognitive (mental) flexibility, attention, planning, and working memory. The primary purposes for any assessment are to provide an understanding of an individual's functioning, as well as his or her specific strengths and weaknesses; to assist in differential diagnosis; and to inform intervention. Thus best practice would suggest that the choice of which executive functions to assess should depend upon the referral question, potential diagnostic conclusions, and subsequent assessment results.

MANIFESTATION OF EXECUTIVE DYSFUNCTION IN COMMON CHILDHOOD DISORDERS

Instead of asking what executive functions should be measured, astute clinicians might ask why it is important to measure executive functions and what executive functions have to do with an individual's ability to function in a home, school, or employment setting. Evans (2009) states that executive functions enable individuals to deal with problems that arise in everyday life and to cope with new situations; they are the cognitive skills required to identify and achieve personal goals, and to modify actions when required. Interest in executive functions has resulted in greater study of executive functions in applied settings, and thus the importance of executive functioning to success in intellectual and social environments has been increasingly recognized (Han, Delis, & Holdnack, 2008). Good executive functioning in children or adolescents rarely warrants concern, but executive dysfunction often results in educational performance deficits that result in referrals for assessment. Executive dysfunction may be the fundamental underlying mechanism or symptom of many childhood disorders.

Delis and colleagues (2007) and Han and colleagues (2008) view executive functioning as a key concept that should be routinely assessed as part of any psychoeducational, psychological, or neuropsychological assessment. Including a component of executive functioning may be appropriate whenever the referral question relates to known or suspected attention-deficit/hyperactivity disorder (ADHD), autism spectrum disorder (ASD), nonverbal learning disability (NVLD), specific learning disability (SLD), traumatic brain injury (TBI), or some other identifiable neurological disorder (e.g., epilepsy or Tourette syndrome) (Barkley, 2000; Brookshire, Levin, Song, & Zhang, 2004; Meltzer & Krishnan, 2007; Ozonoff & Schetter, 2007; Parrish et al., 2007; Shallice et al., 2002; Vaquero, Gomez, Quintero, Gonzalez-Rosa, & Marquez, 2008). To obtain the most informed differential diagnosis during an evaluation, it is necessary to understand how executive dysfunction may be manifested in each of these disorders, but it is also important to note that children with these clinical disorders often exhibit global executive functioning impairments that do not necessarily differentiate clinical groups (P. Anderson, 2002; Ozonoff & Schetter, 2007; Willcutt, Doyle, Nigg, Faraone, & Pennington, 2005).

Children and adolescents with ADHD most noticeably demonstrate difficulties with inhibition and attention (Barkley, 2000; Shallice et al., 2002). They often display difficulties with self-monitoring and vigilance, working memory, organizational skills, and planning (Roth & Saykin, 2004). These deficits may result in the obvious problems of behavioral regulation seen in ADHD, such as difficulties with inhibitory control (frequent impulsive or poorly thought-out behavior), problems with behavioral initiation (inability to independently initiate tasks like homework or chores), or difficulty in sustaining behavior (with resulting failures of task completion). Children and adolescents with ADHD fail to engage in planning or problem solving. They may carry out routine tasks, but if faced with novelty or lack of structure, they are at a loss as to what to do (Evans, 2009). They are seen as easily distracted and disorganized, in that they fail to pay attention to rules, complete work haphazardly, and rarely have the materials needed to complete a given task. Unfortunately, while the behavioral manifestations of ADHD appear consistent with impairments of executive function, tests of executive function do not always differentiate children with ADHD from children without ADHD or with other clinical disorders.

Children and adolescents with ASD may have problems with cognitive flexibility, planning, fluently shifting attention to new or novel tasks, appropriately responding to social cues and regulating social interactions, and recognizing or using nonverbal behaviors (Ozonoff & Schetter, 2007). These deficits are often manifested as difficulty in adapting to environmental changes, resulting in the rigidity and need for sameness seen in many children on the autism spectrum. Poor abstract reasoning skills often result in an inability to understand the subtleties of social interactions. Children with ASD often view things very concretely and may miss the figurative meaning of language involved in sarcasm or jokes. Although executive dysfunction is a significant component of ASD, manifestations of executive dysfunction do not define distinctions in ASD subtypes (Verte, Geurts, Roeyers, Oosterlaan, & Sergeant, 2006).

Executive dysfunction is also often associated with SLD, due to cognitive difficulties that interfere with academic learning; these include problems with self-regulation and monitoring, problem solving, retrieval fluency, cognitive flexibility, or organizing and prioritizing stimuli (Meltzer & Krishnan, 2007). Executive function deficits can have a significant impact on the essential academic skills involved in reading, writing, or mathematics. For example, reading decoding may be affected by difficulties with sustained attention and working memory, which are needed in order to attend to each phoneme, manipulate and apply phonemes using reading rules, and fluently retrieve and remember each phoneme in order to sound out a word (McCloskey, Perkins, & Van Divner, 2009). Writing may be affected by poor graphomotor control, retrieval fluency deficits, or organizational difficulties, resulting in imprecise handwrit-

ing skills, strained writing with limited creativity, and disconnected or dysfluent ideas (McCloskey et al., 2009). In math, problems with working memory, inhibition, and retrieval fluency may affect the ability to recall rote math facts quickly and efficiently, to solve problems requiring mental manipulation, or to switch mental sets in order to solve problems using complex math facts (Bull & Scerif, 2001). Executive dysfunction has also been implicated in NVLD because of the problems with cognitive flexibility, set shifting, adapting to novel situations, working memory, self-regulation, and attentional control that are often seen in the population with NVLD (Stein & Krishnan, 2007).

Problems with executive functioning are also frequently seen in children and adolescents experiencing a variety of neurological conditions, such as TBI, tumors, or seizure disorders. With these disorders, impairment in executive function is often correlated with age of onset, as well as severity and location of injury, seizure activity, or tumor. Global impairments in executive functioning, and critical disruptions in attention and processing speed, are common in these children (Brookshire et al., 2004; Parrish et al., 2007; Vaquero et al., 2008). Han and colleagues (2008) note that executive function deficits are frequent sequelae of moderate and severe TBI and that impairment on a variety of executive measures commonly occurs, suggesting that comprehensive assessment of these functions is warranted for these individuals.

Evaluation of executive functioning is critical to understanding why some children have difficulty with learning and behavior. Han and colleagues (2008) believe that the first step in designing appropriate interventions is to identify the core impairments in executive functioning and to understand how the deficits relate to behavior and learning problems. Various approaches to interventions for executive dysfunction have been developed; however, the evidence base for their effectiveness remains limited, though it is growing slowly. Evans (2009) claims that now is the time to develop and evaluate rehabilitation methods that are clearly set in a theoretical context and can be prescribed on the basis of assessment information.

CONCLUSION

Executive functions appear to be the foundation for human development and the cornerstone for cognition. The study of executive functions is a developing field that is still grappling to describe these functions and their relationship to cognition and behavior. This is made more difficult by a disconnection among theory, assessment, and intervention, as well as by limited research on the developmental nature of executive functions in children, how best to assess these functions, and effective ways to intervene if executive dysfunction is identified. Nevertheless, child clinicians including pediatric neuropsychologists and school psychologists are increasingly focusing on the assessment of executive functions in their assessments. Thus it is important for these clinicians to have appropriate training in administration, scoring, and interpretation of various measures of executive functions; adequate knowledge about what aspects of executive functions are being measured by various tasks in the different instruments; and an understanding of the neurological substrates and developmental trajectories of various executive functions. These issues, as well as the adequacy of measures of intelligence or targeted measures of neurocognitive constructs for measuring executive functioning, need to be discussed in assessment courses within training programs and within the broader field of child assessment in general.

REFERENCES

Alvarez, J. A., & Emory, E. (2006). Executive function and the frontal lobes: A meta-analytic review. *Neuropsychology Review, 16*, 17–42.

Anderson, M. (2008). The concept and development of general intellectual ability. In J. Reed & J. Warner-Rogers (Eds.), *Child neuropsychology: Concepts, theory and practice* (pp. 112–135). Chichester, UK: Wiley-Blackwell.

Anderson, P. (2002). Assessment and development of executive function during childhood. *Child Neuropsychology, 8*, 71–82.

Anderson, V. (2001). Assessing executive functions in children: Biological, psychological and developmental considerations. *Developmental Rehabilitation, 4*, 119–136.

Anderson, V. (2002). Executive functions in children: Introduction. *Child Neuropsychology, 8*, 69–70.

Anderson, V., Anderson, P., Northam, E., Jacobs, R., & Mikiewicz, O. (2002). Relationships between cognitive and behavioral measures of executive functions in children with brain disease. *Child Neuropsychology, 8*, 231–240.

Anderson, V., Levine, H. S., & Jacobs, R. (2002). Executive functioning after frontal lobe injury: A developmental perspective. In R. T. Knight & D. T. Stuss (Eds.), *Principles of frontal lobe functions* (pp. 504–507). New York: Oxford University Press.

Archibald, S. J., & Kerns, K. A. (1999). Identification and description of new tests of executive functioning in children. *Child Neuropsychology, 5*, 115–129.

Ardilla, A. (2008). On the evolutionary origins of executive functions. *Brain and Cognition, 68*(1), 92–99.

Ardilla, A., Pineda, D., & Rosselli, M. (2000). Correlation between intelligence test scores and executive function measures. *Archives of Clinical Neuropsychology, 35*, 31–36.

Ardilla, A., & Surlof, C. (2007). *Dysexecutive syndrome*. San Diego, CA: Medlink Neurology.

Baddeley, A. (1996). Exploring the central executive. *Quarterly Journal of Experimental Psychology, 49A*(1), 5–28.

Baddeley, A. (2000). The episodic buffer: A new component of working memory? *Trends in Cognitive Sciences, 4*, 417–423.

Barkley, R. A. (2000). Commentary on the multimodal treatment study of children with ADHD. *Journal of Abnormal Psychology, 28*, 595–599.

Baron, I. S. (2004). *Neuropsychological evaluation of the child*. New York: Oxford University Press.

Benjamin, M. L. (2004). *Pilot data on the Behavior Rating Inventory of Executive Function (BRIEF) and performance measures of executive function in pediatric traumatic brain injury*. Unpublished master's thesis, University of Florida.

Blair, C. (2006). Toward a revised theory of general intelligence: Further examination of fluid cognitive abilities as unique aspects of human cognition. *Behavioral and Brain Sciences, 29*, 145–153.

Blair, C., Zelazo, P. D., & Greenberg, M. T. (2005). The measurement of executive function in childhood. *Developmental Neuropsychology, 28*, 561–571.

Bradshaw, J. L. (2001). *Developmental disorders of the frontostriatal system: Neuropsychological, neuropsychiatric and evolutionary perspectives*. Hove, UK: Psychology Press.

Brocki, K. C., & Bohlin, G. (2004). Executive functions in children aged 6–13: A dimensional and developmental study. *Developmental Neuropsychology, 26*, 571–593.

Brookshire, B., Levin, H. S., Song, J. X., & Zhang, L. (2004). Components of executive function in typically developing and head-injured children. *Developmental Neuropsychology, 25*(1), 61–83.

Bull, R., & Scerif, G. (2001). Executive functioning as a predictor of children's mathematics ability: Inhibition, switching, and working memory. *Developmental Neuropsychology, 19*, 273–293.

Canivez, G. L. (2008). Orthogonal higher order factor structure of the Stanford–Binet Intelligence Scales—Fifth Edition for children and adolescents. *School Psychology Quarterly, 23*(4), 533–541.

Carlson, N. R. (2004). *Physiology of behavior* (8th ed.). Boston: Pearson/Allyn & Bacon.

Chan, R. C. K., Shum, D., Toulopoulou, T., & Chen, E. Y. H. (2008). Assessment of executive functions: Review of instruments and identification of critical issues. *Archives of Clinical Neuropsychology, 23,* 201–216.

Cheung, A. M., Mitsis, E. M., & Halperin, J. M. (2004). The relationship of behavioral inhibition to executive functions in young adults. *Journal of Clinical and Experimental Neuropsychology, 26,* 393–403.

Cohen, M. J., Riccio, C. A., Kibby, M. Y., & Edmonds, J. E. (2000). Developmental progression of clock face drawing in children. *Child Neuropsychology, 6,* 64–76.

Delis, D. C., Kaplan, E., & Kramer, J. (2001). *Delis–Kaplan Executive Function System.* San Antonio, TX: Psychological Corporation.

Delis, D. C., Lansing, A., Houston, W. S., Wetter, S., Han, S. D., Jacobsen, M., et al. (2007). Creativity lost: The importance of testing higher-level executive functions in school-aged children. *Journal of Psychoeducational Assessment, 25,* 29–40.

DiStefano, C., & Dombrowski, S. C. (2006). Investigating the theoretical structure of the Stanford–Binet—Fifth Edition. *Journal of Psychoeducational Assessment, 24,* 123–136.

Dumont, R., Willis, J. O., & Elliott, C. D. (2009). *Essentials of DAS-II assessment.* Hoboken, NJ: Wiley.

Elliott, C. D. (1983). *British Ability Scales.* Windsor, UK: NFER-Nelson.

Elliott, C. D. (1990). *Differential Ability Scales.* San Antonio, TX: Psychological Corporation.

Elliott, C. D. (2007) *Differential Ability Scales—Second Edition.* San Antonio, TX: Harcourt Assessment.

Elliott, R. (2003). Executive functions and their disorders. *British Medical Bulletin, 65,* 49–59.

Evans, J. J. (2009). Rehabilitation of executive functioning: An overview. In M. Oddy & A. Worthington (Eds.), *The rehabilitation of executive disorders: A guide to theory and practice* (pp. 59–73). Oxford: Oxford University Press.

Flanagan, D. P., Alfonso, V. C., Ortiz, S. O., & Dynda, A. M. (2010). Integrating cognitive assessment in school neuropsychological evaluations. In D. C. Miller (Ed.), *Best practices in school neuropsychology: Guidelines for effective practice, assessment, and evidence-based intervention* (pp. 101–140). Hoboken, NJ: Wiley.

Flanagan, D. P., & Kaufman, A. S. (2009). *Essentials of WISC-IV assessment* (2nd ed.). Hoboken, NJ: Wiley.

Floyd, R. G., McCormack, A. C., Ingram, E. L., Davis, A. E., Bergeron, R., & Hamilton, G. (2006). Relations between the Woodcock Johnson III clinical clusters and measures of executive functions from the Delis–Kaplan Executive Function System. *Journal of Psychoeducational Assessment, 24,* 303–317.

Floyd, R. G., Shaver, R. B., & McGrew, K. S. (2003). Interpretation of the Woodcock–Johnson III Tests of Cognitive Abilities: Acting on evidence. In F. A. Schrank & D. P. Flanagan (Eds.), *WJ III clinical use and interpretation: Scientist-practitioner perspectives* (pp. 29–46). Boston: Academic Press.

Ford, L., Keith, T. Z., Floyd, R. G., Fields, C., & Schrank, F. A. (2003). Using the WJ III Tests of Cognitive Abilities with attention deficit hyperactivity disorder. In F. A. Schrank & D. P. Flanagan (Eds.), *WJ III clinical use and interpretation: Scientist-practitioner perspectives* (pp. 319–344). Boston: Academic Press.

Friedman, N. R., Miyake, A., Corley, R. P., Young, S. E., DeFries, J. C., & Hewitt, J. K. (2006). Not all executive functions are related to intelligence. *Psychological Science, 17,* 172–179.

Fuster, J. M. (2001). The prefrontal cortex—an update: Time is of the essence. *Neuron, 30,* 319–333.

Fuster, J. M. (2002). Frontal lobe and cognitive development. *Journal of Neurocytology, 31,* 373–385.

Gioia, G. A., Isquith, P. K., Guy, S., & Kenworthy, L. (2000). *Behavior Rating Inventory of Executive Function.* Odessa, FL: Psychological Assessment Resources.

Grafman, J. (2006). Human prefrontal cortex: Processes and representations. In J. Risberg & J. Grafman (Eds.), *The frontal lobes: Development, function, and pathology* (pp. 69–91). Cambridge, UK: Cambridge University Press.

Gregg, N., & Coleman, C. (2003). Use of the Woodcock–Johnson III in the diagnosis of learning disabilities. In F. A. Schrank & D. P. Flanagan (Eds.), *WJ III clinical use and interpretation: Scientist-practitioner perspectives* (pp. 125–174). Boston: Academic Press.

Hale, J. B., & Fiorello, C. A. (2004). *School neuropsychology: A practitioner's handbook.* New York: Guilford Press.

Han, S. D., Delis, D. C., & Holdnack, J. A. (2008). Extending the WISC-IV: Executive functioning. In A. Prifitera, D. H. Saklofske, & L. G. Weiss (Eds.), *WISC-IV clinical assessment and intervention* (2nd ed., pp. 497–515). Burlington, MA: Elsevier/Academic Press.

Happaney, K., Zelazo, P. D., & Stuss, D. T. (2004). Development of orbitofrontal function: Current themes and future directions. *Brain and Cognition, 35,* 1–10.

Holdnack, J. A., & Weiss, L. G. (2006). WISC IV Integrated: Beyond the essentials. In L. G. Weiss, D. H. Saklofske, A. Prifitera, & J. A. Holdnack, *WISC-IV: Advanced clinical interpretation* (pp. 201–275). Burlington, MA: Elsevier/Academic Press.

Holdnack, J. A., Weiss, L. G., & Entwistle, P. (2006). Advanced WISC-IV and WISC-IV Integrated interpretation in context with other measures. In L. G. Weiss, D. H. Saklofske, A. Prifitera, & J. A. Holdnack, *WISC-IV: Advanced clinical interpretation* (pp. 275–370). Burlington, MA: Elsevier/Academic Press.

Homack, S., Lee, D., & Ricco, C. A. (2005). Test review: Delis–Kaplan Executive Function System. *Journal of Clinical and Experimental Neuropsychology, 27,* 599–609.

Hughes, C., & Graham, A. (2002). Measuring executive functions in childhood: Problems and solutions. *Child and Adolescent Mental Health, 7,* 131–142.

Hughes, C., & Graham, A. (2008). Executive functions and development. In J. Reed & J. Warner-Rogers (Eds.), *Child neuropsychology: Concepts, theory, and practice* (pp. 264–284). Chichester, UK: Wiley-Blackwell.

Kane, M. J., & Engle, R. W. (2002). The role of prefrontal cortex in working memory capacity, executive attention, and general fluid intelligence: An individual difference perspective. *Psychonomic Bulletin and Review, 9,* 637–671.

Kaufman, A. S., & Kaufman, N. L. (2004). *Kaufman Assessment Battery for Children—Second Edition.* Circle Pines, MN: American Guidance Service.

Kaufman, J. C., Kaufman, A. S., Kaufman-Singer, J., & Kaufman, N. (2005). The Kaufman Assessment Battery for Children—Second Edition and the Kaufman Adolescent and Adult Intelligence Test. In D. P. Flanagan & P. L. Harrison (Eds.), *Contemporary intellectual assessment: Theories, tests, and issues* (2nd ed., pp. 344–370). New York: Guilford Press.

Keith, T. Z., Fine, J. G., Taub, G. E., Reynolds, M. R., & Kranzler, J. H. (2006). Higher-order, multisample, confirmatory factor analysis of the Wechsler Intelligence Scale for Children—Fourth Edition: What does it measure? *School Psychology Review, 30,* 89–119.

Kemp, S. (2007, July). *Introduction to the clinical development and applications of the NEPSY II.* Paper presented at the National School Neuropsychology Conference, Grapevine, TX.

Knight, R. T., & Stuss, D. T. (2002). *Principles of frontal lobe function.* New York: Oxford University Press.

Korkman, M., Kirk, U., & Kemp, S. (2007). *NEPSY II clinical and interpretive manual.* San Antonio, TX: Harcourt Assessment.

Lezak, M. D., Howieson, D. B., & Loring, D. W. (2004). *Neuropsychological assessment* (4th ed.). New York: Oxford University Press.

Lidz, C. (2003). *Early childhood assessment.* New York: Wiley.

Mangeot, S. D., Armstrong, K., Colvin, A. N., Yeates, K. O., & Taylor, H. G. (2002). Long term executive deficits in children with traumatic brain injuries: Assessing using the Behavior Rating Inventory of Executive Function (BRIEF). *Child Neuropsychology, 8,* 271–284.

Maricle, D. E., Johnson, W., & Avirett, E. (2010). Assessing and intervening in children with executive function disorders. In D. C. Miller (Ed.), *Best practices in school neuropsychology: Guidelines for effective practice, assessment, and evidenced-based intervention* (pp. 599–640). Hoboken, NJ: Wiley.

Mays, K. L., Kamphaus, R. W., & Reynolds, C. R. (2009). Applications of the Kaufman Assessment Battery for Children, 2nd Edition in neuropsychological assessment. In C. R. Reynolds & E. Fletcher-Janzen (Eds.), *Handbook of clinical child neuropsychology* (3rd ed., pp. 281–295). New York: Springer.

McCabe, D. P., Roediger, H. L., McDaniel, M. A., Balota, D. A., & Hambrick, D. Z. (2010). The relationship between working memory capacity and executive functioning: Evidence for a common executive attention construct. *Neuropsychology, 24*(2), 222–243.

McCloskey, G., Perkins, L. A., & Van Divner, B. (2009). *Assessment and intervention for executive function difficulties.* New York: Routledge.

McGrew, K. S., & Woodcock, R. W. (2001). *Technical manual: Woodcock–Johnson III Tests of Cognitive Abilities.* Itasca, IL. Riverside.

Meltzer, L., & Krishnan, K. (2007). Executive function difficulties and learning disabilities: Understandings and misunderstandings. In L. Meltzer (Ed.), *Executive function in education* (pp. 77–105). New York: Guilford Press.

Miller, D. C. (2007). *Essentials of school neuropsychological assessment.* Hoboken, NJ: Wiley.

Miller, D. C., & Hale, J. B. (2008). Neuropsychological applications of the WISC-IV and WISC-IV Integrated. In A. Prifitera, D. H. Saklofske, & L. G. Weiss (Eds.), *WISC-IV clinical assessment and intervention* (2nd ed., pp. 445–495). Burlington, MA: Elsevier/Academic Press.

Miyake, A., Friedman, N., Emerson, M., Witzki, A., & Howerter, A. (2000). The unity and diversity of executive functions and their contributions to complex "frontal lobe" tests: A latent variable analysis. *Cognitive Psychology, 41,* 49–100.

Ozonoff, S., & Schetter, P. (2007). Executive dysfunction in autism spectrum disorders: From research to practice. In L. Meltzer (Ed.), *Executive function in education* (pp. 133–160). New York: Guilford Press.

Parrish, J., Geary, E., Jones, J., Seth, R., Hermann, B., & Seidenberg, M. (2007). Executive functioning in childhood epilepsy: Parent-report and cognitive assessment. *Developmental Medicine and Child Neurology, 49,* 412–416.

Read, B. G., & Schrank, F. A. (2003). Qualitative analysis of Woodcock–Johnson III test performance. In F. A. Schrank & D. P. Flanagan (Eds.), *WJ III clinical use and interpretation: Scientist-practitioner perspectives* (pp. 47–91). Boston: Academic Press.

Reynolds, C. R. (2007, July). *Frontal lobe development: What is it and when does it end?* Paper presented at the National School Neuropsychology Conference, Grapevine, TX.

Roberts, A. C., Robbins, T. W., & Weiskrantz, L. (2002). *The prefrontal cortex: Executive and cognitive function.* Oxford: Oxford University Press.

Roid, G. (2003a). *Interpretive manual: Expanded guide to the interpretation of the SB5 test results.* Itasca, IL: Riverside.

Roid, G. (2003b). *Stanford–Binet Intelligence Scales, Fifth Edition.* Itasca, IL: Riverside.

Roid, G., & Barram, R. A. (2004). *Essentials of Stanford–Binet Intelligence Scales (SB5) assessment.* Hoboken, NJ: Wiley.

Romine, C. B., & Reynolds, C. R. (2005). A model of the development of frontal lobe functioning: Findings from a meta-analysis. *Applied Neuropsychology, 12,* 190–201.

Roth, R. M., & Saykin, A. J. (2004). Executive dysfunction in attention deficit hyperactivity disorder: Cognitive and neuroimaging findings. *Psychiatric Clinics of North America, 27*(1), 83–96.

Salthouse, T. (2005). Relations between cognitive abilities and measures of executive functioning. *Neuropsychology, 19,* 532–545.

Sattler, J. M., & Dumont, R. (2008). Wechsler Intelligence Scale for Children—Fourth Edition (WISC-IV): Description. In J. M Sattler, *Assessment of children: Cognitive foundations* (5th ed., pp. 265–315). San Diego, CA: Jerome M. Sattler, Publisher.

Sattler, J. M., Dumont, R., Salerno, J. D., & Roberts-Pittman, B. (2008). Stanford–Binet Intelligence Scales—Fifth Edition (SB5). In J. M. Sattler, *Assessment of children: Cognitive foundations* (5th ed., pp. 565–604). San Diego, CA: Jerome M. Sattler, Publisher.

Sattler, J. M., Dumont, R., Willis, J. O., & Salerno, J. D. (2008). Differential Ability Scales—Second Edition (DAS-II). In J. M. Sattler, *Assessment of children: Cognitive foundations* (5th ed., pp. 605–675). San Diego, CA: Jerome M. Sattler, Publisher.

Shallice, T., Marzocchi, G. M., Coser, S., Del Savio, M., Meuter, R. F., & Rumiati, R. L. (2002). Executive function profile of children with attention deficit hyperactivity disorder. *Developmental Neuropsychology, 21,* 43–71.

Stein, J., & Krishnan, K. (2007). Nonverbal learning disabilities and executive function: The challenges

of effective assessment and teaching. In L. Meltzer (Ed.), *Executive function in education* (pp. 106–132). New York: Guilford Press.

Strauss, E., Sherman, E. M. S., & Spreen, O. (2006). *A compendium of neuropsychological tests: Administration, norms and commentary* (3rd ed.). New York: Oxford University Press.

Stuss, D. T. (2009). Rehabilitation of frontal lobe dysfunction: A working framework. In M. Oddy & A. Worthington (Eds.), *The rehabilitation of executive disorders: A guide to theory and practice* (pp. 3–17). Oxford: Oxford University Press.

Stuss, D. T., & Alexander, M. P. (2000). Executive functions and the frontal lobes: A conceptual view. *Psychological Research, 63,* 289–298.

Sugarman, R. (2002). Evolution and executive functions: Why our toolboxes are empty. *Revista Espanola de Neuropsicologic, 4*(4), 351–377.

Titley, J., & D'Amato, R. C. (2008). Understanding and using the NEPSY II with young children, children, and adolescents. In R. C. D'Amato & L. C. Hartlage (Eds.), *Essentials of neuropsychological assessment* (2nd ed., pp. 149–172). New York: Springer.

Tranel, D., Manzel, K., & Anderson, S. W. (2008). Is the prefrontal cortex important for fluid intelligence?: A neuropsychological study using matrix reasoning. *Clinical Neuropsychology, 22*(2), 242–261.

van Vreen, V., & Carter, C. S. (2002). The timing of action-monitoring processes in the anterior cingulate cortex. *Journal of Cognitive Science, 14,* 593–602.

Vaquero, E., Gomez, C. M., Quintero, E. A., Gonzalez-Rosa, J. J., & Marquez, J. (2008). Differential prefrontal-like deficit in children after cerebellar astrocytoma and meulloblastoma tumor. *Behavioral and Brain Function, 4,* 1–16.

Verte, S., Geurts, H., Roeyers, H., Oosterlaan, J., & Sergeant, J. A. (2006). Executive functioning in children with an autism spectrum disorder: Can we differentiate within the spectrum? *Journal of Autism and Developmental Disorders, 16,* 351–372.

Vriezen, E. R., & Pigott, S. E. (2002). The relationship between parental support on the BRIEF and performance based measures of executive function in children with moderate to severe brain injury. *Child Neuropsychology, 8,* 296–303.

Wechsler, D. (2003). *Wechsler Intelligence Scale for Children—Fourth Edition (WISC-IV).* San Antonio, TX: Psychological Corporation.

Wechsler, D., Kaplan, E., Fein, D., Morris, E., Kramer, J. H., Maerlender, A., et al. (2004). *The Wechsler Intelligence Scale for Children—Fourth Edition Integrated: Technical and interpretive manual.* San Antonio, TX: Harcourt Assessment.

Weiss, L. G., Beal, A. L., Saklofske, D. H., Packiam-

Alloway, T., & Prifitera, A. (2008). Interpretation and intervention with WISC-IV in the clinical assessment context. In A. Prifitera, D. H. Saklofske, & L. G. Weiss (Eds.), *WISC-IV clinical assessment and intervention* (2nd ed., pp. 3–66). Burlington, MA: Elsevier/Academic Press.

Willcutt, E. G., Doyle, A. E., Nigg, J. T., Faraone, S. V., & Pennington, B. F. (2005). Validity of the executive function theory of attention deficit hyperactivity disorder: A meta-analytic review. *Biological Psychiatry, 37,* 1336–1346.

Wood, J. N., & Grafman, J. (2003). Human prefrontal cortex: Processing and representational perspectives. *Nature Reviews Neuroscience, 4,* 139–147.

Woodcock, R. W., McGrew, K. S., & Mather, N. (2001, 2007). *Woodcock–Johnson III Tests of Cognitive Abilities Normative Update.* Rolling Meadows, IL: Riverside.

Zelazo, P. D., Muller, U., Frye, D., & Marcovitch, S. (2003). The development of executive function in early childhood. *Monographs of the Society for Research in Child Development, 68*(3, Serial No. 274).

Zilmer, E. A., Spiers, M. V., & Culbertson, W. C. (2008). *Principles of neuropsychology* (2nd ed.). Belmont, CA: Thomson.

CHAPTER 35

Intelligence Tests in the Context of Emerging Assessment Practices
Problem-Solving Applications

Rachel Brown-Chidsey
Kristina J. Andren

U.S. students take many different types of tests in school. The No Child Left Behind Act (NCLB) of 2001 mandates annual testing in all schools that receive federal aid (Heubert & Hauser, 1999; NCLB, 2001). More recent federal education initiatives, such as Race to the Top, have also required indicators of student performance as a condition of funding (U.S. Department of Education, 2009). These tests are often referred to as *high-stakes* because they may determine whether a student is eligible to move on to the next grade or graduate from high school. As of August 2003, all 50 U.S. states required some form of statewide testing of students (Thurlow, Wiley, & Bielinski, 2003). Currently, 28 states require high school exit exams (Center on Education Policy [CEP], 2010a). Although NCLB does not mandate that a student take a test to be eligible for a high school diploma, it does require states to develop statewide school accountability programs (National Center on Educational Outcomes [NCEO], 2003).

Certain data suggest that requiring such tests may have a positive effect on student learning outcomes. In 2003, the passing rates on Florida's statewide test, the Florida Comprehensive Assessment Test (FCAT), revealed that fewer than half of the state's high school seniors passed the test in most counties (Florida Department of Education,

2003). By 2010, 60% of 10th-grade students passed the FCAT in reading; 84% passed in math. However, of high school seniors who needed to retake the test, passing rates dropped to 16% for reading and 28% for math (Florida Department of Education, 2010). The CEP (2010b) released data showing that in two-thirds of states with sufficient data, reading and math scores for students of different racial and cultural backgrounds have improved over a 3-year period. Still, the fact that many students are not passing high-stakes tests has led to recommendations for review of education policies. New York State Education Commissioner Richard Mills (2003) suggested that New York State allow the passing rate on the Regents Exam to remain at 55, rather than require the higher passing rate of 65. Mills's justification for retaining the lower passing rate was his concern that too many students would fail the exam if the passing score were raised. Mills also noted that additional alternatives for testing students with disabilities were needed.

Despite Mills's concern, assessment policies have actually gone in the other direction. One of the distinguishing features of the recent widespread use of high-stakes tests is that virtually all students are required to participate in such exams (Shriner, 2000; Thurlow et al., 2003). Twenty-seven states prohibit exclusion from statewide testing; of the

23 states where it is permitted, the most common allowance is for medical conditions (Christensen, Lazarus, Crone, & Thurlow, 2008). In contrast to past practice, when students with disabilities were often exempted from state-mandated tests, the current high-stakes testing movement has focused on the importance of having all students—both those with and without disabilities—participate in large-scale, high-stakes tests. In fact, both the 1997 amendments to the original Individuals with Disabilities Education Act and the Individuals with Disabilities Education Improvement Act of 2004 (IDEA 2004) put a heavy emphasis on the participation of students with disabilities in state-mandated testing in general education. The rationale behind the participation of students with disabilities in high-stakes tests is to provide indicators of the students' progress toward individualized education program (IEP) goals, and to provide the students with greater access to postsecondary educational opportunities (Shriner, 2000; Thurlow et al., 2003).

Although the provisions of IDEA 2004 have been in place for several years now, the implications of including students with disabilities in high-stakes tests are not fully understood. The staff of the NCEO has conducted a series of studies related to the effects of participation by students with disabilities in such tests (e.g., Thurlow et al., 2003). As of 2008, all 50 states presented performance data for regular and alternative assessments, and most states reported participation rates of 95% or more for students with IEPs. Preliminary evaluation indicates that students in general are performing at levels lower than desired, and that students with disabilities generally perform at lower levels than other students. Generally, about 30% of students with IEPs perform at a proficient level for reading and math (Altman, Thurlow, & Vang, 2010).

The widespread use of high-stakes tests in U.S. schools has led to cautions about their use. The National Association of School Psychologists (NASP; 2003) has issued a position statement on the use of high-stakes tests in educational decision making; this stipulates that such a test should never be the sole criterion for determining a child's educational future, "including access to educational opportunity, retention or promotion, graduation or receipt of a diploma" (p. 1). The American Psychological Association (APA; 2003) has issued a position statement on the presence of high-stakes tests in schools as well. The APA acknowledges the potential benefit of high-stakes tests for demonstrating the outcomes and efficacy of specific

instructional programs. Like the NASP, however, the APA cautions against using a high-stakes test score as the only measure on which a critical decision about a child's educational future is based. The APA statement calls for additional research into the relationship between student performance on high-stakes tests and other indicators of learning. Despite these cautions from professional organizations, high-stakes tests are more widespread than ever, even with incomplete data from states as to the performance of students with disabilities.

One of the issues facing those who seek to make sense out of high-stakes test data is the extent to which predisposing characteristics of the learners influence their test scores. Specifically, high-stakes tests are designed in part to document the progress that students make in a given program of study or curriculum. The basic premise behind such testing is that those students who have mastered the curriculum should score high enough on the test(s) to move on to the next level of education. Essentially, this follows from the idea that all children can learn. Still, there is abundant evidence of the heterogeneity of learners, and some students have characteristics that prevent them from mastering the program of study.

In cases where a student's particular learning characteristics can be identified as the result of a specific disability, special education services are provided so that all students can have access to education. IDEA 2004 includes 14 specific disability categories. In the 2008–2009 school year, 13% of U.S. students participated in special education, and 39% of students receiving such services were identified as having specific learning disabilities (SLDs) (National Center for Education Statistics, 2010). Notably, this is a drop from 2000, when 46% of students in special education were identified with an SLD. Importantly, under IDEA 2004 and its predecessors, both the definition of an SLD and the process for identifying one have been interpreted to involve the administration of a test of cognitive abilities, such as an IQ test (Peterson & Shinn, 2002). A significant shift in this practice was made available under the 2004 law. This law and its accompanying regulations allow schools to use one of two methods to identify an SLD. Schools can use a formula that calculates the discrepancy between the student's IQ and academic achievement, or it can use data showing whether the student has responded to intervention designed to address a specific learning problem (Brown-Chidsey & Steege, 2010). Many, if not most, of the students currently identified as having

SLDs were identified as such on the basis of discrepancies between their scores on an IQ test and a measure of academic achievement (Peterson & Shinn, 2002; National Center for Education Statistics, 2010). This so-called "discrepancy method" is based on the idea that students with SLDs have at least average intellectual ability but are underperforming in school because of some other learning deficit.

Some students with SLDs have taken high-stakes tests under typical conditions with good results, and the performance of these students is of little concern (Thurlow et al., 2003). Other students with SLDs have done poorly on high-stakes tests under typical conditions, and therefore have been able to take these tests while using accommodations. Anecdotal evidence suggests that some students using accommodations have improved their scores, but others have not.

Interestingly, there are virtually no data on the relationship(s) between IQ scores and high-stakes tests. Despite the extensive use of IQ scores in the identification of the largest subgroup of students receiving special education services in the United States, there has been no systematic evaluation of the connection between the students' general cognitive abilities and their performance on the test(s) that determine whether they are allowed to move forward along the education continuum. Certainly, there are a number of barriers to collecting such data, including the need for parental permission and access to records. Nonetheless, recognition of issues related to IQ and high-stakes testing is important because of the implications both types of tests have for U.S. education policies. This chapter includes a discussion of the use of IQ tests in U.S. education and suggests an alternative method that focuses on specific problem-solving steps to address student learning needs.

CONTEXT OF INTELLIGENCE TESTING IN EDUCATION POLICY

Intelligence (IQ) tests were initially created for the purpose of determining which students would benefit from school-based education and which would not (Gould, 1981; Sattler, 2001). Alfred Binet is credited with creating the first IQ test for use with a school-age population in France (see Wasserman, Chapter 1, this volume). His test was adapted and used in many settings, including U.S. schools. Although it was hoped that IQ tests would help educators make decisions about the best instruc-

tion for different students, the tests have never met that expectation fully. Many studies have shown that all IQ tests have limited reliability (Gould, 1981; Reschly & Grimes, 2002). In addition, other research has shown that the original view of IQ as a fixed trait, immune to instruction, is not accurate (Reschly & Grimes, 2002).

The limits of the reliability of IQ tests have been documented repeatedly (Gould, 1981; Kranzler, 1997; Reschly & Grimes, 2002; Sattler, 2008). Although certain features of IQ appear to be more stable than others (Flanagan, Ortiz, & Alfonso, 2007; Reschly & Grimes, 2002; Sattler, 2008), there is much variability in even average performance on IQ tests. In addition to concerns about the instability of IQ scores, other problems with their use in educational decision making have been identified. The validity of such tests for students from diverse linguistic, cultural, ethnic, and ability backgrounds has been widely challenged (Ortiz & Dynda, 2005; Ortiz & Ochoa, 2005; see also Ortiz, Ochoa, & Dynda, Chapter 22, this volume).

At one time, IQ test scores were widely used in the United States as the sole criteria for determining which students would be enrolled in general education programs and which ones would take remedial classes. This practice was found to be highly discriminatory against certain groups of students, including African American students, and was litigated (e.g., in the well-known case of *Larry P. v. Riles*). For this reason, other ways of identifying aptitude and skills were developed. Many different measures of academic and other skills are widely used in schools for both individualized and large-group assessment. The presence of these skills tests has allowed educators to identify students' levels of performance and then provide instruction to improve the skills of low-achieving students.

Importantly, the premise behind skills and achievement testing is that missing skills can be learned with appropriate instruction. The assumption that instruction can have an impact on academic skills is in contrast to the interpretation of intellectual abilities as fixed traits that vary little over a person's lifetime. What researchers have learned from the use of skills testing followed by teaching and retesting is that certain skills can be improved through instruction (Reschly & Grimes, 2002). A by-product of the test–teach–retest model has been the discovery that IQ scores also improve with certain types of instruction and environmental enrichment (Elliott & Fuchs, 1997; Reschly & Grimes, 2002). Over time, numerous reliable and valid assessment methods have been developed for the purpose of identifying which students need what type of instruction. Many researchers have put forward the case for the superiority of measures other than IQ, such as curriculum-based measurement (CBM), for this task (Brown-Chidsey, Davis, & Maya, 2003; Deno, 1985; Elliott & Fuchs, 1997; Hosp, Hosp, & Howell, 2007; Shinn, 1989, 2005).

The Current Standards-Based Reform Movement

The current national trend toward the use of statewide high-stakes tests as part of standard educational practice is the next chapter in the unfolding story of using assessment to guide instructional decision making. Just as IQ tests were initially intended to help educators identify which students should be in school, high-stakes tests are designed to identify which students are meeting certain learning standards and which ones are not. The current standards-based reform movement is often associated with the publication of the report entitled A Nation at Risk (National Commission on Excellence in Education, 1983). This report, which was commissioned and published by the Reagan administration, deeply criticized the state of U.S. public education. Following the publication of A Nation at Risk, a number of federal- and state-level education reform initiatives were implemented with the goal of (re)establishing higher standards for what U.S. students learn.

The most recent of the federal reform initiatives is the 2001 NCLB, sponsored by the George W. Bush administration. This act goes farther than earlier federal efforts to achieve higher learning outcomes for all public school students because it pins federal education money to the states' plans and success in achieving the NCLB objectives. A revision of the NCLB was proposed to Congress in 2010 by the Obama administration. The Obama administration did provide competitive grant funding through the Race to the Top program (U.S. Department of Education, 2009), and this initiative used assessment criteria similar to those of the NCLB. According to NCLB, all U.S. states must submit plans for implementing and achieving the NCLB goals to the U.S. Department of Education. Those schools that do not meet certain standards may lose funding and/or be taken over by state departments of education until the NCLB goals are met. The way that schools are evaluated in relation to achieving NCLB goals is

through statewide high-stakes tests, which were, for the first time, mandated for students in grades 3–8 (NCLB, 2001).

The NCLB, and its corollary state programs and initiatives, have carried the practice of testing for instructional decision making forward into the 21st century. The current standards-based reform programs have essentially the same purpose as Binet's first IQ scale: determining which students receive access to which educational services. The current high-stakes tests come with far more levels of assessment and decision making than solitary IQ tests administered once, but in the end they are likely to yield similar results. Students who receive passing scores on the high-stakes tests will follow a stepwise progression through the educational system, while students who do not pass will get remedial instruction until or unless they pass the test(s) to earn a diploma or they drop out of school (Special Education Report, 2002; Thurlow & Esler, 2000). In either case, the educational future of all public school students is heavily influenced by the high-stakes tests, in the same way that IQ tests in the past determined students' educational futures.

The NCEO found that, as of 2007, all states had developed procedures for allowing students who receive special education services to have accommodations or take alternative forms of state-mandated tests. However, these policies vary widely across states (Christensen et al., 2008). Similarly, Thurlow and Esler (2000) reported that the process for appealing a failed graduation test for all students, regardless of disability, is nonexistent in most states. Indeed, some states have chosen to lower the criterion for passing the state test rather than to deal with appeals (Education USA, 2001; Mills, 2003). These policy trends suggest the emergence of recognition that high-stakes tests may constitute a significant obstacle to educational access for some students—one that may be challenged through litigation in the future.

Equality of Access to Education

Much of the debate surrounding the use of both IQ measures and high-stakes tests is related to equity. As noted above, IQ tests have been found to have lower reliability and limited validity when used with certain groups of students or under certain conditions (Flanagan, Ortiz, Alfonso, & Dynda, 2008; Lopez, 1997; Ortiz, 2002). Similarly, many critics have argued that group-based high-stakes tests have similarly questionable reliability and validity for certain students. Recent scores on the National Assessment of Educational Progress (NAEP) revealed a large and persistent gap in performance between several groups of students. European American students and students who are not from low-income families tend to score higher than African American, Hispanic, Native American, and low-income students (CEP, 2010b).

Given that a disproportionate number of students from diverse linguistic, cultural, racial, and ability backgrounds tend to live in poverty, high-stakes tests generally reveal that lower-income students are not making satisfactory educational progress. Recent research on the impact of exit exams suggests a negative impact on graduation rates for low-performing students, low-income students, racial minority students, and English-language learners (CEP, 2010a). Although some of the students who do poorly on high-stakes tests may be receiving special education services, special education was not created to provide remedial services to all underperforming students. Thus students who do not pass statewide tests have not typically had recourse to specialized instruction. Although special education was designed to increase access to education for all students, regardless of ability, the use of high-stakes tests may have the effect of reducing educational access. The IDEA 2004 included provisions specifically designed to address the needs of students who do not have a disability but need additional help. By creating a provision that allows schools to use data showing whether a student has responded to intervention, the context of how schools can and should help struggling students is starting to change (Brown-Chidsey, Bronaugh, & McGraw, 2009; Brown-Chidsey & Steege, 2010)

Unlike IQ tests, academic skills tests are designed to reveal the skills that students lack, and then to serve as a starting point for designing instruction by which the students can gain the skills. When joined with high-quality instruction and frequent assessment of progress, such methods have been shown to be very effective (Berninger, 2002; Elliott & Fuchs, 1997; National Center on Response to Intervention, 2011). Often, however, statewide tests of student achievement do not emphasize progress until a target score is met. In addition, the results are returned to schools after a considerable time delay. For example, scores for tests taken in winter or spring may not be sent to the schools until the summer, after the school year has ended (Brown-Chidsey et al., 2003). This time

delay means that the students and their teachers do not get the chance to review the test results and adjust instruction during the school year.

When compared with the initial use of IQ tests over 100 years ago, the shift to wide-scale, large-group testing for the purpose of fine-tuning instruction to meet the needs of individual learners is an improvement. Nonetheless, as currently implemented, state-mandated high-stakes tests may not be meeting the intended goal of improving instruction: The tests are not reliable and valid for all learners, and the results are provided to the students and teachers too late for change to occur. The common thread linking IQ and high-stakes tests is access to education. As noted, IQ tests have been used for many years as a cornerstone of individualized assessment of students to determine special education eligibility. More recently, IQ tests have been criticized as inappropriate indicators of students' aptitudes, and other forms of assessment have been introduced, including tests of student achievement in targeted skills. In isolation, neither IQ tests nor once-a-year statewide tests are effective tools for evaluating student progress. Yet there is evidence that both IQ instruments and high-stakes tests may have unique roles in educational assessment, when used appropriately and in combination with other tools.

ROLE OF INTELLIGENCE TESTING IN ACCESS TO EDUCATION

From their creation, IQ tests were considered to offer unique insight into a student's potential as a learner (Gould, 1981). In time, however, researchers and educators realized that IQ tests were limited in the extent to which they could predict a student's learning potential. Instead, researchers into cognitive assessment turned their attention to understanding a learner's profile (Flanagan et al., 2007; McGrew, Flanagan, Keith, & Vanderwood, 1997). Focusing on cognitive pattern analysis, researchers such as Flanagan, Ortiz, McGrew, and others have suggested that the true usefulness of IQ tests is in their ability to show *how*, not *whether*, a person learns. Nonetheless, others have maintained a position that ipsative analysis and other forms of subtest evaluation are not helpful when it comes to designing instructional interventions for low-achieving students (McDermott & Glutting, 1997; Reschly & Grimes, 2002; Stage, Abbott, Jenkins, & Berninger, 2003). Such research has pointed to other methods for determining which students need additional instruction and what kind (e.g., CBM and performance assessment; Elliott & Fuchs, 1997; Hosp et al., 2007; Howell & Nolet, 2000).

As noted above, an important change was included in IDEA 2004. Instead of requiring an IQ score as well as academic achievement information IDEA 2004 allows schools to document how a student responds to instruction as partial evidence of a learning disability. Since publication of the IDEA regulations (U.S. Department of Education, 2006), the only eligibility area requiring the use of an IQ score is intellectual disability (formerly known as mental retardation). As required by law, IQ scores should always be used alongside a number of other indicators of a student's abilities. For example, in the case of diagnosis of intellectual disability, the IQ score must be accompanied by an assessment of adaptive behavior, as well as other information about how an individual's characteristics fit with the diagnosis (Brown-Chidsey & Steege, 2004).

Problem-Solving Assessment

State-mandated high-stakes tests were implemented with the goal of improving student learning outcomes. Since the implementation of such tests, educators have learned that such data are helpful, but for some students these types of tests occur too infrequently. As a result of the limitations of once-a-year high-stakes testing, current innovations in assessment focus on gathering data about student progress more often and in a way that allows teachers to help students catch up as quickly as possible. This process is often known as a *problem-solving model* of student assessment (Deno, 1985, 2005; Tilly, 2008). Several specific problem-solving models are used for school-based assessment, and they all share the same key features. A model widely used by school psychologists and special educators is one developed by Stan Deno and his colleagues at the University of Minnesota (Deno, 1985). This model has five key problem-solving stages: problem identification, problem definition, exploring solutions, progress monitoring, and problem solution. This model is based on using hypothesis testing to identify the student's area(s) of need, as well as intervention(s) meeting the need(s). At each successive stage of problem solving, a specific hypothesis is tested to learn whether a specific action solves the student's problem(s). In recent

years, applications of this problem-solving model have been developed, implemented, and evaluated within a framework known as *response to intervention* (RTI). RTI refers to a multitier system of student support that offers instructional assistance to all students based on their levels of need. Figure 35.1 provides a graphic representation of one RTI service model.

Most, but not all, RTI service models include three tiers of services for students. These tiers provide students with increasingly specialized instruction if they need it. The pathways between tiers should be fluid and allow students to cross back to less intensive services once they meet certain goals, or to move on to more intensive services if needed. Importantly, and as shown in Figure 35.1, the "doors" between tiers are student data. When an RTI model is in place, no decision about a student's instructional needs and future is made without examining his or her data carefully. In this way, the student's most recent instructional performance guides the planning for the next steps. RTI incorporates problem solving in a systemic way because each tier offers a hypothesized solution as well as data to show whether the hypothesized solution worked. When the student data indicate that the problem is solved, no more intervention is added. But when the data indicate that the student is not yet making adequate progress, a new hypothesis is developed and tested with the addition of specific tier-defined instruction and assessment. How this process unfolds across the three tiers is explained below.

Tier 1: Universal Instruction and Assessment

Tier 1 is the most important part of RTI because it affects all students. Tier 1 includes the core curricula and instructional methods that are used for all students in a school. In essence, this means the instruction in all content areas that students experience every day. Tier 1 is universal because 100% of students participate in it. Each day that a student attends school, he or she is participating in tier 1 of RTI. As shown in Figure 35.1, tier 1 serves to create the foundation on which all the rest of RTI is built. The effectiveness of tier 1 has a direct relationship with how many students will need help at tiers 2 and 3. If tier 1 is strong and effective, fewer students will need support at the other tiers. It is recommended that schools strive to have at least 80% of their students successful

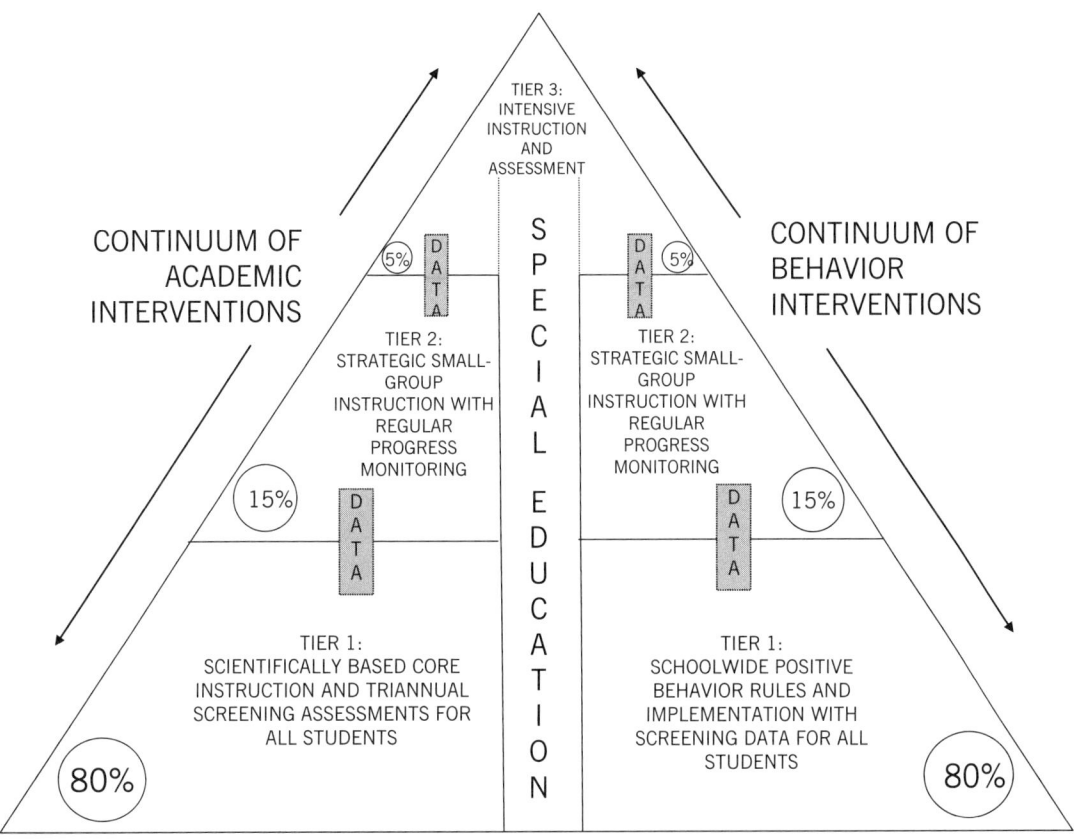

FIGURE 35.1. A model of RTI. From Brown-Chidsey and Steege (2010, p. 5). Copyright 2010 from The Guilford Press. Reprinted by permission.

with tier 1 instruction and assessment alone. Specific guidelines for how to implement and evaluate an effective tier 1 universal program are beyond the scope of this chapter, but many resources are available to assist educators (see Brown-Chidsey & Steege, 2010). In addition to using highly effective core curricula, tier 1 includes conducting brief assessments of all students three times a year. Often referred to as *benchmark screening*, these triannual assessments ensure that teachers know how all of their students are doing and which ones need additional help. The screenings are typically done in the fall, winter, and spring, and use CBM such as oral reading fluency to identify which students need assistance. The benchmark scores, as well as student classroom assessments are used to plan tier 2 instruction for those who need it. Notably, benchmark scores are very different from high-stakes tests like those required under NCLB because they are never used in isolation to make

instructional decisions. Instead, the data are compared with other indicators of student progress to determine a student's instructional needs.

Tier 2: Strategic Instruction and Assessment

Those students who are not making adequate progress with tier 1 instruction alone are provided with tier 2 as well. Importantly, tier 2 is provided *in addition* to tier 1, so that these students get a "double dose" of instruction. The reason for this extra instruction is that research has shown that students who are struggling in one or more areas benefit most when provided with extra instruction (Brown-Chidsey & Steege, 2010). For example, the recommended daily amount of reading instruction for students in kindergarten through third grade is 90 minutes. For a student whose reading scores are below the goal after he or she has received 90 minutes per day over a period of time, an additional 30 minutes per day will be added in tier 2 so that this student can catch up to the goal. The good news is that when tier 2 is added to tier 1, most of the students receiving tier 2 will make strong progress and eventually not need tier 2 any more (Burns & Gibbons, 2008; Jimerson, Burns, & Van Der Heyden, 2008).

In order to know how well the tier 2 instruction is working, regular assessments are needed as part of tier 2 services. Such assessments are a form of progress monitoring and are conducted at least monthly but often weekly. Progress-monitoring assessments use CBM as well and are very brief, taking from 1 to 4 minutes per student to complete. These measures provide immediate feedback to the student and teacher about how well the tier 2 instruction is working. Typically, about 20% of a school's students need tier 2 instruction. Of these, the majority (75% of those in tier 2) will make sufficient progress eventually to exit from tier 2 services. This leaves a very small number of students whose progress is very poor and for whom intensive intervention is needed.

Tier 3: Intensive Instruction and Assessment

For those students not making adequate progress with tier 1 plus tier 2, tier 3 offers intensive intervention. Sometimes tier 3 intervention is provided with a 1:1 student–teacher ratio; at other times, it is given in a very small group of two or three students. Like tier 2, it is provided *in addition* to the other tiers. This means that the student receives the maximum feasible amount of daily instruction. One of the important steps in setting up a multitier system of supports like RTI is to examine the school's daily schedule to make sure that there are times in the day when both tier 2 and tier 3 instruction can happen. Guidance on setting up multitier support schedules can be found in Brown-Chidsey and colleagues (2009). Like students in tier 2, those participating in tier 3 instruction need frequent progress monitoring. Since students at tier 3 have even greater needs than those at tier 2, they need to be monitored at least weekly but sometimes even daily. With tier 3 instruction and assessment, many of these students can make the progress they need to meet specific learning goals. In such cases, tier 3 support is gradually faded back to tier 2 and then tier 1 alone. Of the entire school population, about 5% will need tier 3. For those students who still do not find success with the

combination of tiers 1, 2, and 3, a referral to special education is often the next step. Such a referral reflects the hard work that teachers and specialists have put in to assist the student. It also reflects the need for additional problem solving and possibly other forms of in-depth assessment to determine the nature of the student's school difficulties.

It should be noted that the problem-solving process contained in RTI is all situated in general education. The activities occurring at tiers 1 through 3 all happen before a referral to special education. This is important because it means that RTI involves and supports all students, not just those eligible for special education. As noted, the vast majority of students in a school can be successful with the multiple tiers of support that a system like RTI provides. There will always be a small number of students who have specific disabilities and who need special education. RTI is not intended to prevent students with disabilities from gaining access to special education. Indeed, the opposite is true: RTI is designed to ensure that all students have access to effective and equitable education. By providing successive supports based on student needs, RTI ensures that only those students with disabilities who truly need special education are provided with it.

If a student does not respond to intervention across multiple tiers, the data collected during each tier's activities should be used as part of the comprehensive evaluation process. Such data document the types of interventions used, as well as what growth, if any, has been observed. The nature of the additional assessments to be conducted as part of the comprehensive evaluation will vary a great deal from student to student. For this reason, it is impossible to prescribe a specific battery or set of tests to be used with all students referred for evaluation. Regarding cognitive assessment, the only rule to note is that a standard IQ test is not needed in most cases. As noted above and in other chapters in this volume, the best use of cognitive assessments is based on specific hypothesis testing within a problem-solving process. When multiple tiers of student support have been provided as part of a system like RTI, yet those data indicate that the student has not responded to intervention, a different approach to problem solving is needed. At this stage, the questions become these: Why has the student not responded to intervention, and what permanent supports are needed to ensure that this student can access an effective and equitable education? At this phase, selected cognitive assessments (detailed in other chapters) are likely to be used to document the pervasive nature of the students' learning needs. When the results of these assessments confirm that a student has a learning disability, special education can be provided through an IEP.

A remaining question about how best to support the student is what instruction should be included in the IEP. In other words, how will the instruction in special education be different from what was provided in tiers 1, 2, and 3? In some cases the instruction will not be any different. This is likely to be the case when the student has shown progress, but it is too small to ensure that the student will meet grade-level learning goals. In such cases, the special education instruction includes even more additional intensive instruction in the area(s) of need. In cases where the student's data from tiers 1, 2, and 3 show no growth at all, the IEP will carry forward the hypothesis-testing process of determining the most effective intervention for the student. Once identified, it will be maintained at the level of intensity needed for the student to meet annual learning goals. In both such cases, the benefit of the special education service is that it documents why the student needs such intensive instruction and protects the student's right to effective education.

For all students with disabilities who are required to take high-stakes tests, it is important to determine whether accommodations or modifications are needed in order to obtain a more valid indicator of the students' knowledge and skills (Wasburn-Moses, 2003). Most states have been very strict about the extent and nature of high-stakes test accommodations, but when these are documented and appropriate, alterations to standard testing conditions can be made. Such accommodations and/or modifications should be based on a variety of assessment and evaluation information about a student. It may be the case that information from a cognitive assessment or other individually administered tests can help to document the basis for a student's high-stakes testing accommodations or modifications. For example, some students need extra time to complete the items on high-stakes tests in order to demonstrate their mastery of the learned material. The need for extra time as a result of slower-than-average processing can be documented by providing evidence from a psychological evaluation that has included cognitive measures. Similarly, a psychological evaluation with cognitive information can provide evidence that a student is capable of processing and responding to questions on a test in the expected time, but needs assistive technology in order to produce a response. In both these cases, cognitive testing scores or similar individualized assessment data are appropriate ways to indicate why a student needs accommodations for instruction and assessment. For students whose disabilities are mild enough that they go on to postsecondary education, the documentation of their disabilities is an important step in ensuring that they can access instructional accommodations and modifications in the higher education setting.

AREAS NEEDING MORE RESEARCH

A number of details related to the use of cognitive assessments in an era of multitiered and problem-solving service delivery need to be addressed with future research. It is likely that all U.S. schools will continue to be expected to participate fully in standards-based assessment activities; thus the nature of the questions needing to be addressed by researchers may continue to change over time. Three major lines of research that serve as general starting points for understanding the general effects of standards-driven instructional planning on individual students are discussed below.

Relationship between Cognitive Skills and High-Stakes Tests

As noted above, there is very little research on the actual relationship between cognitive ability scores and students' scores on high-stakes tests. Without even small datasets documenting the relationship between cognitive skills and high-stakes test scores, it is impossible to tell whether students with identified cognitive weaknesses are likely to perform in a certain way on these tests. It may be the case that student performance on high-stakes tests has very little relationship with cognitive scores, and research in this area is desperately needed. Alternatively, there may be a considerable degree of consistency between cognitive and high-stakes test scores. If that is the case, then it seems pertinent to ask this question: How might students' scores on high-stakes tests and other achievement indicators be used to make instructional decisions? Such a practice could reduce the number of cognitive tests given, potentially saving many hours of work and freeing up personnel for other activities—such as implementing and monitoring instruction, or conducting in-depth assessment of students with more complex learning needs.

Accommodations and Alternative Assessments

There is a growing amount of information on the use and effects of accommodations, modifications, and alternative forms of assessment. The NCEO has conducted a number of reviews of states' data about the use of testing accommodations, modifications, and alternative assessments (Thurlow et al., 2003). Although it remains difficult to compare data between and among states, there is an increasing database of students' scores on high-stakes tests under a variety of testing conditions. These data should help to shed light on the extent to which students from diverse backgrounds and experiences are able to succeed on high-stakes tests over time. Similarly, the states themselves are required to collect and report data on student performance on high-stakes tests according to population characteristics and subgroups (e.g., language, race, disability). These data should continue to help policymakers determine whether the use of high-stakes tests is any more useful than previous attempts to identify and address students' learning needs. In particular, it remains to be seen whether high-stakes tests add incremental validity to instructional decisions for students at risk. If data collected as part of multitier student supports is strong enough to show student growth over time, are yearly state-mandated high-stakes tests still needed?

High-Stakes Test Data and Student Improvement

Research on the effects of high-stakes testing on student achievement outcomes has yielded mixed evidence, suggesting possible benefits and negative effects for different groups of students (CEP, 2010a). Similar to the need for disaggregated data about student performance on high-stakes tests, there is a need for longitudinal data about how students in a given testing pool (i.e., a particular state) perform on the newly required tests as instructional adjustments are made. Some states have such data already, and others are making adjustments to state testing requirements to facilitate better reporting and analysis of students' test scores. Another factor likely to influence the nature of states' high stakes tests is the adoption and use of the Common Core Learning Standards. The Common Core was developed by the Council of Chief State School Officers (CCSSO, 2011). It is a uniform core curriculum in the areas of reading and math, and it

was developed in the attempt to make it easier to interpret each state's performance on the only national assessment given in all states: the NAEP. Although selected students from all 50 states complete the NAEP, fairly comparing their scores is impossible because every state has a different set of learning standards. The CCSSO realized that if there was one core set of learning standards for all the states, valid comparisons among states could be conducted. As of 2011, 42 states have formally adopted the proposed Common Core Standards. Six other states (Virginia, Nebraska, Minnesota, North Dakota, Montana, and Washington) have legislation pending to adopt the standards. Alaska and Texas are the only states currently opting out. The time frame for implementing the Common Core has yet to be developed, but once it is in place, scores from the states' high-stakes tests will be able to be reviewed in very new and different ways for all participating states. Not only will comparison of NAEP scores be valid, but how each state's mandated test performs in relation to instruction of the Common Core can be observed. In time, it may be that one Common Assessment will be developed to replace the individual states' high-stakes tests. Over time, these data are also likely to show which instructional programs are most effective in meeting the learning objectives. Once such data are obtained, a thorough review of the role and function of high-stakes tests in regard to student learning outcomes will be necessary.

CONCLUSION

It is very clear that standards-based reform programs are part of the current and future landscape of U.S. public education. Such programs had their origins in criticisms of public education dating from the early 1980s, but have been added to by educators, policymakers, and members of the public who have sought to establish clearer and more challenging educational goals for all students. One of the prominent features of current reform initiatives is the use of high-stakes tests intended to identify which students have met the learning objectives and which have not. There is some evidence that high-stakes tests are related to improved student outcomes, but the data are inconsistent (Thurlow et al., 2003; Viadero, 2003). An additional recent element in the efforts to improve student learning outcomes is the proposed Common Core to provide uniform learning standards across all states.

The current focus on student learning results and on the instruction necessary to achieve them has renewed awareness of the importance of access to education for all students. As noted by Thurlow and Esler (2000), access to a high-quality education has already been identified as a property right by some courts. If equal access to education remains part of U.S. education policy, then it should not be a question of whether cognitive, high-stakes, or other types of tests are used, but rather under what circumstances they are used and for what purposes. For a century now, researchers have argued both the benefits and limitations of cognitive assessments, including IQ tests. With time, a similar body of research will exist for universal screening, progress monitoring, and high-stakes tests. Regardless of the merits or drawbacks of either type of test, what really matters for individual students are how, when, and for what purpose they are used.

As suggested by Reschly and Grimes (2002), there should be a "Surgeon General's warning" on all tests to remind us that every test has limitations, and that no one test should ever be used in isolation to make "high-stakes" decisions about students' educational futures. Instead of expecting any one test to serve as a universal prescription for students' learning needs, educators, parents, policymakers, and the public need to recognize that high-quality assessment comes from the use of a range of evaluation tools over time. Those who are vexed by the current debate over high-stakes testing can learn from the history of IQ testing and research—which shows that no one test will yield all the answers, but that over time a range of indicators can help provide information about what instruction may be most effective in the future.

REFERENCES

Altman, J., Thurlow, M., & Vang, M. (2010). Annual performance report: 2007–2008 state assessment data. Retrieved from *www.cehd.umn.edu/NCEO/OnlinePubs/APRreport2007-2008.pdf*.

American Psychological Association (APA). (2003). Appropriate use of high-stakes testing in our nation's schools. Retrieved from *www.apa.org/pubinfo/testing.html*.

Berninger, V. (2002). Best practices in reading, writing, and math assessment–intervention links: A systems approach for schools, classrooms, and individuals. In A. Thomas & J. Grimes (Eds.), *Best practices in school psychology IV* (pp. 851–866). Bethesda, MD: National Association of School Psychologists.

Brown-Chidsey, R., Bronaugh, L., & McGraw, K. (2009). *RTI in the classroom*. New York: Guilford Press.

Brown-Chidsey, R., Davis, L., & Maya, C. (2003). Sources of variance in curriculum-based measures of silent reading. *Psychology in the Schools, 40,* 363–377.

Brown-Chidsey, R., & Steege, M. W. (2004). Adaptive behavior assessment. In T. S. Watson & C. H. Skinner (Eds.), *Encyclopedia of school psychology* (pp. 14–15). New York: Kluwer Academic/Plenum.

Brown-Chidsey, R., & Steege, M. W. (2010). *Response to intervention: Principles and strategies for effective practice* (2nd ed.). New York: Guilford Press.

Burns, M. K., & Gibbons, K. A. (2008). *Implementing response to intervention in elementary and secondary schools: Procedures to assure scientific-based practices.* New York: Routledge.

Center on Education Policy (CEP). (2010a). State high school tests: Exit exams and other assessments. Retrieved from *www.cep-dc.org*.

Center on Education Policy (CEP). (2010b). State test score trends through 2008–2009, Part 2: Slow and uneven progress in narrowing gaps. Retrieved from *www.cep-dc.org*.

Christensen, L. L., Lazarus, S. S., Crone, M., & Thurlow, M. L. (2008). *2007 state policies on assessment participation and accommodations for students with disabilities* (Synthesis Report No. 69). Minneapolis: University of Minnesota, National Center on Educational Outcomes.

Council of Chief State School Officers (CCSSO). (2010). Common core: State standards initiatives. Retrieved from *www.corestandards.org*.

Deno, S. L. (1985). Curriculum-based measurement: The emerging alternative. *Exceptional Children, 52,* 219–232.

Deno, S. L. (2005). Problem solving assessment. In R. Brown-Chidsey (Ed.), *Assessment for intervention: A problem-solving approach* (pp. 10–42). New York: Guilford Press.

Education USA. (2001). Mass[achusetts] officials mull appeals process for exit exams. *Education USA: The Independent Biweekly News Digest for School Leaders, 43*(20), 1–2.

Elliott, S. N., & Fuchs, L. S. (1997). The utility of curriculum-based measurement and performance assessment as alternatives to traditional intelligence and achievement tests. *School Psychology Review, 26,* 224–233.

Flanagan, D. P., Ortiz, S. , & Alfonso, V. C. (2007). *Essentials of cross-battery assessment* (2nd ed.). Hoboken, NJ: Wiley.

Flanagan, D. P., Ortiz, S. O., Alfonso, V. C., & Dynda, A. M. (2008). Best practices in cognitive assessment: Future directions. In A. Thomas & J. Grimes (Eds.),

Best practices in school psychology V (pp. 633–659). Bethesda, MD: National Association of School Psychologists.

Florida Department of Education. (2003). FCAT 2003 grade 12 passing percent by district. Retrieved from *www.firn.edu/doe/sas/fcat/pdf/grade12pass03.pdf.*

Florida Department of Education. (2010). Florida Comprehensive Assessment Test (FCAT) 2010 state report of district results. Retrieved from *fcat.fldoe.org/mediapacket/2010/default.asp#reports.*

Gould, S. J. (1981). *The mismeasure of man.* New York: Norton.

Heubert, J. P., & Hauser, R. M. (Eds.). (1999). *High stakes: Testing for tracking, promotion, and graduation.* Washington, DC: National Academy Press.

Hosp, J., Hosp, M., & Howell, K. (2007). *The ABCs of CBM.* New York: Guilford Press.

Howell, K. W., & Nolet, V. (2000). *Curriculum-based evaluation: Teaching and decision-making.* Belmont, CA: Thomson Learning.

Individuals with Disabilities Education Act (IDEA) Amendments of 1997, Pub. L. 105-17, 20 U.S.C. § 1400 et seq. (1997).

Individuals with Disabilities Education Improvement Act of 2004 (IDEA 2004), Pub. L. 108–446 20 U.S.C. § 1400 et seq. (2004).

Jimerson, S. R., Burns, M. K., & Van Der Heyden, A. M. (2007). *Handbook of response to intervention: The science and practice of assessment and intervention.* New York: Springer.

Kranzler, J. H. (1997). Educational and policy issues related to the use and interpretation of intelligence tests in the schools. *School Psychology Review, 26,* 150–162.

Lopez, R. (1997). The practical impact of current research and issues in intelligence test interpretation and use for multicultural populations. *School Psychology Review, 26,* 249–254.

McDermott, P. A., & Glutting, J. J. (1997). Informing stylistic learning behavior, disposition, and achievement through ability subtests—or, more illusions or meaning? *School Psychology Review, 26,* 163–175.

McGrew, K. S., Flanagan, D. P., Keith, T. Z., & Vanderwood, M. (1997). Beyond *g:* The impact of Gf-Gc specific cognitive abilities research on the future use and interpretation of intelligence test batteries in the schools. *School Psychology Review, 26,* 189–210.

Mills, R. (2003). Commissioner Mills recommends four major policies on testing to Board of Regents. Retrieved from *www.oms.nysed.gov/press/testing_policy.htm.*

National Association of School Psychologists (NASP). (2003). *Position statement on using large scale assessment for high stakes decisions.* Bethesda, MD: Author.

National Center for Education Statistics. (2010). Condition of education, 2001–2010. Retrieved from *nces.ed.gov/programs/coe/2010/section1/indicator06.asp.*

National Center on Educational Outcomes (NCEO). (2003). Accountability for assessment results in the No Child Left Behind Act: What it means for children with disabilities. Retrieved from *education.umn.edu/NCEO/OnlinePubs/NCLBaccountability.html.*

National Center on Response to Intervention. (2011). The essential components of RTI. Retrieved from *www.rti4success.org.*

National Commission on Excellence in Education. (1983). *A nation at risk: The imperative for educational reform.* Washington, DC: Author.

No Child Left Behind Act (NCLB) of 2001, Pub. L. 107-115, 20 U.S.C. 6301 (2001).

Ortiz, S. O. (2002). Best practices in nondiscriminatory assessment. In A. Thomas & J. Grimes (Eds.), *Best practices in school psychology IV* (pp. 1321–1336). Bethesda, MD: National Association of School Psychologists.

Ortiz, S. O., & Dynda, A. M. (2005). Use of intelligence tests with culturally and linguistically diverse populations. In D. P. Flanagan & P. L. Harrison (Eds.), *Contemporary intellectual assessment: Theories, tests, and issues* (2nd ed., pp. 545–556). New York: Guilford Press.

Ortiz, S. O., & Ochoa, S. H. (2005). Advances in cognitive assessment of culturally and linguistically diverse individuals: A nondiscriminatory interpretive approach. In D. P. Flanagan & P. Harrison (Eds.), *Contemporary intellectual assessment: Theories, tests, and issues* (2nd ed., pp. 234–250). New York: Guilford Press.

Peterson, K. M. H., & Shinn, M. R. (2002). Severe discrepancy models: Which best explains school identification practices for learning disabilities. *School Psychology Review, 31,* 459–476.

Reschly, D. J., & Grimes, J. P. (2002). Best practices in intellectual assessment. In A. Thomas & J. Grimes (Eds.), *Best practices in school psychology IV* (pp. 1337–1350). Bethesda, MD: National Association of School Psychologists.

Sattler, J. M. (2008). *Assessment of children: Cognitive applications* (5th ed.). San Diego, CA: Author.

Shinn, M. R. (Ed.). (1989). *Curriculum-based measurement: Assessing special children.* New York: Guilford Press.

Shinn, M. R. (2005). Identifying and validating academic problems in a problem solving model. In R. Brown (Ed.), *Assessment for intervention: A problem-solving approach* (pp. 219–246). New York: Guilford Press.

Shriner, J. G. (2000). Legal perspectives on school outcomes assessment for students with disabilities. *Journal of Special Education, 33,* 232–239.

Special Education Report. (2002, October 9). Lawyer: failing exam could lead disabled to drop out. *Special Education Report, 28*(21), 8.

Stage, S. A., Abbott, R. D., Jenkins, J. R., & Berninger, V. W. (2003). Predicting response to early reading intervention from Verbal IQ, reading-related language abilities, attention ratings, and Verbal IQ–word reading discrepancy: Failure to validate discrepancy method. *Journal of Learning Disabilities, 36*, 24–33.

Thurlow, M., & Esler, A. (2000). Appeals process for students who fail graduation exams: How do they apply to students with disabilities? (Synthesis Report No. 36). Retrieved from *education.umn.edu/NCEO/OnlinePubs/Synthesis36.html.*

Thurlow, M., Wiley, H. I., & Bielinski, J. (2003). Going public: What 2000–2001 reports tell us about the performance of students with disabilities (Technical Report No. 35). Retrieved from *education. umn.edu/NCEO/OnlinePubs/Technical35.htm.*

Tilly, W. D. (2008). The evolution of school psychology to science-based practice: Problem solving and the three-tiered model. In A. Thomas & J. Grimes (Eds.), *Best practices in school psychology V* (Vol. 1, pp. 17–35). Bethesda, MD: National Association of School Psychologists.

U.S. Department of Education. (2006, August 14). 34 C.F.R. Parts 300 and 301: Assistance to states for the education of children with disabilities and preschool grants for children with disabilities: Final rule. *Federal Register, 71*, 46539–46845.

U.S. Department of Education. (2009). Race to the Top fund. Retrieved from *www2.ed.gov/programs/racetothetop/index.html.*

Viadero, D. (2003). Researchers debate impact of tests. *Education Week, 22*(21), 1–2.

Wasburn-Moses, L. (2003). What every special educator should know about high-stakes testing. *Teaching Exceptional Children, 35*, 12–15.

CHAPTER 36

CHAPTER 36

Intellectual, Cognitive, and Neuropsychological Assessment in Three-Tier Service Delivery Systems in Schools

George McCloskey
James Whitaker
Ryan Murphy
Jane Rogers

From our perspective, intelligence test performance can be interpreted on multiple levels representing successive degrees of aggregated information, as illustrated in Figure 36.1: the global composite score, specific composite scores, subtest scores, item scores, and task-specific cognitive constructs. Each aggregated level of interpretation within the framework masks clinical information that is potentially important to understanding a child's specific pattern of cognitive strengths and weaknesses. In addition, we believe that there are two major conceptual perspectives influencing contemporary intellectual assessment in the schools, referred to here as the *general abilities model* and the *cognitive neuropsychological model*. Each model emphasizes different levels of test interpretation. As shown in Figure 36.1, the general abilities model emphasizes interpretation of a global composite score and/or a handful of specific composite scores. In contrast, the cognitive neuropsychological model primarily emphasizes interpretation at the levels of subtest scores, item scores, and task-

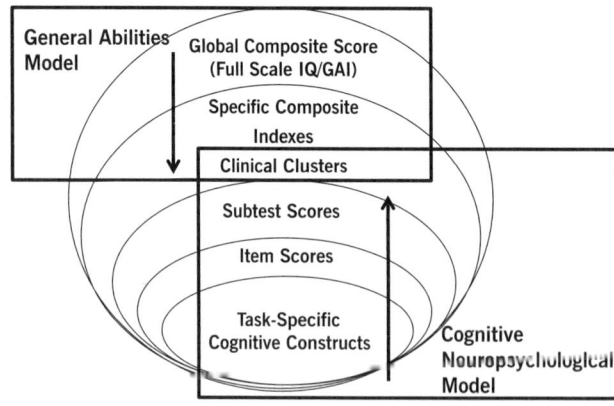

FIGURE 36.1. Interpretive levels coinciding with interpretive models.

specific cognitive constructs, with attention to the specific composite level when such composites represent meaningful clinical clusters (Kamphaus, 2001; Reynolds & French, 2005). Meaningful clinical clusters may or may not be aligned with how test developers create composites in an a priori manner through the use of factor-analytic techniques. In this chapter, the utility of these two models is discussed with special attention to how each does or does not influence assessment at each tier in a three-tier service delivery model, and how each can or cannot be integrated into a three-tier model.

The general abilities model is a traditional approach that has been in use since the inception of the intelligence test early in the 20th century (Jensen, 1998; Sarason, 1975). Proponents of this model often gravitate to the construct of *g* (Spearman, 1904) to explain why general ability is important to assess (Deary, 2001; Gottfredson, 1997, 1998, 2008; Jensen, 1980, 1998; Kamphaus, Winsor, Rowe, & Kim, 2005; Kuncel, Hezlet, & Ones, 2004; McDermott & Glutting, 1997). Over time, *g* has come to be viewed as the quintessential indicator of overall intellectual ability. It is conceptualized as a trait that is stable over time and not easily modified by educational or environmental interventions (Gottfredson, 1997, 1998, 2008; Jensen, 1998).

The general abilities model has guided the development of the intelligence tests currently available for use with school-age children, including the Wechsler Intelligence Scale for Children—Fourth Edition (WISC-IV; Wechsler, 2003); the Stanford–Binet Intelligence Scales, Fifth Edition (SB5; Roid, 2003); the Differential Ability Scales—Second Edition (DAS-II; Elliott, 2007); the Kaufman Assessment Battery for Children—Second Edition (KABC-II; Kaufman & Kaufman, 2004); the Woodcock–Johnson III Tests of Cognitive Abilities (WJ III COG; Woodcock, McGrew, & Mather, 2001); and several others. A general factor tends to emerge in analyses of subtest score data and is found in almost all intelligence tests that tap into a cognitively complex array of abilities (Saklofske, Prifitera, Weiss, Rolfhus, & Zhu, 2005). The prevailing conception of a learning disability as a condition wherein a student's intellectual capacity is significantly greater than the student's academic achievement (i.e., an ability–achievement discrepancy) stems directly from the thinking underlying the general abilities model (Bradley, Danielson, & Hallahan, 2002; Kavale, 2002; Sternberg, Grigorenko, & Bundy, 2001).

A cognitive neuropsychological perspective has emerged more recently from the basic conceptions embodied in clinical neuropsychology; in response to findings in the cognitive neurosciences, including those gleaned from functional magnetic resonance imaging studies and their application to neuropsychology; and in response to advances in the understanding of how children learn and produce academically (Berninger, 1994; Berninger & Richards, 2002; Posner & Rothbart, 2007). Several researchers and clinicians have applied this knowledge to reconceptualize in general the methods used in assessment and intervention in educational settings, including approaches to intellectual assessment (Berninger, 1994; Berninger & Richards, 2002; Hale & Fiorello, 2004; Kaplan, Fein, Morris, Kramer, & Delis, 1999; Levine, 1998; Mapou & Spector, 1995; McCloskey, 2009a, 2009b; Miller, 2007; Pennington, 2009; Reynolds & Fletcher-Janzen, 1997; Sattler & D'Amato, 2002; Temple, 1997), and to generate specific cognitive neuropsychological models (Hale & Fiorello, 2004; Levine, 1998; McCloskey, 2009a; McCloskey, Perkins, & Van Divner, 2009).

The general abilities model has been articulated in this text and elsewhere (Gottfredson, 1997, 1998, 2008; Kamphaus et al., 2005) as a viable approach to conceptualizing intelligence and as an assessment method with clinical utility within educational settings. The argument for the viability and clinical utility of a cognitive neuropsychological model has also been articulated in various sources (Allen, Hulac, & D'Amato, 2005; Berninger & Richards, 2002; Hale & Fiorello, 2004; Hale et al., 2008; Hale & Miller, 2008; Kaplan et al., 1999; McCloskey, 2009a, 2009b; Miller, 2007), but further refinements in the articulation of such a model are needed in order for the benefits of this approach to be fully realized in educational settings. In this chapter, we outline a cognitive neuropsychological model that reflects such refinements, and we contrast its use with the general abilities model in the context of the three-tier service delivery systems currently used in schools.

A COGNITIVE NEUROPSYCHOLOGICAL MODEL OF ASSESSMENT

Within a neuropsychological model of cognition, brain function can be defined and assessed by using a set of psychological constructs collectively referred to here as *cognitive constructs*. These cognitive constructs represent patterns of neural activation within various cortical and subcortical regions of the brain that are involved in the production of perception, thought, action, and the cognitive aspects of emotion (Berninger, 1994; Berninger & Richards, 2002; Levine, 1998; Mapou & Spector, 1995; McCloskey, 2009a; Willis, 2005). Assessment of cognition requires the understanding and use of the following specific cognitive constructs, the definitions of which are provided in Box 36.1: *processes, abilities, lexicons, skills, executive functions, strategies*, and *memory time frames of reference* (*initial registration, working memory, long-term storage*). Additional terms defined in Box 36.1 that are critical for understanding the interaction of cognitive constructs include *sensory processing, motor functioning, processing speed, learning*, and *achievement*.

The cognitive neuropsychological model described here necessitates a more careful use of many terms frequently associated with intellectual assessment. Intellectual capacities have often been described in terms of *abilities, processes*, and *skills*, but these terms are typically used interchangeably in discussions of intelligence and in psychological reports describing the results of an intellectual as-

sessment. In the model described in this chapter, the terms *ability, process*, and *skill* have distinct, noninterchangeable definitions, and each represents a critical component of cognition. In addition to these three core terms, the role of the more recently introduced concept of *executive functions* is defined, and the more traditional but highly ambiguous terms *memory, achievement, learning*, and *strategy* (and the more generalized meaning of the term *ability*) are clarified.

Effective application of tests of cognition requires not just an understanding of the distinctions among the various categories of cognitive constructs, but also an understanding of how the components of cognition interrelate during the occurrence of learning and production, as explained in Box 36.1 (Floyd, 2005; Saklofske et al., 2005). Figures 36.2–36.5 are conceptual diagrams applying the cognitive neuropsychological model to the primary academic domains of oral language, reading, writing, and math, respectively. These diagrams offer a static representation of the cognitive constructs used in these domains. The brief narrative in Box 36.2 offers a description of the dynamic flow of information and the interplay of the cognitive constructs in Figure 36.3 as they are used in reading.

BOX 36.1. Operational Definitions within a Cognitive Neuropsychological Model of Assessment

Processes

Processes are narrow-band cognitive constructs responsible for the organization of input leading to the creation of basic mental representations. Processes thereby provide the basic elements of conscious thought used for academic learning and production, and serve as the springboard for academic skill development. Process deficits can impede learning and production, but often can be bypassed or compensated for (at least to some degree) because of their relatively restricted range of operation. For example, students who have difficulty perceiving and discriminating subword sound units can learn how to decode words and read, despite the phoneme discrimination difficulties that result from this highly specific auditory pro-

cess deficit (Torgesen et al., 1999). In some instances, the effects of process deficits can be significantly reduced if the deficits are addressed during early developmental stages with a good intervention program (e.g., phonemic awareness training for difficulties with subword sound unit discrimination). In these cases, the process deficit may have been due more to underutilization or lack of maturation of intact neural networks than to the presence of damaged neural interconnections; in such cases, early instruction increases the frequency and effectiveness of the use of the process (McCloskey, 2009a). It is possible that basic process deficits resulting from damage to neural networks can be remediated through early childhood intervention as well (McCloskey, 2009a).

Severe basic process deficits can result in learning disabilities involving slowed and/or inconsistent learning and production. Basic processes underlying skill development in one or more academic domains include the following:

(cont.)

- Auditory perception
- Auditory discrimination
- Auditory attention
- Visual perception
- Visual discrimination
- Visual attention
- Kinesthetic perception
- Kinesthetic discrimination
- Kinesthetic attention

Processing

The term *processing* refers to neural activity that involves the coordinated use of one or more processes, almost always in conjunction with the accessing of one or more lexicons (described below) and typically under the direction of one or more executive functions (described below). Because of the manner in which processes are involved in creating mental representations, it is not possible to isolate and measure processes without some involvement from other cognitive constructs. *Processing* therefore refers not only to the integrated process of creating mental representations, but also to the tasks used to assess the effectiveness of processes during the act of creating mental representations.

Basic Motor Functions

Basic motor functions are the fine motor capacities used in the performance of cognitive assessment tasks. All intellectual and cognitive assessment tasks require some form of motor output in order for the adequacy of task performance to be judged. Variations in the adequacy of motor functioning are important to observe and quantify, in order to understand how strengths or weaknesses in motor functioning may be enhancing or impeding learning of academic skills and production with academic tasks.

Processing Speed and Basic Motor Functioning Speed

The term *processing speed* refers to the speed with which one or more processes can be coordinated and applied in the formation of mental representations, often in conjunction with the accessing of lexicons and typically under the direction of one or more executive functions. For all processing speed assessment tasks, processing speed is combined with some form of basic motor function in

order to have an output that can be judged for adequacy of task performance. As a result, all measures of processing speed also are measures of *basic motor functioning speed*.

Abilities

Abilities are broad-band cognitive constructs that operate on the mental representations initially formed through cognitive processing. Abilities enable extended formulation and use of mental representations during learning and production. They include such integral capacities of thought as receptive and expressive language, complex visual–spatial representation and visualization, reasoning with language, reasoning with visual–spatial representations, and reasoning with quantity and idea generation.

Unlike process deficits, which can be bypassed or compensated for, ability deficits constrain learning and production; that is, the degree of ability deficit places an upper limit on the quality (i.e., depth and complexity) of the learning and production. Because of the broad-based effects of ability deficits, compensatory or bypass strategies are typically not very effective in countering ability deficits within relatively short periods of time (McCloskey, 2009a). Severe ability deficits therefore result in cognitive impairments that greatly constrain learning and production, possibly throughout an individual's lifetime (e.g., severe language impairment, severe visual–spatial impairment, severe reasoning impairment).

It should be noted that the word *ability* is also often used to denote the adequacy of a person's use of any or all cognitive constructs, as in "He has the ability to process phonemes," "She demonstrated the ability to retrieve information from long-term storage," or "He demonstrated the ability to decode words." As is clear from these examples, the use of the word *ability* in these statements indicates the individual's facility with the use of the specific cognitive constructs mentioned, rather than indicating the use of a specific mental capacity that has been operationally defined as an ability. Application of the word *ability* in this way results in redundancy when one is discussing specific abilities, as in "He demonstrated the ability to use reasoning abilities."

(cont.)

Lexicons

Lexicons are knowledge bases that are built up gradually through the storage of information during learning and skill acquisition. Once established, a lexicon can be accessed for retrieval of information that can be used in conjunction with processes to form mental representations and to inform new learning or production. Lexicons can range from very basic, narrow forms of knowledge (e.g., the separate phonemes of the English language; how light strikes objects and creates shadows) to very complex forms of knowledge that vary greatly in depth and breadth (how to factor a polynomial; how to put a car engine [specific make and model] together; the influences of 18th-century classical composers on the early development of rock and roll).

Skills (Basic, Complex, Domain-Specific)

Skills are "lexicons under construction" that are acquired through formal or informal formal educational experiences. The term *skill* can be used in a temporal sense to represent what is being learned in the present moment or to represent what was learned in the past or what will be learned in the future. The set of skills to be taught often determines the content of instructional lessons. Skills can be further delineated by content as *basic*, *complex*, or *domain-specific*.

Basic Skills

Basic skills are the skills that form the foundation for all additional skill acquisition. The four broad basic skill domains are oral communication (listening and speaking), reading, writing, and mathematics. Each of these basic skill domains consists of many subdomains or subskills:

- Basic oral communication skills include reflective listening, diction and projection of voice, prosody, and rapid speech production.
- Basic reading skills include sight word recognition, phonological awareness, word decoding, and rapid word recognition.
- Basic writing skills include graphomotor letter, number, and word formation and copying; word spelling; written sentence structure and written sentence formation;

and rapid text production. Basic mathematics skills include computation procedures, basic quantity problem solutions, and rapid application of computation procedures.

Basic skills are the foci of instruction and learning in early elementary school. Basic skill learning represents the building of a set of general lexicons that will enable the application of oral communication, reading, writing, and mathematics to a wide range of subject content areas and to the learning of more complex skills. Skill building is an intermediate state between the immediate experiencing of new information and the retrieval of information from an established lexicon. Skills that have been mastered form distinct lexicons. *Automaticity* refers to the speed with which basic skill lexicons can be accessed and the ease with which information can be retrieved from the lexicon and applied.

Basic skill learning and use rely heavily on effective processing of auditory, visual, and kinesthetic stimuli taken in from the educational environment. Process deficits, therefore, can have a significant negative impact on skill acquisition and use.

Basic skill learning and acquisition also rely heavily on the use of multiple executive functions to cue and direct the new learning and the construction of a new lexicon. Basic skill learning, therefore, is likely to be disrupted when executive function deficits are present.

Complex Skills

Complex skills are oral communication, reading, writing, and mathematics skills that enable a person to take the mental representations formed through the use of basic skills, add new layers of representation, and manipulate all the information to produce relatively complex levels of meaning. Complex skills include extended listening and/or speaking for meaning, reading comprehension, extended written text generation, and applied mathematics problem solving.

Complex skill development and use involve the application of one or more basic skills integrated with the use of one or more abilities and the accessing of one or more lexicons, all under the direction of multiple executive functions. For example, the skill of complex reading comprehension requires the application of the basic skills of word recognition and/or

(cont.)

decoding and reading rate to form in the mind an accurate basic representation of the information on the page. The more complex the grammatical structure of the material being read, the greater the need for involvement of specific language abilities to enable meaningful representation at a deeper level. If the material being read relates to a specific topic, lexicons representing the person's knowledge of the topic will need to be accessed, along with language ability to provide a context for what is being read. If the ideas represented by the words are complex, reasoning abilities will need to be engaged to obtain the highest level of meaning possible from the material. The application of these skills, lexicons, and abilities requires extensive use of executive functions to coordinate the multitasking that must take place during such complex reading comprehension. In addition to the use of multiple basic skills, lexicons, and abilities, application of complex skills very often requires the direction and use of working memory capacities (described below).

Complex skills are the foci of instruction and learning in the upper elementary grades. The development and use of complex skills can be disrupted by inadequate development of, or inadequate use of, basic skills (resulting from the effects of process deficits or lack of direct instruction); by insufficient storage of information in lexicons; by constraints imposed by inadequate or underdeveloped abilities; by constraints imposed by inadequate or underutilized working memory capacity; and/ or by constraints imposed by inadequate or underutilized executive functions.

Domain-Specific Skills

Domain-specific skills are skills that are developed in specific subject domains and subdomains (e.g., the domain of science and the subdomains of biology, chemistry, physics, etc.). Although basic and complex skills may be involved in learning in these content domains, the skills that are the foci of learning involve the building of lexicons related to the specific area of knowledge. The link between learning and lexicon building in these content areas is apparent in the language used to denote course and learning objectives. Educators speak of increasing a student's knowledge of biology, rather than of increasing or building a student's biology skills. Despite the emphasis on specific content knowledge

storage and retrieval, other lexicons are acquired (e.g., how to use biology or chemistry laboratory equipment) that are more readily perceived as skills.

Strategies

Strategies are learned and stored or newly generated routines that can be applied to increase an individual's efficiency of learning and/or production. Strategies are ways to chain together in a specific order a combination of one or more processes, abilities, skills, and knowledge retrieved from lexicons to enhance learning and production. Strategies also involve the sequential or simultaneous use of executive functions to cue and direct the use of the cognitive constructs involved in the strategies. Like skills, strategies can be taught and learned in formal or informal educational settings or can be self-taught. Strategy development, storage, and use are all cued internally by executive functions or by an external mediating source, such as a teacher or parent.

Executive Functions

Executive functions are a unique category of mental capacities defined by their directive role. Executive functions cue and direct the use of other mental capacities and coordinate multitasking efforts. They can be used to guide all cognitive constructs in all aspects of mental activity. They are not the processes, abilities, lexicons, skills, strategies, or memory states, but rather the mental capacities that orchestrate the use of all these other mental capacities—cueing, directing, and coordinating all other elements of thought to produce coherent learning and production. Although executive functions are intricately involved in learning, the teaching process can mediate or substitute for students' inadequate use of executive functions. Executive function deficits are most noticeable in situations requiring independent or unsupervised production.

Memory: Time Frames of Reference

Memory is very different from the other mental capacities discussed here because different forms of memory actually represents different temporal states of mind in which a person may be using any number of pro-

(cont.)

cesses, abilities, lexicons, skills, or strategies. Memory states are the mind's manifestation of time and space, providing the temporal and spatial contexts—a time signature—for all perception, emotion, cognition, and action.

The three major time-related memory states are:

- Initial registration of information in the immediate moment; the experience of "now."
- Retrieval from long-term storage; going back in time to recall previous "immediate" moments.
- Holding and manipulating information in mind; extending the immediate moment into the future, projecting possible immediate moments into the future, or creating scenarios for future immediate moments.

These memory states enable a person to have a psychological sense of now (immediate memory or initial registration of stimuli), the past (retrieval from long-term storage), and the future (holding and manipulating mental representations beyond the immediate moment or projecting mental activity various distances beyond the immediate moment).

Memory cannot be experienced or assessed outside the context of one or more processes, abilities, lexicons, skills, or strategies. What defines a memory state is what a person is doing at any given point in time.

A *memory deficit* refers to inadequate use of one or more mental capacities within a specific time frame. A person with poor immediate memory has difficulty effectively using processes and lexicons to initially register and briefly hold stimuli. A person with long-term retrieval problems has difficulty assessing information stored in lexicons. A person with working memory problems has difficulty effectively applying abilities, lexicons, skills, or strategies to manipulate information being held in mind.

Although memory deficits are similar to ability deficits, in that both types can have a broad-based impact on learning and production, they are also similar to process deficits, in that both types can often be bypassed or compensated for (at least to some degree).

Lack of memory capacity can greatly obstruct learning and production:

- Poor initial registration constrains how much information can be represented in mind at one time.
- Poor retrieval capacity limits access to lexicons.
- Poor working memory capacity constrains how much information can be held in mind; how long that information can be held; and the extent to which the information being held in mind can be manipulated to enable extended states of learning, problem solving, and production.

Learning

Learning is the building of new lexicons. Whereas simple learning involves building a lexicon through basic skill acquisition, complex learning occurs through the use of processes, skills, and strategies along with the accessing of lexicons and the application of abilities to create a new lexicon or to link multiple lexicons for greater ease of strategy use. Learning can occur on a continuum from being mediated extensively by others to being self-mediated. The greater the self-mediation, the greater the demand for executive function involvement in the learning process.

Production

Production is the observable motor output or the unobservable mental output resulting from attempts to use processes, skills, and strategies; access lexicons; and apply abilities and executive functions to perform a task.

Achievement

Like production, *achievement* is the end result (the product) of the use of processes, skills, and strategies; accessing of lexicons; and application of abilities to perform a task. Assessment of achievement, therefore, often is not simply a matter of assessing skill development (basic, complex, or domain-specific). *Production* is typically referred to as *achievement* in formal educational settings, where production is directed at meeting specific academic goals related in some way to skill development.

(cont.)

Category Boundaries

It is important to note that the boundaries of these categories are somewhat amorphous and changeable. At least theoretically, processes, abilities, and executive functions can be taught and learned, thereby becoming skills. Skills can be stored and retrieved and applied in the immediate moment, making them lexicons. The interrelated and overlapping nature of the category definitions, however, should not deter clinicians from making the important distinctions represented by each of these categories.

BOX 36.2. The Dynamic Interplay of Cognitive Constructs in Reading

Reading does not start with the words on the page. Rather, reading starts in the brain with the accessing of lexicons containing what we already know about how to read—that is, our knowledge of how words sound when they are said and what they look like in print. In young children new to reading, these lexicons are built up through prereading instruction in phonemic awareness, orthographic awareness, and language experience activities (Berninger & Richards, 2002; Dehaene, 2009; Posner & Rothbart, 2007; Shaywitz, 2003; Uhry & Clark, 2005). Once we are engaged with words in print, these lexicons must be accessed and used in conjunction with sensory processes that enable us to see the words on the page (visual processes involved in perceiving and discriminating the shapes on the page in order to create visual mental representations of words) and to hear ourselves say the words (auditory processes involved in perceiving and discriminating the phonemes and syllables in order to create the pronunciations of the words on the page), as well as with basic motor routines that enable us to say the words either orally or subvocally. If the orthographic and phonological awareness lexicons have been constructed and the basic processes and motor capacities are in place, these can be used during the instructional process to learn and store new words (sight recognition skills), to analyze and sound out unfamiliar words (decoding skills), and to learn to do both of these quickly and efficiently (fluency skills). It is important to note that the goal of learning these skills is to enable readers to build part- and whole-word pronunciation lexicons, so that they can apply them independently to read any word they encounter in a text.

Quick and efficient recognition of the words in print, however, is only the first stage of reading. Additional cognitive constructs must be used to link the words being read with their individual meaning and to link the meaning of each word with every other word in a sentence in order to grasp the meaning of each sentence (Berninger, 1994, 1998; Berninger & Richards, 2002). Turning words in print into meaning requires not only the use of language abilities, but the accessing of lexicons that store knowledge of the meanings of words and phrases, as well as lexicons that store knowledge about the topic that the sentence is addressing. Depending on what the words are attempting to communicate, extracting meaning from what is being read also may require the use of reasoning to understand more fully what is being read and/or visual–spatial abilities to "see" what is being read (Dehaene, 2009). Reading also involves the three time frames of reference in varying degrees. The words on the page must be initially registered in the immediate moment; knowledge of words in print and their meanings must be retrieved from long-term storage; and the longer the passage being read, the greater the need to hold and manipulate what is being read in working memory. Finally, all of this mental activity must be cued, directed, and integrated through the use of multiple executive functions working in a coordinated manner (Berninger & Richards, 2002; McCloskey, Perkins, & Van Divner, 2009).

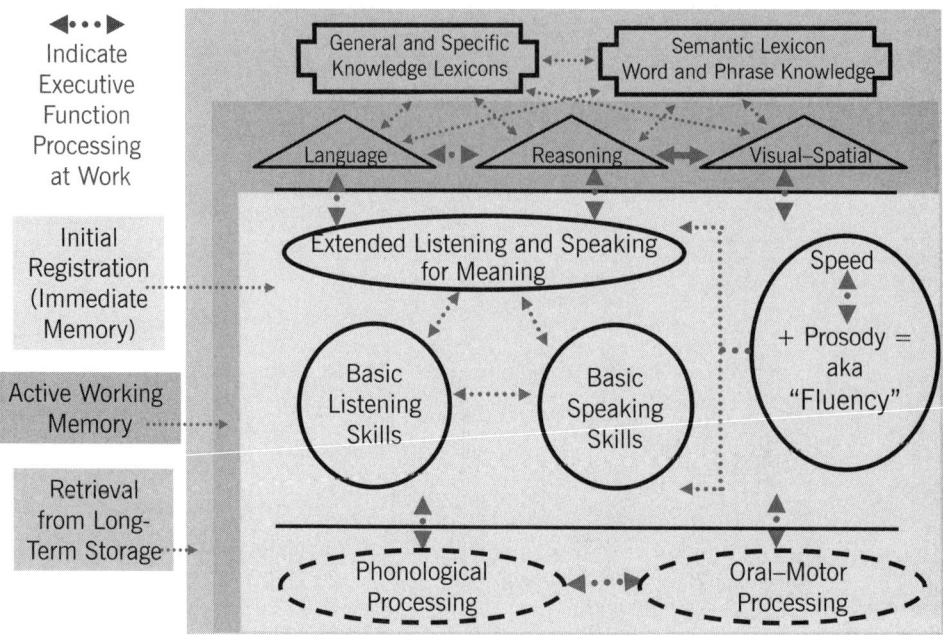

FIGURE 36.2. A cognitive neuropsychological model specifying the cognitive constructs used for listening and speaking. Copyright 2010 by George McCloskey. Reprinted by permission.

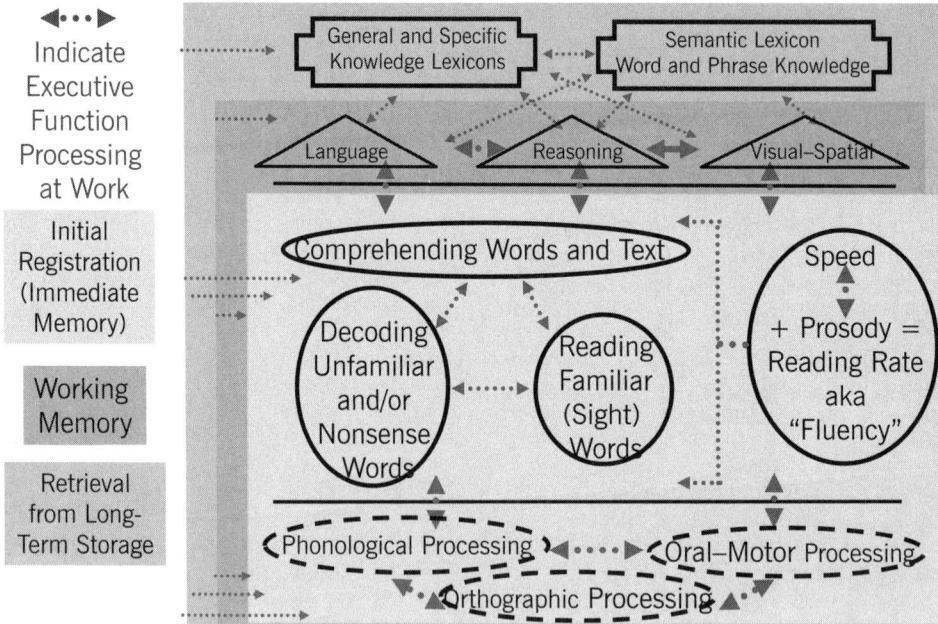

FIGURE 36.3. A cognitive neuropsychological model specifying the cognitive constructs used for reading. Copyright 2010 by George McCloskey. Reprinted by permission.

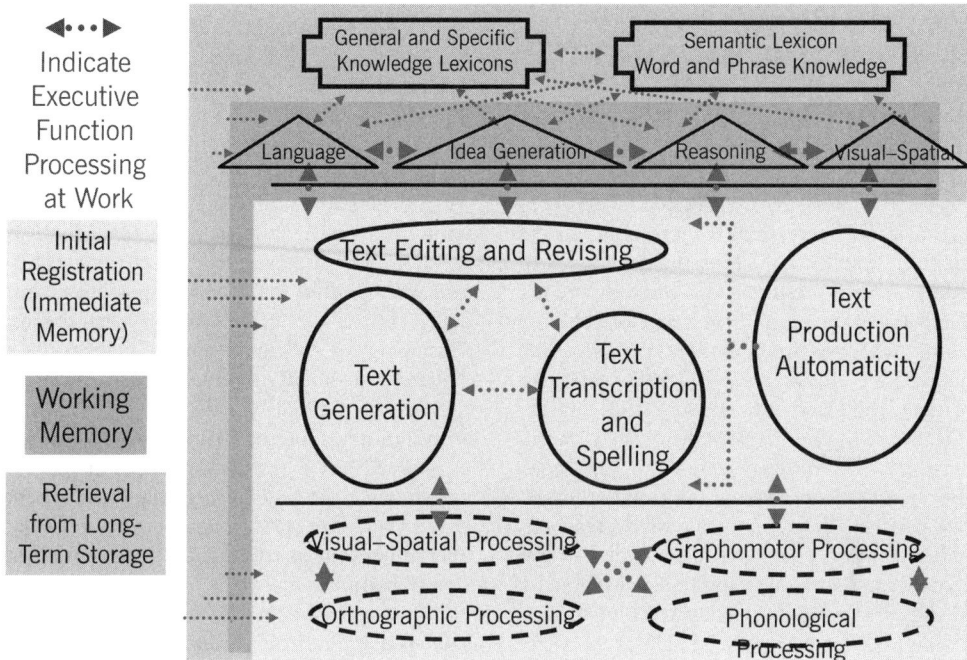

FIGURE 36.4. A cognitive neuropsychological model specifying the cognitive constructs used for writing. Copyright 2010 by George McCloskey. Reprinted by permission.

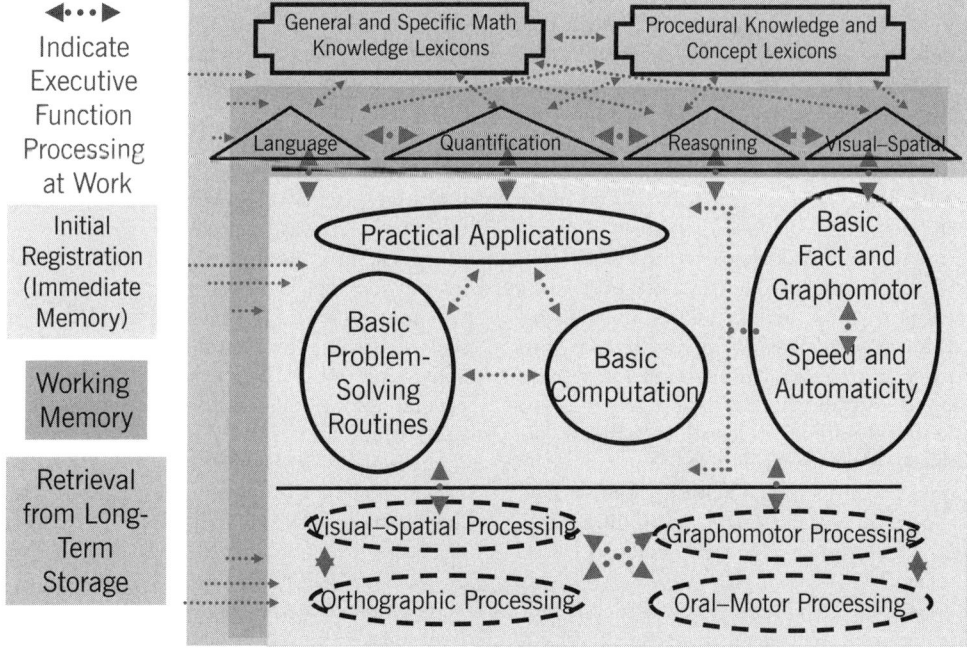

FIGURE 36.5. A cognitive neuropsychological model specifying the cognitive constructs used for doing math. Copyright 2010 by George McCloskey. Reprinted by permission.

COMPARING THE TWO MODELS IN SCHOOL-BASED ASSESSTMENT

In educational settings, the general abilities model is used to interpret intelligence test performance from the perspective of predicting later academic success (Gottfredson, 1997, 1998, 2008; Sternberg et al., 2001; Weinberg, 1989). From this model's perspective, intellectual assessments are conducted because the results can effectively predict academic achievement, and can therefore be used to identify learning disabilities by distinguishing a child who has the capacity to achieve academically from a child who does not have this capacity (Kavale, 2002; Mather & Wendling, 2005; Sternberg et al., 2001). We have been able to apply the general abilities model of interpretation to individual case results to help convince parents, teachers, and administrators that particular students have more academic potential than previously thought, as indicated by the students' relatively high general ability scores. We have also been able to apply this model to convince parents, teachers, and administrators of the substantial educational challenges faced by children with limited cognitive resources, as indicated by the children's extremely low general ability scores.

The limitations of the traditional general abilities model become apparent, however, when professionals who use intelligence tests are much more interested in actively helping a child improve his or her academic achievement than in passively stating current levels of ability in order to predict later levels of academic achievement. When the purpose of assessment is reconceptualized as an effort to characterize a student's pattern of cognitive strengths and weaknesses, to understand how these strengths and weaknesses will affect learning and production, and to understand how instruction can be modified to improve learning and production, the general abilities model falls short. The model also falls short in light of research suggesting that children with learning disabilities are more likely to demonstrate varied than consistent cognitive construct profiles at the subtest level (Fiorello, Hale, McGrath, Ryan, & Quinn, 2001; Fiorello et al., 2007; Flanagan, Alfonso, Ortiz, & Dynda, 2010; Fletcher-Jansen, 2005; Hale & Fiorello, 2004; Miller, 2007). In cases such as this, interpretation at the global composite level can mask clinically meaningful information and lead to inaccurate characterizations of cognitive constructs (Hale & Miller, 2008; Hale et al., 2008; Ka-

plan, 1988; Kaplan et al., 1999; McCloskey, 2009a, 2009b; McCloskey & Maerlender, 2005).

One thing that should be clear from Figures 36.2–36.5 and the discussion of the cognitive neuropsychological model applied to the various academic domains is that listening/speaking, reading, writing, and doing math are extremely complex in nature. Given the multifaceted nature of all these domains, it is not surprising that diagnostic assessment directed at identifying possible cognitive deficits at the root of problems in each domain is a complicated endeavor requiring the use of specialized assessment instrumentation rather than the use of a single intelligence test—even one with multiple subtests. In cases where production is poor within a specific academic domain, the assessment process must determine the extent to which each of these various cognitive constructs is able to perform its role during functioning within that domain.

When contemporary intelligence tests are considered in light of the conceptual model presented in Box 36.1 and the context of diagnostic assessment, it is apparent that such tests consist of multiple tasks (each of which represents a complex amalgam of many of the constructs described in the cognitive neuropsychological model), but that the ways in which the tasks are combined is not consistent with the cognitive models depicted in Figures 36.2–36.5. This lack of alignment with the academic domain models greatly reduces or completely nullifies their usefulness in the diagnostic process (Alfonso, Flanagan, & Radwan, 2005). The primary reason for this state of affairs is the fact that development of contemporary intelligence tests has been dictated primarily by the general abilities model rather than the cognitive neuropsychological model.

The statistical techniques (mostly factor analysis) used to organize intelligence test tasks into composites for interpretation according to the general abilities model often obscure the distinctions necessary for effective understanding and interpretation of the cognitive constructs that a person may use to complete these tasks (Flanagan & Kaufman, 2009; Hale & Miller, 2008; Hale et al., 2008; McCloskey, 2009a, 2009b; McCloskey & Maerlender, 2005). Table 36.1 illustrates the obfuscation created by the general abilities model: It examines the cognitive constructs required to perform tasks that have been aggregated to form a general ability composite. The inadequacy of the general abilities model for diagnostic purposes becomes even clearer when the general ability composites are disaggregated into their component subtests (Watkins, Glutting, & Youngstrom, 2005). Table 36.2 attempts to align the subtests of multiple intelligence tests with the cognitive construct components of the cognitive neuropsychological model as applied to each of the basic academic domains. As reflected in Table 36.2, the intelligence tests commonly used in schools today assess very few of the cognitive constructs related to performance in all four academic domains. Because the intelligence tests in use today have been based on the general abilities model rather than a cognitive neuropsychological model, they are not well suited to the diagnostic process that is at the heart of psychoeducational assessment in the schools, especially as it occurs at tier 3 (Mather & Wendling, 2005).

TABLE 36.1. Analysis of the Cognitive Constructs That May Be Involved in Performance of the Individual Items of Each Subtest within the Verbal Comprehension Index within the Full Scale IQ of the WISC-IV

Interpretive level	Score/index/subtest/capacity		
Global composite	Full Scale IQ		
Specific composite	Verbal Comprehension Index		
Subtests	SI[a]	VC[b]	CO[c]
Items and task-specific cognitive constructs	Cognitive constructs	Cognitive constructs	Cognitive constructs
Retrieval of verbal knowledge	XX	XXX	X
Reasoning with verbal content	XXX		XXX
Auditory attention	X	X	X
Auditory discrimination	XX	XX	XX
Auditory comprehension	X	X	XX
Auditory processing speed			XX
Initial registration of auditorily presented information	X	X	X
Working memory	X		X
Expressive language production	XX	XXX	XXX
EF—Cueing appropriate consideration of the cognitive constructs and mental effort required to perform the task	XX	XX	XX
EF—Directing auditory perception, discrimination, and comprehension	XX	XX	XX
EF—Directing auditory attention	X	X	X
EF—Directing processing speed			XX
EF—Directing retrieval of verbal information	X	XX	X
EF—Directing reasoning with verbal information	XX		XX
EF—Directing language expression	XX	XX	XX
EF—Directing flexible shifting of reasoning mindset	XXX		XX
EF—Directing working memory	X		X
EF—Recognizing and responding to prompts for more information	X	X	X
EF—Coordinating the use of multiple cognitive constructs simultaneously	XX	XX	XX
EF—Cueing the inhibition of impulsive responding	X	X	X
EF—Cueing the focusing and sustaining of attention to auditory details	X	X	X

Note. XXX, primary capacity targeted for assessment with the task; XX, secondary capacity highly likely to be affecting task performance; X, secondary capacity possibly affecting task performance. EF, executive function.
[a]Similarities.
[b]Vocabulary.
[c]Comprehension.

TABLE 36.2. Alignment of Intellectual Assessment Measures with Academic Skill Domains within a Cognitive Neuropsychological Model

Cognitive construct	Intellectual assessment measure				
	WISC-IV/WISC-IV Integrated/WAIS-IV	SB5	WJ III COG	DAS-II	KABC-II
Academic domain: Listening and speaking					
Processing					
Phonological processing			Sound Blending Incomplete Words		
Oral–motor functioning			Retrieval Fluency		
Lexicons					
Word knowledge	Vocabulary	Vocabulary	Verbal Comprehension	Word Definitions	Riddles
General knowledge	Information		General Information		Verbal Knowledge
Abilities					
Listening comprehension (receptive language)		Verbal Absurdities			Riddles
Oral expression (expressive language)	Vocabulary Comprehension Similarities	Vocabulary Picture Absurdities Verbal Absurdities/Analogies Position and Direction		Word Definitions Verbal Similarities	
Visual–spatial representation of language					
Reasoning with verbal information	Similarities Comprehension	Verbal Absurdities Verbal Analogies		Verbal Similarities	Riddles
Reasoning with verbal/visual–spatial information					
Reasoning with verbal/quantitative information	Arithmetic	Quantitative Reasoning			
Executive functions, strategies, memory time frames of reference					
Executive functions involved in cueing, directing, and coordinating cognitive constructs while performing listening/ speaking tasks					
Strategies applied while performing listening/speaking tasks					

Initial registration of phonology and words	Digit Span—Forward	Memory for Sentences Last Word	Auditory Attention		Number Recall
Holding and manipulating information while listening/speaking	Digit Span—Backward; Letter–Number Sequencing	Memory for Sentences Last Word	Auditory Working Memory		Word Order
Retrieving information from long-term storage while listening/speaking	Vocabulary; Vocabulary Multiple Choice; Information; Information Multiple Choice	Vocabulary	Retrieval Fluency		Verbal Knowledge

Academic domain: Reading

Processing

Phonological processing			Sound Blending; Incomplete Words		
Orthographic processing					
Oral–motor functioning					

Lexicons

Word knowledge	Vocabulary		Verbal Comprehension	Word Definitions	Riddles
General knowledge	Information		General Information		Verbal Knowledge

Abilities

Listening comprehension (receptive language)		Verbal Absurdities			Riddles
Oral expression (expressive language)	Vocabulary; Comprehension; Similarities	Vocabulary; Picture Absurdities; Verbal Absurdities; Verbal Analogies		Word Definitions; Verbal Similarities	
Visual–spatial representation of language		Position and Direction			
Reasoning with verbal information	Similarities; Comprehension	Verbal Absurdities; Verbal Analogies		Verbal Similarities	Riddles
Reasoning with verbal/visual–spatial information				Verbal Similarities	
Reasoning with verbal/quantitative information	Arithmetic	Quantitative Reasoning			

(cont.)

TABLE 36.2. (cont.)

	Intellectual assessment measure				
Cognitive construct	WISC-IV/WISC-IV Integrated/WAIS-IV	SB5	WJ III COG	DAS-II	KABC-II
Academic domain: Listening and speaking (cont.)					
Executive functions, strategies, time frames of reference					
Executive functions involved in cueing, directing, and coordinating cognitive constructs while performing reading tasks					
Strategies applied while performing reading tasks					
Initial registration of phonology and/or orthography	Digit Span—Forward	Memory for Sentences Last Word			Number Recall
Holding and manipulating information while listening and/or while reading	Digit Span—Backward Letter–Number Sequencing	Memory for Sentences Last Word	Auditory Working Memory		Word Order
Retrieving information from long-term storage while listening/speaking and/or while reading	Vocabulary Vocabulary Multiple Choice Information Information Multiple Choice	Vocabulary	Retrieval Fluency		Verbal Knowledge
Academic domain: Writing					
Processing					
Phonological processing			Sound Blending Incomplete Words		
Orthographic processing					
Visual–spatial processing					
Graphomotor functioning	Coding				

866

Ability	Associated subtests
Lexicons	
Word knowledge	Vocabulary; Verbal Comprehension; Word Definitions; Riddles; Verbal Knowledge
General knowledge	Information; General Information; Verbal Knowledge
Abilities	
Listening comprehension (receptive language)	Verbal Absurdities
Oral expression (expressive language)	Vocabulary; Comprehension; Similarities; Picture Absurdities; Verbal Absurdities; Verbal Analogies; Word Definitions; Verbal Similarities
Visual–spatial representation of language	Position and Direction
Reasoning with verbal information	Similarities; Comprehension; Verbal Absurdities; Verbal Analogies; Verbal Similarities; Riddles
Reasoning with verbal/visual–spatial information	Verbal Absurdities; Verbal Analogies
Reasoning with verbal/quantitative information	Arithmetic; Quantitative Reasoning
Executive functions, strategies, time frames of reference	
Executive functions involved in cueing, directing, and coordinating cognitive constructs while performing writing tasks	
Strategies applied while performing writing tasks	
Initial registration of phonology and/or orthography	Digit Span—Forward; Memory for Sentences; Last Word; Number Recall
Holding and manipulating information while writing and reading	Digit Span—Backward; Letter–Number Sequencing; Memory for Sentences; Last Word; Auditory Working Memory; Word Order
Retrieving information from long-term storage while writing and reading	Vocabulary; Vocabulary Multiple Choice; Information; Information Multiple Choice; Verbal Knowledge

(cont.)

TABLE 36.2. (cont.)

	Intellectual assessment measure				
Cognitive construct	WISC-IV/WISC-IV Integrated/WAIS-IV	SB5	WJ III COG	DAS-II	KABC-II
Academic domain: Listening and speaking					
Processing					
Phonological processing					
Orthographic processing			Visual Matching		
Visual–spatial processing					
Oral–motor functioning					
Lexicons					
Word knowledge related to math	Vocabulary	Vocabulary		Word Definitions	
General knowledge related to math	Information				
Abilities					
Listening comprehension (receptive language) related to math tasks		Verbal Absurdities			
Oral expression (expressive language) related to math tasks		Picture Absurdities Verbal Absurdities Verbal Analogies			
Visual–spatial representation of nonverbal information	Block Design Block Design Multiple Choice Elithorn Mazes	Form Patterns	Spatial Relations	Pattern Construction	Triangles Rover
Visual–spatial representation of verbal information		Position and Direction			
Visual–spatial representation of quantity					Block Counting

Cognitive ability	WISC-IV (Integrated)/WAIS-IV	SB5	DAS-II	WJ III COG	KABC-II
Reasoning with verbal/visual–spatial information		Verbal Absurdities, Verbal Analogies			
Reasoning with verbal/quantitative information	Arithmetic	Picture Absurdities			
Reasoning with quantitative information	Arithmetic	Quantitative Reasoning	Sequential and Quantitative Reasoning		
Reasoning with abstract visual information	Matrix Reasoning, Block Design, Elithorn Mazes	Matrices	Matrices, Pattern Construction	Concept Formation, Analysis–Synthesis	Pattern Reasoning, Conceptual Thinking, Rover
Executive functions, strategies, time frames of reference					
Executive functions involved in cueing, directing, and coordinating cognitive constructs while performing math tasks					
Executive functions involved in cueing, directing, and coordinating cognitive constructs while performing visual–spatial tasks	Elithorn Mazes			Planning	Rover
Strategies applied while performing math tasks					
Initial registration of phonology and/or orthography related to numbers	Digit Span—Forward, Visual Digits, Spatial Span—Forward	Block Span			Number Recall
Holding and manipulating information while listening about and/or performing math-related tasks	Arithmetic, Digit Span—Backward, Spatial Span—Backward			Numbers Reversed	Word Order
Retrieving information from long-term storage while listening/speaking about and/or performing math tasks	Arithmetic	Quantitative Reasoning			

Note. WISC-IV (Integrated), Wechsler Intelligence Scale for Children—Fourth Edition (Integrated); WAIS-IV, Wechsler Adult Intelligence Scale—Fourth Edition; SB5, Stanford–Binet Intelligence Scales, Fifth Edition; WJ III COG, Woodcock–Johnson III Tests of Cognitive Abilities; DAS-II, Differential Ability Scales—Second Edition; KABC-II, Kaufman Assessment Battery for Children—Second Edition.

INTELLECTUAL ASSESSMENT IN THE CONTEXT OF THREE-TIER SERVICE DELIVERY SYSTEMS

Three-tier service delivery systems emphasize the need for appropriate instruction, assessment, and intervention at varying levels of intensity. Assessment at tier 1 usually involves the administration of very brief progress-monitoring instruments at regular benchmark intervals for all students in general education, and possibly more frequently for students who are not making progress at the expected levels and/or rates. Students who continue to lag behind despite efforts to alter instruction are referred for tier 2 services. At tier 2, progress-monitoring assessment efforts continue, typically on a more frequent basis than at tier 1. In some instances, diagnostic assessments of some processes and skills are conducted to try to pinpoint a student's academic difficulties more specifically and to identify interventions that might be more likely to enable the student to succeed. Students who continue to struggle at tier 2 for a prolonged period of time despite multiple efforts to alter approaches to instruction are referred for a comprehensive assessment before either their assignment to instruction at tier 3 or their return to tier 2 services with a more specific plan for intervention efforts (Berninger, 1998; Berninger, O'Donnell, & Holdnack, 2008).

Although the results of the assessment may not lead to special education placement, a tier 3 assessment is accompanied by a host of requirements and stipulations associated with federal laws governing consideration of a student for special education placement (e.g., receipt of written permission from the parents allowing an intellectual assessment to be conducted, and a specific time frame within which the assessment must be completed after permission has been received). The nature of a tier 3 referral makes it imperative that the specific cognitive strengths and weaknesses of the student and their impact on learning and production be clearly specified. As noted earlier, although an intellectual assessment guided by the general abilities model may be helpful in identifying overall intellectual capacity, the use of global and specific composites does not permit cognitive strengths and weaknesses to be specified at the level required in a tier 3 assessment.

The need for more specific information about a child's pattern of cognitive strengths and weaknesses associated with one or more specific academic domains makes the cognitive neuropsychological model a better fit for selection and interpretation of assessments at tier 3. As we have noted earlier, however, even when a cognitive neuropsychological model is applied, contemporary intelligence tests are not well suited to the needs of a tier 3 assessment because they do not cover many of the cognitive constructs involved in academic learning and production. Psychologists conducting assessments at tier 3 need to incorporate tasks from a broader array of cognitive test batteries in order to effectively assess all the cognitive constructs associated with one or more academic domains (Berninger, Dunn, & Alper, 2005; Decker, 2008; Hale, Kaufman, Naglieri, & Kavale, 2006; Volker, Lopata, & Cook-Cottone, 2006). Table 36.3 provides examples of the types of tasks from other cognitive tests that could be incorporated into diagnostic assessment work at tier 3.

In recent years, the usefulness of an intellectual assessment even at tier 3 has been questioned (Reschly & Grimes, 2002). If psychologists persist in relying solely on a general abilities model for interpretation of test results, criticisms of the use of intellectual assessments at tier 3 are likely to continue because such assessments lack relevance of the findings to the diagnostic process necessitated at tier 3. Application of a cognitive neuropsychological model at tier 3, however, is likely to lead psychologists away from the use of traditional intellectual assessments in favor of tests that offer more specific information about the cognitive constructs involved in academic learning and production. This will create the potential for more meaningful assessments, which in turn can improve intervention selection (Decker, 2008).

The critical differences between the general abilities model and the cognitive neuropsychological model are most apparent when they are applied to the concept of learning disabilities. As shown in Figure 36.6, current models of learning disabilities—such as those discussed by Hale and Fiorello (2004) and by McCloskey (2009b)—look very different, depending on the model applied in the interpretation of intellectual assessment results. In the general abilities model, the contrast between a global composite score from an intellectual assessment and scores from academic skill measures is central to the identification of a learning disability. In contrast, the cognitive neuropsychological model incorporates at most only a few subtest-level scores or clinically meaningful composite cluster scores from an intellectual assessment and supplements these with cognitive measures of processing, abilities, lexicons, executive functions, mem-

TABLE 36.3. Alignment of Some Specific Cognitive Assessment Measures with the Academic Domain of Reading within a Cognitive Neuropsychological Model

Cognitive construct	Intellectual assessment measure			
	PAL-II	WJ III COG/ACH	NEPSY-II	D-KEFS
Processing				
Phonological and morphological processing	Rhyming Phonemes Syllables Rimes Are They Related? Does It Fit?	Sound Blending Incomplete Words Sound Awareness	Phonological Processing Repetition of Nonsense Words	
Orthographic processing	Receptive Coding			
Oral–motor functioning	RAN Letters RAN Words		Oromotor Sequencing Speeded Naming Part II	CWI Word Reading
Lexicons				
Word knowledge		Verbal Comprehension Reading Vocabulary		
General knowledge		General Information Academic Knowledge		
Abilities				
Listening comprehension (receptive language)	VWM Sentences: Listening Notetaking A	Story Recall Understanding Directions Oral Comprehension	Understanding Directions Narrative Memory	
Oral expression (expressive language)		Story Recall	Narrative Memory	
Visual–spatial representation of language			Understanding Directions	
Reasoning with verbal information				
Reasoning with verbal/visual–spatial information			Animal Sorting	
Reasoning with verbal/quantitative information				
Executive functions, strategies, time frames of reference				
Executive functions involved in cueing, directing, and coordinating cognitive constructs while performing reading tasks	Rapid Automatic Switching Sentence Sense		Auditory Attention and Response Set	CWI Inhibition CWI Inhibition/ Switching
Strategies applied while performing language or reading tasks				Twenty Questions
Initial registration of phonology and/or orthography	All phonological and orthographic processing tasks			

(cont.)

TABLE 36.3. *(cont.)*

Cognitive construct	Intellectual assessment measure			
	PAL-II	WJ III COG/ACH	NEPSY-II	D-KEFS
Holding and manipulating information while listening and/or while reading	VWM Letters VWM Words VWM Sentences	Auditory Working Memory	Understanding Directions Narrative Memory	
Retrieving information from long-term storage while listening/speaking and/or while reading	VWM Letters VWM Words	Retrieval Fluency Story Recall—Delayed	Word Generation	Verbal Fluency

Note. PAL-II, Process Assessment of the Learner—Second Edition; WJ III COG/ACH, Woodcock–Johnson III Tests of Cognitive Abilities/Tests of Achievement; D-KEFS, Delis–Kaplan Executive Function System. RAN, Rapid Automatic Naming; CWI, Color–Word Interference; VWM, Verbal Working Memory.

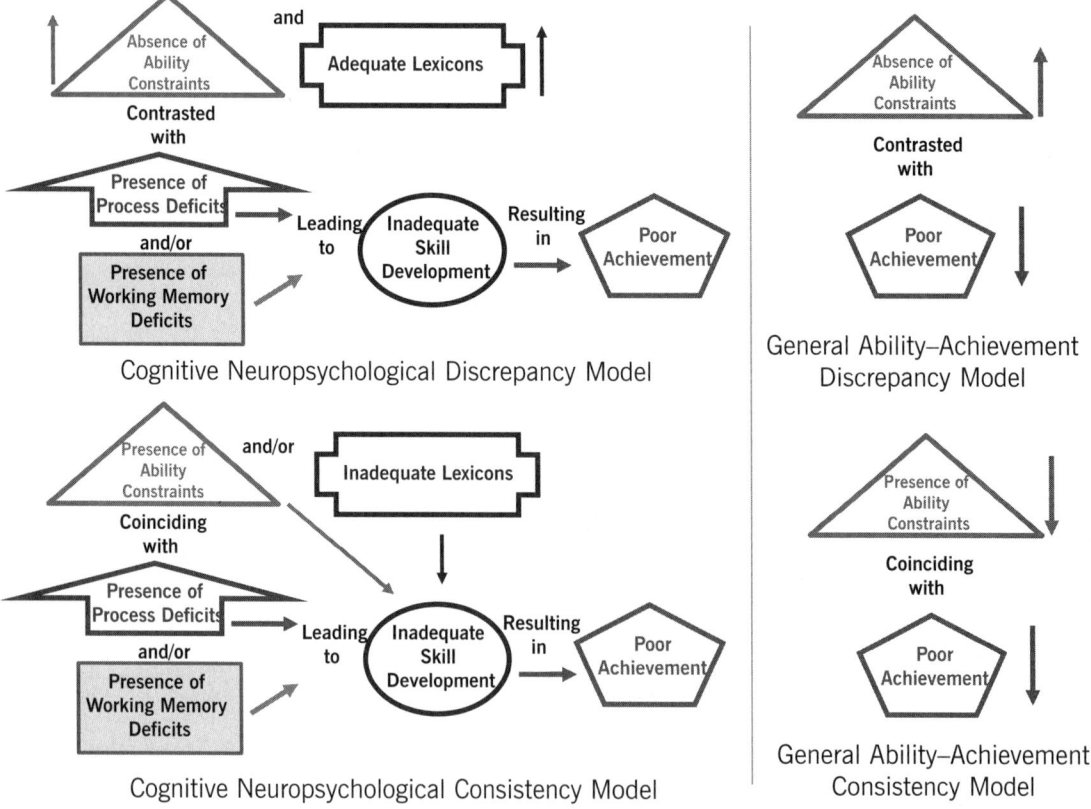

FIGURE 36.6. Models for the identification of learning disabilities, based on different assessment approaches.

ory time frame use, and academic skills measures as dictated by the specific academic difficulties (Berninger et al., 2005).

Applying the General Abilities Model in a Three-Tier System

When the general abilities model is applied across all three levels of a three-tier system, the focus is on predicting which students are likely to succeed and which students are likely to fail. At tiers 1 and 2, the progress-monitoring devices serve as the predictors of the students' later competencies in the academic domains. The need for intellectual assessment at these tiers typically is not even considered, since the progress-monitoring devices are serving as the predictors during the early stages of service delivery. Even at tier 3, the need for an intellectual assessment is questioned when the purpose of such an assessment is the prediction of later academic success. At best, such an assessment at tier 3 offers an indicator of potential for later success from a longer, more reliable intellectual assessment source. In school systems where instruction at tiers 1 and 2 is not particularly strong, many students are referred for what is perceived as a meaningless intellectual assessment at tier 3, simply because it is mandated as part of the process for consideration for placement in special education and for access to some types of tier 3 services. Whether those services are any better than the ones being provided at tiers 1 and 2 seems irrelevant, as the purpose of the assessment process simply seems to be moving the students out of the instructional environments at these tiers and into a tier 3 instructional environment. It should not be surprising that psychologists balk at being involved in such a process and bemoan their role as that of "gatekeepers for special education," with little or no relevance to the general educational process other than at times to specify an arbitrary numerical cutoff for discrepancy between actual achievement and predicted achievement, on the basis of which it will be determined whether a student is or is not placed in a tier 3 special education program (Reschly & Grimes, 2002).

Applying the Cognitive Neuropsychological Model in a Three-Tier System

When a cognitive neuropsychological model is applied, the focus is on characterizing students' cognitive strengths and weaknesses, understanding how these strengths and weaknesses affect learning and production, and understanding how instruction can be modified to improve learning and production. The need for this type of information is apparent at all three tiers. When assessments directly address these needs, parents, teachers, and administrators see the value of a comprehensive assessment for any student who is struggling academically—not simply to get the student placed in a tier 3 program, but to help identify instructional practices that are most likely to help the student improve learning and production. Although the services of psychologists who competently use a cognitive neuropsychological model may be sought after at all three tiers, it is neither possible nor practical to provide every struggling student with a comprehensive assessment. It may, however, be possible to administer to additional students at tier 2 a brief diagnostic battery that addresses most of the capacities in the cognitive neuropsychological model associated with the specific academic area of concern. This type of assessment will at times necessitate the involvement of psychologists in general education assessment below tier 3. The reason for this involvement rests with the need to administer some tasks, such as those involving reasoning with verbal information, that have traditionally been administered only by a psychologist in the context of a comprehensive intellectual assessment. Such diagnostic assessment activity could open the door for academic consultation services that would have an impact on a larger number of students, provided that the psychologist is well trained in diagnostic assessment and research-based instructional programs (Berninger et al., 2005).

The Contrast between the Two Models

With the emphasis on prediction of academic skill levels based on global intellectual assessment results, the general abilities model has little to offer school-based professionals who must identify a student's specific pattern of cognitive strengths and weaknesses and recommend interventions most likely to increase academic skill proficiency. Conversely, the cognitive neuropsychological model can offer a wealth of information about the extent to which a student can effectively process information during initial registration and create adequate mental representations; apply abilities and access lexicons; hold, manipulate, store, and/or retrieve mental representations; and use academic skills—

all cued, directed, and coordinated by executive functions in order to demonstrate adequate academic production. How knowledge of these cognitive constructs can affect educational programming for students is illustrated by the six case profiles shown in Table 36.4. All six of these elementary-school-age students were referred for evaluations by teachers or parents because of suspected reading difficulties. Comparing and contrasting the six cases provides some important insights related to assessment and intervention for reading problems and their relationship to what has traditionally been defined as intellectual ability:

1. The greater the number of process, ability, lexicon, executive function, and memory time frame usage weaknesses identified, the greater the number of reading skill weaknesses, and the poorer the overall level of reading achievement.
2. Although students may be diagnosed with the same type of reading problem, the students' specific patterns of cognitive strengths and weaknesses may vary greatly, thereby necessitating different intervention plans.
3. The amount of time and energy invested, and the diversity of intervention techniques that must be employed, will vary in proportion to the number of cognitive construct weaknesses that are identified.

To illustrate these points, let us consider cases 1–3 in Table 36.4, all of which display the cognitive construct characteristics of developmental phonological dyslexia (DPD) (Berninger & Richards, 2002; Shaywitz, 2003; Temple, 1997; Uhry & Clark, 2005). Although these students' processing profiles look similar, the case 1 student exhibits fewer reading skill and reading achievement weaknesses because she is able to make effective use of her well-developed executive functions, reasoning and language abilities, strategies, lexicons, and working memory time frame—all of which enable her to compensate for (but not completely eradicate) her word-level reading disability.

The case 2 student exhibits more difficulties with reading skills and more inconsistent performance with reading achievement, stemming from the presence of additional weaknesses in the use of executive functions to consistently cue the use of strategies and skills. Note, for example, the additional weaknesses in word recognition fluency and silent reading/comprehension fluency that

reflect an inability to balance speed and accuracy, resulting in a quick work pace that is countered by excessive word-reading error rates. Note also that the weakness in use of strategies is not due to a total lack of knowledge of word- or sentence-level reading strategies, but rather to a failure to cue the use of these learned strategies when the student is reading individual words and sentences (McCloskey et al., 2009; Meltzer, 2010; Swanson, 1993).

The case 3 student exhibits basic reading skill and executive function weaknesses similar to those of the case 2 student, but the additional weaknesses with the use of the working memory time frame experienced by this student are creating difficulties with the more complex skill of reading comprehension, and subsequently are resulting in poorer performance on measures of reading achievement (Berninger & Richards, 2002; Swanson, 1999, 2008).

The critical importance of assessing abilities and lexicons that constrain the act of reading—capacities typically classified as intellectual abilities—becomes more evident when the first three cases (involving only DPD) are contrasted with cases 4–6, in all of which the students exhibit weaknesses in reasoning with verbal information and poor stores of word knowledge and general knowledge. For this reason, these students are designated in Table 36.4 as exhibiting AD (ability deficit). The absence of any processing deficits in the case 4 student, combined with adequate use of executive functions to direct basic word reading and effective use of the working memory time frame, have enabled this student to develop basic reading skills at the word level; however, the ability and lexicon weaknesses are constraining the development of reading comprehension skills at the sentence and passage levels, and are resulting in poor performance on measures of reading achievement.

The case 5 student exhibits ability and lexicon weaknesses similar to those of the case 4 student, but these are joined by a phonological processing weakness that is hindering the development of decoding skills and performance on fluency measures, due to poor use of decoding skills in a manner similar to that of the case 1 student. Unlike that student, however, the case 5 student is exhibiting weaknesses with reading comprehension and poor performance on reading achievement measures, due to reasoning ability and word knowledge lexicon weaknesses. Note that although this student has not stored an adequate amount of knowledge

TABLE 36.4. Cognitive Neuropsychological Profiles of Six Students Referred by Teachers or Parents Due to Concerns about Reading

Cognitive construct	Cognitive construct levels: S = strength, A = adequate, W = weakness					
	Case 1: DPD	Case 2: DPD	Case 3: DPD	Case 4: AD	Case 5: AD/DPD	Case 6: AD/DPD
Processes/processing						
Phonological processing	W	W	W	A	W	W
Orthographic processing	A	A	A	A	A	W
Oral–motor functioning	A	A	A	A	A	W
Executive functions						
Executive functions involved in cueing, directing, and coordinating cognitive constructs while performing reading tasks	S	W	W	A	A	W
Lexicons						
Word knowledge	S	S	S	W	W	W
General knowledge	S	S	S	W	W	W
Abilities						
Listening comprehension (receptive language)	S	S	S	A	A	W
Oral expression (expressive language)	S	S	S	A	A	W
Reasoning with verbal information	S	S	S	W	W	W
Time frames of reference						
Initial registration of phonology (P) and/or orthography (O)	W/P	W/P	W/P	A	W/P	W/P&O
Holding and manipulating information while listening and/or while reading (working memory)	A	A	W	A	A	W
Retrieving information from long-term storage while listening/speaking and/or while reading	S	S	A	W/A	A	W
Strategies						
Strategies applied while performing reading tasks	S	W	W	A	W	W
Reading skills						
Word recognition	A	A/W	W/A	A	A	W
Decoding	W	W	W	A	W	W
Word recognition fluency	A	W	W	A	A	W
Word decoding fluency	W	W	W	A	W	W
Oral reading (passage) fluency	W	W	W	A	W	W
Comprehension	S	S	W/A	W	W	W
Silent reading comprehension/fluency	A	W	W	W	W	W
Reading achievement						
Grade-level group test	A	W/A	W	W	W	W
Grade-level state competency test	A	W/A	W	W	W	W

Note. DPD, developmental phonological dyslexia; AD, ability deficit; AD/DPD, ability deficit/developmental phonological dyslexia.

about words and topics related to school, he is able to recall adequately information that actually has been stored.

The case 6 student exhibits reasoning ability and lexicon weaknesses similar to those of the student in cases 4 and 5, but these are joined by weaknesses in receptive and expressive language abilities, phonological and orthographic processing, and oral–motor functioning, as well as weaknesses in executive functions and inadequate use of all three time frames of reference. The consequent effect on reading is evident in the display of weaknesses for all reading skills and extremely poor performance on measures of reading achievement.

In terms of classification, recommendations for intervention and outlook for improvement, the advantages of a cognitive neuropsychological model over a general abilities model are unequivocal and numerous. The general abilities model would merely specify that an ability–achievement discrepancy exists for the first three students (those with DPD only), and that an ability–achievement consistency exists for the second three students (those with AD or AD/DPD). The cognitive neuropsychological model offers a richer context for understanding the nature of the reading problems in each of these six cases by specifying levels of performance with tasks involving the full array of cognitive constructs involved in the act of reading. As a result, each child's specific pattern of cognitive strengths and weaknesses can be used effectively to specify the nature and number of interventions that are required, as well as the intensity of the intervention efforts needed for improvement of reading skills.

In terms of intervention, the case 1 student represents the least difficulty, as supplemental instruction in decoding skills will probably be sufficient to address the reading skills deficits of this third-grade student (National Institute of Child Health and Human Development, 2000; Shaywitz, 2003; Uhry & Clark, 2005). The case 2 student will also require supplemental instruction in decoding skills, but in addition, the executive function difficulties and failure to use learned strategies for word reading and comprehension will need to be addressed through guided practice in their use when the student is reading sentences and paragraphs. Gradually (likely over the course of 1 or more years), instruction will need to move from guided practice to self-regulated practice in using executive functions to cue and direct word reading and comprehension skill use. Intervention

efforts with this third-grade student will be more challenging and will require more time than those for the case 1 student, and progress is likely to be slower (McCloskey et al., 2009; Swanson, 1993).

The case 3 student will require supplemental interventions similar to those provided for the case 2 student, but will need additional instruction in ways to compensate for poor use of the working memory time frame (Swanson, 1999, 2008). Note that the interventions outlined briefly here relate to supplemental instruction and are not meant to be complete replacements for all elements of a balanced literacy curriculum. All three of these students will need to receive instruction focused on development of vocabulary, comprehension, and fluency, but their cognitive strengths should enable them to benefit from general education instruction of these components of the reading curriculum (NRP, 2000). Because of the students' age, the phonological processing deficits they exhibit are not addressed directly, but the decoding instruction provided reflects a compensation for weak phonological processing (Aylward et al., 2003).

The case 4 student (the one with AD only) represents a very different challenge in terms of intervention because the reading skill weaknesses demonstrated by this student do not stem from deficits in processing, executive functions, strategy use, or memory time frame use, but rather are a result of the student's ability and lexicon weaknesses. For the two students with AD/DPD (cases 5 and 6), interventions are required that take into account deficits in processing, executive functions, strategy use, and memory time frame use, together with the associated specific reading skill deficits, in a manner similar to that described for each of the three students with DPD (cases 1–3). Interventions for the students with AD or with AD/DPD are much more challenging because they also exhibit deficits in reasoning ability, word knowledge, and general knowledge that are constraining reading comprehension (Berninger & Richards, 2002). Intervention efforts will need to be greater in number and will require longer periods of time, given the severity and number of deficits that these students exhibit.

It is important to note that the cognitive construct deficits distinguishing the three students with AD or AD/DPD from the three students with DPD only are the cognitive constructs that have traditionally been associated with intellectual assessment (i.e., cognitive abilities and knowledge lexicons). The intervention challenges presented by the students in cases 4–6 are at the heart of a fundamental ideological debate about intelligence: Do intelligence test scores based on tasks involving reasoning with verbal information and descriptions of word meanings represent innate, immutable intellectual traits or acquired, malleable cognitive constructs? Some psychologists point out that such scores are combining very different cognitive constructs that are better addressed individually (Hale & Fiorello, 2004; Hale & Miller, 2008; McCloskey, 2009a, 2009b). Others might respond that vocabulary represents a crystallized knowledge base that can be increased through academic instruction or self-directed learning, but that reasoning with verbal information represents a more fluid ability and is much more difficult to alter through academic instruction (Flanagan & Kaufman, 2009; Lichtenberger & Kaufman, 2009; McGrew, 2000). Strict adherents of a general abilities model ignore the differences between the two tasks and espouse the view that the composite represented by the combination of these tasks represents a core of relatively innate, immutable verbal ability, or *g* (Gottfredson, 1998; Jensen, 1973, 1998).

When the issue of intervention is raised, however, adherents of a general abilities model and most adherents of a cognitive neuropsychological model tend to behave as if the tasks of reasoning with verbal information and describing the meaning of words both represent innate, immutable traits. Regardless of which model guides the interpretation of intellectual assessments, reports we have reviewed typically do not provide specific recommendations for interventions focused on improving vocabulary knowledge and/or improving reasoning with verbal information. In other words, these capacities tend to be viewed as innate abilities rather than teachable skills. The tendency to view the tasks that are combined to form verbal ability composites as representative of a unitary trait have led some to ignore or deny the role that reasoning with verbal information plays in the development of reading comprehension skills (Fletcher, Lyon, Fuchs, & Barnes, 2007).

Proponents of this viewpoint could point out correctly that no specific, well-researched intervention curriculum has been developed that enables educators to raise the reasoning ability of a student from two standard deviations below the mean to the mean within any reasonable amount of time. This fact fuels the argument that reasoning (whether innate or not) should be discounted as an instructional variable, or even as a source of variability in skill performance, in teaching for acquisition of reading skills. Although no specific intervention program for quickly and dramatically improving reasoning deficits exists at this time, a number of instructional techniques and specific teaching exercises designed to increase reasoning with verbal information have been developed and have been used to improve the academic achievement of students in grades K–12 (Marzano, Pickering, & Pollock, 2001; Sternberg & Grigorenko, 2007). Likewise, teaching strategies and techniques have been developed and used with good results to improve students' vocabulary knowledge and subsequently to raise students' reading achievement levels (Marzano, Pickering, & Pollock, 2004; NRP, 2000). What these instructional techniques are doing, in essence, is reinforcing the idea that a word knowledge lexicon can be built through academic instruction—and most importantly, advancing the idea that reasoning ability can be reframed as a teachable skill.

In order for improvement in reading comprehension skill acquisition and increased scores on reading achievement measures to occur, intervention efforts must attempt to address the reasoning and word knowledge deficits of the three students with AD (cases 4–6) in Table 36.4, and of all other children with similar cognitive construct weaknesses who are currently enrolled in our K–12 schools. This discussion serves to highlight the most important distinction between the general abilities model and the cognitive neuropsychological model: The general abilities model locks the door of opportunity for further cognitive growth by perpetuating the belief that intelligence is an innate, immutable trait, whereas the cognitive neuropsychological model opens this door by advancing the belief that intelligence represents a multifaceted set of cognitive constructs that are malleable and teachable, given the appropriate investment of energy, time, and effort by all stakeholders—students, parents, and educators.

SUMMARY AND CONCLUSIONS

This chapter has described and contrasted two models that can be used to guide the use and interpretation of intellectual assessments. Although the general abilities model may be useful in specific situations where overall level of ability is a central factor in educational programming, the cognitive neuropsychological model holds much greater promise for fulfilling the important diagnostic role of identifying patterns of cognitive strengths and weaknesses and relating these patterns to intervention programming, especially for students with specific learning disabilities and AD. In addition, the cognitive neuropsychological model appears much better suited to addressing assessment needs in the context of the three-tier service delivery systems that are becoming more prevalent in U.S. schools. The assessment demands in school settings necessitate a shift away from a narrow general abilities model focused on predicting achievement. Such a model avoids addressing or highlighting the specific cognitive constructs that may be constraining or impeding academic production, limits interpretation to one or a handful of composite scores, and limits perspectives on intervention by espousing a model implying that intelligence is an innate, immutable trait.

In today's schools, assessment needs to embrace the much broader perspective offered by the cognitive neuropsychological model, which enables assessment of a broad array of cognitive constructs interpreted in the context of their role in learning and production in specific academic domains, and which links results to a broad array of intervention efforts. This sentiment is reflected in a recently published Learning Disabilities Association of America white paper (Hale et al., 2010), which advocates for the assessment and consideration of patterns of cognitive strengths and weaknesses in identification and treatment of learning disabilities. Although contemporary intellectual assessments are not well suited to meeting these assessment needs in the schools, some of the needed instrumentation is available today through various specific cognitive tests of processing, abilities, lexicons, executive functions, memory time frames of reference, and academic skills. Ideally, the shift to a cognitive neuropsychological model would necessitate the development of new cognitive test batteries that directly address the broad array of cognitive constructs specifically involved in listening/speaking, reading, writing, and math.

Psychologists must make a choice as to their role in the use of assessment instruments in the future. To effectively implement a cognitive neuropsychological model such as the one described in this chapter, psychologists working in the schools will need to have a thorough grasp of cutting-edge assessment instrumentation and intervention techniques in reading, writing, and math, for the purposes of diagnosing academic problems and recommending interventions most likely to produce skill growth. Although the field

of school psychology generally claims expertise in this academic skill domain (National Association of School Psychologists, 2006), many school psychologists confess a lack of adequate knowledge in these areas, and some other professionals question whether psychologists really have the knowledge to be involved in such work (Kirby, 2009). If psychologists choose to continue emphasizing the use and interpretation of traditional intelligence tests within a general abilities model, and if they continue to approach ability and lexicon deficits as immutable, irremediable traits, they may find it increasingly more difficult to break out of a meaningless "test and place" model of assessment. Or they may find that their services are no longer needed, as they are being replaced by a cadre of other professionals competently trained in the use and interpretation of a host of processing, ability, and skill tests that are directly related to learning and production in academic domains but do not include the word *intelligence* in their titles.

Alternatively, psychologists can choose to expand their repertoire of assessment skills, incorporating cognitive measures of processing, skills, lexicons, abilities, executive functions, and memory time frames of reference with the occasional handful of intelligence test subtests to provide assessment results that can drive intervention efforts. They can become the leading proponents in a movement to change reasoning ability into a teachable skill, and can become highly knowledgeable about academic intervention programs and the links between assessment and intervention. Concurrently, psychologists can encourage test publishers to increase their efforts to develop more germane cognitive neuropsychological test batteries—ones that directly relate to learning and production in the various academic domains.

Regardless of the choices made by psychologists working in the schools, we predict that the future of assessment belongs to cognitive assessment guided by a cognitive neuropsychological model, rather than intellectual assessment guided by a general abilities model. If the next edition of this text is entitled *Contemporary Cognitive Assessment*, the accuracy of this prediction will be apparent.

REFERENCES

Alfonso, V., Flanagan, D., & Radwan, S., (2005). The impact of the Cattell Horn–Carroll theory on test development and interpretation of cognitive and academic abilities. In D. P. Flanagan & P. L. Harrison

(Eds.), *Contemporary intellectual assessment* (2nd ed., pp. 185–202). New York: Guilford Press.

Allen, T., Hulac, D., & D'Amato, R. C. (2005). The pediatric neurological examination and school neuropsychology. In R. C. D'Amato, E. Fletcher-Janzen, E., & C. Reynolds (Eds.), *Handbook of school neuropsychology* (pp. 145–171). Hoboken, NJ: Wiley.

Aylward, E. H., Richards, T. L., Berninger, V. W., Nagy, W. E., Field, K. M., Grimm, A. C., et al. (2003). Instructional treatment associated with changes in brain activation in children with dyslexia. *Neurology, 61*, 212–219.

Berninger, V. W. (1994). *Reading and writing acquisition: A developmental neuropsychological perspective.* Boulder, CO: Westview Press.

Berninger, V. W. (1998). *Process Assessment of the Learner: Intervention guide.* San Antonio, TX: Psychological Corporation.

Berninger, V. W., Dunn, A., & Alper, T. (2005). Integrated multilevel model for branching assessment, instructional assessment, and profile assessment. In A. Prifitera, D. H. Saklofske, & L. G. Weiss (Eds.), *WISC-IV clinical use and interpretation* (pp. 151–188). Burlington, MA: Elsevier/Academic Press.

Berninger, V. W., O'Donnell, L., & Holdnack, J. (2008). Research supported differential diagnosis of specific learning disabilities and implications for intervention and response to intervention. In A. Prifitera, D. H. Saklofske, & L. G. Weiss (Eds.), *WISC-IV clinical assessment and intervention* (2nd ed., pp. 69–110). Burlington, MA: Elsevier/Academic Press.

Berninger, V. W., & Richards, T. L. (2002). *Brain literacy for educators and psychologists.* Boston: Academic Press.

Bradley, R., Danielson, L., & Hallahan, D. P. (Eds.). (2002). *Identification of learning disabilities: Research to practice.* Mahwah, NJ: Erlbaum.

Deary, I. J. (2001). *Intelligence: A very short introduction.* Oxford: Oxford University Press.

Decker, S. (2008). School neuropsychology consultation in neurodevelopmental disorders. *Psychology in the Schools, 45*(9), 799–811.

Dehaene, S. (2009). *Reading in the brain.* New York: Viking.

Elliott, C. D. (2007). *Differential Ability Scales—Second Edition: Administration and scoring manual.* San Antonio, TX: Harcourt Assessment.

Fiorello, C. A., Hale, J. B., Holdnack, J. A., Kavanagh, J. A., Terrell, J., & Long, L. (2007). Interpreting intelligence tests results for children with disabilities: Is global intelligence relevant? *Applied Neuropsychology, 14*, 2–12.

Fiorello, C. A., Hale, J. B., McGrath, M., Ryan, K., & Quinn, S. (2001). IQ interpretation for children with flat and variable test profiles. *Learning and Individual Differences, 13*, 115–125.

Flanagan, D. P., Alfonso, V., Ortiz, S., & Dynda, A. (2010). Integrating cognitive assessment in school neuropsychological evaluations. In D. Miller (Ed.), *Best practices in school neuropsychology* (pp. 101–140). Hoboken, NJ: Wiley.

Flanagan, D. P., & Kaufman, A. S. (2009). Introduction and overview. In D. P. Flanagan & A. S. Kaufman (Eds.), *Essentials of WISC-IV assessment* (pp. 1–52). Hoboken, NJ: Wiley.

Fletcher, J. M., Lyon, G. R., Fuchs, L. S., & Barnes, M. A. (2007). *Learning disabilities: From identification to intervention.* New York: Guilford Press.

Fletcher-Janzen, E. (2005). The school neuropsychological examination. In R. C. D'Amato, E. Fletcher-Janzen, & C. Reynolds (Eds.), *Handbook of school neuropsychology* (pp. 172–212). Hoboken, NJ: Wiley.

Floyd, R. (2005). Information-processing approaches to interpretation of contemporary intellectual assessment instruments. In D. P. Flanagan & P. L. Harrison (Eds.), *Contemporary intellectual assessment* (2nd ed., pp. 203–233). New York: Guilford Press.

Gottfredson, L. S. (1997). Why g matters: The complexity of everyday life. *Intelligence, 24*, 79–132.

Gottfredson, L. S. (1998). The general intelligence factor. *Scientific American Presents*, pp. 24–29.

Gottfredson, L. S. (2008). Of what value is intelligence? In A. Prifitera, D. H. Saklofske, & L. G. Weiss (Eds.), *WISC-IV clinical assessment and intervention* (2nd ed., pp. 545–564). Burlington, MA: Elsevier/Academic Press.

Hale, J. B., Alfonso, V., Berninger, V., Bracken, B., Christo, C., Clark, E., et al. (2010). Critical issues in response-to-intervention, comprehensive evaluation, and specific learning disabilities identification and intervention: An expert white paper consensus. *Learning Disability Quarterly, 33*(3), 223–236.

Hale, J. B., & Fiorello, C. A. (2004). *School neuropsychology, A practitioner's handbook.* New York: Guilford Press.

Hale, J. B., Fiorello, C. A., Miller, J. A., Wenrich, K., Teodori, A., & Henzel, J. N. (2008). WISC-IV interpretation for specific learning disabilities identification and intervention: A cognitive hypothesis testing approach. In A. Prifitera, D. H. Saklofske, & L. G. Weiss (Eds.), *WISC-IV clinical assessment and intervention* (2nd ed., pp. 111–172). Burlington, MA: Elsevier/Academic Press.

Hale, J. B., Kaufman, A., Naglieri, J. A., & Kavale, K. (2006). Implementation of IDEA: Integrating response to intervention and cognitive assessment methods. *Psychology in the Schools, 43*(7), 753–770.

Hale, J. B., & Miller, D. C. (2008). Neuropsychological applications of the WISC-IV and WISC-IV Integrated. In A. Prifitera, D. H. Saklofske, & L. G. Weiss (Eds.), *WISC-IV clinical assessment and intervention* (2nd ed., pp. 445–496). Burlington, MA: Elsevier/Academic Press.

Jensen, A. R. (1973). *Educability and group differences.* London: Methuen.

Jensen, A. R. (1980). *Bias in mental testing.* New York: Free Press.

Jensen, A. R. (1998). *The g factor: The science of mental ability.* Westport, CT: Praeger.

Kamphaus, R. W. (2001). *Clinical assessment of children's intelligence.* Needham Heights, MA: Allyn & Bacon.

Kamphaus, R. W., Winsor, A. P., Rowe, E. W., & Kim, S. (2005). A history of intelligence test interpretation. In D. P. Flanagan & P. L. Harrison (Eds.), *Contemporary intellectual assessment* (2nd ed., pp. 23–38). New York: Guilford Press.

Kaplan, E. (1988). A process approach to neuropsychological assessment. In T. Boll & B. K. Bryant (Eds.), *Clinical neuropsychology and brain functions: Research, measurement, and practice* (pp. 125–167). Washington, DC: American Psychological Association.

Kaplan, E., Fein, D., Morris, R., Kramer, J. H., & Delis, D. C. (1999). *The WISC-III as a Processing Instrument.* San Antonio, TX: Psychological Corporation.

Kaufman, A. S., & Kaufman, N. L. (2004). *Kaufman Assessment Battery for Children—Second Edition.* Circle Pines, MN: American Guidance Service.

Kavale, K. A. (2002). Discrepancy models in the identification of learning disabilities. In R. Bradley, L. Danielson, & D. Hallahan (Eds.), *Identification of learning disabilities: Research to practice* (pp. 369–407). New York: Routledge.

Kirby, M. W. (2009). Why is the school psychologist involved in the evaluation of struggling readers? *Journal of Educational and Psychological Consultation, 19,* 248–258.

Kuncel, N., Hezlet, S., & Ones, D. (2004). Academic performance, career potential, creativity, and performance: Can one construct predict them all? *Journal of Personality and Social Psychology, 86,* 148–161.

Levine, M. (1998). *Developmental variation and learning disorders.* Cambridge, MA: Educators Publishing Service.

Lichtenberger, E. O., & Kaufman, A. S. (Eds.). (2009). *Essentials of WAIS-IV assessment.* Hoboken, NJ: Wiley.

Mapou, R. L., & Spector, J. (1995). *Clinical neuropsychological assessment: A cognitive approach.* New York: Plenum Press.

Marzano, R. J., Pickering, D. J., & Pollock, J. E. (2001). *Classroom instruction that works: Research-based strategies for increasing student achievement.* Alexandria,

VA: Association for Supervision and Curriculum Development.

Mather, N., & Wendling, B. (2005). Linking cognitive assessment results to academic interventions for students with learning disabilities. In D. P. Flanagan & P. L. Harrison (Eds.), *Contemporary intellectual assessment* (2nd ed., pp. 269–294). New York: Guilford Press.

McCloskey, G. (2009a). Clinical applications I: A neuropsychological approach to interpretation of the WAIS-IV and the use of the WAIS-IV in learning disability assessments. In E. O. Lichtenberger & A. S. Kaufman (Eds.), *Essentials of WAIS-IV assessment* (pp. 208–244). Hoboken, NJ: Wiley.

McCloskey, G. (2009b). The WISC-IV Integrated. In D. P. Flanagan & A. S. Kaufman (Eds.), *Essentials of WISC-IV assessment* (2nd ed., pp. 310–467). Hoboken, NJ: Wiley.

McCloskey, G., & Maerlender, A. (2005). The WISC-IV Integrated. In A. Prifitera, D. H. Saklofske, & L. G. Weiss (Eds.), *WISC-IV clinical use and interpretation: Scientist-practitioner perspectives* (pp. 101–149). Burlington, MA: Elsevier/Academic Press.

McCloskey, G., Perkins, L. A., & Van Divner, B. (2009). *Assessment and intervention for executive function difficulties.* New York: Routledge.

McDermott, P. A., & Glutting, J. J. (1997). Informing stylistic learning behavior, disposition, and achievement through ability subtests—or, more illusions of meaning? *School Psychology Review, 26,* 163–175.

McGrew, K. S. (2000). *Clinical interpretation of the Woodcock–Johnson Tests of Cognitive Ability—Revised.* Boston: Allyn & Bacon.

Meltzer, L. (2010). *Promoting executive function in the classroom.* New York: Guilford Press.

Miller, D. C. (2007). *Essentials of school neuropsychological assessment.* Hoboken, NJ: Wiley.

National Association of School Psychologists. (2006). *School psychology: A blueprint for training and practice III.* Bethesda, MD: Author.

National Institute of Child Health and Human Development. (2000). *Report of the National Reading Panel. Teaching children to read: An evidence-based assessment of the scientific research literature on reading and its implications for reading instruction: Reports of the subgroups* (NIH Publication No. 000-4754). Washington, DC: U.S. Government Printing Office.

Pennington, B. F. (2009). *Diagnosing learning disorders: A neuropsychological framework* (2nd ed.). New York: Guilford Press.

Posner, M. I., & Rothbart, M. K. (2007). *Educating the human brain.* Washington, DC: American Psychological Association.

Reschly, D. J., & Grimes, J. P. (2002). Best practices in intellectual assessment. In A. Thomas & J. Grimes (Eds.), *Best practices in school psychology IV* (pp. 1337–1350). Bethesda, MD: National Association of School Psychologists.

Reynolds, C. R., & Fletcher-Janzen, E. (1997). *Handbook of clinical child neuropsychology* (2nd ed.). New York: Kluwer Academic/Plenum.

Reynolds, C. R., & French, C. L. (2005). The brain as a dynamic organ of information processing and learning. In R. C. D'Amato, E Fletcher-Janzen, & C. Reynolds (Eds.), *Handbook of school neuropsychology* (pp. 86–119). Hoboken, NJ: Wiley.

Roid, G. H. (2003). *Stanford–Binet Intelligence Scales, Fifth Edition: Examiner's manual*. Itasca, IL: Riverside.

Saklofske, D., Prifitera, A., Weiss, L., Rolfhus, E., & Zhu, J. (2005). Clinical interpretation of the WISC-IV FSIQ and GAI. In A. Prifitera, D. H. Saklofske, & L. G. Weiss (Eds.), *WISC-IV clinical use and interpretation*. Burlington, MA: Elsevier/Academic Press.

Sarason, S. (1975). The unfortunate fate of Alfred Binet and school psychology. *Teachers College Record, 77*, 579–592.

Sattler, J. M., & D'Amato, R. C. (2002). Brain injuries: Theory and rehabilitation programs. In J. M. Sattler, *Assessment of children: Behavioral and clinical applications* (4th ed., pp. 431–439). San Diego, CA: Jerome M. Sattler, Publisher.

Shaywitz, S. (2003). *Overcoming dyslexia: A new and complete science-based program for reading problems at any level*. New York: Knopf.

Spearman, C. (1904). "General intelligence," objectively determined and measured. *American Journal of Psychology, 15*, 201–293.

Sternberg, R. J., & Grigorenko, E. L. (2007). *Teaching for successful intelligence to increase student learning and achievement* (2nd ed.). Thousand Oaks, CA: Corwin Press.

Sternberg, R. J., Grigorenko, E. L., & Bundy, D. A. (2001). The predictive value of IQ. *Merrill–Palmer Quarterly, 47*(1), 1–41.

Swanson, H. L. (1993). Working memory in learning disability subgroups. *Journal of Experimental Child Psychology, 56*(1), 87–114.

Swanson, H. L. (1999). Reading comprehension and working memory in learning-disabled readers: Is the phonological loop more important than the executive system? *Journal of Experimental Child Psychology, 72*(1), 1–31.

Swanson, H. L. (2008). Neurosicence and RTI: A complimentary role. In E. Fletcher-Janzen & C. R. Reynolds (Eds.), *Neuropsychological perspectives on learning disabilities in the era of RTI: Recommendations for diagnosis and intervention* (pp. 28–53). Hoboken, NJ: Wiley.

Temple, C. (1997). *Developmental cognitive neuropsychology*. Hove, UK: Psychology Press.

Torgesen, J. K., Wagner, R. K., Rashotte, C. A., Rose, E., Lindamood, P., Conway, T., et al. (1999). Preventing reading failure in young children with phonological processing disabilities: Group and individual responses to instruction. *Journal of Educational Psychology, 91*, 1–15.

Uhry, J. K., & Clark, D. B. (2005). *Dyslexia: Theory and practice of instruction* (3rd ed.). Baltimore: York Press.

Volker, M. A., Lopata, C., & Cook-Cottone, C. (2006). Assessment of children with intellectual giftedness and reading disabilities. *Psychology in the Schools, 43*(8), 855–869

Watkins, M., Glutting, J., & Youngstrom, E. (2005). Issues in subtest profile analysis. In D. P. Flanagan & P. L. Harrison (Eds.), *Contemporary intellectual assessment* (2nd ed., pp. 251–268). New York: Guilford Press.

Wechsler, D. (2003). *Wechsler Intelligence Scale for Children—Fourth Edition (WISC-IV)*. San Antonio, TX: Psychological Corporation.

Weinberg, R. A (1989). Intelligence and IQ: Landmark issues and great debates. *American Psychologist, 44*(2), 98–104.

Willis, W. (2005) Foundations of Developmental Neuroanatomy In C. D'Amato, E. Fletcher-Janzen, & C. Reynolds (Eds.), *Handbook of school neuropsychology* (pp. 41–60). Hoboken, NJ: Wiley.

Woodcock, R. W., McGrew, K. S., & Mather, N. (2001). *Woodcock–Johnson III*. Itasca, IL: Riverside.

The Three-Stratum Theory of Cognitive Abilities

John B. Carroll

The three-stratum theory of cognitive abilities is an expansion and extension of previous theories. It specifies what kinds of individual differences in cognitive abilities exist and how those kinds of individual differences are related to one another. It provides a map of all cognitive abilities known or expected to exist and can be used as a guide to research and practice. It proposes that there are a fairly large number of distinct individual differences in cognitive ability, and that the relationships among them can be derived by classifying them into three different strata: stratum I, "narrow" abilities; stratum II, "broad" abilities; and stratum III, consisting of a single "general" ability.

ORIGIN OF THE THEORY

The theory was developed in the course of a major survey (Carroll, 1993a, 1994) of research over the past 60 or 70 years on the nature, identification, and structure of human cognitive abilities. That research involved the use of the mathematical technique known as *factor analysis*. Necessarily, the work also involved the analysis of correlations among scores on psychological tests and other kinds of assessments of individuals. This is because factor analysis concerns the structure of correlations among such variables—that is, the question of how many *factors* or *latent traits* are indicated by

a set of correlations arranged in a matrix such that all the correlations among variables are shown systematically.

In my survey, I used factor analysis to examine more than 460 sets of data (hereafter, *datasets*) from the relevant literature. In most cases these datasets had been previously analyzed by the original investigators, but I felt it necessary to reanalyze them because I wanted to take advantage of important technical advances in factor-analytic methodology that were not used by the original investigators, usually because they were not yet available at the time of the original data analysis. I also considered it desirable to analyze the datasets in as consistent a way as possible to facilitate making valid general conclusions.

Before beginning my survey, I considered how best to select datasets because it was going to be impossible to reanalyze all of what I estimated as more than 2,000 datasets available in the relevant literature published over the years 1930–1985 (approximately) in many countries—mainly English-speaking countries such as the United States, Canada, Great Britain, and Australia, but also other countries such as France, Germany, Japan, Spain, and even Russia. I established several criteria for selecting datasets: (1) Each dataset should contain a substantial number of variables reflecting performance on cognitive tasks typical of those used in intelligence and aptitude tests or in research in cognitive psychology; (2) the dataset should be based on a substantial number of individuals (preferably more than, say, 100) taken from a defined population of children, adolescents, or adults that had been tested in a consistent way;

After the publication of the first edition of this text, John B. Carroll passed away. Given the importance of his work for nearly every chapter included in the present volume, his chapter from the first edition is reprinted here as the Appendix.

(3) the published form of the dataset should present the matrix of correlations among its variables, thus permitting reanalysis; and (4) sufficient information about the sample and the variables must have been available to permit at least tentative interpretation of the findings.

In the end, more than 480 datasets were selected, but a small number (about 15) turned out to contain mathematical inconsistencies that could not be resolved. Thus reanalysis of these datasets was not feasible. Many of the datasets were from research by prominent investigators of cognitive abilities such as Thurstone (1938), Thurstone and Thurstone (1941), Guilford (1967), Guilford and Hoepfner (1971), Cattell (1971), Horn (1965), and Vernon (1961); for this reason, the three-stratum theory has similarities to certain theories espoused by some of these investigators (e.g., Horn's fluid–crystallized theory) (see Horn & Noll, 1997, and Horn & Blankson, Chapter 3, this volume).

At this point it is necessary to introduce the concept of *stratum* and to describe certain features of the reanalyses performed in my survey. It was probably Thurstone (1947) who created a related concept—the *order* of a factor analysis. A *first-order* factor analysis is the application of factor-analytic techniques directly to a correlation matrix of the original variables in the dataset; it results in one or more *first-order factors*. A *second-order* factor analysis is the application of factor-analytic techniques to the matrix of correlations among the first-order factors (if there are two or more, and if the correlations are other than zero) of a dataset; it results in one or more *second-order factors*. A *third-order* factor analysis is the application of factor-analytic techniques to the matrix of correlations among the second-order factors (if there are two or more) of a dataset; usually it results in a single *third-order factor*, but it could result in more than one such factor. This process could be repeated at still higher orders, but it would rarely be necessary because at each successive order the number of resulting factors becomes ever smaller. (A large number of original variables would be necessary, to permit analysis at the fourth order, for example.)

The concept of order (of a factor, or of a factor analysis) is therefore tied to operations in the application of factor analysis to a particular dataset. Usually, the variables in a dataset are scores on a variety of psychological tests; the factor analysis produces first-order factors that correspond to clusters of tests such that within each cluster, the tests are similar in the contents or psychological processes they involve. A dataset might, for example, yield three first-order factors—one being a "verbal" factor with loadings on vocabulary and reading comprehension tests, another being a "spatial" factor with loadings on formboard and paper-folding tests, and still another being a "memory span" factor with loadings on a series of memory span tests. If these factors are correlated, a second-order factor might be interpreted as a "general intelligence" factor.

Suppose, however, the variables in a dataset are individual test items (e.g., the individual items on a vocabulary test). A first-order factor analysis of the matrix of correlations among vocabulary items might produce one or more factors; if one factor were found, it might indeed be a "vocabulary" or "verbal" factor, but if two or more factors were found, the investigator might be prompted to identify these factors by their different contents (a factor of "literary vocabulary," a factor of "scientific vocabulary," etc.). A second-order factor analysis of the correlations among such factors would probably produce a "general vocabulary" factor, which might be similar to the first-order vocabulary or verbal factor produced in the analysis of a more typical battery of psychological tests. Thus a vocabulary factor might be a first-order factor in one case but a second-order factor in another case. Similarly, a "general" factor might be a second-order factor in one case but a third-order factor in another case.

As factor analysis is essentially a technique of classifying abilities, Cattell (1971) introduced the term *stratum* to help in characterizing factors, in an absolute sense, in terms of the narrowness or breadth of their content. In the conduct of my survey and in interpreting results, I called the first-order factors resulting from analysis of typical sets of psychological tests *factors at the first stratum*, or *stratum I factors*. (Almost all the datasets were composed of typical sets of psychological tests.) *Stratum II factors* were second-order factors from such datasets, and *stratum III factors* were third-order factors from such datasets. Frequently, however, datasets did not produce third-order factors; they produced only one second-order factor, which was often interpretable as a *general* factor similar to the general factor that occurred as a third-order factor in some other datasets. Thus the stratum of a factor is relative to the variety and diversity of the variables covered by it. Sometimes it is the same as the order of a factor, but in other cases it is not; its stratum is assigned in terms of its perceived breadth or narrowness. It is possible that some factors are so narrow or specific (in content) that their stratum is less than 1. This would be the case for highly specific kinds of vocabulary knowledge identified by factor analysis of the items of a vocabulary test, as mentioned previously. For convenience, however, the three-stratum theory omits mention of such narrow factors, of which there could be many.

The three-stratum theory thus postulates that most factors of interest can be classified as being at a certain stratum, and that the total array of cognitive ability factors contains factors at three strata—namely, first, second, and third. At the third or highest stratum is a general factor (often called *g*). The second stratum is composed of a relatively small number (perhaps about 10) of "broad" factors, including *fluid intelligence, crystallized intelligence, general memory and learning, broad visual perception, broad auditory perception, broad retrieval ability, broad cognitive speediness,* and *processing speed.* At the first stratum (or stratum I), there are numerous first-order factors, roughly grouped under the second-stratum factors as shown in Figure A.1. Some are "level" factors in the sense that their scores indicate the level of mastery, along a difficulty scale, that the individual is able to demonstrate. Others are "speed" factors in the sense that their scores indicate the speed with which the individual performs tasks or the individual's rate of learning in learning and memory tasks.

Rationale and Impetus for Generating the Theory

The theory was intended to constitute a provisional statement about the enumeration, identification, and structuring of the total range of cognitive abilities known or discovered thus far. In this way it was expected to replace, expand, or supplement previous theories of the structure of cognitive abilities, such as Thurstone's (1938) theory of primary mental abilities, Guilford's (1967) structure-of-intellect theory, Horn and Cattell's (1966) Gf-Gc theory, or Wechsler's (1974; see also Matarazzo, 1972) theory of verbal and performance components of intelligence.

OPERATIONALIZATION AND APPLICATION OF THE THEORY
Component Parts of the Theory

The theory consists of an enumeration of the cognitive abilities that have been found thus far, with statements concerning the nature and generality of these abilities, the types of tasks that require them, and the types of tests that can be used to measure them. In effect, it also consists of statements about the structure of the abilities in terms of the assignment of abilities to one of three strata of different degrees of generality. Second-order factors subsumed by the third-order general factor are related to each other by virtue of their loadings on the general factor; some of these are more related to the general factor than others. Similarly, first-order factors subsumed by a given second-order factor are related to each other by virtue of their loadings on that second-order factor.

All the abilities covered by the theory are assumed to be "cognitive" in the sense that cognitive processes are critical to the successful understanding and performance of tasks requiring these abilities, most particularly in the *processing of mental information.* In many cases, they go far beyond the kinds of intelligences measured in typical batteries of intelligence tests. The abilities are roughly classified as follows:

Abilities in the domain of language
Abilities in the domain of reasoning
Abilities in the domain of memory and learning
Abilities in the domain of visual perception
Abilities in the domain of auditory reception
Abilities in the domain of idea production
Abilities in the domain of cognitive speed
Abilities in the domain of knowledge and achievement
Miscellaneous domains of ability (e.g., abilities in the sensory domain, attention abilities, cognitive styles, and administrative abilities)

It must be stressed that this theory is only provisional. Further research may suggest that it should be revised, either in small or in radical ways. It is becoming clear that present methods of measuring abilities may not adequately cover all the abilities that exist or that are important in practical life.

Operationalization of the Theory

Thus far, the three-stratum theory has not been operationalized in any formal sense, in terms of either actual batteries of tests or other assessment procedures that are specifically designed to measure the abilities specified by the theory. A detailed description of the theory as it pertains to the different domains of ability, including higher-stratum abilities, can be found in relevant chapters of my

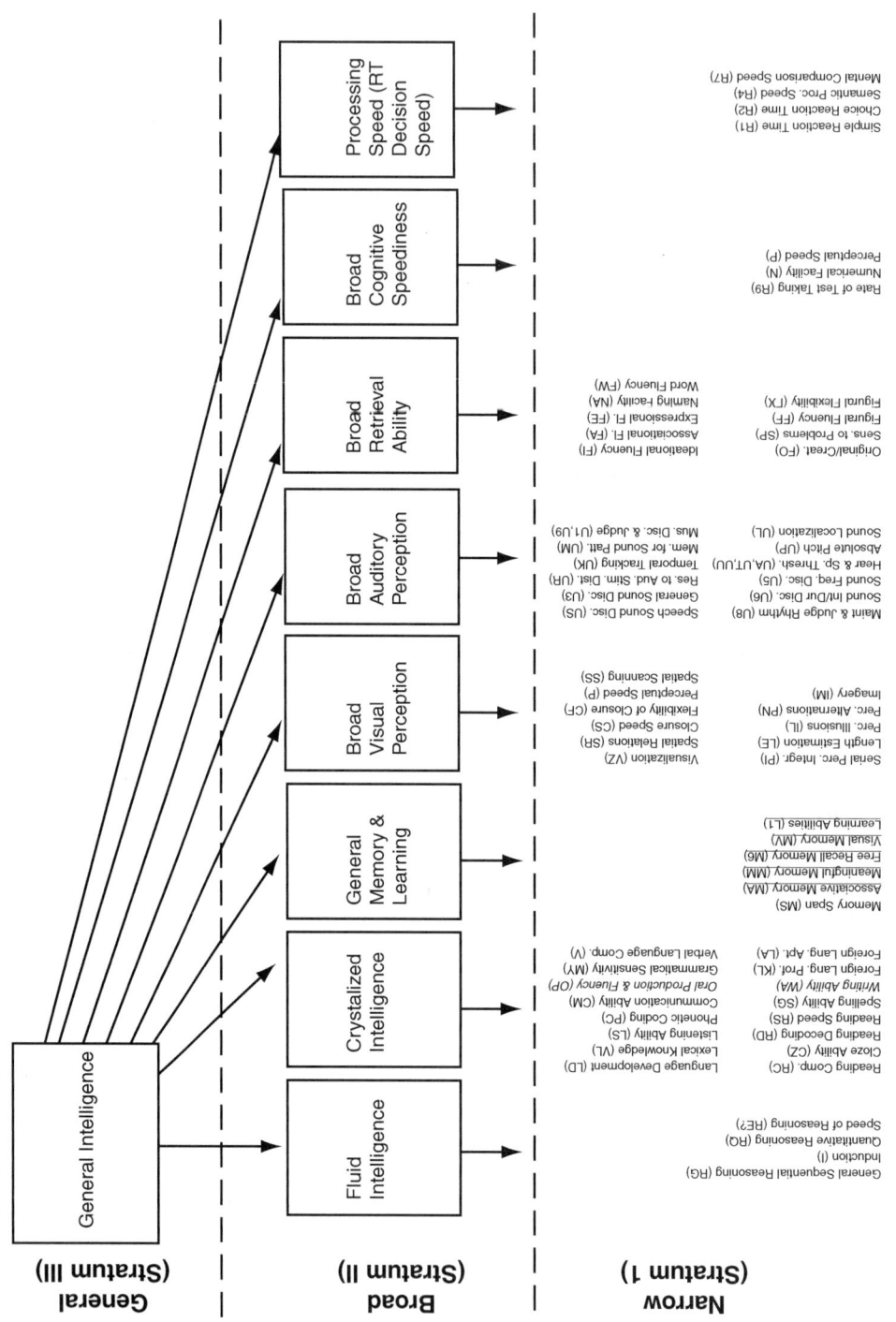

FIGURE A.1. The three-stratum structure of cognitive abilities. From Carroll (1993a). Copyright © 1993 by Cambridge University Press. Adapted and reproduced by permission. *Note:* Stratum I factors are differentiated as "level" (plain type), "speed" (bold type), "speed and level" (italics type), and "rate" (underlined) factors.

book, *Human Cognitive Abilities* (Carroll, 1993a). Most of these chapters describe representative tests or other procedures drawn from research studies or from well-known batteries of tests whereby the relevant factors of ability can be measured. Other sources of information about tests for measuring the abilities specified by the three-stratum theory are handbooks by Jonassen and Grabowski (1993) and Fleishman and Reilly (1992).

Applications of the Theoretical Model for Practice and Research

The three-stratum theory is intended chiefly to provide guidance for further research concerning cognitive abilities and their structure. For example, if new abilities are identified, the theory provides guidance as to where such abilities should fit in the structure already established—whether they are truly new or merely subvarieties of abilities previously identified.

In research, also, the theory plays an important role in presentation of factor-analytic results. Matrices of factor loadings show the loadings of tests (or other variables) on the different factors, at different strata. Most often it is found that a given test has significant loadings (say, greater than .3) on more than one factor; for example, a test might have such a loading on the general factor (at stratum III), a significant loading on one or more of the stratum II factors, and a significant loading on one or more of the stratum I factors. In other cases, a test's significant loadings might occur only on a general factor and one of the stratum I factors. In either case, the display of the test's loadings provides useful information about what the test measures and the extent to which it measures different factors. It is important to realize that the scores of most tests reflect influences of more than one factor, usually factors at different strata.

The theory has similar uses in professional practice. As was mentioned previously, it provides what is essentially a "map" of all known cognitive abilities. Such a map can be used in interpreting scores on the many tests used in individual assessment by clinical psychologists, school psychologists, industrial psychologists, and others. Such scores can be assessed in terms of the abilities they most probably measure. The map also suggests what abilities may need to be assessed in particular cases that require selection of appropriate tests (see Flanagan, Alfonso, & Ortiz, Chapter 19, this volume; Flanagan & McGrew, 1997).

EMPIRICAL SUPPORT FOR THE THEORY

The empirical support for this theory resides in the reanalyses of the more than 460 datasets that were presented in Carroll (1993a), where I offered arguments to justify the procedures I used. The reanalyses themselves were presented in the form of detailed hierarchical orthogonalized factor matrices contained in a set of computer disks (Carroll, 1993b). Reviews of the book have been highly favorable (Brand, 1993; Brody, 1994; Burns, 1994; Eysenck, 1994; Nagoshi, 1994; Sternberg, 1994); thus it would seem that experts in the field have entered no serious objections to the results or the theory. It is possible, however, that more critical reviews will eventually appear, raising questions about certain features of the theory.

Relations with Other Theories

The three-stratum theory is an expansion and extension of most of the previous theories of cognitive abilities—in particular (in rough chronological order), those of Spearman (1927), Thurstone (1938), Vernon (1961), Horn and Cattell (1966; see Horn & Noll, 1997, and Horn & Blankson, Chapter 3, this volume), Hakstian and Cattell (1978), and Gustafsson (1989). Even in 1927, Spearman offered what was essentially a two-stratum theory; the latter authors presented further and more detailed evidence of the hierarchical structure of abilities.

The three-stratum theory differs more radically from the structure-of-intelligence theory offered by Guilford (1967) and Guilford and Hoepfner (1971). These investigators initially did not accept the notion of higher-order factors of intelligence; only in more recent papers did Guilford (1981, 1985) admit the possibility of higher-order factors, and some of Guilford's former colleagues have started to reanalyze his data in terms of higher-order factors (Bachelor, Michael, & Kim, 1994). The three-stratum theory has resemblances to the theory of *multiple intelligences* offered by Gardner (see Chen & Gardner, 1997 and Chapter 5, this volume). The various broad abilities show rough correspondences to Gardner's seven [now eight—Ed.] intelligences; however, Gardner seems not to accept the concept of an overarching general ability, nor does he accept the notion of a hierarchical structure of abilities. Apparently he regards his seven intelligences as being completely independent of each other, despite a plethora of evidence that this is not the case.

BEYOND TRADITIONAL THEORIES OF INTELLIGENCE

The three-stratum theory reflects advances in the behavioral sciences in a number of ways.

The Influence of Recent Advances in Psychometrics

In psychometrics, research over the past 50 years has increasingly emphasized that *intelligence*, or IQ, is not a single thing, but a complex, composite structure of a number of intelligences. A psychometric technique put forward by Schmid and Leiman (1957), the orthogonalization of hierarchical factor matrices, made it possible to formulate more exactly how this composite structure of intelligences could be conceptualized. The Schmid and Leiman technique has become popular only in recent years, but it has become one of the major bases of the three-stratum theory.

Other major bases of the three-stratum theory have been improvements in measurement theory and computational methods. A major advance in measurement theory has been the so-called item response theory (see mainly Lord & Novick, 1968), which presents a model of the relation of ability to test item performance and assists in the design of more valid and reliable ability tests. Although the conduct of a comprehensive factor-analytic study requires large logistic resources in assembling tests, test subjects, and test data, analysis of data has become increasingly easier with the advent of modern high-speed computers, particularly personal computers. The availability of personal computers enormously facilitated the reanalyses of large numbers of datasets in the Carroll (1993a, 1993b) studies.

Influence of Recent Advances in Cognitive Psychology

The three-stratum theory reflects advances in cognitive psychology because these advances make it easier to interpret findings from factor analysis in terms of the properties of cognitive tasks (as represented in the psychological tests studied by factor analysis). Also, cognitive research has made it possible to focus attention on various cognitive tasks

that were largely ignored in psychometrics (e.g., the sentence verification task and category-sorting tasks).

How the Three-Stratum Theory Departs from Traditional Paradigms

Above all, the three-stratum theory emphasizes the multifactorial nature of the domain of cognitive abilities and directs attention to many types of ability usually ignored in traditional paradigms. It implies that individual profiles of ability levels are much more complex than previously thought, but at the same time it offers a way of structuring such profiles, by classifying abilities in terms of strata. Thus a general factor is close to former conceptions of intelligence, whereas second-stratum factors summarize abilities in such domains as visual and spatial perception. Nevertheless, some first-stratum abilities are probably of importance in individual cases, such as the phonetic coding ability that is likely to describe differences between normal and dyslexic readers.

Future Directions in Research and Application

Much work remains to be done in the factor-analytic study of cognitive abilities. The map of abilities provided by the three-stratum theory undoubtedly has errors of commission and omission, with gaps to be filled in by further research, including the development of new types of testing and assessment and the factorial investigation of their relationships with each other and with better-established types of assessment.

The theory needs to be further validated by acquiring information about the importance and relevance of the various abilities it specifies. In this endeavor, cognitive psychology can help by investigating the basic information-processing aspects of such abilities. Developmental and educational psychology can assist by investigating the development, stability, and educability of abilities—not only those such as IQ, which has been studied extensively, but also the other types of abilities in different domains specified by the theory.

Moreover, the three-stratum theory has implications for studies in neuropsychology and human genetics. For example, the theory specifies, on the basis of factor-analytic studies, a certain structure for memory abilities. Does this structure have parallels in theories of brain function (Crick, 1994;

Schacter & Tulving, 1994)? Similarly, the structure of abilities specified by the theory currently says little about the relative roles of genetic and environmental influences on these abilities; such influences can be investigated by considering them in relation to different strata of abilities (Plomin & McClearn, 1993). Thus far, we have a considerable amount of information on the heritability of the third-stratum factor *g*, but relatively little on how much genes influence the development of lower-stratum abilities such as broad visual perception and perceptual speed.

The theory has major implications for practical assessment of individuals in clinical. educational, or industrial settings. It appears to prescribe that individuals should be assessed with regard to the *total range* of abilities the theory specifies. Any such prescription would of course create enormous problems; generally there would not be sufficient time to conduct assessments (by tests, ratings, interviews, personal observations, etc.) of all the abilities that exist. Even if there were, there is a lack of appropriate tests for many abilities. Research is needed to spell out how the assessor can select what abilities need to be tested in particular cases. The conventional wisdom is that abilities close to *g* are the most important to test or assess, but if this policy is followed too strictly, many abilities that are important in particular cases would probably be missed. Only the future will enable us to appreciate these possibilities adequately.

REFERENCES

Bachelor, P., Michael, W. B., & Kim, S. (1994). First-order and higher-order semantic and figural factors in structure-of-intellect divergent production measures. *Educational and Psychological Measurement, 54*, 608–619.

Brand, C. (1993, October 22). The importance of the *g* factor [Review of Carroll, 1993a]. *Times Higher Educational Supplement*, p. 22.

Brody, N. (1994). Cognitive abilities [Review of Carroll, 1993a]. *Psychological Science, 5*, 63, 65–68.

Burns, R. B. (1994). Surveying the cognitive terrain [Review of Carroll, 1993a]. *Educational Researcher, 23*(2), 35–37.

Carroll, J. B. (1993a). *Human cognitive abilities: A survey of factor-analytic studies*. New York: Cambridge University Press.

Carroll, J. B. (1993b). *Human cognitive abilities: A survey of factor-analytic studies*. Appendix B: Hierarchical factor matrix files. New York: Cambridge University Press.

Carroll, J. B. (1994). Cognitive abilities: Constructing a theory from data. In D. K. Detterman (Ed.), *Current topics in human intelligence: Vol. 4. Theories of intelligence* (pp. 43–63). Norwood, NJ: Ablex.

Cattell, R. B. (1971). *Abilities: Their structure, growth, and action*. Boston: Houghton Mifflin.

Chen, J.-Q., & Gardner, H. (1997). Alternative assessment from a multiple intelligences theoretical perspective. In D. P. Flanagan, J. L. Genshaft, & P. L. Harrison (Eds.), *Contemporary intellectual assessment: Theories, tests, and issues* (pp. 105–121). New York: Guilford Press.

Crick, F. (1994). *The astonishing hypothesis: The scientific search for the soul*. New York: Scribner's.

Eysenck, H. J. (1994). [Special review of Carroll, 1993a.] *Personality and Individual Differences, 16*, 199.

Flanagan, D. P., & McGrew, K. S. (1997). A cross-battery approach to assessing and interpreting cognitive abilities: Narrowing the gap between practice and cognitive science. In D. P. Flanagan, J. L. Genshaft, & P. L. Harrison (Eds.), *Contemporary intellectual assessment: Theories, tests, and issues* (pp. 314–325). New York: Guilford Press.

Fleishman, E. A., & Reilly, M. E. (1992). *Handbook of human abilities: Definitions, measurements, and job task requirements*. Palo Alto, CA: Consulting Psychologists Press.

Guilford, J. P. (1967). *The nature of human intelligence*. New York: McGraw-Hill.

Guilford, J. P. (1981). Higher-order structure-of-intellect abilities. *Multivariate Behavioral Research, 16*, 411–435.

Guilford, J. P. (1985). The structure-of-intellect model. In B. B. Wolman (Ed.), *Handbook of intelligence: Theories, measurements, and applications* (pp. 225–266). New York: Wiley.

Guilford, J. P., & Hoepfner, R. (1971). *The analysis of intelligence*. New York: McGraw-Hill.

Gustafsson, J. E. (1989). Broad and narrow abilities in research on learning and instruction. In R. Kanfer, P. L. Ackerman, & R. Cudeck (Eds.), *Abilities, motivation, and methodology: The Minnesota Symposium on Learning and Individual Differences* (pp. 203–237). Hillsdale, NJ: Erlbaum.

Hakstian, A. R., & Cattell, R. B. (1978). Higher-stratum ability structures on a basis of twenty primary abilities. *Journal of Educational Psychology, 70*, 657–669.

Horn, J. L. (1965). *Fluid and crystallized intelligence: A factor analytic study of the structure among primary mental abilities*. Unpublished doctoral dissertation, University of Illinois, Urbana/Champaign.

Horn, J. L., & Cattell, R. B. (1966). Refinement of the theory of fluid and crystallized general intelligences. *Journal of Educational Psychology, 57*, 253–270.

Horn, J. L., & Noll, J. (1997). Human cognitive capabilities: Gf-Gc theory. In D. P. Flanagan, J. L. Genshaft,

& P. L. Harrison (Eds.), *Contemporary intellectual assessment: Theories, tests, and issues* (pp. 53–91). New York: Guilford Press.

Jonassen, D. H., & Grabowski, B. L. (Eds.). (1993). *Handbook of individual differences, learning, and instruction.* Hillsdale, NJ: Erlbaum.

Lord, F. M., & Novick, M. R. (1968). *Statistical theories of mental test scores.* Reading, MA: Addison-Wesley.

Matarazzo, J. D. (1972). *Wechsler's measurement and appraisal of adult intelligence* (5th ed.). Baltimore: Williams & Wilkins.

McGrew, K. S. (1997). Analysis of the major intelligence batteries according to a proposed comprehensive Gf-Gc framework. In D. P. Flanagan, J. L. Genshaft, & P. L. Harrison (Eds.), *Contemporary intellectual assessment: Theories, tests, and issues* (pp. 151–179). New York: Guilford Press.

Nagoshi, C. T. (1994). The factor-analytic guide to cognitive abilities [Review of Carroll, 1993a]. *Contemporary Psychology, 39,* 617–618.

Plomin, R., & McClearn, G. E. (Eds.). (1993). *Nature, nurture, and psychology.* Washington, DC: American Psychological Association.

Schacter, D. L., & Tulving, E. (Eds.). (1994). *Memory systems 1994.* Cambridge, MA: MIT Press.

Schmid, J., & Leiman, J. M. (1957). The development of hierarchical factor solutions. *Psychometrika, 22,* 53–61.

Spearman, C. (1927). *The abilities of man: Their nature and measurement.* New York: Macmillan.

Sternberg, R. J. (1994). 468 factor-analyzed data sets: What they tell us and don't tell us about human intelligence [Review of Carroll, 1993a]. *Psychological Science, 5,* 63–65.

Thurstone, L. L. (1938). *Primary mental abilities* (Psychometric Monographs, No. 1). Chicago: University of Chicago Press.

Thurstone, L. L. (1947). *Multiple factor analysis: A development and expansion of the vectors of mind.* Chicago: University of Chicago Press.

Thurstone, L. L., & Thurstone, T. G. (1941). *Factorial studies of intelligence* (Psychometric Monographs, No. 2). Chicago: University of Chicago Press.

Vernon, P. E. (1961). *The structure of human abilities* (2nd ed.). London: Methuen.

Wechsler, D. (1974). *Wechsler Intelligence Scale for Children—Revised.* New York: Psychological Corporation.

Author Index

Subject Index

Page numbers followed by *f* indicate figure; *n*, note; and *t*, table

908